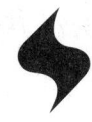

Stedman's

MEDICAL
SPELLER

THIRD EDITION

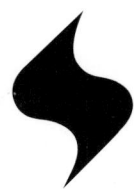

Stedman's MEDICAL SPELLER

THIRD EDITION

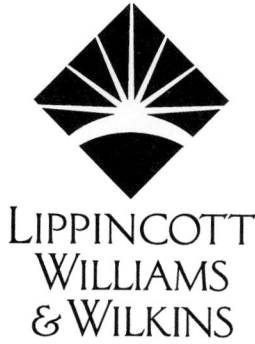

LIPPINCOTT
WILLIAMS
& WILKINS

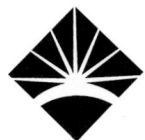

Series Editor: Beverly J. Wolpert
Associate Managing Editor: Trista A. DiPaula
Associate Managing Editor: William A. Howard
Production Manager: Julie K. Stegman
Production Coordinator: Kevin Iarossi
Typesetter: Peirce Graphic Services, Inc.
Printer & Binder: Data Reproductions Corporation

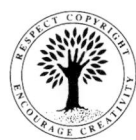

Printed in the United States of America

Third Edition, 2001

Library of Congress Cataloging-in-Publication Data

Stedman's medical speller.—3rd ed.
     p. ; cm. — (Stedman's word book series)
  ISBN 0-7817-3085-6
    1. Medicine—Terminology.   2. English language—Orthography and spelling.
  I. Title: Medical speller. II. Stedman's word books.
    [DNLM: 1. Terminology. W 15 S812 2001]
  R123 .S7 2001
  610'.1'4—dc21

                                      00-063999
                                            01
                           1 2 3 4 5 6 7 8 9 10

Contents

Acknowledgments

Stedman's Medical Speller, Third Edition, is the result of the massive efforts that went into *Stedman's Medical Dictionary, 27th Edition.* We gratefully acknowledge the contributions of the dictionary team to the content of *Stedman's Medical Speller, Third Edition,* including Maureen Barlow, Senior Managing Editor; John H. Dirckx, General Editor; Barb Ferretti, Chief Online Editor; Thomas W. Filardo, M.D., New Terms Editor; and Barbara Werner, Managing Editor; as well as consultants representing 52 medical specialties, numerous proofreaders, database experts, and publishing advisors.

We extend special thanks to Jeanne Bock, CSR, MT, who edited the manuscript, updated appendix material, and created new appendix sections; to Kathryn Mason, CMT, who also edited the manuscript; and to Helen Littrell, CMT, who edited the format to make it consistent with the format of our other published word books. Barb Ferretti played an integral role in the process by updating the database for this reference and by providing a final quality check.

As with all our *Stedman's* word references, this resource incorporates the suggestions and expertise of our many contacts in the medical transcriptionist community. Thanks to all of our advisory board participants, reviewers, and editors; AAMT meeting attendees; and others who have written us with requests and comments—keep talking, and we'll keep listening.

Preface to the Third Edition

Users of *Stedman's Medical Speller, Second Edition,* know that finding answers sometimes can be faster and more convenient with a reference that covers general medical language rather than with a word book that contains only specialty-specific terms. The many requests we received for an updated edition of this word book—our only word book featuring general medical terminology—convinced us to revise this reference.

For *Stedman's Medical Speller, Third Edition,* we have added more oncology, pediatrics, pulmonology, and emergency medicine terms, reflecting the increasing importance of these specialties. We have included the official *Terminologia Anatomica* nomenclature for anatomy terms to the extent that it is currently available—for Gross Anatomy and Neuroanatomy. This reference also includes the *Nomina Anatomica* terms for Gross Anatomy, Neuroanatomy, Embryology, Cytology, and Histology. We have eliminated the appendix sections covering hyphenation and provided other, more useful material, as requested by the users of the previous editions, including ligaments, muscles, and common professional titles. We have also revised and expanded the appendix section covering common prefixes, suffixes, and combining forms, including the meanings of each in an easy-to-follow format.

Unlike our other word books, *Stedman's Medical Speller, Third Edition,* includes only the headwords (main entry terms and subentry terms) from *Stedman's Medical Dictionary, 27th Edition.* We extracted the terms from the "big green" and then fully cross-indexed them for fast and easy look-up. This collection of approximately 125,000 entries builds on a base of about 75,000 medical words, phrases, and acronyms.

We at Lippincott Williams & Wilkins strive to provide you with the most up-to-date and accurate word references available. Your use of this word book will prompt new editions, which we will publish as often as updates and revisions justify. We welcome your suggestions for improvements, changes, corrections, and additions—whatever will make this *Stedman's* product more useful to you. Please complete the postpaid card at the back of this book, and send your recommendations care of "Stedman's" at Lippincott Williams & Wilkins.

Explanatory Notes

Medical transcription is an art as well as a science. Both are needed to correctly interpret the dictation of a physician, whose language is a product of education, training, and experience. This variety in medical language means that there are several acceptable ways to express certain terms, including jargon. *Stedman's Medical Speller, Third Edition* provides variant spellings and phrasings for many terms. These elements, in addition to complete cross-indexing, make *Stedman's Medical Speller, Third Edition* a valuable resource for determining the validity of terms as they are encountered.

Alphabetical Organization

Alphabetization of main entries is letter by letter as spelled, ignoring punctuation, spaces, prefixed numbers, or other characters. Greeks are spelled out and placed in alphabetical order. For example:

acid-fast staining method
acid formaldehyde hematin
acid hematin
alpha-acid glycoprotein

In subentry alphabetization, the abbreviated singular form or the spelled-out plural form of the noun main entry word is ignored.

Format and Style

All main entries are in **boldface** to expedite locating a sought-after term, to enhance distinction between main entries and subentries, and to relieve the textual density of the pages.

Irregular plurals and variant spellings are shown on the same line as the singular or preferred form of the word. For example:

scolex, pl. scoleces

curette, curet

Hyphenation

As a rule of style, multiple eponyms (e.g., Mears-Rubash approach) are hyphenated. Also, hyphens have been added between a manufacturer and one or more eponyms (e.g., Vital-Metzenbaum dissecting scissors). Please note that in many cases, hyphenation is a question of style, not of accuracy, and thus is a matter of choice.

Possessives

Possessive forms have been dropped in this reference for the sake of consistency and conformance with the guidelines of the American Association for Medical Transcription (AAMT), the American Medical Association (AMA), and other groups. Please note, however, that in many cases, retaining the possessive, like hyphenating, is a question of style, not of accuracy, and thus is also a matter of choice. To form the possessive of a word, simply add the apostrophe or apostrophe "s" to the end of the word.

Cross-indexing

The word list is in an index-like main entry-subentry format that contains two combined alphabetical listings:

(1) A *noun* main entry-subentry organization, which is typical of the A-Z section of medical dictionaries like *Stedman's*:

bubo
    bullet b.
    malignant b.
    virulent b.

hand
    drop h.
    ghoul h.
    opera-glass h.

(2) An *adjective* main entry-subentry organization, which lists words and phrases as you hear them. The main entries are the adjectives or modifiers in a multiword term. The subentries are the nouns around which the terms are constructed and to which the adjectives or modifiers pertain:

bipolar
    b. cautery
    b. disorder
    b. taxis

Hamman
    H. disease
    H. murmur
    H. sign

This format provides the user with more than one way to locate and identify a multiword term. For example:

acne
    halogen a.

halogen
    h. acne

clamp
    Fogarty c.
    gingival c.

Fogarty
    F. balloon
    F. clamp

This format also allows the user to see together all terms that contain a particular descriptor, as well as all types, kinds, or variations of a noun entity. For example:

birth
> b. amputation
> b. canal
> cross b.
> b. palsy
> premature b.

clasp
> c. arm
> bar c.
> circumferential c.
> extended c.
> c. guideline

Wherever possible, abbreviations are separately defined and cross-referenced. For example:

RBC
> red blood cell

red
> r. blood cell (RBC)

cell
> red blood c. (RBC)

α (*var. of* alpha)
    alpha particle
A
    adenine
       A band
       A bile
       A cell
       A chain
       A disk
       A fiber
       A wave
°A
A⁻
A
    absorbance
a
    absorptivity
A₂ thalassemia
AA
    amino acid
aa
    arteriae
āā
    ANA
AAA
    aaa disease
Aad
    alpha-aminoadipic acid
AAF
    2-acetylaminofluorene
Aagenaes syndrome
AAMC
    Association of American Medical
      Colleges
AAR
    antigen-antibody reaction
Aaron sign
Aarskog-Scott syndrome
**A1, A2 segment of anterior cerebral
  artery**
AASH
    adrenal androgen-stimulating hormone
AAV
    adenoassociated virus
Ab
    antibody
abacterial thrombotic endocarditis
Abadie sign of tabes dorsalis
abampere
abapical pole
abarognosis
abarticular gout
abasia
    atactic a.
    ataxic a.
abasia-astasia
abasic
abatement
    sound a.
abatic
abaxial, abaxile
Abbé condenser

Abbe flap
Abbott
    A. artery
    A. stain for spores
    A. tube
abciximab
ABC lead
abcoulomb
A.B.C. process
abdomen
    acute a.
    carinate a.
    navicular a.
    a. obstipum
    pendulous a.
    protuberant a.
    scaphoid a.
    surgical a.
abdominal
    a. angina
    a. aorta
    a. aortic plexus
    a. apoplexy
    a. aura
    a. ballottement
    a. canal
    a. cavity
    a. dropsy
    a. external oblique muscle
    a. fibromatosis
    a. fissure
    a. fistula
    a. guarding
    a. hernia
    a. hysterectomy
    a. hysteropexy
    a. hysterotomy
    a. internal oblique muscle
    a. lymph node
    a. migraine
    a. muscle deficiency syndrome
    a. myomectomy
    a. nephrectomy
    a. ostium of uterine tube
    a. pad
    a. part of aorta
    a. part of esophagus
    a. part of pectoralis major muscle
    a. part of peripheral autonomic
      plexuses and ganglia
    a. part of thoracic duct
    a. part of ureter
    a. pool
    a. pregnancy
    a. pressure
    a. pulse
    a. reflex
    a. region
    a. respiration
    a. ring
    a. sac
    a. salpingectomy

abdominal *(continued)*
    a. salpingotomy
    a. section
    a. testis
    a. typhoid
    a. zone
abdominocardiac reflex
abdominocentesis
abdominocyesis
abdominocystic
abdominogenital
abdominohysterectomy
abdominohysterotomy
abdominojugular reflux
abdominopelvic
    a. cavity
    a. splanchnic nerve
abdominoperineal resection (APR)
abdominoplasty
abdominoscopy
abdominoscrotal
abdominothoracic arch
abdominovaginal hysterectomy
abdominovesical
abduce
abducens
    a. eminence
    a. nerve
    a. nucleus
    a. oculi
abducent nerve [CN VI]
abduct
abduction
abductor
    a. digiti minimi muscle of foot
    a. digiti minimi muscle of hand
    a. hallucis muscle
    a. muscle
    a. muscle of great toe
    a. muscle of little finger
    a. muscle of little toe
    a. pollicis brevis muscle
    a. pollicis longus muscle
    a. spasmodic dysphonia
Abegg rule
Abell-Kendall method
Abelson murine leukemia virus
abembryonic
abenteric
Abernethy
    A. fascia
aberrant
    a. artery
    a. bile duct
    a. bundle
    a. complex
    a. duct
    a. ductule
    a. ganglion
    a. goiter
    a. hemoglobin
    a. obturator artery
    a. regeneration
    a. ventricular conduction

aberration
    chromatic a.
    chromosome a.
    color a.
    coma a.
    curvature a.
    dioptric a.
    distortion a.
    lateral a.
    longitudinal a.
    mental a.
    meridional a.
    monochromatic a.
    newtonian a.
    optic a.
    spherical a.
    ventricular a.
aberrometer
abetalipoproteinemia
    normotriglyceridemic a.
abeyance
abfarad
ABG
    arterial blood gas
abhenry
ability
abiotic
abiotrophy
abirritation
abl
ablastemic
ablastin
ablate
ablation
    electrode catheter a.
    endometrial a.
    laparoscopic uterosacral nerve a.
ABLB
    alternate binaural loudness balance
        ABLB test
ablepharia
abluent
ablution
abnerval
abneural
abnormal
    a. cleavage of cardiac valve
    a. correspondence
    a. occlusion
    a. ST segment
abnormality
    neuronal migration a.
    snowman a.
ABO
    ABO antigen
    ABO blood group
    ABO factor
    ABO hemolytic disease of the
        newborn
abohm
aborad, aboral
abort
aborted
    a. ectopic pregnancy
    a. systole

aborticide
abortient
abortifacient
abortigenic
abortion
    ampullar a.
    complete a.
    criminal a.
    elective a.
    habitual a.
    illegal a.
    incomplete a.
    induced a.
    inevitable a.
    infected a.
    menstrual extraction a.
    missed a.
    a. rate
    recurrent a.
    septic a.
    spontaneous a.
    therapeutic a.
    threatened a.
    tubal a.
abortionist
abortive
    a. neurofibromatosis
    a. transduction
abortus bacillus
aboulia
ABP
    androgen binding protein
ABPA
    allergic bronchopulmonary aspergillosis
ABR
    auditory brainstem response
abrachia
abrachiocephaly, abrachiocephalia
abrade
abraded wound
Abrahams sign
Abrams heart reflex
abrasion
    brush burn a.
    gingival a.
    tooth a.
abrasiveness
abrasive strip
abreact
abreaction
    motor a.
abrin
abruption
abruptio placentae
Abrus
abscess
    acute a.
    alveolar a.
    amebic a.
    apical a.
    apical periodontal a.
    appendiceal a.
    Bartholin a.
    Bezold a.
    bicameral a.

    bone a.
    Brodie a.
    bursal a.
    caseous a.
    cheesy a.
    cholangitic a.
    chronic a.
    cold a.
    crypt a.
    dental a.
    dentoalveolar a.
    diffuse a.
    Douglas a.
    dry a.
    Dubois a.
    embolic a.
    fecal a.
    follicular a.
    gas a.
    gingival a.
    gravitation a.
    gummatous a.
    hematogenous a.
    hot a.
    hypostatic a.
    ischiorectal a.
    lateral alveolar a.
    lateral periodontal a.
    mastoid a.
    metastatic a.
    migrating a.
    miliary a.
    Munro a.
    orbital a.
    otitic a.
    palatal a.
    pancreatic a.
    parafrenal a.
    parametric a.
    paranephric a.
    parapharyngeal a.
    parotid a.
    Pautrier a.
    pelvic a.
    perforating a.
    periapical a.
    periappendiceal a.
    periarticular a.
    pericemental a.
    pericoronal a.
    perinephric a.
    periodontal a.
    perirectal a.
    peritonsillar a.
    periureteral a.
    periurethral a.
    phlegmonous a.
    Pott a.
    premammary a.
    psoas a.
    pulp a.
    pyemic a.
    radicular a.
    residual a.
    retrobulbar a.

abscess *(continued)*
    retrocecal a.
    retropharyngeal a.
    ring a.
    root a.
    satellite a.
    septicemic a.
    stellate a.
    stercoral a.
    sterile a.
    stitch a.
    subdiaphragmatic a.
    subepidermal a.
    subhepatic a.
    subperiosteal a.
    subphrenic a.
    subungual a.
    sudoriferous a.
    suture a.
    thymic a.
    Tornwaldt a.
    tropical a.
    tuboovarian a.
    verminous a.
    wandering a.
    worm a.
abscissa
abscission
absconsio
abscopal effect
absence
    pure a.
    a. seizure
    simple a.
absente febre (abs. feb.)
absent state
abs. feb.
    absente febre
Absidia
absinthe
absinthin
absinthium
absinthol
absolute
    a. agraphia
    a. alcohol
    a. cell increase
    a. dehydration
    a. glaucoma
    a. hemianopia
    a. humidity
    a. hydration
    a. hyperopia
    a. intensity threshold acuity
    a. leukocytosis
    a. oil
    a. pressure
    a. refractory period
    a. scale
    a. scotoma
    a. system of unit
    a. temperature (T)
    a. terminal innervation ratio
    a. threshold

    a. unit
    a. viscosity
    a. zero
absorb
absorbable
    a. gelatin film
    a. gelatin sponge
    a. surgical suture
absorbance *(A)*
    specific a.
absorbancy index
absorbed dose
absorbefacient
absorbency
absorbent
    a. cotton
    a. point
    a. system
    a. vessel
absorber head
absorption
    a. band
    a. cell
    a. chromatography
    a. coefficient
    a. collapse
    cutaneous a.
    disjunctive a.
    electron resonance a.
    external a.
    a. fever
    fluorescent treponemal antibody a.
    (FTA-ABS)
    interstitial a.
    a. line
    parenteral a.
    pathologic a.
    percutaneous a.
    photoelectric a.
    a. spectrum
absorptive cell of intestine
absorptivity *(a)*
    molar a.
abstinence
    a. symptom
    a. syndrome
abstract
    a. intelligence
    structured a.
    a. thinking
abstraction
abstriction
abterminal
γ-Abu
    gamma-aminobutyric acid
abulia
abulic
abundance
abuse
    child a.
    drug a.
    elder a.
    sexual a.
    spousal a.
    substance a.

abutment
    auxiliary a.
    ball and socket a.
    dovetail stress-broken a.
    intermediate a.
    isolated a.
    splinted a.
ABVD
    Adriamycin, bleomycin, vinblastine, dacarbazine
abvolt
abzyme
AC
    alternating current
Ac
    actinium
aC
    arabinosylcytosine
a.c.
    ante cibum
AC/A
    accommodative convergence-accommodation ratio
acacia
acalculia
acampsia
acantha
acanthamebiasis
Acanthamoeba **medium**
acanthella
acanthesthesia
Acanthia lectularia
acanthion
Acanthocephala
acanthocephaliasis
Acanthocheilonema
acanthocyte
acanthocytosis with chorea
acanthoid
acantholysis
acanthoma
    clear cell a.
acanthopodia
acanthor
acanthosis
    glycogenic a.
    a. nigricans
acanthotic
acanthrocyte
acanthrocytosis
acapnia
acapnial alkalosis
acarbose
acardia
acardiac
acardius
    a. acephalus
    a. amorphus
    a. anceps
acariasis
    psoroptic a.
    sarcoptic a.
acaricide
acarid
Acaridae

acaridan
Acarina
acarine
acarodermatitis urticarioides
acaroid
acarology
acarophobia
Acarus
    A. *balatus*
    A. *folliculorum*
    A. *gallinae*
    A. *hordei*
    A. *rhizoglypticus hyacinthi*
    A. *scabei*
acaryote
acatalasemia
acatalasia
acathectic
acathexia
acathexis
acathisia
acaudal
acaudate
ACC
    anodal closure contraction
accelerans
accelerant
accelerated
    a. conduction
    a. eruption
    a. hypertension
    a. reaction
    a. rejection
acceleration
    angular a.
    linear a.
    radial a.
accelerator
    a. factor
    a. fiber
    a. globulin (AcG)
    linear a. (LINAC)
    a. nerve
    proserum prothrombin conversion a. (PPCA)
    prothrombin a.
    serum a.
    serum prothrombin conversion a. (SPCA)
accelerin
accelerometer
accentuator
acceptor
    hydrogen a.
    a. RNA
    a. site
    a. splicing site
accès pernicieux
access opening
accessorius willisii
accessory
    a. adrenal
    a. atrium
    a. auricle

accessory *(continued)*
    a. branch of middle meningeal artery
    a. breast
    a. canal
    a. cartilage
    a. cell
    a. cephalic vein
    a. chromosome
    a. cuneate nucleus
    a. flexor muscle of foot
    a. flocculus
    a. gland
    a. hemiazygos vein
    a. lacrimal gland
    a. lymph node
    a. meningeal artery
    a. meningeal branch
    a. meningeal branch of middle meningeal artery
    a. molecule
    a. nasal cartilage
    a. nerve [CN XI]
    a. nerve lymph node
    a. nerve trunk
    a. nipple
    a. nuclei of optic tract
    a. obturator artery
    a. olivary nuclei
    a. organ
    a. organ of the eye
    a. pancreas
    a. pancreatic duct
    a. parotid gland
    a. phrenic nerve
    a. placenta
    a. plantar ligament
    a. process of lumbar vertebra
    a. quadrate cartilage
    a. root of tooth
    a. saphenous vein
    a. sign
    a. spleen
    a. structure
    a. suprarenal gland
    a. symptom
    a. thyroid
    a. thyroid gland
    a. tragus
    a. tubercle
    a. vertebral vein
    a. visual apparatus
    a. visual structure
    a. volar ligament
accident
    cardiac a.
    cerebrovascular a. (CVA)
    a. neurosis
    serum a.
accidental
    a. host
    a. hypothermia
    a. image
    a. murmur
    a. myiasis
    a. parasite
    a. symptom
accident-prone
acclimating fever
acclimation
acclimatization
accolé form
accommodation
    amplitude of a.
    a. of eye
    histologic a.
    negative a.
    a. of nerve
    a. phosphene
    positive a.
    range of a.
    a. reflex
    relative a.
accommodative
    a. asthenopia
    a. convergence
    a. convergence-accommodation ratio (AC/A)
    a. insufficiency
    a. strabismus
accompanying
    a. vein
    a. vein of hypoglossal nerve
accomplice
accouchement forcé
accoucheur hand
accrementition
accretio cordis
accretionary growth
accretion line
accrochage
accumulation
    a. analysis
    a. disease
accuracy
ACD
    acid-citrate-dextrose
ACE
    angiotensin-converting enzyme
acebutolol
aceclidine
acedapsone
acedia
acefylline piperazine
ACEI
    angiotensin-converting enzyme inhibitor
acellular
acelom
acelomate, acelomatous
acenocoumarin
acenocoumarol
acentric
    a. chromosome
    a. fragment
acephalgic migraine
acephalia, acephalism
acephaline
acephalobrachia
acephalocardia

acephalocheiria, acephalochiria
acephalocyst
acephalogasteria
acephalopodia
acephalorrhachia
acephalothoracia
acephalous
acephalus
    a. acormus
    a. dibrachius
    a. dipus
    a. monobrachius
    a. monopus
    a. sympus
acephaly
acerola
acervulus
acestoma
acesulfame
aceta (*pl. of* acetum)
acetabula (*pl. of* acetabulum)
acetabular
    a. artery
    a. branch
    a. fossa
    a. labrum
    a. lip
    a. margin
    a. notch
acetabulectomy
acetabuloplasty
acetabulum, pl. **acetabula**
acetal
    a. phosphatidate
    a. phosphatide
acetaldehyde
    activated a.
acetamide
2-acetamidofluorene
acetaminophen
acetaminosalol
acetarsol
acetarsone
acetate
    active a.
    a. kinase
    a. replacement factor
    a. thiokinase
acetate-CoA ligase
acetazolamide
acetenyl
acetic
    a. aldehyde
    a. amide
    a. fermentation
    a. solution
acetic acid
    a. a. amide
    diluted a. a.
    glacial a. a.
aceticoceptor
acetify
acetimeter
acetoacetate decarboxylase
acetoacetic acid

acetoacetyl-CoA
    acetoacetyl-CoA reductase
    acetoacetyl-CoA thiolase
acetoacetyl-coenzyme A
acetoacetyl-succinic thiophorase
acetohexamide
acetohydroxamic acid
acetoin
acetokinase
acetol
acetolysis
acetomenaphthone
acetometer
acetone
    a. body
    a. chloroform
    a. compound
    a. fixative
    a. test
acetone-insoluble antigen
acetonemia
acetonemic
acetonitrile
acetonuria
acetoorcein stain
acetophenazine maleate
acetophenetidin
acetosoluble albumin
acetosulfone sodium
acetowhitening
acetrizoate sodium
acetum, pl. **aceta**
aceturate
acetyl
    a. chloride
    a. phosphate
    a. transacylase
    a. value
acetyl-activating enzyme
acetyladenylate
2-acetylaminofluorene (AAF)
acetylase
***N*-acetylaspartate**
acetylation
acetylcarbromal
***O*-acetylcarnitine**
acetylcholine (ACH, Ach)
    a. chloride
acetylcholinesterase
acetyl-CoA
    a.-CoA acetyltransferase
    a.-CoA acylase
    a.-CoA acyltransferase
    a.-CoA carboxylase
    a.-CoA deacylase
    a.-CoA:α-glucosaminide
      acetyltransferase
    a.-CoA hydrolase
    a.-CoA ligase
    a.-CoA synthetase
    a.-CoA thiolase
acetyl-coenzyme A
acetylcysteine
acetyldigitoxin
acetyldigoxin

N-acetylglucosamine
N-acetylglutamate (NAG)
acetylmethadol
N-acetylneuraminic acid (NeuAc)
acetylornithine deacetylase
3-acetylpyridine
acetylsalicylic acid
N¹-acetylsulfanilamide
N⁴-acetylsulfanilamide
acetyl sulfisoxazole
acetyltannic acid
acetyltransferase
AcG
    accelerator globulin
ACH, Ach
    acetylcholine
achalasia
    a. of the cardia
    cricopharyngeal a.
    esophageal a.
    a. of the upper sphincter
Achard syndrome
Achard-Thiers syndrome
ache
    bone a.
    stomach a.
acheilia
acheilous, achilous
acheiria, achiria
acheiropody, achiropody
acheirous, achirous
Achenbach syndrome
achievement
    a. age
    a. motive
    a. quotient
    a. test
Achilles
    A. bursa
    A. reflex
    A. tendon
    A. tendon reflex
achillobursitis
achillotenotomy
achilous (*var. of* acheilous)
achiral
achiria (*var. of* acheiria)
achiropody (*var. of* acheiropody)
achirous (*var. of* acheirous)
achlorhydria
achlorhydric anemia
achlorophyllous
Acholeplasma, pl. *Acholeplasmata*
    A. axanthum
    A. laidlawii
acholia
acholic
acholuria
acholuric jaundice
achondrogenesis
    Type IA, IB, II a.
achondroplasia
    homozygous a.
achondroplastic
    a. dwarfism

achordal
achordate
achoresis
Achorion
achrestic anemia
achroacyte
achrodextrin
achromacyte
achromasia
achromat
achromatic
    a. apparatus
    a. lens
    a. objective
    a. threshold
    a. vision
achromatin
achromatinic
achromatism
achromatocyte
achromatolysis
achromatophil
achromatophilia
achromatopsia, achromatopsy
    atypical a.
    complete a.
    incomplete a.
    typical a.
achromatosis
achromatous
achromaturia
achromia parasitica
achromic
Achromobacter
achromocyte
achromophil
achromophilic, achromophilous
achromotrichia
achroodextrin
achylia
    a. gastrica
    a. pancreatica
achylous
acicular
acid
    acrylic a.
    a. agglutination
    a. alcohol
    allantoic a.
    bile a.
    Brønsted a.
    a. carboxypeptidase
    a. cell
    complementary ribonucleic a.
    (cRNA)
    conjugate a.
    cysteine sulfinic a.
    a. deoxyribonuclease
    a. dextran
    a. dextrin
    dibasic a.
    a. dyspepsia
    a. etch cemented splint
    fatty acid
    a. fuchsin

a. gland
glutamic a. (Glu)
a. indigestion
inorganic a.
a. intoxication
Lewis a.
a. maltase
monobasic a.
organic a.
a. oxide
a. perfusion test
a. phosphatase
a. phosphatase test for semen
polybasic a.
a. radical
a. reaction
a. red 87
a. red 91
a. reflux test
a. rigor
a. salt
a. seromucoid
a. stain
a. sulfate
a. tartrate
a. tide
unspecified amino a. (Xaa)
a. wave
wax a.
acid-ash diet
acid-base
a.-b. balance
a.-b. equilibrium
acid-citrate-dextrose (ACD)
acidemia
acid-etched restoration
acid-fast
a.-f. bacillus (AFB)
acidic
a. amino acid
a. dye
acidified serum test
acidify
acidity
total a.
acidophil, acidophile
a. adenoma
a. cell
a. granule
acidophilic leukocyte
acidophilus milk
acidosis
carbon dioxide a.
compensated a.
compensated respiratory a.
diabetic a.
hypercapnic a.
hyperchloremic a.
lactic a.
metabolic a.
primary renal tubular a.
renal tubular a.
respiratory a.
secondary renal tubular a.

starvation a.
uncompensated a.
acidotic
aciduria
aciduric
acinar
a. carcinoma
a. cell
a. cell tumor
Acinetobacter calcoaceticus
acini (*pl. of* acinus)
acinic
a. cell adenocarcinoma
a. cell carcinoma
aciniform
acinose
acinotubular gland
acinous
a. cell
a. gland
a-c interval
acinus, pl. **acini**
liver a.
pulmonary a.
Rappaport a.
ackee poisoning
acknemia (*var. of* acnemia)
aclasia
aclasis
tarsoepiphyseal a.
acme
acne
a. artificialis
bromide a.
a. cachecticorum
a. ciliaris
a. conglobata
a. cosmetica
cystic a.
a. fulminans
a. generalis
halogen a.
a. hypertrophica
iodide a.
a. keloid
a. medicamentosa
a. necrotica miliaris
a. neonatorum
pomade a.
a. punctata
a. pustulosa
a. rosacea
simple a.
steroid a.
tar a.
tropical a.
a. varioliformis
a. venenata
a. vulgaris
acneform, acneiform
acnemia, acknemia, aknemia
ACNM
American College of Nuclear Medicine
ACNP
American College of Nuclear Physicians

acokanthera
acolous
aconitase
aconitate hydratase
aconite
cis-**aconitic acid**
aconitine
acorea
acorn-tipped catheter
Acosta disease
acoustic
  a. agraphia
  a. aphasia
  a. area
  a. cell
  a. crest
  a. enhancement
  a. impedance
  a. lemniscus
  a. lens
  a. meatus
  a. nerve
  a. neurilemoma
  a. neurinoma
  a. neuroma
  a. papilla
  a. pressure
  a. radiation
  a. reference level
  a. reflex
  a. schwannoma
  a. shadow
  a. spot
  a. stimulation test
  a. stria
  a. teeth
  a. tetanus
  a. tolerance
  a. trauma hearing loss
  a. tubercle
  a. tumor
  a. vesicle
acousticofacial ganglion
acousticopalpebral reflex
acousticophobia
acoustics
acoustic surround
ACP
  acyl carrier protein
ACP-acetyltransferase
ACP-malonyltransferase
ACPS
  acrocephalosyndactyly
acquired
  a. agammaglobulinemia
  a. centric relation
  a. character
  a. cuticle
  a. drive
  a. eccentric relation
  a. enamel cuticle
  a. epileptic aphasia
  a. hemolytic anemia
  a. hemolytic icterus
  a. hyperlipoproteinemia

  a. hypogammaglobulinemia
  a. ichthyosis
  a. immunity
  a. immunodeficiency syndrome
   (AIDS)
  a. leukoderma
  a. megacolon
  a. methemoglobinemia
  a. nevus
  a. pellicle
  a. reflex
  a. sensitivity
  a. toxoplasmosis
  a. tufted angioma
acquisition
  gradient-recalled a. in the steady
   state (GRASS)
ACR
  American College of Radiology
acral
  a. lentiginous melanoma
Acrania
acrania
acranial
acranius
Acrel ganglion
Acremonium
acribometer
acridine
  acridine dye
  acridine orange
  acridine yellow
  tetramethyl a.
acrid poison
acriflavine
acrimonia
acrimony
acrinol
acrisorcin
acritical
acroagnosis
acroanesthesia
acroarthritis
acroasphyxia
acroataxia
acroblast
acrobrachycephaly
acrocentric chromosome
acrocephalia
acrocephalic
acrocephalopolysyndactyly
acrocephalosyndactyly (ACPS)
  type I, II, III, V a.
acrocephalous
acrocephaly
acrochordon
acrocinesia, acrocinesis
acrocontracture
acrocyanosis
acrocyanotic
acrodermatitis
  a. chronica atrophicans
  a. continua
  a. enteropathica

papular a. of childhood
    a. perstans
acrodermatosis
acrodont
acrodynia
acrodynic erythema
acrodysesthesia
acrodysostosis
acroesthesia
acrofacial
    a. dysostosis
    a. syndrome
acrogenous
acrogeria
acrognosis
acrohyperhidrosis
acrohyperkeratosis
    focal a.
acrokeratoelastoidosis
acrokeratosis
    paraneoplastic a.
acrokinesia
acromegalia
acromegalic gigantism
acromegalogigantism
acromegaloidism
acromegaly
acromelalgia
acromelia
acromelic dwarfism
acromesomelia
acromesomelic dwarfism
acrometagenesis
acromial
    a. anastomosis of the
      thoracoacromial artery
    a. angle
    a. arterial network
    a. artery
    a. articular facies of clavicle
    a. articular surface of clavicle
    a. branch of suprascapular artery
    a. branch of thoracoacromial artery
    a. end of clavicle
    a. extremity of clavicle
    a. facet of clavicle
    a. part of deltoid muscle
    a. plexus
    a. process
    a. reflex
acromicria
acromioclavicular
    a. disk
    a. joint
    a. ligament
acromiocoracoid
acromiohumeral
acromion presentation
acromioplasty
acromioscapular
acromiothoracic artery
acromphalus
acromyotonia
acromyotonus
acroosteolysis

acropachy
acropachyderma
acroparesthesia syndrome
acropetal
acrophobia
acropigmentation
acropleurogenous
acropustulosis
    infantile a.
acroscleroderma
acrosclerosis
acrosin
acrosomal
    a. cap
    a. granule
    a. vesicle
acrosome
acrosomin
acrospiroma
    eccrine a.
acroteric
Acrotheca
acrotheca
acrotic
acrotism
acrotrophodynia
acrotrophoneurosis
acrylate
acrylic
    a. acid
    a. resin
    a. resin base
    a. resin tooth
    a. resin tray
ACT
    activated clotting time
ACTH
    adrenocorticotropic hormone
    big ACTH
    little ACTH
    ACTH stimulation test
ACTH-producing adenoma
actin
    F-a.
    a. filament
    G-a.
acting out
actinic
    a. cheilitis
    a. conjunctivitis
    a. dermatitis
    a. granuloma
    a. keratitis
    a. keratosis
    a. porokeratosis
    a. prurigo
    a. ray
    a. reticuloid
actinide element
actinium (Ac)
    a. emanation
actinobacillosis
Actinobacillus
    A. actinomycetemcomitans
    A. lignieresii

actinohematin
Actinomadura
   A. africana
   A. latina
   A. madurae
   A. pelliertieri
actinomycelial
Actinomyces
   A. bovis
   A. israelii
   A. naeslundii
   A. odontolyticus
   A. viscosus
Actinomycetaceae
Actinomycetales
actinomycetes
actinomycetoma
actinomycin
   a. A, C, D, F_1
actinomycosis
actinomycotic appendicitis
Actinomyxidia
actinophage
actinophytosis
Actinopoda
actinosin
actinotherapy
action
   ball valve a.
   calorigenic a.
   cumulative a.
   a. current
   a. potential
   salt a.
   sparing a.
   specific a.
   specific dynamic a. (SDA)
   thermogenic a.
   a. tremor
activated
   a. acetaldehyde
   a. amino acid
   a. atom
   a. carbon dioxide
   a. carboxylic acid
   a. charcoal
   a. choline
   a. clotting time (ACT)
   a. fatty acid
   a. glucose
   a. glycol aldehyde
   a. hydrogen
   a. macrophage
   a. partial thromboplastin time
   (aPTT)
   a. resin
   a. sludge
   a. sludge method
   a. state
activation
   amino acid a.
   a. analysis
   EEG a.
   feedback a.

feed-forward a.
gene a.
activator
   catabolite gene a. (CGA)
   plasminogen a.
   polyclonal a.
   tissue plasminogen a.
active
   a. acetate
   a. aldehyde
   a. anaphylaxis
   a. carbon dioxide
   a. caries
   a. center
   a. congestion
   a. electrode
   a. formaldehyde
   a. formate
   a. formyl
   a. glycoaldehyde
   a. hyperemia
   a. immunity
   a. immunization
   a. inflammation
   a. labor
   a. length-tension curve
   a. methionine
   a. methyl
   a. movement
   a. mutant
   a. placebo
   a. principle
   a. prophylaxis
   a. psychoanalysis
   a. pyruvate
   a. repressor
   a. site
   a. splint
   a. succinate
   a. sulfate
   a. transport
   a. treatment
   a. vasoconstriction
   a. vasodilation
activin
activity
   blocking a.
   a. coefficient
   a.'s of daily living scale (ADL)
   insulinlike a. (ILA)
   intrinsic sympathomimetic a. (ISA)
   nonsuppressible insulinlike a.
   (NSILA)
   optic a.
   plasma renin a. (PRA)
   pulseless electrical a. (PEA)
   specific a.
   triggered a.
actomyosin
   platelet a.
actual cautery
Acuaria spiralis
acuity
   absolute intensity threshold a.
   resolution a.

spatial a.
stereoscopic a.
Vernier a.
visibility a.
visual a. (V)
aculeate
acumentin
acuminate
acuology
acupressure
acupuncture anesthesia
acusis
acute
a. abdomen
a. abscess
a. adrenocortical insufficiency
a. African sleeping sickness
a. alcoholism
a. angle
a. anterior poliomyelitis
a. appendicitis
a. ascending paralysis
a. ataxia
a. bacterial endocarditis
a. brachial radiculitis
a. bulbar poliomyelitis
a. cellular rejection
a. chalazion
a. cholecystitis
a. chorea
a. compression triad
a. contagious conjunctivitis
a. crescentic glomerulonephritis
a. cutaneous leishmaniasis
a. decubitus ulcer
a. delirium
a. disseminated encephalomyelitis
a. epidemic conjunctivitis
a. epidemic leukoencephalitis
a. febrile neutrophilic dermatosis
a. fibrinous pericarditis
a. fulminating meningococcal
septicemia
a. fulminating meningococcemia
a. glaucoma
a. goiter
a. hallucinatory paranoia
a. hemorrhagic conjunctivitis
a. hemorrhagic encephalitis
a. hemorrhagic glomerulonephritis
a. hemorrhagic leukoencephalitis
a. hemorrhagic pancreatitis
a. histoplasmosis
a. idiopathic polyneuritis
a. inclusion body encephalitis
a. infectious nonbacterial
gastroenteritis
a. inflammation
a. inflammatory demyelinating
polyradiculoneuropathy
a. inflammatory polyneuropathy
a. intermittent porphyria
a. interstitial nephritis
a. interstitial pneumonia
a. interstitial pneumonitis

a. invasive aspergillosis
a. isolated myocarditis
a. lead poisoning
a. lobar nephrosis
a. lymphocytic leukemia (ALL)
a. malaria
a. mania
a. massive liver necrosis
a. mercury poisoning
a. motor axonal neuropathy
a. multifocal placoid pigment
epitheliopathy
a. necrotizing encephalitis
a. necrotizing hemorrhagic
encephalomyelitis
a. necrotizing hemorrhagic
leukoencephalitis
a. necrotizing myelitis
a. necrotizing ulcerative gingivitis
(ANUG)
a. nephritis
a. nephrosis
a. organic brain syndrome
a. parenchymatous hepatitis
a. phase protein
a. phase reactant
a. phase reaction
a. phase response
a. physiology and chronic health
evaluation (APACHE)
a. porphyria
a. poststreptococcal
glomerulonephritis
a. primary hemorrhagic
meningoencephalitis
a. promyelocytic leukemia
a. pulmonary alveolitis
a. pyelonephritis
a. radiation syndrome
a. recurrent rhabdomyolysis
a. reflex bone atrophy
a. respiratory distress syndrome
a. retinal necrosis (ARN)
a. rheumatic arthritis
a. rhinitis
a. rickets
a. scalp cellulitis
a. schizophrenia
a. schizophrenic episode
a. sensory motor axonal neuropathy
a. situational reaction
a. splenic tumor
a. stress reaction
a. transverse myelitis
a. trypanosomiasis
a. urticaria
a. viral conjunctivitis
a. yellow atrophy of the liver
acyanotic
acyclic compound
acycloguanosine
acyclovir
**acyl-ACP dehydrogenase, acyl-ACP
reductase**
acyl-activating enzyme

acyladenylate
n-acylamino acid
acylation
acylcarnitine
acyl carrier protein (ACP)
acyl-CoA
    acyl-coenzyme A
      acyl-CoA dehydrogenase (NADPH)
      acyl-CoA synthetase
acyl-coenzyme A (acyl-CoA)
1-acylglycerol-3-phosphate acyltransferase
    (*var. of* lysophosphatidic acid
    acyltransferase)
acyl-malonyl-ACP synthase
acylmercaptan bond
N-acylsphingosine
acyltransferase
acystia
A.D.
    auris dexter
ADA
    American Dental Association
adacrya
adactylous
Adair-Koshland-Némethy-Filmer model
    (AKNF)
adamantine membrane
adamantinoma
    a. of long bone
    pituitary a.
Adam's apple
adamsite (DM)
Adams-Stokes
    A.-S. disease
    A.-S. syncope
    A.-S. syndrome
adansonian classification
adaptation
    dark a.
    a. disease
    light a.
    photopic a.
    reality a.
    retinal a.
    scotopic a.
    social a.
    a. syndrome of Selye
adapter, adaptor
    a. hypothesis
adaptive
    a. behavior
    a. behavior scale
    a. enzyme
    a. hypertrophy
adaptometer
adaptor (*var. of* adapter)
adaxial
ADC
    AIDS dementia complex
ADCC
    antibody-dependent cell-mediated
    cytotoxicity
add.
    adde
adde (add.)

adder
addict
addiction
    alcohol a.
addictive drug
Addis
    A. count
    A. test
Addison
    A. anemia
    A. clinical plane
    A. disease
Addison-Biermer disease
addisonian
    a. anemia
    a. crisis
    a. syndrome
addition
    a. compound
    a. mutation
addition-deletion mutation
additive
    a. effect
    a. model
additivity
    causal a.
    interlocal a.
    intralocal a.
addressin
    a. ligand
adducent
adducin
adduct
adduction
adductor
    a. brevis muscle
    a. canal
    a. compartment of thigh
    a. hallucis muscle
    a. hiatus
    a. longus muscle
    a. magnus muscle
    a. minimus muscle
    a. muscle
    a. muscle of great toe
    a. muscle of thumb
    a. pollicis muscle
    a. reflex
    a. spasmodic dysphonia
    a. tubercle of femur
Ade
    adenine
adelomorphous
adenalgia
adendric
adendritic
adenectomy
adenectopia
adenemphraxis
Aden fever
adeniform
adenine (A, Ade)
    a. arabinoside
    a. deaminase
    a. deoxyribonucleotide

a. nucleotide
a. phosphoribosyltransferase
a. sulfate
adenitis
mesenteric a.
adenization
adenoacanthoma
adenoameloblastoma
adenoassociated virus (AAV)
adenoblast
adenocarcinoma
acinic cell a.
alveolar a.
a. in Barrett esophagus
bronchiolar a.
bronchioloalveolar a.
clear cell a.
mesonephric a.
mucoid a.
papillary a.
renal a.
a. in situ
adenocystoma
adenocyte
adenodiastasis
adenodynia
adenofibroma
adenofibrosis
adenogenous
adenohypophysial
adenohypophysis
adenohypophysitis
lymphocytic a.
adenoid
a. cystic carcinoma
a. facies
a. tissue
a. tumor
adenoidal-pharyngeal-conjunctival (A-P-C)
a.-p.-c. virus
adenoidectomy
adenoiditis
adenolipoma
adenolipomatosis
symmetric a.
adenolymphocele
adenolymphoma
adenoma
acidophil a.
ACTH-producing a.
adnexal a.
adrenocortical a.
apocrine a.
basal cell a.
basophil a.
bronchial a.
bronchial mucous gland a.
canalicular a.
chromophobe a.
chromophobic a.
colloid a.
embryonal a.
eosinophil a.
follicular a.
Fuchs a.

gonadotropin-producing a.
growth hormone–producing a.
hepatic a.
hepatocellular a.
Hürthle cell a.
invasive pituitary a.
lactating a.
macrofollicular a.
mammosomatotroph cell a.
microfollicular a.
monomorphic a.
nephrogenic a.
a. of nipple
null-cell a.
oncocytic a.
oxyphil a.
papillary cystic a.
papillary a. of large intestine
pituitary a.
pleomorphic a.
polypoid a.
prolactin-producing a.
prostatic a.
renal cortical a.
sebaceous a.
a. sebaceum
thyrotropin-producing a.
tubular a.
undifferentiated cell a.
villous a.
adenomatoid
a. odontogenic tumor
adenomatosis
erosive a. of nipple
familial multiple endocrine a.
fibrosing a.
multiple endocrine a.
pulmonary a.
adenomatous
a. goiter
a. hyperplasia
a. polyp
a. polyposis coli
adenomegaly
adenomere
adenomyoma
adenomyosis uteri
adenopathy
adenophlegmon
Adenophorasida
Adenophorea
adenosalpingitis
adenosarcoma
müllerian a.
adenosatellite virus
adenose
adenosine (Ado)
a. 3′,5′-cyclic monophosphate (cAMP)
a. cyclic phosphate
a. 3′,5′-cyclic phosphate phosphodiesterase
a. deaminase
a. diphosphate
a. 5′-diphosphate (ADP)

adenosine *(continued)*
    a. kinase
    a. monophosphate (AMP)
    a. nucleosidase
    a. phosphate
    a. 3′-phosphate
    a. 5′-phosphate
    a. 3′-phosphate 5′-phosphosulfate (PAPS)
    a. 5′-phosphosulfate (APS)
    a. tetraphosphate
    a. triphosphatase (ATPase)
    a. triphosphate
    a. 5′-triphosphate (ATP)
adenosine 5′-phosphosulfate (APS)
    adenosine 5′-phosphosulfate kinase
adenosis
    blunt duct a.
    fibrosing a.
    microglandular a.
    sclerosing a.
adenosquamous carcinoma
adenosyl
adenosylcobalamin
S-**adenosyl-L-homocysteine**
S-**adenosyl-L-methionine (AdoMet, SAM)**
adenotomy
adenotonsillectomy
adenous
Adenoviridae
adenovirus
    canine a. 1
adenylate
    a. cyclase
    a. kinase
adenyl cyclase
adenylic acid
    cyclic a. a.
    a. a. deaminase
    a. a. kinase
adenylosuccinase
    a. lyase
adenylosuccinate
    a. synthase
adenylosuccinic acid (sAMP)
adenylyl cyclase
adenylylosuccinate
    a. lyase
    a. synthase
adenylylosuccinic acid
adenylylsulfate kinase
adeps
    a. lanae
    a. renis
adequal cleavage
adequate stimulus
adermia
ADH
    antidiuretic hormone
adherence
    immune a.
    a. syndrome
adherent
    a. leukoma

    a. pericardium
    a. placenta
adhering junctions
adhesin
adhesio, pl. **adhesiones**
    a. interthalamica
adhesiolysis
adhesion
    amnionic a.
    a. dyspepsia
    fibrinous a.
    fibrous a.
    interthalamic a.
    a. molecule
    a. phenomenon
    primary a.
    secondary a.
    a. test
adhesiones (*pl. of* adhesio)
adhesiotomy
adhesive
    a. absorbent dressing
    a. arachnoiditis
    a. atelectasis
    a. bandage
    a. capsulitis
    a. inflammation
    a. otitis
    a. pericarditis
    a. peritonitis
    a. phlebitis
    a. pleurisy
    a. tape
    a. vaginitis
adhib.
    adhibendus
adhibendus (adhib.)
adiabatic
adiadochocinesia
adiadochocinesis
adiadochokinesis
adiaphoresis
adiaphoretic
adiaphoria
adiaspiromycosis
adiaspore
adiastole
adiathermancy
Adie
    A. pupil
    A. syndrome
adiemorrhysis
Adinida
adipes
adiphenine hydrochloride
adipic acid
Adipiodone
adipocellular
adipoceratous
adipocere
adipocyte
adipogenesis
adipogenic
adipogenous
adipoid

adipokinetic hormone
adipokinin
adipometer
adiponecrosis
adiposalgia
adipose
    a. capsule
    a. cell
    a. degeneration
    a. fold of the pleura
    a. fossa
    a. infiltration
    a. tissue
    a. tumor
adiposis
    a. cerebralis
    a. dolorosa
    a. orchica
    a. tuberosa simplex
    a. universalis
adiposity
adiposogenital
    a. degeneration
    a. dystrophy
    a. syndrome
adiposuria
adipsia, adipsy
aditus
    a. ad antrum
    a. ad antrum mastoideum
    a. ad aqueductum cerebri
    a. ad infundibulum
    a. ad saccum peritonei minorem
    a. glottidis inferior
    a. glottidis superior
    laryngeal a.
    a. laryngis
    a. to mastoid antrum
    a. orbitae
    a. pelvis
adjacent angle
adjustable
    a. articulator
    a. axis face-bow
    a. occlusal pivot
adjustment
    a. disorder
    occlusal a.
adjuvant
    a. chemotherapy
    Freund complete a.
    Freund incomplete a.
    a. vaccine
ADL
    activities of daily living scale
adlerian
    a. psychoanalysis
    a. psychology
Adler test
ad lib
    ad libitum
ad libitum (ad lib)
adm.
    admove
admaxillary gland

admedial, admedian
adminiculum, pl. **adminicula**
    a. lineae albae
admittance
admov.
    admove
admove (adm., admov.)
adnerval
adneural
adnexa, sing. **adnexum**
    a. oculi
    a. uteri
adnexal
    a. adenoma
    a. carcinoma
adnexectomy
adnexitis
adnexopexy
adnexum (*sing. of* adnexa)
Ado
    adenosine
adolescence
adolescent
    a. albuminuria
    a. crisis
    a. medicine
    a. round back
AdoMet
    s-adenosyl-l-methionine
adonis
adonitol
adoptive
    a. immunity
    a. immunotherapy
ADP
    adenosine 5′-diphosphate
    ADP ribosylation
ADPase
adrenal
    accessory a.
    a. androgen
    a. androgen-stimulating hormone
      (AASH)
    a. apoplexy
    a. body
    a. capsule
    a. cortex
    a. cortex injection
    a. cortical carcinoma
    a. cortical syndrome
    a. crisis
    a. gland
    a. hermaphroditism
    a. hypertension
    a. leukodystrophy
    Marchand a.
    a. rest
    a. virilism
    a. virilizing syndrome
    a. weight factor
adrenalectomy
adrenaline
    a. oxidase
    a. reversal
adrenalism

adrenalitis
adrenalone
adrenalopathy
adrenarche
adrenergic
  a. amine
  a. blockade
  a. fiber
  a. neuronal blocking agent
  a. neurotransmitter
  a. receptor
adrenic
adrenoceptive
adrenoceptor
adrenocortical
  a. adenoma
  a. hormone
  a. insufficiency
adrenocorticoid
adrenocorticomimetic
adrenocorticotropic, adrenocorticotrophic
  a. hormone (ACTH)
  a. peptide
  a. releasing factor
adrenocorticotropin
adrenogenic, adrenogenous
adrenogenital syndrome
adrenoleukodystrophy (ALD)
adrenolytic
adrenomedullary hormone
adrenomegaly
adrenomimetic amine
adrenomyeloneuropathy
adrenopathy
adrenopause
adrenoprival
adrenoreactive
adrenoreceptor
adrenosterone
adrenotoxin
adrenotropic, adrenotrophic
  a. hormone
adrenotropin
Adriamycin, bleomycin, vinblastine, dacarbazine (ABVD)
ad sat
  ad saturatum
ad saturatum (ad sat)
Adson
  A. forceps
  A. maneuver
  A. test
adsorb
adsorbate
adsorbent
adsorption
  a. chromatography
  immune a.
  a. theory of narcosis
adsternal
adterminal
adult
  a. foveomacular retinal dystrophy
  a. hypophosphatasia
  a. lactase deficiency

  a. medulloepithelioma
  a. pseudohypertrophic muscular dystrophy
  a. respiratory distress syndrome (ARDS)
  a. rickets
  a. T-cell leukemia (ATL)
  a. T-cell lymphoma
  a. tuberculosis
  a. type
adulterant
adulteration
adultomorphism
adult-onset diabetes
advanced
  a. life support
  a. multiple-beam equalization radiography (AMBER)
advance directive
advancement
  capsular a.
  a. flap
  tendon a.
adventitia
adventitial
  a. cell
  a. neuritis
adventitious
  a. albuminuria
  a. breath sound
  a. bursa
  a. cyst
adverse reaction
adversive movement
adynamia episodica hereditaria
adynamic ileus
A-E amputation
Aeby plane
Aedes
  A. aegypti
  A. albopictus
  A. atlanticus
  A. caballus
  A. dorsalis
  A. leucocelaenus
  A. melanimon
  A. mitchellae
  A. nigromaculis
  A. polynesiensis
  A. sollicitans
  A. taeniorhynchus
  A. triseriatus
  A. trivittatus
  A. variegatus
  A. vexans
Aelurostrongylus
aequorin
aerate
aerendocardia
aerial
  a. mycelium
  a. sickness
Aerobacter
aerobe
  obligate a.

aerobic
  a. dehydrogenase
  a. respiration
aerobiology
aerobioscope
aerobiosis
aerobiotic
aerocele
Aerococcus
aerocolpos
aerodermectasia
aerodontalgia
  primary a.
  secondary a.
aerodontia
aerodynamic
  a. size
  a. theory
aerodynamics
aerogastria
  blocked a.
aerogen
aerogenesis
aerogenic, aerogenous
  a. tuberculosis
aeromedicine
aeromonad
Aeromonas
  A. *hydrophila*
aeroodontalgia
aeroodontodynia
aeropause
aerophagia, aerophagy
aerophil, aerophile
aerophilic, aerophilous
aerophobia
aeropiesotherapy
aeroplankton
aerosialophagy
aerosinusitis
aerosis
aerosol
  a. generator
  respirable a.
aerosolization
aerospace medicine
aerotherapeutics, aerotherapy
aerotitis media
aerotonometer
aesculapian
aesculin
aestival
aestivoautumnal fever
AFA fixative
AFB
  acid-fast bacillus
afebrile
afetal
affect
  blunted a.
  a. displacement
  a. display
  flat a.
  a. hunger

  inappropriate a.
  labile a.
  a. memory
  a. spasm
affection
affective
  a. disorder
  a. personality
  a. psychosis
  a. tone
affectivity
affectomotor
afferent
  a. fiber
  a. glomerular arteriole
  a. loop syndrome
  a. lymphatic
  a. nerve
  a. vessel
affinity
  a. antibody
  a. chromatography
  a. column
  residual a.
affinous
affirmation
affusion
AFH
  anterior facial height
afibrillar cementum
afibrinogenemia
  congenital a.
Afipia
aflatoxicosis
aflatoxin
AFORMED
  alternating failure of response,
    mechanical, to electrical depolarization
    AFORMED phenomenon
AFP
  alpha-fetoprotein
African
  A. endomyocardial fibrosis
  A. furuncular myiasis
  A. hemorrhagic fever
  A. histoplasmosis
  A. sleeping sickness
  A. tick-bite fever
  A. tick fever
  A. trypanosomiasis
afterbirth
aftercare
afterchroming
aftercontraction
aftercurrent
afterdischarge
aftereffect
aftergilding
afterimage
  negative a.
  positive a.
afterimpression
afterload
  ventricular a.

afterloading
    a. radiation
    a. screw
aftermovement
afterpain
afterperception
afterpotential
    diastolic a.
    positive a.
aftersensation
aftersound
aftertaste
aftertouch
aftosa
afunctional occlusion
A/G
    albumin-globulin
    A/G ratio
Ag
    antigen
agalactia
agalactorrhea
agalactosis
agalactous
agamete
agamic
agammaglobulinemia
    acquired a.
    Bruton a.
    secondary a.
    Swiss type a.
    transient a.
    X-linked a.
agamocytogeny
Agamofilaria
agamogenesis
agamogenetic
agamogony
Agamomermis culicis
agamont
agamous
aganglionic
aganglionosis
agapism
agar
    bile salt a.
    birdseed a.
    blood a.
    Bordet-Gengou potato blood a.
    brain-heart infusion a.
    chocolate a.
    cholera a.
    cornmeal a.
    Czapek solution a.
    EMB a.
    Endo a.
    eosin-methylene blue a.
    MacConkey a.
    Mueller-Hinton a.
    Novy and MacNeal blood a.
    nutrient a.
    oatmeal-tomato paste a.
    potato dextrose a.
    rice-Tween a.
    Sabouraud dextrose a.

    serum a.
    Thayer-Martin a.
    yeast extract a.
agaric
    a. acid
    deadly a.
    fly a.
Agaricus
agaropectin
agarose
Ag-AS stain
agastric
agastroneuria
AGC
    automatic gain control
age
    achievement a.
    anatomical a.
    basal a.
    Binet a.
    bone a.
    childbearing a.
    chronologic a.
    developmental a. (DA)
    emotional a.
    gestational a.
    menstrual a.
    mental a. (MA)
    physical a.
    physiologic a.
agene process
agenesis
    gonadal a.
    müllerian a.
    renal a.
    thymic a.
agenitalism
agenosomia
agent
    adrenergic neuronal blocking a.
    alkylating a.
    alpha-adrenergic blocking a.
    antianxiety a.
    antidyskinetic a.
    antifoaming a.
    antipsychotic a.
    atypical antipsychotic a.
    bacteriostatic a.
    beta-adrenergic receptor blocking a.
    Bittner a.
    blister a.
    blocking a.
    calcium channel-blocking a.
    chimpanzee coryza a. (CCA)
    cholinergic a.
    contrast a.
    cycle-specific a.
    delta a.
    Eaton a.
    embedding a.
    enterokinetic a.
    F a.
    fertility a.
    foamy a.
    ganglionic blocking a.

high osmolar contrast a. (HOCA)
initiating a.
inotropic a.
LDH a.
low osmolar contrast a. (LOCA)
luting a.
mood stabilizing a.
neuroleptic a.
neuromuscular blocking a.
non–cycle-specific a.
nondepolarizing neuromuscular
  blocking a.
nonionic contrast a.
Norwalk a.
A. Orange
Pittsburgh pneumonia a.
promoting a.
psychotropic a.
reovirus-like a.
sclerosing a.
slow channel-blocking a.
sympathetic a.
transforming a.
TRIC a.
typical antipsychotic a.

agerasia
age-related macular degeneration
age-specific rate
ageusia
ageustia
agger, pl. **aggeres**
a. nasi
a. perpendicularis
a. valvae venae
agglomerate, agglomerated
agglomeration
agglutinant
agglutinate
agglutinating antibody
agglutination
acid a.
bacteriogenic a.
cold a.
cross a.
false a.
group a.
immune a.
indirect a.
nonimmune a.
passive a.
spontaneous a.
a. test
agglutinative thrombus
agglutinin
blood group a.
chief a.
cold a.
cross-reacting a.
flagellar a.
group a.
H a.
immune a.
incomplete a.
major a.
minor a.

O a.
partial a.
plant a.
saline a.
somatic a.
warm a.
agglutinogen
blood group a.
T a.
agglutinogenic
agglutinophilic
agglutogen
agglutogenic
aggrecan
aggregate
a. anaphylaxis
a. gland
proteoglycan a.
aggregated
a. lymphatic follicles of small
  intestine
a. lymphatic follicles of vermiform
  appendix
a. lymphatic nodule
a. lymphoid nodule
a. lymphoid nodule of small
  intestine
aggregation
familial a.
aggregometer
aggressin
aggression
aggressive
a. angiomyxoma
a. infantile fibromatosis
a. instinct
aging
clonal a.
agitated depression
agitolalia
agitophasia
aglomerular
aglossia
aglossia-adactylia syndrome
aglossostomia
aglucon
aglutition
aglycon, aglycone, pl. **aglyca**
aglycosuria
aglycosuric
agmen, pl. **agmina**
a. peyerianum
agminate gland
agnathia
agnathous
agnea
agnogenic myeloid metaplasia
agnosia
auditory a.
color a.
finger a.
gustatory a.
localization a.
olfactory a.
optic a.

agnosia *(continued)*
    position a.
    tactile a.
    visual a.
    visual-spatial a.
agomphious
agomphosis, agomphiasis
agonadal
agonal
    a. clot
    a. infection
    a. leukocytosis
    a. rhythm
    a. thrombus
agonist
agony
agoraphobia
agoraphobic
agouti
-agra
agraffe
agrammatica
agrammatism
agrammatologia
agranular
    a. cortex
    a. endoplasmic reticulum
    a. leukocyte
agranulocyte
agranulocytic angina
agranulocytosis
agranuloplastic
agraphia
    absolute a.
    acoustic a.
    amnemonic a.
    atactic a.
    constructional a.
    literal a.
    motor a.
    musical a.
    verbal a.
agraphic
agretope
ague
    brass founder's a.
AGUS
    atypical glandular cell of undetermined
      significance
agyiophobia
agyria
AH
    AH conduction time
    AH interval
ahaustral
AHG
    antihemophilic globulin
aHyl
    allohydroxylysine
ahylognosia
Aicardi syndrome
aichmophobia
AID
    programmable hearing aid

AIDS
    acquired immunodeficiency syndrome
      AIDS dementia
      AIDS dementia complex (ADC)
AIDS-related
    AIDS-r. complex (ARC)
    AIDS-r. virus (ARV)
AILD
    angioimmunoblastic lymphadenopathy
      with dysproteinemia
aIle
    alloisoleucine
ailurophobia
ainhum
AIR
    5-aminoimidazole ribose 5-phosphate
air
    alveolar a.
    a. bladder
    a. bronchogram
    a. cell
    a. cell of auditory tube
    complemental a.
    complementary a.
    a. conduction
    a. contrast barium enema
    a. contrast enema
    a. dose
    a. embolism
    functional residual a.
    a. hunger
    liquid a.
    minimal a.
    a. pollution
    reserve a.
    residual a.
    a. sac
    a. sickness
    a. splint
    supplemental a.
    a. syringe
    a. thermometer
    tidal a.
    a. tube
    a. vesicle
    vitiated a.
air-bone gap
airborne infection
airbrasive technique
air-conditioner lung
air-gap
    a.-g. radiography
    a.-g. technique
airplane splint
airport malaria
airsickness
air-slaked lime
airspace
airspace-filling pattern
airtrapping
airway
    anatomic a.
    conducting a.
    Guedel a.
    lower a.

neurogenic a.
a. pattern
a. pressure release ventilation
a. resistance
respiratory a.
upper a.
Airy disk
Ajellomyces
    A. capsulatum
    A. dermatitidis
ajmaline
ajowan oil
Akabane virus
A-K amputation
akamushi disease
akanthion
akaryocyte
akaryote
akathisia
akembe
Akerlund deformity
akinesia
    a. algera
    a. amnestica
akinesic
akinesis
akinesthesia
akinetic
    a. mutism
    a. seizure
akiyami
aklomide
aknemia (*var. of* acnemia)
AKNF
    Adair-Koshland-Némethy-Filmer model
Al
    aluminum
ALA
    delta-aminolevulinic acid
Ala
ala, pl. **alae**
    a. auris
    a. central lobule
    a. cerebelli
    a. cinerea
    a. cristae galli
    a. of crista galli
    a. of ilium
    ala lingulae cerebelli
    a. lobulis centralis
    a. major ossis sphenoidalis
    a. minor ossis sphenoidalis
    a. nasi
    a. of nose
    a. orbitalis
    a. ossis ilii
    a. sacralis
    a. of sacrum
    a. temporalis
    a. of vomer
    a. vomeris
alacrima
alactic oxygen debt
alae (*pl. of* ala)
Alagille syndrome

alalia
alalic
Aland Island albinism
alanine
    a. aminotransferase (ALT)
    a.-glyoxylate aminotransferase
    a.-oxomalonate aminotransferase
    a. racemase
    a. transaminase
β-alanine
β-alanine-pyruvate aminotransferase
alanosine
Alanson amputation
alantin
alantol
alant starch
alanyl
alar
    a. artery of nose
    a. chest
    a. fold of intrapatellar synovial fold
    a. lamina of neural tube
    a. ligament
    a. part of nasalis muscle
    a. plate of neural tube
    a. process
    a. spine
ALARA
    as low as reasonably achievable
alarmone
alarm reaction
alaryngeal speech
alastrim
alba
Albarran
    A. gland
    A. test
    A. y Dominguez tubule
albedo
Albers-Schönberg
    A.-S. disease
Albert
    A. stain
    A. suture
albicans, pl. **albicantia**
albiduria
albidus
Albini
    A. nodule
albinism
    Åland Island a.
    cutaneous a.
    Forsius-Eriksson a.
    Nettleshop-Falls a.
    ocular a.
    ocular a. 1, 2, 3
    ocular a. with late-onset
      sensorineural deafness
    ocular a. with sensorineural
      deafness
    oculocutaneous a.
    rufous a.
albino
    a. rat
albinotic

albinuria
Albinus muscle
albocinereous
Albrecht bone
Albright
    A. disease
    A. hereditary osteodystrophy
    A. syndrome
albuginea
albugineotomy
albugineous
albumen
albumin
    a. A, B
    acetosoluble a.
    Bence Jones a.
    blood a.
    bovine serum a. (BSA)
    dried human a.
    egg a.
    a. Ghent
    iodinated ^{131}I human serum a.
    iodinated ^{125}I serum a.
    macroaggregated a. (MAA)
    a. Mexico
    a. Naskapi
    native a.
    normal human serum a.
    Patein a.
    plasma a.
    radioiodinated serum a. (RISA)
    a. Reading
    serum a.
    a. tannate
albuminate
albuminaturia
albumin-globulin (A/G)
albumin-globulin ratio (A/G ratio)
albuminiferous
albuminiparous
albuminized iron
albuminocytologic dissociation
albuminogenous
albuminoid
albuminolysis
albuminoptysis
albuminorrhea
albuminous
    a. cell
    a. degeneration
    a. gland
    a. swelling
albuminuria
    adolescent a.
    adventitious a.
    a. of athletes
    Bamberger a.
    benign a.
    cardiac a.
    colliquative a.
    cyclic a.
    dietetic a.
    digestive a.
    essential a.
    false a.

    febrile a.
    functional a.
    intermittent a.
    lordotic a.
    neuropathic a.
    orthostatic a.
    physiologic a.
    postrenal a.
    postural a.
    prerenal a.
    recurrent a.
    regulatory a.
    transient a.
albuminuric retinitis
albuterol
Alcaligenes
alcapton
alcaptonuria, alkaptonuria
Alcian blue
alclofenac
alclometasone
Alcock canal
alcogel
alcohol
    absolute a.
    acid a.
    a. acid
    a. addiction
    a. amnestic syndrome
    anhydrous a.
    bile a.
    dehydrated a.
    a. dehydrogenase
    a. dehydrogenase (acceptor)
    a. dehydrogenase (NADP$^+$)
    denatured a.
    dihydric a.
    dilute a.
    a. diuresis
    fatty a.
    grain a.
    methyl a.
    monohydric a.
    multiple a.
    polyoxyethylene a.
    primary a.
    pyroligneous a.
    rubbing a.
    secondary a.
    sugar a.
    tertiary a.
    trihydric a.
    unsaturated a.
    wax a.
    a. withdrawal delirium
alcoholate
alcohol-glycerin fixative
alcoholic
    a. cardiomyopathy
    a. cirrhosis
    a. deterioration
    a. extract
    a. fermentation
    a. hyalin
    a. hyaline body

a. myocardiopathy
a. pneumonia
a. polyneuropathy
a. psychoses
a. tincture
a. withdrawal tremor
alcoholism
acute a.
chronic a.
alcoholization
alcoholophobia
alcoholysis
alcuronium chloride
ALD
adrenoleukodystrophy
aldadiene
aldaric acid
aldehol
aldehyde
activated glycol aldehyde
active a.
angular a.
a. dehydrogenase (acylating)
a. dehydrogenase (NAD$^+$)
a. dehydrogenase (NAD(P)$^+$)
a. fuchsin
a. reaction
a. reductase
aldehyde-lyase
Alder
A. anomaly
A. body
aldimine
alditol
aldobiuronic acid
aldocortin
aldohexose
aldoketomutase
aldolase
aldol condensation
aldonic acid
aldopentose
aldose
a. 1-epimerase
a. mutarotase
a. reductase
aldoside
aldosterone antagonist
aldosteronism
idiopathic a.
primary a.
secondary a.
aldosteronogenesis
aldotetrose
aldotriose
aldoxime
Aldrich syndrome
aldrin
alecithal ovum
Alectorobius talaje
alemmal
Aleppo boil
aleukemia

aleukemic
a. leukemia
a. myelosis
aleukemoid
aleukia
aleukocytic
aleukocytosis
aleurioconidium
aleuriospore
aleuron
aleuronate
aleuronoid
Alexander
A. disease
A. hearing impairment
A. law
alexia
incomplete a.
motor a.
musical a.
optic a.
sensory a.
visual a.
alexic
alexin unit
alexithymia
alfacalcidol
alfentanil hydrochloride
ALG
antilymphocyte globulin
algae
blue-green a.
algal
algaroba
algefacient
algesia
algesic
algesichronometer
algesimeter
algesiogenic
algesiometer
algesthesia
algesthesis
algestone acetophenide
algetic
algicide
algid
a. malaria
a. pernicious fever
a. stage
algin
alginate
algiomotor
algiomuscular
algiovascular
algodystrophy
algogenesis, algogenesia
algogenic
algoid cell
algolagnia
algology
algometer
algometry
algophilia
algophobia

algorithm
algoscopy
algospasm
algovascular
alible
Alice in Wonderland syndrome
alicyclic compound
alienation
alienia
aliform
alignment
    a. curve
    a. mark
aliment
alimentary
    a. apparatus
    a. canal
    a. diabetes
    a. glycosuria
    a. hyperinsulinism
    a. lipemia
    a. osteopathy
    a. pentosuria
    a. system
    a. tract
    a. tract smear
alimentation
    forced a.
    parenteral a.
    rectal a.
alinasal
alinement
alinjection
aliphatic
    a. acid
    a. compound
alipoid
alipotropic
aliquot
alisphenoid cartilage
alizarin
    a. cyanin
    a. indicator
    a. purpurin
    a. red S
alkadiene
alkalemia
alkali, pl. alkalies
    caustic a.
    a. denaturation test
    a. earth metal
    fixed a.
    a. metal
    a. reserve
    a. therapy
    vegetable a.
alkaline
    a. earth
    a. earth element
    a. milk drip
    a. phosphatase
    a. reaction
    a. reflux gastritis
    a. RNase
    a. tide

    a. toluidine blue O
    a. water
    a. wave
alkaline-ash diet
alkalinity
alkalinization
alkalinuria
alkalitherapy
alkalization
alkalizer
alkaloid
    ergot a.
    fixed a.
    Vinca a.
alkalosis
    acapnial a.
    compensated metabolic a.
    compensated respiratory a.
    metabolic a.
    respiratory a.
    uncompensated a.
alkalotic
alkaluria
alkane
alkanet
alkannan
alkannin
alkapton
alkaptonuria (*var. of* alcaptonuria)
alkatriene
alkavervir
alkene
alkenyl
alk-1-enyl
alk-1-enylglycerophospholipid
alkide
alkyl
    arylated a.
alkylamine
alkylating agent
alkylation
ALL
    acute lymphocytic leukemia
allachesthesia
allantoate deiminase
allantochorion
allantoenteric diverticulum
allantogenesis
allantoic
    a. acid
    a. bladder
    a. cyst
    a. diverticulum
    a. fluid
    a. sac
    a. stalk
    a. vesicle
allantoid membrane
allantoidoangiopagous twin
allantoidoangiopagus
allantoin
allantoinase
allantoinuria
allantois
allaxis

allele
  codominant a.
  silent a.
allelic
  a. exclusion
  a. gene
allelism
allelocatalysis
allelocatalytic
allelochemicals
allelomorph
allelomorphic
allelomorphism
allelotaxis
allelotaxy
Allen-Doisy
  A.-D. test
  A.-D. unit
Allen-Masters syndrome
Allen test
allergen
allergenic extract
allergic
  a. bronchopulmonary aspergillosis
    (ABPA)
  a. conjunctivitis
  a. contact dermatitis
  a. coryza
  a. eczema
  a. extract
  a. granulomatosis
  a. granulomatous angiitis
  a. inflammation
  a. purpura
  a. reaction
  a. rhinitis
  a. salute
allergist
allergization
allergized
allergology
allergosis
allergy
  atopic a.
  bacterial a.
  cold a.
  contact a.
  delayed a.
  drug a.
  immediate a.
  latent a.
  physical a.
  polyvalent a.
Allescheria boydii
allesthesia
allethrins
allethrolone
Allgrove syndrome
allied
  a. health professional
  a. reflex
alligation
alligator
  a. forceps
  a. skin

Allis forceps
alliteration
allium
all or none
all or none law
allo-
alloalbuminemia
alloantibody
alloantigen
allobarbital
allocentric
allochiria, allocheiria
allocholesterol
allochroic
allochroism
allocortex
allodeoxycholic acid
allodiploid
allodynia
alloerotism
alloesthesia
allogamy
allogenic, allogeneic
  a. antigen
  a. graft
  a. inhibition
allogotrophia
allograft rejection
allogroup
allohexaploid
allohydroxylysine (aHyl)
alloimmune
alloisoleucine (aIle)
alloisomer
allokeratoplasty
allokinesis
allolactose
allolalia
allomeric function
allomerism
allometron
allomones
allomorphism
allongement
allopath
allopathic keratoplasty
allopathist
allopathy
allopentaploid
allophanic acid
allophasis
allophenic
allophore
allophthalmia
alloplasia
alloplast
alloplasty
alloploid
alloploidy
allopolyploid
allopolyploidy
allopregnane
allopsychic
allopurinol
allorhythmia

allorhythmic
allose
allosensitization
allosome
    paired a.'s
    unpaired a.
allosteric
    a. enzyme
    a. site
allosterism, allostery
allotetraploid
allotherm
allothreonine (aThr)
allotope
allotopia
allotransplantation
allotriodontia
allotriosmia
allotriploid
allotrope
allotrophic
allotropic
allotropism, allotropy
allotype
    Gm a.
    InV a.
    Km a.
allotypic
    a. determinant
    a. marker
allowance
    recommended daily a. (RDA)
alloxan diabetes
alloxantin
alloxuremia
alloxuria
alloy
    chrome-cobalt a.
    eutectic a.
    gold a.
    Raney a.
    silver-tin a.
all-*trans*-retinal
allspice oil
allyl
    a. alcohol
    a. cyanide
    a. isothiocyanate
    a. sulfide
allylamine
allylestrenol
allylmercaptomethylpenicillin
***N*-allylnormorphine**
allysine
Almeida disease
Almén test for blood
almond oil
    bitter almond a. o.
aloe
aloe-emodin
aloetin
alogia
aloin
alopecia
    a. adnata

    androgenic a.
    a. areata
    a. capitis totalis
    cicatricial a.
    a. congenitalis
    congenital sutural a.
    female pattern a.
    a. hereditaria
    a. leprotica
    a. liminaris frontalis
    lipedematous a.
    male pattern a.
    a. marginalis
    a. medicamentosa
    moth-eaten a.
    a. mucinosa
    patterned a.
    postoperative pressure a.
    postpartum a.
    a. prematura
    premature a.
    a. presenilis
    pressure a.
    scarring a.
    a. senilis
    a. symptomatica
    a. syphilitica
    a. totalis
    a. toxica
    traction a.
    traumatic a.
    a. triangularis
    a. triangularis congenitalis
    a. universalis
alopecic
Alpers disease
alpha, α
    a. angle
    a. blocker
    a. blocking
    a. cell of anterior lobe of hypophysis
    a. cell of pancreas
    a. chain disease
    a. error
    a. fetoprotein
    a. fiber
    a. granule
    a. granule
    a. helix
    a. hemolysin
    a. methyl dopa
    a. particle (α)
    a. radiation
    a. ray
    a. rhythm
    a. substance
    A. tests
    a. thalassemia
    a. thalassemia intermedia
    a. unit
    a. wave
alpha-acetolactic acid
alpha-*N*-acetylgalactosaminidase
alpha-*N*-acetylglucosaminidase

alpha$_1$-acid glycoprotein
alpha-actinin
alpha-adrenergic
    -a. blocking agent
    -a. receptor
alpha-adrenoceptor antagonist
alpha-allocortol
alpha-allocortolone
alpha-allopregnanediol
alpha-amanitin
alpha-amino acid
alpha-aminoadipic acid (Aad)
alpha-aminoisobutyric acid
alpha-amino-β-ketoadipic acid
alpha amylase
alpha$_1$-antichymotrypsin
alpha$_1$-antitrypsin
    alpha$_1$-a. deficiency
    alpha$_1$-a. deficiency panniculitis
alpha-chymotrypsin-induced glaucoma
alpha-cortol
alpha-cortolone
alpha-dextrin endo-1,6-alpha-glucosidase
4,5-alpha-dihydrocortisol
1alpha,25-dihydroxycholecalciferol
alphadione
alpha-farnesene
alpha-fetoprotein (AFP)
9alpha-fluorocortisol
9alpha-fluorohydrocortisone acetate
alpha-fucosidase
alpha-D-galactosidase
1,4-alpha-D-glucan 6-alpha-D-
    glucosyltransferase
1,4-alpha-D-glucan-branching enzyme
alpha-glucan-branching glycosyltransferase
alpha-glucan phosphorylase
alpha-D-glucosidase
alpha-glucosidase inhibitor
alpha-heavy-chain disease
alpha-hemolytic streptococci
Alphaherpesvirinae
3alpha-hydroxy-5alpha-pregnan-20-one
7alpha-hydroxycholesterol
alpha-hydroxyethylthiamin pyrophosphate
alpha-L-iduronidase
alpha-keto
    a.-k. acid dehydrogenase
    a.-k. acid dehydrogenase complex
alpha-ketodecarboxylase
alpha-ketoglutaramic acid
alpha-ketoglutarate
alpha-ketoglutarate dehydrogenase
    complex
alpha-ketosuccinamic acid
alpha-lactyl-thiamin pyrophosphate
alpha-naphthylthiourea (ANTU)
L-alpha-narcotine
alpha$_2$-neuraminoglycoprotein
alpha-phenoxyethylpenicillin potassium
alpha-phenoxypropylpenicillin potassium
alpha$_1$PI
alphaprodine
alpha-ribazole
alpha-sarcin

alphasone acetophenide
alpha-T
alpha-tocopherol
Alphavirus
alpidem
Alpine scurvy
Alport syndrome
alprazolam
alprenolol hydrochloride
alprostadil
ALS
    amyotrophic lateral sclerosis
alseroxylon
Alström syndrome
ALT
    alanine aminotransferase
ALT:AST ratio
Altemeier operation
alteration
    modal a.
    qualitative a.
    quantitative a.
alterative inflammation
altercursive intubation
alteregoism
alternans
    auditory a.
    auscultatory a.
    concordant a.
    cycle length a.
    discordant a.
    electrical a.
Alternaria
alternate
    a. binaural loudness balance
      (ABLB)
    a. binaural loudness balance test
    a. cover test
    a. day strabismus
    a. hemianesthesia
alternating
    a. current (AC)
    a. failure of response, mechanical,
      to electrical depolarization
      (AFORMED)
    a. hemiplegia
    a. light test
    a. mydriasis
    a. pulse
    a. strabismus
    a. tremor
alternation
    cardiac a.
    concordant a.
    discordant a.
    electrical a. of heart
    a. of generations
    mechanical a. of the heart
alternative
    a. hypothesis
    a. inheritance
    a. medicine
    a. splicing
    a. tremor

alternator
alternis horis (alt. hor.)
alternocular
Alteromonas
    A. putrefaciens
althea
Altherr
alt. hor.
    alternis horis
altitude
    a. chamber
    a. disease
    a. erythremia
    a. sickness
altitudinal hemianopia
Altmann
    A. anilin-acid fuchsin stain
    A. fixative
    A. granule
    A. theory
Altmann-Gersh method
altrose
alu-equivalent family
alu family
alum
    burnt a.
    cake a.
    chrome a.
    dried a.
    exsiccated a.
    ferric a.
    whey a.
    a. whey
alum-hematoxylin
alumina
    hydrated a.
aluminated
aluminon
aluminosis
aluminum (Al)
    a. acetate
    a. acetotartrate
    a. acetylsalicylate
    a. ammonium sulfate
    a. aspirin
    a. bismuth oxide
    a. carbonate, basic
    a. chlorate nonahydrate
    a. chloride hexahydrate
    a. diacetate
    a. group
    a. hydrate
    a. hydroxide
    a. hydroxide gel
    a. hydroxychloride
    a. magnesium silicate
    a. monostearate
    a. nicotinate
    a. oleate
    a. oxide
    a. penicillin
    a. phenolsulfonate
    a. phosphate
    a. phosphate gel
    a. potassium sulfate

    a. salicylate, basic
    a. salicylate, basic, soluble
    a. silicate
    a. subacetate
    a. sulfate octadecahydrate
Alu sequence
alvei (*pl. of* alveus)
alveoalgia
alveolalgia
alveolar
    a. abscess
    a. adenocarcinoma
    a. air
    a. angle
    a. arch of mandible
    a. arch of maxilla
    a. atrophy
    a. body
    a. bone
    a. border
    a. canal of maxilla
    a. cell
    a. cell carcinoma
    a. crest
    a. dead space
    a. duct
    a. duct emphysema
    a. foramina of maxilla
    a. gas
    a. gas equation
    a. gingiva
    a. gland
    a. hydatid cyst
    a. index
    a. macrophage
    a. mucosa
    a. osteitis
    a. part of mandible
    a. pattern
    a. periosteum
    a. point
    a. pore
    a. process of maxilla
    a. ridge
    a. sac
    a. septum
    a. soft part sarcoma
    a. supporting bone
    a. ventilation ($\dot{V}A$)
    a. yoke
alveolar-arterial oxygen difference
alveolate
alveolectomy
alveoli (*pl. of* alveolus)
alveolingual
alveolitis
    acute pulmonary a.
    chronic fibrosing a.
    cryptogenic fibrosing a.
    extrinsic allergic a.
    fibrosing a.
alveolo-
alveolobuccal
    a. groove
    a. sulcus

alveolocapillary
    a. block
    a. membrane
alveoloclasia
alveolodental
    a. canal
    a. ligament
    a. membrane
alveololabial
    a. groove
    a. sulcus
alveololabialis
alveololingual
    a. groove
    a. sulcus
alveolonasal line
alveolopalatal
alveoloplasty
    interradicular a.
    intraseptal a.
alveoloschisis
alveolotomy
alveolus, pl. **alveoli**
    a. dentalis, pl. alveoli dentales
    pulmonary a.
    alveoli pulmonis
alveoplasty
alveus, pl. **alvei**
    a. hippocampi
    a. of hippocampus
    a. urogenitalis
ALW
    arch-loop-whorl system
alymphia
alymphocytosis
alymphoplasia
    Nezelof type of thymic a.
    thymic a.
Alzheimer
    A. dementia
    A. disease
    A. sclerosis
    A. type I, II astrocyte
alzyme
Am
    americium
am
    ammeter
AMA
    American Medical Association
amacrine cell
Amadori rearrangement
amadou
amalgam
    a. carrier
    a. matrix
    pin a.
    spherical a.
    a. strip
    a. tattoo
amalgamate
amalgamation
amalgamator

Amanita
    A. *muscaria*
    A. *phalloides*
amantadine hydrochloride
Am antigen
amara
amaranth solution
amaranthum
amarine
amaroid
amaroidal
amarum
amastia
amastigote
amathophobia
amatoxin
amaurosis
    a. congenita of Leber
    a. fugax
    pressure a.
    toxic a.
amaurotic
    a. cat eye
    a. mydriasis
    a. nystagmus
    a. pupil
amaxophobia
ambageusia
ambenonium chloride
AMBER
    advanced multiple-beam equalization
    radiography
amber
    a. codon
    a. mutant
    a. mutation
    a. suppressor
Amberg lateral sinus line
ambergris
ambidexterity
ambidextrism
ambidextrous
ambient cistern
ambiguity
    genital a.
ambiguous
    a. atrioventricular connection
    a. external genitalia
    a. genitalia
ambiguus nucleus
ambilateral
ambilevous
ambisexual
ambisinister
ambisinistrous
ambivalence
ambivalent
ambivert
amblygeustia
amblyogenic period
Amblyomma
    A. *americanum*
    A. *cajennense*
    A. *hebraeum*

Amblyomma (continued)
   A. maculatum
   A. variegatum
amblyopia
   anisometropic a.
   deprivation a.
   a. ex anopsia
   hysterical a.
   meridional a.
   nocturnal a.
   nutritional a.
   pattern distortion a.
   refractive a.
   sensory a.
   strabismic a.
   suppression a.
   tobacco-alcohol a.
   toxic a.
amblyopic
amblyoscope
   major a.
   Worth a.
amboceptor unit
ambomalleal
ambrosin
Ambu bag
ambucetamide
ambulance
ambulatory, ambulant
   a. anesthesia
   a. automatism
   a. edema
   a. erysipelas
   a. plague
   a. schizophrenia
   a. surgery
   a. typhoid
ambuphylline
amcinonide
ameba, pl. **amebae, amebas**
amebacide
amebaism
amebas (pl. of ameba)
amebiasis
   canine a.
   a. cutis
   hepatic a.
   pulmonary a.
amebic
   a. abscess
   a. colitis
   a. dysentery
   a. granuloma
   a. vaginitis
amebicidal
amebicide
amebiform
amebiosis
amebism
amebocyte
ameboid
   a. cell
   a. movement
ameboididity

ameboidism
ameboma
amebula, pl. **amebulae**
amebule
ameburia
amelanotic melanoma
amelia
amelioration
ameloblast
ameloblastic
   a. adenomatoid tumor
   a. fibroma
   a. fibrosarcoma
   a. layer
   a. odontoma
   a. sarcoma
ameloblastoma
   pigmented a.
   pituitary a.
ameloblastomatous craniopharyngioma
amelodental junction
amelogenesis imperfecta
amelogenins
amenia
amenorrhea
   dietary a.
   emotional a.
   exercise-induced a.
   hyperprolactinemic a.
   hypophysial a.
   hypothalamic a.
   lactation a.
   ovarian a.
   pathologic a.
   physiologic a.
   postpartum a.
   primary a.
   secondary a.
   traumatic a.
amenorrhea-galactorrhea syndrome
amenorrheal
amenorrheic
amentia
   nevoid a.
   phenylpyruvic a.
amential
American
   A. College of Nuclear Medicine
     (ACNM)
   A. College of Nuclear Physicians
     (ACNP)
   A. College of Radiology (ACR)
   A. Dental Association (ADA)
   A. Law Institute formulation
   A. Law Institute rule
   A. leishmaniasis
   A. Medical Association (AMA)
   A. National Standards Institute
     (ANSI)
   A. Red Cross
   A. Sign Language (ASL)
   A. tarantula
   A. trypanosomiasis
americium (Am)
amerism

A

ameristic
Ames
    A. assay
    A. test
amethopterin
ametria
ametriodinic acid
ametropia
    axial a.
    index a.
    refractive a.
ametropic
amiantaceous
amianthoid
amicrobic
amicroscopic
amidase
amide
    angiotensin a.
    nicotinic acid a.
    a. oxime
    primary a.
    secondary a.
    substituted a.
    tertiary a.
amidine
amidinohydrolases
amidinotransferases
amido black 10B
amidohydrolase
amidonaphthol red
amidopyrine
Amidostomum anseris
amidoximes
amidoxyl
amikacin sulfate
amiloride hydrochloride
amimia
aminacrine hydrochloride
aminate
amination
amine, quaternary ammonium ion
    adrenergic a.
    adrenomimetic a.
    biogenic a.
    a. oxidase (copper-containing)
    a. oxidase (flavin-containing)
    pressor a.
    primary a.
    secondary a.
    sympathetic a.
    sympathomimetic a.
    tertiary a.
    vasoactive a.
aminergic
amino
    a. acid activating enzyme
    a. acid activation
    a. acid analysis
    a. acid reagent
    a. sugar
amino acid (AA)
    acidic a. a.
    activated a. a.
    basic a. a.

    a. a. dehydrogenases
    dibasic a. a.
    essential a. a.
    nonessential a. a.
    nonpolar a. a.
    a. a. oxidase
    polar a. a.
aminoacidemia
aminoacid-tRNA ligases
aminoaciduria
    hyperbasic aminoaciduria
9-aminoacridine
5-aminoacridine hydrochloride
9-aminoacridine hydrochloride
aminoacyl adenylate
aminoacylase
aminoacyl-tRNA
    aminoacyl-tRNA ligases
    aminoacyl-tRNA synthetases
aminoadipic delta-semialdehyde synthase
aminobenzene
o-aminobenzoic acid
p-aminobenzoic acid (PABA)
D(-)-α-aminobenzylpenicillin
4-aminobutyrate pathway
aminocaproic acid
aminocarbonyl
aminocitric acid
2-amino-2-deoxy-D-galactose
aminoglutethimide
aminoglycoside
p-aminohippuric acid (PAH)
    p.-a. a. synthase
5-aminoimidazole ribose 5′-phosphate (AIR)
5-aminoimidazole ribotide
5-aminoimidazole-4-*N*-succinocarboxamide ribonucleotide
β-aminoisobutyrate:pyruvate aminotransferase
aminolysis
aminometradine
aminometramide
6-aminopenicillanic acid (6-APS)
aminopenicillin
aminopeptidase
aminopeptidase (cytosol)
aminopeptidase (microsomal)
aminophenazone
aminophylline
aminopromazine
aminopropionic acid
p-aminopropiophenone (PAPP)
aminopterin
6-aminopurine
4-aminopyridine
aminopyrine
aminorex
p-aminosalicylic acid (PAS, PASA)
amino-terminal
aminotransferase
aminotriazole
aminotripeptidase
aminuria
amiodarone hydrochloride

amithiozone
amitosis
amitotic
amitriptyline hydrochloride
amitrole
amlodipine
ammeter (am)
Ammon
    A. fissure
    A. horn
    A. prominence
ammonemia, ammoniemia
ammonia
    a. assimilation
    a. detoxication
    a. fixation
ammoniac
ammoniacal urine
ammonia-lyases
ammoniated
    a. mercuric chloride
    a. mercury
    a. tincture
ammoniemia (*var. of* ammonemia)
ammonium
    a. benzoate
    a. carbonate
    a. chloride
    dibasic a. phosphate
    a. ferric sulfate
    a. ichthosulfonate
    a. iodide
    a. mandelate
    a. molybdate
    monobasic a. phosphate
    a. nitrate
ammoniuria
ammonolysis
ammonotelia
ammonotelic
ammonotelism
amnemonic agraphia
amnesia
    anterograde a.
    emotional a.
    lacunar a.
    localized a.
    posthypnotic a.
    retrograde a.
    transient global a.
    traumatic a.
amnesiac
amnestic
    a. aphasia
    a. syndrome
amniocardiac vesicle
amniocele
amniocentesis
amniochorial, amniochorionic
amnioembryonic junction
amniogenesis
amniogenic cell
amniography
amnio-hook
amnioinfusion

amnioma
amnion
    a. nodosum
    a. ring
amnionic
    a. adhesion
    a. amputation
    a. band
    a. band syndrome
    a. cavity
    a. corpuscle
    a. duct
    a. ectoderm
    a. fluid
    a. fluid embolism
    a. fluid index
    a. fluid syndrome
    a. fold
    a. raphe
    a. sac
amnionitis
amniorrhea
amniorrhexis
amnioscope
amnioscopy
Amniota
amniotic
amniotome
amniotomy
amobarbital
A-mode
amodiaquine hydrochloride
Amoeba
    A. buccalis
    A. coli
    A. dentalis
    A. dysenteriae
    A. histolytica
    A. proteus
amoebapore
Amoebotaenia
amok
amorph
amorphagnosia
amorphia, amorphism
amorphosynthesis
amorphous
    a. fraction of adrenal cortex
    a. hydroxyapatite
    a. insulin zinc suspension
    a. phosphorus
    a. selenium plate
    a. silicon
amorphus
amoxapine
amoxicillin
AMP
    adenosine monophosphate
    cyclic AMP
    AMP deaminase
AMPA receptor
amperage
Ampère postulate
amperometry
ampheclexis

A

amphetamine
    a. (4-chlorophenoxy)acetate
    a. phosphate
    a. sulfate
d-**amphetamine phosphate**
d-**amphetamine sulfate**
amphiarthrodial
amphiarthrosis
amphiaster
amphibolic fistula
amphicelous
amphicentric
amphichroic
amphichromatic
amphicyte
amphid
amphidiploid
amphikaryon
amphileukemic
Amphimerus
amphimicrobe
amphimictic
amphimixis
amphinucleolus
amphion
Amphioxus
amphipathic
amphiphilic
amphiphobic
amphiprotic solvent
amphistome
amphitrichate, amphitrichous
amphitypy
amphixenosis
amphochromatophil, amphochromatophile
amphochromophil, amphochromophile
amphocyte
ampholyte
amphomycin
amphophil
amphophile
amphophilic, amphophilous
amphoric
    a. rale
    a. resonance
    a. respiration
    a. voice
    a. voice sound
amphoriloquy
amphorophony
amphoteric
    a. electrolyte
    a. element
    a. reaction
amphotericin, amphotericin B
amphotropic virus
ampicillin
ampl.
    amplus
amplexus
amplification
    genetic a.
    linear a.

amplifier
    a. host
    image a.
amplitude
    a. of accommodation
    a. of convergence
    a. of pulse
amplus (ampl.)
ampoule
amprotropine phosphate
ampule, ampul
ampulla, pl. **ampullae**
    biliaropancreatic a.
    a. biliaropancreatica
    bony ampullae of semicircular canal
    a. canaliculi lacrimalis
    a. chyli
    a. of ductus deferens
    a. ductus deferentis
    a. ductus lacrimalis
    duodenal a.
    a. duodeni
    a. of duodenum
    a. of gallbladder
    Henle a.
    hepatopancreatic a.
    a. hepatopancreatica
    a. of lacrimal canaliculus
    a. lactifera
    lactiferous a.
    a. of lactiferous duct
    a. membranacea, pl. ampullae
      membranaceae ductuum
      semicircularium
    membranous a.
    membranous ampullae of the
      semicircular duct
    a. of milk duct
    ampullae osseae canalium
      semicircularium
    osseous a.
    phrenic a.
    rectal a.
    a. recti
    a. of rectum
    Thoma a.
    a. tubae uterinae
    a. of uterine tube
    a. of Vater
ampullar
    a. abortion
    a. pregnancy
ampullary
    a. aneurysm
    a. crest
    a. crest of semicircular duct
    a. crus of semicircular duct
    a. cupula
    a. fold of uterine tube
    a. groove
    a. membranous limb of semicircular
      duct
    a. sulcus
    a. type of renal pelvis
ampullitis

ampullula
amputation
>A-E a.
>A-K a.
>Alanson a.
>amnionic a.
>aperiosteal a.
>B-E a.
>Bier a.
>B-K a.
>bloodless a.
>Callander a.
>Carden a.
>central a.
>cervical a.
>Chopart a.
>cinematic a.
>cineplastic a.
>circular a.
>congenital a.
>a. in continuity
>double flap a.
>dry a.
>Dupuytren a.
>eccentric a.
>elliptical a.
>excentric a.
>Farabeuf a.
>flap a.
>flapless a.
>forequarter a.
>Gritti-Stokes a.
>guillotine a.
>Guyon a.
>Hancock a.
>Hey a.
>hindquarter a.
>immediate a.
>intermediate a.
>interscapulothoracic a.
>intrauterine a.
>Jaboulay a.
>kineplastic a.
>Kirk a.
>knee disarticulation a.
>a. knife
>Krukenberg a.
>Le Fort a.
>linear a.
>Lisfranc a.
>Mackenzie a.
>major a.
>Malgaigne a.
>Mikulicz-Vladimiroff a.
>minor a.
>multiple a.
>a. neuroma
>oblique a.
>osteoplastic a.
>pathologic a.
>Pirogoff a.
>primary a.
>pulp a.
>quadruple a.
>racket a.

>rectangular a.
>root a.
>secondary a.
>spontaneous a.
>Stokes a.
>subastragalar a.
>subperiosteal a.
>Syme a.
>tarsotibial a.
>transverse a.
>traumatic a.
>Tripier a.
>Vladimiroff-Mikulicz a.

amputee
amrinone lactate
Amsel criteria
Amsler
>A. chart
>A. grid
>A. test

Amsterdam syndrome
amu
>atomic mass unit

amuck
amusia
>instrumental a.
>motor a.
>sensory a.
>vocal a.

Amussat
>A. valve
>A. valvula

amychophobia
Amycolatopsis orientalis subsp. *lurida*
amyelencephalia
amyelencephalic
amyelencephalous
amyelia
amyelic
amyelinated
amyelination
amyelinic
amyeloic, amyelonic
amyelous
amygdala, pl. amygdalae
>a. cerebelli

amygdalase
amygdalin
amygdaline
amygdaloclaustral area
amygdaloid
>a. body
>a. complex
>a. fossa
>a. nucleus
>a. tubercle

amygdalopiriform transition area
amygdalose
amygdaloside
amyl
>a. alcohol
>a. hydrate
>a. nitrite
>tertiary a. alcohol
>a. valerate

A

amylaceous corpuscle
amylase
amylase-creatinine clearance ratio
amylasuria
amylemia
amylene
    a. chloral
    a. hydrate
amylic fermentation
amylin
amylodextrin
amylogenesis
amylogenic body
amylo-1,4:1,6-glucantransferase
amyloglucosidase
amylo-1,6-glucosidase
amyloid
    a. angiopathy
    a. corpuscle
    a. degeneration
    a. kidney
    a. nephrosis
    a. protein
    a. tumor
amyloidoma
amyloidosis
    a. of aging
    chronic amyloidosis
    a. cutis
    familial a.
    focal a.
    hereditary a.
    lichen a.
    lichenoid a.
    light chain-related a.
    macular a.
    a. of multiple myeloma
    nodular a.
    primary a.
    renal a.
    secondary a.
    senile a.
amylolysis
amylolytic
amylomaltase
amylopectin
    a. 6-glucanohydrolase
    a. 1,6-glucosidase
amylopectinosis
amylophagia
amyloplast
amylopsin
amylorrhea
amylose
amylosuria
amylo-(1,4→1,6)-transglucosidase, amylo-
(1,4→1,6)-transglucosylase
amylum
amyluria
amyoesthesia, amyoesthesis
amyoplasia
    a. congenita
amyostasia
amyostatic
amyosthenia

amyosthenic
amyotaxy, amyotaxia
amyotonia congenita
amyotrophia
amyotrophic lateral sclerosis (ALS)
amyotrophy
    diabetic a.
    hemiplegic a.
    neuralgic a.
    progressive spinal a.
amyous
amyxorrhea
ANA (āā)
    antinuclear antibody
Anabaena
anabiosis
anabiotic cell
anabolic steroid
anabolism
anabolite
anacamptometer
anacatadidymus (*var. of* anakatadidymus)
anacatesthesia
anacidity
anaclasis
anaclitic
    a. depression
    a. psychotherapy
anacrotic
    a. limb
    a. pulse
anacrotism
anacusis
anadenia ventriculi
anadicrotism
anadidymus
anadipsia
anadrenalism
anadromous
anaerobe
    facultative a.
    obligate a.
anaerobic
    a. cellulitis
    a. dehydrogenase
    a. pneumonia
    a. respiration
anaerobiosis
Anaeroboplasma
anaerogenic
anaerophyte
anaeroplasty
anagen effluvium
anagenesis
anagenetic
anagestone acetate
anagogy
anakatadidymus, anacatadidymus
anákhré
anakmesis
anakusis
anal
    a. atresia
    a. canal
    a. cleft

anal *(continued)*
    a. column
    a. crypt
    a. cushion
    a. duct
    a. erotism
    a. fascia
    a. fissure
    a. fistula
    a. gland
    a. membrane
    a. orifice
    a. pecten
    a. phase
    a. pit
    a. plate
    a. reflex
    a. region
    a. sinus
    a. skin tag
    a. sphincter
    a. transitional zone
    a. triangle
    a. valves
    a. verge
analbuminemia
analeptic enema
analgesia
    conduction a.
    inhalation a.
    patient-controlled a. (PCA)
    spinal a.
analgesic
    a. cuirass
    a. nephritis
    a. nephropathy
analgesimeter
analgetic
anality
anallergic
analog
    enzyme a.
analogous
analogue
analphalipoproteinemia
analysand
analysis, pl. **analyses**
    accumulation a.
    activation a.
    amino acid a.
    bite a.
    blood gas a.
    bradykinetic a.
    breath a.
    cephalometric a.
    character a.
    cluster a.
    content a.
    decision a.
    didactic a.
    discriminant a.
    displacement a.
    distributive a.
    Downs a.

    ego a.
    Fourier a.
    gastric a.
    intention-to-treat a.
    interaction process a.
    Kaplan-Meier a.
    linkage a.
    Northern blot a.
    occlusal a.
    path a.
    pedigree a.
    percept a.
    qualitative a.
    quantitative a.
    regression a.
    saturation a.
    segregation a.
    sequential a.
    Southern blot a.
    survival a.
    training a.
    transactional a.
    a. of variance (ANOVA)
    volumetric a.
    Western blot a.
    zoo blot a.
analyst
analyte
analytic, analytical
    a. chemistry
    a. psychiatry
    a. psychology
    a. sensitivity
    a. specificity
    a. study
    a. therapy
analyzer, analyzor
    batch a.
    centrifugal fast a.
    continuous flow a.
    discrete a.
    kinetic a.
    pulse height a.
    wave a.
analyzing rod
anamnesis
anamnestic
    a. reaction
    a. response
anamnionic, anamniotic
Anamniota
anamorph
anamorphosis
ananastasia
anancasm
anancastia
anancastic
anandria
anangioplasia
anangioplastic
ANAP
    anionic neutrophil-activating peptide
anaphase lag
anaphia
anaphoresis

anaphoretic
anaphrodisiac
anaphylactic
    a. antibody
    a. intoxication
    a. reaction
    a. shock
anaphylactogen
anaphylactogenesis
anaphylactogenic
anaphylactoid
    a. crisis
    a. purpura
    a. shock
anaphylatoxin inactivator
anaphylaxis
    active a.
    aggregate a.
    antiserum a.
    chronic a.
    generalized a.
    inverse a.
    local a.
    passive a.
    passive cutaneous a.
    reversed a.
    reversed passive a.
    systemic a.
anaphylotoxin
anaplasia
anaplastic
    a. astrocytoma
    a. carcinoma
    a. cell
    a. large cell lymphoma
    a. oligodendroglioma
anaplastology
anaplerosis
anaplerotic reaction
anapophysis
anaptic
anarithmia
anarthria
anarthritic rheumatoid disease
anasarca
    fetoplacental a.
anasarcous
anastigmatic
anastigmats
anastole
anastomose
anastomosing
    a. fiber
    a. vessel
anastomosis, pl. **anastomoses**
    acromial a. of the thoracoacromial
      artery
    arteriolovenular a.
    a. arteriolovenularis
    a. arteriovenosa
    arteriovenous a. (ava)
    Béclard a.
    bevelled a.
    Billroth I, II a.
    Braun a.

    calcaneal a.
    cavopulmonary a.
    Clado a.
    conjoined a.
    crucial a.
    cruciate a.
    cubital a.
    Damus-Stancel-Kaye a.
    elliptical a.
    end-to-end a.
    Galen a.
    genicular a.
    Hofmeister-Pólya a.
    Hoyer a.
    Hyrtl a.
    intermesenteric arterial a.
    intestinal a.
    isoperistaltic a.
    Jacobson a.
    Martin-Gruber a.
    microvascular a.
    patellar a.
    portacaval a.
    portal-systemic a.
    postcostal a.
    Potts a.
    precapillary a.
    precostal a.
    pulmonary artery a.
    ranine a.
    Riolan a.
    Roux-en-Y a.
    Schmidel a.
    sequential a.
    Sucquet a.
    Sucquet-Hoyer a.
    terminoterminal a.
    transureteroureteral a.
    ureteroileal a.
    ureterosigmoid a.
    ureteroureteral a.
anastomotic
    a. branch
    a. branch of middle meningeal
      artery with lacrimal artery
    a. fiber
    a. stricture
    a. ulcer
    a. vein
    a. vessel
anastral
anatomic
    a. airway
    a. dead space
    a. pathology
    a. position
    a. snuffbox
    a. sphincter
    a. tooth
    a. tubercle
    a. wart
anatomical
    a. age
    a. conjugate
    a. crown

anatomical *(continued)*
    a. element
    a. internal os of uterus
    a. neck of humerus
    a. root
anatomicomedical
anatomicopathologic
anatomicosurgical
anatomist
anatomy
    applied a.
    artificial a.
    artistic a.
    clastic a.
    clinical a.
    comparative a.
    dental a.
    descriptive a.
    developmental a.
    functional a.
    general a.
    gross a.
    living a.
    macroscopic a.
    medical a.
    microscopic a.
    pathologic a.
    physiologic a.
    plastic a.
    practical a.
    radiologic a.
    regional a.
    special a.
    surface a.
    surgical a.
    systematic a.
    systemic a.
    topographic a.
    transcendental a.
    ultrastructural a.
anatopism
anatoxic
anatoxin
anatricrotic
anatricrotism
anatripsis
anatriptic
anatrophic nephrotomy
anaxon, anaxone
anazoturia
ANCA
    antineutrophil cytoplasmic antibody
AnCC
    anodal closure contraction
ancestor
    leading a.
anchorage
    cervical a.
    a. dependence
    extraoral a.
    intermaxillary a.
    intramaxillary a.
    intraoral a.
    multiple a.

    occipital a.
    reciprocal a.
    reinforced a.
    simple a.
    stationary a.
anchorin
anchoring
    a. fibril
    a. villus
anchor splint
anchusin
ancillary port
ancipital, ancipitate, ancipitous
ancon
anconad
anconal, anconeal
    a. fossa
anconeus
    a. muscle
anconoid
ancrod
Ancylostoma
    A. braziliense
    A. caninum
    A. ceylanicum
    A. dermatitis
    A. duodenale
    A. tubaeforme
ancylostomatic
ancylostomiasis
    cutaneous a.
ancyroid
Andernach ossicles
Andersch
    A. ganglion
    A. nerve
Anders disease
Andersen disease
Anderson
    A. and Goldberger test
    A. splint
Anderson-Collip test
Andes virus
andira
Andral decubitus
andrenosterone
andriatrics, andriatry
androgen
    adrenal a.
    a. binding protein (ABP)
    a. insensitivity syndrome
    a. resistance syndrome
    a. unit
androgenesis
androgenic
    a. alopecia
    a. hormone
    a. zone
androgenous
androgynism
androgynoid
androgynous
androgyny

android
> a. obesity
> a. pelvis

andrology
andromedotoxin
andromorphous
andropathy
andropause
androphobia
androstane
androstanediol
androstanedione
androstene
androstenediol
androstenedione
androstenol
androstenolone
androsterone
anecdotal
anechoic chamber
anelectrotonic
anelectrotonus
Anel method
anemia
> achlorhydric a.
> achrestic a.
> acquired hemolytic a.
> Addison a.
> addisonian a.
> angiopathic hemolytic a.
> aplastic a.
> asiderotic a.
> autoimmune hemolytic a.
> *Bartonella* a.
> Belgian Congo a.
> Biermer a.
> brickmaker's a.
> chlorotic a.
> congenital aplastic a.
> congenital dyserythropoietic a.
> congenital hemolytic a.
> congenital hypoplastic a.
> congenital nonregenerative a.
> Cooley a.
> cow milk a.
> deficiency a.
> Diamond-Blackfan a.
> dilution a.
> dimorphic a.
> diphyllobothrium a.
> drepanocytic a.
> dyshemopoietic a.
> Ehrlich a.
> elliptocytary a.
> elliptocytotic a.
> erythroblastic a.
> erythronormoblastic a.
> essential a.
> Faber a.
> false a.
> familial hypoplastic a.
> familial microcytic a.
> familial pyridoxine-responsive a.
> Fanconi a.
> fish tapeworm a.

> folic acid deficiency a.
> goat's milk a.
> a. gravis
> ground itch a.
> Heinz body a.
> hemolytic a.
> hemolytic a. of newborn
> hemorrhagic a.
> hookworm a.
> hypochromic microcytic a.
> hypoferric a.
> hypoplastic a.
> infectious a.
> iron deficiency a.
> isochromic a.
> lead a.
> leukoerythroblastic a.
> local a.
> macrocytic achylic a.
> macrocytic a. of pregnancy
> macrocytic a. tropical
> malignant a.
> Marchiafava-Micheli a.
> megaloblastic a.
> megalocytic a.
> metaplastic a.
> microangiopathic hemolytic a.
> microcytic a.
> microdrepanocytic a.
> milk a.
> mountain a.
> myelopathic a.
> myelophthisic a.
> neonatal a.
> a. neonatorum
> normochromic a.
> normocytic a.
> nutritional macrocytic a.
> osteosclerotic a.
> pernicious a.
> physiologic a.
> polar a.
> posthemorrhagic a.
> primary erythroblastic a.
> primary refractory a.
> pure red cell a.
> radiation a.
> refractory a.
> scorbutic a.
> secondary refractory a.
> sickle cell a.
> sideroachrestic a.
> sideroblastic a.
> slaty a.
> spastic a.
> spherocytic a.
> splenic a.
> spur cell a.
> target cell a.
> toxic a.
> traumatic a.
> tropical a.
> unstable hemoglobin hemolytic a.

anemic
> a. anoxia

anemic *(continued)*
    a. halo
    a. hypoxia
    a. infarct
    a. murmur
anemometer
anemonol
anemophobia
anemotrophy
anencephalia
anencephalic
anencephalous
anencephaly
    partial a.
anenterous
anenzymia
anephric
anepiploic
anergia
anergic leishmaniasis
anergy
    negative a.
    nonspecific a.
    positive a.
    specific a.
aneroid manometer
anerythroplasia
anerythroplastic
anerythroregenerative
anesthecinesia
anesthekinesia
anesthesia
    acupuncture a.
    ambulatory a.
    axillary a.
    balanced a.
    basal a.
    block a.
    brachial a.
    caudal a.
    cervical a.
    circle absorption a.
    closed a.
    compression a.
    conduction a.
    continuous epidural a.
    continuous spinal a.
    crossed a.
    dental a.
    diagnostic a.
    differential spinal a.
    dissociated a.
    dissociative a.
    a. dolorosa
    electric a.
    endotracheal a.
    epidural a.
    extradural a.
    field block a.
    fractional epidural a.
    fractional spinal a.
    general a.
    girdle a.
    glove a.

    gustatory a.
    high spinal a.
    hyperbaric spinal a.
    hypobaric spinal a.
    hypotensive a.
    hypothermic a.
    hysterical a.
    infiltration a.
    inhalation a.
    insufflation a.
    intercostal a.
    intramedullary a.
    intranasal a.
    intraoral a.
    intraosseous a.
    intraspinal a.
    intratracheal a.
    intravenous regional a.
    isobaric spinal a.
    local a.
    low spinal a.
    a. machine
    nerve block a.
    nonrebreathing a.
    open drop a.
    outpatient a.
    painful a.
    paracervical block a.
    paravertebral a.
    patient-controlled a.
    peridural a.
    periodontal a.
    presacral a.
    pressure a.
    pudendal a.
    rebreathing a.
    a. record
    rectal a.
    refrigeration a.
    regional a.
    retrobulbar a.
    sacral a.
    saddle block a.
    segmental a.
    spinal a.
    splanchnic a.
    stocking a.
    subarachnoid a.
    surgical a.
    tactile a.
    therapeutic a.
    thermal a.
    thermic a.
    to-and-fro a.
    topical a.
    total spinal a.
    traumatic a.
    unilateral a.
    visceral a.
anesthesiologist
anesthesiology
anesthetic
    a. circuit
    a. depth
    a. ether

flammable a.
a. gas
general a.'s
a. index
inhalation a.
intravenous a.
a. leprosy
local a.'s
primary a.
secondary a.
a. shock
spinal a.
topical a.
a. vapor
volatile a.

anesthetist
certified registered nurse a. (CRNA)
anesthetization
anesthetize
anestrous ovulation
anestrum
anestrus
anethopath
anetoderma
Jadassohn-Pellizzari a.
Schweninger-Buzzi a.
aneuploid
aneuploidy
partial a.
aneurine
a. hydrochloride
a. pyrophosphate
aneurolemmic
aneurysm
ampullary a.
a. by anastomosis
aortic sinus a.
arteriosclerotic a.
arteriovenous a.
atherosclerotic a.
axial a.
benign bone a.
Bérard a.
berry a.
cardiac a.
Charcot-Bouchard a.
cirsoid a.
compound a.
congenital cerebral a.
consecutive a.
coronary artery a.
cylindroid a.
diffuse a.
dissecting a.
ductal a.
ectatic a.
false a.
fusiform a.
hernial a.
infraclinoid a.
intracavernous a.
intracranial a.
miliary a.
mural aneurysm
mycotic a.

a. needle
Park a.
peripheral a.
phantom a.
Pott a.
pulmonary artery a.
racemose a.
Rasmussen a.
a. of the right ventricle or right
ventricular outflow patch
ruptured a.
saccular a.
sacculated a.
serpentine a.
a. of sinus of Valsalva
supraclinoid a.
syphilitic a.
traumatic a.
true a.
tubular a.
varicose a.
ventricular a.
a. of the ventricular portion of the
membranous septum
aneurysmal
a. bone cyst
a. bruit
a. cough
a. murmur
a. sac
a. varix
aneurysmatic
aneurysmectomy
aneurysmoplasty
aneurysmorrhaphy
aneurysmotomy
ANF
antinuclear factor
angelica root
Angelman syndrome
Angelucci syndrome
angel wing
Anger
Anger camera
angiectasia
congenital dysplastic a.
angiectasis
angiectatic
angiectopia
angiitis, angitis
allergic granulomatous a.
consecutive a.
frosted branch a.
hypersensitivity a.
necrotizing a.
angina
abdominal a.
a. abdominis
agranulocytic a.
crescendo a.
a. cruris
a. decubitus
a. of effort
false a.
Heberden a.

angina *(continued)*
    hypercyanotic a.
    intestinal a.
    a. inversa
    Ludwig a.
    lymphatic a.
    a. lymphomatosa
    neutropenic a.
    a. pectoris
    a. pectoris decubitus
    a. pectoris sine dolore
    a. pectoris vasomotoria
    preinfarction a.
    Prinzmetal a.
    reflex a.
    a. sine dolore
    a. spuria
    unstable a.
    variant a. pectoris
    vasomotor a.
    a. vasomotoria
    Vincent a.
    walk-through a.
anginal
anginiform
anginoid
anginophobia
anginose, anginous
    a. scarlatina
angioarchitecture
angioblast
angioblastic
    a. cell
    a. cyst
angioblastoma of Nakagawa
angiocardiography
    exercise radionuclide a.
    gated radionuclide a.
    radionuclide a.
angiocardiokinetic, angiocardiocinetic
angiocardiopathy
angiocholitis
angiocyst
angioderm
angiodysgenetic myelomalacia
angiodysplasia
angiodystrophy, angiodystrophia
angioedema
    hereditary a.
angioelephantiasis
angioendotheliomatosis
    proliferating systematized a.
angiofibrolipoma
angiofibroma
    juvenile a.
angiofibrosis
angiofollicular mediastinal lymph node hyperplasia
angiogenesis factor
angiogenic
angioglioma
angiogliomatosis
angiogliosis

angiogram
    projection a.
angiographic
angiography
    biplane a.
    a. catheter
    cerebral a.
    closed a.
    coronary a.
    digital subtraction a. (DSA)
    fluorescein a.
    indocyanine green a.
    interventional a.
    magnetic resonance a. (MRA)
    magnification a.
    MR a.
    open a.
    radionuclide a.
    scintigraphic a.
    selective a.
    therapeutic a.
angiohyalinosis
angiohypertonia
angiohypotonia
angioid streak
angioimmunoblastic lymphadenopathy with dysproteinemia (AILD)
angioinvasive
angiokeratoma
    diffuse a.
    Fordyce a.
    Mibelli a.
angiokeratosis
angioleiomyoma
angiolipofibroma
angiolipoma
angiolith
angiolithic
    a. degeneration
    a. sarcoma
angiologia
angiology
angiolymphoid hyperplasia with eosinophilia
angiolysis
angioma
    acquired tufted a.
    capillary a.
    cavernous a.
    cherry a.
    petechial a.
    a. serpiginosum
    spider a.
    superficial a.
    telangiectatic a.
    a. venosum racemosum
    venous a.
angiomatoid
angiomatosis
    bacillary a.
    cephalotrigeminal a.
    cerebroretinal a.
    congenital dysplastic a.
    cutaneomeningospinal a.
    encephalotrigeminal a.

oculoencephalic a.
telangiectatic a.
angiomatous
angiomegaly
angiomyocardiac
angiomyofibroma
angiomyolipoma
angiomyoma
angiomyopathy
angiomyosarcoma
angiomyxoma
aggressive a.
angioneurectomy
angioneuropathy
angioneurotic edema
angioneurotomy
angioosteohypertrophy syndrome
angioparalysis
angioparesis
angiopathic
a. hemolytic anemia
a. neurasthenia
angiopathy
amyloid a.
cerebral amyloid a.
congophilic a.
giant cell hyaline a.
angiophacomatosis, angiophakomatosis
angioplany
angioplasty
a. balloon
percutaneous transluminal a.
percutaneous transluminal
coronary a. (PTCA)
angiopoiesis
angiopoietic
angiorrhaphy
angiosarcoma
angioscope
angioscopy
angioscotoma
angioscotometry
angiosis
angiosome
angiospasm
angiospastic
angiostenosis
angiostrongylosis
Angiostrongylus
A. *cantonensis*
A. *costaricensis*
A. *malaysiensis*
angiotelectasia
angiotelectasis
angiotensin
a. amide
angiotensin I, II, III
a. receptor
a. receptor blocker
angiotensinase
angiotensin-converting
a.-c. enzyme (ACE)
a.-c. enzyme inhibitor (ACEI)
angiotensinogen
angiotensinogenase

angiotensin precursor
angiotomy
angitis (*var. of* angiitis)
angle
acromial a.
acute a.
adjacent a.
alpha a.
alveolar a.
anorectal a.
a. of antetorsion
a. of anteversion
a. of aperture
apical a.
axial a.
basilar a.
Bennett a.
beta a.
biorbital a.
Broca basilar a.
Broca facial a.
buccal a.
buccoocclusal a.
cardiodiaphragmatic a.
cardiohepatic a.
cardiophrenic a.
carrying a.
cavity line a.
cavosurface a.
cephalic a.
cephalomedullary a.
cerebellopontile a.
cerebellopontine a.
A. classification of malocclusion
a. of convergence
costal a.
costophrenic a.
costovertebral a.
costoxiphoid a.
craniofacial a.
critical a.
cusp a.
Daubenton a.
a. of declination
a. of deviation
disparity a.
duodenojejunal a.
a. of eccentricity
a. of emergence
epigastric a.
ethmoid a.
facial a.
a. of femoral torsion
filtration a.
flip a.
Frankfort-mandibular incisor a.
frontal a. of parietal bone
a. of Fuchs
gamma a.
hypsiloid a.
impedance a.
a. of incidence
incident a.
incisal guide a.
a. of inclination

angle *(continued)*
    inferior a. of scapula
    infrasternal a.
    iridocorneal a.
    a. of iris
    Jacquart facial a.
    a. of jaw
    kappa a.
    lateral a. of eye
    lateral a. of scapula
    lateral a. of uterus
    limiting a.
    line a.
    Louis a.
    Lovibond a.
    Ludwig a.
    lumbosacral a.
    a. of mandible
    mastoid a. of parietal bone
    maxillary a.
    medial a. of eye
    mesial a.
    metafacial a.
    meter a.
    a. of mouth
    neck-shaft a.
    occipital a. of parietal bone
    olfactory a.
    ophryospinal a.
    parietal a.
    pelvivertebral a.
    phrenopericardial a.
    Pirogoff a.
    point a.
    a. of polarization
    pontine a.
    pubic a.
    Q a.
    Quatrefages a.
    Ranke a.
    a. recession
    a. of reflection
    refracting a. of a prism
    a. of refraction
    a. of retroversion
    a. of rib
    Rolando a.
    Serres a.
    S-N-A a.
    S-N-B a.
    sphenoid a.
    sphenoidal a. of parietal bone
    sternal a.
    sternoclavicular a.
    subcostal a.
    subpubic a.
    substernal a.
    superior a. of scapula
    sylvian a.
    tentorial a.
    Topinard facial a.
    a. of torsion
    urethrovesical a.
    venous a.
    Virchow a.
    Virchow-Holder a.
    visual a.
    Vogt a.
    Weisbach a.
    Welcker a.
    xiphocostal a.
    y-a.

angle-closure glaucoma
angor
    a. animi
    a. pectoris
Ångström
    Ångström law
    Ångström scale
    Ångström unit
Anguillula
angular
    a. acceleration
    a. aldehyde
    angular sphincter
    a. aperture
    a. artery
    a. cheilitis
    a. conjunctivitis
    a. convolution
    a. curvature
    a. gyrus
    a. incisure
    a. methyl
    a. notch
    a. spine
    a. stomatitis
    a. vein
angulation
    apex anterior a.
    apex posterior a.
angulus, pl. **anguli**
    a. acromii
    a. costae
    a. frontalis ossis parietalis
    a. inferior scapulae
    a. infrasternalis
    a. iridis
    a. iridocornealis
    a. lateralis scapulae
    a. mandibulae
    a. mastoideus ossis parietalis
    a. occipitalis ossis parietalis
    a. oculi lateralis
    a. oculi medialis
    a. oculi nasalis
    a. oculi temporalis
    a. oris
    a. pontocerebellaris
    a. sphenoidalis ossis parietalis
    a. sterni
    a. subpubicus
    a. superior scapulae
anhaphia
anhedonia
anhepatic jaundice
anhepatogenous jaundice
anhidrosis
anhidrotic ectodermal dysplasia

A

anhistic, anhistous
anhydrase
    carbonic a.
anhydration
anhydride
3,6-anhydrogalactose
anhydrogitalin
anhydroleucovorin
anhydrosugar
anhydrous
    a. alcohol
    a. chloral
    a. lanolin
ani (*pl. of* anus)
aniacinamidosis
aniacinosis
anicteric
    a. hepatitis
    a. leptospirosis
    a. virus hepatitis
anidean
anideus
    embryonic a.
anidous
anileridine
anilide
anilinction, anilinctus
aniline
    a. blue
    a. fuchsin
anilingus
anilinism
anilinophil, anilinophile
anilinophilous
anilism
anima
animal
    a. black
    a. charcoal
    cold-blooded a.
    control a.
    conventional a.
    a. dextran
    a. force
    a. graft
    Houssay a.
    a. magnetism
    a. model
    normal a.
    a. pole
    a. protein factor (APF)
    a. psychology
    sentinel a.
    a. soap
    a. starch
    a. toxin
    a. viruses
    warm-blooded a.
    a. wax
animalcule
animation
    suspended a.
animatism
animism
animus

AN interval
anion
    a. exchange
    a. exchanger
    a. gap
anion-exchange resin
anionic
    a. detergent
    a. neutrophil-activating peptide
      (ANAP)
anionotropy
aniridia
anisakiasis
anisakid
Anisakidae
Anisakis
anisate
anise
aniseikonia
anisic acid
anisindione
anisoaccommodation
anisochromasia
anisochromatic
anisocoria
    essential a.
    physiologic a.
    simple a.
    simple-central a.
anisocytosis
anisodactylous
anisodactyly
anisogamy
anisognathous
anisokaryosis
anisole
anisomastia
anisomelia
anisometropia
anisometropic amblyopia
anisopiesis
anisorrhythmia
anisosphygmia
anisosthenic
anisotonic
anisotropic
    a. disk
    a. lipid
anisotropine methylbromide
Anitschkow
    A. cell
    A. myocyte
ankle
    a. bone
    a. clonus
    a. jerk
    a. joint
    a. reflex
    a. region
ankle-foot orthosis
ankyloblepharon
ankylodactyly, ankylodactylia
ankyloglossia superior syndrome
ankylomele
ankylosed tooth

ankylosing
 a. hyperostosis
 a. spondylitis
ankylosis
 artificial a.
 bony a.
 dental a.
 extracapsular a.
 false a.
 fibrous a.
 intracapsular a.
 spurious a.
 true a.
Ankylostoma
ankylostomiasis
ankylotic
ankyrin
ankyroid
anlage, pl. **anlagen**
anneal
annealing
 a. lamp
 a. tray
annectent gyrus
Annelida
annelids
annellide
annelloconidium
annexa
annexal
annexin
annihilation radiation
annotto
annular
annulate lamellae
annuloaortic ectasia
annuloplasty ring
annulorrhaphy
annulospiral
 a. ending
 a. organ
annulus
AnOC
 anodal opening contraction
anochromasia
anociassociation
anococcygeal
 a. body
 a. ligament
 a. nerve
anocutaneous line
anodal
 a. closure contraction (ACC, AnCC)
 a. current
 a. opening contraction (AnOC, AOC)
anode
 a. ray
 rotating a.
anoderm
anodic
anodontia
 partial a.
anodontism
anodyne

anoetic
anogenital
 a. band
 a. raphe
anomalad
anomaloscope
anomalous
 a. atrioventricular excitation
 a. complex
 a. conduction
 a. mitral arcade
 a. pulmonary venous connection, total or partial
 a. retinal correspondence
 a. trichromatism
 a. uterus
 a. viscosity
anomaly
 Alder a.
 Aristotle a.
 Chédiak-Steinbrinck-Higashi a.
 developmental a.
 Ebstein a.
 eugnathic a.
 Freund a.
 Hegglin a.
 May-Hegglin a.
 morning glory a.
 Pelger-Huët nuclear a.
 Peters a.
 Rieger a.
 Shone a.
 Uhl a.
 urogenital sinus a.
 vertebral defects, anal atresia, tracheoesophageal fistula with esophageal atresia, and radial and renal a.'s (VATER)
anomer
anomeric carbon
anomia
anomic aphasia
anomie
anonychia, anonychosis
anonyma
anonymous vein
Anopheles
 A. aconitus
 A. albimanus
 A. albitarsus
 A. annularis
 A. annulipes
 A. aquasalis
 A. arabiensis
 A. aztecus
 A. balabacensis
 A. barbirostris
 A. bellator
 A. brunnipes
 A. campestris
 A. crucians
 A. cruzi
 A. culicifacies
 A. darlingi
 A. flavirostris

A. *fluviatilis*
A. *freeborni*
A. *funestus*
A. *gambiae*
A. *jeyporiensis*
A. *karwari*
A. *kweiyangensis*
A. *labranchiae*
A. *lesteri*
A. *leucosphyrus*
A. *maculatus*
A. *maculipennis*
A. *messeae*
A. *minimus*
A. *pseudopunctipennis*
A. *quadrimaculatus*
A. *stephensi*
A. *sundaicus*
A. *superpictus*

anophelicide
anophelifuge
Anophelinae
anopheline
Anophelini
anophelism
anophthalmia
anophthalmos
anoplasty
Anoplocephala
A. *perfoliata*
Anoplura
anorchia
anorchism
anorectal
a. angle
a. flexure
a. junction
a. lymph node
a. spasm
a. syndrome
anorectic, anoretic
anorectoperineal muscle
anorexia nervosa
anorexiant
anorexic
anorexigenic
anorgasmy, anorgasmia
anoscope
Bacon a.
anosigmoidoscopy
anosmia
anosmic
anosodiaphoria
anosognosia
anosognosic
a. epilepsy
a. seizure
anospinal center
anosteoplasia
anostosis
anotia
ANOVA
analysis of variance
anovesical

anovular
a. menstruation
a. ovarian follicle
anovulation
anovulational menstruation
anovulatory cycle
anoxemia test
anoxia
anemic a.
anoxic a.
diffusion a.
histotoxic a.
a. neonatorum
oxygen affinity a.
stagnant a.
anoxic anoxia
ANP
atrial natriuretic peptide
ANP clearance receptor
Anrep
A. effect
A. phenomenon
ANS
anterior nasal spine
ansa, pl. **ansae**
a. cervicalis
Haller a.
Henle a.
a. hypoglossi
lenticular a.
a. lenticularis
ansae nervorum spinalium
peduncular a.
a. peduncularis
Reil a.
a. sacralis
a. subclavia
Vieussens a.
ansate
anserine
a. bursa
a. bursitis
ANSI
American National Standards Institute
ansiform lobule
ansoparamedian fissure
ansotomy
ant
black imported fire a.
fire a.
harvester a.
red imported fire a.
velvet a.
antacid
antagonism
bacterial a.
antagonist
aldosterone a.
alpha-adrenoceptor a.
associated a.
beta-adrenoreceptor a.
calcium a.
competitive a.
enzyme a.
folic acid a.

antagonist *(continued)*
    5-hydroxytryptamine a.
    insulin a.
    leukotriene receptor a.
    muscarinic a.
    opioid a.
antagonistic
    a. muscle
    a. reflex
antalgesia
antalgic gait
antalkaline
antaphrodisiac
antaphroditic
antarthritic
antasthenic
antasthmatic
antatrophic
antazoline hydrochloride
antebrachial
    a. fascia
    a. flexor retinaculum
antebrachium
antecardium
antecedent
    plasma thromboplastin a. (PTA)
    a. sign
ante cibum (a.c.)
antecubital space
antefebrile
anteflex
anteflexion of iris
antegonial notch
antegrade
    a. block
    a. cardioplegia
    a. conduction
    a. cystography
    a. pyelography
    a. urography
antemortem
    a. clot
    a. thrombus
antenatal diagnosis
antepartum
anteposition
antepyretic
anterior
    a. abdominal cutaneous branch of intercostal nerve
    a. acoustic stria
    a. ampullary nerve
    a. amygdaloid area
    a. antebrachial nerve
    a. antebrachial region
    a. aphasia
    a. apprehension test
    a. arch of atlas
    a. articular surface of dens
    a. asynclitism
    a. atlanto-occipital membrane
    a. auricular branch of superficial temporal artery
    a. auricular groove

    a. auricular muscle
    a. auricular nerve
    a. auricular vein
    a. axillary fold
    a. axillary line
    a. axillary lymph node
    a. basal branch
    a. basal branch of superior basal vein (of right and left inferior pulmonary veins)
    a. basal segmental artery
    a. basal segment [S VIII]
    a. basal vein
    a. belly of digastric muscle
    a. border
    a. border of body of pancreas
    a. border of eyelids
    a. border of fibula
    a. border of lung
    a. border of pancreas
    a. border of radius
    a. border of testis
    a. border of tibia
    a. border of ulna
    a. brachial region
    a. branch
    a. branch of the renal artery
    a. (bronchopulmonary) segment [S III]
    a. canaliculus of chorda tympani
    a. cardiac vein
    a. carpal region
    a. cecal artery
    a. central convolution
    a. central gyrus
    a. centriole
    a. cerebellar notch
    a. cerebral artery
    a. cerebral vein
    a. cervical intertransversarii muscle
    a. cervical intertransverse muscle
    a. cervical lymph node
    a. cervical region
    a. chamber cleavage syndrome
    a. chamber of eyeball
    a. chamber trabecula
    a. choroidal artery
    a. choroiditis
    a. ciliary artery
    a. ciliary vein
    a. circumflex humeral artery
    a. circumflex humeral vein
    a. clear space
    a. clinoid process
    a. column
    a. column of medulla oblongata
    a. commissure of the larynx
    a. communicating artery
    a. compartment of arm
    a. compartment of forearm
    a. compartment of leg
    a. compartment of thigh
    a. component of force
    a. condyloid canal of occipital bone
    a. condyloid foramen

Got a Good Word for STEDMAN'S?

Help us keep STEDMAN'S products fresh and up-to-date with new words and new ideas! How can we make your STEDMAN'S product the best medical word reference possible for you?

Do we need to add or revise any items? Is there a better way to organize the content?

Be specific! Fill in the lines below with your thoughts and recommendations and FAX the page to **ATTENTION STEDMAN'S, 410.528.4153**.

You are our most important contributor, and we want to know what's on your mind. Thanks!

Please tell us a little bit about yourself:

Name/Title: _____

Company: _____

Address: _____

City/State/Zip: _____

Day Telephone No.: (_____) _____

E-mail Address: _____

TERMS YOU BELIEVE ARE INCORRECT:

Appears as: Suggested revision:

_____   _____

_____   _____

_____

NEW TERMS/WORDS YOU WOULD LIKE US TO ADD:

_____

_____

Other comments:

_____

_____

_____

May we quote you?   ☐ Yes   ☐ No

All done? Great, just FAX this page to the attention of STEDMAN'S at 410.528.4153 or MAIL the page to us at:

ATTN: STEDMAN'S
Lippincott Williams & Wilkins
P.O. Box 17344
Baltimore, MD 21298-9595

OR enter your information
ONLINE at **www.stedmans.com**

Thanks again!

BUSINESS REPLY MAIL

FIRST CLASS   PERMIT NO. 724   BALTIMORE, MD

ATTN: STEDMAN'S
LIPPINCOTT WILLIAMS & WILKINS
PO BOX 17344
BALTIMORE   MD   21298-9595

A

a. conjunctival artery
a. corneal dystrophy
a. coronary periarterial plexus
a. corticospinal tract
a. costotransverse ligament
a. cranial base
a. cranial fossa
a. cruciate ligament
a. crural nerve
a. crural region
a. crus of stapes
a. cubital region
a. curvature
a. cusp of left atrioventricular valve
a. cusp of mitral valve
a. cusp of right atrioventricular valve
a. cusp of tricuspid valve
a. cutaneous branch of femoral nerve
a. cutaneous branch of iliohypogastric nerve
a. cutaneous branch of intercostal nerve
a. cutaneous nerve of abdomen
a. deep cervical lymph node
a. division of (trunk of) brachial plexus
a. elastic layer
a. embryotoxon
a. epithelium of cornea
a. ethmoidal air cell
a. ethmoidal artery
a. ethmoidal cell
a. ethmoidal nerve
a. external arcuate fiber
a. extremity of caudate nucleus
a. extremity of spleen
a. facial height (AFH)
a. facial vein
a. fascicle of palatopharyngeus muscle
a. fasciculus proprius
a. femoral cutaneous nerve
a. focal point
a. fontanelle
a. fovea
a. funiculus
a. gastric branch of anterior vagal trunk
a. glandular branch of superior thyroid artery
a. gray column
a. gray commissure
a. ground bundle
a. guide
a. horn
a. horn cell
a. humeral circumflex artery
a. hypothalamic area
a. hypothalamic nucleus
a. hypothalamic region
a. inferior cerebellar artery
a. inferior iliac spine
a. inferior renal segment

a. inferior segmental artery of kidney
a. intercondylar area of tibia
a. intercostal artery
a. intercostal branch of internal thoracic artery
a. intercostal vein
a. intermediate groove
a. intermediate sulcus
a. interosseous artery
a. interosseous nerve
a. interpositus nucleus
a. interventricular artery
a. interventricular branch of left coronary artery
a. interventricular groove
a. interventricular sulcus
a. intestinal portal
a. intraoccipital joint
a. intraoccipital synchondrosis
a. jugular lymph node
a. jugular vein
a. junction line
a. knee region
a. labial artery
a. labial branch of deep external pudendal artery
a. labial commissure
a. labial nerve
a. labial vein
a. lacrimal crest
a. lateral malleolar artery
a. lateral nasal branch of anterior ethmoidal artery
a. layer of rectus sheath
a. layer of thoracolumbar fascia
a. ligament of fibular head
a. ligament of Helmholtz
a. ligament of malleus
a. limb of internal capsule
a. limb of stapes
a. limiting lamina
a. limiting layer of cornea
a. limiting ring
a. lingual gland
a. lip of external os of uterus
a. lip of uterine os
a. lobe of hypophysis
a. longitudinal ligament
a. lunate lobule
a. margin
a. medial malleolar artery
a. median fissure of medulla oblongata
a. median fissure of spinal cord
a. median line
a. mediastinal artery
a. mediastinal lymph node
a. mediastinoscopy
a. mediastinotomy
a. mediastinum
a. medullary velum
a. megalophthalmos
a. meningeal artery

anterior (*continued*)

a. meningeal branch (of anterior ethmoidal artery)
a. meniscofemoral ligament
a. myocardial infarction
a. naris
a. nasal spine (ANS)
a. nasal spine of maxilla
a. neuropore
a. notch of auricle
a. notch of cerebellum
a. notch of ear
a. nuclei of thalamus
a. nucleus
a. nucleus of trapezoid body
a. occlusion
a. ocular segment
a. olfactory nucleus
a. palatine arch
a. palatine foramen
a. palpebral margin
a. paracentral gyrus
a. parietal artery
a. parolfactory sulcus
a. part
a. part of anterior commissure of brain
a. part of diaphragmatic surface of liver
a. part of fornix of vagina
a. part of pons
a. part of tongue
a. pectoral cutaneous branch of intercostal nerve
a. pelvic exenteration
a. perforated substance
a. perforating artery
a. periventricular nucleus
a. peroneal artery
a. pillar of fauces
a. pillar of fornix
a. piriform gyrus
a. pituitary
a. pituitary gonadotropin
a. pole of eyeball
a. pole of lens
a. pontomesencephalic vein
a. portion of left medial segment IV of liver
a. and posterior radicular artery
a. and posterior superior pancreaticoduodenal artery
a. and posterior vestibular veins
a. primary division
a. process of malleus
a. pyramid
a. pyramidal fasciculus
a. pyramidal tract
a. quadrigeminal body
a. ramus of cervical nerve
a. ramus of lateral sulcus of cerebrum
a. ramus of lumbar nerve
a. ramus of sacral nerve

a. ramus of spinal nerve
a. ramus of thoracic nerve
a. raphespinal tract
a. recess
a. recess of tympanic membrane
a. rectus muscle of head
a. region of arm
a. region of elbow
a. region of forearm
a. region of knee
a. region of leg
a. region of neck
a. region of thigh
a. region of wrist
a. rhinoscopy
a. rhizotomy
a. root of spinal nerve
a. sacrococcygeal ligament
a. sacroiliac ligament
a. sacrosciatic ligament
a. scalene muscle
a. scleritis
a. sclerotomy
a. scrotal branch of deep external pudendal artery
a. scrotal nerve
a. scrotal vein
a. segment
a. segmental artery
a. semicircular canal
a. septal branch of anterior ethmoidal artery
a. serratus muscle
a. sinus
a. spinal artery
a. spinocerebellar tract
a. spinothalamic tract
a. staphyloma
a. sternoclavicular ligament
a. superficial cervical lymph node
a. superior alveolar artery
a. superior alveolar branch of infraorbital nerve
a. superior alveolar nerve
a. superior dental artery
a. superior iliac spine
a. superior renal segment
a. superior segmental artery of kidney
a. supraclavicular nerve
a. surface
a. surface of arm
a. surface of cornea
a. surface of elbow
a. surface of eyelid
a. surface of forearm
a. surface of iris
a. surface of kidney
a. surface of leg
a. surface of lens
a. surface of lower limb
a. surface of maxilla
a. surface of patella
a. surface of petrous part of temporal bone

a. surface of prostate
a. surface of radius
a. surface of suprarenal gland
a. surface of thigh
a. surface of ulna
a. surface of uterus
a. symblepharon
a. synechia
a. talar articular surface of calcaneus
a. talofibular ligament
a. talotibial ligament
a. tarsal tendinous sheath
a. tegmental decussation
a. temporal artery
a. temporal branch
a. thalamic radiation
a. thalamic tubercle
a. thoracic region
a. thoracotomy
a. tibial artery
a. tibial bursa
a. tibial compartment syndrome
a. tibial lymph node
a. tibial muscle
a. tibial nerve
a. tibial node
a. tibial recurrent artery
a. tibial vein
a. tibiofibular ligament
a. tibiotalar ligament
a. tibiotalar part of deltoid ligament
a. tibiotalar part of medial ligament of ankle joint
a. tooth
a. transverse temporal gyrus
a. triangle of neck
a. trigeminothalamic tract
a. tubercle of atlas
a. tubercle of cervical vertebrae
a. tubercle of thalamus
a. tympanic artery
a. urethra
a. urethral valve
a. urethritis
a. uveitis
a. vein of septum pellucidum
a. vertebral vein
a. vestibular artery
a. vitrectomy
a. wall of middle ear
a. wall of stomach
a. wall of tympanic cavity
a. wall of vagina
a. white commissure
anterior/lateral/posterior glandular branch of superior thyroid artery
anterodorsal nucleus of thalamus
anteroexternal
anterofacial dysplasia
anterograde
a. amnesia
a. block
a. conduction
a. memory

anteroinferior
a. myocardial infarction
a. surface of pancreas
anterointernal
anterolateral
a. central artery
a. column of spinal cord
a. cordotomy
a. fontanelle
a. groove
a. myocardial infarction
a. striate artery
a. sulcus
a. surface of arytenoid cartilage
a. surface of shaft of humerus
a. system
a. thalamostriate artery
a. tract
a. tractotomy
anteromedial
a. central artery
a. central branch
a. frontal branch of callosomarginal artery
a. intermuscular septum
a. nucleus
a. nucleus of thalamus
a. surface of shaft of humerus
a. thalamostriate artery
anteromedian
a. groove
anteroposterior
a. diameter of the pelvic inlet
a. dysplasia
a. projection
anteroposterior facial dysplasia (*var. of* anterofacial dysplasia)
anteroseptal myocardial infarction
anterosuperior surface of body of pancreas
anterotic
anteroventral nucleus of thalamus
antesystole
anteversion
anteverted
anthelix
anthelminthic
anthelmintic
anthelone
a. E, U
antheridium
anthiolimine
anthocyanins
Anthomyia
A. canicularis
anthracemia
anthracene
anthracic
anthracin
anthracosilicosis
anthracosis
anthracotic tuberculosis
anthracycline
anthralin
anthramucin

anthranilic acid
anthraniloyl
anthrapurpurin
9,10-anthraquinone
anthrax
    cerebral a.
    cutaneous a.
    intestinal a.
    pulmonary a.
    a. septicemia
    a. toxin
anthrone
anthropobiology
anthropocentric
anthropogenesis
anthropogenic, anthropogenetic
anthropogeny
anthropogony
anthropography
Anthropoidea
anthropoid pelvis
anthropology
    applied a.
    criminal a.
    cultural a.
    physical a.
anthropometer
anthropometric
anthropometry
anthropomorphism
anthroponomy
anthroponotic cutaneous leishmaniasis
anthropopathy
anthropophilic
anthropophobia
anthroposcopy
anthroposomatology
anthropozoonosis
antiacid
antiadrenergic
antiagglutinin
antialexin
antiallergic
antialopecia factor
antianaphylaxis
antiandrogen
antianemic
    a. factor
    a. principle
antiangiogenesis factor
antiantibody
antiantitoxin
antianxiety agent
antiarachnolysin
antiarrhythmic
antiarthritic
antiasthmatic
antiautolysin
antibacterial
anti-basement
    a. membrane antibody
    a. membrane glomerulonephritis
    a. membrane nephritis
antibechic

antiberiberi
    a. factor
    a. vitamin
antibiont
antibiosis
antibiotic
    broad-spectrum a.
    a. enterocolitis
    peptide a.
    a. resistant
    a. sensitivity
    a. sensitivity test
    transport a.
antibiotin
anti–black-tongue factor
antiblennorrhagic
antibody (Ab)
    affinity a.
    agglutinating a.
    anaphylactic a.
    anti-basement membrane a.
    anticardiolipin a.
    antiidiotype a.
    anti-MAG a.
    antineutrophil cytoplasmic a.
      (ANCA)
    antinuclear a. (ANA)
    antiphospholipid a.
    antithyroglobulin a.
    avidity a.
    bivalent a.
    blocking a.
    blood group a.
    catalytic a.
    cell-bound a.
    CF a.
    chimeric a.
    cold a.
    cold-reactive a.
    complement-fixing a.
    complete a.
    cross-reacting a.
    cytophilic a.
    cytotropic a.
    a. deficiency disease
    a. deficiency syndrome
    epitope for a monoclonal a.
    a. excess
    fluorescent a.
    Forssman a.
    heterocytotropic a.
    heterogenetic a.
    heterophil a.
    heterophile a.
    HMB-45 a.
    homocytotropic a.
    human antimouse a. (HAMA)
    idiotypic a.
    immobilizing a.
    incomplete a.
    inhibiting a.
    lymphocytotoxic a.
    monoclonal a. (MAB, MoAb)
    natural a.
    neutralizing a.

nonprecipitable a.
nonprecipitating a.
normal a.
P-K a.
polyclonal a.
Prausnitz-Küstner a.
precipitating a.
reaginic a.
ricin-blocked a.
treponema-immobilizing a.
treponemal a.
univalent a.
Vi a.
Wassermann a.
antibody-combining site
antibody-dependent cell-mediated cytotoxicity (ADCC)
antibrachial
antibrachium
antibromic
anticalculous
anticardiolipin antibody
anticarious
anticathexis
anticephalalgic
anticholagogue
anticholinergic
anticholinesterase
anticipate
anticipation
anticlinal
anticnemion
anticoagulant
lupus a.
a. therapy
anticoding strand
anticodon
anticomplement
anticomplementary
a. factor
a. serum
anticontagious
anticonvulsant
anticonvulsive
anticurare
anticus
anticytotoxin
antidepressant
tetracyclic a.
triazolopyridine a.
tricyclic a.
antidermatitis factor
antidiabetic
antidiarrheal, antidiarrhetic
anti-D immunoglobulin
antidiuresis
antidiuretic hormone (ADH)
antidotal
antidote
chemical a.
mechanical a.
physiologic a.
universal a.
antidromic
antidysenteric

antidyskinetic agent
antidysrhythmic
antidysuric
antiemetic
antienergic
antienzyme
antiepileptic
antiepithelial serum
antiestrogen
antifebrile
antifibrillatory
antifibrinolysin
antifibrinolytic
antifoaming agent
antifolic
antifungal
anti-G
antigen (Ag)
ABO a.
acetone-insoluble a.
allogenic a.
Am a.
Au a.
Aus a.
Australia a.
Be^a a.
Becker a.
Bi a.
Bile a.
blood group a.
By a.
CA 125 a.
CA 15-3 a.
CA 19-9 a.
capsular a.
carcinoembryonic a. (CEA)
Casoni a.
C carbohydrate a.
CDE a.
cholesterinized a.
Chr^a a.
class I, II, III a.
cluster of differentiation (CD) a.
common a.
complete a.
conjugated a.
D a.
delta a.
Dharmendra a.
Di a.
Duffy a.
epithelial membrane a. (EMA)
a. excess
flagellar a.
Forssman a.
Fy a.
G a.
Ge a.
Gerbich a.
Gm a.
Good a.
Gr a.
group a.
H a.
H-2 a.

antigen *(continued)*
He a.
heart a.
hepatitis-associated a. (HAA)
hepatitis B core a. (HB$_c$Ab, HB$_c$Ag)
hepatitis B e a. (HB$_e$Ab, HBe)
hepatitis B surface a. (HB$_s$Ab)
heterogeneic a.
heterogenetic a.
heterophil a.
heterophile a.
hexon a.
histocompatibility a.
HL-A a.
Ho a.
homologous a.
Hu a.
human leukocyte a. (HLA)
H-Y a.
I a.
incomplete a.
a. interferon
InV group a.
Jk a.
Jobbins a.
Js a.
K a.
Km a.
Kveim a.
Kveim-Siltzbach a.
Lan a.
Le a.
leukocyte common a.
Levay a.
Lu a.
lymphocyte function associated a. (LFA)
lymphogranuloma venereum a.
Lyt a.
M a.
M$_1$ a., M^c a., M^g a., M$_2$ a.
Mitsuda a.
MNSs a.
Mu a.
mumps skin test a.
O a.
oncofetal a.
organ-specific a.
Ot a.
P a.
partial a.
penton a.
a. peptide
pollen a.
private a.
proliferating cell nuclear a.
prostate-specific a. (PSA)
public a.
R a.
Rh a.
Rhus toxicodendron a.
Rhus venenata a.
S a.

sensitized a.
shock a.
Sm a.
soluble a.
somatic a.
species-specific a.
specific a.
Stobo a.
Streptococcus M a.
Sw^a a.
Swann a.
T a.
Tac a.
T-dependent a.
theta a.
thymus-independent a.
tissue-specific a.
Tj a.
Tr^a a.
transplantation a.
tumor a.
tumor-associated a.
tumor-specific transplantation a. (TSTA)
a. unit
V a.
Vel a.
Ven a.
Vi a.
Vw a.
Webb a.
Wright a. (Wr^a)
Xg a.
Yt^a a.
antigen-antibody
a.-a. complex
a.-a. reaction (AAR)
antigen-binding site
antigenemia
antigenic
a. competition
a. complex
a. determinant
a. drift
a. shift
antigenicity
antigenome
antigen-presenting cell
antigen-responsive cell
antigen-sensitive cell
antiglobulin test
antigonorrheic
antigravity muscle
anti-G suit
anti-HB$_c$
anti-HB$_s$
anti-HB$_e$
antihelix
antihelminthic
antihemagglutinin
antihemolysin
antihemolytic
antihemophilic
a. factor A, B
a. globulin (AHG)

a. globulin A, B
a. plasma
antihemorrhagic
a. factor
a. vitamin
antihistamine
antihistaminic
antihormone
antihuman
a. globulin
a. globulin test
antihydropic
antihypertensive
antihypnotic
antihypotensive
antiicteric
antiidiotype
a. antibody
a. autoantibody
antiinflammatory
antiinsulin
antiketogenesis
antiketogenic
anti–kidney serum nephritis
antileukocidin
antileukotoxin
antileukotriene
antilewisite
antilipotropic
antilithic
antilobium
antiluteogenic
antilymphocyte
a. globulin (ALG)
a. serum
antilysin
anti-MAG antibody
antimalarial
antimere
antimesenteric
antimetabolite
antimetropia
antimicrobial spectrum
antimitotic
antimongoloid
antimonid
antimonous oxide
anti-Monson curve
antimony (Sb)
a. chloride
a. dimercaptosuccinate
a. oxide
a. potassium tartrate
a. sodium gluconate
a. sodium tartrate
a. sodium thioglycollate
tartrated a.
a. thioglycollamide
a. trichloride
a. trioxide
antimonyl
anti-müllerian hormone
antimuscarinic
antimutagen
antimutagenic

antimyasthenic
antimycotic
antinauseant
antineoplastic
antineoplaston
antineuritic
a. factor
a. vitamin
antineurotoxin
antineutrophil cytoplasmic antibody (ANCA)
antiniad
antinial
antinion
antinomy
antinuclear
a. antibody (ANA)
a. factor (ANF)
antiodontalgic
antioncogene
antioxidant
antipain
antiparallel strand
antiparasitic
antipedicular
antipediculotic
antipellagra factor
antiperiodic
antiperistalsis
antiperistaltic
antipernicious anemia factor (APA)
antiperspirant
antiphagocytic
antiphlogistic
antiphobic
antiphospholipid antibody
antiplasmin
antiplatelet
antipneumococcic
antipodal cone
antipode
optic a.
antiport
antiporter
anti-Pr cold autoagglutinin
antiprecipitin
antiprogestin
antiprothrombin
antipruritic
antipsychotic agent
antipurine
antipyogenic
antipyresis
antipyretic
antipyrimidine
antipyrine
a. acetylsalicylate
a. salicylacetate
a. salicylate
antipyrotic
antirabies serum
antirachitic vitamin
antireflection coating
antireticular cytotoxic serum
antirheumatic

antiricin
antiruminant
anti-S
antischistosomal
antiscorbutic vitamin
antiseborrheic
antisecretory
antisense
    a. DNA
    a. RNA
    a. strand
    a. therapy
antisepsis
antiseptic dressing
antiserum
    a. anaphylaxis
    blood group a.
    heterologous a.
    homologous a.
    monovalent a.
    nerve growth factor a.
    NGF a.
    polyvalent a.
    specific a.
antishock garment
antisialagogue
antisideric
antisocial
    a. personality
    a. personality disorder
antispasmodic
antistaphylococcic
antistaphylolysin
antisteapsin
antisterility
    a. factor
    a. vitamin
antistreptococcic
antistreptokinase
antistreptolysin
antitac
antitermination protein
antitetanic
antithenar
antithrombin
    a. III
    normal a.
    a. test
antithyroglobulin antibody
antithyroid
antitonic
antitoxic serum
antitoxigen
antitoxin
    bivalent gas gangrene a.
    bothropic a.
    Bothrops a.
    botulinum a.
    botulism a.
    bovine a.
    Crotalus a.
    despeciated a.
    diphtheria a.
    dysentery a.
    gas gangrene a.

    normal a.
    pentavalent gas gangrene a.
    plant a.
    a. rash
    scarlet fever a.
    staphylococcus a.
    tetanus a.
    tetanus and gas gangrene a.
    tetanus-perfringens a.
    a. unit
antitoxinogen
antitragicus muscle
antitragohelicine fissure
antitragus
antitreponemal
antitrismus
antitrope
antitropic
antitrypsic
antitrypsin
    alpha$_1$-a.
    a. deficiency
antitryptic index
antitumor
    a. enzyme
    a. protein
antitumorigenesis
antitussive
antityphoid
antivenene unit
antivenereal
antivenin
antiviral
    a. immunity
    a. protein (AVP)
antivitamin
antivivisection
antixerophthalmic
antixerotic
Antoni
    A. type A, B neurilemoma
Anton syndrome
antra (*pl. of* antrum)
antral
    a. follicle
    a. lavage
    a. pouch
    a. sphincter
antrectomy
antronasal
antrophose
antropyloric
antroscope
antroscopy
antrostomy
    intraoral a.
antrotomy
antrotonia
antrotympanic
antrum, pl. antra
    a. auris
    cardiac a.
    a. cardiacum
    antra ethmoidalia
    follicular a.

a. of Highmore
mastoid a.
a. mastoideum
maxillary a.
pyloric a.
a. pyloricum
tympanic a.
Valsalva a.

ANTU
alpha-naphthylthiourea
Antyllus method
ANUG
acute necrotizing ulcerative gingivitis
anular
a. band
a. cartilage
a. cataract
a. ligament
a. ligament of radius
a. ligament of stapes
a. ligament of trachea
a. lipid
a. pancreas
a. part of fibrous digital sheath of
digits of hand and foot
a. placenta
a. plexus
a. pulley
a. scleritis
a. scotoma
a. sphincter
a. staphyloma
a. stricture
a. synechia
anulus, pl. **anuli**
a. abdominalis
a. ciliaris
a. conjunctivae
a. femoralis
a. fibrocartilagineus membranae
tympani
a. fibrosus
a. fibrosus dexter/sinister cordis
a. fibrosus disci intervertebralis
a. fibrosus of intervertebral disk
a. of fibrous sheath
Haller a.
a. hemorrhoidalis
a. inguinalis profundus
a. inguinalis superficialis
a. iridis
a. iridis major
a. iridis minor
a. lymphaticus cardiae
a. lymphoideus pharyngis
a. ovalis
a. tendineus communis
a. tympanicus
a. umbilicalis
a. urethralis
Vieussens a.
a. of Zinn
anuria
anuric
anus, pl. **ani**

Bartholin a.
a. cerebri
imperforate a.
a. vesicalis
vesicalis a.
vestibular a.
vulvovaginal a.
anvil sound
anxiety
a. attack
castration a.
a. disorder
a. dream
free-floating a.
a. hysteria
a. neurosis
noetic a.
a. reaction
separation a.
situation a.
a. syndrome
a. tension state
anxiolytic
anxious delirium
AOC
anodal opening contraction
Aonchotheca
aorta, pl. **aortae**
abdominal a.
a. abdominalis
a. angusta
a. ascendens
ascending a.
buckled a.
a. descendens
descending a.
dynamic a.
kinked a.
overriding a.
primitive a.
pseudocoarctation of the a.
shaggy a.
thoracic a.
a. thoracica
ventral a.
aortal
aortalgia
aortarctia
aortartia
aortectasis, aortectasia
aortectomy
aortic
a. arch
a. arch syndrome
a. area (of auscultation)
a. atresia
a. bifurcation
a. body
a. body tumor
a. bulb
a. coarctation
a. curtain
a. dissection
a. dwarfism
a. facies

aortic *(continued)*
    a. foramen
    a. glomera
    a. hiatus
    a. impression of left lung
    a. incompetence
    a. insufficiency
    a. isthmus
    a. knob
    a. knuckle
    a. lymphatic plexus
    a. murmur
    a. nerve
    a. nipple
    a. notch
    a. opening
    a. orifice
    a. ostium
    a. reflex
    a. regurgitation
    a. sac
    a. septal defect
    a. sinus
    a. sinus aneurysm
    a. spindle
    a. stenosis
    a. sulcus
    a. valve
    a. vestibule
    a. window
aortico-left ventricular tunnel
aorticopulmonary
    a. septal defect
    a. window
aorticorenal ganglia
aortic-pulmonic window
aortitis
    giant cell a.
    syphilitic a.
aortoannular ectasia
aortocoronary bypass
aortogram
aortography
    retrograde a.
    translumbar a.
aortoiliac
    a. bypass
    a. occlusive disease
aortopathy
aortopexy
aortoplasty
aortoptosia, aortoptosis
aortopulmonary
    a. septum
    a. window
aortorenal bypass
aortorrhaphy
aortosclerosis
aortostenosis
aortotomy
AP
    area postrema
APA
    antipernicious anemia factor

APACHE
    acute physiology and chronic health
      evaluation
      APACHE score
apallesthesia
apallic
    a. state
    a. syndrome
apancreatic
aparalytic
aparathyreosis
aparathyroidism
apareunia
apathetic thyrotoxicosis
apathism
apathy
apatite calculus
A-pattern
    A-p. esotropia
    A-p. exotropia
    A-p. strabismus
A-P-C
    adenoidal-pharyngeal-conjunctival
      A-P-C virus
APC
    phenacetin
APC compound
ape
    a. fissure
    a. hand
apellous
apenteric
apepsinia
aperiodic biopolymer
aperiosteal amputation
aperistalsis
aperitive
apertognathia
apertometer
Apert syndrome
apertura, pl. **aperturae**
    a. aqueductus cerebri
    a. aqueductus mesencephali
    a. canaliculi cochleae
    a. canaliculi vestibuli
    a. lateralis ventriculi quarti
    a. mediana ventriculi quarti
    a. pelvis inferior
    a. pelvis minoris
    a. pelvis superior
    a. piriformis
    a. sinus frontalis
    a. sinus sphenoidalis
    a. thoracis inferior
    a. thoracis superior
    a. tympanica canaliculi chordae
      tympani
aperture
    angular a.
    a. diaphragm
    external acoustic a.
    external a. of cochlear canaliculus
    external a. of vestibular aqueduct
    frontal sinus a.
    inferior pelvic a.

inferior thoracic a.
laryngeal a.
lateral a. of fourth ventricle
a. of mastoid antrum
median a. of fourth ventricle
numerical a.
a. of orbit
piriform a.
posterior nasal a.
sphenoidal sinus a.
superior pelvic a.
superior thoracic a.
tympanic a. of canaliculus

apex, pl. **apices**
a. anterior angulation
a. of arytenoid cartilage
a. of auricle
a. auriculae
a. beat
a. capitis fibulae
a. cartilaginis arytenoideae
a. cordis
a. cornus posterioris
a. cuspidis dentis
a. of cusp of tooth
a. of dens
a. dentis
a. of head of fibula
a. of heart
a. impulse
a. linguae
a. of lung
a. nasi
a. of nose
a. of orbit
a. ossis sacri
a. partis petrosae ossis temporalis
a. of patella
a. patellae
a. of petrous part of temporal bone
a. pneumonia
a. posterior angulation
a. of posterior horn
a. prostatae
a. of prostate
a. pulmonis
a. radicis dentis
root a.
a. of sacrum
a. satyri
a. of tongue
a. of (urinary) bladder
a. vesicae

apexcardiogram
apexcardiography
apexification
apexigraph
APF
    animal protein factor
Apgar score
aphagia
aphakia
aphakic
a. eye
a. glaucoma

aphalangia
aphasia
acoustic a.
acquired epileptic a.
amnesic a.
amnestic a.
anomic a.
anterior a.
associative a.
ataxic a.
auditory a.
Broca a.
conduction a.
crossed a.
expressive a.
fluent a.
functional a.
global a.
graphic a.
graphomotor a.
impressive a.
jargon a.
mixed a.
motor a.
nominal a.
nonfluent a.
pathematic a.
posterior a.
psychosensory a.
pure a.
receptive a.
semantic a.
sensory a.
syntactical a.
total a.
transcortical a.
visual a.
Wernicke a.

aphasiac, aphasic
aphasiologist
aphasiology
aphasmid
Aphasmidia
apheliotropism
apheresis
aphilopony
aphonia
hysterical a.
nonorganic a.
a. paralytica
spastic a.

aphonic pectoriloquy
aphonous
aphotesthesia
aphrasia
aphrodisia
aphrodisiac
aphrodisiomania
aphtha, pl. **aphthae**
Bednar a.
herpetiform a.
a. major
Mikulicz a.
a. minor
recurrent scarring a.

aphthoid
aphthosis
aphthous stomatitis
Aphthovirus
aphylactic
aphylaxis
apical
    a. abscess
    a. angle
    a. area
    a. axillary lymph node
    a. branch of inferior lobar branch
      of right pulmonary artery
    a. branch of right superior
      pulmonary vein
    a. cap
    a. complex
    a. dendrite
    a. dental foramen
    a. ectodermal ridge
    a. foramen of tooth
    a. gland
    a. granuloma
    a. infarction
    a. infection
    a. ligament of dens
    a. lordotic projection
    a. periodontal abscess
    a. periodontal cyst
    a. periodontitis
    a. pneumonia
    a. process
    a. segmental artery
    a. segmental artery of superior
      lobar artery of right lung
    a. segment [S I]
    a. space
    a. vein
apical-aortic conduit
apicalis
apicectomy
apiceotomy
apices (*pl. of* apex)
apicis
apicoectomy
apicolocator
apicolysis
Apicomplexa
apicoposterior
    a. artery
    a. branch of left superior
      pulmonary vein
    a. segment [SI + SII]
    a. vein
apicostome
apicostomy
apicotomy
apiculate
apiculus
apicurettage
apinealism
apiphobia
apituitarism
aplacental
aplanatic lens

aplanatism
aplasia
    congenital a. of thymus
    a. cutis congenita
    germinal a.
    gonadal a.
    pure red cell a.
aplastic
    a. anemia
    a. lymph
apleuria
apnea
    central a.
    deglutition a.
    induced a.
    obstructive sleep a.
    sleep a.
    sleep-induced a.
apnea-hypopnea index
apneic
    a. oxygenation
    a. pause
apneumia
apneusis
apneustic breathing
apo
   apoenzyme
apobiosis
apochromatic
    a. lens
    a. objective
apocrine
    a. adenoma
    a. carcinoma
    a. chromhidrosis
    a. gland
    a. hidrocystoma
    a. metaplasia
    a. miliaria
    a. sweat gland
apocrustic
apodal
apodia
apodous
apody
apoenzyme (apo)
apoferritin
apogamia, apogamy
apogee
apoinducer
apo-2L
apolar
    a. bond
    a. cell
    a. interaction
apolipoprotein
    a. A-I, A-II, A-IV
    a. B
    a. B-100
    a. B-48
    a. C-I, C-II, C-III
    a. D
    a. E
apomixia
apomorphine hydrochloride

aponeurectomy
aponeurogenic ptosis
aponeurorrhaphy
aponeurosis, pl. aponeuroses
    bicipital a.
    a. bicipitalis
    Denonvilliers a.
    epicranial a.
    a. epicranialis
    extensor a.
    a. of external oblique muscle
    a. of insertion
    a. of internal oblique muscle
    a. of investment
    a. linguae
    lingual a.
    a. musculi bicipitis brachii
    a. of origin
    a. palatina
    palatine a.
    palmar a.
    a. palmaris
    Petit a.
    a. pharyngea
    plantar a.
    a. plantaris
    Sibson a.
    temporal a.
    thoracolumbar a.
    a. of vastus muscle
aponeurositis
aponeurotic
    a. fibroma
    a. reflex
aponeurotome
aponeurotomy
apophylaxis
apophysary point
apophysial, apophyseal
    a. fracture
    a. point
apophysis, pl. apophyses
    basilar a.
    a. conchae
    a. helicis
    lenticular a.
    temporal a.
apophysitis
    calcaneal a.
    a. tibialis adolescentium
Apophysomyces
apoplasmia
apoplectic cyst
apoplectiform
apoplexy
    abdominal a.
    adrenal a.
    bulbar a.
    functional a.
    heat a.
    labyrinthine a.
    neonatal a.
    pituitary a.
    spinal a.
    uteroplacental a.

apoprotein
apoptosis
aporepressor
aposome
apostaxis
aposthia
apostilb
apothanasia
apothecaries weight
apothecary
apothem, apotheme
apoxesis
apozem, apozema
apparatus
    accessory visual a.
    achromatic a.
    alimentary a.
    attachment a.
    Barcroft-Warburg a.
    Beckmann a.
    Benedict-Roth a.
    branchial a.
    central a.
    chromatic a.
    chromidial a.
    dental a.
    digestive a.
    a. digestorius
    genitourinary a.
    Golgi a.
    Haldane a.
    hyoid a.
    a. hyoideus
    juxtaglomerular a.
    Kirschner a.
    Kjeldahl a.
    lacrimal a.
    a. lacrimalis
    a. ligamentosus colli
    a. ligamentosus weitbrechti
    masticatory a.
    mental a.
    pyriform a.
    a. respiratorius
    respiratory a.
    Roughton-Scholander a.
    Scholander a.
    self-contained underwater
      breathing a. (SCUBA)
    subneural a.
    a. suspensorius lentis
    Taylor a.
    Tiselius a.
    urinary a.
    urogenital a.
    a. urogenitalis
    Van Slyke a.
    vestibular a.
    Warburg a.
apparent
    a. origin
    a. viscosity
appendage
    atrial a.
    auricular a.

appendage *(continued)*
    drumstick a.
    epiploic a.
    a. of eye
    a. of the fetus
    left auricular a.
    right auricular a.
    a. of skin
    testicular a.
    uterine a.
    vermiform a.
    vesicular a. of epoophoron
appendalgia
appendectomy
    auricular a.
appendical
appendiceal abscess
appendicectasis
appendicectomy
appendices (*pl. of* appendix)
appendicism
appendicitis
    actinomycotic a.
    acute a.
    bilharzial a.
    chronic a.
    focal a.
    foreign-body a.
    gangrenous a.
    left-sided a.
    lumbar a.
    obstructive a.
    perforating a.
    recurrent a.
    relapsing a.
    stercoral a.
    subperitoneal a.
    suppurative a.
    verminous a.
appendicocele
appendicolith
appendicolithiasis
appendicolysis
appendicostomy
appendicovesicostomy
appendicular
    a. artery
    a. colic
    a. lymph node
    a. muscle
    a. skeleton
    a. vein
appendix, pl. **appendices**
    appendices adiposae coli
    auricular a.
    a. ceci
    a. of epididymidis
    a. epididymidis
    epiploic a.
    a. epiploica, pl. appendices epiploicae
    fatty a. of colon
    a. fibrosa hepatis
    fibrous a. of liver
    Morgagni a.

    omental a.
    appendices omentales
    a. of testis
    a. testis
    a. of the testis
    a. ventriculi laryngis
    vermiform a.
    a. vermiformis
    vesicular appendices of uterine tube
    a. vesiculosa, pl. appendices vesiculosae
apperception
apperceptive mass
appersonation, appersonification
appestat
appetite juice
appetitive behavior
applanation tonometer
applanometry
apple
    apple jelly nodule
    apple oil
    bitter a.
appliance
    craniofacial a.
    edgewise a.
    extraoral fracture a.
    Hawley a.
    intraoral fracture a.
    labiolingual a.
    light wire a.
    obturator a.
    orthodontic a.
    ribbon arch a.
    Roger Anderson pin fixation a.
    surgical a.
    universal a.
applicand.
    applicandus
applicandus (applicand.)
applicator
applied
    a. anatomy
    a. anthropology
    a. chemistry
appliqué form
apposition
    bayonet a.
    a. suture
appositional growth
approach
    facial recess a.
    idiographic a.
    infratemporal a.
    middle fossa a.
    nomothetic a.
    posterior fossa a.
    regressive-reconstructive a.
    retrosigmoid a.
    transcochlear a.
    translabyrinthine a.
approach-approach conflict
approach-avoidance conflict
AP projection
approximal surface of tooth

approximate
approximation
    steady state a.
    a. suture
APR
    abdominoperineal resection
apractagnosia
apractic
apragmatism
apraxia
    constructional a.
    cortical a.
    gait a.
    ideokinetic a.
    ideomotor a.
    innervation a.
    limb-kinetic a.
    motor a.
    ocular motor a.
    transcortical a.
    verbal a.
apraxic
apricot kernel oil
aproctia
aprofen, aprofene, aprophen
aprosody
aprosopia
aprotinin
APS
    adenosine 5′-phosphosulfate
6-APS
    6-aminopenicillanic acid
aptitude test
aPTT
    activated partial thromboplastin time
Apt test
APUD
    a. cell
apurinic acid
apyknomorphous
apyrase
apyretic typhoid
apyrexia
apyrexial
apyrimidinic acid
aq.
    aqua
aq. bull.
    aqua bulliens
aq. dest.
    aqua destillata
aq. ferv.
    aqua fervens
aq. frig.
    aqua frigida
aqua, pl. **aquae (aq.)**
    a. bulliens (aq. bull.)
    a. destillata (aq. dest.)
    a. fervens (aq. ferv.)
    a. frigida (aq. frig.)
    a. regalis
    a. regia
aquacobalamin
aquagenic pruritus
aquaphobia

aquapuncture
Aquaspirillum
aquatic
aqueduct
    cerebral a.
    a. of cerebrum
    cochlear a.
    Cotunnius a.
    fallopian a.
    sylvian a.
    a. veil
    vestibular a.
aqueductal intubation
aqueductus
    a. cerebri
    a. cochleae
    a. cotunnii
    a. fallopii
    a. mesencephali
    a. sylvii
    a. vestibuli
aqueous
    a. chamber
    a. flare
    a. humor
    a. influx phenomenon
    a. phase
    a. solution
    a. vaccine
    a. vein
aquiparous
aquocobalamin
aquo-ion
aquosity
Ar
    argon
Ara
    arabinose
ara-
arab-
araban
arabic
    a. acid
arabin
arabinoadenosine
arabinocytidine
arabinofuranosyladenine
arabinofuranosylcytosine
arabinose (Ara)
    a. 5-phosphate
    a. 5-phosphate 2-epimerase
arabinoside
arabinosis
arabinosuria
arabinosyladenine
arabinosylcytosine (aC, araC)
arabitol
AraC
    cytosine arabinoside
araC
    arabinosylcytosine
arachic acid
arachidic acid
arachidonic acid
arachidonic acid cascade

arachis oil
arachnephobia
Arachnia
    A. propionica
Arachnida
arachnidism
    necrotic a.
arachnodactyly
arachnoid
    a. of brain
    cranial a. mater
    a. cyst
    a. foramen
    a. granulation
    a. mater
    a. mater cranialis
    a. mater encephali
    a. mater and pia mater
    a. membrane
    a. of spinal cord
    a. spinalis
    spinal a. mater
    a. trabecula
    a. villi
arachnoidal granulation
arachnoidea
    arachnoidea mater spinalis
    a. encephali
    a. mater, arachnoides
    a. mater cranialis
    a. mater encephali
arachnoides (*var. of* arachnoidea mater)
arachnoiditis
    adhesive a.
    neoplastic a.
    obliterative a.
arachnolysin
arachnophobia
aralkyl
Aran-Duchenne disease
araneism
Arantius
    A. ligament
    A. nodule
    A. ventricle
araphia
arbor, pl. **arbores**
    a. vitae
    a. vitae uteri
arborescent
arborization block
arborize
arboroid
arborvirus
arbovirus
ARC
    AIDS-related complex
arc
    auricular a.
    bregmatolambdoid a.
    crater a.
    flame a.
    interauricular a.
    longitudinal a. of skull
    mercury a.

    nasobregmatic a.
    naso-occipital a.
    a. perimeter
    pulmonary a.
    reflex a.
    Riolan a.
arcade
    anomalous mitral a.
    arterial a.
    Flint a.
    intestinal arterial a.
    lower dental a.
    mandibular dental a.
    marginal a.
    maxillary dental a.
    pancreaticoduodenal arterial a.
    Riolan a.
    upper dental a.
Arcanobacterium haemolyticum
arcate
arc-flash conjunctivitis
arch
    abdominothoracic a.
    alveolar a. of mandible
    alveolar a. of maxilla
    anterior a. of atlas
    anterior palatine a.
    a. of the aorta
    aortic a.
    arterial a. of colon
    arterial a. of ileum
    arterial a. of jejunum
    arterial a. of lower eyelid
    arterial a. of upper eyelid
    axillary a.
    a. bar
    branchial a.
    carpal a.
    coracoacromial a.
    Corti a.
    cortical a. of kidney
    costal a.
    a. of cricoid cartilage
    crural a.
    deep crural a.
    deep palmar (arterial) a.
    deep palmar venous a.
    dental a.
    dorsal carpal arterial a.
    dorsal venous a. of foot
    double aortic a.
    expansion a.
    fallen a.
    fallopian a.
    femoral a.
    a. of the foot
    a. form
    glossopalatine a.
    Gothic a.
    Haller a.
    hemal a.
    hyoid a.
    iliopectineal a.
    inferior dental a.
    inferior palpebral (arterial) a.

jugular venous a.
labial a.
Langer a.
lateral longitudinal a. of foot
lateral lumbocostal a.
a. length
a. length deficiency
lingual a.
longitudinal a. of foot
malar a.
mandibular a.
medial longitudinal a. of foot
medial lumbocostal a.
nasal a.
nasal venous a.
neural a. of vertebra
a. of the palate
palatoglossal a.
palatopharyngeal a.
pharyngeal a.
pharyngopalatine a.
plantar arterial a.
plantar venous a.
popliteal a.
posterior a. of atlas
posterior palatine a.
postoral a.
primitive costal a.
pubic a.
ribbon a.
subcostal a.
superciliary a.
superficial palmar (arterial) a.
superficial palmar venous a.
superior dental a.
superior palpebral arterial a.
supraorbital a.
tarsal a.
tendinous a.
tendinous a. of levator ani muscle
tendinous a. of pelvic fascia
tendinous a. of soleus muscle
a. of thoracic duct
transverse a. of foot
Treitz a.
vertebral a.
visceral a.
W-a.
wire a.
a. wire
zygomatic a.
archaeocerebellum
archaeus
archaic
archaic-paralogical thinking
arched crest
archenteric canal
archenteron
archeocerebellum
archeokinetic
archetype
archeus
archicerebellum
archicortex
archil

archin
archipallium
architectonics
architecture
    bone a.
arch-loop-whorl system (ALW)
archwire
arciform
    a. artery
    a. vein of kidney
Arcobacter butzleri
arcon articulator
arctation
arcual
arcuate
    a. artery of foot (inconstant)
    a. artery of kidney
    a. crest
    a. crest of arytenoid cartilage
    a. eminence
    a. fasciculus
    a. fiber
    a. fiber of cerebrum
    a. line
    a. line of ilium
    a. line of rectus sheath
    a. nucleus
    a. nucleus of thalamus
    a. popliteal ligament
    a. pubic ligament
    a. scotoma
    a. uterus
    a. vein of kidney
    a. zone
arcuation
arcus
    a. adiposus
    a. alveolaris mandibulae
    a. alveolaris maxillae
    a. anterior atlantis
    a. aortae
    a. cartilaginis cricoideae
    a. cornealis
    a. costalis
    a. costarum
    a. dentalis inferior
    a. dentalis mandibularis
    a. dentalis maxillaris
    a. dentalis superior
    a. ductus thoracici
    a. glossopalatinus
    a. iliopectineus
    a. inguinalis
    a. juvenilis
    a. lipoides
    a. lumbocostalis lateralis
    a. lumbocostalis medialis
    a. marginalis coli
    a. palatini
    a. palatoglossus
    a. palatopharyngeus
    a. palmaris profundus
    a. palmaris superficialis
    a. palpebralis inferior
    a. palpebralis superior

arcus *(continued)*
a. pedis longitudinalis
a. pedis longitudinalis pars lateralis
a. pedis longitudinalis pars medialis
a. pedis transversalis
a. plantaris profundus
a. posterior atlantis
a. pubis
a. raninus
a. senilis
a. superciliaris
a. tarseus
a. tendineus
a. tendineus fasciae pelvis
a. tendineus musculi levatoris ani
a. tendineus musculi solei
a. tendineus of obturator fascia
a. tendineus of pelvic diaphragm
a. unguium
a. venosus dorsalis pedis
a. venosus juguli
a. venosus palmaris profundus
a. venosus palmaris superficialis
a. venosus plantaris
a. vertebrae
a. volaris profundus
a. volaris superficialis
a. zygomaticus

ardent
a. fever
a. spirit

ardor

ARDS
adult respiratory distress syndrome

area, pl. **areae**
acoustic a.
a. acustica
amygdaloclaustral a.
a. amygdaloclaustralis
a. amygdaloidea anterior
amygdalopiriform transition a.
anterior amygdaloid a.
anterior hypothalamic a.
anterior intercondylar a. of tibia
aortic a. (of auscultation)
apical a.
association areas
auditory a.
bare a. of liver
bare a. of stomach
basal seat a.
Broca parolfactory a.
Brodmann areas
a. of cardiac dullness
catchment a.
a. centralis
a. cochleae
cochlear a.
Cohnheim a.
contact a.
cribriform a. of the renal papilla
a. cribrosa papillae renalis
denture-bearing a.
denture foundation a.

denture-supporting a.
dermatomic a.
dorsal hypothalamic a.
embryonal a.
embryonic a.
entorhinal a.
excitable a.
facial nerve a.
Flechsig a.
frontal a.
fronto-orbital a.
fusion a.
gastric a.
a. gastrica
germinal a.
a. germinativa
Head a.
a. hypothalamica dorsalis
a. hypothalamica intermedia
a. hypothalamica lateralis
a. hypothalamica posterior
a. hypothalamica rostralis
impression a.
inferior vestibular a.
insular a.
a. intercondylaris anterior tibiae
a. intercondylaris posterior tibiae
intermediate hypothalamic a.
Kiesselbach a.
a. of Laimer
Laimer-Haeckerman a.
lateral hypothalamic a.
lateral inferior hepatic a.
lateral superior hepatic a.
Little a.
macular a.
Martegiani a.
mitral a.
motor a.
a. nervi facialis
a. nuda hepatis
olfactory a.
oval a. of Flechsig
Panum a.
parastriate a.
a. parolfactoria
a. parolfactoria Brocae
parolfactory a.
pear-shaped a.
peristriate a.
piriform a.
Pitres a.
postcentral a.
post dam a.
posterior hypothalamic a.
posterior intercondylar a. of tibia
posterior palatal seal a.
a. postrema (AP)
precentral a.
precommissural septal a.
prefrontal a.
premotor a.
preoptic a.
a. preoptica
prestriate a.

A

pretectal a.
primary visual a.
pulmonary a.
relief a.
rest a.
retention a.
retrochiasmatic a.
a. retrochiasmatica
Rolando a.
secondary aortic a.
secondary visual a.
sensorial a.
sensorimotor a.
sensory a.
septal a.
silent a.
skip a.
somesthetic a.
stress-bearing a.
striate a.
a. subcallosa
subcallosal a.
superior vestibular a.
supporting a.
tissue-bearing a.
a. transitionis amygdalopiriformis
tricuspid a.
trigger a.
a. under the curve (AUC)
vagus a.
vestibular a.
a. vestibularis
a. vestibularis inferior
a. vestibularis superior
visual a.
V-shaped a. of esophagus
Wernicke a.
areatus, areata
Areca
arecaidine
arecaine
arecoline
areflexia
detrusor a.
arenaceous
Arenaviridae
Arenavirus
areola, pl. **areolae**
a. of breast
a. mammae
a. of nipple
a. papillaris
a. umbilicus
areolar
a. choroiditis
a. choroidopathy
a. gland
a. tissue
a. tubercle
a. venous plexus
areometer
Arg
arginine
argasid
Argasidae

Argas reflexus
argentaffin, argentaffine
a. cell
a. granule
argentation
argentic
argentine
Argentinean hemorrhagic fever
Argentine hemorrhagic fever virus
argentophil
argentophile
argentous
argentum
arginase
arginine (Arg)
a. deiminase
a. glutamate
a. hydrochloride
a. oxytocin
a. phosphate
a. vasopressin
a. vasotocin
argininosuccinase
argininosuccinate lyase
argininosuccinic acid
argininosuccinicaciduria
arginosuccinate lyase deficiency
arginyl
argipressin
argon (Ar)
a. laser
Argyll Robertson pupil
argyria
argyric
argyrism
argyrol
argyrophil
argyrophile
argyrophilic
a. cell
a. fiber
arhinencephaly (*var. of* arrhinencephaly)
arhinia
Arias-Stella
A.-S. effect
A.-S. phenomenon
A.-S. reaction
ariboflavinosis
aristolochic acid
aristotelian method
Aristotle
A. anomaly
arithmetic mean
arithmomania
Arizona hinshawii
Arlt
A. operation
A. sinus
arm
bar clasp a.
a. bone
brawny a.
circumferential clasp a.
clasp a.
dynein a.

arm (*continued*)
nuchal a.
a. phenomenon
reciprocal a.
retention a.
retentive circumferential clasp a.
stabilizing circumferential clasp a.
armamentarium
Armanni-Ebstein
A.-E. change
A.-E. kidney
armarium
armed
a. macrophage
a. rostellum
Armillifer armillatus
Armitage-Doll model
armored heart
armor heart
armpit
Army
A. Alpha test
A. Beta test
A. General Classification Test
ARN
acute retinal necrosis
Arndt law
Arneth
A. classification
A. count
A. formula
A. index
A. stage
arnica
Arnold
A. body
A. bundle
A. canal
A. ganglion
A. nerve
A. tract
Arnold-Chiari
A.-C. deformity
A.-C. malformation
A.-C. syndrome
aromatase inhibitor
aromatic
a. D-amino acid decarboxylase
a. ammonia spirit
a. bitters
a. castor oil
a. compound
a. series
a. water
arotinoid
arousal
a. function
a. reaction
aroyl
arrack
arrector, pl. **arrectores**
a. muscle of hair
a. pili muscle

arrest
a. of active phase dystocia
cardiac a.
cardioplegic a.
cardiopulmonary a.
circulatory a.
deep hypothermic a.
a. of descent dystocia
epiphysial a.
heart a.
a. of labor
maturation a.
a. signal
sinus a.
arrested
a. dental caries
a. tuberculosis
arrhaphia
arrhenic
Arrhenius
A. doctrine
A. equation
A. law
Arrhenius-Madsen theory
arrhenoblastoma
arrhinencephaly, arhinencephaly, arrhinencephalia
arrhinia
arrhythmia
cardiac a.
continuous a.
juvenile a.
nonphasic sinus a.
phasic sinus a.
respiratory a.
sinus a.
arrhythmic
arrhythmogenic
arrival
dead on a. (DOA)
arrow
a. point tracing
a. poison
arrowroot
Arruga forceps
arsacetin
arsenamide
arsenate
arseniasis
arsenic (As)
a. acid
a. fast
a. pigmentation
a. trihydride
a. trioxide
white a.
arsenical
a. keratosis
a. polyneuropathy
arsenicalism
arsenide
arsenious
arsenium
arseniuret
arseniureted hydrogen

arsenotherapy
arsenous
>arsenous acid
>arsenous hydride
>arsenous oxide

arsenoxide
arsine
arsonic acid
arsonium
arsphenamine
arsthinol
artefact (*var. of* artifact)
artemether
Artemisia annua
artemisinin
arterenol
arteria, pl. **arteriae**
>a. acetabuli
>arteriae alveolares superiores anteriores
>a. alveolaris inferior
>a. alveolaris superior posterior
>a. anastomotica auricularis magna
>a. anastomotica magna
>a. angularis
>a. aorta
>a. appendicularis
>arteriae arcuatae renis
>a. arcuata (pedis)
>a. articularis azygos
>a. ascendens
>arteriae atriales
>a. auditiva interna
>a. auricularis posterior
>a. auricularis profunda
>a. axillaris
>a. basilaris
>a. brachialis
>a. brachialis superficialis
>a. buccalis
>a. bulbi penis
>a. bulbi urethrae
>a. bulbi vaginae
>a. bulbi vestibuli
>a. calcarina
>a. callosa mediana
>a. callosomarginalis
>a. canalis pterygoidei
>arteriae caroticotympanicae (arteriae carotidis internae)
>a. carotis communis
>a. carotis externa
>a. carotis interna
>a. caudae pancreatis
>a. cecalis anterior
>a. cecalis posterior
>a. celiaca
>arteriae centrales anterolaterales
>arteriae centrales anteromediales
>arteriae centrales posterolaterales
>arteriae centrales posteromediales
>a. centralis brevis
>a. centralis retinae
>a. cerebri anterior
>a. cerebri media

>a. cerebri posterior
>a. cervicalis ascendens
>a. cervicalis profunda
>a. cervicalis superficialis
>a. cervicovaginalis
>a. choroidea anterior
>a. choroidea posterior
>arteriae ciliares anteriores
>arteriae ciliares posteriores longae
>a. ciliaris posterior brevis
>arteriae circumferentiales brevis
>a. circumflexa femoris lateralis
>a. circumflexa femoris medialis
>a. circumflexa humeri anterior
>a. circumflexa humeri posterior
>a. circumflexa iliaca profunda
>a. circumflexa iliaca superficialis
>a. circumflexa scapulae
>a. cochlearis communis
>a. cochlearis propria
>a. colica dextra
>a. colica media
>a. colica sinistra
>a. collateralis media
>a. collateralis radialis
>a. collateralis ulnaris inferior
>a. collateralis ulnaris superior
>a. collicularis
>a. comes nervi phrenici
>a. comitans nervi ischiadici
>a. comitans nervi mediani
>a. commissuralis mediana
>a. communicans anterior
>a. communicans posterior
>a. conjunctivalis anterior
>a. conjunctivalis posterior
>a. coronaria dextra
>a. coronaria sinistra
>arteriae corticales radiatae
>a. cremasterica
>a. cystica
>a. deferentialis
>a. descendens genus
>arteriae digitales palmares propriae
>arteriae digitales plantares propriae
>a. digitalis dorsalis
>a. digitalis palmaris communis
>a. digitalis palmaris propria
>a. digitalis plantaris communis
>a. digitalis plantaris propria
>a. dorsalis clitoridis
>a. dorsalis nasi
>a. dorsalis pedis
>a. dorsalis penis
>a. dorsalis scapulae
>a. ductus deferentis
>arteriae encephali
>a. epigastrica inferior
>a. epigastrica superficialis
>a. epigastrica superior
>a. episcleralis
>a. ethmoidalis anterior
>a. ethmoidalis posterior
>a. facialis
>a. femoralis

arteria *(continued)*
- a. fibularis
- a. flexurae dextrae
- a. frontalis
- a. frontobasalis lateralis
- a. frontobasalis medialis
- a. gastrica dextra
- arteriae gastricae breves
- a. gastrica posterior
- a. gastrica sinistra
- a. gastroduodenalis
- a. gastroepiploica dextra
- arteriae gastroepiploicae
- a. gastroepiploica sinistra
- arteriae gastro-omentales
- a. gastroomentalis dextra
- a. gastroomentalis sinistra
- a. genus inferior lateralis
- a. genus inferior medialis
- a. genus media
- a. glutea inferior
- a. glutea superior
- a. gyri angularis
- arteriae helicinae penis
- arteriae helicinae uteri
- a. hepatica communis
- a. hepatica propria
- a. hyaloidea
- a. hypogastrica
- a. hypophysialis inferior
- a. hypophysialis superior
- arteriae ileales
- a. ileocolica
- a. iliaca communis
- a. iliaca externa
- a. iliaca interna
- a. iliolumbalis
- a. inferior anterior cerebelli
- a. inferior lateralis genus
- a. inferior medialis genus
- a. inferior posterior cerebelli
- a. infraorbitalis
- arteriae insulares
- arteriae intercostales posteriores I et II
- arteriae intercostales posteriores III-XI
- arteriae intercostales posteriores prima et secunda
- a. intercostalis suprema
- arteriae interlobares renis
- arteriae interlobulares
- a. interlobulares (hepatis)
- a. interlobulares (renis)
- a. intermesenterica
- a. interossea anterior
- a. interossea communis
- a. interossea posterior
- a. interossea recurrens
- a. interossea volaris
- arteriae intestinales
- arteriae intrarenales
- a. ischiadica, a. ischiatica
- arteriae jejunales

- a. juxtacolica
- arteriae labiales anteriores
- a. labialis inferior
- a. labialis superior
- a. labyrinthi
- a. lacrimalis
- a. laryngea inferior
- a. laryngea superior
- a. lienalis
- a. ligamenti teretis uteri
- a. lingualis
- a. lingularis
- a. lingularis inferior
- a. lingularis superior
- arteriae lobares inferiores
- arteriae lobares inferior et superior
- arteriae lobares superiores
- a. lobaris media
- a. lobaris media pulmonis dextri
- a. lobi caudati
- arteriae lumbales
- arteriae lumbales imae
- a. lusoria
- arteriae malleolares posteriores laterales
- arteriae malleolares posteriores mediales
- a. malleolaris anterior lateralis
- a. malleolaris anterior medialis
- a. mammaria interna
- arteriae mammillares
- a. marginalis coli
- a. masseterica
- a. maxillaris
- a. maxillaris externa
- a. media genus
- a. mediana
- arteriae medullares segmentales
- arteriae membri inferioris
- arteriae membri superioris
- a. meningea anterior
- a. meningea media
- a. meningea posterior
- a. mentalis
- a. mesenterica inferior
- a. mesenterica superior
- a. metacarpalis dorsalis
- a. metacarpalis palmaris
- a. metatarsalis
- a. metatarsalis dorsalis
- a. metatarsalis plantaris
- arteriae musculares (arteriae ophthalmicae)
- a. musculophrenica
- arteriae nasales posteriores laterales
- a. nasalis posterior septi
- a. nasi externa
- arteriae nervorum
- a. nutricia
- a. nutriciae femoris
- arteriae nutriciae humeri
- a. nutricia tibiae
- a. nutricia ulnae
- a. nutriens femoris
- a. nutriens fibulae

A

a. nutriens humeri
a. nutriens radii
a. nutriens tibiae
a. nutriens tibialis
a. nutriens ulnae
a. obturatoria
a. obturatoria accessoria
a. occipitalis
a. occipitalis lateralis
a. occipitalis medialis
a. ophthalmica
a. orbitofrontalis lateralis
a. orbitofrontalis medialis
a. ovarica
a. palatina ascendens
a. palatina descendens
a. palatina major
a. palatina minor
arteriae palpebrales (laterales et
  mediales)
a. pancreatica dorsalis
a. pancreatica inferior
a. pancreatica magna
a. pancreaticoduodenalis inferior
a. pancreaticoduodenalis superior
  (anterior et posterior)
a. paracentralis
arteriae parietales (laterales et
  mediales)
a. parietalis anterior
a. parietalis posterior
arteriae parieto-occipitales
arteriae perforantes anteriores
arteriae perforantes arteriae
  profundae femoris
arteriae perforantes penis
arteriae perforantes radiatae (renis)
a. pericallosa
a. pericardiacophrenica
a. perinealis
a. peronea
a. pharyngea ascendens
a. phrenica inferior
a. phrenica superior
a. plantaris lateralis
a. plantaris medialis
a. plantaris profunda arteriae
  dorsalis pedis
a. plantaris profundus
a. polaris frontalis
a. polaris temporalis
arteriae pontis
a. poplitea
a. precunealis
a. prepancreatica
a. princeps pollicis
a. profunda brachii
a. profunda clitoridis
a. profunda femoris
a. profunda linguae
a. profunda penis
a. pterygomeningealis
arteriae pudendae externae
a. pudenda interna
a. pulmonalis

a. pulmonalis dextra
a. pulmonalis sinistra
a. quadrigeminalis
a. radialis
a. radialis indicis
arteriae radiculares (anterior et
  posterior)
a. radicularis magna
a. radii nutricia
a. ranina
a. rectalis inferior
a. rectalis media
a. rectalis superior
a. recurrens
a. recurrens radialis
a. recurrens tibialis anterior
a. recurrens tibialis posterior
a. recurrens ulnaris
a. renalis
arteriae renis
a. retinae centralis
a. retroduodenalis
arteriae sacrales laterales
a. sacralis mediana
a. scapularis descendens
a. scapularis dorsalis
a. segmentalis anterior
a. segmentalis apicalis
a. segmentalis basalis anterior
a. segmentalis basalis lateralis
a. segmentalis basalis medialis
a. segmentalis lateralis
a. segmentalis medialis
a. segmentalis posterior
a. segmentalis superior
a. segmenti anterioris inferioris renis
a. segmenti anterioris superioris
  renis
arteriae segmenti hepaticae
a. segmenti inferioris renis
a. segmenti posterioris renis
a. segmenti superioris renis
arteriae sigmoideae
a. spermatica interna
a. sphenopalatina
a. spinalis anterior
a. spinalis posterior
a. splenica
a. striata medialis distalis
a. stylomastoidea
a. subclavia
a. subcostalis
a. sublingualis
a. submentalis
a. subscapularis
a. sulci centralis
a. sulci postcentralis
a. sulci precentralis
a. superior cerebelli
a. superior lateralis genus
a. superior medialis genus
a. suprachiasmatica
a. supraduodenalis
a. supraoptica
a. supraorbitalis

arteria *(continued)*
    arteriae suprarenales superiores
    a. suprarenalis inferior
    a. suprarenalis media
    a. suprascapularis
    a. supratrochlearis
    arteriae surales
    a. tarsea lateralis
    a. tarsea medialis
    a. temporalis anterior
    a. temporalis intermedia
    a. temporalis media
    a. temporalis posterior
    a. temporalis profunda
    a. temporalis superficialis
    a. testicularis
    arteriae thalamostriatae anterolaterales
    arteriae thalamostriatae
      anteromediales
    a. thoracica interna
    a. thoracica lateralis
    a. thoracica superior
    a. thoracoacromialis
    a. thoracodorsalis
    a. thyroidea ima
    a. thyroidea inferior
    a. thyroidea superior
    a. tibialis anterior
    a. tibialis posterior
    a. transversa cervicis
    a. transversa colli
    a. transversa faciei
    a. tuberis cinerei
    a. tympanica anterior
    a. tympanica inferior
    a. tympanica posterior
    a. tympanica superior
    a. ulnaris
    a. umbilicalis
    a. uncalis
    a. urethralis
    a. uterina
    a. vaginalis
    arteriae ventriculares
    a. vertebralis
    a. vesicalis inferior
    a. vesicalis superior
    a. vestibularis anterior
    a. vestibuli
    a. vestibulocochlearis
    a. vitellina
    a. volaris indicis radialis
    a. zygomatico-orbitalis
arteria ischiatica *(var. of* arteria
  ischiadica)
arterial
    a. arcade
    a. arch of colon
    a. arch of ileum
    a. arch of jejunum
    a. arch of lower eyelid
    a. arch of upper eyelid
    a. blood
    a. blood gas (ABG)

    a. bulb
    a. canal
    a. capillary
    a. circle of cerebrum
    a. cone
    a. duct
    a. flap
    a. forceps
    a. groove
    a. hyperemia
    a. hypotension
    a. ligament
    a. line
    a. murmur
    a. nephrosclerosis
    a. plexus
    a. sclerosis
    a. segment of kidney
    a. spider
    a. switch operation
    a. tension
    a. thoracic outlet syndrome
    a. vein
    a. wave
arterialization
arteriectasia
arteriectasis
arteriectomy
arterioatony
arteriocapillary sclerosis
arteriococcygeal gland
arteriogram
arteriographic
arteriography
    bronchial a.
    cerebral a.
arteriola, pl. arteriolae
    a. glomerularis afferens
    a. glomerularis efferens
    a. maculae medius
    a. macularis inferior
    a. macularis superior
    a. medialis retinae
    a. nasalis retinae inferior
    a. nasalis retinae superior
    arteriolae rectae
    a. temporalis retinae inferior
    a. temporalis retinae superior
arteriolar
    a. nephrosclerosis
    a. network
    a. sclerosis
arteriole
    afferent glomerular a.
    capillary a.
    efferent glomerular a.
    inferior macular a.
    inferior nasal a. of retina
    inferior temporal retinal a.
    medial a. of retina
    middle macular a.
    superior macular a.
    superior nasal retinal a.
    superior temporal retinal a.
arteriolith

arteriolitis
    necrotizing a.
arteriology
arteriolonecrosis
arteriolonephrosclerosis
arteriolosclerosis
arteriolosclerotic kidney
arteriolovenous
arteriolovenular
    a. anastomosis
    a. bridge
arteriomalacia
arteriometer
arteriomotor
arteriomyomatosis
arterionephrosclerosis
arteriopalmus
arteriopathy
    hypertensive a.
    plexogenic pulmonary a.
arterioplania
arterioplasty
arteriopressor
arteriorrhaphy
arteriorrhexis
arteriosclerosis
    coronary a.
    hyperplastic a.
    hypertensive a.
    medial a.
    Mönckeberg a.
    nodular a.
    a. obliterans
    peripheral a.
    senile a.
arteriosclerotic
    a. aneurysm
    a. gangrene
    a. kidney
    a. retinopathy
arteriospasm
arteriostenosis
arteriotomy
arteriovenous
    a. anastomosis (ava)
    a. aneurysm
    a. carbon dioxide difference
    a. fistula
    a. nicking
    a. oxygen difference
    a. shunt
arteritis
    brachiocephalic a.
    coronary a.
    cranial a.
    extracranial a.
    giant cell a.
    granulomatous a.
    Heubner a.
    Horton a.
    intracranial granulomatous a.
    neurocranial granulomatous a.
    a. nodosa
    a. obliterans
    obliterating a.
    rheumatic a.
    rheumatoid a.
    Takayasu a.
    temporal a.
artery
    Abbott a.
    aberrant a.
    aberrant obturator a.
    accessory meningeal a.
    accessory obturator a.
    acetabular a.
    acromial a.
    acromiothoracic a.
    a. of Adamkiewicz
    alar a. of nose
    angular a.
    a. of angular gyrus
    anterior basal segmental a.
    anterior cecal a.
    anterior cerebral a.
    anterior choroidal a.
    anterior ciliary a.
    anterior circumflex humeral a.
    anterior communicating a.
    anterior conjunctival a.
    anterior ethmoidal a.
    anterior humeral circumflex a.
    anterior inferior cerebellar a.
    anterior inferior segmental a. of
      kidney
    a. of anterior inferior segment of
      kidney
    anterior intercostal a.
    anterior interosseous a.
    anterior interventricular a.
    anterior labial a.
    anterior lateral malleolar a.
    anterior medial malleolar a.
    anterior mediastinal a.
    anterior meningeal a.
    anterior parietal a.
    anterior perforating a.
    anterior peroneal a.
    anterior and posterior radicular a.
    anterior and posterior superior
      pancreaticoduodenal a.
    anterior segmental a.
    anterior spinal a.
    anterior superior alveolar a.
    anterior superior dental a.
    anterior superior segmental a. of
      kidney
    a. of anterior superior segment of
      kidney
    anterior temporal a.
    anterior tibial a.
    anterior tibial recurrent a.
    anterior tympanic a.
    anterior vestibular a.
    anterolateral central a.
    anterolateral striate a.
    anterolateral thalamostriate a.
    anteromedial central a.
    anteromedial thalamostriate a.
    apical segmental a.

artery *(continued)*
apical segmental a. of superior lobar artery of right lung
apicoposterior a.
appendicular a.
arciform a.
arcuate a. of foot (inconstant)
arcuate a. of kidney
ascending cervical a.
ascending palatine a.
ascending pharyngeal a.
atrial a.
a. to atrioventricular node
axillary a.
azygos a. of vagina
basilar a.
brachial a.
a. of brain
bronchial a.
buccal a.
buccinator a.
buckled innominate a.
a. of bulb of penis
a. of bulb of vestibule
calcaneal a.
calcarine a.
a. of calf
callosomarginal a.
caroticotympanic a. (of internal carotid artery)
carotid a.
carpal a.
caudal pancreatic a.
a. of caudate lobe
cavernous a.
cecal a.
celiac a.
central a. of retina
central retinal a.
central sulcal a.
a. of central sulcus
cerebellar a.
cerebral a.
a. of cerebral hemorrhage
cervicovaginal a.
Charcot a.
chief a. of thumb
circumflex femoral a.
circumflex fibular a.
circumflex humeral a.
circumflex iliac a.
circumflex scapular a.
coiled a. of the uterus
colic a.
collateral digital a.
collicular a.
comitant a. of median nerve
common carotid a.
common cochlear a.
common hepatic a.
common iliac a.
common interosseous a.
common palmar digital a.
common plantar digital a.

communicating a.
companion a. to sciatic nerve
conjunctival a.
coronary a.
cortical radiate a.
costocervical a.
cremasteric a.
cricothyroid a.
cystic a.
deep a. of arm
deep auricular a.
deep brachial a.
deep cervical a.
deep circumflex iliac a.
deep a. of clitoris
deep epigastric a.
deep lingual a.
deep a. of penis
deep plantar a.
deep temporal a.
deep a. of thigh
deep a. of tongue
deferential a.
descending genicular a.
descending a. of knee
descending palatine a.
descending scapular a.
digital collateral a.
distal medial striate a.
distributing a.
dolichoectatic a.
dorsal a. of clitoris
dorsal digital a.
dorsal a. of foot
dorsal interosseous a.
dorsalis pedis a.
dorsal metacarpal a.
dorsal metatarsal a.
dorsal nasal a.
dorsal a. of nose
dorsal pancreatic a.
dorsal a. of penis
dorsal scapular a.
dorsal thoracic a.
a. of Drummond
a. to ductus deferens
elastic a.
end a.
episcleral a.
esophageal a.
external carotid a.
external iliac a.
external mammary a.
external maxillary a.
external nasal a.
external a. of nose
external spermatic a.
facial a.
femoral nutrient a.
fibular a.
fibular nutrient a.
first and second posterior intercostal a.
frontal a.
frontopolar a.

A

gastric a.
gastroduodenal a.
gastroepiploic a.
gastroomental a.
genicular a.
glaserian a.
great anastomotic a.
greater palatine a.
greater pancreatic a.
great radicular a.
great segmental medullary a.
great superior pancreatic a.
helicine a. of penis
helicine a. of the uterus
hepatic a.
hepatic a. proper
a. of Heubner
Heubner a.
highest intercostal a.
highest thoracic a.
humeral a.
humeral nutrient a.
hyaloid a.
hypogastric a.
ileal a.
ileocolic a.
iliac a.
iliolumbar a.
inferior alveolar a.
inferior dental a.
inferior epigastric a.
inferior gluteal a.
inferior hemorrhoidal a.
inferior hypophysial a.
inferior internal parietal a.
inferior labial a.
inferior laryngeal a.
inferior lateral genicular a.
inferior lingular a.
inferior lobar a.
inferior medial genicular a.
inferior mesenteric a.
inferior pancreatic a.
inferior pancreaticoduodenal a.
inferior phrenic a.
inferior rectal a.
inferior segmental a. of kidney
a. of inferior segment of kidney
inferior and superior lobar a.'s
inferior suprarenal a.
inferior thyroid a.
inferior tympanic a.
inferior ulnar collateral a.
inferior vesical a.
infraorbital a.
infrascapular a.
innominate a.
insular a.
intercostal a.
interlobar a.
interlobar a. of kidney
interlobular a.
interlobular a. of kidney
interlobular a. of liver
intermediate temporal a.

internal auditory a.
internal carotid a.
internal iliac a.
internal mammary a.
internal maxillary a.
internal pudendal a.
internal spermatic a.
internal thoracic a.
intestinal a.
intrarenal a.
jejunal a.
juxtacolic a.
a. of kidney
Kugel anastomotic a.
a. of labyrinth
labyrinthine a.
lacrimal a.
lateral basal segmental a.
lateral circumflex femoral a.
lateral circumflex a. of thigh
lateral femoral circumflex a.
lateral frontobasal a.
lateral inferior genicular a.
lateral malleolar a.
lateral and medial palpebral a.
lateral and medial parietal a.
lateral nasal a.
lateral occipital a.
lateral orbitofrontal a.
lateral plantar a.
lateral sacral a.
lateral segmental a.
lateral splanchnic a.
lateral striate a.
lateral superior genicular a.
lateral tarsal a.
lateral thoracic a.
left anterior descending a.
left colic a.
left coronary a.
left gastric a.
left gastroepiploic a.
left gastroomental a.
left hepatic a.
left marginal a.
left pulmonary a.
lenticulostriate a.
lesser palatine a.
lienal a.
lingual a.
lingular a.
long central a.
long posterior ciliary a.
long thoracic a.
a. of lower limb
lowest lumbar a.
lowest thyroid a.
lumbar a.
macular a.
mammillary a.
marginal a. of colon
masseteric a.
mastoid a.
maxillary a.
medial basal segmental a.

artery *(continued)*

medial circumflex femoral a.
medial circumflex a. of thigh
medial collateral a.
medial commisural a.
medial femoral circumflex a.
medial frontobasal a.
medial inferior genicular a.
medial malleolar a.
medial occipital a.
medial orbitofrontal a.
medial plantar a.
medial segmental a.
medial striate a.
medial superior genicular a.
medial tarsal a.
median callosal a.
median commissural a.
median sacral a.
mediastinal a.
medium a.
medullary a. of brain
medullary spinal a.
mental a.
metatarsal a.
middle cerebral a.
middle colic a.
middle collateral a.
middle genicular a.
middle hemorrhoidal a.
middle lobar a.
middle lobar a. of right lung
middle meningeal a.
middle rectal a.
middle sacral a.
middle suprarenal a.
middle temporal a.
muscular a.
muscular a. (of ophthalmic artery)
musculophrenic a.
mylohyoid a.
myometrial arcuate a.
myometrial radial a.
a. needle
Neubauer a.
nutrient a.
nutrient a. of femur
nutrient a. of fibula
nutrient a. of humerus
nutrient a. of radius
nutrient a. of the tibia
nutrient a. of ulna
obturator a.
occipital a.
omphalomesenteric a.
ophthalmic a.
orbital a.
orbitofrontal a.
ovarian a.
palmar interosseous a.
palmar metacarpal a.
paracentral a.
paramedian a.
parent a.

parietooccipital a.
a. of penis
perforating a. of hand
perforating a. (of deep femoral artery)
perforating a. (of foot)
perforating a. (of internal thoracic artery)
perforating a. of penis
perforating radiate a. (of kidney)
pericallosal a.
pericardiacophrenic a.
perineal a.
peroneal a.
pipestem a.
plantar metatarsal a.
polar frontal a.
polar temporal a.
a. of pons
pontine a.
popliteal a.
postcentral sulcal a.
a. of postcentral sulcus
posterior alveolar a.
posterior auricular a.
posterior basal segmental a.
posterior cecal a.
posterior cerebral a.
posterior choroidal a.
posterior circumflex humeral a.
posterior communicating a.
posterior conjunctival a.
posterior dental a.
posterior descending coronary a.
posterior ethmoidal a.
posterior gastric a.
posterior humeral circumflex a.
posterior inferior cerebellar a.
posterior intercostal a. 1–11
posterior interosseous a.
posterior interventricular branch of right coronary a.
posterior labial a.
posterior lateral nasal a.
posterior mediastinal a.
posterior meningeal a.
posterior pancreaticoduodenal a.
posterior parietal a.
posterior peroneal a.
posterior segmental a.
a. of posterior segment of kidney
posterior septal a. of nose
posterior spinal a.
posterior superior alveolar a.
posterior temporal a.
posterior tibial recurrent a.
posterior tympanic a.
posterolateral central a.
posteromedial central a.
precentral sulcal a.
a. of precentral sulcus
precuneal a.
prepancreatic a.
pre-rolandic a.
princeps cervicis a.

princeps pollicis a.
principal a. of thumb
profunda brachii a.
profunda femoris a.
proper cochlear a.
proper palmar digital a.
proper plantar digital a.
proximal medial striate a.'s
a. of pterygoid canal
pterygomeningeal a.
pubic a.
pulmonary a.
a. of pulp
pyloric a.
quadrigeminal a.
radial collateral a.
radial index a.
radialis indicis a.
radial recurrent a.
ranine a.
recurrent a. of Heubner
recurrent interosseous a.
recurrent radial a.
recurrent ulnar a.
renal a.
retroduodenal a.
right colic a.
right coronary a.
right descending pulmonary a.
  (RDPA)
right flexural a.
right gastric a.
right gastroepiploic a.
right gastroomental a.
right hepatic a.
right pulmonary a.
rolandic sulcal a.
a. of round ligament of uterus
a. to sciatic nerve
screw a.
scrotal a.
segmental a. of kidney
segmental a. of liver
segmental medullary a.
septal a.
sheathed a.
short central a.
short circumferential a.
short gastric a.
short posterior ciliary a.
sigmoid a.
a. to the sinoatrial (S-A) node
sinuatrial nodal a.
sinuatrial node a.
sinus node a.
small a.
somatic a.
sphenopalatine a.
spinal a.
spiral modiolar a.
splenic a.
stapedial a.
sternal a.
sternomastoid a.
straight a.

stylomastoid a.
subclavian a.
subcostal a.
sublingual a.
submental a.
subscapular a.
sulcal a.
superficial brachial a.
superficial cervical a.
superficial circumflex iliac a.
superficial epigastric a.
superficial external pudendal a.'s
superficial palmar a.
superficial temporal a.
superficial volar a.
superior cerebellar a.
superior epigastric a.
superior gluteal a.
superior hemorrhoidal a.
superior hypophysial a.
superior intercostal a.
superior internal parietal a.
superior labial a.
superior laryngeal a.
superior lateral genicular a.
superior lingular a.
superior lobar a.
superior medial genicular a.
superior mesenteric a.
superior phrenic a.
superior rectal a.
superior segmental a.
superior segmental a. of kidney
a. of superior segment of kidney
superior suprarenal a.
superior thoracic a.
superior thyroid a.
superior tympanic a.
superior ulnar collateral a.
superior vesical a.
suprachiasmatic a.
supraduodenal a.
supraoptic a.
supraorbital a.
suprascapular a.
supratrochlear a.
supreme intercostal a.
sural a.
a. to tail of pancreas
terminal a.
testicular a.
thoracoacromial a.
thoracodorsal a.
thyroid ima a.
tibial nutrient a.
transverse cervical a.
transverse facial a.
transverse a. of neck
transverse pancreatic a.
transverse scapular a.
a. of tuber cinereum
ulnar recurrent a.
umbilical a.
uncal a.
a. of upper limb

artery *(continued)*
    urethral a.
    uterine a.
    vaginal a.
    a. to vas deferens
    venous a.
    ventral splanchnic a.
    ventricular a.'s
    vertebral a.
    vestibulocochlear a.
    vidian a.
    vitelline a.
    volar interosseous a.
    Zinn a.
    zygomatico-orbital a.
arthral
arthralgia
    intermittent a.
    periodic a.
    a. saturnina
arthralgic
arthrectomy
arthresthesia
arthritic
    a. atrophy
    a. calculus
    a. general pseudoparalysis
arthritis, pl. **arthritides**
    acute rheumatic a.
    chronic absorptive a.
    chylous a.
    a. deformans
    degenerative a.
    enteropathic a.
    filarial a.
    gonococcal a.
    gonorrheal arthritis
    gouty a.
    hemophilic a.
    hypertrophic a.
    Jaccoud a.
    juvenile chronic a.
    juvenile rheumatoid a.
    Lyme a.
    a. mutilans
    neuropathic a.
    a. nodosa
    ochronotic a.
    proliferative a.
    psoriatic a.
    pyogenic a.
    reactive a.
    rheumatoid a.
    septic a.
    suppurative a.
Arthrobacter
arthrocentesis
arthrochondritis
arthroclasia
arthroconidium
Arthroderma
arthrodesis
    triple a.
arthrodia

arthrodial
    a. articulation
    a. cartilage
    a. joint
arthrodynia
arthrodynic
arthrodysplasia
arthroendoscopy
arthroereisis
arthrogenous
arthrogram
arthrography
arthrogryposis multiplex congenita
arthrokatadysis
arthrolith
arthrolithiasis
arthrologia
arthrology
arthrolysis
arthrometer
arthrometry
arthroophthalmopathy
    hereditary progressive a.
arthropathia psoriatica
arthropathology
arthropathy
    diabetic a.
    Jaccoud a.
    long-leg a.
    neuropathic a.
    static a.
    tabetic a.
arthroplasty
    Charnley hip a.
    gap a.
    interposition a.
    intracapsular temporomandibular
     joint a.
    total joint a.
arthropneumoradiography
arthropod
Arthropoda
arthropodiasis
arthropodic, arthropodous
arthropyosis
arthrorisis
arthrosclerosis
arthroscope
arthroscopy
arthrosis
    temporomandibular a.
arthrospore
arthrostomy
arthrosynovitis
arthrotome
arthrotomy
arthrotropic
arthrotyphoid
Arthus
    A. phenomenon
    A. reaction
articular
    a. branch
    a. capsule
    a. cartilage

a. cavity
a. chondrocalcinosis
a. circumference of head of radius
a. circumference of head of ulna
a. corpuscle
a. crepitus
a. crescent
a. crest
a. disk
a. disk of acromioclavicular joint
a. disk of distal radioulnar joint
a. disk of sternoclavicular joint
a. disk of temporomandibular joint
a. eminence of temporal bone
a. facet
a. facet of head of fibula
a. facet of head of rib
a. facet of lateral malleolus
a. facet of medial malleolus
a. facet of radial head
a. facet of tubercle of rib
a. fossa of temporal bone
a. fracture
a. gout
a. labrum
a. lamella
a. lip
a. margin
a. meniscus
a. muscle
a. muscle of elbow
a. muscle of knee
a. nerve
a. pit of head of radius
a. process
a. rheumatism
a. sensibility
a. surface
a. surface of acromion
a. surface of arytenoid cartilage
a. surface of mandibular fossa of temporal bone
a. surface on calcaneus for cuboid bone
a. surface of patella
a. tubercle of temporal bone
a. vascular circle
a. vascular network
a. vascular network of elbow
a. vascular network of knee
a. vascular plexus

articulare
articularis

a. cubiti muscle
a. genus muscle

articulate
articulated skeleton
articulating paper
articulatio, pl. **articulationes**

a. acromioclavicularis
a. atlantoaxialis lateralis
a. atlantoaxialis mediana
a. atlanto-occipitalis
a. bicondylaris
a. calcaneocuboidea

a. capitis costae
a. carpi
articulationes carpi
articulationes carpometacarpales
a. carpometacarpalis pollicis
a. cartilaginis
articulationes cinguli membri inferioris
articulationes cinguli membri superioris
articulationes cinguli pectoralis
articulationes cinguli pelvici
a. complexa
a. composita
a. condylaris
articulationes costochondrales
a. costotransversaria
articulationes costovertebrales
a. cotylica
a. coxae
a. coxofemoralis
articulationes cranii
a. cricoarytenoidea
a. cricothyroidea
a. cubiti
a. cuneonavicularis
a. cylindrica
a. dentoalveolaris
a. ellipsoidea
a. fibrosa
a. genus
a. glenohumeralis
a. humeri
a. humeroradialis
a. humeroulnaris
a. incudomallearis
a. incudostapedia
articulationes intercarpales
articulationes interchondrales
articulationes intercuneiformes
articulationes intermetacarpales
articulationes intermetatarsales
articulationes interphalangeae manus
articulationes interphalangeae pedis
articulationes intertarseae
a. lumbosacralis
a. mandibularis
articulationes manus
a. mediocarpalis
articulationes membri inferioris liberi
articulationes membri superioris liberi
articulationes metacarpophalangeae
articulationes metatarsophalangeae
articulationes ossiculorum auditoriorum
articulationes ossiculorum auditus
a. ossis pisiformis
a. ovoidalis
articulationes pedis
a. plana
a. radiocarpalis
a. radioulnaris distalis
a. radioulnaris proximalis
a. sacrococcygea

articulatio *(continued)*
    a. sacroiliaca
    a. sellaris
    a. simplex
    a. spheroidea
    a. sternoclavicularis
    articulationes sternocostales
    a. subtalaris
    a. synovialis
    a. talocalcanea
    a. talocalcaneonavicularis
    a. talocruralis
    a. tarsi transversa
    articulationes tarsometatarsales
    a. temporomandibularis
    articulationes thoracis
    a. tibiofibularis
    a. trochoidea
    articulationes zygapophysiales
articulation
    arthrodial a.
    atlantooccipital a.
    balanced a.
    bicondylar a.
    cartilaginous a.
    compound a.
    condylar a.
    confluent a.
    cricoarytenoid a.
    cricothyroid a.
    cuneonavicular a.
    dental a.
    a. disorder
    distal radioulnar a.
    a. of foot
    glenohumeral a.
    a. of hand
    humeral a.
    humeroradial a.
    incudomalleolar a.
    incudostapedial a.
    interchondral a.
    intermetatarsal a.
    interphalangeal a.
    intertarsal a.
    metacarpophalangeal a.
    metatarsophalangeal a.
    peg-and-socket a.
    a. of pisiform bone
    proximal radioulnar a.
    radiocarpal a.
    sacroiliac a.
    spheroid a.
    sternocostal a.
    superior tibial a.
    talocrural a.
    temporomandibular a.
    tibiofibular a.
    transverse tarsal a.
    trochoid a.
articulator
    adjustable a.
    arcon a.
    non-arcon a.

articulatory
articulostat
articulus
artifact, artefact
    chemical shift a.
    thermal a.
artifactitious
artifactual
artificial
    a. active immunity
    a. anatomy
    a. ankylosis
    a. Carlsbad salt
    a. crown
    a. dentition
    a. eye
    a. fever
    a. heart
    a. insemination
    a. intelligence
    a. kidney
    a. Kissingen salt
    a. melanin
    a. membrane rupture
    a. pacemaker
    a. passive immunity
    a. pneumothorax
    a. pupil
    a. radioactivity
    a. respiration
    a. selection
    a. sphincter
    a. stone
    a. tears
    a. ventilation
    a. Vichy salt
Artiodactyla
artistic anatomy
ARV
    AIDS-related virus
arycorniculate synchondrosis
aryepiglottic
    a. fold
    a. muscle
    a. part of oblique arytenoid muscle
aryl acylamidase
arylamidase
arylarsonic acid
arylated alkyl
arylsulfatase
    a. A deficiency
    a. B deficiency
arytenoepiglottidean fold
arytenoid
    a. cartilage
    a. dislocation
    a. gland
    a. subluxation
    a. swelling
arytenoidal articular surface of cricoid
arytenoidectomy
arytenoideus
arytenoiditis
arytenoidopexy

AS
> auris sinistra

As
> arsenic

asafetida

Asarum
> a. canadense
> a. europaeum

asbestoid

asbestos
> a. body
> a. corn
> a. liner
> a. wart

asbestosis

ascariasis

ascaricide

ascarid

Ascaridae

Ascaridata

Ascaridida

Ascarididae

Ascarididea

Ascaridoidea

ascaridole

Ascaridorida

Ascaris
> *A. equorum*
> *A. lumbricoides*

Ascaroidea

ascaron

Ascarops strongylina

ascendens

ascending
> a. aorta
> a. branch
> a. branch of the inferior mesenteric artery
> a. branch of superficial cervical artery
> a. cervical artery
> a. cholangitis
> a. colon
> a. current
> a. degeneration
> a. frontal convolution
> a. frontal gyrus
> a. lumbar vein
> a. myelitis
> a. neuritis
> a. palatine artery
> a. paralysis
> a. parietal convolution
> a. parietal gyrus
> a. part of aorta
> a. part of duodenum
> a. part of trapezius muscle
> a. pharyngeal artery
> a. pharyngeal plexus
> a. process
> a. pyelonephritis
> a. ramus of lateral sulcus of cerebrum

ascensus

ascertainment
> a. bias
> complete a.
> incomplete a.
> single a.
> total a.
> truncate a.

Aschelminthes

Ascher
> A. aqueous influx phenomenon
> A. syndrome

Aschner
> A. phenomenon
> A. reflex

Aschner-Dagnini reflex

Aschoff
> A. body
> A. cell
> A. nodule

asci (*pl. of* ascus)

ascites
> a. adiposus
> chyliform a.
> a. chylosus
> chylous a.
> fatty a.
> gelatinous a.
> hemorrhagic a.
> milky a.
> pseudochylous a.

ascitic

ascitogenous

ascocarp

ascogenous

ascogonium

Ascoli
> A. reaction
> A. test

Ascomycetes

ascomycetous

Ascomycota

ascorbase

ascorbate

ascorbate-cyanide test

ascorbic acid

ascorbyl palmitate

ascospore

ASCUS
> atypical squamous cell of undetermined significance

ascus, pl. **asci**

asecretory

Aselli
> A. gland
> A. pancreas

asepsis

aseptate

aseptic
> a. fever
> a. necrosis
> a. surgery

asepticism

asequence

asexual
> a. dwarfism

asexual *(continued)*
    a. generation
    a. reproduction
ash
    bone a.
Ashby method
ashen
    a. tuber
    a. tubercle
    a. wing
Asherman syndrome
ash-leaf macule
Ashman phenomenon
ashy dermatosis
asialism
asialoglycoprotein receptor
Asian influenza
Asiatic
    A. cholera
    A. schistosomiasis
asiderotic anemia
asitia
Askanazy cell
Ask-Upmark kidney
ASL
    American Sign Language
**as low as reasonably achievable
    (ALARA)**
Asn
asocial
asoma, pl. **asomata**
Asp
    aspartic acid
aspalasoma
asparaginase
    Erwinia L-a.
asparagine
    a. ligase
    a. synthetase
asparaginyl
Asparagus
aspartame
aspartase
aspartate
    a. aminotransferase (AST)
    a. ammonia-lyase
    a. carbamoyltransferase
    a. 1-decarboxylase
    a. 4-decarboxylase
    a. kinase
    a. transaminase
aspartic acid (Asp, Asx)
aspartyl
aspartylglycosamine
aspartylglycosaminidase
aspartylglycosaminuria
aspect
    facial a.
    frontal a.
    lateral a.
    occipital a.
    superior a.
    vertical a.
Asperger disorder

aspergillic acid
aspergillin
aspergilloma
aspergillosis
    acute invasive a.
    allergic bronchopulmonary a.
        (ABPA)
    chronic necrotizing a.
    disseminated a.
Aspergillus
    A. clavatus
    A. flavus
    A. fumigatus
    A. nidulans
    A. niger
    A. terreus
aspermatogenic sterility
aspermia
aspersion
aspheric lens
asphygmia
asphyxia
    cyanotic a.
    local a.
    symmetric a.
    traumatic a.
asphyxial
asphyxiant
asphyxiate
asphyxiating
    a. thoracic chondrodystrophy
    a. thoracic dysplasia
    a. thoracic dystrophy
asphyxiation
Aspiculuris tetraptera
aspidin
aspidinol
aspidium
aspidosamine
aspidospermine
aspirate
aspirating needle
aspiration
    a. biopsy
    meconium a.
    a. pneumonia
aspirator
    vacuum a.
    water a.
aspirin
asplenia
    functional a.
    a. syndrome
    a. with cardiovascular anomalies
asplenic
asporogenous
asporous
asporulate
Assam fever
assassin bug
assay
    Ames a.
    biologic a.
    clonogenic a.
    competitive binding a.

complement binding a.
double antibody sandwich a.
EAC rosette a.
enzyme-linked immunosorbent a.
  (ELISA)
Grunstein-Hogness a.
hemizona a.
hemolytic plaque a.
immunochemical a.
immunoradiometric a.
indirect a.
Jerne plaque a.
Lowry-Folin a.
Lowry protein a.
radioreceptor a.
Raji cell radioimmune a.

assertive
a. conditioning
a. training

assessment
health risk a. (h.r.a.)

Assézat triangle

assident
a. sign
a. symptom

assimilable

assimilation
ammonia a.
a. pelvis
reproductive a.
a. sacrum

assist-control ventilation

assisted
a. cephalic delivery
a. circulation
a. reproductive technology
a. respiration
a. ventilation

assistive movement

Assmann tuberculous infiltrate

associate
paired a.'s

associated
a. antagonist
a. movement

association
American Dental A. (ADA)
American Medical A. (AMA)
A. of American Medical Colleges
  (AAMC)
a. area
CHARGE a.
clang a.
a. constant
a. cortex
dream a.
a. fiber
free a.
genetic a.
independent practice a. (IPA)
loose a.
a. mechanism
a. system
a. test

a. time
a. tract

associationism

associative
a. aphasia
a. reaction
a. strength

assortative mating

assortment
independent a.

assumption

AST
aspartate aminotransferase

astasia

astasia-abasia

astatic seizure

astatine (At)

asteatosis cutis

astemizole

aster
sperm a.

astereognosis

asterion

asteriosaponins

asteriotoxins

asterixis

asternal

asternia

Asterococcus

asteroid
a. body
a. hyalosis

asthenia
neurocirculatory a.

asthenic
a. personality
a. personality disorder

asthenopia
accommodative a.
muscular a.
nervous a.

asthenopic

asthenospermia

asthenozoospermia

asthma
atopic a.
bronchial a.
bronchitic a.
cardiac a.
catarrhal a.
cotton-dust a.
a. crystal
dust a.
extrinsic a.
food a.
hay a.
intrinsic a.
miller a.
miner's a.
nervous a.
reflex a.
spasmodic a.
steam-fitter's a.
stripper's a.

asthma *(continued)*
    summer a.
    triad a.
asthmatic bronchitis
asthmatoid wheeze
asthma-weed
asthmogenic
astigmatic
    a. dial
    a. lens
astigmatism
    a. against the rule
    compound hyperopic a.
    compound myopic a.
    corneal a.
    hyperopic a.
    irregular a.
    lenticular a.
    mixed a.
    myopic a.
    a. of oblique pencil
    regular a.
    simple hyperopic a.
    simple myopic a.
    a. with the rule
astigmatometry, astigmometry
astigmia
Astler-Coller classification
astomatous
astomia
astomous
astragalar
astragalectomy
astragalocalcanean
astragalofibular
astragaloscaphoid
astragalotibial
Astragalus
astral fiber
astrapophobia
astriction
astringent
astroblast
astroblastoma
astrocele
astrocyte
    Alzheimer type I, II a.
    fibrillary a.
    fibrous a.
    gemistocytic a.
    protoplasmic a.
    reactive a.
astrocytoma
    anaplastic a.
    cerebellar a.
    desmoplastic cerebral a.
    fibrillary a.
    gemistocytic a.
    grade I, II, III, IV a.
    juvenile cerebellar a.
    low grade a.
    pilocytic a.
    piloid astrocytoma

    protoplasmic a.
    subependymal giant cell a.
astrocytosis cerebri
astroependymoma
astroglia cell
astroid
astrokinetic
astrosphere
Astrovirus
Astwood test
asverin
Asx
    aspartic acid
asyllabia
asylum
asymbolia
asymmetric
    a. chondrodystrophy
    a. disulfide
    a. fetal growth restriction
    a. motor neuropathy
asymmetry
asymptomatic neurosyphilis
asymptotic
asynchronous pulse generator
asynclitism
    anterior a.
    posterior a.
    a. of the skull
asynechia
asynergia
asynergic
asynergy
asynesia, asynesis
asystematic
asystole
asystolia
asystolic
At
    astatine
ata
    atmosphere absolute
atabrine hydrochloride
atactic
    a. abasia
    a. agraphia
atactilia
ataractic
ataraxia
ataraxic
atavism
atavistic epiphysis
ataxia
    acute a.
    Briquet a.
    Bruns a.
    cerebellar a.
    chronic a.
    a. cordis
    Friedreich a.
    gluten a.
    hereditary cerebellar a.
    hereditary spinal a.
    hysterical a.
    kinetic a.

Leyden a.
locomotor a.
Marie a.
motor a.
optic a.
respiratory a.
sensory a.
spinal a.
spinocerebellar a.
static a.
a. telangiectasia
a. telangiectasia syndrome
vasomotor a.
vestibulocerebellar a.
ataxiadynamia
ataxiagram
ataxiagraph
ataxiameter
ataxiaphasia
ataxia-telangiectasia
ataxic
a. abasia
a. aphasia
a. breathing
a. dysarthria
a. gait
a. paramyotonia
a. paraplegia
ataxiophobia
ataxy
A/T cloning
atelectasis
adhesive a.
cicatrization a.
a. of the middle ear
nonobstructive a.
passive a.
patchy a.
platelike a.
primary a.
relaxation a.
resorption a.
rounded a.
secondary a.
segmental a.
subsegmental a.
atelectatic rale
atelia
ateliosis
ateliotic dwarfism
atelopidtoxin
atenolol
athelia
atherectomy
coronary a.
directional a.
athermancy
athermanous
athermosystaltic
atheroembolism
atherogenesis
atherogenic
atheroma
atheromatous
a. degeneration

a. embolism
a. plaque
atherosclerosis
atherosclerotic aneurysm
atherosis
atherothrombosis
atherothrombotic
athetoid
athetosic, athetotic
athetosis
double congenital a.
posthemiplegic a.
athlete's
a. foot
a. heart
athletic heart
aThr
allothreonine
athrepsia
athrepsy
athrocytosis
athrombia
athymia
athymism
athyrea
athyroidism
athyrosis
athyrotic
ATL
adult T-cell leukemia
atlantad
atlantal
atlantic part of vertebral artery
atlantoaxial joint
atlantodidymus
atlantoepistrophic
atlantooccipital
a. articulation
a. joint
a. membrane
atlantoodontoid
atlas
atloaxoid
atlodidymus
atloid
atlooccipital
atm
atmolysis
atmometer
atmos
atmosphere
a. absolute (ata)
ICAO standard a.
standard a.
atmospheric pressure
atmospherization
Atmungsferment
atom
activated a.
Bohr a.
excited a.
halogen a. (X)
ionized a.
labeled a.
nuclear a.

atom *(continued)*
 quaternary carbon a.
 radioactive a.
 recoil a.
 stripped a.
 tagged a.
atomic
 a. absorption spectrophotometry
 a. core
 a. heat
 a. mass unit (amu)
 a. number (Z)
 a. theory
 a. volume
 a. weight (at. wt., AW)
atomism
atomistic psychology
atomization
atomizer
atonia
atonic
 a. bladder
 a. dyspepsia
 a. ectropion
 a. entropion
 a. epiphora
 a. seizure
atonicity
atony
 postpartum a.
 uterine a.
atopen
atopic
 a. allergy
 a. asthma
 a. cataract
 a. dermatitis
 a. eczema
 a. keratoconjunctivitis
 a. reagin
Atopobium
atopognosia, atopognosis
atopy
atoxic
ATP
 adenosine 5′-triphosphate
 ATP citrate lyase
 ATP citrate (*pro*-3*S*)-lyase
 ATP cobalamin adenoxyltransferase
 ATP-diphosphatase
 ATP sulfurylase
ATPase
 adenosine triphosphatase
atrabiliary capsule
atractosylidic acid
atractylic acid
atractyligenin
atractylin
atracurium besylate
atraumatic
 a. needle
 a. suture
atrepsy

atresia
 anal a.
 a. ani
 aortic a.
 biliary a.
 bronchial a.
 choanal a.
 esophageal a.
 a. folliculi
 intestinal a.
 a. iridis
 laryngeal a.
 pulmonary artery a.
 tricuspid a.
 vaginal a.
atresic teratosis
atretic
 a. corpus luteum
 a. ovarian follicle
atretoblepharia
atretocystia
atretogastria
atretopsia
atria (*pl. of* atrium)
atrial
 a. anastomotic branch of circumflex branch of left coronary artery
 a. appendage
 a. artery
 a. auricle
 a. auricula
 a. bigeminy
 a. branch
 a. capture
 a. capture beat
 a. chaotic tachycardia
 a. complex
 a. diastole
 a. dissociation
 a. echo
 a. extrasystole
 a. fibrillation
 a. flutter
 a. fusion beat
 a. gallop
 a. kick
 a. myxoma
 a. natriuretic factor
 a. natriuretic peptide (ANP)
 a. septal defect
 a. septostomy
 a. sound
 a. standstill
 a. synchronous pulse generator
 a. systole
 a. transport function
 a. triggered pulse generator
 a. ventricular canal defect
atrial-well technique
atrichia
atrichosis
atriomegaly
atrionector
atriopeptin
atrioseptoplasty

atrioseptostomy
> balloon a.

atriosystolic murmur

atriotomy

atrioventricular (AV)
> a. band
> a. block
> a. bundle
> a. canal
> a. canal cushion
> a. conduction (AVC)
> a. connection
> a. dissociation (AVD)
> a. extrasystole
> a. gradient
> a. groove
> a. interval
> a. junctional bigeminy
> a. junctional rhythm
> a. junctional tachycardia
> a. nodal branch
> a. node
> a. septum
> a. sulcus
> a. valve

atriplicism

atrium, pl. **atria**
> accessory a.
> a. cordis dextrum
> a. cordis sinistrum
> a. dextrum cordis
> a. glottidis
> a. of heart
> a. of lateral ventricle
> left a. of heart
> a. meatus medii
> a. meatus medii nasalis
> a. of middle nasal meatus
> nasal a.
> a. pulmonale
> right a. of heart
> a. sinistrum cordis
> a. ventriculi lateralis
> a. ventriculus lateralis

Atropa

atrophia
> a. cutis
> a. maculosa varioliformis cutis
> a. pilorum propria

atrophic
> a. excavation
> a. gastritis
> a. glossitis
> a. heterochromia
> a. inflammation
> a. kidney
> a. pharyngitis
> a. rhinitis
> a. thrombosis
> a. vaginitis

atrophie blanche

atrophied

atrophoderma
> a. albidum
> a. diffusum

> a. maculatum
> a. neuriticum
> a. of Pasini and Pierini
> senile a.
> a. senilis
> a. striatum

atrophodermatosis

atrophy
> acute reflex bone a.
> acute yellow a. of the liver
> alveolar a.
> arthritic a.
> blue a.
> brown a.
> Buchwald a.
> central areolar choroidal a.
> cerebellar a.
> choroidal vascular a.
> congenital cerebellar a.
> congenital microvillus a.
> cyanotic a.
> cyanotic a. of the liver
> dentatorubral cerebellar a. with
>   polymyoclonus
> disuse a.
> dominant optic a.
> essential progressive a. of iris
> facioscapulohumeral a.
> familial spinal muscular a.
> fatty a.
> geographic retinal a.
> gingival a.
> gyrate a. of choroid and retina
> Hoffmann muscular a.
> horizontal a.
> infantile progressive spinal
>   muscular a.
> ischemic muscular a.
> juvenile spinal muscular a.
> Kjer optic a.
> Leber hereditary optic a.
> linear a.
> macular a.
> marantic a.
> multiple system a.
> muscular a.
> myopathic a.
> neurogenic a.
> neurotrophic a.
> nutritional type cerebellar a.
> olivopontocerebellar a.
> periodontal a.
> peroneal muscular a.
> Pick a.
> postmenopausal a.
> pressure a.
> primary idiopathic macular a.
> primary macular a. of skin
> progressive choroidal a.
> progressive circumscribed cerebral a.
> progressive infantile spinal
>   muscular a.
> progressive spinal muscular a.
> pulp a.
> red a.

atrophy *(continued)*
    scapulohumeral a.
    senile a.
    spinal muscular a.
    spinal muscular a., type I, II, III
    striate a. of skin
    Sudeck a.
    traction a.
    transneuronal a.
    trophoneurotic a.
    villous a.
    Vulpian a.
    Werdnig-Hoffmann muscular a.
    yellow a. of the liver
    Zimmerlin a.

atropine
    a. methonitrate
    a. methylbromide
    a. sulfate
    a. test

atropinic
atropinism
atropinization
atroscine
atrotoxin
attached
    a. cranial section
    a. craniotomy
    a. gingiva

attachment
    a. apparatus
    bar clip a.
    bar-sleeve a.
    epithelial a.
    epithelial a. of Gottlieb
    frictional a.
    internal a.
    key a.
    keyway a.
    muscle-tendon a.
    parallel a.
    pericemental a.
    precision a.
    slotted a.

attack
    brain a.
    drop a.
    heart a.
    panic a.
    a. rate
    salaam a.
    transient ischemic a. (TIA)
    uncinate a.
    vagal a.
    vasovagal a.

attar of rose
attending
    a. physician
    a. staff
    a. surgeon

attention
    a. deficit hyperactivity disorder
    a. span

attenuant

attenuate
attenuated
    a. tuberculosis
    a. vaccine
    a. virus

attenuation
    a. compensation
    interaural a.

attenuator
attic
    tympanic a.

atticomastoid
atticotomy
attitude
    emotional a.
    fetal a.
    passional a.

attitudinal reflex
attollens
    a. aurem
    a. auriculam
    a. oculi

attractin
attraction
    capillary a.
    chemical a.
    magnetic a.
    neurotropic a.
    a. sphere

attrahens
attributable risk
attrition
at. wt.
    atomic weight

atypia
atypical
    a. absence seizure
    a. achromatopsia
    a. antipsychotic agent
    a. endometrial hyperplasia
    a. facial neuralgia
    a. fibroxanthoma
    a. gingivitis
    a. glandular cell of undetermined significance (AGUS)
    a. lipoma
    a. measles
    a. melanocytic hyperplasia
    a. mycobacteria
    a. pneumonia
    a. pseudocholinesterase
    a. squamous cell of undetermined significance (ASCUS)
    a. trigeminal neuralgia
    a. verrucous endocarditis

atypism
A.U.
    auris uterque

Au
    gold
        Au antigen
        Au blood group

Aub-DuBois table
Auberger blood group
Aubert phenomenon

A

AUC
>   area under the curve

Auchmeromyia
>   *a. luteola*

¹⁹⁸Au colloid
audile
audioanalgesia
audiogenic seizure
audiogram
>   pure tone a.
>   speech a.

audiologist
audiology
audiometer
>   automatic a.
>   Békésy a.
>   pure-tone a.
>   speech a.

audiometric
audiometrist
audiometry
>   automatic a.
>   behavioral observation a.
>   Békésy a.
>   cortical a.
>   diagnostic a.
>   screening a.

audiovisual
audit
audition
>   chromatic a.

auditive
auditory
>   a. agnosia
>   a. alternans
>   a. aphasia
>   a. area
>   a. aura
>   a. brainstem response (ABR)
>   a. canal
>   a. capsule
>   a. cortex
>   a. fatigue
>   a. feedback
>   a. field
>   a. ganglion
>   a. hair
>   a. hallucination
>   a. hyperesthesia
>   a. lemniscus
>   a. localization
>   a. nerve
>   a. neuropathy
>   a. nucleus
>   a. oculogyric reflex
>   a. organ
>   a. ossicle
>   a. pathway
>   a. pit
>   a. placode
>   a. pore
>   a. process
>   a. prosthesis
>   a. receptor cell
>   a. stria

>   a. string
>   a. threshold
>   a. tooth
>   a. tract
>   a. tube
>   a. vesicle

Auenbrugger sign
Auer
>   A. body
>   A. rod

Auerbach
>   A. ganglia
>   A. plexus

Aufrecht sign
Auger electron
augmentation mammaplasty
augmented
>   a. histamine test
>   a. lead

augmentor
>   a. fiber
>   a. nerve

augnathus
Aujeszky disease virus
aura, pl. **aurae**
>   abdominal a.
>   auditory a.
>   experiential a.
>   gustatory a.
>   intellectual a.
>   kinesthetic a.
>   olfactory a.
>   reminiscent a.
>   somatosensory a.
>   visual a.

aural
>   a. myiasis
>   a. vertigo

auramine O fluorescent stain
auranofin
aureolic acid
aures (*pl. of* auris)
auriasis
auric
auricle
>   accessory a.
>   atrial a.
>   cervical a.
>   left a.
>   a. of left atrium
>   ligament of a.
>   a. (of atria)
>   right a.
>   a. of right atrium

auricula, pl. **auriculae**
>   atrial a.
>   auriculae atrii
>   a. atrii dextra
>   a. atrii sinistra

auricular
>   a. appendage
>   a. appendectomy
>   a. appendix
>   a. arc
>   a. branch of occipital artery

auricular *(continued)*
  a. branch of posterior auricular artery
  a. branch of vagus nerve
  a. canaliculus
  a. cartilage
  a. complex
  a. extrasystole
  a. fibrillation
  a. fissure
  a. flutter
  a. ganglion
  a. index
  a. ligament
  a. muscle
  a. notch
  a. point
  a. reflex
  a. standstill
  a. surface of ilium
  a. surface of sacrum
  a. systole
  a. tachycardia
  a. triangle
  a. tubercle
  a. vein
auriculare, pl. **auricularia**
auricularis
  a. anterior muscle
  a. posterior muscle
  a. superior muscle
auriculocranial
auriculoinfraorbital plane
auriculopalpebral reflex
auriculopressor reflex
auriculotemporal
  a. nerve
  a. nerve syndrome
auriculoventricular
  a. groove
  a. interval
aurid, pl. **aurides**
auriform
aurin
aurintricarboxylic acid
auris, pl. **aures**
  a. dexter (A.D.)
  a. externa
  a. interna
  a. media
  a. sinistra (AS)
  a. uterque (A.U.)
aurochromoderma
auromercaptoacetanilid
aurone
auropalpebral reflex
aurotherapy
aurothioglucose
aurothioglycanide
aurum
Aus antigen
ausculatory triangle
auscultate, auscult

auscultation
  direct a.
  immediate a.
  mediate a.
auscultatory
  a. alternans
  a. gap
  a. percussion
  a. sound
Auspitz sign
aussage test
Austin Flint
  A. F. murmur
  A. F. phenomenon
Australia antigen
Australian
  A. bat Lyssavirus
  A. Q fever
  A. tick typhus
  A. X disease
  A. X disease virus
  A. X encephalitis
autacoid substance
autecic, autecious
autemesia
authenticity
authoritarian personality
authority figure
autism
  early infantile a.
  infantile a.
autistic
  a. disorder
  a. parasite
autoactivation
autoagglutination
autoagglutinin
  anti-Pr cold a.
  cold a.
autoallergic
autoallergization
autoallergy
autoanalysis
autoanalyzer
  sequential multichannel a. (SMA)
autoanaphylaxis
autoantibody
  antiidiotype a.
  cold a.
  Donath-Landsteiner cold a.
  hemagglutinating cold a.
  idiotype a.
  warm a.
autoanticomplement
autoantigen
autoassay
autoaugmentation
autoblast
autocatalysis
autocatalytic
autocatheterization, autocatheterism
autochthonous
  a. idea
  a. malaria
  a. parasite

autoclasis, autoclasia
autoclave
autocoid
autocrine hypothesis
autocystoplasty
autocytolysin
autocytolysis
autocytotoxin
autodermic
autodigestion
autodiploid
autodrainage
autoecholalia
autoerotic
autoeroticism
autoerotism
autoerythrocyte
    a. sensitization
    a. sensitization syndrome
autofluoroscope
autogamous
autogamy
autogeneic graft
autogenesis
autogenetic, autogenic
autogenous
    a. control
    a. keratoplasty
    a. union
    a. vaccine
autognosis
autograft
autografting
autogram
autographism
autohemagglutination
autohemolysin
autohemolysis test
autohexaploid
autohypnosis
autohypnotic
autohypnotism
autoimmune
    a. disease
    a. hemolytic anemia
    a. neonatal thrombocytopenia
    a. thyroiditis
autoimmunity
autoimmunization
autoimmunocytopenia
autoinfection
autoinfusion
autoinoculable
autoinoculation
autointoxicant
autointoxication
autoisolysin
autokeratoplasty
autokinesia, autokinesis
autokinetic effect
autolesion
autologous
    a. graft
    a. protein
autolysate

autolyse
autolysin
autolysis
autolytic enzyme
autolyze
automallet
automated
    a. differential leukocyte counter
    a. lamellar keratectomy
automatic
    a. audiometer
    a. audiometry
    a. auditory brainstem response
    a. beat
    a. condenser
    a. contraction
    a. epilepsy
    a. gain control (AGC)
    a. plugger
automatism
    ambulatory a.
    immediate posttraumatic a.
automatograph
automixis
automnesia
automotor seizure
automysophobia
autonomic
    a. division of nervous system
    a. epilepsy
    a. ganglia
    a. imbalance
    a. motor neuron
    a. nerve
    a. nerve fiber
    a. nervous system
    a. neurogenic bladder
    a. nucleus
    a. part of peripheral nervous system
    a. plexus
    a. seizure
autonomotropic
autonomous psychotherapy
autonomy
    functional a.
autooxidation
autooxidizable
autoparenchymatous metaplasia
autopathic
autopentaploid
autopepsia
autophagia
autophagic vacuole
autophagolysosome
autophagy
autophobia
autophony
autoplastic graft
autoploid
autoploidy
autoplugger
autopod
autopodium, pl. autopodia
autopoisonous
autopolymerizing resin

autopolymer resin
autopolyploid
autopolyploidy
autoprotolysis
    a. constant of water (K_w)
autopsy
    verbal a.
autoradiogram
autoradiograph
autoradiography
    paper a.
autoreceptor
autoregulation
    heterometric a.
    homeometric a.
autoreinfection
autoreproduction
autorrhaphy
autoscopic phenomenon
autosensitize
autosepticemia
autoserotherapy
autoserum therapy
autosite
autosmia
autosomal gene
autosomatognosis
autosomatognostic
autosome
autosuggestibility
autosuggestion
autosynnoia
autosynthesis
autotelic
autotemnous
autotetraploid
autotherapy
autotomy
autotopagnosia
autotoxemia
autotoxic
autotoxicosis
autotoxin
autotransfusion
autotransplant
autotransplantation
autotriploid
autotroph
autotrophic
autotrophy
    carbon a.
    nitrogen a.
    sulfur a.
autovaccination
autoxidation
autozygous
autumn fever
auxanogram
auxanographic method
auxanography
auxanology
auxesis
auxetic growth
auxiliary abutment
auxiliomotor

auxilytic
auxocardia
auxochrome
auxodrome
auxoflore
auxogluc
auxotonic
auxotox
auxotroph
auxotrophic
    a. mutant
    a. strain
AV
    atrioventricular
        AV block
        AV conduction
        AV difference
        AV dissociation
        AV interval
        AV junction
        AV junctional rhythm
        AV junctional tachycardia
        AV node
        AV shunt
        AV strabismus syndrome
        AV valves
ava
    arteriovenous anastomosis
available arch length
avalanche conduction
avalvular
avascularization
avascular necrosis
AVC
    atrioventricular conduction
AVD
    atrioventricular dissociation
Avellis syndrome
avenin
average
    a. flow rate
    a. pulse magnitude
    pure-tone a.
avermectins
aversion therapy
aversive
    a. behavior
    a. conditioning
    a. control
    a. stimulus
    a. training
aVF
    electrocardiographic lead
Aviadenovirus
avian
    a. encephalomyelitis virus
    a. influenza virus
    a. lymphomatosis virus
    a. neurolymphomatosis virus
    a. pneumoencephalitis virus
    a. sarcoma
    a. viral arthritis virus
aviation medicine
aviator's disease
avidin

avidity antibody
Avipoxvirus
avirulent
avitaminosis
    conditioned a.
avivement
aVL
    electrocardiographic lead
Avogadro
Avogadro
    A. constant
    A. hypothesis
    A. law
    A. number (N_A)
    A. postulate
avoidance
    a. conditioning
    a. training
avoidance-avoidance conflict
avoidant
    a. disorder of adolescence
    a. disorder of childhood
    a. personality
    a. personality disorder
avoirdupois
AVP
    antiviral protein
aVR
    electrocardiographic lead
avulsed wound
avulsion
    a. fracture
    nerve a.
    root a.
    tooth a.
AW
    atomic weight
ax
    axis
axenic
axerophthol
axes (*pl. of* axis)
axial
    a. ametropia
    a. aneurysm
    a. angle
    a. cataract
    a. current
    a. filament
    a. hyperopia
    a. illumination
    a. muscle
    a. myopia
    a. neuritis
    a. pattern flap
    a. plane
    a. plate
    a. point
    a. projection
    a. section
    a. skeleton
    a. surface
    a. view
    a. walls of the pulp chamber
axialis

axifugal
axil
axile corpuscle
axilla, pl. **axillae**
    a. thermometer
axillary
    a. anesthesia
    a. arch
    a. arch muscle
    a. artery
    a. cavity
    a. fascia
    a. fold
    a. fossa
    a. gland
    a. hair
    a. line
    a. lymphatic plexus
    a. lymph node
    a. nerve
    a. region
    a. sheath
    a. space
    a. sweat gland
    a. thermometer
    a. thoracotomy
    a. triangle
    a. vein
axio-
axiobuccal
axiobuccogingival
axioincisal
axiolabial
axiolabiolingual plane
axiolingual
axiolinguocervical
axiolinguoclusal
axiolinguogingival
axiomesial
axiomesiocervical
axiomesiodistal plane
axiomesiogingival
axiomesioincisal
axion
axioocclusal
axioplasm
axiopodium, pl. **axiopodia**
axiopulpal
axioversion
axipetal
axiramificate
axis, pl. **axes (ax)**
    basibregmatic a.
    basicranial a.
    basifacial a.
    biauricular a.
    celiac a.
    cephalocaudal a.
    cerebrospinal a.
    condylar a.
    conjugate a.
    a. corpuscle
    craniofacial a.
    a. deviation
    electrical a.

axis (*continued*)
    embryonic a.
    encephalomyelonic a.
    external a. of eye
    a. externus bulbi oculi
    facial a.
    axes of Fick
    hinge a.
    instantaneous electrical a.
    internal a. of eye
    a. internus bulbi oculi
    a. of lens
    a. lentis
    a. ligament of malleus
    long a.
    long a. of body
    mandibular a.
    mean electrical a.
    neural a.
    neutral a. of straight beam
    normal electrical a.
    opening a.
    optic a.
    a. opticus
    orbital a.
    pelvic a.
    a. pelvis
    a. of pelvis
    principal optic a.
    pupillary a.
    rotational a.
    sagittal a.
    secondary a.
    a. shift
    a. of symmetry
    thoracic a.
    thyroid a.
    a. traction
    transporionic a.
    transverse horizontal a.
    vertical a.
    visual a.
    Y-a.
axis-traction forceps
axoaxonic synapse
axodendritic synapse
axofugal
axograph
axolemma
axolysis
axon
    a. degeneration
    a. hillock
    a. loss polyneuropathy
    a. reflex
    a. terminal
axonal
    a. degeneration
    a. polyneuropathy
    a. terminal bouton
axoneme
axonography
axonopathy
axonotmesis

axopetal
axoplasm
axoplasmic transport
axopodium, pl. **axopodia**
axosomatic synapse
axostyle
axotomy
ayahuasca
Ayala
    A. index
    A. quotient
Ayerza
    A. disease
    A. syndrome
Ayre brush
azacrine
azacyclonol hydrochloride
9-azafluorene
8-azaguanine
azamethonium bromide
azaperone
azapetine phosphate
azapirone
azaribine
azaserine
azaspirodecanedione
azatadine maleate
azathioprine
6-azathymine
6-azauridine (AZUR)
azeotrope
    halothane-ether a.
azeotropic
azide
azidothymidine (AZT)
azin dye
azlocillin sodium
azo
    a. dye
    a. itch
azobilirubin
azocarmine
    a. B, G
    a. dye
azoic
azole
azolitmin
azoospermia
azophloxin
azoprotein
Azorean disease
azosulfamide
azotemia
    nonrenal a.
    prerenal a.
azotemic
azothermia
azotobacter nuclease
azoturia
azovan blue
AZT
    azidothymidine
Aztec ear
aztreonam
azul

AZUR
    6-azauridine
azure
    a. A, B, C
    a. I, II
    a. lunula of nail
azuresin
azurophil, azurophile
    a. granule
azurophilia
azygoesophageal recess

azygogram
azygography
azygos
    a. artery of vagina
    a. continuation (of the inferior vena cava)
    a. fissure
    a. lobe of right lung
    a. vein
azygous

β (*var. of* beta)
B
  boron
    B bile
    B cell
    B cell co-receptor
    B cell differentiating factor
    B cell differentiation/growth factor
    B cell receptor
    B cell stimulatory factor 2
    B chain
    B fiber
    B lymphocyte
    B virus
    B wave
b
  barn
B19 virus
B6 bronchus sign
Ba
  barium
Babbitt metal
Babcock tube
Babesia
    B. *divergens*
    B. *microti*
Babesiella
Babesiidae
babesiosis
  human b.
Babès node
Babinski
    B. phenomenon
    B. reflex
    B. sign
    B. syndrome
baby
  blue b.
  blueberry muffin b.
  b. bottle syndrome
  collodion b.
  test-tube b.
  b. tooth
bacampicillin hydrochloride
baccate
Baccelli sign
bacciform
Bachelor of Dental Science (BDSc)
Bachelor of Dental Surgery (BDS)
Bachelor of Surgery (ChB)
Bachmann bundle
Bachman-Pettit test
Bachman test
Bacillaceae
bacillar
bacillary
    b. angiomatosis
    b. dysentery
    b. layer
bacille Calmette-Guérin (BCG)
bacillemia
bacilliform

bacillin
bacillomyxin
bacillosis
bacilluria
Bacillus
    B. *anthracis*
    B. *anthracis* toxin
    B. *brevis*
    B. *cereus*
    B. *circulans*
    B. *hemolyticus*
    B. *histolyticus*
    B. *megaterium*
    B. *polymyxa*
    B. *pumilis*
    B. *sphaericus*
    B. *subtilis*
    B. *subtilis* ribonuclease
    B. *thuringiensis*
bacillus
  abortus b.
  acid-fast b. (AFB)
  Battey b.
  blue pus b.
  Bordet-Gengou b.
  Calmette-Guérin b.
  b. Calmette-Guérin vaccine
  cholera b.
  coliform b.'s
  colon b.
  comma b.
  Döderlein b.
  Ducrey b.
  dysentery b.
  Eberth b.
  Flexner b.
  Friedländer b.
  gas b.
  grass b.
  Hansen b.
  hay b.
  Hofmann b.
  influenza b.
  Kitasato b.
  Klebs-Loeffler b.
  Koch b.
  Koch-Weeks b.
  lactic acid b.
  leprosy b.
  Loeffler b.
  Moeller grass b.
  Morgan b.
  Much b.
  necrosis b.
  paracolon b.
  paradysentery b.
  paratyphoid b.
  plague b.
  Shiga b.
  Shiga-Kruse b.
  tubercle b.
  typhoid b.

B

bacillus *(continued)*
  Vincent b.
  Weeks b.
  Welch b.
  Whitmore b.
bacitracin
back
  adolescent round b.
  b. cross
  b. of foot reflex
  hollow b.
  b. mutation
  poker b.
  b. pressure
  saddle b.
  b. table procedure
  b. tooth
  b. vertex power
backache
back-action plugger
backboard splint
backbone
backcross
backflow
  pyelovenous b.
background
  b. level
  b. radiation
backing
back-knee
backprojection
backscatter
backtracking
backward
  b. curvature
  b. heart failure
backwash ileitis
baclofen
Bacon anoscope
bacteremia
bacteria
  blue-green b.
  cell wall–defective b.
  coryneform b.
bacterial
  b. allergy
  b. antagonism
  b. capsule
  b. cast
  b. cystitis
  b. encephalitis
  b. endarteritis
  b. endocarditis
  b. food poisoning
  b. growth
  b. hemolysin
  b. interference
  b. peliosis
  b. pericarditis
  b. photosynthesis
  b. plaque
  b. pneumonia
  b. toxin
  b. translocation

  b. vaginosis
  b. vegetations
  b. virus
bactericholia
bactericidal
bactericide
  specific b.
bacterid
bacteriemia
bacterioagglutinin
bacteriochlorin
bacteriochlorophyll
bacteriocidal
bacteriocide
bacteriocidin
bacteriocin
bacteriocin factor
bacteriocinogen
bacteriocinogenic plasmid
bacteriofluorescin
bacteriogenic agglutination
bacteriogenous
bacterioid
bacteriologic
bacteriological
bacteriologist
bacteriology
  systematic b.
bacteriolysin
bacteriolysis
bacteriolytic serum
bacteriolyze
bacteriopexy
bacteriophage
  defective b.
  filamentous b.
  b. immunity
  mature b.
  b. plaque
  b. resistance
  temperate b.
  typhoid b.
  b. typing
  vegetative b.
  virulent b.
bacteriophagia
bacteriophagology
bacteriopheophorbin
bacteriophytoma
bacterioprotein
bacteriopsonin
bacteriosis
bacteriospermia
bacteriostasis
bacteriostat
bacteriostatic agent
bacteriotoxic
bacteriotropic substance
bacteriotropin
bacteriotrypsin
Bacterium
bacterium
  blue-green b.
  endoteric b.
  exoteric b.

lysogenic b.
pyogenic b.
bacteriuria
bacteroid
Bacteroidaceae
Bacteroides
    B. *bivius*
    B. *capillosus*
    B. *corrodens*
    B. *disiens*
    B. *distasonis*
    B. *fragilis*
    B. *furcosus*
    B. *melaninogenicus*
    B. *nodosus*
    B. *oralis*
    B. *oris*
    B. *pneumosintes*
    B. *praeacutus*
    B. *putredinis*
    B. *splanchnicus*
    B. *thetaiotamicron*
    B. *ureolyticus*
bacteroidosis
baculiform
Baculoviridae
baculovirus
Baehr-Lohlein lesion
Baelz disease
BAER
    brainstem auditory evoked response
Baer law
Baermann concentration
Baeyer theory
bag
    Ambu b.
    breathing b.
    colostomy b.
    Douglas b.
    nuclear b.
    Politzer b.
    reservoir b.
    b. ventilation
    b. of waters
bagassosis
Bagdad boil
Baggenstoss change
Bagolini test
Baillarger
    B. band
    B. line
Bailliart ophthalmodynamometer
Bainbridge reflex
baked tongue
Baker
    B. acid hematein
    B. cyst
    B. pyridine extraction
baker
    b.'s eczema
    b.'s itch
baking soda
BAL
    British anti-Lewisite
    bronchoalveolar lavage

Balamuth aqueous egg yolk infusion medium
Balamuthia
balance
    acid-base b.
    nitrogen b.
    occlusal b.
    phonetic b.
    b. theory
    Wilhelmy b.
balanced
    b. anesthesia
    b. articulation
    b. bite
    b. diet
    b. occlusion
    b. polymorphism
    b. translocation
balancing
    b. contact
    b. occlusal surface
    b. side
    b. side condyle
balanic hypospadias
Balanites aegyptiaca
balanitic epispadias
balanitis
    b. circumscripta plasmacellularis
    b. diabetica
    plasma cell b.
    b. xerotica obliterans
balanoplasty
balanoposthitis
balantidial dysentery
balantidiasis
Balantidium
    B. *coli*
    B. *suis*
balantidosis
balanus
Balbani ring
baldness
    common b.
    congenital b.
    male pattern b.
bald tongue
Balint syndrome
Balkan
    B. beam
    B. frame
    B. nephropathy
    B. splint
ball
    chondrin b.
    food b.
    b. of the foot
    fungus b.
    B. operation
    b. and socket abutment
    b. and socket joint
    b. thrombus
    b. valve
    b. valve action
    b. variance
Ballance sign

B

ballerina-foot pattern
ballism
ballismus
ballistocardiogram
ballistocardiograph
ballistocardiography
ballistophobia
balloon
    angioplasty b.
    b. atrioseptostomy
    b. catheter
    b. cell
    b. cell nevus
    b. counter pulsation
    detachable b.
    intraaortic b.
    b. septostomy
    b. sickness
ballooning degeneration
balloon-tip catheter
ballottable
ballottement
    abdominal b.
    renal b.
ballpoint pen technique
ball-valve thrombus
balm
    b. of Gilead
    mountain b.
    sweet b.
balneotherapeutics, balneotherapy
Baló disease
balsam
    Canada b.
    b. of copaiba
    Mecca b.
    b. of Peru
    Tolu b.
balsamic
BALT
    bronchus-associated lymphoid tissue
Baltic myoclonus disease
Bamberger
    B. albuminuria
    B. disease
    B. sign
Bamberger-Marie
    B.-M. disease
    B.-M. syndrome
Bamberger-Pins-Ewart sign
bamboo
    b. hair
    b. spine
bamifylline hydrochloride
bamipine
banana sign
bancroftian filariasis
bancroftiasis
bancroftosis
band
    A b.
    absorption b.
    amnionic b.
    anogenital b.
    anular b.

    atrioventricular b.
    Baillarger b.
    Bechterew b.
    Broca diagonal b.
    b. cell
    b. centrifugation
    chromosome b.
    Clado b.
    b. of colon
    contraction b.
    diagonal b.
    Essick cell b.
    Gennari b.
    b. of Giacomini
    H b.
    His b.
    Hunter-Schreger b.
    I b.
    iliotibial b.
    b. of Kaes-Bechterew
    Ladd b.
    Lane b.
    longitudinal b.'s of cruciform
      ligament of atlas
    M b.
    Mach b.
    Maissiat b.
    matrix b.
    Meckel b.
    moderator b.
    Muehrcke b.
    b. neutrophil
    oligoclonal b.
    orthodontic b.
    pecten b.
    Q b.'s
    Reil b.
    silastic b.
    Simonart b.
    Soret b.
    uncus b. of Giacomini
    ventricular b. of larynx
    Z b.
    zonular b.
bandage
    adhesive b.
    Barton b.
    capeline b.
    circular b.
    b. contact lens
    cravat b.
    crucial b.
    demigauntlet b.
    Desault b.
    elastic b.
    Esmarch b.
    figure-of-8 b.
    four-tailed b.
    gauntlet b.
    gauze b.
    Gibney fixation b.
    Gibson b.
    hammock b.
    immovable b.
    Martin b.

B

oblique b.
plaster b.
roller b.
scarf b.
Scultetus b.
spica b.
spiral b.
suspensory b.
T-b.
triangular b.
Velpeau b.
bandbox resonance
banding
BrDu-b.
high-resolution b.
NOR-b.
prometaphase b.
pulmonary artery b.
reverse b.
bandpass filter
band-shaped keratopathy
bandwidth
bandy-leg
bane
Bang disease
banisterine
Bankart lesion
Bannwarth syndrome
Banti
B. disease
B. syndrome
baptitoxine
bar
arch b.
b. of bladder
clasp b.
b. clasp
b. clasp arm
b. clip attachments
connector b.
b. joint denture
labial b.
lingual b.
median b. of Mercier
Mercier b.
occlusal rest b.
palatal b.
Passavant b.
sternal b.
terminal b.
baragnosis
Bárány
B. caloric test
B. sign
barba
barbaloin
barbed broach
barber
b.'s itch
b.'s pilonidal sinus
barbiero
barbital
barbiturate
barbituric acid

barbiturism
barbotage
barbula hirci
Barclay-Baron disease
Barcoo vomit
Barcroft-Warburg
B.-W. apparatus
B.-W. technique
Bardet-Biedl syndrome
Bardinet ligament
bare
b. area of liver
b. area of stomach
b. lymphocyte syndrome
baresthesia
baresthesiometer
bariatric
bariatrics
baric
baricity
barilla
baritosis
barium (Ba)
b. chloride
b. enema
b. hydroxide
b. meal
b. monoxide
b. oxide
b. sulfate
b. sulfide
b. swallow
bark
cinchona b.
cotton-root b.
Peruvian b.
Barkan
B. membrane
B. operation
Barkman reflex
Barkow ligament
Barlow
B. disease
B. maneuver
B. syndrome
B. test
Barmah Forest virus
barn (b)
Barnes
B. curve
B. zone
baroceptor
barognosis
barograph
barometric pressure (P_B)
barometrograph
barophilic
baroreceptor nerve
baroreflex
baroscope
barosinusitis
barostat
barotaxis
barotitis media

barotrauma
    otic b.
    sinus b.
barotropism
Barraquer
    B. disease
    B. method
Barr chromatin body
barrel
    b. chest
    b. distortion
barrel-shaped thorax
barren
Barré sign
Barrett
    B. epithelium
    B. esophagus
    B. metaplasia
    B. syndrome
barrier
    blood-air b.
    blood-aqueous b.
    blood-brain b. (BBB)
    blood-cerebrospinal fluid b.
    blood-CSF b.
    blood-testis b.
    blood-thymus b.
    b. contraceptive
    incest b.
    placental b.
bar-sleeve attachments
Barth
    B. hernia
    B. syndrome
Bartholin
    B. abscess
    B. anus
    B. cyst
    B. cystectomy
    B. duct
    B. gland
bartholinitis
Barton
    B. bandage
    B. forceps
    B. fracture
Bartonella
    B. anemia
    B. bacilliformis
    B. henselae
    B. quintana
Bartonellaceae
bartonellosis
Bart syndrome
Bartter syndrome
Baruch law
baruria
barye
baryta water
basad
basal
    b. age
    b. anesthesia
    b. body
    b. body temperature

    b. bone
    b. cell
    b. cell adenoma
    b. cell epithelioma
    b. cell hyperplasia
    b. cell layer
    b. cell nevus
    b. cell nevus syndrome
    b. cell papilloma
    b. cistern
    b. corpuscle
    b. crest of cochlear duct
    b. diet
    b. encephalocele
    b. ganglion
    b. gland
    b. granule
    b. joint reflex
    b. lamina
    b. lamina of choroid
    b. lamina of ciliary body
    b. lamina of cochlear duct
    b. lamina of neural tube
    b. laminar drusen
    b. lamina of semicircular duct
    b. layer of choroid
    b. layer of ciliary body
    b. linear drusen
    b. membrane of semicircular duct
    b. metabolic rate (BMR)
    b. metabolism
    b. nuclei
    b. nucleus of Ganser
    b. part
    b. part of left and right inferior pulmonary artery
    b. part of occipital bone
    b. plate of neural tube
    b. ridge
    b. rod
    b. seat
    b. seat area
    b. skull fracture
    b. sphincter
    b. squamous cell carcinoma
    b. striation
    b. substantia
    b. surface
    b. tentorial branch of internal carotid artery
    b. tuberculosis
    b. vein
    b. vein of Rosenthal
basalis
basaloid
    b. carcinoma
    b. cell
basal ration
base
    acrylic resin b.
    anterior cranial b.
    b. of arytenoid cartilage
    b. of bladder
    b. of brain
    Brønsted b.

cavity preparation b.
cement b.
b. of cochlea
b. composition
cranial b.
b. deficit
denture b.
dissociation constant of a b. (K_b)
b. excess
external b. of skull
b. of heart
hexone b.
histone b.
b. hospital
b. of hyoid bone
b. increase at low levels
internal b. of skull
Lewis b.
b. line
b. of lung
b. of mandible
b. material
b. of metacarpal
b. metal
metal b.
b. of metatarsal
methamphetamine b.
b. of modiolus of cochlea
nucleic acid b.
ointment b.
b. pair
b. of patella
b. of phalanx
b. of phalanx of foot
b. of phalanx of hand
b. plate
pressor b.
b. projection
b. of prostate
purine b.
pyrimidine b.
record b.
b. of renal pyramid
b. of sacrum
Schiff b.
shellac b.
b. of skull
b. of stapes
temporary b.
tinted denture b.
b. of tongue
tooth-borne b.
trial b.
b. units
vegetable b.
b. view
wobble b.
baseball finger
basedoid
Basedow
B. disease
B. goiter
B. pseudoparaplegia
basedowian

baseline
Reid b.
b. tonus
b. variability of fetal heart rate
basement
b. lamina
b. membrane
baseplate
stabilized b.
b. wax
base-stacking
bas-fond
Basham mixture
basialis
basialveolar
basibregmatic axis
basic
b. amino acid
basic metal
b. diet
b. dye
b. electrical rhythm (BER)
b. esotropia
b. exotropia
b. fuchsin
b. fuchsin-methylene blue stain
b. life support
b. oxide
b. personality
b. personality type
b. protein
b. reaction
b. salt
basicity
basicranial
b. axis
b. flexure
basicranium
basidia (*pl. of* basidium)
Basidiobolus
Basidiomycetes
Basidiomycota
basidiospore
basidium, pl. **basidia**
basifacial axis
basihyal
basihyoid
basilar, basilaris
b. angle
b. apophysis
b. artery
b. bone
b. cartilage
b. cell
b. crest of cochlear duct
b. fibrocartilage
b. impression
b. index
b. invagination
b. lamina
b. leptomeningitis
b. membrane of cochlear duct
b. meningitis
b. migraine
b. papilla

basilar *(continued)*
    b. part
    b. part of occipital bone
    b. part of pons
    b. pontine sulcus
    b. process
    b. process of occipital bone
    b. prognathism
    b. sinus
    b. sulcus
    b. venous plexus
    b. vertebra
basilateral
basilemma
basilicus
basilic vein
basin
    emesis b.
    kidney b.
    pus b.
basinasal line
basioccipital bone
basiocciput
basioglossus
basion
basipetal
basipharyngeal canal
basiphobia
basis
    b. cartilaginis arytenoideae
    b. cerebri
    b. cochleae
    b. cordis
    b. cranii
    b. cranii externa
    b. cranii interna
    b. mandibulae
    b. modioli cochleae
    b. ossis metacarpalis
    b. ossis metatarsalis
    b. ossis sacri
    b. patellae
    b. pedunculi
    b. phalangis
    b. phalangis manus
    b. phalangis pedis
    b. pontis
    b. prostatae
    b. pulmonis
    b. pyramidis renis
    b. stapedis
basisphenoid bone
basisquamous carcinoma
basitemporal
basivertebral vein
basket
    b. cell
    fibrillar b.
    b. nucleus
    Stokes b.
    stone b.
Basle Nomina Anatomica (BNA)
basocyte
basocytopenia

basocytosis
basoerythrocyte
basoerythrocytosis
basolateral amygdaloid nucleus
basomedial amygdaloid nucleus
basometachromophil,
    basometachromophile
basopenia
basophil, basophile
    b. adenoma
    b. cell of anterior lobe of
      hypophysis
    b. granule
    b. substance
    tissue b.
basophilia
    Grawitz b.
    punctate b.
basophilic
    b. degeneration
    b. leukemia
    b. leukocyte
    b. leukocytosis
    b. leukopenia
    b. substance
basophilism
    Cushing pituitary b.
basoplasm
basosquamous carcinoma
Bassen-Kornzweig syndrome
Bassini
    B. herniorrhaphy
    B. operation
Bassler sign
Bassora gum
bassorin
Bastedo sign
bastokinin
bat
    b. ear
    vampire b.
batch
    b. analyzer
    b. culture
bath
    colloid b.
    contrast b.
    douche b.
    dousing b.
    electric b.
    electrotherapeutic b.
    Greville b.
    hafussi b.
    hydroelectric b.
    immersion b.
    b. itch
    light b.
    Nauheim b.
    needle b.
    oil b.
    b. pruritus
    sand b.
    sitz b.
    water b.
bathing trunk nevus

B

bathochromic
bathoflore
bathophobia
bathyanesthesia
bathycardia
bathyesthesia
bathygastry
bathyhyperesthesia
bathyhypesthesia
Batista procedure
batrachotoxin
Batson plexus
Batten disease
Batten-Mayou disease
battered
    b. child syndrome
    b. spouse syndrome
battery
    Halstead-Reitan b.
Battey bacillus
Battista operation
battle
    b. fatigue
    B. sign
battledore placenta
Bauer
    B. chromic acid leucofuchsin stain
    B. syndrome
Bauer-Kirby test
Bauhin
    B. gland
    B. valve
Baumé scale
Baumès symptom
Baumgarten
    B. gland
    B. vein
bauxite pneumoconiosis
bay
    celomic b.
    lacrimal b.
bayberry bark
bayesian hypothesis
Bayes theorem
Bayley Scale of Infant Development
baylisascariasis
Baylisascaris
    B. procyonis
bayonet
    b. apposition
    b. forceps
    b. hair
Bayou virus
Bazett formula
Bazex syndrome
Bazin disease
BBB
    blood-brain barrier
BBC
    bromobenzylcyanide
BBOT
    2,5-bis5-t-butylbenzoxazol-2-ylthiophene
BCG
    bacille calmette-guerin
      BCG vaccine

BCL-2
BCNU
    carmustine
bdellin
Bdellovibrio
BDS
    Bachelor of Dental Surgery
BDSc
    Bachelor of Dental Science
Be
    beryllium
beaded hair
beading of the rib
beaked pelvis
beaker cell
beak sign
Beale cell
beam
    Balkan b.
    cantilever b.
    continuous b.
    electron b.
    restrained b.
    simple b.
B-E amputation
bean
Be^a antigen
beard
bearing
    central b.
bearing down
bearing-down pain
beat
    apex b.
    atrial capture b.
    atrial fusion b.
    automatic b.
    combination b.
    coupled b.'s
    dependent b.
    Dressler b.
    dropped b.
    echo b.
    ectopic b.
    escape b.
    forced b.
    fusion b.
    heart b.
    interference b.
    mixed b.
    paired b.'s
    parasystolic b.
    premature b.
    pseudofusion b.
    reciprocal b.
    retrograde b.
    summation b.
    ventricular fusion b.
beat-to-beat variability of fetal heart
rate
Beau line
Beauvaria
becanthone hydrochloride
Bechterew
    B. band

Bechterew *(continued)*
  B. disease
  B. nucleus
  B. sign
Bechterew-Mendel reflex
Beck
  B. method
  B. triad
Becker
  B. antigen
  B. disease
  B. muscular dystrophy
  B. nevus
  B. stain for spirochetes
Becker-type tardive muscular dystrophy
Beckmann apparatus
Beckwith-Wiedemann syndrome
Béclard
  B. anastomosis
  B. hernia
  B. triangle
beclomethasone dipropionate
becquerel (Bq)
  b. ray
bed
  b. of breast
  capillary b.
  fracture b.
  Gatch b.
  mud b.
  nail b.
  parotid b.
  b. of parotid gland
  b. rest
  b. sore
  b. of stomach
  water b.
bedbug
bedlam
Bednar
  B. aphtha
  B. tumor
bedside radiography
bedsore
bedwetting
beech oil
beechwood
  b. sugar
  b. tar
beer
  b. heart
  B. knife
  B. law
Beer-Lambert law
beeswax
  white b.
bee toxin
beet sugar
beeturia
Beevor sign
Begg light wire differential force technique
Béguez César disease

behavior
  adaptive b.
  appetitive b.
  aversive b.
  b. chain
  coronary-prone b.
  b. disorder
  health b.
  hookean b.
  hostile b.
  b. modification
  molar b.
  molecular b.
  obsessive b.
  operant b.
  passive-aggressive b.
  b. reflex
  respondent b.
  ritualistic b.
  target b.
  b. therapy
  type A, B b.
behavioral
  b. epidemic
  b. genetics
  b. health
  b. manifestation
  b. medicine
  b. observation audiometry
  b. pathogen
  b. psychology
  b. science
behaviorism
behaviorist
behavioristic psychology
Behçet
  B. disease
  B. syndrome
behenic acid
behind-the-ear hearing aid
Behr
  B. disease
  B. syndrome
Behring law
BEI
  butanol-extractable iodine
BEI test
bejel
Békésy
  B. audiometer
  B. audiometry
belching
belemnoid
Belgian Congo anemia
bell
  b. clapper deformity
  B. law
  B. muscle
  B. palsy
  B. phenomenon
  B. respiratory nerve
  b. sound
  B. spasm
  b. stage

B

belladonna
- b. extract
- b. tincture

belladonnine
bell-crowned
belle indifférence
Bellini
- B. duct
- B. ligament

Bell-Magendie law
bellmetal resonance
bellows murmur
bell-shaped crown
belly
- anterior b. of digastric muscle
- b. button
- b. of digastric muscle
- frontal b. of occipitofrontalis muscle
- inferior b. of omohyoid b.
- occipital b. of occipitofrontalis muscle
- b. of omohyoid muscle
- posterior b. of digastric muscle
- prune b.
- superior b. of omohyoid muscle

bellyache
belonephobia
Belsey
- B. fundoplication
- B. Mark operation
- B. procedure

belt test
bel unit
bemegride
ben
- bene

benactyzine hydrochloride
Bence Jones
- B. J. albumin
- B. J. myeloma
- B. J. protein
- B. J. proteinuria
- B. J. reaction

Bence Jones cylinder
bench testing
bendazac
Bender
- B. Visual Motor Gestalt test

bending fracture
bendrofluazide
bendroflumethiazide
bends
bene (ben)
- bene (well)

beneceptor
Benedek reflex
Benedict
- B. solution
- B. test for glucose

Benedict-Hopkins-Cole reagent
Benedict-Roth
- B.-R. apparatus
- B.-R. calorimeter

Benedikt syndrome
beneficence

benign
- b. albuminuria
- b. bone aneurysm
- b. cementoblastoma
- b. childhood epilepsy with centrotemporal spike
- b. coital cephalalgia
- b. congenital hypotonia
- b. dry pleurisy
- b. dyskeratosis
- b. essential tremor
- b. exertional headache
- b. familial chorea
- b. familial chronic pemphigus
- b. familial icterus
- b. fructosuria
- b. giant lymph node hyperplasia
- b. glycosuria
- b. hypertension
- b. infantile myoclonus
- b. inoculation lymphoreticulosis
- b. inoculation reticulosis
- b. juvenile melanoma
- b. lymphadenosis
- b. lymphocytoma cutis
- b. lymphoepithelial lesion
- b. lymphoma of the rectum
- b. mesenchymoma
- b. mesothelioma
- b. mesothelioma of genital tract
- b. migratory glossitis
- b. monoclonal gammopathy
- b. mucosal pemphigoid
- b. myalgic encephalomyelitis
- b. myoclonus of infancy
- b. neonatal convulsion
- b. nephrosclerosis
- b. paroxysmal peritonitis
- b. paroxysmal positional vertigo
- b. paroxysmal torticollis of infancy
- b. prostatic hyperplasia
- b. prostatic hypertrophy
- b. rheumatoid nodule
- b. stupor
- b. tertian fever
- b. tertian malaria
- b. tumor

benne oil
Bennett
- B. angle
- B. fracture
- B. movement

Bennhold Congo red stain
benoxaprofen
benperidol
benserazide
Bensley specific granule
bentiromide test
bentonite flocculation test
benzalacetophenone
benzalcoumaran-3-one
benzaldehyde
benzalkonium chloride
benz[a]anthracene
benzanthrene

benzene
    b. bromide
    b. nucleus
    b. ring
benzeneamine
(γ)-benzene hexachloride
benzestrol
benzethonium chloride
benzidine test
benzimidazole
benzin, benzine
benzindamine hydrochloride
benziodarone
benzoate
benzoated
benzocaine
benzodiazepine
benzoic
    benzoic acid
    benzoic aldehyde
benzoin
benzoinated lard
benzol
benzomorphan
benzonatate
benzopurpurin 4B
1,4-benzoquinone
benzoquinonium chloride
benzoresinol
benzosulfimide
benzothiadiazides
benzoxiquine
benzoxyline
benzoyl
    b. chloride
    b. hydrate
    b. peroxide
benzoylecgonine
benzoylpas calcium
benzperidol
benzphetamine hydrochloride
benzpyrene
benzpyrinium bromide
benzquinamide
benzstigminum bromidum
benzthiazide
benztropine mesylate
benzydamine hydrochloride
benzyl
    b. alcohol
    b. benzoate
    b. benzoate-chlorophenothane-ethyl
      aminobenzoate
    b. carbinol
    b. cinnamate
    b. fumarate
    b. mandelate
    b. penicillin
    b. succinate
benzylic
benzylidene
benzylisoquinolines
benzyloxycarbonyl (Z)
benzylpenicillin
bephenium hydroxynaphthoate

BER
    basic electrical rhythm
Beradinelli syndrome
Bérard aneurysm
Berardinelli syndrome
Béraud valve
berberine
bereavement
Berger
    B. cell
    B. disease
    B. focal glomerulonephritis
    B. rhythm
    B. space
Bergmann
    B. cord
    B. fiber
Bergman sign
Bergmeister papilla
Berg stain
beriberi, beri beri
    dry b.
    b. heart
    infantile b.
    ship b.
    wet b.
Berkefeld filter
berkelium (Bk)
Berlin
    B. blue
    B. edema
berloque dermatitis
Bernard
    B. canal
    B. duct
    B. puncture
Bernard-Cannon homeostasis
Bernard-Horner syndrome
Bernard-Sergent syndrome
Bernard-Soulier
    B.-S. disease
    B.-S. syndrome
Bernays sponge
Bernhardt
    B. disease
    B. formula
Bernhardt-Roth syndrome
Bernheim syndrome
Bernoulli
    B. distribution
    B. effect
    B. law
    B. principle
    B. theorem
    B. trial
Bernstein test
berry
    b. aneurysm
    b. cell
    B. ligament
Berson test
Berthelot reaction
Berthollet law
Bertiella studeri
bertiellosis

Bertin
- B. bone
- B. column
- B. ligament
- B. ossicle

berylliosis
beryllium (Be)
- b. granuloma

Besnier-Boeck-Schaumann
- B.-B.-S. disease
- B.-B.-S. syndrome

Besnier prurigo
Besnoitiidae
best
- B. carmine stain
- B. disease
- b. frequency

bestiality
besylate
beta, β
- b. angle
- b. blocker
- b. cell of anterior lobe of hypophysis
- b. cell of pancreas
- b. corynebacteriophage
- b. error
- b. fiber
- b. granule
- b. hemolysin
- b. hemolysis
- b. particle
- b. phage
- b. radiation
- b. ray
- b. rhythm
- b. sheet
- B. test
- b. thalassemia
- b. wave

beta-adrenergic
- -a. receptor
- -a. receptor blocking agent

beta-adrenoreceptor antagonist
beta-allocortol
beta-allocortolone
beta-allopregnanediol
beta-aminoisobutyric acid
beta-amylase
beta-aspartyl(acetylglucosamine)
beta,beta-dimethylcysteine
beta-carotene-cleavage enzyme
beta-carotene 15,15'-dioxygenase
beta-chlorovinyldichloroarsine
betacism
beta-cortol
beta-cortolone
betacyanin
betacyaninuria
beta-cystathionase
beta-farnesene
beta-fructofuranosidase
beta-D-galactosidase
beta-galactosylceramidase
beta-glucocerebrosidase

beta-D-glucosidase
beta-D-glucuronidase
beta-*d*-glucuronidase deficiency
beta-HCG
beta-hemolytic streptococci
Betaherpesvirinae
betahistine hydrochloride
beta-human chorionic gonadotropin
beta-hydroxy-beta-methylglutaryl-CoA (HMG-CoA)
beta-hydroxybutyric acid
beta-hydroxyisobutyric acid
beta-hydroxypropionic acid
beta-hydroxypropionic aciduria
3beta-hydroxysteroid sulfatase
betaine
- b. aldehyde
- b. hydrochloride

betaine-aldehyde dehydrogenase
beta-ketoacyl-ACP reductase
beta-ketoacyl-ACP synthase
beta-ketohydrogenase
beta-ketoreductase
beta-ketothiolase
beta-lactam
beta-lactamase
beta-lactamase inhibitors
betalain
beta-mercaptoethanol
betamethasone
betanidine sulfate
betanin
beta-oxidation-condensation theory
beta⁺ positron
beta-T
beta-thionase
beta-tocopherol
betatron
beta-tyrosinase
betaxolol hydrochloride
betazole hydrochloride
betel
- betel nut
- b. cancer

bethanechol chloride
bethanidine sulfate
Bethesda
- B. classification
- B. system
- B. unit

Bethesda-Ballerup Group
Betke-Kleihauer test
Bettendorff test
betula
- b. oil

Betz cell
Beuren syndrome
Bevan-Lewis cell
bevel
- cavosurface b.
- reverse b.

bevelled anastomosis
bevonium methyl sulfate
bezoar

Bezold
>B. abscess
>B. ganglion

Bezold-Jarisch reflex

B$_T$ factor

BGP
>bone gla protein

BHA
>butylated hydroxyanisole

bhang

BH interval

BHN
>Brinell hardness number

BHT
>butylated hydroxytoluene

bi
>B. antigen
>b. bi reaction

Bial test

Bianchi nodule

biarticular

bias
>ascertainment b.
>cross-level b.
>recall b.
>reporting b.
>response b.
>sampling b.

biasterionic

biauricular axis

biaxial joint

bib.
>bibe

bibe (bib.)
>b. (drink)

bibliomania

bibulous

bicameral abscess

bicanalicular sphincter

BICAP cautery

bicapsular

bicarbonate
>standard b.

bicardiogram

bicellular

bicephalus

biceps
>b. brachii muscle
>b. femoris muscle
>b. femoris reflex
>b. muscle of arm
>b. muscle of thigh

Bichat
>B. canal
>B. fat-pad
>B. fissure
>B. fossa
>B. ligament
>B. membrane
>B. protuberance
>B. tunic

bicho

biciliate

bicipital
>b. aponeurosis

>b. fascia
>b. groove
>b. rib
>b. ridge
>b. tuberosity

bicipitoradial bursa

Bickel ring

biclonal
>b. gammopathy
>b. peak

biclonality

biconcave lens

bicondylar
>b. articulation
>b. joint

biconvex lens

bicornous, bicornate, bicornuate
>b. uterus

bicoudate catheter

bicron

bicuculline

bicuspid
>b. aortic valve
>b. tooth
>b. valve

bicuspidization

b.i.d.
>bis in die

bidactyly

bidet

bidirectional
>b. replication
>b. ventricular tachycardia

bidiscoidal placenta

BIDS
>brittle hair, impaired intellect, decreased
>fertility, short stature

biduous

Biebl loop

Biebrich scarlet red

Biederman sign

Bielschowsky
>B. disease
>B. sign
>B. stain

Biemond syndrome

Bier
>B. amputation
>B. hyperemia
>B. method

Biermer
>B. anemia
>B. disease

Biesiadecki fossa

bifascicular

bifid
>bifid cranium
>b. epiglottis
>b. penis
>b. rib
>b. thumb
>b. tongue
>b. uterus
>b. uvula

Bifidobacterium
    B. bifidum
    B. dentium
bifidus factor
bifocal
    b. lens
    b. spectacles
biforate uterus
bifoveal fixation
bifunctional
bifurcated ligament
bifurcate ligament
bifurcatio
    b. aortae
    b. tracheae
    b. trunci pulmonalis
bifurcation
    b. of aorta
    aortic b.
    b. lymph node
    b. of pulmonary trunk
    b. of trachea
    tracheal b.
big ACTH
Bigelow
    B. ligament
    B. septum
bigemina
bigeminal
    b. body
    b. pulse
    b. rhythm
bigemini
bigeminum
bigeminy
    atrial b.
    atrioventricular junctional b.
    escape-capture b.
    nodal b.
    reciprocal b.
    ventricular b.
bigerminal
bigitalin
biglycan
bikunin
bilabe
bilaminar blastoderm
bilateral
    b. hermaphroditism
    b. left-sidedness
    b. medial orbital ecchymosis
    b. pleurisy
    b. synchrony
bilateralism
bile
    A b.
    b. acid
    b. acid tolerance test
    b. alcohol
    B. antigen
    B b.
    C b.
    b. capillary
    b. cyst
    b. duct

    b. esculin test
    b. gastritis
    b. papilla
    b. peritonitis
    b. pigment
    b. pigment hemoglobin
    b. salt
    b. salt agar
    b. solubility test
    b. thrombus
    white b.
bileaflet valve
Bilharzia
bilharzial
    b. appendicitis
    b. dysentery
    b. granuloma
bilharziasis
bilharzioma
bilharziosis
biliaropancreatic ampulla
biliary
    b. atresia
    b. calculus
    b. canaliculus
    b. cirrhosis
    b. colic
    b. duct
    b. ductule
    b. dyskinesia
    b. fistula
    b. gland
    b. steatorrhea
    b. xanthomatosis
bilifaction
biliferous
bilification
biligenesis
biligenic
bilin, biline
bilious
    b. headache
    b. pneumonia
    b. remittent fever
    b. remittent malaria
    b. typhoid of Griesinger
    b. vomit
biliousness
bilirachia
bilirubin
    conjugated b.
    delta b.
    direct reacting b.
    b. encephalopathy
    indirect reacting b.
    b. UDPglucuronyltransferase
    unconjugated b.
bilirubinemia
bilirubinglobulin
bilirubin-glucuronoside
    glucuronosyltransferase
bilirubinoids
bilirubinuria
bilitherapy
biliuria

B

biliverdin, biliverdine
Billings method
billion
    parts per b. (ppb)
Bill maneuver
billowing mitral valve syndrome
Billroth
    B. cord
    B. I, II anastomosis
    B. I, II operation
    B. venae cavernosae
bilobate, bilobed
bilobectomy
bilobular
bilocular, biloculate
    b. femoral hernia
    b. joint
    b. stomach
bimalleolar fracture
bimanual
    b. palpation
    b. percussion
    b. version
bimastoid
bimaxillary
    b. dentoalveolar protrusion
    b. protrusion
    b. protrusive occlusion
bimodal
bimolecular
binangle chisel
binary
    b. combination
    b. complex
    b. digit
    b. fission
    b. nomenclature
    b. process
binasal hemianopia
binaural
    b. alternate loudness balance test
    b. stethoscope
bind
    double b.
binder
    obstetric b.
    T-b.
binding
    b. constant
    b. energy
Binet
    B. age
    B. scale
    B. test
Binet-Simon scale
Bingham
    B. flow
    B. model
    B. plastic
Bing reflex
binocular
    b. fixation
    b. heterochromia
    b. loupe
    b. microscope

    b. ophthalmoscope
    b. parallax
    b. rivalry
    b. vision
binomial distribution
binomial nomenclature (*var. of* binary nomenclature)
binotic
Binswanger
    B. disease
    B. encephalopathy
binuclear
binucleate
binucleolate
bioacoustics
bioactive
bioassay
bioastronautics
bioavailability
bioburden
biocatalyst
biocenosis
biochemical
    b. genetics
    b. metastasis
    b. modulation
    b. oxygen demand (BOD)
    b. pathway
    b. pharmacology
    b. profile
biochemistry
biochemorphic
biochrome
biocidal
bioclimatology
biocompatibility
biocybernetics
biocytin
biocytinase
biodegradable
biodegradation
biodynamic
biodynamics
bioecology
bioelectric potential
bioelement
bioenergetics
bioengineering
biofeedback
    EMG b.
bioflavonoids
biogenesis
    mitochondrial b.
biogenetic law
biogenic amine
biogeochemistry
biogravics
bioinformatics
bioinstrument
biokinetics
biologic, biological
    b. assay
    b. chemistry
    b. coefficient
    b. control

B

b. evolution
b. half-life
b. hemolysis
b. immunotherapy
b. psychiatry
b. response modifier
b. sampling
b. standard unit
b. time
b. valve
b. vector
biologist
biology
cellular b.
molecular b.
oral b.
pharmaceutical b.
radiation b.
bioluminescence
biolysis
biolytic
biomacromolecule
biomass
biomaterial
biome
biomechanics
dental b.
biomedical
b. engineering
b. model
biomembrane
biometer
biometrical school
biometrician
biometry fetal
biomicroscope
biomicroscopy
Biomphalaria
bion
Biondi-Heidenhain stain
bionecrosis
bionic
bionics
bionomics
bionomy
biophage
biophagism
biophagous
biophagy
biopharmaceutics
biophylactic
biophylaxis
biophysical profile
biophysics
cellular b.
dental b.
medical b.
molecular b.
radiation b.
bioplasm
bioplasmic
biopolymer
aperiodic b.
periodic b.

biopsy
aspiration b.
brush b.
chorionic villus b.
endoscopic b.
excision b.
fine needle b.
fine needle aspiration b. (FNA)
incision b.
needle b.
b. needle
open b.
punch b.
sentinal node b.
shave b.
sponge b.
trephine b.
wedge b.
biopsychology
biopsychosocial model
biopterin
bioptome
biorbital angle
biorheology
biorhythm
biosafety
biosis
biosocial
biospectrometry
biospectroscopy
biospeleology
biosphere
biostatics
biostatistics
biosynthesis
biosynthetic
biosystem
Biot
B. breathing
B. breathing sign
B. respiration
biota
biotaxis
biotechnology
biotelemetry
biotest
biotic
b. community
b. factor
b. potential
biotics
biotin
b. carboxylase
b. oxidase
biotinidase deficiency
biotinides
biotinyllysine
biotope
biotoxicology
biotoxin
biotransformation
biotype
biovar
biovular
bipalatinoid

biparasitism
biparental
biparietal diameter
biparous
bipartite
    b. uterus
    b. vagina
biped
bipedal
bipedicle flap
bipennate, bipenniform
    b. muscle
biperforate
biperiden
biphasic
    b. insulin
    b. response
biphenamine hydrochloride
biphenotypic
biphenotypy
biphenyl
    polychlorinated b. (PCB)
biplane angiography
bipolar
    b. cautery
    b. cell
    b. disorder
    b. lead
    b. neuron
    b. psychosis
    b. version
Bipolaris
    B. australiensis
    B. hawaiiensis
    B. spicifera
bipotentiality
biramous
Birbeck granule
birch
    b. tar
    b. tar oil
Birch-Hirschfeld stain
bird
    b. face
    b. shot retinochoroiditis
    B. sign
    b. unit
bird-breeder's
    b.-b. disease
    b.-b. lung
birdseed agar
bird's nest filter
birefringence
birefringent
Birnaviridae
Birnavirus
birotation
birth
    b. canal
    b. certificate
    b. control
    b. defect
    b. fracture

    b. palsy
    premature b.
    b. rate
    b. trauma
    b. weight
birthing center
birthmark
    strawberry b.
bisacodyl
bisacromial
bisalbuminemia
bisaxillary
bisbenzylisoquinoline alkaloids
2,5-bis(5-*t*-butylbenzoxazol-2-yl)thiophene
    (BBOT)
Bischof myelotomy
biscuit-bake
biscuit bite
biscuit-firing
bisdequalinium chloride
bis in die (b.i.d.)
bisexual
bisferient
bisferious pulse
Bishop
    B. score
    B. sphygmoscope
bishydroxycoumarin
bisiliac
Biskra
    B. boil
    B. button
Bismarck
    B. brown R
    B. brown Y
bismuth
    b. aluminate
    b. ammonium citrate
    b. carbonate
    b. chloride oxide
    b. citrate
    b. hydroxide
    b. iodide
    b. line
    b. oxide
    b. oxycarbonate
    b. oxychloride
    b. oxynitrate
    b. salicylate
    b. sodium tartrate
    b. sodium triglycollamate
    b. subcarbonate
    b. subgallate
    b. subnitrate
    b. subsalicylate
    b. tribromophenate
    b. tribromophenol
    b. trichloride
    b. triiodide
bismuthosis
bismuthyl
    b. carbonate
    b. chloride

B

bisoxatin acetate
1,4-bis(5-phenyloxazol-2-yl)benzene
 (POPOP)
1,3-bisphosphoglycerate (1,3-P₂Gri)
2,3-bisphosphoglycerate (2,3-P₂Gri)
    2,3-b. mutase
bisphosphonates
bistephanic
bisteroid
bistoury
bistratal
bisulfate
bisulfide
bisulfite
bit
bitartrate
bitch
bite
    b. analysis
    balanced b.
    biscuit b.
    close b.
    closed b.
    deep b.
    edge-to-edge b.
    end-to-end b.
    b. fork
    b. gauge
    jumping the b.
    locked b.
    normal b.
    open b.
    b. plane
    rest b.
    b. rim
    working b.
bitemporal hemianopia
biteplate, biteplane
bitewing
    b. film
    b. radiograph
bithermal caloric test
bithionol
biting
    b. louse
    b. pressure
    b. strength
bitolterol mesylate
Bitot spot
bitrochanteric
bitropic
bitter
    b. almond oil
    b. apple
    aromatic b.'s
    b. orange peel
    b. orange peel, dried
    b. orange peel, fresh
    b. orange peel oil
    b. peptide
    b. principle
    b. tonic
    b. water
Bittner
    B. agent

B. milk factor
B. virus
Bittorf reaction
biundulant meningoencephalitis
biuret
    b. reaction
    b. reagent
    b. test
bivalence, bivalency
bivalent
    b. antibody
    b. chromosome
    b. gas gangrene antitoxin
bivalve speculum
biventer
    b. cervicis
    b. lobule
    b. mandibulae
biventral lobule
biventricular
bixin
Bixler type hypertelorism
bizygomatic
Bizzozero
    B. corpuscle
    B. red cell
Bjerrum
    B. scotoma
    B. screen
    B. sign
Björk-Shiley valve
Björnstad syndrome
Bk
    berkelium
B-K amputation
BK virus
black
    bone b.
    b. box
    b. cataract
    B. classification
    B. Creek Canal virus
    b. currant rash
    b. death
    b. eye
    b. fever
    B. formula
    b. hairy tongue
    b. heel
    b. imported fire ant
    b. lead
    b. line
    b. lung
    b. measles
    b. mustard
    b. piedra
    b. plague
    b. root
    b. sickness
    b. spore
    b. tarantula
    b. tongue
    b. urine
    b. vomit
black-dot ringworm

blackout
    visual b.
blackwater fever
bladder
    air b.
    allantoic b.
    atonic b.
    autonomic neurogenic b.
    b. calculus
    b. compliance
    b. ear
    gall b.
    hyperreflexic b.
    hypertonic b.
    ileal b.
    kidneys, ureters, b. (KUB)
    neurogenic b.
    neuropathic b.
    nonneurogenic neurogenic b.
    poorly compliant b.
    pseudoneurogenic b.
    b. reflex
    reflex neurogenic b.
    b. schistosomiasis
    b. stone
    swim b.
    trabeculated b.
    uninhibited neurogenic b.
    unstable b.
    urinary b.
bladderworm
blade bone
bladevent
Blagden law
Blainville ear
Blalock-Hanlon operation
Blalock shunt
Blalock-Taussig
    B.-T. operation
    B.-T. shunt
bland
    b. diet
    b. embolism
    b. infarct
Blandin gland
blank
blanket
    mucus b.
    b. suture
blas
Blasius duct
blast
    b. cell
    b. crisis
    b. injury
blastema
    metanephric b.
    nephric b.
blastemic
blastic
blastocele
blastocelic
blastocoele
blastocoelic
Blastoconidium

blastocyst
Blastocystis
    B. hominis
blastocyte
blastoderm
    bilaminar b.
    embryonic b.
    extraembryonic b.
    trilaminar b.
blastoderma
blastodermic, blastodermal
    b. disk
    b. layer
    b. vesicle
blastodisk
blastogenesis
blastogenetic, blastogenic
blastolysis
blastolytic
blastoma
blastomere
blastomerotomy
blastomogenic
Blastomyces dermatitidis
blastomycetic dermatitis
blastomycin
blastomycosis
    Brazilian b.
    cutaneous b.
    North American b.
    South American b.
    systemic b.
blastoneuropore
blastophore
blastopore
blastoporic canal
Blastoschizomyces
    B. capitatus
blastospore
blastotomy
blastula
blastular
blastulation
Blatin syndrome
Blatta
Blattella
Blattidae
bleached wax
bleaching powder
blear eye
bleary eye
bleb
    filtering b.
    pulmonary b.
bleed
bleeder
bleeding
    dysfunctional uterine b.
    occult b.
    b. polyp
    b. time
blemish
blending inheritance
blennadenitis
blennemesis

blennogenic
blennogenous
blennoid
blennophthalmia
blennorrhagic
blennorrhea
 b. conjunctivalis
 inclusion b.
 b. neonatorum
blennorrheal
blennostasis
blennostatic
blennuria
bleomycin sulfate
blepharadenitis
blepharal
blepharectomy
blepharedema
blepharitis
 b. acarica
 b. angularis
 ciliary b.
 demodectic b.
 b. follicularis
 marginal b.
 b. marginalis
 meibomian b.
 b. parasitica
 pediculous b.
 b. phthiriatica
 posterior b.
 pustular b.
 b. rosacea
 seborrheic b.
 b. sicca
 staphylococcal b.
 b. ulcerosa
blepharoadenitis
blepharoadenoma
blepharochalasis
blepharoclonus
blepharocoloboma
blepharoconjunctivitis
blepharodiastasis
blepharokeratoconjunctivitis
blepharon
blepharophimosis
blepharoplast
blepharoplastic
blepharoplasty
blepharoplegia
blepharoptosis, blepharoptosia
 b. adiposa
 false b.
blepharospasm, blepharospasmus
blepharostat
blepharostenosis
blepharosynechia
blepharotomy
blighted ovum
blind
 b. boil
 b. enema
 b. fistula
 b. foramen of frontal bone

 b. foramen of the tongue
 b. gut
 b. headache
 b. loop syndrome
 b. nasotracheal intubation
 b. passage
 b. spot
 b. study
 b. test
blinding
 b. disease
 b. glare
blindness
 change b.
 color b.
 cortical b.
 day b.
 eclipse b.
 flash b.
 flight b.
 functional b.
 hysterical b.
 legal b.
 letter b.
 mind b.
 music b.
 night b.
 note b.
 object b.
 psychic b.
 river b.
 sight b.
 sign b.
 snow b.
 solar b.
 taste b.
 text b.
 word b.
blink
 b. reflex
 b. response
blister
 b. agent
 blood b.
 fever b.
 fly b.
 fracture b.
 sucking b.
blistering
 b. collodion
 b. distal dactylitis
bloat
bloating
Bloch reaction
Bloch-Sulzberger
 B.-S. disease
 B.-S. syndrome
block
 alveolocapillary b.
 b. anesthesia
 antegrade b.
 anterograde b.
 arborization b.
 atrioventricular b.
 AV b.

B

block *(continued)*
    bone b.
    bundle-branch b.
    complete AV b.
    conduction b.
    congenital heart b.
    depolarizing b.
    b. design test
    divisional b.
    entrance b.
    epidural b.
    exit b.
    fascicular b.
    field b.
    first-degree AV b.
    heart b.
    incomplete atrioventricular b.
    interatrial b.
    intraatrial b.
    intraventricular b. (IVB)
    IV b.
    Mobitz type of atrioventricular b.
    nerve b.
    nondepolarizing b.
    partial heart b.
    periinfarction b.
    phase I, II b.
    protective b.
    pupillary b.
    retrograde b.
    reverse pupillary b.
    S-A b.
    second-degree AV b.
    sinoatrial b.
    sinoauricular b.
    sinus b.
    spinal b.
    stellate b.
    suprahisian b.
    third-degree AV b.
    unidirectional b.
    b. vertebrae
    Wenckebach b.
    Wolff-Chaikoff b.

blockade
    adrenergic b.
    cholinergic b.
    ganglionic b.
    myoneural b.
    narcotic b.
    sympathetic b.
    virus b.

blocked
    b. aerogastria
    b. reading frame

blocker
    alpha b.
    angiotensin receptor b.
    beta b.
    calcium channel b.

blocking
    b. activity
    b. agent

    alpha b.
    b. antibody
block-out
Blocq disease
Blom-Singer valve
blood
    b. agar
    b. albumin
    arterial b.
    b. bank
    b. blister
    b. calculus
    b. capillary
    b. cast
    b. cell
    b. circulation
    b. clot
    cord b.
    b. corpuscle
    b. count
    b. crisis
    b. crystal
    b. cyst
    b. disk
    b. dust
    b. dyscrasia
    b. gas
    b. gas analysis
    b. group
    b. group agglutinin
    b. group agglutinogen
    b. group antibody
    b. group antigen
    b. group antiserum
    b. group-specific substance A and B
    b. group substance
    b. group system
    b. island
    b. islet
    laky b.
    b. lymph
    mixed venous b. ($\bar{v}$)
    b. mote
    occult b.
    b. pH
    b. plasma
    b. plasma fraction
    b. plastid
    b. plate
    b. poisoning
    b. pool imaging
    b. pressure (BP)
    b. relative
    b. serum
    sludged b.
    b. spot
    b. substitute
    b. sugar
    b. tumor
    b. type
    b. urea nitrogen (BUN)
    venous b.
    b. vessel

b. volume nomogram
whole b.
blood-air barrier
blood-aqueous barrier
blood-brain barrier (BBB)
blood-cerebrospinal fluid barrier
blood count
complete b. c. (CBC)
differential white b. c.
Schilling b. c.
blood-CSF barrier
blood group
private b. g.
bloodless
b. amputation
b. decerebration
b. operation
b. phlebotomy
bloodletting
general b.
local b.
bloodshot
bloodstream
blood-testis barrier
blood-thymus barrier
blood-vascular system
blood vessel
choroid b. v.
intrapulmonary b. v.
retinal b. v.
bloodworm
Bloom syndrome
blot
Western b.
blotch
Blount-Barber disease
Blount disease
blowfly
blowout
blowout fracture
b. pipette
blubber finger
blue
b. atrophy
b. baby
b. cataract
b. cone monochromatism
b. dextran
b. diaper syndrome
b. disease
b. dome cyst
b. dot sign
b. edema
eosin-methylene b. (EMB)
Evans b.
b. fever
b. line
b. nevus
b. ointment
postpartum b.'s
b. pus
b. pus bacillus
b. rubber-bleb nevi
b. sclera
b. spot

b. toe syndrome
b. vision
blueberry muffin baby
blue-green
b.-g. algae
b.-g. bacteria
b.-g. bacterium
bluetongue virus
Blumberg sign
Blumenau nucleus
Blumenbach clivus
Blumer shelf
blunt duct adenosis
blunted affect
blunt-end
b.-e. ligation
blunt-ended DNA
blush
tumor b.
BLV
bovine leukemia virus
B-mode
BMR
basal metabolic rate
BNA
Basle Nomina Anatomica
board
institutional review b. (IRB)
boat
b. conformation
b. form
bobbing
inverse ocular b.
ocular b.
bobierrite
BOC, *t*-BOC, Boc
t-butoxycarbonyl
Bochdalek
B. foramen
B. ganglion
B. gap
B. muscle
B. valve
Bock
B. ganglion
B. nerve
Bockhart impetigo
BOD
biochemical oxygen demand
Bodansky unit
Bödecker index
Bodian copper-PROTARGOL stain
Bodo
B. caudatus
B. saltans
B. urinarius
body
acetone b.
adrenal b.
alcoholic hyaline b.
Alder b.
alveolar b.
amygdaloid b.
amylogenic b.
anococcygeal b.

body *(continued)*

anterior quadrigeminal b.
aortic b.
Arnold b.
asbestos b.
Aschoff b.
asteroid b.
Auer b.
Barr chromatin b.
basal b.
bigeminal b.
b. of bladder
brassy b.
b. of breast
Cabot ring b.
Call-Exner b.
carotid b.
b. of caudate nucleus
cavernous b. of anal canal
cavernous b. of clitoris
cavernous b. of penis
b. cavity
cell b.
central b.
central fibrous b.
chromaffin b.
chromatin b.
ciliary b.
Civatte b.
b. of clavicle
b. of clitoris
coccygeal b.
colloid b.
compressible cavernous b.
conchoidal b.
b. of corpus callosum
Councilman hyaline b.
Cowdry type A inclusion b.
Cowdry type B inclusion b.
creola b.
cyanobacteriumlike b.
cytoid b.
cytoplasmic inclusion b.
Deetjen b.
demilune b.
dense b.
Döhle b.
Donovan b.
b. dysmorphic disorder
Ehrlich inner b.
elementary b. (E.B., EB)
b. of epididymis
epithelial b.
fat b.
fat b. of cheek
fat b. of ischioanal fossa
fat b. of ischiorectal fossa
fat b. of orbit
b. of femur
ferruginous b.
b. of fibula
foreign b.
b. of fornix
fruiting b.

fuchsin b.
b. of gallbladder
Gamna-Favre b.
Gamna-Gandy b.
Gandy-Gamna b.
geniculate b.
glass b.
glomus b.
Golgi b.
Guarnieri b.
Halberstaedter-Prowazek b.
Hassall b.
Hassall-Henle b.
Heinz b.
Heinz-Ehrlich b.
hematoxylin b.
hematoxyphil b.
Herring b.
Highmore b.
Howell-Jolly b.
b. of humerus
hyaline b.
hyaline b. of pituitary
hyaloid b.
b. of hyoid bone
b. of ilium
b. image
inclusion b.
b. of incus
infrapatellar fat b.
intercarotid b.
intermediate b. of Flemming
b. of ischium
Jaworski b.
Jolly b.
juxtaglomerular b.
juxtarestiform b.
ketone b.
Lafora b.
Lallemand b.
b. language
lateral geniculate b.
b. of lateral ventricle
L-D b.
LE b.
Leishman-Donovan b.
Lewy b.
Lieutaud b.
Lindner b.
loose b.
Luse b.
Luys b.
Mallory b.
malpighian b.
b. of mammary gland
mammillary b.
b. of mandible
b. mass index
b. of maxilla
b. mechanics
medial geniculate b.
melon-seed b.
b. of metacarpal
metachromatic b.
b. of metatarsal

Michaelis-Gutmann b.
Miyagawa b.
molluscum b.
Mooser b.
multilamellar b.
multivesicular b.
myelin b.
b. of nail
Negri b.
nerve cell b.
neuroepithelial b.
Nissl b.
nodular b.
nu b.
nuclear inclusion b.
Odland b.
olivary b.
orbital fat b.
pacchionian b.
pampiniform b.
b. of pancreas
Pappenheimer b.
paraaortic b.
parabasal b.
paranephric b.
paranuclear b.
paraphysial b.
paraterminal b.
Paschen b.
b. of penis
perineal b.
b. of phalanx
Pick b.
pineal b.
b. plethysmograph
polar b.
polyhedral b.
pontobulbar b.
posterior quadrigeminal b.
Prowazek b.
Prowazek-Greeff b.
psammoma b.
psittacosis inclusion b.
pubic b.
b. of pubic bone
b. of pubis
purine b.
quadrigeminal b.
b. of radius
Renaut b.
residual b.
residual b. of Regaud
rest b.
restiform b.
b. of rib
rice b.
b. righting reflex
Rushton b.
Russell b.
sand b.
Sandström b.
Savage perineal b.
Schaumann b.
b. schema
sclerotic b.

segmenting b.
b. of sphenoid
spongy b. of penis
b. stalk
b. of sternum
b. of stomach
striate b.
suprarenal b.
b. of sweat gland
Symington anococcygeal b.
b. of talus
b. of thigh bone
threshold b.
thyroid b.
b. of tibia
tigroid b.
b. of tongue
trachoma b.
trapezoid b.
Trousseau-Lallemand b.
tuffstone b.
turbinated b.
tympanic b.
b. of ulna
ultimobranchial b.
b. of uterus
vaccine b.
Verocay b.
b. of vertebra
vertebral b.
Virchow-Hassall b.
vitreous b.
Weibel-Palade b.
wolffian b.
Wolf-Orton b.
Y b.
yellow b.
zebra b.
Zuckerkandl b.

body burden
body-weight ratio
Boeck
B. disease
B. and Drbohlav Locke-egg-serum medium
B. sarcoid
Boehmer hematoxylin
Boerhaave
B. syndrome
bogbean
Bogros
B. serous membrane
B. space
Bohn nodule
Bohr
B. atom
B. effect
B. equation
B. magneton (μ_B)
B. theory
boil
Aleppo b.
Bagdad b.
Biskra b.
blind b.

boil (*continued*)
    date b.
    Delhi b.
    Jericho b.
    Madura b.
    Oriental b.
    salt water b.
    tropical b.
boilermaker's hearing loss
boiling point (b.p.)
bol
    bolus
boldin
boldine dimethyl ether
boldo
boldoglucin
boldus
Boley gauge
Bolivian
    B. hemorrhagic fever
    B. hemorrhagic fever virus
Boll cell
Bollinger granule
Bollman
Bolognini symptom
bolometer
bolus (bol)
    b. dressing
    intravenous b.
bombard
Bombay
    B. phenomenon
    B. trait
bomb calorimeter
bombesin
bond
    acylmercaptan b.
    apolar b.
    conjugated double b.'s
    coordinate covalent b.
    disulfide b.
    double b.
    electrostatic b.
    energy-rich b.
    eupeptide b.
    heteropolar b.
    high energy phosphate b.
    hydrogen b.
    hydrophobic b.
    isopeptide b.
    noncovalent b.
    peptide b.
    semipolar b.
    single b.
    triple b.
bonding
bone
    b. abscess
    b. ache
    b. age
    Albrecht b.
    alveolar b.
    alveolar supporting b.
    ankle b.

b. architecture
arm b.
b. ash
basal b.
basilar b.
basioccipital b.
basisphenoid b.
Bertin b.
b. black
blade b.
b. block
b. block fusion
breast b.
Breschet b.
brittle b.
bundle b.
calcaneal b.
calf b.
b. canaliculus
cancellous b.
capitate b.
carpal b.
cartilage b.
b. cell
central b.
central b. of ankle
b. charcoal
cheek b.
b. chip
coccygeal b.
collar b.
compact b.
b. conduction
convoluted b.
b. corpuscle
cortical b.
coxal b.
cranial b.
b. of cranium
cubital b.
cuboid b.
cuneiform b.
b. cyst
b. density
dermal b.
b. of digits
dorsal talonavicular b.
ear b.
elbow b.
endochondral b.
epactal b.
epihyal b.
epipteric b.
episternal b.
ethmoid b.
exoccipital b.
facial b.
first cuneiform b.
flank b.
b. flap
flat b.
Flower b.
b. of foot
foot b.
b. forceps

fourth turbinated b.
frontal b.
funny b.
b. Gla protein
Goethe b.
b. graft
greater multangular b.
hamate b.
heel b.
heterotopic b.
highest turbinated b.
hip b.
hollow b.
hooked b.
hyoid b.
iliac b.
incarial b.
incisive b.
b. infarct
b. of inferior limb
inferior turbinated b.
innominate b.
intermaxillary b.
intermediate cuneiform b.
interparietal b.
irregular b.
ischial b.
b. island
jaw b.
jugal b.
Krause b.
lacrimal b.
lamellar b.
lateral cuneiform b.
lenticular b.
lentiform b.
lesser multangular b.
lingual b.
long b.
b. of lower limb
lunate b.
malar b.
marble b.
b. marrow
b. marrow dose
b. marrow embolism
b. marrow transplantation
mastoid b.
b. matrix
medial cuneiform b.
membrane b.
mesethmoid b.
metacarpal b. [I–V]
metatarsal b. [I–V]
middle cuneiform b.
middle turbinated b.
multangular b.
nasal b.
navicular b.
navicular b. of hand
nonlamellar b.
occipital b.
orbicular b.
palatine b.
parietal b.

pelvic b.
perichondral b.
periosteal b.
periotic b.
peroneal b.
petrosal b.
petrous b.
b. phosphate
ping-pong b.
pipe b.
Pirie b.
pisiform b.
b. plate
pneumatic b.
pneumatized b.
postsphenoid b.
preinterparietal b.
premaxillary b.
presphenoid b.
pubic b.
pyramidal b.
replacement b.
b. resorption
reticular b.
rider's b.
Riolan b.
sacred b.
b. salt
scaphoid b.
b. sclerosis
scroll b.
second cuneiform b.
semilunar b.
b. sensibility
septal b.
sesamoid b.
shin b.
short b.
b. sialoprotein 1
sieve b.
b. of skull
sphenoid b.
sphenoidal turbinated b.
spongy b.
b. of superior limb
superior turbinated b.
suprainterparietal b.
suprasternal b.
supreme turbinated b.
sutural b.
tail b.
tarsal b.
temporal b.
thigh b.
third cuneiform b.
three-cornered b.
b. tissue
tongue b.
trabecular b.
trapezium b.
trapezoid b.
triangular b.
triquetrum b.
turbinated b.
tympanic b.

bone *(continued)*
    tympanohyal b.
    unciform b.
    upper jaw b.
    b. of upper limb
    Vesalius b.
    b. of visceral cranium
    b. wax
    wedge b.
    wormian b.
    woven b.
    yoke b.
    zygomatic b.
bonelet
bone-salt
Bonhoeffer sign
Bonnet capsule
Bonnet-Dechaume-Blanc syndrome
Bonney test
Bonnier syndrome
Bonwill triangle
bony
    b. ampulla of semicircular canal
    b. ankylosis
    b. crepitus
    b. heart
    b. labyrinth
    b. limb of semicircular canal
    b. nasal septum
    b. palate
    b. part of external acoustic meatus
    b. part of nasal septum
    b. part of pharyngotympanic tube
    b. part of skeletal system
    b. semicircular canal
Böök syndrome
BOOP
    bronchiolitis obliterans with organizing
      pneumonia
booster
    b. dose
    b. response
boot
    Gibney b.
    Unna b.
boracic acid
borate
borated
borax
borborygmus, pl. **borborygmi**
Bordeaux mixture
border
    alveolar b.
    anterior b.
    anterior b. of body of pancreas
    anterior b. of eyelid
    anterior b. of fibula
    anterior b. of lung
    anterior b. of pancreas
    anterior b. of radius
    anterior b. of testis
    anterior b. of tibia
    anterior b. of ulna
    brush b.

b. cell
ciliary b. of iris
denture b.
b.'s of eyelid
fibular (peroneal) b. of foot
free b.
free b. of nail
free b. of ovary
frontal b.
frontal b. of parietal bone
frontal b. of sphenoid bone
hidden b. of nail
inferior b.
inferior b. of body of pancreas
inferior b. of liver
inferior b. of lung
inferior b. of pancreas
inferior b. of spleen
inner b. of iris
interosseous b.
interosseous b. of fibula
interosseous b. of radius
interosseous b. of tibia
interosseous b. of ulna
b. of iris
lacrimal b. of maxilla
lambdoid b. of occipital bone
lateral b.
lateral b. of foot
lateral b. of forearm
lateral b. of humerus
lateral b. of kidney
lateral b. of nail
lateral b. of scapula
mastoid b. of occipital bone
medial b.
medial b. of foot
medial b. of forearm
medial b. of humerus
medial b. of kidney
medial b. of scapula
medial b. of suprarenal gland
medial b. of tibia
mesovarian b. of ovary
b. molding
nasal b. of frontal bone
occipital b.
occipital b. of parietal bone
occipital b. of temporal bone
occult b. of nail
outer b. of iris
parietal b.
parietal b. of frontal bone
parietal b. of sphenoid bone
parietal b. of squamous part of
  temporal bone
parietal b. of temporal bone
peroneal b. of foot
posterior b. of eyelid
posterior b. of fibula
posterior b. of petrous part of
  temporal bone
posterior b. of radius
posterior b. of testis
posterior b. of ulna

proximal b. of nail
pupillary b. of iris
radial b. of forearm
right b. of heart
sagittal b. of parietal bone
b. seal
sphenoidal b. of temporal bone
squamosal b.
squamosal b. of parietal bone
squamous b.
squamous b. of parietal bone
squamous b. of sphenoid bone
striated b.
superior b.
superior b. of body of pancreas
superior b. of pancreas
superior b. of petrous part of
  temporal bone
superior b. of scapula
superior b. of spleen
superior b. of suprarenal gland
tibial b. of foot
b. tissue movement
ulnar b. of forearm
b. of uterus
ventral b.
vermilion b.
vertebral b. of scapula
zygomatic b. of greater wing of
  sphenoid bone

borderline
b. case
b. hypertension
b. leprosy
b. ovarian tumor
b. personality
b. personality disorder

Bordetella
B. *bronchiseptica*
B. *hinzii*
B. *holmesii*
B. *parapertussis*
B. *pertussis*

Bordet-Gengou
B.-G. bacillus
B.-G. phenomenon
B.-G. potato blood agar

Bordet and Gengou reaction
boric acid
borism
Börjeson-Forssman-Lehmann syndrome
Borna disease virus
bornane
Bornholm
B. disease
B. disease virus

Born method of wax plate
  reconstruction
boroglycerin
boroglycerol
boron (B)
Borrel blue stain
Borrelia
B. *afzelii*
B. *anserina*

B. *burgdorferi*
B. *burgdorferi sensu lato*
B. *burgdorferi sensu stricto*
B. *caucasica*
B. *crocidurae*
B. *duttonii*
B. *garinii*
B. *hermsii*
B. *hispanica*
B. *latyschewii*
B. *mazzottii*
B. *parkeri*
B. *persica*
B. *recurrentis*
B. *turicatae*
B. *venezuelensis*

borreliosis
Lyme b.

Borst-Jadassohn type intraepidermal
  epithelioma
BOR syndrome
bosch yaws
Bosin disease
boss
bosselated
bosselation
Boston
B. exanthema
B. opium

Botallo
B. duct
B. foramen
B. ligament

botfly
head b.
human b.
skin b.
warble b.

bothria (*pl. of* bothrium)
bothriocephaliasis
Bothriocephalus
B. *cordatus*
B. *latus*
B. *mansoni*
B. *mansonoides*

bothrium, pl. **bothria**
bothropic antitoxin
Bothrops antitoxin
botryoid
b. odontogenic cyst
b. sarcoma

Botryomyces
botryomycosis
botryomycotic
bots
ox b.
sheep b.

Böttcher
B. canal
B. cell
B. crystal
B. ganglion
B. space

bottle
Mariotte b.

B

bottle *(continued)*
    wash-b.
    Woulfe b.
botulin
botulinogenic
botulinum antitoxin
botulinus toxin
botulism
    b. antitoxin
    wound b.
botulismotoxin
botulogenic
boubas
Bouchard disease
bouche de tapir
Bouchut tube
bougie
    b. à boule
    bulbous b.
    Eder-Pustow b.
    elastic b.
    elbowed b.
    filiform b.
    following b.
    Hurst b.
    Maloney b.
    Savary b.
    tapered b.
    wax-tipped b.
    whip b.
bougienage
bouillon
Bouin fixative
boulimia
boundary lamina
bound water
bouquet
    b. fever
    Riolan b.
Bourgery ligament
Bourneville disease
Bourneville-Pringle disease
bouton
    axonal terminal b.
    b. de Baghdad
    b. de Biskra
    b. d'Orient
    b. en chemise
    b.'s en passage
    synaptic b.
    terminal b.
    b. terminaux
boutonneuse fever
boutonnière deformity
Bovicola
Bovie
bovine
    b. antitoxin
    b. brucellosis
    b. colloid
    b. ketosis
    b. leukemia virus (BLV)
    b. leukosis virus
    b. papular stomatitis virus

    b. rhinoviruses
    b. serum albumin (BSA)
    b. spongiform encephalopathy (BSE)
    b. virus diarrhea virus
bow
    Cupid's b.
    Logan b.
Bowditch
    B. effect
    B. law
bowel
    b. bypass
    b. bypass syndrome
    large b.
    b. movement
    small b.
    b. sound
Bowen
    B. disease
    B. precancerous dermatosis
bowenoid
    b. cell
    b. papulosis
Bowie stain
bowleg, bow-leg
Bowles-type stethoscope
Bowman
    B. capsule
    B. disk
    B. gland
    B. layer
    B. membrane
    B. muscle
    B. probe
    B. space
Bowman-Birk inhibitor
box
    black b.
    brain b.
    CAAT b.
    Hogness b.
    b. jelly
    Pribnow b.
    Skinner b.
    TATA b.
    view b.
boxer's
    b. ear
    b. fracture
boxing wax
Boyd communicating perforation vein
Boyden
    B. meal
    B. sphincter
Boyer
    B. bursa
    B. cyst
Boyle law
Bozeman
    B. operation
    B. position
Bozeman-Fritsch catheter
Bozzolo sign
BP
    blood pressure

B

bronchopleural
    BP fistula
b.p.
    boiling point
Bq
    becquerel
Br
    bromine
Braasch
    B. bulb
    B. catheter
brace
    cast b.
    Taylor back b.
brachia (*pl. of* brachium)
brachial
    b. anesthesia
    b. artery
    b. autonomic plexus
    b. birth palsy
    b. fascia
    b. gland
    b. lymph node
    b. muscle
    b. neuritis
    b. plexitis
    b. plexus
    b. plexus injury
    b. plexus neuropathy
    b. vein
brachialgia statica paresthetica
brachialis muscle
brachiocephalic
    b. (arterial) trunk
    b. arteritis
    b. lymph node
brachiocrural
brachiocubital
brachiogram
brachioradial
    b. muscle
    b. reflex
brachioradialis muscle
brachium, pl. **brachia**
    b. colliculi inferioris
    b. colliculi superioris
    b. conjunctivum cerebelli
    b. of inferior colliculus
    inferior quadrigeminal b.
    b. pontis
    b. quadrigeminum inferius
    b. quadrigeminum superius
    b. of superior colliculus
    superior quadrigeminal b.
Bracht maneuver
Bracht-Wächter lesion
brachybasia
brachybasocamptodactyly
brachybasophalangia
brachycardia
brachycephalia
brachycephalic
brachycephalism
brachycephalous
brachycephaly

brachycheilia, brachychilia
brachycnemic, brachyknemic
brachycranic
brachydactylia
brachydactylic
brachydactyly
brachyesophagus
brachyfacial
brachyglossal
brachygnathia
brachygnathous
brachykerkic
brachyknemic (*var. of* brachycnemic)
brachymelia
brachymesophalangia
brachymetacarpalia, brachymetacarpalism
brachymetacarpia
brachymetapody
brachymetatarsia
brachymorphic
brachyodont
brachyonychia
brachypellic pelvis
brachypelvic
brachyphalangia
brachypodous
brachyprosopic
brachyrhinia
brachyrhynchus
brachyskelic
brachystaphyline
brachysyndactyly
brachytelephalangia
brachytherapy
    high-dose-rate b.
    interstitial b.
    remote afterloading b.
    stereotactic b.
brachytype
bracing
bracket
Bradbury-Eggleston syndrome
Bradford frame
brady-
bradyarrhythmia
bradyarthria
bradycardia
    central b.
    essential b.
    fetal b.
    idiopathic b.
    marked fetal b.
    mild fetal b.
    nodal b.
    postinfectious b.
    sinus b.
    vagal b.
    ventricular b.
bradycardiac
bradycardic
bradycinesia
bradycrotic
bradydiastole
bradyesthesia
bradyglossia

bradykinesia
bradykinetic analysis
bradykininogen
bradykinin-potentiating peptide
bradykinin potentiator B
bradylalia
bradylexia
bradylogia
bradypepsia
bradyphagia
bradyphasia
bradyphemia
bradypnea
bradypsychia
bradyrhythmia
bradyspermatism
bradysphygmia
bradystalsis
bradytachycardia syndrome
bradyteleocinesia
bradyteleokinesis
bradyuria
bradyzoite
braille
Brailsford
Brailsford-Morquio disease
brain
    b. attack
    b. box
    b. cicatrix
    b. concussion
    b. congestion
    b. contusion
    b. death
    b. edema
    b. laceration
    b. lipid
    b. mantle
    b. murmur
    b. potential
    B. reflex
    b. sand
    split b.
    b. stem
    b. sugar
    b. swelling
    visceral b.
    b. wave
    b. wave complex
    b. wave cycle
braincase
brain-heart infusion agar
brainstem
    b. auditory evoked potential
    b. auditory evoked response
    (BAER)
    b. evoked response (BSER)
    b. glioma
    b. hemorrhage
brainwashing
bran
branch
    accessory meningeal b.
    accessory meningeal b. of middle
      meningeal artery

accessory b. of middle meningeal
  artery
acetabular b.
acromial b. of suprascapular artery
acromial b. of thoracoacromial
  artery
anastomotic b.
anastomotic b. of middle meningeal
  artery with lacrimal artery
b. to angular gyrus
anterior b.
anterior abdominal cutaneous b. of
  intercostal nerve
anterior auricular b. of superficial
  temporal artery
anterior basal b.
anterior basal b. of superior basal
  vein (of right and left inferior
  pulmonary veins)
anterior cutaneous b. of femoral
  nerve
anterior cutaneous b. of
  iliohypogastric nerve
anterior cutaneous b. of intercostal
  nerve
anterior gastric b. of anterior vagal
  trunk
anterior glandular b. of superior
  thyroid artery
anterior intercostal b. of internal
  thoracic artery
anterior interventricular b. of left
  coronary artery
anterior labial b. of deep external
  pudendal artery
anterior lateral nasal b. of anterior
  ethmoidal artery
anterior/lateral/posterior glandular b.
  of superior thyroid artery
anterior meningeal b. (of anterior
  ethmoidal artery)
anterior pectoral cutaneous b. of
  intercostal nerve
anterior b. of the renal artery
anterior scrotal b. of deep external
  pudendal artery
anterior septal b. of anterior
  ethmoidal artery
anterior superior alveolar b. of
  infraorbital nerve
anterior temporal b.
anteromedial central b.
anteromedial frontal b. of
  callosomarginal artery
apical b. of inferior lobar branch
  of right pulmonary artery
apical b. of right superior
  pulmonary vein
apicoposterior b. of left superior
  pulmonary vein
articular b.
ascending b.
ascending b. of the inferior
  mesenteric artery

ascending b. of superficial cervical artery

atrial b.

atrial anastomotic b. of circumflex branch of left coronary artery

atrioventricular nodal b.

b. to atrioventricular node

auricular b. of occipital artery

auricular b. of posterior auricular artery

auricular b. of vagus nerve

b. of auriculotemporal nerve to tympanic membrane

basal tentorial b. of internal carotid artery

bronchial b. of thoracic aorta

buccal b. of facial nerve

calcaneal b.

calcarine b. of medial occipital artery

capsular b. of intrarenal artery

capsular b. of renal artery

carotid b. of glossopharyngeal nerve (CN IX)

carotid sinus b.

caudate b. of left branch of portal vein

cavernous b. of cavernous part of internal carotid artery

cavernous sinus b. of internal carotid artery

celiac b. of posterior vagal trunk

celiac b. of vagus nerve

cervical b. of facial nerve

choroid b.

cingular b. of callosomarginal artery

circumferential pontine b. of pontine artery

circumflex fibular b. (of posterior tibial artery)

circumflex b. of left coronary artery

circumflex peroneal b. of posterior tibial artery

circumflex b. of posterior tibial artery

clavicular b. of thoracoacromial artery

clivus b. of cerebral part of internal carotid artery

cochlear b. of labyrinthine artery

cochlear b. of vestibulocochlear artery

colic b. of ileocolic artery

collateral b. of intercostal nerve

collateral b. of posterior intercostal artery 3–11

communicating b.

communicating b. of anterior interosseous nerve with ulnar nerve

communicating b. of auriculotemporal nerve with facial nerve

communicating b. of chorda tympani to lingual nerve

communicating b. of chorda tympani with lingual nerve

communicating b. of facial nerve with glossopharyngeal nerve

communicating b. of facial nerve with tympanic plexus

communicating b. of fibular artery

communicating b. of glossopharyngeal nerve with auricular branch of vagus nerve

communicating b. of intermediate nerve with tympanic plexus

communicating b. of internal laryngeal nerve with recurrent laryngeal nerve

communicating b. of lacrimal nerve with zygomatic nerve

communicating b. of lingual nerve with hypoglossal nerve

communicating b. of median nerve with ulnar nerve

communicating b. of nasociliary nerve with ciliary ganglion

communicating b. of otic ganglion to auriculotemporal nerve

communicating b. of otic ganglion to chorda tympani

communicating b. of otic ganglion with chorda tympani

communicating b. of otic ganglion with medial pterygoid nerve

communicating b. of otic ganglion with meningeal branch of mandibular nerve

communicating b. of peroneal artery

communicating b. of radial nerve with ulnar nerve

communicating b. of spinal nerve

communicating b. of superficial radial nerve with ulnar nerve

communicating b. of superior laryngeal nerve with recurrent laryngeal nerve

communicating b. of sympathetic trunk

communicating b. of tympanic plexus with auricular branch of vagus nerve

cricothyroid b. of superior thyroid artery

cutaneous b. of anterior branch of obturator nerve

cutaneous b. of mixed nerve

cutaneous b. of obturator nerve

deep b.

deep b. of the lateral plantar nerve

deep b. of the medial circumflex femoral artery

deep b. of the medial plantar artery

deep palmar b. of ulnar artery

deep plantar b. of dorsalis pedis artery

branch (*continued*)

deep b. of radial nerve
deep b. of the superior gluteal
artery
deep b. of the transverse cervical
artery
deep b. of the ulnar nerve
deltoid b.
dental b.
descending b.
descending anterior b.
descending b. of anterior segmental
artery of left and right lungs
descending b. of hypoglossal nerve
descending b. of lateral circumflex
femoral artery
descending b. of medial circumflex
femoral artery
descending b. of occipital artery
descending posterior b.
descending b. of posterior segmental
artery of left and right lungs
descending b. of superficial cervical
artery
digastric b. of facial nerve
dorsal b.
dorsal carpal b. of radial artery
dorsal carpal b. of ulnar artery
dorsal b. of first and second
posterior intercostal artery
dorsal lingual b. of lingual artery
dorsal b. of the lumbar artery
dorsal b. of the posterior intercostal
artery 3–11
dorsal b. of the posterior intercostal
veins 4–11
dorsal b. of the subcostal artery
dorsal b. of the superior intercostal
artery
dorsal b. of the ulnar nerve
duodenal b. of anterior superior
pancreaticoduodenal artery
duodenal b. of posterior superior
pancreaticoduodenal artery
epiploic b.
esophageal b.
esophageal b. of the inferior
thyroid artery
esophageal b. of the left gastric
artery
esophageal b. of the recurrent
laryngeal nerve
esophageal b. of the thoracic aorta
esophageal b. of thoracic ganglia
esophageal b. of the vagus nerve
external nasal b. of infraorbital
nerve
external b. of superior laryngeal
nerve
external b. of trunk of accessory
nerve
femoral b. of genitofemoral nerve
frontal b. of middle meningeal
artery

frontal b. of superficial temporal
artery
ganglionic b. of internal carotid
artery
ganglionic b. of lingual nerve
ganglionic b. of lingual nerve to
sublingual ganglion
ganglionic b. of lingual nerve to
submandibular ganglion
ganglionic b. of maxillary nerve
ganglionic b. of maxillary nerve to
pterygopalatine ganglion
gastric b. of anterior vagal trunk
gastric b. of posterior vagal b.
genital b. of genitofemoral nerve
genital b. of iliohypogastric nerve
glandular b.
glandular b. of facial artery
glandular b. of inferior thyroid
artery
glandular b. of submandibular
ganglion
b. of glossopharyngeal nerve to
stylopharyngeus muscle
hepatic b. of anterior vagal trunk
hepatic b. of vagus nerve
faucial b. of lingual nerve
iliac b. of iliolumbar artery
iliacus b. of iliolumbar artery
inferior b.
inferior cervical cardiac b. of vagus
nerve
inferior dental b. of inferior dental
plexus
inferior gingival b. of inferior
dental plexus
inferior labial b. of facial artery
inferior labial b. of mental nerve
inferior lingular b. of lingular
branch of left pulmonary artery
inferior b. of oculomotor nerve
inferior b. of pubic bone
inferior b. of superior gluteal artery
inferior b. of transverse cervical
nerve
infrahyoid b. of superior thyroid
artery
infrapatellar b. of saphenous nerve
inguinal b. of deep external
pudendal artery
interganglionic b. of sympathetic
trunk
intermediate atrial b. of left
coronary artery
intermediate atrial b. of right
coronary artery
intermediate b. of hepatic artery
proper
intermediate temporal b. of lateral
occipital artery
intermediomedial frontal b. of
callosomarginal artery
b. to internal capsule, genu
b. to internal capsule, posterior
limb

b. to internal capsule, retrolentiform limb

b. of internal carotid artery to trigeminal ganglion

internal nasal b.

internal b. of superior laryngeal nerve

internal b. of trunk of accessory nerve

interventricular septal b. of left/right coronary artery

joint b.

labial b. of mental nerve

laryngopharyngeal b. of superior cervical ganglion

lateral b.

lateral abdominal/pectoral cutaneous b. of intercostal nerve

lateral b. of artery of tuber cinereum

lateral atrial b. of left coronary artery

lateral atrial b. of right coronary artery

lateral basal b.

lateral calcaneal b. of sural nerve

lateral costal b. of internal thoracic artery

lateral cutaneous b.

lateral cutaneous b. of intercostal nerve

lateral cutaneous b. of ventral primary ramus of thoracic spinal nerve

lateral malleolar b. of fibular peroneal artery

lateral mammary b.

lateral mammary b. of lateral cutaneous branch of intercostal nerve

lateral mammary b. of lateral cutaneous branch of thoracic spinal nerve

lateral mammary b. of lateral thoracic artery

lateral and medial posterior choroidal b. of posterior cerebral artery

lateral medullary b. of intracranial part of vertebral artery

lateral nasal b. of anterior ethmoidal nerve

lateral nasal b. of facial artery

lateral b. of pontine artery

lateral b. of posterior ramus of spinal nerve

lateral sacral b. of median sacral artery

left b.

left b. of hepatic artery proper

lingual b.

lingual b. of facial nerve

b. of lingual nerve to isthmus of fauces

lumbar b. of iliolumbar artery

mammary b.

marginal atrial b. of right coronary artery

marginal b. of cingulate sulcus

marginal mandibular b. of facial nerve

marginal b. of parietooccipital sulcus

marginal b. [TA] of cingulate sulcus

marginal tentorial b. of internal carotid artery

mastoid b. of occipital artery

mastoid b. of posterior auricular artery

mastoid b. of posterior tympanic artery

medial b.

medial b. of artery of tuber cinereum

medial basal b. of pulmonary artery

medial calcaneal b. of tibial nerve

medial crural cutaneous b. of saphenous nerve

medial cutaneous b. of dorsal branch of posterior intercostal artery

medial malleolar b. of posterior tibial artery

medial mammary b.

medial medullary b. of vertebral artery

medial nasal b. of anterior ethmoidal nerve

medial b. of pontine artery

medial b. of posterior branch of spinal nerve

medial b. of posterior rami of spinal nerve

mediastinal b.

mediastinal b. of internal thoracic artery

mediastinal b. of thoracic aorta

meningeal b.

meningeal b. of cavernous part of internal carotid artery

meningeal b. of cerebral part of internal carotid artery

meningeal b. of internal carotid artery

meningeal b. of (intracranial part of) vertebral artery

meningeal b. of mandibular nerve

meningeal b. of maxillary nerve

meningeal b. of occipital artery

meningeal b. of ophthalmic nerve

meningeal b. of spinal nerve

meningeal b. of vagus nerve

mental b. of inferior alveolar artery

mental b. of mental nerve

middle lobe b. of right superior pulmonary vein

middle meningeal b. of maxillary nerve

B

branch (continued)

middle superior alveolar b. of infraorbital nerve

middle temporal b. of insular part of middle cerebral artery

middle temporal b. of lateral occipital artery

b. migration

muscular b.

mylohyoid b. of inferior alveolar artery

nasal septal b. of superior labial branch of facial artery

obturator b. of pubic branch of inferior epigastric vein

occipital b.

b. of oculomotor nerve to ciliary ganglion

omental b.

orbital b. of maxillary nerve

orbital b. of middle meningeal artery

orbital b.'s of pterygopalatine ganglion

ovarian b. of uterine artery

palmar b. of anterior interosseous nerve

palmar carpal b. of radial artery

palmar carpal b. of ulnar artery

palmar b. of median nerve

palmar b. of ulnar nerve

palpebral b. of infratrochlear nerve

pancreatic b.

paracentral b. of callosomarginal artery

paracentral b. of pericallosal artery

paramedian pontine b. of pontine artery

parietal b.

parietal b. of medial occipital artery

parietal b. of middle meningeal artery

parietal b. of superficial temporal artery

parietooccipital b. of anterior cerebral artery

parietooccipital b. of posterior cerebral artery

parotid b.

pectoral and abdominal anterior cutaneous b. of intercostal nerve

pectoral b.'s of thoracoacromial artery

perforating b.'s

perforating b. of anterior interosseous artery

perforating b. of fibular artery

perforating b.'s of internal thoracic artery

perforating b.'s (of palmar metacarpal arteries)

perforating b.'s (of plantar metatarsal arteries)

perforating b. of peroneal artery

pericardial b. of phrenic nerve

pericardial b.'s of thoracic aorta

perineal b. of posterior cutaneous nerve of thigh

perineal b. of posterior femoral cutaneous nerve

peroneal communicating b.

petrosal b. of middle meningeal artery

pharyngeal b.

pharyngeal b. of the artery of pterygoid canal

pharyngeal b. of the ascending pharyngeal artery

pharyngeal b. of descending palatine artery

pharyngeal b. of glossopharyngeal nerve

pharyngeal b. of inferior thyroid artery

pharyngeal b. of pterygopalatine ganglion

pharyngeal b. of recurrent laryngeal nerve

pharyngeal b. of vagus nerve

phrenicoabdominal b. of phrenic nerve

posterior b.

posterior basal b.

posterior gastric b. of posterior vagal trunk

posterior glandular b. of superior thyroid artery

posterior b. of great auricular nerve

posterior inferior nasal b. of greater palatine nerve

posterior b. of inferior pancreaticoduodenal artery

posterior labial branch of internal perineal b.

posterior labial b. of perineal artery

posterior b. of lateral cerebral sulcus

posterior b. of medial antebrachial cutaneous nerve

posterior b. of medial cutaneous nerve of forearm

posterior b. of obturator artery

posterior b. of obturator nerve

posterior b. of recurrent ulnar artery

posterior b. of renal artery

posterior b. of right branch of portal vein

posterior b. of right hepatic duct

posterior b. of right superior pulmonary vein

posterior scrotal b. of internal pudendal artery

posterior scrotal b. of perineal artery

posterior septal b. of nose

posterior septal b. of sphenopalatine artery

posterior b. of spinal nerve

posterior superior alveolar b.'s of maxillary nerve

posterior superior lateral nasal b. of maxillary nerve

posterior superior lateral nasal b. of pterygopalatine ganglion

posterior superior medial nasal b. of maxillary nerve

posterior superior medial nasal b. of pterygopalatine ganglion

posterior b. of superior thyroid artery

posterior temporal b. of middle cerebral artery

posterior b. of ulnar recurrent artery

posterior vestibular b. of vestibulocochlear artery

posteromedial frontal b. of callosomarginal artery

precuneal b. of anterior cerebral artery

prelaminar b. of spinal branch of dorsal branch of posterior intercostal artery

prostatic b. of inferior vesical artery

prostatic b. of middle rectal artery

pterygoid b. of maxillary artery

pterygoid b. of posterior deep temporal artery

pubic b. of inferior epigastric artery

pubic b. of inferior epigastric vein

pubic b. of obturator artery

pulmonary b. of autonomic nervous system

pulmonary b. of pulmonary nerve plexus

pyloric b. of anterior vagal trunk

recurrent meningeal b. of spinal nerve

recurrent b. of spinal nerve

renal b. of lesser splanchnic b.

renal b. of vagus nerve

right b.

right atrial b. of right coronary artery

right b. of hepatic artery proper

right marginal b.

right b. of portal vein

saphenous b. of descending genicular artery

b.'s of segmental bronchi

septal b.'s

sinuatrial nodal b. of right coronary artery

b. to sinuatrial node

sinuatrial (S-A) nodal b. of right coronary artery

spinal b.

splenic b. of splenic artery

stapedial b. of posterior tympanic artery

stapedial b. of stylomastoid artery

sternal b. of internal thoracic artery

sternocleidomastoid b. of occipital artery

sternocleidomastoid b. of superior thyroid artery

stylohyoid b. of facial nerve

stylopharyngeal b. of glossopharyngeal nerve

subendocardial b. of atrioventricular bundle

subscapular b. of axillary artery

superficial b.

superficial b. of the lateral plantar nerve

superficial b. of medial circumflex femoral artery

superficial b. of the medial plantar artery

superficial palmar b. of radial artery

superficial b. of the radial nerve

superficial b. of the superior gluteal artery

superficial temporal b. of auriculotemporal nerve

superficial b. of the transverse cervical artery

superficial b. of the ulnar nerve

superior b.

superior cervical cardiac b. of vagus nerve

superior dental b. of superior dental plexus

superior gingival b. of superior dental plexus

superior labial b. of facial artery

superior labial b. of infraorbital nerve

superior lingular b. of lingular branch of superior lobar left pulmonary artery

superior b. of the oculomotor nerve

superior b. of the pubic bone

superior b. of the right and left inferior pulmonary veins

superior b. of the superior gluteal artery

superior b. of the transverse cervical nerve

superior vermian b. of superior cerebellar artery

suprahyoid b. of lingual artery

sural communicating b. of common fibular nerve

sural communicating b. of common peroneal nerve

sympathetic b. to submandibular ganglion

temporal b. of facial nerve

tentorial basal b. of internal carotid artery

tentorial marginal b. of cavernous part of internal carotid artery

terminal b. of middle cerebral artery

B

branch (*continued*)
    thoracic cardiac b. of thoracic ganglia
    thoracic cardiac b. of vagus nerve
    thoracic pulmonary b. of thoracic ganglia
    thymic b. of internal thoracic artery
    thyrohyoid b. of ansa cervicalis
    tonsillar b. of the facial artery
    tonsillar b. of glossopharyngeal nerve
    tonsillar b. of lesser palatine nerve
    tracheal b.
    transverse b. of lateral femoral circumflex artery
    b. to trigeminal ganglion
    tubal b.
    tubal b. of ovarian artery
    tubal b. of the tympanic plexus
    tubal b. of the uterine artery
    ulnar communicating b. of superficial radial nerve
    ulnar b. of medial antebrachial cutaneous nerve
    ureteral b.
    ureteric b.
    ureteric b. of the inferior suprarenal artery
    ureteric b. of the ovarian artery
    ureteric b. of the patent part of umbilical artery
    ureteric b. of the renal artery
    ureteric b. of the testicular artery
    ventral b.
    vestibular b. of labyrinthine artery
    zygomatic b. of facial nerve
    zygomaticofacial b. of zygomatic nerve
    zygomaticotemporal b. of zygomatic nerve

branched
    b. calculus
    b. chain ketoaciduria
    b. chain ketonuria

brancher
    b. deficiency glycogenosis
    b. glycogen storage disease

branchia, pl. **branchiae**

branchial
    b. apparatus
    b. arch
    b. cartilage
    b. cleft
    b. cleft cyst
    b. cyst
    b. efferent column
    b. fissure
    b. fistula
    b. groove
    b. mesoderm
    b. pouch

branching
    b. enzyme
    b. factor

    false b.
    b. type of renal pelvis

branchiogenic, branchiogenous

branchiomere

branchiomeric muscle

branchiomerism

branchiomotor nucleus

branchiootorenal
    b. dysplasia
    b. syndrome

brandy nose

Branhamella
    B. catarrhalis

Branham sign

branny desquamation

Brasdor

Brasdor method

brass
    b. founder's ague
    b. founder's fever

brassy
    b. body
    b. cough

BRAT diet

Braun anastomosis

Braune
    B. muscle
    B. valve

brawny
    b. arm
    b. edema
    b. scleritis

Braxton
    B. Hicks contraction
    B. Hicks sign

Brazelton Neonatal Behavioral Assessment Scale

brazilein

Brazilian
    B. blastomycosis
    B. hemorrhagic fever
    B. pemphigus
    B. purpuric fever
    B. spotted fever

brazilin

Brazil wax

brazing

BRCA1 gene

BRCA2 gene

BrDu
    bromodeoxyuridine

bread-and-butter pericardium

bread pill

break
    double-strand b.
    b. shock
    single-strand b.

breakaway phenomenon (*var. of* breakoff phenomenon)

breakbone fever

breakdown
    nervous b.

breakoff phenomenon

breakpoint

breakthrough

breast
    accessory b.
    b. bone
    chicken b.
    funnel b.
    irritable b.
    male b.
    b. pang
    pigeon b.
    b. pump
    supernumerary b.
breath
    b. analysis
    liver b.
    b. sound
    b. test
    uremic b.
breath-holding
    b.-h. test
breathing
    apneustic b.
    ataxic b.
    b. bag
    Biot b.
    bronchial b.
    glossopharyngeal b.
    intermittent positive pressure b.
     (IPPB)
    mouth b.
    positive-negative pressure b. (PNPB)
    pursed lips b.
    b. reserve
    shallow b.
    stertorous b.
Breda disease
bredouillement
breech
    b. delivery
    b. extraction
    b. presentation
breeding
bregma
bregmatic fontanelle
bregmatolambdoid arc
bregmocardiac reflex
brei
bremsstrahlung
Brenner tumor
Breschet
    B. bone
    B. canal
    B. hiatus
    B. sinus
    B. vein
Brescia-Cimino fistula
Breslow thickness
bretylium tosylate
brevetoxins (BTX)
Brevibacterium
brevicollis
brevis
Brewer infarct
brewers' yeast
brickdust deposit
Bricker operation

brickmaker's anemia
bridge
    arteriolovenular b.
    cantilever b.
    caudolenticular gray b.
    cell b.
    b. corpuscle
    cystine b.
    cytoplasmic b.
    dentin b.
    disulfide b.
    extension b.
    fixed b.
    Gaskell b.
    intercellular b.
    myocardial b.
    removable b.
    salt b.
    transcapsular gray b.
    Wheatstone b.
bridgework
bridging hepatic necrosis
bridle
    b. of clitoris
    b. stricture
    b. suture
brief psychotherapy
Brigg test
Bright disease
brightness difference threshold
Brill disease
brilliant
    b. cresyl blue
    b. green
    b. vital red
    b. yellow
Brill-Zinsser disease
brim
    pelvic b.
Brimacombe fragment
brimstone
brindle
Brinell hardness number (BHN)
Briquet
    B. ataxia
    B. disease
    B. syndrome
brisement
Brissaud
    B. disease
    B. infantilism
    B. reflex
Brissaud-Marie syndrome
bristle cell
British
    B. anti-Lewisite (BAL)
    B. gum
    B. Pharmacopoeia
    B. thermal unit
brittle
    b. bone
    b. diabetes
    b. hair, impaired intellect, decreased
     fertility, short stature (BIDS)

B

broach
        barbed b.
        smooth b.
broad
        b. beta disease
        b. fascia
        b. ligament of the uterus
        b. spectrum
Broadbent
        B. law
        B. sign
broadest muscle of back
broad-spectrum
        b.-s. antibiotic
Broca
        B. aphasia
        B. basilar angle
        B. center
        B. diagonal band
        B. facial angle
        B. field
        B. fissure
        B. formula
        B. parolfactory area
        B. pouch
        B. visual plane
Brock
        B. operation
        B. syndrome
Brockenbrough sign
brocresine
Brödel bloodless line
Brodie
        B. abscess
        B. bursa
        B. disease
        B. fluid
        B. knee
        B. ligament
Brodmann areas
Broesike fossa
bromate
bromated
bromazepam
bromazine hydrochloride
bromcresol
        b. green
        b. purple
bromelain, bromelin
bromhexine hydrochloride
bromhidrosis
bromic
bromide acne
bromidrosiphobia
bromidrosis
brominated
bromindione
bromine (Br)
        b. water
bromism, brominism
bromobenzylcyanide (BBC)
bromocresol green
bromocriptine
bromodeoxyuridine (BrDu)
bromoderma

bromodiphenhydramine hydrochloride
bromohyperhidrosis, bromohyperidrosis
bromophenol blue
bromosulfophthalein
5-bromouracil
brompheniramine maleate
bromphenol
        b. blue
        b. test
Brompton cocktail
bromsulfophthalein
bromsulphalein test
bromthymol blue
broncatar
bronchi (*pl. of* bronchus)
bronchia
bronchial
        b. adenoma
        b. arteriography
        b. artery
        b. asthma
        b. atresia
        b. branch of thoracic aorta
        b. breathing
        b. breath sound
        b. bud
        b. calculus
        b. fremitus
        b. gland
        b. mucosa
        b. mucous gland adenoma
        b. pneumonia
        b. polyp
        b. respiration
        b. stenosis
        b. tube
        b. vein
        b. voice
bronchic cell
bronchiectasia sicca
bronchiectasis
        congenital b.
        cylindrical b.
        cystic b.
        dry b.
        saccular b.
        varicose b.
bronchiectatic
bronchiloquy
bronchiogenic
bronchiolar
        b. adenocarcinoma
        b. carcinoma
        b. exocrine cell
bronchiole
        respiratory b.
        terminal b.
bronchiolectasia
bronchiolectasis
bronchioli (*pl. of* bronchiolus)
bronchiolitis
        constrictive b.
        exudative b.
        b. fibrosa obliterans
        b. obliterans

b. obliterans with organizing
pneumonia (BOOP)
proliferative b.
bronchioloalveolar
b. adenocarcinoma
b. carcinoma
bronchiolopulmonary
bronchiolus, pl. **bronchioli**
bronchioli respiratorii
b. terminalis
bronchiostenosis
bronchitic asthma
bronchitis
asthmatic b.
Castellani b.
chronic b.
croupous b.
fibrinous b.
hemorrhagic b.
b. obliterans
obliterative b.
plastic b.
pseudomembranous b.
putrid b.
bronchium
bronchoalveolar
b. carcinoma
b. fluid
b. lavage (BAL)
bronchoaortic constriction
bronchobiliary fistula
bronchocavernous
bronchocavitary fistula
bronchocele
bronchoconstriction
bronchoconstrictor
bronchodilatation
bronchodilation
bronchodilator
bronchoedema
bronchoesophageal
b. fistula
b. muscle
bronchoesophageus muscle
bronchoesophagology
bronchoesophagoscopy
bronchofiberscope
bronchogenic
b. carcinoma
b. cyst
bronchogram
air b.
bronchography
tantalum b.
broncholith
broncholithiasis
bronchomalacia
bronchomediastinal (lymphatic) trunk
bronchomotor
bronchomycosis
bronchophony
whispered b.
bronchoplasty
bronchopleural (BP)
b. fistula

bronchopleural-cutaneous fistula
bronchopneumonia
postoperative b.
tuberculous b.
bronchopulmonary
b. dysplasia
b. lymph node
b. segment
b. sequestration
b. spirochetosis
bronchorrhaphy
bronchorrhea
bronchoscope
bronchoscopic
b. brush
b. smear
bronchoscopy
bronchospasm
bronchospasmolytic
bronchospirochetosis
bronchospirography
bronchospirometer
bronchospirometry
bronchostaxis
bronchostenosis
bronchostomy
bronchotomy
bronchotracheal
bronchovesicular
b. breath sound
b. respiration
bronchus, pl. **bronchi**
eparterial b.
hyparterial b.
intermediate b.
b. intermedius
intrasegmental b.
bronchi intrasegmentales
left main b.
lobar b.
bronchi lobares
b. lobaris inferior
b. lobaris medius
b. lobaris superior
mucoid impaction of b.
primary b.
b. principalis dexter
b. principalis sinister
right main b.
segmental b.
b. segmentalis
stem b.
**bronchus-associated lymphoid tissue
(BALT)**
Brønsted
B. acid
B. base
B. theory
brontophobia
bronze
b. baby syndrome
b. diabetes
bronzed
b. diabetes

B

bronzed *(continued)*
> b. disease
> b. skin

brood
> b. capsule
> b. cell

Brooke
> B. ileostomy
> B. tumor

brother complex
brotizolam
Broviac catheter
brown
> b. adipose tissue
> b. atrophy
> b. edema
> b. fat
> b. induration of the lung
> b. layer
> b. lung
> b. pellicle
> b. stria
> B. syndrome
> b. tumor

Brown-Adson forceps
Brown-Brenn stain
brownian
> b. motion
> b. movement

brownian-Zsigmondy movement
Browning vein
Brown-Séquard
> B.-S. paralysis
> B.-S. syndrome

brow presentation
Brucella
> *B. abortus*
> *B. canis*
> *B. melitensis*
> *B.* strain 19 vaccine
> *B. suis*

Brucellaceae
brucellergin
brucellin
brucellosis
> bovine b.

Bruce protocol
Bruch
> B. gland
> B. membrane

brucine
Bruck disease
Brücke
> B. muscle
> B. tunic

Brücke-Bartley phenomenon
Brudzinski sign
Brug filariasis
Brugia
> *B. malayi*

bruise
bruissement
bruit
> aneurysmal b.

> carotid b.
> b. de canon
> b. de claquement
> b. de cuir neuf
> b. de diable
> b. de frolement
> b. de galop
> b. de la roue de moulin
> b. de lime
> b. de rappel
> b. de Roger
> b. de scie
> b. de scie ou de rape
> b. de soufflet
> b. de tabourka
> b. de tambour
> b. de triolet
> Roger b.
> systolic b.
> thyroid b.
> Traube b.

Brunn
> B. membrane
> B. nest
> B. reaction

Brunner gland
Bruns
> B. ataxia
> B. nystagmus

Brunschwig operation
brush
> Ayre b.
> b. biopsy
> b. border
> bronchoscopic b.
> b. burn
> b. burn abrasion
> b. catheter
> denture b.
> Haidinger b.
> b. heap structure
> Kruse b.
> polishing b.

Brushfield spot
Brushfield-Wyatt disease
brushite
Bruton agammaglobulinemia
bruxism
Bryant traction
BSA
> bovine serum albumin

BSE
> bovine spongiform encephalopathy

BSER
> brainstem evoked response

BSP test
Bt$_2$cAMP
BTU
> british thermal unit

BTX
> brevetoxins

buaki
buba madre
bubas braziliana
bubble gum dermatitis

bubbling rale
bubo
>bullet b.
>chancroidal b.
>indolent b.
>malignant b.
>parotid b.
>primary b.
>tropical b.
>venereal b.
>virulent b.

bubonalgia
bubonic plague
bubonulus
bucardia
bucca, pl. **buccae**
buccal
>b. angle
>b. artery
>b. branch of facial nerve
>buccal node
>b. caries
>b. cavity
>b. curve
>b. digestion
>b. embrasure
>b. fat-pad
>b. flange
>b. gingiva
>b. gland
>b. lymph node
>b. nerve
>b. occlusion
>b. pit
>b. region
>b. root of tooth
>b. smear
>b. surface
>b. tablet
>b. vestibule

buccinator
>buccinator artery
>b. crest
>b. muscle
>b. nerve
>b. node

buccoaxial
buccoaxiocervical
buccoaxiogingival
buccocervical ridge
buccoclusal
buccodistal
buccogingival ridge
buccolabial
buccolingual
>b. diameter
>b. dimension
>b. relation

buccomesial
bucconasal membrane
bucconeural duct
buccooclusal angle
buccopharyngeal
>b. fascia
>b. membrane

>b. part of superior pharyngeal
>   constrictor

buccopulpal
buccoversion
buccula
Büchner
>B. extract
>B. funnel

buchu
Buchwald atrophy
buck
>B. extension
>B. fascia
>b. tooth
>B. traction

buckbean
bucket-handle
>b.-h. incision
>b.-h. tear

buckled
>b. aorta
>b. innominate artery

buckthorn polyneuropathy
Bucky diaphragm
buclizine hydrochloride
buclosamide
bucrylate
bud
>bronchial b.
>end b.
>b. fission
>gustatory b.
>limb b.
>liver b.
>lung b.
>median tongue b.
>metanephric b.
>periosteal b.
>b. stage
>syncytial b.
>tail b.
>taste b.
>tooth b.
>ureteric b.
>vascular b.

Budd-Chiari syndrome
buddeized milk
Budde process
budding
Budd syndrome
Budge center
Budin obstetrical joint
Buerger disease
bufadienolide
bufagenins
bufagins
bufanolide
bufenolide
buffalo
>b. hump
>b. neck
>b. type

buffer
>b. capacity
>dipolar b.

buffer *(continued)*
    b. index
    b. pair
    b. value
    b. value of the blood
    zwitterionic b.
buffered crystalline penicillin G
buffy
    b. coat
    b. coat concentration
bufogenins
Bufonidae
buformin
bufotenine
bufotoxin
bug
    assassin b.
buggery
bulb
    aortic b.
    arterial b.
    Braasch b.
    carotid b.
    b. of corpus spongiosum
    dental b.
    duodenal b.
    end b.
    b. of eye
    hair b.
    b. of hair
    jugular b.
    b. of jugular vein
    Krause end b.'s
    b. of occipital horn
    olfactory b.
    b. of penis
    b. of posterior horn of lateral
      ventricle of brain
    Rouget b.
    speech b.
    taste b.
    b. of urethra
    b. of vestibule
bulbar
    b. apoplexy
    b. conjunctiva
    b. corticonuclear fiber
    b. myelitis
    b. palsy
    b. paralysis
    b. pulse
    b. ridge
    b. septum
bulbi (*pl. of* bulbus)
bulbitis
bulbocapnine
bulbocavernosus
    b. muscle
    b. reflex
bulboid corpuscle
bulbomimic reflex
bulbonuclear
bulbopontine
bulboreticulospinal tract

bulbosacral system
bulbospinal
bulbospongiosus muscle
bulbourethral gland
bulbous bougie
bulboventricular
    b. loop
    b. ridge
bulbus, pl. **bulbi**
    b. aortae
    b. cordis
    b. cornus posterioris
    b. duodeni
    b. oculi
    b. olfactorius
    b. penis
    b. pili
    b. urethrae
    b. venae jugularis
    b. vestibuli vaginae
bulesis
bulging eye disease
bulimia nervosa
bulimic
Bulinus
bulkage
bulk modulus
bulky
    b. disease
    b. lymphadenopathy
bull.
bulla, pl. **bullae**
    ethmoidal b.
    b. ethmoidalis
    intraepidermal b.
    pulmonary b.
    subepidermal b.
bulldog
    b. forceps
    b. head
bullectomy
bullet
    b. bubo
    b. forceps
bull neck
bullous
    b. congenital ichthyosiform
      erythroderma
    b. edema
    b. edema vesicae
    b. emphysema
    b. impetigo of newborn
    b. keratopathy
    b. myringitis
    b. pemphigoid
bull's-eye maculopathy
bumetanide
Bumke pupil
BUN
    blood urea nitrogen
bunamidine hydrochloride
bundle
    aberrant b.
    anterior ground b.
    Arnold b.

atrioventricular b.
Bachmann b.
b. bone
comma b. of Schultze
Flechsig ground b.
Gantzer accessory b.
Gierke respiratory b.
ground b.
Held b.
Helie b.
Helweg b.
His b.
Hoche b.
hooked b. of Russell
Keith b.
Kent b.
Kent-His b.
Killian b.
Krause respiratory b.
lateral ground b.
lateral proprius b.
left b. of atrioventricular bundle
Lissauer b.
Loewenthal b.
longitudinal pontine b.
medial forebrain b.
medial longitudinal b.
Monakow b.
muscle b.
neurovascular b. of Walsh
oblique b. of pons
olfactory b.
olivocochlear b.
Pick b.
posterior longitudinal b.
precommissural b.
predorsal b.
b. of Rasmussen
Rathke b.
retroflex b. of Meynert
right b. of atrioventricular bundle
Schütz b.
solitary b.
tendon b.
Türck b.
uncinate b. of Russell
Vicq d'Azyr b.
bundle-branch block
bungarotoxins
bungpagga
bunion
bunionectomy
Keller b.
Mayo b.
Bunnell suture
bunodont
bunolol hydrochloride
bunolophodont
bunoselenodont
Bunostomum
B. phlebotomum
B. trigonocephalum
Bunsen
B. burner
B. solubility coefficient

Bunsen-Roscoe law
Bunyamwera
B. fever
B. virus
Bunyaviridae
bunyavirus encephalitis
buoyant density
buphthalmia, buphthalmos, buphthalmus
bupivacaine
buprenorphine hydrochloride
bupropion hydrochloride
bur
cross-cut b.
b. drill
end-cutting b.
finishing b.
fissure b.
inverted cone b.
round b.
Burchard-Liebermann reaction
Burdach
B. column
B. fasciculus
B. nucleus
B. tract
burden
clinical b.
genetic b.
global b. of disease
Burdwan fever
buret, burette
Bürger-Grütz
B.-G. disease
B.-G. syndrome
Burger triangle
Burgundy pitch
buried
b. flap
b. penis
b. suture
Burkholderia
B. cepacia
B. mallei
B. pseudomallei
Burkitt lymphoma
Burlew
B. disk
B. wheel
burn
brush b.
chemical b.
first-degree b.
flash b.
full-thickness b.
mat b.
partial-thickness b.
radiation b.
B. and Rand theory
rope b.
second-degree b.
superficial b.
thermal b.
third-degree b.
burners
burner syndrome

B

Burnett syndrome
burning
- b. drops sign
- b. foot syndrome
- b. mouth syndrome
- b. tongue
- b. tongue syndrome
- b. vulva syndrome

burnisher
burnout
Burns
- B. falciform process
- B. ligament
- B. space

burnt alum
Burow
- B. solution
- B. triangle
- B. vein

Burow
burr cell
burrow
burrowing hair
bursa, pl. **bursae**
- Achilles b.
- b. achillis
- b. of acromion
- adventitious b.
- b. anserina
- anserine b.
- anterior tibial b.
- bicipitoradial b.
- b. bicipitoradialis
- Boyer b.
- Brodie b.
- b. of calcaneal tendon
- Calori b.
- coracobrachial b.
- b. cubitalis interossea
- deep infrapatellar b.
- b. of extensor carpi radialis brevis muscle
- b. fabricii
- b. of Fabricius
- Fleischmann b.
- b. of gastrocnemius
- bursae of gastrocnemius
- gluteofemoral b.
- gluteus medius bursae
- gluteus minimus b.
- b. of great toe
- b. of hyoid
- iliac b.
- b. iliopectinea
- iliopectineal b.
- inferior subtendinous b. of biceps femoris
- infracardiac b.
- infrahyoid b.
- b. infrahyoidea
- b. infrapatellaris profunda
- infraspinatus b.
- intermuscular gluteal b.
- b. intermuscularis musculorum gluteorum

- interosseous cubital b.
- interosseous b. of elbow
- b. intratendinea olecrani
- intratendinous b. of elbow
- intratendinous olecranon b.
- b. ischiadica musculi glutei maximi
- b. ischiadica musculi obturatoris interni
- ischial b.
- laryngeal b.
- lateral malleolar subcutaneous b.
- lateral malleolus b.
- b. of latissimus dorsi
- Luschka b.
- medial malleolar subcutaneous b.
- b. of Monro
- b. mucosa
- b. musculi bicipitis femoris superior
- b. musculi coracobrachialis
- b. musculi extensoris carpi radialis brevis
- b. musculi piriformis
- b. musculi semimembranosi
- b. musculi tensoris veli palatini
- bursae of obturator internus
- b. of olecranon
- omental b.
- b. omentalis
- ovarian b.
- b. ovarica
- b. pharyngea
- pharyngeal b.
- b. of piriformis
- b. of popliteus
- prepatellar b.
- b. quadrati femoris
- radial b.
- retrocalcaneal b.
- retrohyoid b.
- b. retrohyoidea
- rider's b.
- sartorius bursae
- sciatic b. of gluteus maximus
- b. of semimembranosus muscle
- semimembranous b.
- subacromial b.
- b. subacromialis
- subcoracoid b.
- b. subcutanea acromialis
- b. subcutanea calcanea
- b. subcutanea infrapatellaris
- b. subcutanea malleoli lateralis
- b. subcutanea malleoli medialis
- b. subcutanea olecrani
- b. subcutanea prepatellaris
- b. subcutanea prominentiae laryngeae
- b. subcutanea trochanterica
- b. subcutanea tuberositatis tibiae
- subcutaneous acromial b.
- subcutaneous calcaneal b.
- subcutaneous infrapatellar b.
- subcutaneous b. of the laryngeal prominence
- subcutaneous b. of lateral malleolus
- subcutaneous b. of medial malleolus

subcutaneous olecranon b.
subcutaneous prepatellar b.
subcutaneous b. of teres major
subcutaneous b. of tibial tuberosity
subcutaneous b. of tuberosity of
tibia
subdeltoid b.
b. subdeltoidea
b. subfascialis prepatellaris
subfascial prepatellar b.
subhyoid b.
sublingual b.
b. sublingualis
subscapular b.
b. subtendineae musculi gastrocnemii
bursae subtendineae musculi
gastrocnemii
bursae subtendineae musculi sartorii
b. subtendinea iliaca
b. subtendinea musculi bicipitis
femoris inferior
b. subtendinea musculi infraspinati
b. subtendinea musculi latissimus
dorsi
b. subtendinea musculi obturatoris
interni
b. subtendinea musculi subscapularis
b. subtendinea musculi teretis
majoris
b. subtendinea musculi tibialis
anterioris
b. subtendinea musculi trapezii
b. subtendinea musculi tricipitis
brachii
b. subtendinea prepatellaris
subtendinous bursae of
gastrocnemius muscle
subtendinous iliac b.
subtendinous b. of iliacus
subtendinous b. of infraspinatus
subtendinous b. of latissimus dorsi
subtendinous prepatellar b.
subtendinous b. of sartorius
subtendinous b. of subscapularis
subtendinous b. of tibialis anterior
subtendinous b. of trapezius
subtendinous b. of triceps brachii
superior b. of biceps femoris
suprapatellar b.
b. suprapatellaris
synovial b.
b. synovialis
synovial trochlear b.
b. tendinis calcanei
b. of tendo calcaneus
b. of tensor veli palatine
b. of teres major
tibial intertendinous b.
b. of trapezius
triceps b.
trochanteric b.
b. trochanterica
bursae trochantericae musculi glutei
medii

b. trochanterica musculi glutei
maximi
b. trochanterica musculi glutei
minimi
trochanteric bursae of gluteus
medius
trochanteric bursae of gluteus
minimus
trochlear synovial b.
ulnar b.
bursal
b. abscess
b. cyst
b. synovitis
bursectomy
bursitis
anserine b.
calcific b.
ischial b.
olecranon b.
prepatellar b.
subacromial b.
subdeltoid b.
bursolith
bursopathy
bursotomy
burst
respiratory b.
b. size
bursula
b. testium
Burton line
Buruli ulcer
Busacca nodule
Buschke disease
Buschke-Ollendorf syndrome
bush yaws
buspirone hydrochloride
Busquet disease
busulfan
busulphan
butabarbital
butacaine sulfate
butamben
butane
butanoic acid
butanol
butanol-extractable
b.-e. iodine (BEI)
b.-e. iodine test
butanoyl
butaperazine
butaverine
butethamate
butethamine hydrochloride
buthiazide
buthionine sulfoximine
butoconazole nitrate
butopyronoxyl
butorphanol tartrate
butoxamine hydrochloride
t-**butoxycarbonyl (BOC,** *t*-**BOC, Boc)**
butriptyline hydrochloride
butt

B

butter
    b. of antimony
    b. of bismuth
    cacao b.
    cocoa b.
    b. stool
    b. of tin
    b. yellow
    b. of zinc
butterfly
    b. eruption
    b. fragment
    b. lung
    b. patch
    b. pattern
    b. rash
    b. vertebra
buttermilk
buttocks
button
    Biskra b.
    Murphy b.
    Oriental b.
    peritoneal b.
    b. suture
buttonhole
    b. iridectomy
    b. stenosis
buttress plate
butyl
    b. alcohol
    b. aminobenzoate
    primary b. alcohol
    secondary b. alcohol
    tertiary b. alcohol
butylated
    b. hydroxyanisole (BHA)
    b. hydroxytoluene (BHT)
tert-**butyloxycarbonyl (tBoc)**
butylparaben
butyraceous
butyrate

butyrate-CoA ligase
butyric
    b. acid
    normal b.
γ-butyrobetaine
butyrocholinesterase
butyroid
butyrometer
butyrophenone
butyrous
butyryl
butyrylcholine esterase
butyryl-CoA
    butyryl-CoA synthetase
buyo cheek cancer
Buzzard maneuver
Bwamba
    B. fever
    B. virus
By antigen
Byars flap
Byler disease
bypass
    aortocoronary b.
    aortoiliac b.
    aortorenal b.
    bowel b.
    cardiopulmonary b.
    coronary artery b.
    extraanatomic b.
    extracranial-intracranial b.
    femoropopliteal b.
    gastric b.
    jejunoileal b.
    left heart b.
    partial ileal b.
    right heart b.
byproduct material
byssinosis
bystander lysis
byte
Byzantine arch palate

C
>coulomb
>large calorie
>>C bile
>>C carbohydrate antigen
>>C cell
>>C chain
>>C factor
>>C fiber
>>C gene
>>C group viruses
>>C terminus
>>C value
>>C wave

C1
>>C1 esterase
>>C1 esterase inhibitor

^{12}C
>carbon-12

^{14}C
>carbon-14

^{13}C
>carbon-13

^{11}C
>carbon-11

c
>curie

c̄
>cum

CA
>carcinoma
>croup-associated

CA 125
Ca
>cathode

^{47}Ca
>calcium-47

^{45}Ca
>calcium-45

ca.
CA 125 antigen
CA 15-3 antigen
CA 19-9 antigen
caapi
CAAT box
cabbage
>c. goiter
>c. tree

Cabot-Locke murmur
Cabot ring body
cacao
>c. butter
>c. oil

CaCC
>cathodal closure contraction

cachectic
>c. diarrhea
>c. edema
>c. endocarditis
>c. fever
>c. pallor

cachectin

cachet
cachexia
>c. aphthosa
>c. aquosa
>diabetic neuropathic c.
>hypophyseal c.
>c. hypophyseopriva
>hypophysial c.
>malarial c.
>pituitary c.
>c. strumipriva
>c. thyroidea
>c. thyropriva

cachinnation
cacodyl
cacodylate
cacodylic acid
cacogeusia
cacomelia
cacoplastic
cacosmia
cactinomycin
cacumen, pl. **cacumina**
cacuminal
cadaver
cadaveric
>c. rigidity
>c. spasm

cadaverine
cadaverous
caddis worm
cade oil
cadherin
cadmium (Cd)
CaDTe
caduca
caduceus
caecum
caeruleun nucleus
caerulospinal tract
café au lait spot
cafe coronary
caffearine
caffeine
>c. citrate
>c. hydrate
>c. and sodium salicylate

caffeinism
Caffey
>C. disease
>C. syndrome

Caffey-Kempe syndrome
Caffey-Silverman syndrome
cage
>thoracic c.

Cagot ear
Cain complex
c-a interval (*var. of* cardioarterial interval)
caisson
>c. disease
>c. sickness

C

Cajal
    C. astrocyte stain
    C. cell
Cajal
cajeput oil
cajeputol, cajuputol
cake
    c. alum
    c. kidney
Cal
   large calorie
cal
   small calorie
Calabar
    C. bean
    C. swelling
calabash curare
calamine
calamus scriptorius
calcaneal, calcanean
    c. anastomosis
    c. apophysitis
    c. arterial network
    c. artery
    c. articular surface of talus
    c. bone
    c. branch
    c. gait
    c. petechia
    c. process of cuboid
    c. region
    c. sulcus
    c. tendon
    c. tuber
    c. tubercle
    c. tuberosity
calcanei (*pl. of* calcaneus)
calcaneoapophysitis
calcaneoastragaloid
calcaneocavus
calcaneocuboid
    c. joint
    c. ligament
calcaneodynia
calcaneofibular ligament
calcaneonavicular ligament
calcaneoscaphoid
calcaneotibial ligament
calcaneovalgocavus
calcaneovalgus
calcaneovarus
calcaneum
calcaneus, pl. **calcanei**
calcar
    c. avis
    c. femorale
    c. pedis
    c. sclera
calcareous
    c. corpuscle
    c. degeneration
    c. infiltration
    c. metastasis
    c. pancreatitis

calcarine
    c. artery
    c. branch of medial occipital artery
    c. fasciculus
    c. fissure
    c. spur
    c. sulcus
calcariuria
calcergy
calces (*pl. of* calx)
calcicosis
calcic water
calcidiol 1α-hydroxylase, 25-hydroxycholecalciferol 1α-hydroxylase
calcifediol
calciferol
calciferous
calcific
    c. bursitis
    c. nodular aortic stenosis
    c. pancreatitis
calcification
   dystrophic c.
   eggshell c.
   c. line of Retzius
   metastatic c.
   Mönckeberg medial c.
   pathologic c.
   pulp c.
calcified cartilage
calcify
calcifying
    c. epithelial odontogenic tumor
    c. and keratinizing odontogenic cyst
    c. odontogenic cyst
calcigerous
calcination
calcine
calcined magnesia
calcineurin
calcinosis
    c. circumscripta
    c. cutis
   dystrophic c.
    c. intervertebralis
    c., Raynaud phenomenon, esophageal motility disorder, sclerodactyly and telangiectasia (CREST)
   reversible c.
   tumoral c.
    c. universalis
calcinuric diabetes
calciokinesis
calciokinetic
calciol
calciorrhachia
calciostat
calciotraumatic
calcipectic
calcipenia
calcipenic
calcipexic
calcipexis, calcipexy
calciphilia
calciphylaxis

calciprivia
calciprivic
calcite
calcitetrol
calcitonin gene-related peptide (CGRP)
calcitriol
calcium
    c. alginate
    c. aminosalicylate
    c. antagonist
    c. benzoylpas
    c. bromide
    c. carbide
    c. carbimide
    c. carbonate
    c. caseinate
    c. channel blocker
    c. channel-blocking agent
    c. chloride
    citrated c. carbimide
    crude c. sulfide
    c. cyanamide
    dibasic c. phosphate
    c. folinate
    c. glubionate
    c. gluceptate
    c. glucoheptonate
    c. gluconate
    c. glycerophosphate
    c. gout
    c. group
    c. hippurate
    c. hydroxide
    c. hypophosphite
    c. iodate
    c. iodobehenate
    c. ipodate
    c. lactate
    c. lactophosphate
    c. leucovorin
    c. levulinate
    c. mandelate
    milk of c.
    c. monohydrogen phosphate
    c. oxalate
    c. oxide
    c. pantothenate
    precipitated c. carbonate
    c. propionate
    c. pump
    c. pyrophosphate deposition disease
      (CPPD)
    racemic c. pantothenate
    c. rigor
    c. saccharate
    secondary c. phosphate
    c. sign
    c. stearate
    c. sulfate
    c. sulfite
    tertiary c. phosphate
    tribasic c. phosphate

    c. trisodium pentetate
    c. tungstate
calcium-45 (^{45}Ca)
calcium-47 (^{47}Ca)
calciuria
calcophorous
calcospherite
calcspar
calculated
    c. mean organism (CMO)
    c. serum osmolality
calculosis
calculus, pl. **calculi**
    apatite c.
    arthritic c.
    biliary c.
    bladder c.
    blood c.
    branched c.
    bronchial c.
    cerebral c.
    coral c.
    cystine c.
    dendritic c.
    dental c.
    encysted c.
    fibrin c.
    gastric c.
    hematogenetic c.
    hemic c.
    infection c.
    intestinal c.
    lacrimal c.
    mammary c.
    matrix c.
    metabolic c.
    mulberry c.
    nasal c.
    oxalate c.
    pancreatic c.
    pharyngeal c.
    pleural c.
    pocketed c.
    preputial c.
    primary renal c.
    prostatic c.
    pulp c.
    renal c.
    salivary c.
    secondary renal c.
    serumal c.
    staghorn c.
    struvite c.
    subgingival c.
    supragingival c.
    C. Surface Index (CSI)
    tonsillar c.
    urethral c.
    urinary c.
    uterine c.
    vesical c.
    weddellite c.
    whewellite c.
Caldani ligament
caldesmon

C

Caldwell
    C. projection
    C. view
Caldwell-Luc operation
Caldwell-Moloy classification
calefacient
calf, pl. **calves**
    c. bone
    c. pump
calf-bone
caliber
calibrate
calibration
    c. curve
    c. interval
calibrator
caliceal diverticulum
calicectasis
calicectomy
calices (*pl. of* calix)
caliciform
    c. cell
    c. ending
calicine
Caliciviridae
Calicivirus
calicoplasty
calicotomy
caliculus, pl. **caliculi**
    c. gustatorius
    c. ophthalmicus
caliectasis
California
    C. encephalitis
    C. psychological inventory test
    C. virus
californium (Cf)
calioplasty
caliorrhaphy
caliotomy
caliper micrometer
calisthenics
calix, pl. **calices**
    major calices
    minor calices
    calices renales majores
    calices renales minores
Calkins sign
Callahan method
Callander amputation
Call-Exner body
Calliphora
Callison fluid
Callitroga
callosal
    c. convolution
    c. gyrus
    c. sulcus
callose
callosity
callosomarginal
    c. artery
    c. fissure
    c. sulcus
callous

callus
    central c.
    definitive c.
    ensheathing c.
    medullary c.
    permanent c.
    provisional c.
    temporary c.
calmative
Calmette-Guérin
    C.-G. bacillus
    C.-G. vaccine
Calmette test
calmodulin
Calodium
calomel
    c. electrode
    vegetable c.
calor
Calori bursa
caloric
    c. intake
    c. nystagmus
    c. test
    c. value
calorie
    gram c.
    large c. (C, Cal)
    mean c.
    small c. (cal)
calorific
calorigenic action
calorimeter
    Benedict-Roth c.
    bomb c.
calorimetric
calorimetry
    direct c.
    indirect c.
caloritropic
calory
Calot triangle
calpains
calsequestrin
calumba
calumbin
calusterone
calvaria, pl. **calvariae**
calvarial
    c. hook
calvarium
Calvé-Perthes disease
calves (*pl. of* calf)
calvities
calx, pl. **calces**
calyceal
calyces (*pl. of* calyx)
calyciform ending
calycine
calycle, calyculus
Calymmatobacterium granulomatis
calyx, pl. **calyces**
CAM
    cell adhesion molecule
cambendazole

cambium layer
camera, pl. **camerae**
    Anger c.
    c. anterior bulbi
    camerae bulbi
    gamma c.
    multiformat c.
    c. oculi anterior
    c. oculi major
    c. oculi minor
    c. oculi posterior
    c. posterior bulbi
    c. postrema
    retinal c.
    scintillation c.
    c. vitrea
    c. vitrea bulbi
    vitreous c.
camerostome
camisole
camomile
CAMP
    CAMP factor
    CAMP test
cAMP
    adenosine 3′,5′-cyclic monophosphate
    camp fever
    camp hospital
    cAMP phosphodiesterase
    cAMP receptor protein (CRP)
Campbell
    C. ligament
    C. sound
Camper
    C. chiasm
    C. fascia
    C. ligament
    C. line
    C. plane
camphene
camphor
    cantharis c.
    c. liniment
    monobromated c.
    tar c.
    thyme c.
camphoraceous
camphorated
    c. menthol
    c. oil
    c. phenol
campi foreli
campimeter
camplodactyly
campothecins
camptocormia
camptodactyly, camptodactylia
camptomelia
camptomelic
    c. dwarfism
    c. syndrome
camptospasm
camptothecin
Campylobacter
    C. coli

    C. concisus
    C. fetus
    C. fetus subsp. *jejuni*
    C. hyointestinalis
    C. jejuni
    C. lari
    C. pylori
    C. sputorum
campylobacteriosis
Canada
    C. balsam
    C. snakeroot
    C. turpentine
canadine
canal
    abdominal c.
    accessory c.
    adductor c.
    Alcock c.
    alimentary c.
    alveolar c. of maxilla
    alveolodental c.
    anal c.
    anterior condyloid c. of occipital bone
    anterior semicircular c.
    archenteric c.
    Arnold c.
    arterial c.
    atrioventricular c.
    auditory c.
    basipharyngeal c.
    Bernard c.
    Bichat c.
    birth c.
    blastoporic c.
    bony semicircular c.
    Böttcher c.
    Breschet c.
    carotid c.
    carpal c.
    caudal c.
    central c.
    central c. of cochlea
    central c. of spinal cord
    central c. of the vitreous
    cervical c.
    cervicoaxillary c.
    ciliary c.
    Civinini c.
    Cloquet c.
    cochlear c.
    condylar c.
    condyloid c.
    Corti c.
    Cotunnius c.
    craniopharyngeal c.
    deferent c.
    dental c.
    dentinal c.
    diploic c.
    Dorello c.
    Dupuytren c.
    ear c.
    endodermal c.

C

canal (*continued*)
endometrial c.
facial c.
fallopian c.
femoral c.
Ferrein c.
Fontana c.
galactophorous c.
Gartner c.
gastric c.
greater palatine c.
gubernacular c.
c. of Guyon
Guyon c.
gynecophoric c.
Hannover c.
haversian c.
Hensen c.
c. of Hering
Hirschfeld c.
Holmgrén-Golgi c.
c. of Hovius
Hoyer c.
Huguier c.
Hunter c.
hyaloid c.
hypoglossal c.
incisive c.
incisor c.
inferior dental c.
infraorbital c.
inguinal c.
interdental c.
interfacial c.
Jacobson c.
Kürsteiner c.
lateral c.
lateral semicircular c.
Laurer c.
Lauth c.
Leeuwenhoek c.
lesser palatine c.
c. for lesser palatine nerve
longitudinal c. of modiolus
Löwenberg c.
mandibular c.
marrow c.
mental c.
musculotubal c.
nasolacrimal c.
neural c.
neurenteric c.
notochordal c.
c. of Nuck
nutrient c.
obturator c.
optic c.
palatovaginal c.
parturient c.
pelvic c.
pericardioperitoneal c.
persistent atrioventricular c.
Petit c.
pharyngeal c.
c. for pharyngotympanic (auditory) tube
pleural c.
pleuropericardial c.
pleuroperitoneal c.
portal c.
posterior semicircular c.
pterygoid c.
pterygopalatine c.
pudendal c.
pulp c.
pyloric c.
Rivinus c.
root c. of tooth
Rosenthal c.
sacral c.
Santorini c.
c. of Scarpa
Schlemm c.
semicircular c.
semicircular c. of bony labyrinth
small c. of chorda tympani
Sondermann c.
spinal c.
spiral c. of cochlea
spiral c. of modiolus
Stilling c.
subsartorial c.
Sucquet c.
Sucquet-Hoyer c.
tarsal c.
temporal c.
c. for tensor tympani muscle
Theile c.
tubotympanic c.
tympanic c.
uniting c.
uterovaginal c.
van Horne c.
Velpeau c.
vertebral c.
vesicourethral c.
vestibular c.
vidian c.
Volkmann c.
vomerine c.
vomerobasilar c.
vomerorostral c.
vomerovaginal c.
Walther c.
Wirsung c.
canales (*pl. of* canalis)
canalicular
c. adenoma
c. duct
c. sphincter
canaliculi (*pl. of* canaliculus)
canaliculitis
canaliculization
canaliculus, pl. **canaliculi**
anterior c. of chorda tympani
auricular c.
biliary c.
bone c.
caroticotympanic canaliculi

canaliculi caroticotympanici
c. chordae tympani
c. of chorda tympani
c. cochleae
cochlear c.
canaliculi dentales
c. innominatus
intercellular c.
intracellular c.
lacrimal c.
c. lacrimalis
mastoid c.
c. mastoideus
posterior c. of chorda tympani
c. reuniens
secretory c.
Thiersch canaliculi
tympanic c.
c. tympanicus
canalis, pl. **canales**
c. adductorius
canales alveolares corporis maxillae
c. analis
c. caroticus
c. carpi
c. centralis medullae spinalis
c. cervicis uteri
c. condylaris
canales diploici
c. femoralis
c. gastricus
c. hyaloideus
c. hypoglossalis
canales incisivi
c. infraorbitalis
c. inguinalis
canales longitudinales modioli
c. mandibulae
c. musculotubarius
c. nasolacrimalis
c. nervi facialis
c. nervi petrosi superficialis minoris
c. nutricius
c. obturatorius
c. opticus
canales palatini minores
c. palatinus major
c. palatovaginalis
c. pterygoideus
c. pudendalis
c. pyloricus
c. radicis dentis
c. reuniens
c. sacralis
canales semicircularis anterior
canales semicircularis lateralis
canales semicircularis ossei
canales semicircularis posterior
c. spiralis cochleae
c. spiralis modioli
c. umbilicalis
c. vertebralis
c. vomerorostralis
c. vomerovaginalis
canalization

Canavan
C. disease
C. sclerosis
canavanase
canavanine
Canavan-van Bogaert-Bertrand disease
cancellated
cancellous
c. bone
c. tissue
cancellus, pl. **cancelli**
cancer
c. antigen 125 test
betel c.
buyo cheek c.
chimney sweep's c.
colloid c.
conjugal c.
c. à deux
c. en cuirasse
epidermoid c.
epithelial c.
familial c.
c. family
glandular c.
hereditary nonpolyposis colorectal c.
kang c.
kangri c.
mouse c.
mule-spinner's c.
paraffin c.
pipe-smoker's c.
pitch-worker's c.
scar c.
scar c. of the lung
stump c.
telangiectatic c.
cancerophobia
cancerous
cancra (*pl. of* cancrum)
cancriform
cancroid
cancrum, pl. **cancra**
c. nasi
c. oris
candela (cd)
candicans
candicidin
Candida
C. albicans
C. glabrata
C. parapsilosis
C. tropicalis
candidemia
candidiasis
candidosis
candle
candle-meter
candle-power
cane sugar
canicola fever
Canidae
canine
c. adenovirus 1
c. amebiasis

canine *(continued)*
    c. carcinoma 1
    c. distemper virus
    c. eminence
    c. fossa
    c. leishmaniasis
    c. prominence
    c. spasm
    c. tooth
caniniform
canister
canities
    canities c.
    c. circumscripta
    rapid c.
canker
    c. sore
    water c.
cannabidiol
cannabinoid
cannabinol
cannabis
cannabism
Cannizzaro reaction
cannon
    C. point
    C. ring
    c. sound
    C. theory
    c. wave
cannonball pulse
Cannon-Bard theory
cannula
    Hasson c.
    Karman c.
    laparoscopic c.
    perfusion c.
    washout c.
cannulation, cannulization
Cantelli sign
cantering rhythm
canthal hypertelorism
cantharidal collodion
cantharidate
cantharides (*pl. of* cantharis)
cantharidic acid
cantharidin
cantharis, pl. **cantharides**
    c. camphor
canthectomy
canthi (*pl. of* canthus)
canthitis
cantholysis
canthomeatal plane
canthoplasty
canthorrhaphy
canthotomy
canthus, pl. **canthi**
    external c.
    internal c.
    lateral c.
    medial c.

cantilever
    c. beam
    c. bridge
Cantor tube
CaOC
    cathodal opening contraction
caoutchouc pelvis
CAP
    catabolite gene activator protein
cap
    acrosomal c.
    apical c.
    cervical c.
    chin c.
    cradle c.
    dental c.
    duodenal c.
    enamel c.
    head c.
    metanephric c.
    phrygian c.
    pyloric c.
    c. splint
    c. stage
capacitance
capacitation
capacitor
capacity
    buffer c.
    carrying c.
    cranial c.
    diffusing c.
    forced vital c. (FVC)
    functional residual c. (FRC)
    heat c.
    inspiratory c.
    iron-binding c. (IBC)
    maximum breathing c. (MBC)
    oxygen c.
    residual c.
    respiratory c.
    thermal c.
    total lung c.
    vital c.
capactin
CAPD
    continuous ambulatory peritoneal dialysis
capeline bandage
Capgras
    C. phenomenon
    C. syndrome
capillarectasia
Capillaria
    C. granuloma
    C. hepatica
    C. philippinensis
capillariasis
    intestinal c.
capillariomotor
capillarioscopy
capillaritis
capillarity
capillaron
capillaropathy
capillaroscopy

capillary
   c. angioma
   arterial c.
   c. arteriole
   c. attraction
   c. bed
   bile c.
   blood c.
   c. circulation
   continuous c.
   c. drainage
   fenestrated c.
   c. fracture
   c. fragility
   c. fragility test
   c. hemangioma
   c. hemangioma of infancy
   c. lake
   c. lamina of choroid
   c. loop
   lymph c.
   c. nevus
   c. permeability factor
   c. pulse
   c. resistance test
   sinusoidal c.
   c. vein
   venous c.
   c. vessel
   c. zone electrophoresis (CZE)
Capim virus
capita (*pl. of* caput)
capitate bone
capitation
capitellum
capitopedal
capitular joint
capitulum, pl. **capitula**
   c. humeri
   c. of humerus
Caplan
   C. nodule
   C. syndrome
Capnocytophaga
   C. canimorsus
capnogram
capnograph
capnometry
capon-comb unit
capon unit
capping
   direct pulp c.
   indirect pulp c.
   c. protein
Capps reflex
caprate
capreomycin sulfate
***n*-capric acid**
capriloquism
caprin
caprine
Capripoxvirus
caprizant
caproate
***n*-caproic acid**

caproyl
caproylate
caprylate
caprylic acid
capsaicin
capsicin
capsicum
capsid
capsomer, capsomere
capsula, pl. **capsulae**
   c. adiposa perirenalis
   c. adiposa renis
   c. articularis
   c. articularis cricoarytenoidea
   c. articularis cricothyroidea
   c. bulbi
   c. cordis
   c. externa
   c. extrema
   c. fibrosa
   c. fibrosa glandulae thyroideae
   c. fibrosa perivascularis
   c. fibrosa renis
   c. glomeruli
   c. interna
   c. lentis
   c. lienis
   c. vasculosa lentis
capsular
   c. advancement
   c. antigen
   c. branch of intrarenal artery
   c. branch of renal artery
   c. cataract
   c. cirrhosis of liver
   c. flap pyeloplasty
   c. ligament
   c. precipitation reaction
   c. space
capsulation
capsule
   adipose c.
   adrenal c.
   articular c.
   atrabiliary c.
   auditory c.
   bacterial c.
   Bonnet c.
   Bowman c.
   brood c.
   cartilage c.
   c. cell
   cricoarytenoid articular c.
   c. of cricoarytenoid joint
   cricothyroid articular c.
   c. of cricothyroid joint
   Crosby c.
   crystalline c.
   external c.
   extreme c.
   eye c.
   fatty renal c.
   fibrous c.
   fibrous articular c.
   fibrous c. of kidney

C

capsule *(continued)*
  fibrous c. of liver
  fibrous c. of parotid gland
  fibrous c. of spleen
  fibrous c. of thyroid gland
  c. forceps
  Gerota c.
  Glisson c.
  glomerular c.
  internal c.
  joint c.
  c. of lens
  lens c.
  lenticular c.
  malpighian c.
  Müller c.
  nasal c.
  optic c.
  otic c.
  perirenal fat c.
  perivascular fibrous c.
  radiotelemetering c.
  seminal c.
  suprarenal c.
  Tenon c.
capsulectomy
capsulitis
  adhesive c.
  hepatic c.
capsulolenticular cataract
capsuloplasty
capsulorrhaphy
capsulorrhexis
capsulotome
capsulotomy
  renal c.
captopril
capture
  atrial c.
  electron c.
  K c.
  ventricular c.
capture-recapture method
Capuron point
caput, pl. **capita**
  c. angulare quadrati labii superioris
  c. breve
  c. breve musculi bicipitis brachii
  c. breve musculi bicipitis femoris
  c. costae
  c. epididymidis
  c. epididymis
  c. femoris
  c. fibulae
  c. gallinaginis
  c. humerale
  c. humerale musculi flexoris carpi ulnaris
  c. humerale musculi pronatoris teretis
  c. humeri
  c. humeroulnare musculi flexoris digitorum superificialis

  c. infraorbitale quadrati labii superioris
  c. laterale
  c. laterale musculi gastrocnemii
  c. laterale musculi tricipitis brachii
  c. longum
  c. longum musculi bicipitis brachii
  c. longum musculi bicipitis femoris
  c. longum musculi tricipitis brachii
  c. mallei
  c. mandibulae
  c. mediale
  c. mediale musculi gastrocnemii
  c. mediale musculi tricipitis brachii
  c. medusae
  c. nuclei caudati
  c. obliquum
  c. obliquum musculi adductoris hallucis
  c. obliquum musculi adductoris pollicis
  c. ossis femoris
  c. ossis metacarpalis
  c. ossis metatarsalis
  c. pancreatis
  c. phalangis (manus et pedis)
  c. profundum musculi flexoris pollicis brevis
  c. quadratum
  c. radii
  c. stapedis
  c. succedaneum
  c. superficiale musculi flexoris pollicis brevis
  c. tali
  c. transversum
  c. transversum musculi adductoris hallucis
  c. transversum musculi adductoris pollicis
  c. ulnae
  c. ulnare
  c. ulnare musculi flexoris carpi ulnaris
  c. ulnare musculi pronatoris teretis
  c. zygomaticum quadrati labii superioris
Carabelli tubercle
caramel
caramiphen ethanedisulfonate
caramiphen hydrochloride
Caraparu virus
carate
carbachol
carbacrylamine resin
carbadox
carbamate kinase
carbamazepine
carbamic acid
carbamide
carbamino compound
carbaminohemoglobin
carbamoate
carbamoyl
carbamoylaspartate dehydrase

N-carbamoylaspartic acid
carbamoylation
carbamoylcarbamic acid
N-carbamoylglutamic acid
carbamoyl phosphate synthetase
carbamoyltransferase
carbamoylurea
carbamyl
carbamylation
carbamylcholine chloride
carbanion
carbapenem
carbaril
carbarsone
carbaryl
carbazide
carbazochrome salicylate
carbazole
carbazotic acid
carbenicillin disodium
carbenium
carbetapentane citrate
carbhemoglobin
carbide
carbidopa
carbimazole
carbinol
carbinoxamine maleate
carbo
    charcoal
carbobenzoxy- (Cbz)
carbocation
carbogen
carbohemoglobin
carbohydrate
    c. loading
    c. metabolism
    c. utilization test
carbohydrate-induced hyperlipemia
carbohydraturia
carbohydrazide
carbolate
carbolated
carbol fuchsin
carbol-fuchsin paint
carbolic acid
carbolize
carbol-thionin stain
carboluria
carbomer
carbometry
carbomycin
carbon
    activated c. dioxide
    active c. dioxide
    anomeric c.
    c. autotrophy
    c. bisulfide
    c. cycle
    c. dichloride
    c. dioxide
    c. dioxide acidosis
    c. dioxide combining power
    c. dioxide content
    c. dioxide cycle

    c. dioxide electrode
    c. dioxide elimination ($\dot{V}_{CO2}$)
    c. dioxide-free water
    c. dioxide snow
    c. disulfide
    c. disulfide poisoning
    c. monoxide (CO)
    c. monoxide hemoglobin
    c. monoxide poisoning
    c. tetrachloride
carbon-11 (^{11}C)
carbon-12 (^{12}C)
carbon-13 (^{13}C)
carbon-14 (^{14}C)
carbonate
    c. dehydratase
    c. dehydratase inhibitor
    c. hydro-lyase
carbonated water
carbonic
    c. acid
    c. acid gas
    c. anhydrase
    c. anhydrase II deficiency syndrome
    c. anhydrase inhibitor
    c. anhydride
    c. water
carbonium
carbonmonoxy myoglobin
carbonometer
carbonometry
carbonuria
carbonyl
carboplatin
carboprost tromethamine
carboxamide
carboximide
N-carboxyanhydrides
carboxycathepsin
carboxydismutase
4-carboxyglutamic acid (Gla)
carboxyhemoglobin (HbCO)
carboxyhemoglobinemia
carboxyl
carboxylase
carboxylation
carboxylic acid
    activated c. a.
    c. a. ester
carboxyltransferases
carboxymethylcellulose
carboxymethyl radical (CM-)
carboxypeptidase
    c. A, B, C, G
    acid c.
    serine c.
carboxyterminal
N-carboxyurea
carbromal
carbuncle
    kidney c.
    renal c.
carburet
carbutamide
carbuterol hydrochloride

C

carcase
carcass
carcinoembryonic antigen (CEA)
carcinogen
    complete c.
carcinogenesis
    field c.
carcinogenic
carcinogenicity
carcinoid
    c. flush
    c. syndrome
    c. tumor
carcinolytic
carcinoma, pl. **carcinomas (CA)**
    acinar c.
    acinic cell c.
    adenoid cystic c.
    adenosquamous c.
    adnexal c.
    adrenal cortical carcinoma
    alveolar cell c.
    anaplastic c.
    apocrine c.
    basaloid c.
    basal squamous cell c.
    basisquamous c.
    basosquamous c.
    c. of the breast
    bronchiolar c.
    bronchioloalveolar c.
    bronchoalveolar c.
    bronchogenic c.
    canine c. 1
    clear cell c.
    clear cell c. of kidney
    clear cell c. of salivary gland
    cloacogenic c.
    colloid c.
    cuboid c.
    cylindromatous c.
    cystic c.
    duct c.
    ductal c.
    embryonal c.
    endometrioid c.
    epidermoid c.
    epithelial myoepithelial c.
    c. ex pleomorphic adenoma
    fibrolamellar liver cell c.
    follicular carcinoma
    giant cell c.
    giant cell c. of thyroid gland
    glandular c.
    hepatocellular c.
    Hürthle cell c.
    inflammatory c.
    intraductal c.
    intraepidermal c.
    intraepithelial c.
    invasive c.
    juvenile c.
    kangri burn c.
    large cell c.
    latent c.

lateral aberrant thyroid c.
    leptomeningeal c.
    liver cell c.
    lobular c.
    lobular c. in situ
    medullary c.
    medullary c. of breast
    medullary c. of thyroid
    meningeal c.
    metaplastic c.
    metastatic c.
    microinvasive c.
    mucinous c.
    mucoepidermoid c.
    nasopharyngeal c.
    noninfiltrating lobular c.
    oat cell c.
    occult c.
    oncocytic c.
    oxyphilic c.
    papillary c.
    polymorphous low-grade c. of
      salivary gland
    primary c.
    primary neuroendocrine c. of the
      skin
    c. of the prostate
    renal cell c.
    sarcomatoid c.
    scar c.
    scirrhous c.
    secondary c.
    secretory c.
    signet-ring cell c.
    c. in situ (CIS)
    small cell c.
    spindle cell c.
    squamous cell c.
    sweat gland c.
    terminal duct c.
    trabecular c.
    transitional cell c.
    tubular c.
    urothelial c.
    V-2 c.
    verrucous c.
    villous c.
    wolffian duct c.
    yolk sac c.
carcinomatosis
    leptomeningeal c.
    lymphangitic c.
    meningeal c.
carcinomatous
    c. encephalomyelopathy
    c. implant
    c. myelopathy
    c. myopathy
    c. neuromyopathy
    c. pericarditis
carcinophobia
carcinosarcoma
carcinostatic
carcoma
cardamom

Carden amputation
cardenolide
cardia
cardiac
    c. accident
    c. albuminuria
    c. alternation
    c. aneurysm
    c. antrum
    c. arrest
    c. arrhythmia
    c. asthma
    c. ballet
    c. catheter
    c. cirrhosis
    c. competence
    c. contractility
    c. cycle
    c. decompression
    c. depressor reflex
    c. diuretic
    c. dropsy
    c. dyspnea
    c. dysrhythmia
    c. edema
    c. failure
    c. fibrous skeleton
    c. ganglia
    c. gating
    c. gland
    c. gland of esophagus
    c. gland of stomach
    c. glycoside
    c. heterotaxia
    c. histiocyte
    c. hormone
    c. impression of diaphragmatic
      surface of liver
    c. impression on lung
    c. impulse
    c. incompetence
    c. index
    c. infarction
    c. insufficiency
    c. jelly
    c. liver
    c. lung
    c. lymphatic ring
    c. mapping
    c. massage
    c. monitor
    c. murmur
    c. muscle
    c. muscle tissue
    c. muscle wrap
    c. neurosis
    c. notch
    c. notch of left lung
    c. opening
    c. orifice
    c. output
    c. part of stomach
    c. plexus
    c. polyp
    c. prominence

    c. reserve
    c. segment
    c. shock
    c. skeleton
    c. souffle
    c. sound
    c. standstill
    c. syncope
    c. tamponade
    c. telemetry
    c. tube
    c. valve prosthesis
    c. valvular incompetence
    c. vein
cardial
    c. notch
    c. orifice
    c. part of stomach
cardialgia
cardiataxia
cardiatelia
cardiectasia
cardiectomy
cardiectopia
cardinal
    c. ligament
    c. ocular movement
    c. point
    c. symptom
    c. vein
carding
cardioaccelerator
cardioactive
cardioangiography
cardioaortic
Cardiobacterium
    c. hominis
    c. violaceum
cardiocele
cardiochalasia
cardiodiaphragmatic angle
cardiodiosis
cardiodynamics
cardiodynia
cardioesophageal
    c. junction
    c. relaxation
cardiofacial syndrome
cardiogenesis
cardiogenic
    c. plate
    c. shock
cardiogram
    esophageal c.
cardiograph
cardiography
    ultrasonic c.
    ultrasound c.
cardiohemothrombus
cardiohepatic
    c. angle
    c. triangle
cardiohepatomegaly
cardioid condenser
cardioinhibitory

C

cardiokymogram
cardiokymograph
cardiokymography
cardiolipin
cardiologist
cardiology
cardiolysis
cardiomalacia
cardiomegaly
    glycogen c.
    glycogenic c.
cardiometry
cardiomotility
cardiomuscular
cardiomyopathy
    alcoholic c.
    congestive c.
    dilated c.
    familial hypertrophic c.
    hypertrophic c.
    idiopathic c.
    peripartum c.
    postpartum c.
    primary c.
    restrictive c.
    secondary c.
cardiomyoplasty
cardiomyotomy
cardionatrin
cardionecrosis
cardionector
cardionephric
cardioneural
cardioneurosis
cardioomentopexy
cardiopaludism
cardiopath
cardiopathia nigra
cardiopathy
cardiophobia
cardiophone
cardiophony
cardiophrenia
cardiophrenic angle
cardioplasty
cardioplegia
    antegrade c.
    retrograde c.
cardioplegic arrest
cardioptosia
cardiopulmonary
    c. arrest
    c. bypass
    c. murmur
    c. resuscitation (CPR)
    c. splanchnic nerve
    c. transplantation
cardiopyloric
cardiorenal
cardiorespiratory murmur
cardiorrhaphy
cardiorrhexis
cardioscope
cardioselective
cardioselectivity

cardiospasm
cardiosphygmograph
cardiotachometer
cardiothoracic ratio
cardiothrombus
cardiothyrotoxicosis
cardiotomy
cardiotonic
cardiotoxic myolysis
cardiotoxin
cardiovalvulitis
cardiovascular
    c. radiology
    c. syphilis
    c. system
cardiovasculare
cardiovasculorenal
cardioversion
cardiovert
cardioverter
Cardiovirus
carditis
    rheumatic c.
care
    comprehensive medical c.
    end-of-life c.
    health c.
    intensive c.
    managed c.
    medical c.
    primary medical c.
    secondary medical c.
    tertiary medical c.
Carey Coombs murmur
caribi
carica
caries
    active c.
    arrested dental c.
    buccal c.
    cemental c.
    compound c.
    dental c.
    distal c.
    fissure c.
    incipient c.
    interdental c.
    mesial c.
    nursing bottle c.
    occlusal c.
    pit c.
    pit and fissure c.
    primary c.
    proximal c.
    radiation c.
    recurrent c.
    root c.
    secondary c.
    senile dental c.
    smooth surface c.
carina, pl. carinae
    c. fornicis
    c. of trachea
    c. tracheae
    tracheal c.

c. urethralis vaginae
urethral c. of vagina
c. vaginae
carinal lymph node
carinate abdomen
cariogenesis
cariogenic
cariogenicity
cariology
cariostatic
carious
carisoprodate
carisoprodol
carissin
Carlen tube
carmalum
Carman sign
carminate
carminative
carmine
lithium c.
Schneider c.
carminic acid
carminophil, carminophile, carminophilous
Carmody
Carmody-Batson operation
carmustine (BCNU)
carnassial tooth
carnauba wax
carneous
c. degeneration
c. mole
carnes (*pl. of* caro)
Carnett sign
Carney complex
carnification
carnitine
c. acetyltransferase
c. acylcarnitine translocase
c. deficiency
c. palmitoyltransferase
Carnivora
carnivore
carnivorous
carnosinase
carnosine
carnosinemia
carnosity
Carnoy fixative
caro, pl. **carnes**
c. quadrata sylvii
carob flour
Caroli
C. disease
C. syndrome
carotenase
carotenemia
carotene oxidase
carotenoderma
carotenoid
carotenoid
carotenoprotein
carotenosis cutis
carotic

caroticoclinoid ligament
caroticotympanic
c. artery (of internal carotid artery)
c. canaliculi
c. nerve
carotid
c. artery
c. body
c. body tumor
c. branch of glossopharyngeal nerve (CN IX)
c. bruit
c. bulb
c. canal
c. duct
c. endarterectomy
c. foramen
c. ganglion
c. groove
c. pulse
c. sheath
c. shudder
c. sinus
c. sinus branch
c. sinus nerve
c. sinus reflex
c. sinus syncope
c. sinus syndrome
c. sinus test
c. sulcus
c. triangle
c. tubercle
c. wall of middle ear
c. wall of tympanic cavity
carotid-cavernous fistula
carotidynia
carotinemia
carotinosis cutis
carotodynia
carpal
c. arch
c. artery
c. articular surface of radius
c. bone
c. canal
c. groove
c. joint
c. tendinous sheath
c. tunnel
c. tunnel syndrome
carpectomy
Carpenter syndrome
Carpentier-Edwards valve
carphenazine maleate
carpi (*pl. of* carpus)
carp mouth
carpocarpal
Carpoglyphus
carpometacarpal
c. joint
c. joint of thumb
c. ligament dorsal and palmar
carpopedal spasm
carpoptosia

carpoptosis
carpus, pl. **carpi**
    c. curvus
carrageen, carragheen
carrageenan, carrageenin
carre-four sensitif
Carrel-Lindbergh pump
Carrel treatment
carrier
    amalgam c.
    c. cell
    convalescent c.
    c. electrophoresis
    genetic c.
    hydrogen c.
    incubatory c.
    latent c.
    manifesting c.
    c. screening
    c. state
    c. strain
    translocation c.
carrier-free
Carrington disease
Carrión disease
Carr-Price
    C.-P. reaction
    C.-P. test
Carr-Purcell experiment
carrying
    c. angle
    c. capacity
carry-over
car sickness
cartesian nomogram
carthamus
cartilage
    accessory c.
    accessory nasal c.
    accessory quadrate c.
    c. of acoustic meatus
    alisphenoid c.
    anular c.
    arthrodial c.
    articular c.
    arytenoid c.
    c. of auditory tube
    auricular c.
    basilar c.
    c. bone
    branchial c.
    calcified c.
    c. capsule
    c. cell
    cellular c.
    ciliary c.
    circumferential c.
    conchal c.
    connecting c.
    corniculate c.
    costal c.
    cricoid c.
    cuneiform c.
    diarthrodial c.
    c. of ear

    elastic c.
    ensiform c.
    ensisternum c.
    epiglottic c.
    epiphysial c.
    falciform c.
    floating c.
    greater alar c.
    Huschke c.
    hyaline c.
    hypsiloid c.
    interosseous c.
    intervertebral c.
    intraarticular c.
    intrathyroid c.
    investing c.
    Jacobson c.
    c. knife
    c. lacuna
    c. of larynx
    lateral c. of nose
    lesser alar c.
    loose c.
    Luschka c.
    major alar c.
    mandibular c.
    c. matrix
    meatal c.
    Meckel c.
    Meyer c.
    minor alar c.
    Morgagni c.
    nasal septal c.
    c. of nasal septum
    c. of nose
    ossifying c.
    parachordal c.
    paraseptal c.
    parenchymatous c.
    periotic c.
    permanent c.
    pharyngeal c.
    c. of pharyngotympanic tube
    precursory c.
    primordial c.
    quadrangular c.
    Reichert c.
    reticular c.
    retiform c.
    Santorini c.
    Seiler c.
    semilunar c.
    septal nasal c.
    sesamoid c. of cricopharyngeal
      ligament
    sesamoid c. of larynx
    sesamoid c. of nose
    slipping rib c.
    c. space
    sternal c.
    supra-arytenoid c.
    tarsal c.
    temporary c.
    thyroid c.
    tracheal c.

triangular c.
triquetrous c.
triticeal c.
tubal c.
uniting c.
vomerine c.
vomeronasal c.
Weitbrecht c.
Wrisberg c.
xiphoid c.
Y c.
yellow c.
Y-shaped c.
cartilage-hair hypoplasia
cartilagines (*pl. of* cartilago)
cartilaginoid
cartilaginous
    c. articulation
    c. joint
    c. neurocranium
    c. part of external acoustic meatus
    c. part of nasal septum
    c. part of pharyngotympanic tube
    c. part of skeletal system
    c. septum
    c. tissue
    c. viscerocranium
cartilago, pl. **cartilagines**
    cartilagines alares minores
    c. alaris major
    c. articularis
    c. arytenoidea
    c. auriculae
    c. corniculata
    c. costalis
    c. cricoidea
    c. cuneiformis
    c. epiglottica
    c. epiphysialis
    cartilagines laryngis
    c. meatus acustici
    cartilagines nasales accessoriae
    cartilagines nasi
    c. nasi lateralis
    c. septi nasi
    c. sesamoidea laryngis
    c. sesamoidea ligamentum
      cricopharyngeum
    c. thyroidea
    cartilagines tracheales
    c. triticea
    c. tubae auditivae
    c. vomeronasalis
caruncle
    lacrimal c.
    Morgagni c.
    Santorini major c.
    Santorini minor c.
    urethral c.
caruncula, pl. **carunculae**
    hymenal c.
    c. hymenalis
    c. lacrimalis
    c. myrtiformis
    c. salivaris

    sublingual c.
    c. sublingualis
Carus
    C. circle
    C. curve
carvacrol
Carvallo sign
carvedilol
carver
caryophyllum
caryophyllus
caryotheca
Casal necklace
casamino acid
cascade stomach
cascara
    c. amara
    c. sagrada
case
    borderline c.
    c. control study
    c. fatality rate
    c. fatality ratio
    index c.
    c. management
    trial c.
caseation necrosis
casein
    iodinated c.
    c. iodine
    plant c.
caseinate
caseinogen
caseo-iodine
caseose
caseous
    c. abscess
    c. degeneration
    c. necrosis
    c. osteitis
    c. pneumonia
    c. rhinitis
    c. tubercle
Casoni
    C. antigen
    C. intradermal test
    C. skin test
cassava starch
Casselberry position
Casser
    C. fontanelle
    C. perforated muscle
casserian
cassette
    c. mutagenesis
    susceptibility c.
cassia
    c. bark
    c. cinnamon
    c. fistula
    c. oil
cast
    bacterial c.
    blood c.
    c. brace

C

cast (*continued*)
    coma c.
    decidual c.
    dental c.
    diagnostic c.
    epithelial c.
    false c.
    fatty c.
    fibrinous c.
    granular c.
    hair c.
    halo c.
    hyaline c.
    investment c.
    master c.
    mucous c.
    red blood cell c.
    red cell c.
    refractory c.
    renal c.
    spica c.
    spurious c.
    tube c.
    urinary c.
    waxy c.
    white blood cell c.
    white cell c.
Castellani
    C. bronchitis
    C. paint
Castile soap
casting
    centrifugal c.
    ceramo-metal c.
    c. flask
    gold c.
    c. ring
    vacuum c.
    c. wax
Castle intrinsic factor
Castleman disease
castor bean
castor oil
    aromatic c. o.
castrate
castration
    c. anxiety
    c. cell
    c. complex
    functional c.
casualty
CAT
    computerized axial tomography
    cat unit
catabasial
catabiotic
catabolic
catabolism
catabolite
    c. gene activator (CGA)
    c. gene activator protein (CAP)
    c. repression
catachronobiology
catacrotic pulse

catacrotism
catadicrotic pulse
catadicrotism
catadidymus
catadioptric
catadromous
catagen
catagenesis
catalase
catalatic reaction
catalepsy
cataleptic
cataleptoid
catalysis
    contact c.
    surface c.
catalyst
    inorganic c.
    negative c.
    organic c.
    Raney c.
catalytic
    c. antibody
    c. center
catalyze
catalyzer
catamenial pneumothorax
catamnesis
catamnestic
catapasm
cataphoresis
cataphoretic
cataplasia, cataplasis
cataplasm
cataplectic
cataplexy
cataract
    anular c.
    atopic c.
    axial c.
    black c.
    blue c.
    capsular c.
    capsulolenticular c.
    central c.
    cerulean c.
    complete c.
    complicated c.
    concussion c.
    congenital c.
    copper c.
    coralliform c.
    coronary c.
    cortical c.
    crystalline c.
    cuneiform c.
    cupuliform c.
    dendritic c.
    diabetic c.
    disk-shaped c.
    electric c.
    embryonic c.
    embryopathic c.
    fibrinous c.
    fibroid c.

floriform c.
furnacemen's c.
fusiform c.
galactose c.
glassworker's c.
glaucomatous c.
gray c.
hard c.
hook-shaped c.
hypermature c.
hypocalcemic c.
immature c.
infantile c.
infrared c.
intumescent c.
juvenile c.
lamellar c.
c. lens
life-belt c.
mature c.
membranous c.
Morgagni c.
myotonic c.
c. needle
nuclear c.
overripe c.
perinuclear c.
peripheral c.
pisciform c.
polar c.
posterior subcapsular c.
progressive c.
punctate c.
pyramidal c.
radiation c.
reduplicated c.
ripe c.
rubella c.
saucer-shaped c.
secondary c.
sedimentary c.
senile c.
siderotic c.
soft c.
spindle c.
c. spoon
stationary c.
stellate c.
subcapsular c.
sugar c.
sunflower c.
sutural c.
tetany c.
total c.
toxic c.
traumatic c.
umbilicated c.
vascular c.
zonular c.
cataracta
c. adiposa
c. brunescens
c. cerulea
c. electrica

c. fibrosa
c. nigra
cataractogenesis
cataractogenic
cataract-oligophrenia syndrome
cataractous
cataria
catarrh
nasal c.
vernal c.
catarrhal
c. asthma
c. fever
c. gastritis
c. inflammation
c. ophthalmia
catastalsis
catastaltic
catastasis
catastrophe theory
catastrophic reaction
catatonia
excited c.
periodic c.
stuporous c.
catatonic, catatoniac
c. dementia
c. excitement
c. pupil
c. rigidity
c. schizophrenia
c. stupor
catatrichy
catatricrotic
catatricrotism
catatropic image
cat-bite
c.-b. disease
c.-b. fever
catchment area
cat-cry syndrome
catechase
catechin
catechinic acid
catechol
c. 1,2-dioxygenase
c. 2,3-dioxygenase
c. estrogen
c.-*O*-methyltransferase
c. oxidase
c. oxidase (dimerizing)
catecholamines
catechuic acid
catechu nigrum
categorical trait
catelectrotonus
catenate
catenating
catenin
catenoid
catenulate
caterpillar
c. cell
c. dermatitis
dermatitis-causing c..

C

caterpillar *(continued)*
c. rash
saddleback c.
stinging c.
caterpillar-hair ophthalmia
catgut
chromic c.
silverized c.
c. suture
Catha edulis
Catharanthus alkaloid
catharsis
cathartic
cathectic
cathemoglobin
cathepsin
catheter
acorn-tipped c.
angiography c.
balloon c.
balloon-tip c.
bicoudate c.
c. bicoudé
Bozeman-Fritsch c.
Braasch c.
Broviac c.
brush c.
cardiac c.
central venous c.
c. coiling sign
conic c.
c. coudé
c. à demeure
de Pezzer c.
double-channel c.
elbowed c.
c. embolus
eustachian c.
female c.
c. fever
Fogarty embolectomy c.
Foley c.
c. gauge
Gouley c.
c. guide
Hickman c.
indwelling c.
intracardiac c.
Malecot c.
Nélaton c.
olive-tipped c.
pacing c.
Pezzer c.
Phillips c.
pigtail c.
prostatic c.
pulmonary artery c.
Robinson c.
self-retaining c.
spiral tip c.
Swan-Ganz c.
two-way c.
vertebrated c.

whistle-tip c.
winged c.
catheterization
clean intermittent bladder c. (CIC)
catheterize
catheterostat
cathexis
cathodal
c. closure contraction (CaCC, CCC)
c. opening contraction (CaOC, COC)
c. opening tetanus (COTe)
cathode (Ca)
c. ray
c. ray oscilloscope (CRO)
c. ray tube (CRT)
cathodic
catholysis
cation
c. exchange
c. exchanger
cation-anion difference
cation-exchange resin
cationic detergent
cationogen
catlin, catling
catnep, catnip
catochus
catoptric
catscratch
c. disease (CSD)
c. fever
cat's cry syndrome
cat's eye
c. e. pupil
c. e. syndrome
Cattell Infant Intelligence Scale
Catu virus
cauda, pl. **caudae**
c. epididymidis
c. epididymis
c. equina
c. equina syndrome
c. fasciae dentatae
c. helicis
c. nuclei caudati
c. pancreatis
c. striati
caudad
caudal
c. anesthesia
c. canal
c. flexure
c. ligament
c. neuropore
c. neurosecretory system
c. pancreatic artery
c. pharyngeal complex
c. pontine reticular nucleus
c. retinaculum
c. sheath
c. transtentorial herniation
c. transverse fissure
c. vertebrae
caudalis

caudate
  c. branch of left branch of portal vein
  c. lobe
  c. nucleus
  c. process
caudatolenticular
caudatum
caudocephalad
caudolenticular gray bridge
caul
cauliflower ear
causal
  c. additivity
  c. independence
  c. indication
  c. treatment
causalgia
causality
cause
  constitutional c.
  exciting c.
  necessary c.
  precipitating c.
  predisposing c.
  proximate c.
  specific c.
  sufficient c.
caustic
  c. alkali
  c. potash
  c. soda
cauterant
cauterization
cauterize
cautery
  actual c.
  BICAP c.
  bipolar c.
  chemical c.
  cold c.
  c. conization
  electric c.
  gas c.
  c. knife
  monopolar c.
cava (*pl. of* cavum)
cavagram
caval
  c. fold
  c. opening of diaphragm
  c. valve
cave
  c. sickness
  trigeminal c.
cavea thoracis
caveola, pl. **caveolae**
cavern
  c. of corpora cavernosa
  c. of corpus spongiosum
caverna, pl. **cavernae**
  cavernae corporis spongiosi
  cavernae corporum cavernosorum
caverniloquy

cavernitis
  fibrous c.
cavernositis
cavernous
  c. angioma
  c. artery
  c. body of anal canal
  c. body of clitoris
  c. body of penis
  c. branch of cavernous part of internal carotid artery
  c. groove
  c. hemangioma
  c. lymphangiectasis
  c. nerve of clitoris
  c. nerve of penis
  c. nervous plexus
  c. part of internal carotid artery
  c. plexus of clitoris
  c. plexus of conchae
  c. plexus of penis
  c. rale
  c. resonance
  c. respiration
  c. rhonchus
  c. sinus
  c. sinus branch of internal carotid artery
  c. sinus syndrome
  c. space
  c. space of corpora cavernosa
  c. space of corporus spongiosum
  c. tissue
  c. transformation of portal vein
  c. vein of penis
  c. voice
  c. voice sound
Cavia
  C. porcellus
caviar lesion
CA virus
cavitary
cavitas, pl. **cavitates**
  c. abdominalis
  c. abdominis et pelvis
  c. articularis
  c. conchae
  c. coronae
  c. coronalis
  c. cranii
  c. dentis
  c. glenoidalis
  c. glenoidalis scapulae
  c. infraglottica
  c. infraglotticum
  c. laryngis
  c. medullaris
  c. nasi
  c. oris
  c. oris propria
  c. pelvina
  c. pelvis
  c. pericardiaca
  c. peritonealis
  c. pharyngis

C

cavitas *(continued)*
    c. pleuralis
    c. pulparis
    c. thoracis
    c. tympanica
    c. uteri
cavitation
cavitis
cavity
    abdominal c.
    abdominopelvic c.
    amnionic c.
    articular c.
    axillary c.
    body c.
    buccal c.
    cleavage c.
    c. of concha
    c. of corpora cavernosa
    c. of corpus spongiosum
    cotyloid c.
    cranial c.
    crown c.
    ectoplacental c.
    ectotrophoblastic c.
    epamniotic c.
    epidural c.
    glenoid c.
    glenoid c. of scapula
    greater peritoneal c.
    head c.
    idiopathic bone c.
    inferior laryngeal c.
    infraglottic c.
    intermediate laryngeal c.
    intracranial c.
    laryngeal c.
    c. of larynx
    lesser peritoneal c.
    c. line angle
    c. liner
    c. margin
    Meckel c.
    medullary c.
    c. of middle ear
    nasal c.
    nephrotomic c.
    oral c.
    oral c. proper
    orbital c.
    pelvic c.
    pericardial c.
    peritoneal c.
    perivisceral c.
    pharyngonasal c.
    c. of pharynx
    pleural c.
    pleuroperitoneal c.
    c. preparation
    c. preparation base
    c. preparation form
    primitive perivisceral c.
    pulmonary c.
    pulp c.

    pulp c. of crown
    Retzius c.
    segmentation c.
    c. of septum pellucidum
    somite c.
    splanchnic c.
    subarachnoid c.
    subdural c.
    subgerminal c.
    superior laryngeal c.
    thoracic c.
    c. of tooth
    trigeminal c.
    tympanic c.
    uterine c.
    c. of uterus
    visceral c.
    c. wall
cavogram
cavography
cavopulmonary
    c. anastomosis
    c. shunt
cavosurface
    c. angle
    c. bevel
cavum, pl. **cava**
    c. abdominis
    c. articulare
    c. conchae
    c. coronale
    c. dentis
    c. douglasi
    c. epidurale
    c. infraglotticum
    c. laryngis
    c. mediastinale
    c. medullare
    c. nasi
    c. oris
    c. pelvis
    c. pericardii
    c. peritonei
    c. pharyngis
    c. pleurae
    c. psalterii
    c. retzii
    c. septum pellucidum
    c. subarachnoideum
    c. subdurale
    c. thoracis
    c. trigeminale
    c. tympani
    c. uteri
    c. vergae
    c. vesicouterinum
Cb
    columbium
C-banding stain
CBC
    complete blood count
CBF
    cerebral blood flow
CBG
    corticosteroid-binding globulin

Cbl
cobalamin
CB lead
Cbz
carbobenzoxy-
CC
chief complaint
cc
cubic centimeter
CCA
chimpanzee coryza agent
CCC
cathodal closure contraction
CCDM
Control of Communicable Diseases Manual
CCK
cholecystokinin
CCNU
lomustine
CCU
coronary care unit
CD
circular dichroism
cluster of differentiation
CD 54
intercellular adhesion molecule-1
CD^{50}
curative dose
Cd
cadmium
cd
candela
CD4/CD8 count
CDC
Centers for Disease Control and Prevention
CDE
CDE antigen
CDE blood group
cDNA
complementary DNA
cDNA clone
cDNA library
CDP
cytidine 5′-diphosphate
CDP-choline
cytidine diphosphocholine
CDP-glyceride
cytidine diphosphoglyceride
CDP-sugar
cytidine diphosphosugar
Ce
cerium
CEA
carcinoembryonic antigen
ceasmic teratosis
cebocephaly
ceca (*pl. of* cecum)
cecal
c. artery
c. fold
c. foramen of frontal bone
c. foramen of the tongue
c. hernia

c. recess
c. volvulus
cecectomy
Cecil urethroplasty
cecitis
cecocentral scotoma
cecocolostomy
cecofixation
cecoileostomy
cecopexy
cecoplication
cecorrhaphy
cecosigmoidostomy
cecostomy
cecotomy
cecoureterocele
cecropin
cecum, pl. **ceca**
cupular c. of the cochlear duct
c. cupulare
intestinal c.
vestibular c. of the cochlear duct
c. vestibulare
cedar
c. leaf oil
c. wood oil
Cedecea
Ceelen-Gellerstedt syndrome
cefaclor
cefadroxil
cefamandole nafate
cefazolin
cefonicid disodium
cefoperazone sodium
ceforanide
cefotaxime sodium
cefotetan disodium
cefoxitin sodium
ceftazidime sodium
ceftizoxime sodium
ceftriaxone disodium
cel
celenteron
celery seed
celestine blue B
Celestin tube
celiac
c. (arterial) trunk
c. artery
c. axis
c. branch of posterior vagal trunk
c. branch of vagus nerve
c. disease
c. ganglia
c. lymph node
c. plexus
c. plexus reflex
c. rickets
c. sprue
c. syndrome
celiacoduodenal part of suspensory ligament of duodenum
celiagra
celiocentesis
celiomyalgia

C

celiomyositis
celioparacentesis
celiopathy
celiorrhaphy
celioscopy
celiotomy
  c. incision
  vaginal c.
celitis
cell
  A c.
  absorption c.
  absorptive c. of intestine
  accessory c.
  acid c.
  acidophil c.
  acinar c.
  acinous c.
  acoustic c.
  c. adhesion molecule (CAM)
  adipose c.
  adventitial c.
  air c.
  air c. of auditory tube
  albuminous c.
  algoid c.
  alpha c. of anterior lobe of
    hypophysis
  alpha c. of pancreas
  alveolar c.
  amacrine c.
  ameboid c.
  amniogenic c.
  anabiotic c.
  anaplastic c.
  angioblastic c.
  Anitschkow c.
  anterior ethmoidal c.
  anterior ethmoidal air c.
  anterior horn c.
  antigen-presenting c.
  antigen-responsive c.
  antigen-sensitive c.
  apolar c.
  APUD c.
  argentaffin c.
  argyrophilic c.
  Aschoff c.
  Askanazy c.
  astroglia c.
  A-type nevus c.
  atypical glandular c. of
    undetermined significance (AGUS)
  atypical squamous c. of
    undetermined significance (ASCUS)
  auditory receptor c.
  B c.
  balloon c.
  band c.
  basal c.
  basaloid c.
  basilar c.
  basket c.
  basophil c. of anterior lobe of
    hypophysis

  beaker c.
  Beale c.
  Berger c.
  berry c.
  beta c. of anterior lobe of
    hypophysis
  beta c. of pancreas
  Betz c.
  Bevan-Lewis c.
  bipolar c.
  Bizzozero red c.
  blast c.
  blood c.
  c. body
  Boll c.
  bone c.
  border c.
  Böttcher c.
  Bowenoid c.
  c. bridge
  bristle c.
  bronchic c.
  bronchiolar exocrine c.
  brood c.
  B-type nevus c.
  burr c.
  C c.
  Cajal c.
  caliciform c.
  capsule c.
  carrier c.
  cartilage c.
  castration c.
  caterpillar c.
  c. center
  centroacinar c.
  chalice c.
  chief c.
  chief c. of corpus pineale
  chief c. of parathyroid gland
  chief c. of stomach
  chromaffin c.
  chromophobe c. of anterior lobe of
    hypophysis
  Clara c.
  Clarke c.
  Claudius c.
  clear c.
  cleavage c.
  cleaved c.
  clonogenic c.
  clue c.
  cochlear hair c.
  column c.
  commissural c.
  compound granule c.
  cone c. of retina
  connective tissue c.
  contrasuppressor c.
  Corti c.
  crescent c.
  C-type nevus c.
  c. culture
  c. cycle
  cytomegalic c.

cytotoxic c.
cytotrophoblastic c.
D c.
dark c.
daughter c.
Davidoff c.
decidual c.
decoy c.
deep c.
Deiters c.
delta c. of anterior lobe of
  hypophysis
delta c. of pancreas
dendritic c.
c. determination
Dogiel c.
dome c.
Downey c.
dust c.
effector c.
egg c.
embryonic c.
enamel c.
end c.
endodermal c.
endothelial c.
enterochromaffin c.
enteroendocrine c.
entodermal c.
ependymal c.
epidermic c.
epithelial reticular c.
epithelioid c.
erythroid c.
ethmoid air c.
ethmoidal c.
external pillar c.
exudation c.
Fañanás c.
fasciculata c.
fat c.
fat-storing c.
Ferrata c.
flame c.
foam c.
follicular epithelial c.
follicular ovarian c.
foreign body giant c.
formative c.
foveolar c. of stomach
fuchsinophil c.
fusiform c. of cerebral cortex
c. fusion
G c.
gamma c. of pancreas
ganglion c.
ganglion c. of dorsal spinal root
ganglion c. of retina
Gaucher c.
gemistocytic c.
germ c.
germinal c.
ghost c.
giant c.
Gierke c.

gitter c.
glia c.
glitter c.
globoid c.
glomerulosa c.
goblet c.
Golgi c.
Golgi epithelial c.
Goormaghtigh c.
granule c.
granule c. of connective tissue
granulosa c.
granulosa lutein c.
great alveolar c.
guanine c.
gustatory c.
gyrochrome c.
hair c.
hairy c.
Haller c.
heart failure c.
HeLa c.
helmet c.
helper c.
HEMPAS c.
Hensen c.
heteromeric c.
hilus c.
hobnail c.
Hofbauer c.
horizontal c. of Cajal
horizontal c. of retina
horny c.
Hortega c.
host c.
Hürthle c.
c. hybridization
I c.
immunologically activated c.
immunologically competent c.
c. inclusion
inclusion c.
indifferent c.
inducer c.
innocent bystander c.
intercapillary c.
interdigitating reticulum c.
internal pillar c.
interstitial c.
irritation c.
islet c.
Ito c.
Jurkat c.
juvenile c.
juxtaglomerular c.
K c.
karyochrome c.
keratinized c.
killer c.
Kulchitsky c.
Kupffer c.
lacis c.
Langerhans c.
Langhans c.
Langhans-type giant c.

cell *(continued)*
  LE c.
  Leishman chrome c.
  lepra c.
  Leydig c.
  light c. of thyroid
  c. line
  lining c.
  Lipschütz c.
  littoral c.
  Loevit c.
  lupus erythematosus c.
  luteal c.
  lutein c.
  lymph c.
  lymphoid c.
  lymphokine activated killer c.
  (LAK)
  M c.
  macroglia c.
  malpighian c.
  Marchand wandering c.
  c. marker
  marrow c.
  Martinotti c.
  mast c.
  mastoid c.
  mastoid air c.
  c. matrix
  c. membrane
  memory B c.
  memory T c.
  Merkel tactile c.
  mesangial c.
  mesenchymal c.
  mesoglial c.
  mesothelial c.
  Mexican hat c.
  Meynert c.
  microfold c.
  microglia c.
  microglial c.
  middle ethmoidal c.
  middle ethmoidal air c.
  midget bipolar c.
  migratory c.
  Mikulicz c.
  mirror-image c.
  mitral c.
  monocytoid c.
  mossy c.
  mother c.
  motor c.
  mucoalbuminous c.
  mucoserous c.
  mucous c.
  mucous neck c.
  Müller radial c.
  multipolar c.
  mural c.
  myeloid c.
  myoepithelial c.
  myoid c.
  Nageotte c.

  natural killer c.
  nerve c.
  c. nest
  neurilemma c.
  neuroendocrine transducer c.
  neuroepithelial c.
  neuroglia c.
  neurolemma c.
  neurosecretory c.
  nevus c.
  Niemann-Pick c.
  NK c.
  nonclonogenic c.
  null c.
  nurse c.
  oat c.
  OKT c.
  olfactory receptor c.
  oligodendroglia c.
  Onodi c.
  Opalski c.
  c. organelle
  osseous c.
  osteochondrogenic c.
  osteogenic c.
  osteoprogenitor c.
  oxyntic c.
  oxyphil c.
  P c.
  packed human blood c.
  Paget c.
  pagetoid c.
  Paneth granular c.
  parafollicular c.
  paraganglionic c.
  paraluteal c.
  paralutein c.
  parenchymal c.
  parenchymatous c. of corpus pineale
  parent c.
  parietal c.
  peptic c.
  pericapillary c.
  peripolar c.
  perithelial c.
  peritubular contractile c.
  permissive c.
  pessary c.
  phalangeal c.
  photo c.
  photoreceptor c.
  physaliphorous c.
  Pick c.
  pigment c.
  pigment c. of iris
  pigment c. of retina
  pigment c. of skin
  pillar c.
  pillar c. of Corti
  pineal c.
  plasma c.
  c. plate
  pluripotent c.
  polar c.
  polychromatic c.

polychromatophil c.
posterior ethmoidal c.
posterior ethmoidal air c.
pregnancy c.
pregranulosa c.
prickle c.
primary embryonic c.
primitive reticular c.
primordial germ c.
prolactin c.
pseudo-Gaucher c.
pseudounipolar c.
pseudoxanthoma c.
pulpar c.
Purkinje c.
pus c.
pyramidal c.
pyrrhol c.
pyrrol c.
Raji c.
reactive c.
red blood c. (rbc)
Reed c.
Reed-Sternberg c.
Renshaw c.
resting c.
resting wandering c.
restructured c.
reticular c.
reticularis c.
reticuloendothelial c.
rhagiocrine c.
Rieder c.
rod nuclear c.
rod c. of retina
Rolando c.
rosette-forming c.
c. sap
sarcogenic c.
satellite c.
satellite c. of skeletal muscle
scavenger c.
Schilling band c.
Schultze c.
Schwann c.
segmented c.
sensitized c.
sensory c.
septal c.
seromucous c.
serous c.
Sertoli c.
sex c.
Sézary c.
shadow c.
sickle c.
signet ring c.
silver c.
skein c.
small cleaved c.
smudge c.
somatic c.
sperm c.
spider c.
spindle c.

spine c.
splenic c.
spur c.
squamous c.
squamous alveolar c.
stab c.
staff c.
standard c.
stellate c. of cerebral cortex
stellate c. of liver
stem c.
Sternberg c.
Sternberg-Reed c.
stichochrome c.
c. strain
strap c.
supporting c.
suppressor c.
c. surface marker
surface mucous c. of stomach
sustentacular c.
sympathetic formative c.
sympathicotropic c.
sympathochromaffin c.
synovial c.
T c.
Tγ c.
Tμ c.
tactile c.
tanned red c.
target c.
tart c.
taste c.
T cytotoxic c. (Tc)
TDTH c.
tendon c.
theca lutein c.
theca c. of stomach
T helper c. (Th)
T helper subset 1 c.
T helper subset 2 c.
Tiselius electrophoresis c.
Toker c.
totipotent c.
touch c.
Touton giant c.
transducer c.
c. transformation
transitional c.
tubal air c.
tufted c.
tunnel c.
Türk c.
tympanic air c.
type I, II c.
Tzanck c.
undifferentiated c.
unipolar c.
vasoformative c.
veil c.
veiled c.
vestibular hair c.
Virchow c.
virus-transformed c.
visual receptor c.

C

cell *(continued)*
    vitreous c.
    c. wall
    c. wall–defective bacteria
    wandering c.
    Warthin-Finkeldey c.
    wasserhelle c.
    water-clear c. of parathyroid
    white blood c. (WBC)
    WI-38 c.
    wing c.
    yolk c.
    zymogenic c.
cella, pl. **cellae**
    c. media
cell-bound antibody
cellicolous
cell-mediated
    c.-m. immunity (CMI)
    c.-m. reaction
cellobiase
cellobiose
cellohexose
celloidin
cellon
cellona
cellula, pl. **cellulae**
    cellulae coli
    cellulae ethmoidales
    cellulae ethmoidales anteriores
    cellulae ethmoidales mediae
    cellulae ethmoidales posteriores
    cellulae mastoideae
    cellulae pneumaticae tubae auditivae
    cellulae tympanicae
cellular
    c. biology
    c. biophysics
    c. blue nevus
    c. cartilage
    c. embolism
    c. immune theory
    c. immunity
    c. immunity deficiency syndrome
    c. immunodeficiency with abnormal immunoglobulin synthesis
    c. infiltration
    c. mosaicism
    c. pathology
    c. polyp
    c. spill
    c. tenacity
    c. tumor
cellularity
cellulase
cellule
cellulicidal
cellulifugal
cellulin
cellulipetal
cellulite
cellulitis
    acute scalp c.
    anaerobic c.

    dissecting c.
    eosinophilic c.
    gangrenous c.
    necrotizing c.
    orbital c.
    pelvic c.
    periorbital c.
    preseptal c.
celluloid strip
cellulosan
cellulose
    c. acetate
    c. acetate phthalate
    O-diethylaminoethyl c.
    microcrystalline c.
    oxidized c.
    c. tape technique
    TEAE-c.
    O-(triethylaminoethyl) c.
cellulosic acid
celom
    extraembryonic c.
celoma
celomic
    c. bay
    c. metaplasia theory of endometriosis
celophlebitis
celoscope
celoscopy
celosomia
CELO virus
Celovirus
celozoic
Celsius scale
cement
    c. base
    composite dental c.
    copper phosphate c.
    c. corpuscle
    dental c.
    c. disease
    glass ionomer c.
    inorganic dental c.
    intercellular c.
    c. line
    modified zinc oxide-eugenol c.
    organic dental c.
    polycarboxylate c.
    resin c.
    silicate c.
    tooth c.
    unmodified zinc oxide-eugenol c.
    zinc phosphate c.
cemental
    cemental caries
    c. dysplasia
cementation
cementicle
cementification
cementing substance
cementoblast
cementoblastoma
    benign c.
cementoclasia

cementoclast
cementocyte
cementodentinal junction
cementoenamel junction
cementogenesis
cementoma
    gigantiform c.
    true c.
cementoossifying fibroma
cementum
    afibrillar c.
    c. hyperplasia
    primary c.
    secondary c.
cenesthesia
cenesthesic, cenesthetic
cenocyte
cenocytic
cenosite
cenotrope
censor
censoring
census
center
    active c.
    anospinal c.
    birthing c.
    Broca c.
    Budge c.
    catalytic c.
    cell c.
    chondrification c.
    ciliospinal c.
    community mental health c.
    dentary c.
    diaphysial c.
    C.'s for Disease Control and
      Prevention (CDC)
    epiotic c.
    expiratory c.
    feeding c.
    germinal c. of Flemming
    inspiratory c.
    Kerckring c.
    medullary c.
    microtubule-organizing c.
    motor speech c.
    ossific c.
    ossification c.
    c. of ossification
    primary ossification c.
    primary c. of ossification
    reaction c.
    respiratory c.
    c. of ridge
    c. of rotation
    satiety c.
    secondary c. of ossification
    secondary ossification c.
    semioval c.
    sensory speech c.
    speech c.
    sphenotic c.
    vasomotor c.

    vital c.
    Wernicke c.
centesis
centibar
centigrade scale
centigram
centile
centiliter
centimeter (cm)
    cubic c. (cc)
centimeter-gram-second
    c.-g.-s. system (CGS)
    c.-g.-s. unit
centimorgan (cM)
centinormal
centipede
centipoise
centra (*pl. of* centrum)
centrad
centrage
central
    c. amputation
    c. amygdaloid nucleus
    c. angiospastic retinopathy
    c. apnea
    c. apparatus
    c. areolar choroidal atrophy
    c. areolar choroidal dystrophy
    c. areolar choroidal sclerosis
    c. artery of retina
    c. axillary lymph node
    c. bearing
    c. body
    c. bone
    c. bone of ankle
    c. bradycardia
    c. callus
    c. canal
    c. canal of cochlea
    c. canal of spinal cord
    c. canal of the vitreous
    c. cataract
    c. chromatolysis
    c. cloudy corneal dystrophy of
      François
    c. complex
    c. cord syndrome
    c. core disease
    c. crystalline corneal dystrophy of
      Snyder
    c. deafness
    c. dogma
    C. European tick-borne encephalitis
      virus
    C. European tick-borne fever
    c. excitatory state
    c. fibrous body
    c. ganglioneuroma
    c. gray substance
    c. gyrus
    c. illumination
    c. implantation
    c. incisor
    c. inhibition
    c. lacteal

C

central *(continued)*
   c. and lateral intermediate substance
   c. lateral nucleus of thalamus
   c. limit theorem
   c. lobule
   c. lobule of cerebellum
   c. mesenteric lymph node
   c. necrosis
   c. nervous system (CNS)
   c. neuritis
   c. nucleus
   c. ossifying fibroma
   c. osteitis
   c. palmar space
   c. paralysis
   c. part of lateral ventricle
   c. pit
   c. placenta previa
   c. pneumonia
   c. pontine myelinolysis
   c. retinal artery
   c. retinal fovea
   c. retinal vein
   c. scotoma
   c. serous choroidopathy
   c. serous retinopathy
   c. spindle
   c. sulcal artery
   c. sulcus
   c. sulcus of insula
   c. superior mesenteric lymph node
   c. tegmental fasciculus
   c. tegmental tract
   c. tendon of diaphragm
   c. tendon of perineum
   c. terminal electrode
   c. thalamic radiation
   c. transactional core
   c. type neurofibromatosis
   c. vein of liver
   c. vein of suprarenal gland
   c. venous catheter
   c. venous pressure (CVP)
   c. vision
central-bearing
   c.-b. point
   c.-b. tracing device
centralis
centralization phenomenon
centrally active phenethylamine derivative related to amphetamine and methamphetamine (MDMA)
centre médian de Luys
centrencephalic epilepsy
centriacinar emphysema
centric
   c. contact
   c. fusion
   c. interocclusal record
   c. jaw relation
   c. occlusion
   c. position
centriciput

centrifugal
   c. casting
   c. current
   c. fast analyzer
   c. nerve
centrifugalization
centrifugalize
centrifugation
   band c.
   density gradient c.
   zone c.
centrifuge
centrilobular emphysema
centriole
   anterior c.
   distal c.
   posterior c.
   proximal c.
centripetal
   c. current
   c. nerve
centroacinar cell
centroblast
Centrocestus
centrocyte
centrofacial lentiginosis
centrokinesia
centrokinetic
centrolecithal
   c. egg
   c. ovum
centromedian nucleus
centromere banding stain
centromeric index
centronuclear myopathy
centroplasm
centrosome
centrosphere
centrostaltic
centrum, pl. **centra**
   c. medianum
   c. medullare
   c. ossificationis
   c. ossificationis primarium
   c. ossificationis secundarium
   c. ovale
   c. semiovale
   c. tendineum diaphragmatis
   c. tendineum perinei
   c. of a vertebra
   Vicq d'Azyr c. semiovale
   Vieussens c.
   Willis c. nervosum
Centruroides
centum
cenuris, coenuris
cenurosis, cenuriasis
cephaeline
Cephaelis
cephalad
cephalalgia
   benign coital c.
   histaminic c.
   Horton c.
cephaledema

cephalemia
cephalexin
cephalhematocele
cephalhematoma
cephalhydrocele
cephalic
    c. angle
    c. arterial rami
    c. curve
    c. flexure
    c. index
    c. pole
    c. presentation
    c. replacement
    c. tetanus
    c. triangle
    c. vein
    c. vein of forearm
    c. version
cephalin
cephaline
cephalitis
cephalization
cephalocaudal axis
cephalocele
cephalocentesis
cephalochord
cephalodactyly
    Vogt c.
cephalodidymus
cephalodiprosopus
cephalodynia
cephalogenesis
cephaloglycin
cephalogram
cephalogyric
cephalohematocele
cephalohematoma
cephalohemometer
cephalomedullary angle
cephalomegaly
cephalomelus
cephalomeningitis
cephalometer
cephalometric
    c. analysis
    c. radiograph
    c. tracing
cephalometrics
cephalometry
    ultrasonic c.
cephalomotor
Cephalomyia
cephalont
cephalooculocutaneous telangiectasia
cephaloorbital index
cephalopagus
cephalopalpebral reflex
cephalopelvic disproportion
cephalopelvimetry
cephalopharyngeus
cephaloridine
cephalorrhachidian
cephalosporanic acid

cephalosporin
    c. C, N, P
cephalosporinase
Cephalosporium
cephalostat
cephalothin
cephalothoracic
cephalothoracopagus
    c. asymmetros
    c. disymmetros
    c. monosymmetros
cephalotome
cephalotomy
cephalotoxin
cephalotribe
cephalotrigeminal angiomatosis
cephamycins
cephapirin sodium
cephradine
ceptor
    chemical ceptor
    contact ceptor
    distance ceptor
cera
ceraceous
ceramidase
ceramide
    c. dihexoside
    c. lactosidase
    c. lactoside
    c. lactoside lipidosis
    c. 1-phosphorylcholine
    c. saccharide
ceramo-metal casting
cerasin
cerate
ceratin
cerato-
ceratocricoid
    c. ligament
    c. muscle
ceratoglossus muscle
ceratohyal
ceratopharyngeal
    c. part of middle constrictor muscle of pharynx
    c. part of middle pharyngeal constrictor (muscle) of pharynx
Ceratophyllidae
Ceratophyllus
    C. punjatensis
cercaria, pl. cercariae
cerci (*pl. of* cercus)
cerclage
cercocystis
cercomer
cercomonad
Cercomonas
Cercopithecoidea
cercopithecrine herpesvirus
Cercopithecus
cercus, pl. cerci
cerea flexibilitas
cerebella (*pl. of* cerebellum)

cerebellar
  c. artery
  c. astrocytoma
  c. ataxia
  c. atrophy
  c. cortex
  c. cyst
  c. falx
  c. fissure
  c. fossa
  c. frenulum
  c. gait
  c. nucleus
  c. pyramid
  c. rigidity
  c. speech
  c. sulci
  c. syndrome
  c. tentorium
  c. tonsil
  c. vein
cerebellin
cerebellitis
cerebellohypothalamic fiber
cerebellolental
cerebellomedullary
  c. cistern
  c. malformation syndrome
cerebelloolivary fiber
cerebellopontile angle
cerebellopontine
  c. angle
  c. angle syndrome
  c. angle tumor
  c. cisternography
  c. recess
cerebellorubral tract
cerebellospinal fiber
cerebellothalamic tract
cerebellum, pl. **cerebella**
cerebra (*pl. of* cerebrum)
cerebral
  c. amyloid angiopathy
  c. angiography
  c. anthrax
  c. aqueduct
  c. arterial circle
  c. arteriography
  c. artery
  c. blood flow (CBF)
  c. calculus
  c. cladosporiosis
  c. compression
  c. cortex
  c. cranium
  c. death
  c. decompression
  c. decortication
  c. diataxia
  c. dominance
  c. dysplasia
  c. edema
  c. falx
  c. fissure
  c. flexure

  c. gigantism
  c. gyrus
  c. hemisphere
  c. hemorrhage
  c. hernia
  c. index
  c. lacuna
  c. layer of retina
  c. lipidosis
  c. lobe
  c. localization
  c. malaria
  c. palsy
  c. part of arachnoid
  c. part of dura mater
  c. part of internal carotid artery
  c. peduncle
  c. porosis
  c. rheumatism
  c. sinus
  c. sphingolipidosis
  c. sulcus
  c. surface
  c. tetanus
  c. thrombosis
  c. trigone
  c. tuberculosis
  c. vein
  c. ventricle
  c. vesicle
  c. vomiting
cerebration
cerebriform
cerebritis
  suppurative c.
cerebrocuprein
cerebrohepatorenal syndrome
cerebroma
cerebromalacia
cerebromeningitis
cerebron
cerebronic acid
cerebropathia
cerebropathy
cerebrophysiology
cerebroretinal angiomatosis
cerebrosclerosis
cerebroside
  c. lipidosis
  c. lipoidosis
  c.-sulfatase
  c. sulfatidase
cerebrosidosis
cerebrospinal
  c. axis
  c. fever
  c. fluid (CSF)
  c. fluid otorrhea
  c. fluid rhinorrhea
  c. index
  c. meningitis
  c. nematodiasis
  c. pressure
  c. system
cerebrosterol

cerebrotendinous xanthomatosis
cerebrotomy
cerebrovascular
    c. accident (CVA)
    c. disease
cerebrum, pl. **cerebra**
cerecloth
Cerenkov radiation
ceresin
cerin
Cerithidea
cerium (Ce)
    c. oxalate
ceroid lipofuscinosis
ceroplasty
cerosin
cerotinic acid
certifiable
certification
certified
    C. Medical Assistant (CMA)
    C. Medical Transcriptionist (CMT)
    c. milk
    c. nurse-midwife (CNM)
    c. pasteurized milk
    c. reference material (CRM)
    c. registered nurse anesthetist
      (CRNA)
certify
cerulean cataract
cerulein
ceruloplasmin
cerumen
    inspissated c.
    c. inspissatum
ceruminal
ceruminolytic
ceruminoma
ceruminosis
ceruminous gland
ceruse
cerveau isolé
cervical
    c. amputation
    c. anchorage
    c. anesthesia
    c. aortic knuckle
    c. auricle
    c. branch of facial nerve
    c. canal
    c. cap
    c. compression syndrome
    c. disk syndrome
    c. diverticulum
    c. duct
    c. dysplasia
    c. enlargement
    c. enlargement of spinal cord
    c. fibrositis
    c. flexure
    c. fusion syndrome
    c. gland
    c. gland of uterus
    c. hydrocele
    c. hygroma

    c. hyperesthesia
    c. iliocostal muscle
    c. interspinales muscle
    c. interspinal muscle
    c. intraepithelial neoplasia
    c. ligament of uterus
    c. line
    c. longissimus muscle
    c. loop
    c. lordosis
    c. margin
    c. margin of tooth
    c. myelogram
    c. myositis
    c. myospasm
    c. nerve [C1–C8]
    c. nystagmus
    c. orthosis
    c. part of esophagus
    c. part of internal carotid artery
    c. part of spinal cord
    c. part of thoracic duct
    c. part of vertebral artery
    c. pleura
    c. plexus
    c. pregnancy
    c. rib
    c. rib and band syndrome
    c. rotator muscle
    c. segment of spinal cord [C1–C8]
    c. sinus
    c. smear
    c. splanchnic nerve
    c. spondylosis
    c. tension syndrome
    c. triangle
    c. vein
    c. vertebra [C1–C7]
    c. vesicle
    c. zone
    c. zone of tooth
cervicalis ascendens
cervicectomy
cervices (*pl. of* cervix)
cervicitis
cervico-
cervicoaxillary canal
cervicobrachial
cervicobuccal
cervicodynia
cervicofacial
cervicography
cervicolabial
cervicolingual
cervicolinguoaxial
cervicolumbar phenomenon
cervicooccipital
cervicooculoacoustic syndrome
cervicoplasty
cervicoscopy
cervicothoracic
    c. ganglion
    c. orthosis
    c. transition
cervicotomy

C

cervicovaginal artery
cervicovesical
cervilaxin
cervix, pl. **cervices**
 c. of the axon
 c. columnae posterioris
 c. dentis
 strawberry c.
 c. of tooth
 c. uteri
 c. of uterus
 c. vesicae urinariae
ceryl
cesarean
 c. hysterectomy
 c. operation
 c. section
cesium (Cs)
Cestan-Chenais syndrome
Cestoda
Cestodaria
cestode, cestoid
cestodiasis
Cestoidea
cetaceum
cetalkonium chloride
cethexonium bromide
cetostearyl alcohol
cetraria
cetrimonium bromide
cetyl
 c. alcohol
 c. palmitate
cetylpyridinium chloride
cetyltrimethylammonium bromide
cevadilla
cevadine
cevitamic acid
Ceylon
 C. cinnamon
 C. moss
CF
 citrovorum factor
  CF antibody
  CF lead
  CF test
Cf
 californium
CFF
 critical fusion frequency
CG
 chorionic gonadotropin
CGA
 catabolite gene activator
cGMP
 cyclic guanosine 3,5-monophosphate
CGP
 chorionic growth hormone-prolactin
CGRP
 calcitonin gene-related peptide
CGS
 centimeter-gram-second system
  CGS unit
CH
 crown-heel length

Chaddock
 C. reflex
 C. sign
Chadwick sign
chaeta
chafe
Chagas-Cruz disease
Chagas disease
chagasic myocardiopathy
chagoma
Chagres virus
chain
 A c.
 B c.
 behavior c.
 C c.
 cold c.
 electron-transport c.
 c. ganglia
 ganglionic c.
 H c.
 heavy c.
 J c.
 L c.
 light c.
 long c.
 ossicular c.
 c. reaction
 c. reflex
 respiratory c.
 short c.
 side c.
chain-compensated spirometer
chaining
chair form
chalasia
chalasis
chalaza
chalazion, pl. **chalazia**
 acute c.
 collar-stud c.
chalcone
chalcosis lentis
chalice cell
chalicosis
chalk
 French c.
 prepared c.
chalkitis
challenge diet
chalone
chalybeate water
chamber
 altitude c.
 anechoic c.
 anterior c. of eyeball
 aqueous c.
 counting c.
 decompression c.
 c. of eyeball
 high altitude c.
 hyperbaric c.
 ionization c.
 posterior c. of eyeball
 postremal c. of eyeball

pulp c.
relief c.
Sandison-Clark c.
sinuatrial c.
vitreous c.
vitreous c. of eye
Zappert counting c.
Chamberlain
C. line
C. procedure
Chamberlen forceps
chamecephalic
chamecephalous
chameprosopic
chamfer
chamomile
Champy fixative
Chance fracture
chancre
hard c.
mixed c.
monorecidive c.
c. redux
soft c.
sporotrichositic c.
tularemic c.
chancriform syndrome
chancroid
chancroidal bubo
chancrous
chandelier sign
Chandler syndrome
change
Armanni-Ebstein c.
Baggenstoss c.
c. blindness
Crooke hyaline c.
fatty c.
c. of life
mitral valve prolapse, aortic anomalies, skeletal and skin c.'s (MASS)
c., organomegaly, endocrinopathy, monoclonal gammopathy, and skin changes (POEMS)
polyneuropathy, organomegaly, endocrinopathy, monoclonal gammopathy, and skin c.'s (POEMS)
reactive c.
trophic c.
channel
ion c.
ligand-gated c.
transnexus c.
voltage-gated c.
channelopathies
Chantemesse reaction
chaos
mathematical c.
c. theory
chaotic
c. heart
c. rhythm
chaotropic

chaotropism
CHAP
cyclophosphamide, hexamethylmelamine, doxorubicin (Adriamycin), and cisplatin
chaperone
chappa
chapped
character
acquired c.
c. analysis
c. armor
classifiable c.
compound c.
denumerable c.
discrete c.
c. disorder
dominant c.
inherited c.
mendelian c.
c. neurosis
primary sex c.
recessive c.
secondary sex c.
sex-linked c.
unit c.
characteristic
c. curve
c. emission
c. frequency
c. radiation
receiver operating c. (ROC)
characterization
denture c.
characterizing group
charas
charbon
charcoal (carbo)
activated c.
animal c.
bone c.
medicinal c.
vegetable c.
wood c.
Charcot
C. artery
C. disease
C. gait
C. intermittent fever
C. joint
C. syndrome
C. triad
C. vertigo
Charcot-Böttcher crystalloid
Charcot-Bouchard aneurysm
Charcot-Leyden crystal
Charcot-Marie-Tooth disease
Charcot-Neumann crystal
Charcot-Robin crystal
Charcot-Weiss-Baker syndrome
Chargaff rule
CHARGE
C. association
C. syndrome
charge
elementary c. (e)

C

charge (continued)
- c. nurse
- c. transfer
- c. transfer complex
- c. transfer system

charlatan

charlatanism

Charles law

charley horse

Charnley hip arthroplasty

Charrière scale

chart
- Amsler c.
- isometric c.
- Levey-Jennings c.
- Pickles c.
- quality control c.
- Tanner growth c.
- Walker c.

Charters method

charting

Chassaignac
- C. space
- C. tubercle

Chauffard syndrome

chaulmoogra oil

Chaussier
- C. line
- C. sign

Chayes method

ChB
- Bachelor of Surgery

ChD
- Doctor of Surgery

Cheadle disease

Cheatle slit

check
- c. ligament of odontoid
- c. ligaments of eyeball, medial and lateral
- c. ligaments of medial and lateral rectus muscles

checkbite

checkerberry oil

Chédiak-Higashi
- C.-H. disease
- C.-H. syndrome

Chédiak-Steinbrinck-Higashi
- C.-S.-H. anomaly
- C.-S.-H. syndrome

cheek
- c. bone
- c. muscle
- c. tooth

cheese
- c. maggot
- c. worker's lung

cheesy
- c. abscess
- c. pus

cheilalgia, chilalgia

cheilectomy, chilectomy

cheilectropion, chilectropion

cheilion

cheilitis, chilitis
- actinic c.
- angular c.
- commissural c.
- contact c.
- c. exfoliativa
- c. glandularis
- c. granulomatosa
- impetiginous c.
- solar c.
- c. venenata
- Volkmann c.

cheilognathoglossoschisis

cheilognathopalatoschisis

cheilognathouranoschisis

cheilophagia, chilophagia

cheiloplasty

cheilorrhaphy, chilorrhaphy

cheilosis, chilosis

cheilotomy, chilotomy

cheiralgia paresthetica

cheirarthritis

cheirognostic

cheirokinesthesia

cheirokinesthetic

cheirology, chirology

cheiromegaly, chiromegaly

cheiropodalgia

cheiropompholyx

cheirospasm

chelate

chelation

chelicera, pl. **chelicerae**

chelidon

cheloid

chemexfoliation

chemiatry

chemical
- c. antidote
- c. attraction
- c. burn
- c. cautery
- c. ceptor
- c. complexity
- c. conjunctivitis
- c. depilatory
- c. dermatitis
- c. diabetes
- c. energy
- c. equation
- c. evolution
- c. formula
- c. kinetics
- c. knife
- c. modification
- c. peeling
- c. peritonitis
- c. pneumonia
- c. potential
- c. pregnancy
- c. prophylaxis
- c. ray
- "c." thyroidectomy
- c. repair
- c. sampling

c. sense
c. shift
c. shift artifact
c. solution
c. sympathectomy
c. taxonomy
chemically
  chemically cured resin
  c. pure (c.p.)
chemicocautery
chemiluminescence
chemiosmotic theory
chemiotaxis
chemise
chemist
chemistry
  analytic c.
  applied c.
  biologic c.
  clinical c.
  combinatorial c.
  ecologic c.
  epithermal c.
  inorganic c.
  macromolecular c.
  medicinal c.
  nuclear c.
  organic c.
  pharmaceutical c.
  physiologic c.
  radiopharmaceutical c.
  synthetic c.
chemoattractant
chemoautotroph
chemoautotrophic
chemobiodynamics
chemocautery
chemoceptor
chemodectoma
chemodectomatosis
chemodifferentiation
chemoheterotroph
chemoheterotrophic
chemoimmunology
chemokine
chemokinesis
chemokinetic
chemolithotroph
chemolithotrophic
chemolithotrophy
chemoluminescence
chemolysis
chemonucleolysis
chemoorganotroph
chemoorganotrophic
chemopallidectomy
chemopallidothalamectomy
chemopallidotomy
chemoprevention
chemoprophylaxis
chemoreception
chemoreceptive
chemoreceptor
  medullary c.
  peripheral c.

chemoreflex
chemoresistance
chemoresponse
chemosensation
chemosensitive
chemoserotherapy
chemosis
chemosmosis
chemostat
chemosurgery
  Mohs c.
chemosynthesis
chemotactic
chemotaxis
  negative c.
  positive c.
chemothalamectomy
chemothalamotomy
chemotherapeutic index
chemotherapeutics
chemotherapy
  adjuvant c.
  combination c.
  consolidation c.
  cytostatic c.
  cytotoxic c.
  induction c.
  intensification c.
  salvage c.
chemotic
chemotransmitter
chemotroph
chemotropism
Cheney syndrome
chenodeoxycholic acid
chenodiol
chenopodium
cherry
  c. angioma
  c. juice
cherry-red
  c.-r. spot
  c.-r. spot myoclonus syndrome
cherubic facies
cherubism
chest
  alar c.
  barrel c.
  flail c.
  flat c.
  foveated c.
  funnel c.
  c. index
  keeled c.
  c. lead
  phthinoid c.
  pigeon c.
  pterygoid c.
  c. radiology
  c. wall
Chevalier-Jackson dilator
chevron incision
chewing
  c. cycle
  c. force

Cheyne-Stokes
> C.-S. psychosis
> C.-S. respiration

chi
> c. sequence
> c. structure

Chian turpentine

Chiari
> C. disease
> C. II syndrome
> C. net

Chiari-Budd syndrome

Chiari-Frommel syndrome

chiasm
> Camper c.
> optic c.
> tendinous c. of the digital tendons

chiasma, pl. chiasmata
> c. opticum
> c. syndrome
> c. tendinum

chiasmapexy

chiasmatic
> c. cistern
> c. groove
> c. sulcus

Chicago disease

chicken
> c. breast
> c. embryo lethal orphan virus
> c. fat clot

chickenpox
> c. immune globulin (human)
> c. immunoglobulin
> c. virus

Chick-Martin test

chicle

chief
> c. agglutinin
> c. artery of thumb
> c. cell
> c. cell of corpus pineale
> c. cell of parathyroid gland
> c. cell of stomach
> c. complaint (CC)

Chievitz
> C. layer
> C. organ

chigger

chigoe

chikungunya virus

Chilaiditi syndrome

chilalgia (*var. of* cheilalgia)

chilblain
> c. lupus
> c. lupus erythematosus

CHILD

child
> c. abuse
> c. psychiatry
> c. psychology

childbearing age

childbed fever

childbirth

childhood
> c. absence epilepsy
> c. epilepsy with occipital paroxysms
> c. hypophosphatasia
> c. muscular dystrophy
> c. schizophrenia
> c. tuberculosis
> c. type tuberculosis

CHILD syndrome

Chilean saltpeter

chilectomy (*var. of* cheilectomy)

chilectropion (*var. of* cheilectropion)

chilitis (*var. of* cheilitis)

chill
> smelter's c.'s

chilomastigiasis

Chilomastix

chilomastosis

chilophagia (*var. of* cheilophagia)

Chilopoda

chilopodiasis

chilorrhaphy (*var. of* cheilorrhaphy)

chilosis (*var. of* cheilosis)

chilotomy (*var. of* cheilotomy)

chimera
> radiation c.

chimeric
> c. antibody
> c. molecule

chimerism

chimney sweep's cancer

chimpanzee coryza agent (CCA)

chin
> c. cap
> double c.
> c. jerk
> c. muscle
> c. reflex

Chinese
> C. cinnamon
> C. ginger
> C. restaurant syndrome
> C. wax

chiniofon

chinoleine

chip
> bone c.
> c. syringe

chip-blower

chiral crystal

chirality

chirarthritis

chirognostic

chirokinesthesia

chirology (*var. of* cheirology)

chiromegaly (*var. of* cheiromegaly)

chiropodalgia

chiropodist

chiropody

chiropompholyx

chiropractic
> Doctor of C. (DC)

chiropractor

Chiropsalmus quadrumanus

Chiroptera

chiroscope
chirospasm
chirurg.
    chirurgicalis
chirurgeon
chirurgery
Chirurgiae
    Magister C. (MC, MCh)
chirurgical
chirurgicalis (chirurg.)
chisel
    binangle c.
chi-square
    c.-s. distribution
    c.-s. test
chitin
chitinase
chitinous
chitobiose
chitosamine
chiufa
CHL
    crown-heel length
Chlamydia
    C. pneumoniae (TWAR)
    C. psittaci
    C. trachomatis
chlamydia, pl. **chlamydiae**
Chlamydiaceae
chlamydial
chlamydiosis
chlamydoconidium
Chlamydophrys
Chlamydozoon
chloasma bronzinum
chlophedianol hydrochloride
chloracetic acid
chloracne
chloral
    c. alcoholate
    anhydrous c.
    c. betaine
    c. hydrate
m-chloral
p-chloral
chloralism
α-chloralose
chlorambucil
chloramine
    c. B, T
chloraminophene
chloramiphene
chloramphenicol
    c. acetyl transferase
    c. palmitate
    c. sodium succinate
chlorate
chlorazanil
chlorazene
chlorazol black E
chlorbenzoxamine
chlorbenzoxyethamine
chlorbetamide
chlorbutol
chlorcyclizine hydrochloride

chlordane
chlordantoin
chlordiazepoxide hydrochloride
chloremia
chlorethene homopolymer
chlorguanide hydrochloride
chlorhexidine hydrochloride
chlorhydria
chloric acid
chloride
    carbamylcholine c.
    c. shift
chloridimetry
chloridometer
chloriduria
chlorin
chlorinated
    c. lime
    c. paraffin
chlorindanol
chlorine
    c. group
    c. water
chloriodized oil
chloriodoquin
chlorisondamine chloride
chlorite
chlormadinone acetate
chlormerodrin
chlormezanone
chloroacetic acid
chloroacetophenone
chloroambucil
chloroanemia
chloroazodin
o-chlorobenzalmalononitrile
chlorobutanol
chlorocresol
chlorocruorin
chloroethane
chloroethylene
chloroform
    acetone c.
chloroformism
chloroguanide hydrochloride
chlorohemin crystal
chloroma
p-chloromercuribenzoate (*p*-CMB, PCMB, *p*CMB)
chloromethane
chlorometry
chloropenia
chloropercha method
chlorophenol
    o-c.
    p-c.
chlorophenothane
chlorophyll
    c. *a, b, c, d*
    c. esterase
    c. unit
    water-soluble c. derivatives
chlorophyllase
chlorophyllide, chlorophyllid
chloropicrin

C

chloroplast
chloroprednisone
chloroprocaine hydrochloride
chloroprocaine penicillin O
chloropsia
chloropyramine
chloroquine
chlorosis
chlorothen citrate
chlorothiazide sodium
chlorothymol
chlorotic anemia
chlorotrianisene
chlorotriazine dye
chlorous acid
chlorozotocin
chlorphenesin carbamate
chlorphenindione
chlorpheniramine maleate
chlorphenol red
chlorphenoxamine
chlorphentermine hydrochloride
chlorproguanil hydrochloride
chlorpromazine hydrochloride
chlorpropamide
chlorprothixene
chlorquinaldol
chlortetracycline
chlorthalidone
chlorthenoxazin
chlorthymol
chloruresis
chloruretic
chloruria
chlorzoxazone
choana, pl. choanae
    primary c.
    primitive c.
    secondary c.
choanal
    c. atresia
    c. polyp
choanate
choanoflagellate
choanoid
choanomastigote
Choanotaenia infundibulum
chocolate
    c. agar
    c. cyst
Chodzko reflex
choke
choked disk
chokes
cholagogic
cholagogue
cholaic acid
cholalic acid
cholane, 5β-cholane
cholaneresis
cholangeitis
cholangiectasis
cholangiocarcinoma
cholangioenterostomy
cholangiofibrosis

cholangiogastrostomy
cholangiogram
cholangiography
    cystic duct c.
    intravenous c.
    percutaneous c.
    percutaneous transhepatic c. (PTHC)
cholangiole
cholangiolitic hepatitis
cholangiolitis
cholangioma
cholangiopancreatography
    endoscopic retrograde c. (ERCP)
cholangioscopy
cholangiostomy
cholangiotomy
cholangitic abscess
cholangitis
    ascending c.
    c. lenta
    primary sclerosing c.
    recurrent pyogenic c.
cholanic acid
cholanopoiesis
cholanopoietic
cholanthrene
cholascos
cholate
    c. ligase
    c. synthetase
    c. thiokinase
cholecalciferol
cholechromopoiesis
cholecyst
cholecystagogic
cholecystagogue
cholecystatony
cholecystectasia
cholecystectomy
cholecystenterostomy
cholecystenterotomy
cholecystic
cholecystis
cholecystitis
    acute c.
    chronic c.
    emphysematous c.
    xanthogranulomatous c.
cholecystoduodenal fistula
cholecystoduodenostomy
cholecystogastrostomy
cholecystogram
cholecystography
cholecystoileostomy
cholecystojejunostomy
cholecystokinase
cholecystokinetic
cholecystokinin (CCK)
cholecystolithiasis
cholecystolithotripsy
cholecystomy
cholecystopaque
cholecystopathy
cholecystopexy
cholecystorrhaphy

cholecystosonography
cholecystostomy
cholecystotomy
    laparoscopic c.
choledoch
    c. duct
choledochal
    c. cyst
    c. sphincter
choledochectomy
choledochendysis
choledochiarctia
choledochitis
choledochocholedochostomy
choledochoduodenal junction
choledochoduodenostomy
choledochoenterostomy
choledochojejunostomy
choledocholith
choledocholithiasis
choledocholithotomy
choledocholithotripsy
choledocholithotrity
choledochoplasty
choledochorrhaphy
choledochostomy
choledochotomy
choledochous
choledochus
choleglobin
cholehematin
cholehemia
choleic
choleic acid
cholelith
cholelithiasis
cholelithotomy
cholelithotripsy
cholelithotrity
cholemesis
cholemia
cholemic
cholepathia spastica
choleperitonitis
cholepoiesis
cholepoietic
cholera
    c. agar
    Asiatic c.
    c. bacillus
    c. infantum
    c. morbus
    pancreatic c.
    c. sicca
    c. toxin
    typhoid c.
    c. vaccine
choleragen
choleraic diarrhea
choleraphage
cholera-red reaction
choleresis
choleretic
cholerheic
choleric jaundice

choleriform
cholerigenic
cholerigenous
cholerine
choleroid
cholerrhagia
cholerrhagic
cholescintigraphy
cholestane
cholestanol
cholestanone
cholestasia
cholestasis
    intrahepatic c. of pregnancy
    c. of pregnancy
cholestatic
    c. hepatitis
    c. hepatosis icterus gravidarum
    c. jaundice
cholesteatoma
cholesteatomatous
cholestenone
cholesteremia
cholesterinemia
cholesterinized antigen
cholesterinosis
cholesterinuria
cholesterol
    c. cleft
    c. embolism
    c. ester storage disease, cholesteryl
      ester storage disease
    c. ester transport protein
    c. granuloma
cholesterolemia
cholesterologenesis
cholesterolosis
cholesteroluria
cholesteryl ester storage disease (*var. of*
    cholesterol ester storage disease)
cholestyramine resin
choleuria
cholic acid
cholicele
choline
    c. acetylase
    c. acetyltransferase
    activated c.
    c. chloride
    c. dihydrogen citrate
    c. esterase I, II
    c. kinase
    c. phosphatase
    c. phosphate cytidylyltransferase
    c. phosphokinase
    c. salicylate
    c. theophyllinate
cholinephosphotransferase
cholinergic
    c. agent
    c. blockade
    c. fiber
    c. neurotransmitter
    c. receptor
    c. urticaria

C

cholinester
cholinesterase
    "e"-type c.
    c. inhibitor
    nonspecific c.
    c. reactivator
    specific c.
    "s"-type c.
    true c.
cholinoceptive
cholinolytic
cholinomimetic
cholinoreactive
cholinoreceptors
cholistine sulphomethate sodium
chololithiasis
choloplania
cholopoiesis
cholorrhea
choloscopy
cholothorax
choloyl
choluria
cholyl-coenzyme A
    cholyl-coenzyme A synthetase
chondral
chondralloplasia
chondrectomy
chondrification center
chondrify
chondrin ball
chondritis
    costal c.
chondroblast
chondroblastoma
chondrocalcin
chondrocalcinosis
    articular c.
chondroclast
chondrocostal
chondrocranium
chondrocyte
    isogenous c.
chondrodermatitis nodularis chronica helicis
chondrodysplasia
    c. calcificans congenita
    Nance-Sweeney c.
    c. punctata
    rhizomelic c. punctata
chondrodystrophic dwarfism
chondrodystrophy
    asphyxiating thoracic c.
    asymmetric c.
    hereditary deforming c.
    hypoplastic fetal c.
    myotonic c.
    c. with sensorineural deafness (OSMED)
chondroectodermal dysplasia
chondrofibroma
chondrogenesis
chondroglossus muscle

chondroid
    c. syringoma
    c. tissue
chondroitin
    c. sulfate A. B, C
chondrology
chondrolysis
chondroma
    extraskeletal c.
    juxtacortical c.
    periosteal c.
chondromalacia
    c. fetalis
    generalized c.
    c. of larynx
    c. patellae
    systemic c.
chondromatosis
    synovial c.
chondromatous
chondrome
chondromere
chondromyxoid fibroma
chondromyxoma
chondronectin
chondroosseous
chondroosteodystrophy
chondropathy
chondropharyngeal
    c. part of middle constrictor muscle of pharynx
    c. part of middle pharyngeal constrictor muscle of pharynx
chondropharyngeus
chondrophyte
chondroplast
chondroplasty
chondroporosis
chondrosarcoma
chondrosin, chondrosine
chondroskeleton
chondrosternal
chondrosternoplasty
chondrotome
chondrotomy
chondrotrophic
chondroxiphoid ligament
chondrus
CHOP
    cyclophosphamide, doxorubicin (Adriamycin), vincristine, prednisone
Chopart
    C. amputation
    C. joint
chorda, pl. chordae
    c. arteriae umbilicalis
    c. chirurgicalis
    c. dorsalis
    false chordae tendineae
    c. magna
    c. obliqua membranae interosseae antebrachii
    c. saliva
    c. spermatica
    c. spinalis

chordae tendineae cordis
chordae tendineae falsae
chordae tendineae of heart
chordae tendineae spuriae
c. tympani
c. umbilicalis
c. vertebralis
c. vocalis
chordae willisii
chordal
chorda-mesoderm
Chordata
chordate
chordee
chorditis vocalis inferior
chordoma
chordoskeleton
chorea
c.-acanthocytosis
acanthocytosis with c.
acute c.
benign familial c.
chronic progressive c.
dancing c.
degenerative c.
electric c.
fibrillary c.
c. gravidarum
habit c.
hemilateral c.
Henoch c.
hereditary c.
Huntington c.
hysterical c.
juvenile c.
laryngeal c.
c. minor
Morvan c.
posthemiplegic c.
procursive c.
rheumatic c.
rhythmic c.
saltatory c.
senile c.
Sydenham c.
choreal
choreic movement
choreiform
choreoathetoid
choreoathetosis
congenital c.
choreoid
chorioadenoma destruens
chorioallantoic
c. graft
c. membrane
c. placenta
chorioallantois
chorioamnionic placenta
chorioamnionitis
chorioangioma
chorioangiomatosis
chorioangiosis
choriocapillaris
choriocapillary layer

choriocarcinoma
choriocele
chorioepithelioma
choriogonadotropin
chorioid-, chorioido-
choriomammotropin
choriomeningitis
lymphocytic c.
chorion
c. frondosum
c. laeve
previllous c.
primitive c.
shaggy c.
smooth c.
chorionic
c. ectoderm
c. gonadotropic hormone
c. gonadotropin (CG)
c. gonadotropin unit
c. "growth hormone-prolactin"
c. plate
c. sac
c. villi
c. villus biopsy
chorioretinal
chorioretinitis sclopetaria
chorioretinopathy
chorista
choristoblastoma
choristoma
choroid
c. blood vessel
c. branch
choroid capillary layer
c. enlargement
c. fissure
c. glomus
c. line
c. membrane
c. plexus
c. plexus of fourth ventricle
c. plexus of lateral ventricle
c. plexus of third ventricle
c. skein
c. vein
c. vein of eye
choroidal
c. fissure
c. neovascularization
c. ring
c. vascular atrophy
choroidea
choroideremia
choroiditis
anterior c.
areolar c.
diffuse c.
disseminated c.
exudative c.
juxtapupillary c.
metastatic c.
multifocal c.
posterior c.
proliferative c.

C

choroiditis *(continued)*
    suppurative c.
    vitiliginous c.
choroidocyclitis
choroidopathy
    areolar c.
    central serous c.
    Doyne honeycomb c.
    geographic c.
    helicoid c.
    myopic c.
    serpiginous c.
choroidosis
choroplethic map
Chotzen syndrome
Chr^a antigen
Christchurch chromosome
Christensen-Krabbe disease
Christian
    C. disease
    C. syndrome
Christison formula
Christmas
    C. disease
    C. factor
chromaffin
    c. body
    c. cell
    c. reaction
    c. system
    c. tissue
    c. tumor
chromaffinoma
chromaffinopathy
chroman, chromane
chromanol
chromaphil
chromate
    sodium c. Cr 51
    c. stain for lead
chromatic
    c. aberration
    c. apparatus
    c. audition
    c. fiber
    c. granule
    c. spectrum
    c. vision
chromatid
chromatin
    c. body
    heteropyknotic c.
    c. network
    c. nucleolus
    oxyphil c.
    c. particle
    sex c.
chromatinolysis
chromatinorrhexis
chromatism
chromatogenous
chromatogram
chromatograph
chromatographic

chromatography
    absorption c.
    adsorption c.
    affinity c.
    column c.
    fast protein liquid c. (FPLC)
    gas c.
    gas-liquid c. (GLC)
    gel filtration c.
    high-performance liquid c.
    high-pressure liquid chromatography (HPLC)
    ion exchange c.
    liquid-liquid c.
    paper c.
    c. paper
    partition c.
    reversed phase c.
    thin-layer c. (TLC)
    two-dimensional c.
chromatoid
chromatokinesis
chromatolysis
    central c.
    retrograde c.
    transsynaptic c.
chromatolytic
chromatometer
chromatopectic
chromatopexis
chromatophil
chromatophilia
chromatophilic, chromatophilous
chromatophobia
chromatophore
chromatophorotropic
chromatoplasm
chromatopsia
chromatosome
chromatotropism
chromaturia
chrome
    c. alum
    c. alum hematoxylin-phloxine stain
    c. red
    c. ulcer
    c. yellow
chrome-cobalt alloy
chromene
chromenol
chromesthesia
chromhidrosis
    apocrine c.
chromic
    c. acid
    c. catgut
    c. phosphate ^{32}P colloidal suspension
chromidia (*pl. of* chromidium)
chromidial
    c. apparatus
    c. net
    c. substance
chromidiation

chromidiosis
chromidium, pl. chromidia
chromidrosis
chromium trioxide
Chromobacterium
    c. violaceum
chromoblast
chromoblastomycosis
chromocenter
chromocyte
chromogen
    Porter-Silber c.
chromogenesis
chromogenic
chromogranin
chromoisomerism
chromolipid
chromolysis
chromomere
chromometer
chromomycosis
chromone
chromonema, pl. chromonemata
chromonychia
chromopectic
chromopexis
chromophil, chromophile
    c. granule
    c. substance
chromophilia
chromophilic, chromophilous
chromophobe
    c. adenoma
    c. cell of anterior lobe of
    hypophysis
    c. granule
chromophobia
chromophobic adenoma
chromophore
chromophoric, chromophorous
chromophototherapy
chromoplast
chromoplastid
chromoprotein
chromosomal
    c. breakage syndrome
    c. deletion
    c. gap
    c. instability syndrome
    c. region
    c. RNA
    c. trait
chromosome
    c. aberration
    accessory c.
    acentric c.
    acrocentric c.
    c. band
    bivalent c.
    Christchurch c.
    derivative c.
    dicentric c.
    double minute c.
    fragile X c.
    giant c.

    heterotypical c.
    homologous c.
    lampbrush c.
    late replicating c.
    c. map
    c. mapping
    marker c.
    metacentric c.
    mitochondrial c.
    c. mosaicism
    nonhomologous c.
    nucleolar c.
    odd c.
    c. pair
    c. pairing
    Philadelphia c. (Ph1)
    polytene c.
    c. puff
    ring c.
    c. satellite
    sex c.
    submetacentric c.
    telocentric c.
    translocation c.
    unpaired c.
    W c.
    c. walking
    X c.
    Y c.
    yeast artificial c. (YAC)
    Z c.
chromotherapy
chromotoxic
chromotrichia
chromotrichial
chromotrope 2R
chromotropic acid
chronaxia
chronaxie
chronaximeter
chronaximetry
chronaxis
chronaxy
chronic
    c. abscess
    c. absorptive arthritis
    c. acholuric jaundice
    c. actinic keratopathy
    c. active hepatitis
    c. active inflammation
    c. active liver disease
    c. adrenocortical insufficiency
    c. African sleeping sickness
    c. alcoholism
    c. allograft rejection
    c. amyloidosis
    c. anaphylaxis
    c. anterior poliomyelitis
    c. appendicitis
    c. ataxia
    c. atrophic polychondritis
    c. atrophic thyroiditis
    c. atrophic vulvitis
    c. bacillary diarrhea
    c. bronchitis

C

chronic *(continued)*
   c. bullous dermatosis of childhood
   c. cholecystitis
   c. cicatrizing enteritis
   c. constrictive pericarditis
   c. cutaneous leishmaniasis
   c. cystic mastitis
   c. desquamative gingivitis
   c. diffuse sclerosing osteomyelitis
   c. discoid lupus erythematosus
   c. eczema
   c. endemic fluorosis
   c. eosinophilic pneumonia
   c. familial icterus
   c. familial jaundice
   c. familial polyneuritis
   c. fibrosing alveolitis
   c. fibrosing pancreatitis
   c. fibrous thyroiditis
   c. focal sclerosing osteomyelitis
   c. follicular conjunctivitis
   c. glaucoma
   c. glomerulonephritis
   c. granulocytic leukemia
   c. granulomatous disease
   c. hemorrhagic villous synovitis
   c. hypertensive disease
   c. hypertrophic vulvitis
   c. hyperventilation syndrome
   c. idiopathic jaundice
   c. idiopathic xanthomatosis
   c. inflammatory demyelinating
    polyneuropathy (CIDP)
   c. interstitial hepatitis
   c. interstitial salpingitis
   c. lead poisoning
   c. lymphadenoid thyroiditis
   c. lymphocytic lymphoma
   c. lymphocytic thyroiditis
   c. malaria
   c. mediastinal histoplasmosis
   c. mercury poisoning
   c. mountain sickness
   c. myelocytic leukemia
   c. myelogenous leukemia (CML)
   c. myeloid leukemia
   c. necrotizing aspergillosis
   c. nephritis
   c. nonleukemic myelosis
   c. obstructive pulmonary disease
    (COPD)
   c. pancreatitis
   c. persistent hepatitis
   c. persisting hepatitis
   c. pleurisy
   c. posterior laryngitis
   c. progressive chorea
   c. progressive external
    ophthalmoplegia (CPEO)
   c. progressive syphilitic
    meningoencephalitis
   c. pyelonephritis
   c. relapsing pancreatitis
   c. rheumatism
   c. rhinitis
   c. shock
   c. soroche
   c. subglottic laryngitis
   c. tamponade
   c. trypanosomiasis
   c. ulcer
   c. ulcerative proctitis
   c. urticaria
   c. vertigo
chronicity
chronobiology
chronognosis
chronograph
chronologic age
chronometry
   mental c.
chronooncology
chronopharmacology
chronophobia
chronophotograph
chronotaraxis
chronotherapy
chronotropic
chronotropism
   negative c.
   positive c.
chroococcals
chrysanthemum-carboxylic acids
Chrysaora quinquecirrha
chrysarobin
chrysazine
chrysiasis
chrysocyanosis
chrysoidin
Chrysomyia
Chrysops
Chrysosporium parvum
chrysotherapy
chunking
Churg
Churg-Strauss syndrome
chutta
Chvostek sign
chylangioma
chylaqueous
chyle
   c. cistern
   c. corpuscle
   c. cyst
   c. fistula
   c. peritonitis
   c. vessel
chylemia
chylidrosis
chylifaction
chylifactive
chyliferous
chylification
chyliform ascites
chylocele
   parasitic c.
chylocyst

chylomediastinum
chylomicron, pl. **chylomicra**
  c. retention disease
chylomicron
chylomicronemia
chylopericardium
chyloperitoneum
chylophoric
chylopleura
chylopneumothorax
chylopoiesis
chylopoietic
chylorrhea
chylosis
chylothorax
chylous
  c. arthritis
  c. ascites
  c. hydrothorax
  c. urine
chyluria
chymase
chyme
chymification
chymopapain
chymopoiesis
chymorrhea
chymosin
chymosinogen
chymostatin
chymotropic pigment
chymotrypsin
chymotrypsinogen
chymous
chymus
chytide
Ci
  curie
Ciaccio
  C. gland
  C. stain
Cianca syndrome
cib.
  cibus
cibophobia
cibus (cib.)
CIC
  clean intermittent bladder catheterization
  completely in the canal hearing aid
cicatrectomy
cicatrices (*pl. of* cicatrix)
cicatricial
  c. alopecia
  c. conjunctivitis
  c. ectropion
  c. entropion
  c. horn
cicatricotomy
cicatrisotomy
cicatrix, pl. **cicatrices**
  brain c.
  filtering c.
  meningocerebral c.
  vicious c.
cicatrizant

cicatrization atelectasis
ciclopiroxolamine
cicutoxin
CIDP
  chronic inflammatory demyelinating
  polyneuropathy
cigarette drain
cigarette-paper scar
ciguatera
ciguatoxin
cilastatin sodium
cilia (*pl. of* cilium)
ciliary
  c. blepharitis
  c. body
  c. border of iris
  c. canal
  c. cartilage
  c. crown
  c. disk
  c. dyskinesis
  c. fold
  c. ganglion
  c. ganglionic plexus
  c. gland
  c. ligament
  c. margin of iris
  c. movement
  c. muscle
  c. part of retina
  c. poliosis
  c. process
  c. ring
  c. staphyloma
  c. wreath
  c. zone
  c. zonule
ciliastatic
Ciliata
ciliated epithelium
ciliates
ciliectomy
ciliocytophthoria
ciliogenesis
Ciliophora
cilioretinal
cilioscleral
ciliospinal
  c. center
  c. reflex
ciliotoxicity
cilium, pl. **cilia**
Cillobacterium
cimetidine
Cimex
  c. hemipterus
  c. lectularius
Cimino
cIMP
  cyclic inosine 3,5-monophosphate
cinanesthesia
cinanserin hydrochloride
cinchol
cinchona bark
cinchonic

cinchonine
cinchonism
cinchophen
cinclisis
cineangiocardiography
cinefluorography
cinefluoroscopy
cinegastroscopy
cinematic amputation
cinematics
cineol
cineole
cinephotomicrography
cineplastic amputation
cineplastics
cineradiography
cinerea
cinereal
cineritious
cineroentgenography
cineseismography
cinetoplasm
cinetoplasma
cingula (*pl. of* cingulum)
cingular branch of callosomarginal
  artery
cingulate
    c. convolution
    c. gyrus
    c. herniation
    c. sulcus
cingulectomy
cingulotomy
cingulum, pl. cingula
    c. dentis
    c. membri inferioris
    c. membri superioris
    c. pectorale
    c. pelvici
    c. rest
    c. of tooth
cinnamaldehyde
cinnamate
cinnamein
cinnamene
cinnamic
    c. acid
    c. alcohol
    c. aldehyde
cinnamon
    cassia c.
    Ceylon c.
    Chinese c.
    c. oil
    Saigon c.
cinnamylic acid
cinnarizine
cinnipirine
cinocentrum
cinoxacin
cinoxate
cion
ciprofloxacin hydrochloride
cirantin
circadian rhythm

Circe effect
circellus venosus hypoglossi
circhoral
circinate
    c. retinitis
    c. retinopathy
circle
    c. absorption anesthesia
    arterial c. of cerebrum
    articular vascular c.
    Carus c.
    cerebral arterial c.
    closed c.
    defensive c.
    greater arterial c. of iris
    Haller c.
    Huguier c.
    least confusion c.
    lesser arterial c. of iris
    major arterial c. of iris
    minor arterial c. of iris
    Pagenstecher c.
    Ridley c.
    rolling c.
    semi-closed c.
    vascular c.
    vascular c. of optic nerve
    venous c. of mammary gland
    vicious c.
    Vieth-Müller c.
    c. of Willis
    Zinn vascular c.
circuit
    anesthetic c.
    Papez c.
    reverberating c.
    signal-processing c.
circular
    c. amputation
    c. bandage
    c. dichroism (CD)
    c. fiber
    c. folds of small intestine
    c. layer of detrusor muscle of
    urinary bladder
    c. layer of muscle coat of small
    intestine
    c. layer of muscular coat
    c. layer of muscular tunics
    c. layer of tympanic membrane
    c. reaction
    c. sinus
    c. sulcus of insula
    c. sulcus of Reil
circulation
    assisted c.
    blood c.
    capillary c.
    collateral c.
    compensatory c.
    cross c.
    embryonic c.
    enterohepatic c.
    extracorporeal c.
    fetal c.

greater c.
hypophysial portal c.
hypothalamohypophysial portal c.
lesser c.
lymph c.
placental c.
portal hypophysial c.
pulmonary c.
Servetus c.
systemic c.
thebesian c.
c. time
circulatory
c. arrest
c. collapse
c. system
circulus, pl. **circuli**
c. arteriosus cerebri
c. arteriosus halleri
c. arteriosus iridis major
c. arteriosus iridis minor
c. articularis vasculosus
major c. arteriosus of iris
minor c. arteriosus of iris
c. vasculosus nervi optici
c. venosus halleri
c. venosus ridleyi
c. zinnii
circumalveolar fixation
circumanal gland
circumarticular
circumaxillary
circumbulbar
circumcise
circumcision
female c.
circumcorneal
circumductio
circumduction gait
circumference
articular c. of head of radius
articular c. of head of ulna
circumferentia
c. articularis capitis radii
c. articularis capitis ulnae
circumferential
c. cartilage
c. clasp
c. clasp arm
c. fibrocartilage
c. implantation
c. lamella
c. pontine branch of pontine artery
c. wiring
circumflex
c. branch of left coronary artery
c. branch of posterior tibial artery
c. femoral artery
c. fibular artery
c. fibular branch (of posterior tibial artery)
c. humeral artery
c. iliac artery
c. nerve

c. peroneal branch of posterior tibial artery
c. scapular artery
c. scapular vein
c. vein
circumgemmal
circumintestinal
circumlental
circummandibular fixation
circumnuclear
circumocular
circumoral
circumorbital
circumrenal
circumscribed
c. craniomalacia
c. peritonitis
c. posterior keratoconus
c. pyocephalus
circumscriptus
circumsporozoite protein
circumstantiality
circumvallate papillae
circumvascular
circumventricular organ
circumvolute
circumzygomatic
c. fixation
c. wiring
circus
c. movement
c. rhythm
cirrhogenic
cirrhogenous
cirrhonosus
cirrhosis
alcoholic c.
biliary c.
capsular c. of liver
cardiac c.
congestive c.
cryptogenic c.
fatty c.
Glisson c.
Hanot c.
juvenile c.
Laënnec c.
necrotic c.
nutritional c.
periportal c.
pigment c.
pigmentary c.
pipe stem c.
portal c.
posthepatitic c.
postnecrotic c.
primary biliary c.
pulmonary c.
stasis c.
syphilitic c.
toxic c.
cirrhotic
cirrose, cirrous
cirrus, pl. **cirri**

C

cirsoid
    c. aneurysm
    c. varix
cirsomphalos
cirsophthalmia
CIS
   carcinoma in situ
    c. phase
cis-**acting**
    cis-a. locus
    cis-a. protein
cis **configuration**
cisplatin
   cyclophosphamide,
    hexamethylmelamine, doxorubicin
    (Adriamycin), and c. (CHAP)
cistern
    ambient c.
    basal c.
    cerebellomedullary c.
    c. of chiasm
    chiasmatic c.
    chyle c.
    c. of cytoplasmic reticulum
    c. of great cerebral vein
    interpeduncular c.
    c. of lamina terminalis
    lateral cerebellomedullary c.
    c. of lateral cerebral fossa
    lumbar c.
    c. of nuclear envelope
    Pecquet c.
    pericallosal c.
    pontine c.
    pontocerebellar c.
    posterior cerebellomedullary c.
    prepontine c.
    quadrigeminal c.
    subarachnoid c.
    superior c.
    Sylvian c.
cisterna, pl. **cisternae**
    c. ambiens
    c. basalis
    c. caryothecae
    c. cerebellomedullaris lateralis
    c. cerebellomedullaris posterior
    c. chiasmatica
    c. chiasmatis
    c. chyli
    c. cruralis
    c. fossae lateralis cerebri
    c. interpeduncularis
    c. laminae terminalis
    c. lumbalis
    c. magna
    c. pericallosa
    c. perilymphatica
    c. pontis
    c. pontocerebellaris
    c. quadrigeminalis
    cisternae subarachnoideae
    subsurface c.
    terminal cisternae
    c. venae magnae cerebri

cisternal puncture
cisternography
    cerebellopontine c.
    radionuclide c.
cis/trans **test**
cistron
cisvestism, cisvestitism
Citellus
cito disp.
citral
citrase, citratase
citrate
    c. aldolase
    ATP c. (*pro-3S*)-lyase
    c. intoxication
    c. lyase
    c. synthase
citrate-cleavage enzyme
citrated calcium carbimide
citric
    c. acid
    c. acid cycle
citrin
Citrobacter
    C. amalonatica
    C. diversus
    C. freundii
    C. koseri
citronella
citronellal
citrovorum factor (CF)
citrulline
citrullinemia
citrullinuria
Civatte body
Civinini
    C. canal
    C. ligament
    C. process
CJD
    creutzfeldt-jakob disease
CK
    creatine kinase
Cl
cladiosis
Clado
    C. anastomosis
    C. band
    C. ligament
    C. point
Cladorchis watsoni
cladosporiosis
    cerebral c.
Cladosporium
    C. carrionii
    C. cladosporioides
    C. werneckii
    C. (Xylohypha) bantianum
Clagett procedure for empyema
clairvoyance
Claisen condensation
clamoxyquin hydrochloride
clamp
    c. connection
    Cope c.

Crafoord c.
Crile c.
Fogarty c.
c. forceps
Gant c.
Gaskell c.
gingival c.
Kelly c.
Kocher c.
liver-shod c.
Mikulicz c.
Mixter c.
Mogen c.
mosquito c.
Ochsner c.
patch c.
Payr c.
Potts c.
Rankin c.
right angle c.
rubber dam c.
rubber-shod c.

clamshell
c. incision
c. thoracotomy
clang association
clapotage, clapotement
Clapton line
Clara cell
clarificant
clarification
Clark
C. electrode
C. level
C. weight rule
Clarke
C. cell
C. column
C. nucleus
Clarke-Hadfield syndrome
clasmatocyte
clasmatosis
clasp
c. arm
bar c.
c. bar
circumferential c.
continuous c.
extended c.
c. guideline
Roach c.
clasping reflex
clasp-knife
c.-k. effect
c.-k. rigidity
c.-k. spasticity
class
c. I, II, III antigen
c. I,II molecule
c. switch
c. switching
classic
c. cervical rib syndrome
c. choroidal neovascularization

c. hemophilia
c. migraine
classical
c. cesarean section
c. conditioning
c. genetics
classifiable character
classification
adansonian c.
Angle c. of malocclusion
Arneth c.
Astler-Coller c.
Bethesda c.
Black c.
Caldwell-Moloy c.
Cummer c.
DeBakey c.
Denver c.
Dukes c.
FAB c.
French-American-British c.
Gell and Coombs C.
International Labour Organization C.
Jansky c.
Kennedy c.
Kiel c.
Lancefield c.
Lennert c.
Lukes-Collins c.
multiaxial c.
New York Heart Association c.
Rappaport c.
REAL c.
Runyon c.
Rye c.
Salter-Harris c. of epiphysial plate
injuries
Tessier c.
clastic anatomy
clastogen
clastogenic
clathrate crystal
clathrin
Clauberg
C. test
C. unit
Claude syndrome
claudication
intermittent c.
neurogenic c.
claudicatory
Claudius
C. cell
C. fossa
claustra (*pl. of* claustrum)
claustral layer
claustrophobia
claustrophobic
claustrum, pl. **claustra**
c. gutturis
c. oris
c. virginale
clausura
clava
claval

C

clavate papillae
clavi (*pl. of* clavus)
Claviceps purpurea
clavicle
clavicula, pl. **claviculae**
clavicular
    c. articular facet of acromion
    c. branch of thoracoacromial artery
    c. facet
    c. head of pectoralis major muscle
    c. notch of sternum
    c. part of deltoid muscle
    c. part of pectoralis major muscle
    c. percussion
claviculus, pl. **claviculi**
clavipectoral
    c. fascia
    c. triangle
clavulanic acid
clavus, pl. **clavi**
claw
    c. foot
    c. hand
clawfoot
clawhand
Claybrook sign
clay shoveler's fracture
CLB
    cyanobacterialike
cleaning
    ultrasonic c.
clean intermittent bladder catheterization (CIC)
cleansing cream
clear
    c. cell
    c. cell acanthoma
    c. cell adenocarcinoma
    c. cell carcinoma
    c. cell carcinoma of kidney
    c. cell carcinoma of salivary gland
    c. cell hidradenoma
    c. layer of epidermis
    c. liquid diet
clearance
    p-aminohippurate c.
    creatinine c.
    endogenous creatinine c.
    exogenous creatinine c.
    free water c.
    interocclusal c.
    inulin c.
    isotope c.
    maximum urea c.
    mucociliary c.
    occlusal c.
    osmolal c.
    standard urea c.
    urea c.
clearer
clearing
    c. factor
    c. medium
cleavage
    abnormal c. of cardiac valve

    adequal c.
    c. cavity
    c. cell
    complete c.
    determinate c.
    discoidal c.
    c. division
    enamel c.
    equal c.
    equatorial c.
    holoblastic c.
    hydrolytic c.
    incomplete c.
    indeterminate c.
    c. line
    meridional c.
    meroblastic c.
    phosphoroclastic c.
    c. product
    progressive c.
    pudendal c.
    c. site
    c. spindle
    subdural c.
    superficial c.
    thioclastic c.
    total c.
    unequal c.
    yolk c.
cleaved cell
cleaver
    enamel c.
cleft
    anal c.
    branchial c.
    cholesterol c.
    complete posterior laryngeal c.
    facial c.
    first visceral c.
    gill c.
    gingival c.
    gluteal c.
    c. hand
    hyobranchial c.
    hyomandibular c.
    intergluteal c.
    interneuromeric c.
    Larrey c.
    laryngotracheoesophageal c.
    c. lip
    Maurer c.
    median maxillary anterior alveolar c.
    natal c.
    c. nose
    oblique facial c.
    occult posterior laryngeal c.
    c. palate
    partial cricoid c.
    partial posterior laryngeal c.
    posterior laryngeal c.
    pudendal c.
    residual c.
    Schmidt-Lanterman c.
    c. spine

subdural c.
submucous laryngeal c.
synaptic c.
c. tongue
total cricoid c.
urogenital c.
visceral c.

cleidagra, clidagra
cleidal
cleidocostal
cleidocranial
 c. dysostosis
 c. dysplasia, clidocranial dysplasia
cleidotomy
cleistothecium
Cleland
 C. nomenclature
 C. reagent
clemastine
clenched fist sign
cleoid
cleptoparasite
clerical spectacles
Clevenger fissure
CLIA
 Clinical Laboratory Improvement
  Amendments
click
 ejection c.
 mitral c.
 c. syndrome
 systolic c.
clicking
 c. rale
 c. tinnitus
clidagra (*var. of* cleidagra)
clidal
clidinium bromide
clidocostal
clidocranial
 clidocranial dysostosis
clidocranial dysplasia (*var. of*
 cleidocranial dysplasia)
clidocranial dysplasia (*var. of*
 cleidocranial dysplasia)
client-centered therapy
climacophobia
climacteric
 c. syndrome
climacterium
climatic
 c. droplike keratopathy
climatology
climatotherapy
climax
climbing fiber
climograph
clindamycin
cline
clinic
clinical
 c. anatomy
 c. burden
 c. chemistry
 c. crown

c. depression
c. diagnosis
c. end point
c. epidemiology
c. eruption
c. fitness
c. genetics
c. indicator
C. Laboratory Improvement
 Amendments (CLIA)
c. lethal
c. medicine
c. nurse specialist
c. path
c. pathology
c. pharmacologist
c. pharmacology
c. pharmacy
c. practice guidelines
c. psychology
c. recording
c. root of tooth
c. sensitivity
c. spectrometry
c. spectroscopy
c. thermometer
c. trial

clinician
clinicopathologic
clinocephalic
clinocephalous
clinocephaly
clinodactyly
clinography
clinoid process
clioquinol
clioxanide
clip
 c. forceps
 wound c.
clipped speech
clithrophobia
clition
clitoral recession
clitoridean
clitoridectomy
clitoriditis
clitoris, pl. **clitorides**
clitorism
clitoritis
clitoromegaly
clitoroplasty
clival
clivus, pl. **clivi**
 Blumenbach c.
 c. branch of cerebral part of
  internal carotid artery
 c. ocularis
CL lead
cloaca
 ectodermal c.
 endodermal c.
 persistent c.
cloacal
 c. exstrophy

C

cloacal (*continued*)
 c. membrane
 c. plate
 c. theory
cloacogenic carcinoma
clobazam
clobetasol propionate
clocortolone
clofazimine
clofenamide
clofibrate
clogestone acetate
clomacran phosphate
clomegestone acetate
clomiphene
 c. citrate
 c. test
clomipramine hydrochloride
clonal
 c. aging
 c. deletion theory
 c. expansion
 c. selection theory
clonazepam
clone
 cDNA c.
 genomic c.
clonic
 c. convulsion
 c. seizure
clonicity
clonicotonic
clonidine
 c. growth hormone stimulation test
 c. hydrochloride
cloning
 A/T c.
 positional c.
 c. vector
clonism
clonogenic
 c. assay
 c. cell
clonograph
clonorchiasis
clonorchiosis
Clonorchis sinensis
clonus
 ankle c.
 toe c.
 wrist c.
clopamide
Cloquet
 C. canal
 C. hernia
 C. septum
 C. space
clorazepate
clorprenaline hydrochloride
close bite
closed
 c. anesthesia
 c. angiography
 c. bite

 c. chain compound
 c. chest massage
 c. circle
 c. circuit method
 c. comedo
 c. dislocation
 c. drainage
 c. head injury
 c. hospital
 c. laparoscopy
 c. loop obstruction
 c. reading frame
 c. reduction of fractures
 c. skull fracture
 c. surgery
 c. system
closed-angle glaucoma
closing
 c. contraction
 c. membrane
 c. snap
 c. volume
clostridia (*pl. of* clostridium)
clostridial myonecrosis
clostridiopeptidase
 c. A, B
Clostridium
 C. bifermentans
 C. botulinum
 C. butyricum
 C. cadaveris
 C. carnis
 C. chauvoei
 C. cochlearium
 C. difficile
 C. fallax
 C. haemolyticum
 C. histolyticum
 C. histolyticum collagenase
 C. histolyticum proteinase B
 C. innominatum
 C. nigrificans
 C. novyi
 C. oedematiens
 C. parabotulinum
 C. paraputrificum
 C. perfringens
 C. perfringens alpha toxin
 C. perfringens beta toxin
 C. perfringens enterotoxin
 C. perfringens epsilon toxin
 C. perfringens iota toxin
 C. ramosum
 C. septicum
 C. sordellii
 C. sphenoides
 C. sporogenes
 C. tertium
 C. tetani
 C. thermosaccharolyticum
 C. welchii
clostridium, pl. **clostridia**
clostripain
closure
 flask c.

c. principle
velopharyngeal c.
closylate
clot
agonal c.
antemortem c.
blood c.
chicken fat c.
currant jelly c.
laminated c.
passive c.
postmortem c.
c. retraction time
clotrimazole
clottage
clotting
c. factor
c. time
clouding of consciousness
Cloudman melanoma
cloudy
c. swelling
c. urine
clove oil
cloverleaf
c. model
c. skull
c. skull syndrome
cloxacillin sodium
clozapine
CLQ
cognitive laterality quotient
club
c. foot
c. hair
c. hand
c. moss
clubbed
c. digit
c. finger
c. penis
clubbing
hereditary c.
clubfoot
clubhand
radial c.
ulnar c.
clue cell
clump
clumping
cluneal
clunes
clupanodonic acid
cluster
c. analysis
c. of differentiation (CD) antigen
egg c.
c. headache
c. sample
cluster of differentiation (CD)
cluttering
Clutton joint
clysis
clyster

CM-
carboxymethyl radical
Cm
curium
cM
centimorgan
cm
centimeter
CMA
Certified Medical Assistant
p-**CMB**
p-chloromercuribenzoate
cmc
critical micelle concentration
CM-cellulose
CMG
cystometrogram
CMI
cell-mediated immunity
CML
chronic myelogenous leukemia
CMO
calculated mean organism
CMP
cytidine 5′-monophosphate
c-mp1
CMT
Certified Medical Transcriptionist
CMV
controlled mechanical ventilation
cnemial
cnemis
cnida, pl. **cnidae**
cnidocyst
Cnidospora
Cnidosporidia
CNM
certified nurse-midwife
CNS
central nervous system
CO
carbon monoxide
Co
cobalt
coccygeal
^{60}**Co**
cobalt-60
^{58}**Co**
cobalt-58
^{57}**Co**
cobalt-57
CoA
coenzyme A
coacervate
coacervation
coadaptation
coagglutination
coagula (*pl. of* coagulum)
coagulable
coagulant
coagulate
coagulation
disseminated intravascular c. (DIC)
c. factor
c. necrosis

C

coagulation (*continued*)
    c. time
    c. vitamin
coagulative
coagulopathy
    consumption c.
coagulum, pl. **coagula**
coal
    c. oil
    c. tar
    c. tar naphtha
    c. worker's pneumoconiosis
co-alcoholic
co-alcoholism
coalescence
coapt
coaptation
    c. splint
    c. suture
coarct
coarctate
coarctation
    aortic c.
    reversed c.
coarctectomy
coarctotomy
coarse
    c. dispersion
    c. tremor
CoAS–
    coenzyme A radical
CoASH
    reduced coenzyme A
coat
    buffy c.
    muscular c.
    muscular c. of bronchi
    muscular c. of colon
    muscular c. of ductus deferens
    muscular c. of esophagus
    muscular c. of female urethra
    muscular c. of gallbladder
    muscular c. of intermediate part of
      male urethra
    muscular c. of large intestine
    muscular c. of male urethra
    muscular c. of pharynx
    muscular c. of prostatic urethra
    muscular c. of rectum
    muscular c. of small intestine
    muscular c. of spongy part of male
      urethra
    muscular c. of stomach
    muscular c. of trachea
    muscular c. of ureter
    muscular c. of urinary bladder
    muscular c. of uterine tube
    muscular c. of uterus
    muscular c. of vagina
    sclerotic c.
    serous c.
    serous c. of peritoneum
coated
    c. pit

    c. tongue
    c. vesicle
coating
    antireflection c.
CoA transferase
Coats disease
cobalamin (Cbl)
    ATP c. adenoxyltransferase
    c. concentrate
cobalt (Co)
cobalt-57 (^{57}Co)
cobalt-58 (^{58}Co)
cobalt-60 (^{60}Co)
cobaltous chloride
Cobb
    C. method
    C. syndrome
cobbler's suture
cobra
    c. hemotoxin
    c. toxin
    c. venom cofactor
    c. venom factor
cobrotoxin
cobyric acid
cobyrinamide
cobyrinic acid
COC
    cathodal opening contraction
coca
cocaine
    crack c.
    c. hydrochloride
cocainization
cocarboxylase
cocarcinogen
cocarde reaction
Coccaceae
coccal
cocci (*pl. of* coccus)
Coccidia
coccidia (*pl. of* coccidium)
coccidial
Coccidiasina
coccidioidal granuloma
Coccidioides
coccidioidin test
coccidioidoma
coccidioidomycosis
    disseminated c.
    primary c.
    primary extrapulmonary c.
    secondary c.
    subclinical c.
coccidiosis
coccidiostat
coccidium, pl. **coccidia**
coccinella
coccinellin
coccobacillary
coccobacillus
coccoid
cocculin
coccus, pl. **cocci**

Neisser c.
Weichselbaum c.
coccycephaly
coccydynia
coccygeal (Co)
c. body
c. bone
c. cornu
c. dimple
c. fistula
c. foveola
c. ganglion
c. gland
c. horn
c. joint
c. ligament
c. muscle
c. nerve [Co]
c. part of spinal cord
c. plexus
c. segment of spinal cord [Co]
c. sinus
c. vertebrae [Co1–Co4]
c. whorl
coccygectomy
coccyges (*pl. of* coccyx)
coccygeus muscle
coccygodynia
coccygotomy
coccyodynia
coccyx, pl. **coccyges**
Cochin China diarrhea
cochineal
cochlea, pl. **cochleae**
membranous c.
cochlear
c. aqueduct
c. area
c. branch of labyrinthine artery
c. branch of vestibulocochlear artery
c. canal
c. canaliculus
c. cupula
c. drill-out
c. duct
c. dysplasia
c. ganglion
c. hair cell
c. implant
c. joint
c. labyrinth
c. microphonic
c. nerve
c. nuclei
c. part of vestibulocochlear nerve
c. potential
c. prosthesis
c. recess
c. root of VIII nerve
c. window
cochleare
c. amplum
c. magnum
c. medium

c. modicum
c. parvum
cochleariform process
cochleate
cochleitis
cochleo-orbicular reflex
cochleopalpebral reflex
cochleopupillary reflex
cochleosacculotomy
cochleostapedial reflex
cochleotopic
cochleovestibular
Cochliomyia
C. americana
C. hominivorax
Cochrane collaboration
cocillana
cockade reaction (*var. of* cocarde
reaction)
Cockayne
C. disease
C. syndrome
Cockett communicating perforating vein
cocktail
Brompton c.
Philadelphia c.
Rivers c.
cocoa butter
coconsciousness
coconut sound
coconversion
coctolabile
coctostabile
coctostable
code
genetic c.
soundex c.
codeine
c. phosphate
c. sulfate
Codex medicamentarius
codfish vertebrae
coding
place c.
c. sequence
c. strand
cod liver oil
Codman
C. triangle
C. tumor
codogenic
codominant
c. allele
c. gene
c. inheritance
c. trait
codon
amber c.
initiating c.
initiation c.
nonsense c.
ochre c.
opal c.
punctuation c.
start c.

C

codon *(continued)*
    stop c.
    termination c.
    umber c.
coefficient
    absorption c.
    activity c.
    biologic c.
    Bunsen solubility c.
    c. of consanguinity
    correlation c.
    creatinine c.
    diffusion c.
    distribution c.
    economic c.
    extinction c.
    extraction c.
    filtration c.
    Hill c.
    hygienic laboratory c.
    c. of inbreeding
    isotonic c.
    c. of kinship
    lethal c.
    linear absorption c.
    Long c.
    molar absorption c.
    molar extinction c.
    Ostwald solubility c.
    oxygen utilization c.
    partition c.
    permeability c.
    phenol c.
    Poiseuille viscosity c.
    reflection c.
    c. of relationship
    reliability c.
    respiratory c.
    Rideal-Walker c.
    sedimentation c.
    selection c. (*s*)
    specific absorption c.
    temperature c.
    ultrafiltration c.
    c. of variation (CV)
    velocity c.
    c. of viscosity
Coelenterata
coelenterate
coelom
coelomic metaplasia
coenesthesia
coenocyte
coenocytic
coenuris *(var. of* cenuris)
coenurosis
Coenurus
    C. cerebralis
    C. serialis
coenzyme
    c. A (CoA)
    c. A radical (CoAS–)
    c. F
    c. factor

    c. Q (CoQ)
    c. R
    reduced c. A (CoASH)
coeur en sabot
Coe virus
coevolution
cofactor
    cobra venom c.
    molybdenum c.
    platelet c. I, II
coffee-ground vomit
Coffey suspension
Coffin-Lowry syndrome
Coffin-Siris syndrome
Cogan
    C. dystrophy
    C. syndrome
Cogan-Reese syndrome
cognition
cognitive
    c. development
    c. dissonance
    c. dissonance theory
    c. laterality quotient (CLQ)
    c. psychology
    c. therapy
cogwheel
    c. ocular movement
    c. phenomenon
    c. respiration
    c. rigidity
cohesion
cohesive gold
Cohnheim
    C. area
    C. field
cohoba
cohort study
coil
    detector c.
    c. gland
    random c.
    surface c.
coiled artery of the uterus
coin
    c. lesion of lung
    c. test
coincidental evolution
coin-counting
cointegrate structure
coital headache
Coiter muscle
coition
coitophobia
coitus
    c. interruptus
    c. reservatus
Cokeromyces
cola
colchicine
Colchicum corm
cold
    c. abscess
    c. agglutination
    c. agglutinin

c. agglutinin syndrome
c. allergy
c. antibody
c. autoagglutinin
c. autoantibody
c. bend test
c. cautery
c. chain
c. cream
c. cure resin
c. erythema
c. gangrene
head c.
c. hemagglutinin disease
c. hemolysin
c. knife conization
c. light
c. nodule
c. pack
c. pressor test
rose c.
c. snare
c. sore
c. stage
c. urticaria
c. virus
cold-blooded animal
cold-curing resin
cold-reactive antibody
cold-rigor point
cold-sensitive
c.-s. enzyme
c.-s. mutant
Cole-Cecil murmur
colectasia
colectomy
Coleoptera
coleoptosis
coleotomy
colestipol
colet.
coletur
coletur (colet.)
colibacillosis
colibacillus, pl. **colibacilli**
colic
appendicular c.
c. artery
biliary c.
c. branch of ileocolic artery
copper c.
Devonshire c.
gallstone c.
gastric c.
hepatic c.
c. impression on liver
c. impression of spleen
infantile c.
c. intussusception
lead c.
c. lymph node
meconial c.
menstrual c.
ovarian c.
painter's c.

pancreatic c.
Poitou c.
renal c.
salivary c.
saturnine c.
c. sphincter
c. surface of spleen
c. tenia
tubal c.
ureteral c.
uterine c.
c. vein
vermicular c.
zinc c.
colica
colicin
colicinogeny
colicky
colicoplegia
coliform bacilli
colimycin
colinearity
colipase
coliphage
coliplication
colipuncture
colistimethate sodium
colistin
c. sulfate
c. sulfomethate sodium
colitis
amebic c.
collagenous c.
c. cystica profunda
c. cystica superficialis
granulomatous c.
hemorrhagic c.
mucous c.
myxomembranous c.
pseudomembranous c.
ulcerative c.
uremic c.
colitose
colla (*pl. of* collum)
collaboration
Cochrane c.
collacin
collagen
c. disease
c. fiber
c. fibril
c. helix
c. implantation
c. injection
type I, II, III, IV c.
collagenase
c. A
Clostridium histolyticum c.
c. I
microbial c.
collagenation
collagenic
collagenization
collagenolytic

C

collagenosis
    reactive perforating c.
collagenous
    c. colitis
    c. fiber
    c. pneumoconiosis
collagen-vascular disease
collapse
    absorption c.
    circulatory c.
    c. of dental arch
    massive c.
    pressure c.
    pulmonary c.
    c. therapy
collapsing pulse
collar
    c. bone
    c. incision
    renal c.
collared flagellate
collarette
collar-stud chalazion
collastin
collateral
    c. branch of intercostal nerve
    c. branch of posterior intercostal
    artery 3–11
    c. circulation
    c. digital artery
    c. eminence
    c. fissure
    c. hyperemia
    c. inheritance
    c. ligament
    c. sulcus
    c. trigone
    c. vessel
collectin
collective unconscious
college
    Association of American
    Medical C.'s (AAMC)
Colles
    C. fascia
    C. fracture
    C. ligament
    C. space
Collet-Sicard syndrome
collicular artery
colliculectomy
colliculus, pl. **colliculi**
    c. of arytenoid cartilage
    c. cartilaginis arytenoideae
    facial c.
    c. facialis
    c. inferior
    inferior c.
    inferior nasal c.
    seminal c.
    c. seminalis
    c. superior
    superior c.
    c. urethralis

Collier
    C. lung
    C. tract
    C. tucked lid sign
colligation
colligative
collimation
collimator
colliotomy
colliquation
colliquative
    c. albuminuria
    c. diarrhea
    c. necrosis
Collis-Belsey
    C.-B. fundoplication
    C.-B. procedure
Collis gastroplasty
collision tumor
Collis-Nissen fundoplication
collodion
    c. baby
    blistering c.
    cantharidal c.
    flexible c.
    hemostatic c.
    iodized c.
    salicylic acid c.
    styptic c.
    c. vesicans
collodium
colloid
    c. adenoma
    c. bath
    c. body
    bovine c.
    c. cancer
    c. carcinoma
    c. corpuscle
    c. cyst
    c. degeneration
    dispersion c.
    emulsion c.
    c. goiter
    hydrophil c.
    hydrophilic c.
    hydrophobic c.
    irreversible c.
    lyophilic c.
    lyophobic c.
    c. milium
    protective c.
    c. pseudomilium
    reversible c.
    stable c.
    styptic c.
    suspension c.
    c. system
    c. theory of narcosis
    thyroid c.
    unstable c.
colloidal
    c. dispersion
    c. gel
    c. gold reaction

c. gold test
c. metal
c. radioactive gold
c. silicon dioxide
c. silver iodide
c. solution
colloidin
colloidoclasia
colloidoclasis
colloidoclastic
colloidogen
colloxylin
collum, pl. **colla**
c. anatomicum humeri
c. chirurgicum humeri
c. costae
c. dentis
c. femoris
c. fibulae
c. folliculi pili
c. glandis
c. humeri
c. mallei
c. mandibulae
c. ossis femoris
c. radii
c. scapulae
c. tali
c. vesicae
c. vesicae biliaris
c. vesicae felleae
collutorium
collutory
collyrium
coloboma
c. of choroid
Fuchs c.
c. iridis
c. lentis
c. lobuli
macular c.
c. of optic nerve
c. palpebrale
c. of vitreous
colobomatous microphthalmia
colocentesis
colocolic
colocolostomy
colocutaneous fistula
colocynth
colocystoplasty
coloenteritis
colohepatopexy
coloileal fistula
cololysis
colominic acid
colon
c. ascendens
ascending c.
c. bacillus
c. cutoff sign
c. descendens
descending c.
giant c.
iliac c.

irritable c.
lead-pipe c.
c. pelvinum
sigmoid c.
c. sigmoideum
spastic c.
stove-pipe c.
transverse c.
c. transversum
colonalgia
colonic
c. diverticulum
c. fistula
c. smear
colonization
genetic c.
colonogram
colonometer
colonopathy
fibrosing c.
colonorrhagia
colonorrhea
colonoscope
colonoscopy
colony
daughter c.
filamentous c.
H c.
lenticular c.
mother c.
mucoid c.
O c.
rough c.
smooth c.
spheroid c.
colony-forming unit
colony-stimulating factor
colopathy
colopexostomy
colopexotomy
colopexy
colophony
coloplication
coloproctitis
coloproctostomy
coloptosia
coloptosis
colopuncture
color
c. aberration
c. agnosia
c. blindness
complementary c.
confusion c.
c. constancy
extrinsic c.
c. hearing
intrinsic c.
c. match
opponent c.
primary c.
pure c.
c. radical
reflected c.
saturated c.

C

color *(continued)*
    c. scotoma
    c. sense
    simple c.
    c. solid
    c. spectrum
    structural c.
    c. taste
    tone c.
    c. triangle
Colorado
    C. tick fever
    C. tick fever virus
color-contrast microscope
colorectal
colorectitis
colorectostomy
colored vision (VC)
colorimeter
    Duboscq c.
colorimetric
    c. caries susceptibility test
    c. titration
colorimetry
colorrhagia
colorrhaphy
colorrhea
coloscopy
colosigmoidostomy
colostomy bag
colostrorrhea
colostrous
colostrum corpuscle
colotomy
Colour Index
colovaginal fistula
colovesical fistula
colpatresia
colpectasia
colpectasis
colpectomy
colpocele
colpocleisis
colpocystoplasty
colpocystotomy
colpocystoureterotomy
colpodynia
colpohysterectomy
colpohysteropexy
colpohysterotomy
colpomicroscope
colpomicroscopy
colpomycosis
colpomyomectomy
colpoperineoplasty
colpoperineorrhaphy
colpopexy
colpoplasty
colpopoiesis
colpoptosia
colpoptosis
colporectopexy
colporrhaphy
colporrhexis

colposcope
colposcopy
colpospasm
colpostat
colpostenosis
colpostenotomy
colposuspension
colpotomy
colpoureterotomy
colpoxerosis
Coltivirus
Colubridae
Columbia
    C. Mental Maturity Scale
    C. S. K. virus
columbium (Cb)
columella, pl. **columellae**
    c. cochleae
    c. nasi
column
    affinity c.
    anal c.
    anterior c.
    anterior gray c.
    anterior c. of medulla oblongata
    anterolateral c. of spinal cord
    Bertin c.
    branchial efferent c.
    Burdach c.
    c. cell
    c. chromatography
    Clarke c.
    dorsal c. of spinal cord
    c. of fornix
    general somatic afferent c.
    general somatic efferent c.
    general visceral afferent c.
    general visceral efferent c.
    Goll c.
    Gowers c.
    gray c.
    intermediate c.
    intermediolateral cell c. of spinal cord (IML)
    lateral c.
    lateral c. of spinal cord
    Lissauer c.
    Morgagni c.
    posterior c.
    posterior c. of spinal cord
    rectal c.
    renal c.
    Rolando c.
    rugal c. of vagina
    Sertoli c.
    special somatic afferent c.
    special visceral efferent c.
    spinal c.
    c. of Spitzka-Lissauer
    splanchnic afferent c.
    splanchnic efferent c.
    Stilling c.
    Türck c.
    vaginal c.

ventral white c.
vertebral c.

columna, pl. **columnae**
columnae anales
c. anterior
columnae carneae
c. fornicis
columnae griseae
c. intermedia
c. lateralis
c. posterior
columnae renales
columnae rugarum
c. vertebralis

columnar
c. epithelium
c. layer

columnella, pl. **columnellae**

colypeptic

coma
c. aberration
c. cast
delayed c. after hypoxia
diabetic c.
hepatic c.
hyperosmolar (hyperglycemic) nonketotic c.
hypoglycemic c.
hypoventilation c.
Kussmaul c.
metabolic c.
c. scale
thyrotoxic c.
trance c.
uremic c.
c. vigil

comatose

combat neurosis

combination
c. beat
binary c.
c. chemotherapy
new c.
c. oral contraceptive
c. restoration

combinatorial chemistry

combined
c. fat- and carbohydrate-induced hyperlipemia
c. glaucoma
c. immunodeficiency
c. immunodeficiency syndrome
c. method
c. pregnancy
c. sclerosis
c. system disease
c. version

combining weight

comblike septum

combustible

combustion
c. equivalent
slow c.
spontaneous c.

Comby sign

comedo, pl. **comedos, comedones**
closed c.
open c.
solar c.

comedocarcinoma

comedogenic

comedonecrosis

comedones (*pl. of* comedo)

comedos (*pl. of* comedo)

comes, pl. **comites**

comet
c. tail sign

comfort zone

comitance

comitant
c. artery of median nerve
c. strabismus

comites (*pl. of* comes)

comma
c. bacillus
c. bundle of Schultze
c. tract of Schultze

command hallucination

commando
c. operation
c. procedure

commemorative sign

commensalism
epizoic c.

commensal parasite

comminuted
c. skull fracture

comminution

commission
Enzyme C. of the International Union of Biochemistry (EC)
Nuclear Regulatory C.

commissura, pl. **commissurae**
c. alba anterior
c. alba posterior
c. anterior
c. anterior grisea
c. bulborum
c. cinerea
c. colliculorum inferiorum
c. colliculorum superiorum
c. epithalamica
c. fornicis
c. grisea
c. grisea anterior
c. grisea posterior
c. habenularum
c. hippocampi
c. labiorum
c. labiorum anterior
c. labiorum posterior
c. lateralis palpebrum
c. medialis palpebrum
c. palpebrarum lateralis
c. palpebrarum medialis
c. posterior
c. supraoptica dorsalis
c. ventralis alba

C

commissural
c. cell
c. cheilitis
c. fiber
c. myelotomy

commissure
anterior gray c.
anterior labial c.
anterior c. of the larynx
anterior white c.
c. of bulbs
c. of cerebral hemispheres
dorsal supraoptic c.
c. of fornix
Ganser c.
gray c.
Gudden c.
c. of habenulae
habenular c.
hippocampal c.
c. of inferior colliculus
labial c.
lateral palpebral c.
c. of lips
medial palpebral c.
Meynert c.
posterior gray c.
posterior labial c.
posterior c. of the larynx
c. of superior colliculus
ventral white c.
c. of vestibular bulb
Wernekinck c.
white c.

commissurotomy
mitral c.

commisural pit
commitment
common
c. antigen
c. baldness
c. basal vein
c. bile duct
c. cardinal vein
c. carotid artery
c. carotid nervous plexus
c. cochlear artery
c. cold virus
c. crus of semicircular duct
c. facial vein
c. fibular nerve
c. flexor sheath of hand
c. hepatic artery
c. hepatic duct
c. iliac artery
c. iliac lymph node
c. iliac vein
c. interosseous artery
c. membranous limb of membranous
semicircular duct
c. membranous limb of semicircular
duct
c. migraine
c. modiolar vein
c. opsonin

c. palmar digital artery
c. palmar digital nerve
c. peroneal nerve
c. peroneal tendon sheath
c. plantar digital artery
c. plantar digital nerve
c. salt
c. tendinous ring of extraocular
muscle
c. variable immunodeficiency
c. vehicle c.
c. wart

commotio
c. cerebri
c. retinae

communicable disease
communicans, pl. **communicantes**
communicating
c. artery
c. branch
c. branch of anterior interosseous
nerve with ulnar nerve
c. branch of auriculotemporal nerve
with facial nerve
c. branch of chorda tympani to
lingual nerve
c. branch of chorda tympani with
lingual nerve
c. branch of facial nerve with
glossopharyngeal nerve
c. branch of facial nerve with
tympanic plexus
c. branch of fibular artery
c. branch of glossopharyngeal nerve
with auricular branch of vagus
nerve
c. branch of intermediate nerve
with tympanic plexus
c. branch of internal laryngeal
nerve with recurrent laryngeal
nerve
c. branch of lacrimal nerve with
zygomatic nerve
c. branch of lingual nerve with
hypoglossal nerve
c. branch of median nerve with
ulnar nerve
c. branch of nasociliary nerve with
ciliary ganglion
c. branch of otic ganglion to
auriculotemporal nerve
c. branch of otic ganglion to
chorda tympani
c. branch of otic ganglion with
chorda tympani
c. branch of otic ganglion with
medial pterygoid nerve
c. branch of otic ganglion with
meningeal branch of mandibular
nerve
c. branch of peroneal artery
c. branch of radial nerve with
ulnar nerve
c. branch of spinal nerve

c. branch of superficial radial nerve with ulnar nerve
c. branch of superior laryngeal nerve with recurrent laryngeal nerve
c. branch of sympathetic trunk
c. branch of tympanic plexus with auricular branch of vagus nerve
c. hematoma
c. hydrocele
c. hydrocephalus
c. junction
c. ramus of sympathetic trunk

communication
human c.
simultaneous c.
total c.

community
biotic c.
c. dentistry
c. health nurse
c. medicine
c. mental health center
c. nurse
c. psychiatry
c. psychology
therapeutic c.

community-acquired pneumonia
comorbidity
compact
c. bone
c. substance

compacta
compages thoracis
companion
c. artery to sciatic nerve
c. lymph node of accessory nerve
c. vein

comparascope
comparative
c. anatomy
c. medicine
c. pathology
c. physiology
c. psychology

comparator microscope
compartimentum
c. antebrachii anterius
c. antebrachii extensorum
c. antebrachii flexorum
c. antebrachii posterius
c. brachii anterius
c. brachii extensorum
c. brachii flexorum
c. brachii posterius
c. cruris
c. cruris anterius
c. cruris extensorum
c. cruris fibularium
c. cruris flexorum
c. cruris laterale peroneorum
c. cruris posterius
c. femoris adductorum
c. femoris anterius
c. femoris extensorum

c. femoris flexorum
c. femoris mediale
c. femoris posterius

compartment
adductor c. of thigh
anterior c. of arm
anterior c. of forearm
anterior c. of leg
anterior c. of thigh
dorsiflexor c. of leg
extensor c. of arm
extensor c. of forearm
extensor c. of leg
extensor c. of thigh
fibular c. of leg
flexor c. of arm
flexor c. of forearm
flexor c. of leg
flexor c. of thigh
lateral c. of leg
medial c. of thigh
nonplasmatic c.
peroneal c. of leg
plantarflexor c. of leg
plasmatic c.
posterior c. of arm
posterior c. of forearm
posterior c. of leg
posterior c. of thigh
c. syndrome
c. of thigh for extensors of hip joint
c. of thigh for extensors of knee
c. of thigh for flexors of hip
c. of thigh for flexors of knee

compartmentation
compatibility
compatible
compensated
c. acidosis
c. glaucoma
c. metabolic alkalosis
c. respiratory acidosis
c. respiratory alkalosis

compensating
c. curve
c. emphysema
c. ocular

compensation
attenuation c.
depth c.
gene dosage c.
c. neurosis
time-gain c.

compensatory
c. circulation
c. emphysema
c. hypertrophy
c. hypertrophy of the heart
c. pause
c. polycythemia

competence
cardiac c.
immunologic c.

competing risk

C

competition
    antigenic c.
competitive
    c. antagonist
    c. binding assay
    c. inhibition
competitor DNA
complaint
    chief c. (CC)
complement
    c. binding assay
    c. chemotactic factor
    c. factor I
    c. fixation
    heparin c.
    c. pathway
    c. system
    c. unit
complemental air
complementarity
    c. determining region
complementary
    c. air
    c. color
    c. DNA (cDNA)
    c. hypertrophy
    c. medicine
    c. ribonucleic acid (cRNA)
    c. role
    c. strand
    c. structure
complementation
    intergenic c.
    intragenic c.
complement-fixation
    c.-f. reaction
    c.-f. test
complement-fixing antibody
complete
    c. abortion
    c. achromatopsia
    c. androgen insensitivity syndrome
    c. antibody
    c. antigen
    c. ascertainment
    c. atrioventricular dissociation
    c. AV block
    c. AV dissociation
    c. blood count (CBC)
    c. carcinogen
    c. cataract
    c. cleavage
    c. denture
    c. denture impression
    c. disinfectant
    c. fistula
    c. hemianopia
    c. hernia
    c. iridoplegia
    c. mastoidectomy
    c. medium
    c. metamorphosis
    c. posterior laryngeal cleft

    c. tetanus
    c. transduction
completely in the canal hearing aid (CIC)
complex
    aberrant c.
    AIDS dementia c. (ADC)
    AIDS-related c. (ARC)
    alpha-keto acid dehydrogenase c.
    amygdaloid c.
    anomalous c.
    antigen-antibody c.
    antigenic c.
    apical c.
    atrial c.
    auricular c.
    binary c.
    brain wave c.
    brother c.
    Cain c.
    Carney c.
    castration c.
    caudal pharyngeal c.
    central c.
    charge transfer c.
    Diana c.
    diphasic c.
    EAHF c.
    Eisenmenger c.
    Electra c.
    electrocardiographic c.
    c. endometrial hyperplasia
    enzyme-substrate c.
    equiphasic c.
    father c.
    c. febrile convulsion
    femininity c.
    c. fracture
    Ghon c.
    Golgi c.
    H-2 c.
    histocompatibility c.
    HLA c.
    immune c.
    inferiority c.
    inferior olivary c.
    iron-dextran c.
    isodiphasic c.
    j-g c.
    Jocasta c.
    c. joint
    junctional c.
    juxtaglomerular c.
    K c.
    α-ketoglutarate dehydrogenase c.
    Lear c.
    c. learning process
    c. locus
    MAC c.
    major histocompatibility c. (MHC)
    mediator c.
    membrane attack c.
    Meyenburg c.
    Michaelis c.
    minor histocompatibility c.

monophasic c.
c. motor seizure
multienzyme c.
c. odontoma
Oedipus c.
ostiomeatal c.
c. partial seizure
persecution c.
c. pleural effusion
c. precipitated epilepsy
primary c.
pyruvate dehydrogenase c.
QRS c.
Ranke c.
ribosome-lamella c.
Shone c.
sicca c.
c. sound
spike and wave c.
superiority c.
superior olivary c.
symptom c.
synaptinemal c.
synaptonemal c.
Tacaribe c. of viruses
ternary c.
triple symptom c.
VATER c.
ventricular c.
ventrobasal c.

complexion
complexity
chemical c.
complexus
c. olivaris inferior
c. stimulans cordis
compliance
c. of bladder
bladder c.
detrusor c.
dynamic c. of lung
c. of heart
specific c.
static c.
thoracic c.
ventilatory c.
complicated
c. cataract
c. migraine
complication
component
anterior c. of force
c. of complement
c. of force
c. management
c. of mastication
c. of occlusion
plasma thromboplastin c. (PTC)
secretory c.
composite
c. dental cement
c. flap
c. graft
c. joint
c. resin

composition
base c.
modeling c.
compos mentis
compound
acetone c.
c. action potential
acyclic c.
addition c.
alicyclic c.
aliphatic c.
c. aneurysm
APC c.
aromatic c.
c. articulation
carbamino c.
c. caries
c. character
closed chain c.
condensation c.
conjugated c.
cyclic c.
c. cyst
c. dislocation
c. eye
c. flap
genetic c.
c. gland
glycosyl c.
c. granule cell
heterocyclic c.
c. heterozygote
high-energy c.
homocyclic c.
c. hyperopic astigmatism
impression c.
inclusion c.
inorganic c.
isocyclic c.
c. joint
Kendall c.
c. lens
c. lipid
meso c.
methonium c.
c. microscope
modeling c.
c. myopic astigmatism
c. nevus
nonpolar c.
c. odontoma
open chain c.
organic c.
polar c.
c. pregnancy
c. presentation
c. protein
Reichstein c.
c. restoration
ring c.
c. skull fracture
Wintersteiner c. F
comprehension
comprehensive medical care

compress
    graduated c.
    wet c.
compressed
    c. sponge
    c. tablet
    c. yeast
compressible cavernous body
compression
    c. anesthesia
    c. of brain
    cerebral c.
    c. cyanosis
    c. limiting
    c. molding
    c. neuropathy
    c. paralysis
    c. plate
    c. plating
    c. retinopathy
    c. syndrome
    c. thrombosis
    c. of tissue
    wide dynamic range c.
compressive
    c. myelopathy
    c. nystagmus
    c. strength
compressor
    c. urethra
    c. urethra muscle
    c. venae dorsalis penis
compressorium
Compton
    C. effect
    C. scatter
Compton scattering
compulsion
compulsive
    c. idea
    c. neurosis
    c. personality
computed
    c. perimetry
    c. radiography
    c. tomography (CT)
computer
    c. model
    c. simulation
computerized axial tomography (CAT)
conA, con A
    concanavalin a
conalbumin
conanine
CO_2 narcosis
conarium
conation
conative
conatus
concameration
concanavalin A (conA, con A)
concatamer
concatenate
Concato disease

concave
    c. lens
    c. mirror
concavity
concavoconcave lens
concavoconvex lens
concealed
    c. conduction
    c. hemorrhage
    c. hernia
    c. penis
concentrated human red blood corpuscle
concentration
    Baermann c.
    buffy coat c.
    critical micelle c. (cmc)
    fecal c.
    formalin-ether sedimentation c.
    formalin-ethyl acetate
      sedimentation c.
    c. gradient
    gravity c.
    M c.
    mean corpuscular hemoglobin c.
      (MCHC)
    microhematocrit c.
    minimal alveolar c.
    minimal anesthetic c. (MAC)
    minimal inhibitory c. (MIC)
    molar c.
    normal c. (N)
    c. × time (CxT)
    zinc sulfate flotation c.
concentric
    c. fibroma
    c. hypertrophy
    c. lamella
concept
    c. formation
    no-threshold c.
    self-c.
concepti (*pl. of* conceptus)
conception
    imperative c.
    retained products of c.
conceptual
conceptus, pl. **concepti**
concerted
    c. evolution
    c. model
concha, pl. **conchae**
    c. of auricle
    c. auriculae
    c. bullosa
    c. of ear
    highest c.
    inferior nasal c.
    middle nasal c.
    Morgagni c.
    c. nasalis inferior
    c. nasalis media
    c. nasalis superior
    c. nasalis suprema
    Santorini c.
    c. santorini

sphenoidal c.
conchae sphenoidales
superior nasal c.
supreme c.
supreme nasal c.
conchal
    c. cartilage
    c. crest
    c. crest of body of maxilla
    c. crest of palatine bone
conchoidal body
concomitance
concomitant
    c. immunity
    c. strabismus
    c. symptom
concordance rate
concordant
    c. alternans
    c. alternation
    c. atrioventricular connection
    c. changes electrocardiogram
concrement
concrescence
concrete
    c. oil
    c. operation
    c. thinking
concretio cordis
concretion
concretization
concurrent
    c. disinfection
    c. validity
concussion
    brain c.
    c. cataract
    c. myelitis
    spinal c.
    spinal cord c.
condensation
    aldol c.
    Claisen c.
    c. compound
condense
condensed milk
condenser
    Abbé c.
    automatic c.
    cardioid c.
    dark-field c.
    paraboloid c.
condensing
    c. enzyme
    c. osteitis
condition
    fibrocystic c. of the breast
conditional-lethal mutant
conditionally lethal mutant
conditional probability
conditioned
    c. avitaminosis
    c. hemolysis
    c. insomnia
    c. reflex (CR)

    c. response
    c. stimulus
conditioning
    assertive c.
    aversive c.
    avoidance c.
    classical c.
    escape c.
    higher order c.
    instrumental c.
    operant c.
    pavlovian c.
    respondent c.
    second-order c.
    skinnerian c.
    c. therapy
    trace c.
condom
conductance
conduct disorder
conducting
    c. airway
    c. system of heart
conduction
    aberrant ventricular c.
    accelerated c.
    air c.
    c. analgesia
    c. anesthesia
    anomalous c.
    antegrade c.
    anterograde c.
    c. aphasia
    atrioventricular c. (AVC)
    AV c.
    avalanche c.
    c. block
    bone c.
    concealed c.
    decremental c.
    delayed c.
    forward c.
    intraatrial c.
    intraventricular c.
    nerve c.
    orthograde c.
    Purkinje c.
    retrograde VA c.
    saltatory c.
    sinoventricular c.
    supernormal c.
    supranormal c.
    synaptic c.
    VA c.
    ventricular c.
    ventriculoatrial c. (VAC)
conductive
    c. hearing impairment
    c. heat
conductivity
    hydraulic c.
conductor
conduit
    apical-aortic c.
    ileal c.

C

conduplicate
conduplicato corpore
condurango
condylar
    c. articulation
    c. axis
    c. canal
    c. emissary vein
    c. fossa
    c. guidance
    c. guidance inclination
    c. guide
    c. hinge position
    c. joint
    c. process of mandible
condylarthrosis
condyle
    balancing side c.
    c. cord
    c. of humerus
    lateral c.
    lateral c. of femur
    lateral c. of tibia
    mandibular c.
    medial c.
    medial c. of femur
    medial c. of tibia
    occipital c.
    c. path
    working side c.
condylectomy
condylion
condyloid
    c. canal
    c. process
condyloma, pl. **condylomata**
    c. acuminatum
    flat c.
    giant c.
    c. latum
condylomatous
condylotomy
condylus
    c. humeri
    c. lateralis
    c. lateralis femoris
    c. lateralis tibiae
    c. medialis
    c. medialis femoris
    c. medialis tibiae
    c. occipitalis
cone
    antipodal c.
    arterial c.
    c. cell of retina
    c. degeneration
    c. disk
    c. down
    c. dystrophy
    elastic c.
    c. fiber
    c. granule
    gutta-percha c.
    Haller c.
    implantation c.

    c. of light
    long-wavelength-sensitive c. (l-cone)
    medullary c.
    nerve growth c.
    ocular c.
    Politzer luminous c.
    pulmonary c.
    retinal c.
    silver c.
    theca interna c.
    twin c.
    vascular c.
    c. vision
cone-rod retinal dystrophy
conessi
conessine
conexus, pl. **conexus**
    c. intertendineus
confabulation
confectio, pl. **confectiones**
confection
confertus
confidence interval
confidentiality
configuration
    cis c.
confinement
    estimated date of c. (EDC)
conflict
    approach-approach c.
    approach-avoidance c.
    avoidance-avoidance c.
    c. of interest
    interpersonal c.
    intrapersonal c.
    role c.
confluence of sinus
confluens
    c. sinuum
confluent
    c. articulation
    c. and reticulate papillomatosis
    c. smallpox
confocal microscope
conformation
    boat c.
    envelope c.
conformational map
conformer
confounding
confrontation method
confusional
confusion color
congener
congenerous
congenic strain
congenital
    c. adrenal hyperplasia
    c. afibrinogenemia
    c. amputation
    c. aplasia of thymus
    c. aplastic anemia
    c. atonic pseudoparalysis
    c. baldness
    c. bronchiectasis

c. cataract
c. cerebellar atrophy
c. cerebral aneurysm
c. choreoathetosis
c. conus
c. diaphragmatic hernia
c. dyserythropoietic anemia
c. dysphagocytosis
c. dysplastic angiectasia
c. dysplastic angiomatosis
c. ectodermal defect
c. ectodermal dysplasia
c. elephantiasis
c. epulis of newborn
c. erythropoietic porphyria
c. facial diplegia
c. fibrosis of the extraocular
  muscles
c. generalized fibromatosis
c. glaucoma
c. heart block
c. hemolytic anemia
c. hemolytic icterus
c. hemolytic jaundice
c. hereditary endothelial dystrophy
c. hip dysplasia
c. hydrocele
c. hydrocephalus
c. hypophosphatasia
c. hypoplastic anemia
c. hypothyroidism
c. ichthyosiform erythroderma
c. lobar emphysema
c. lymphedema
c. megacolon
c. methemoglobinemia
c. microvillus atrophy
c. myxedema
c. nevus
c. nonregenerative anemia
c. nystagmus
c. pancytopenia
c. paramyotonia
c. pneumonia
c. pulmonary arteriovenous fistula
c. pyloric stenosis
c. rubella syndrome
c. selective glucose and galactose
  malabsorption
c. spastic paraplegia
c. stridor
c. sutural alopecia
c. syphilis
c. torticollis
c. total lipodystrophy
c. toxoplasmosis
c. valve
c. virilizing adrenal hyperplasia
congenitus
congested
congestion
active c.
brain c.
functional c.
hypostatic c.

passive c.
physiologic c.
venous c.
congestive
c. cardiomyopathy
c. cirrhosis
c. heart failure
c. splenomegaly
conglobate
conglobation
conglomerate
conglutinant
conglutination
conglutinin
Congo
C. red
C. red paper
Congolian red fever
congophilic angiopathy
congruent point
congruous hemianopia
coni (*pl. of* conus)
conic, conical
c. catheter
c. cornea
c. lobule of epididymis
c. papillae
conidia (*pl. of* conidium)
conidial
Conidiobolus
conidiogenous
conidiophore
Phialophore-type c.
conidium, pl. **conidia**
coniine
coniofibrosis
coniolymphstasis
coniometer
coniophage
coniosis
coniotomy
conium
conization
cautery c.
cold knife c.
conjoined
c. anastomosis
c. asymmetric twin
c. equal twin
c. nerve root
c. symmetric twin
c. tendon
c. unequal twin
conjoint
c. tendon
c. therapy
conjugal cancer
conjugant
conjugata
c. anatomica
c. diagonalis
c. externa
c. recta
c. vera

conjugate
    c. acid
    c. acid-base pair
    anatomical c.
    c. axis
    c. deviation of the eye
    diagonal c.
    c. diameter of pelvic inlet
    c. diameter of pelvic outlet
    c. division
    effective c.
    external c.
    false c.
    c. foci
    folic acid c.
    c. foramen
    c. gaze
    internal c.
    median c.
    c. movement of eye
    c. nystagmus
    obstetric c.
    obstetric c. of pelvic outlet
    c. of pelvic inlet
    c. of pelvic outlet
    c. point
    straight c.
    true c.
conjugated
    c. antigen
    c. bilirubin
    c. compound
    c. double bonds
    c. estrogen
    c. hapten
    c. protein
conjugation
conjugative plasmid
conjunctiva, pl. **conjunctivae**
    bulbar c.
    palpebral c.
conjunctival
    c. artery
    c. cul-de-sac
    c. fornix
    c. gland
    c. layer of bulb
    c. layer of eyelid
    c. reflex
    c. ring
    c. sac
    c. varix
    c. vein
conjunctive
conjunctiviplasty
conjunctivitis
    actinic c.
    acute contagious c.
    acute epidemic c.
    acute hemorrhagic c.
    acute viral c.
    allergic c.
    angular c.
    arc-flash c.
    c. arida

    chemical c.
    chronic follicular c.
    cicatricial c.
    diphtherial c.
    follicular c.
    giant papillary c.
    gonococcal c.
    gonorrheal c.
    granular c.
    hyperacute purulent c.
    inclusion c.
    infantile purulent c.
    larval c.
    ligneous c.
    c. medicamentosa
    membranous c.
    molluscum c.
    Moraxella c.
    necrotic infectious c.
    neonatal c.
    Parinaud c.
    Pascheff c.
    phlyctenular c.
    pseudomembranous c.
    purulent c.
    simple c.
    snow c.
    spring c.
    squirrel plague c.
    swimming pool c.
    toxicogenic c.
    trachomatous c.
    tularemic c.
    c. tularensis
    vernal c.
    welder's c.
conjunctivochalasis
conjunctivodacryocystorhinostomy
conjunctivodacryocystostomy
conjunctivoplasty
conjunctivorhinostomy
connectin
connecting
    c. cartilage
    c. stalk
    c. tubule
connection
    ambiguous atrioventricular c.
    anomalous pulmonary venous c., total or partial
    atrioventricular c.
    clamp c.
    concordant atrioventricular c.
    discordant atrioventricular c.
    double inlet atrioventricular c.
    intertendinous c. of extensor digitorum
    marrow-mesenchyme c.
    partial anomalous pulmonary venous c.
    total anomalous pulmonary venous c. (TAPVC)
    univentricular c.
connective
    c. tissue

c. tissue cell
c. tissue group
c. tumor
connective-tissue disease
connector
c. bar
major c.
minor c.
nonrigid c.
rigid c.
stress-broken c.
Connell suture
connexin 26
connexins, connexons
connexus intertendinei musculi extensoris
digitorum
Conn syndrome
conoid
c. ligament
c. process
Sturm c.
c. tubercle
conomyoidin
conquinine
Conradi
C. disease
C. line
Conradi-Hünermann
C.-H. disease
C.-H. syndrome
consanguineous
consanguinity
conscious
consciousness
clouding of c.
double c.
field of c.
consecutive
c. aneurysm
c. angiitis
c. esotropia
consensual
c. light reflex
c. reaction
c. validation
conservation of energy
conservative
c. replication
c. treatment
conserve
consistency principle
consolidant
consolidation chemotherapy
consonating rale
conspecific
conspicuity
constancy
color c.
object c.
c. phenomenon
constant
association c.
autoprotolysis c. of water (K_w)
Avogadro c.
binding c.

c. coupling
decay c.
diffusion c.
disintegration c.
dissociation c. (K, K_d)
dissociation c. of an acid (K_a)
dissociation c. of a base (K_b)
dissociation c. of an inhibitor (K_i)
dissociation c. of water (K_w)
equilibrium c. (K_{eq})
Faraday c.
c. field equation
flotation c. (S_f)
gas c.
Hill c.
c. infusion pump
Michaelis c. (K_m)
Michaelis-Menten c.
molar gas c. (R)
newtonian c. of gravitation
permeability c.
Planck c. (h)
radioactive c.
rate c. (k)
c. region
sedimentation c.
specificity c.
time c.
transformation c.
velocity c.
constellation
constipate
constipated
constipation
constitution
constitutional
c. cause
c. formula
c. hepatic dysfunction
c. hirsutism
c. psychology
c. reaction
c. symptom
c. thrombopathy
constitutive
c. enzyme
c. heterochromatin
constrictio
c. bronchoaortica esophagea
c. diaphragmatica esophagea
c. partis thoracicae esophagea
c. pharyngoesophagealis
c. phrenica esophagea
constriction
bronchoaortic c.
diaphragmatic c. of esophagus
esophageal c.
inferior esophageal c.
middle esophageal c.
pharyngoesophageal c.
primary c.
pyloric c.
c. ring
secondary c.
thoracic c. of esophagus

C

constriction (*continued*)
    upper esophageal c.
    c.'s of ureter
constrictive
    c. bronchiolitis
    c. endocarditis
    c. pericarditis
constrictor
constructional
    c. agraphia
    c. apraxia
construct validity
consultand
    dummy c.
consultant
consultation
consulting staff
consumption
    c. coagulopathy
    oxygen c. (Q_O, Q_{O2}, $\dot{V}_{O2}$)
consumptive
contact
    c. allergy
    c. area
    balancing c.
    c. catalysis
    centric c.
    c. ceptor
    c. cheilitis
    deflective occlusal c.
    c. dermatitis
    c. hypersensitivity
    c. hysteroscope
    c. illumination
    c. inhibition
    initial c.
    interceptive occlusal c.
    c. lens
    c. point
    premature c.
    proximal c.
    proximate c.
    c. surface of tooth
    c. with reality
    working c.
contactant
contagion
    psychic c.
contagious
    c. disease
    c. ecthyma
    c. ecthyma (pustular dermatitis)
      virus of sheep
    c. pustular dermatitis
    c. pustular stomatitis virus
contagiousness
contagium
contained disk herniation
containment
contaminant
contaminate
contamination
content
    c. analysis

    carbon dioxide c.
    GC c.
    latent c.
    manifest c.
    c. validity
contig
    c. map
contiguity
    spatial c.
    temporal c.
contiguous
continence
continent
contingency table
continued fever
continuenter remedia (cont. rem.)
continuity
continuous
    c. ambulatory peritoneal dialysis
      (CAPD)
    c. arrhythmia
    c. bar retainer
    c. beam
    c. capillary
    c. clasp
    c. culture
    c. epidural anesthesia
    c. eruption
    c. flow analyzer
    c. interleaved sampling
    c. loop wiring
    c. murmur
    c. otoacoustic emission
    c. passive motion (CPM, cpm)
    c. phase
    c. positive airway pressure (CPAP)
    c. positive pressure ventilation
      (CPPV)
    c. random variable
    c. reinforcement schedule
    c. spectrum
    c. spinal anesthesia
    c. suture
    c. tremor
    c. variation
    c. wave laser
contour
    flange c.
    gingival c.
    gum c.
    height of c.
    c. line of Owen
contraangle
contraaperture
contrabevel
contraception
    emergency hormonal c.
    postcoital c.
contraceptive
    barrier c.
    combination oral c.
    c. device
    intrauterine c. device (IUCD)
    oral c.
    c. sponge

contract
contracted
    c. foot
    c. kidney
    c. pelvis
contractile
    c. stricture
    c. vacuole
contractility
    cardiac c.
contraction
    after-c.
    anodal closure c. (ACC, AnCC)
    anodal opening c. (AnOC, AOC)
    automatic c.
    c. band
    c. band necrosis
    Braxton Hicks c.
    cathodal closure c. (CaCC, CCC)
    cathodal opening c. (CaOC, COC)
    closing c.
    escape c.
    escape ventricular c.
    fibrillary c.
    front-tap c.
    Gowers c.
    hourglass c.
    hunger c.'s
    idiomuscular c.
    isometric c.
    isotonic c.
    myotatic c.
    opening c.
    paradoxical c.
    postural c.
    premature c.
    reflex detrusor c.
    c. stress test
    tetanic c.
    tonic c.
    uterine c.
contractual
    c. psychiatry
    c. psychotherapy
contractural diathesis
contracture
    c. deformity
    Dupuytren c.
    fixed c.
    functional c.
    ischemic c. of the left ventricle
    organic c.
    Volkmann c.
contrafissura
contraindicant
contraindication
contralateral
    c. hemiplegia
    c. partner
    c. reflex
    c. routing of signal
    c. sign
contrast
    c. agent

    c. bath
    c. echocardiography
    c. enema
    c. enhancement
    c. material
    c. medium
    c. sensitivity
    c. sensitivity testing
    simultaneous c.
    c. stain
    successive c.
contrasuppressor cell
contrecoup injury of brain
cont. rem.
    continuenter remedia
control
    c. animal
    autogenous c.
    automatic gain c. (AGC)
    aversive c.
    biologic c.
    birth c.
    C. of Communicable Diseases Manual (CCDM)
    c. experiment
    c. gene
    c. group
    idiodynamic c.
    negative c.
    own c.
    positive c.
    quality c.
    reflex c.
    c. release suture
    social c.
    stimulus c.
    synergic c.
    c. syringe
    time-varied gain c. (TGC)
    tonic c.
    vestibulo-equilibratory c.
controlled
    c. hypotension
    c. mechanical ventilation (CMV)
    c. respiration
    c. substance
    c. ventilation
contusion
    brain c.
    scalp c.
conular
Conus
conus, pl. **coni**
    c. arteriosus
    congenital c.
    distraction c.
    c. elasticus
    coni epididymidis
    c. medullaris
    myopic c.
    pulmonary c.
    supertraction c.
    coni vasculosi
convalescence

C

convalescent
c. carrier
c. serum
convallaria
convection
convective heat
convenience form
conventional
c. animal
c. sign
c. thoracoplasty
c. tomography
convergence
accommodative c.
amplitude of c.
angle of c.
c. excess
far point of c.
c. insufficiency
near point of c.
negative c.
c. nucleus of Perlia
positive c.
range of c.
unit of c.
convergence-retraction nystagmus
convergent
c. evolution
c. squint
c. strabismus
converging meniscus
conversion
c. disorder
c. electron
c. hysteria
c. hysteria neurosis
c. reaction
conversive heat
convertase
convertin
convex
high c.
c. lens
low c.
c. mirror
convexity
cortical c.
convexobasia
convexoconcave lens
convexoconvex lens
convolute
convoluted
c. bone
c. gland
c. part of kidney lobule
c. seminiferous tubule
c. tubule of kidney
convolution
angular c.
anterior central c.
ascending frontal c.
ascending parietal c.
callosal c.
cingulate c.
first temporal c.

hippocampal c.
inferior frontal c.
inferior temporal c.
middle frontal c.
middle temporal c.
posterior central c.
second temporal c.
superior frontal c.
superior temporal c.
supramarginal c.
third temporal c.
transitional c.
transverse temporal c.'s
Zuckerkandl c.
convulsant
c. threshold
convulsion
benign neonatal c.
clonic c.
complex febrile c.
febrile c.
hysterical c.
hysteroid c.
immediate posttraumatic c.
infantile c.
salaam c.
tetanic c.
tonic c.
convulsive
c. seizure
c. state
c. therapy
c. tic
cooing murmur
Cooke speculum
cooled-knife method
Cooley anemia
Coolidge tube
Coomassie brilliant blue R-250
Coombs
C. murmur
C. serum
C. test
Cooper
C. fascia
C. hernia
C. herniotome
C. ligament
cooperative enzyme
cooperativity
c. model
negative c.
positive c.
Cooperia
C. bisonis
C. curticei
C. fieldingi
C. oncophora
C. pectinata
C. punctata
C. spatulata
Cooper-Rand artificial larynx
coordinate covalent bond
coordination
co-ossification

co-ossify
copaiba
COPD
  chronic obstructive pulmonary disease
cope
Cope clamp
copepod
Copepoda
copia element
coping
   transfer c.
copolymer
   c.-1
   c. resin
copper (Cu)
   c. arsenite
   c. bichloride
   c. cataract
   c. chloride
   c. citrate
   c. colic
   c. dichloride
   c. nose
   c. pennies
   c. phosphate cement
   c. protein
   c. sulfate
   c. sulfate method
copper-64 (^{64}Cu)
copper-67 (^{67}Cu)
copperas
copperhead
Coppet law
copra itch
coprecipitation
copremesis
coproantibody
coprolalia
coprolith
coprology
coproma
coprophagia
coprophagous
coprophagy
coprophil
coprophile
coprophilia
coprophilic
coprophobia
coprophrasia
coproplanesia
coproporphyria
   hereditary c.
coproporphyrin
coproporphyrinogen oxidase
coprostane
3β-coprostanol
epi-coprostanol
coprostanone
coprostasis
coprostenol
coprosterol
epi-coprosterol
coprostigmastane
coprozoa

coprozoic
coptosis
copula
   His c.
   c. linguae
copulation
copuline
CoQ
   coenzyme Q
coquille
cor
   c. adiposum
   c. biloculare
   c. bovinum
   c. mobile
   c. pendulum
   c. pulmonale
   c. triatriatum
   c. triloculare
   c. triloculare biatriatum
   c. triloculare biventriculare
coracidium
coracoacromial
   c. arch
   c. ligament
coracobrachial
   c. bursa
   c. muscle
coracobrachialis muscle
coracoclavicular ligament
coracohumeral ligament
coracoid
   c. process
   c. tuberosity
coral calculus
coralliform cataract
corallin
   yellow c.
cord
   Bergmann c.
   Billroth c.
   c. blood
   condyle c.
   dental c.
   false tendinous c.
   false vocal c.
   Ferrein c.
   gangliated c.
   genital c.
   germinal c.
   gonadal c.
   gubernacular c.
   hepatic c.
   c. hydrocele
   lateral c. of brachial plexus
   lymph c.
   medial c. of brachial plexus
   medullary c.
   nephrogenic c.
   nuchal c.
   oblique c. of interosseous membrane
     of forearm
   omphalomesenteric c.
   posterior c. of brachial plexus
   psalterial c.

C

cord (*continued*)
    red pulp c.
    rete c.
    sex c.
    spermatic c.
    spinal c.
    splenic c.
    tendinous c.
    testicular c.
    testis c.
    true vocal c.
    c. of tympanum
    umbilical c.
    c. of umbilical artery
    vitelline c.
    vocal c.
    Weitbrecht c.
    Wilde c.
    Willis c.
cordate pelvis
cordectomy
cordial
cordianine
cordiform
    c. pelvis
    c. uterus
cordis
    diastasis c.
cordocentesis
cordon sanitaire
cordopexy
cordotomy
    anterolateral c.
    open c.
    posterior column c.
    spinothalamic c.
    stereotactic c.
Cordylobia
    C. anthropophaga
cordylobiasis
cordy pulse
core
    atomic c.
    central transactional c.
    c. particle
    c. pneumonia
co-receptor
    B cell c.-r.
corectopia
corelysis
coremium
coreoplasty
corepexy
    purse-string c.
corepraxy
    laser c.
    mechanical c.
corepressor
Cori
    C. cycle
    C. disease
    C. ester
coriander
corium, pl. **coria**

corkscrew vessel
corn
    asbestos c.
    c. ergot
    hard c.
    c. oil
    c. smut
    soft c.
    c. sugar
cornea
    conic c.
    c. farinata
    floury c.
    c. plana
    c. urica
    c. verticillata
corneal
    c. astigmatism
    c. corpuscle
    c. decompensation
    c. dystrophy
    c. ectasia
    c. endothelial polymorphism
    c. facet
    c. graft
    c. layer of epidermis
    c. lens
    c. limbus
    c. margin
    c. pannus
    c. reflex
    c. space
    c. spot
    c. staphyloma
    c. transplantation
    c. trepanation
    c. vertex
Cornelia de Lange syndrome
corneoblepharon
corneocyte envelope
corneosclera
corneoscleral
    c. junction
    c. part of trabecular tissue of sclera
Corner-Allen
    C.-A. test
    C.-A. unit
Corner tampon
corneum
corniculate
    c. cartilage
    c. tubercle
corniculopharyngeal ligament
corniculum laryngis
cornification
cornified layer of nail
cornmeal agar
cornoid lamella
cornsilk
cornu, pl. **cornua**
    c. ammonis
    c. anterius
    coccygeal c.
    cornua coccygealia

c. coccygeum
c. cutaneum
cornua of falciform margin of saphenous opening
c. frontale ventriculi lateralis
cornua of hyoid bone
c. inferius
c. inferius cartilaginis thyroideae
c. inferius marginis falciformis hiatus sapheni
c. inferius ventriculi lateralis
c. laterale
cornua of lateral ventricle
c. majus ossis hyoidei
c. minus ossis hyoidei
c. occipitale ventriculi lateralis
c. posterius
c. posterius ventriculi lateralis
sacral c.
c. sacrale
c. of spinal cord
styloid c.
c. superius cartilaginis thyroideae
c. superius marginalis falciformis
c. temporale ventriculi lateralis
cornua of thyroid cartilage
c. uteri
cornual pregnancy
corona, pl. **coronae**
c. capitis
c. ciliaris
c. clinica
c. dentis
c. glandis penis
c. of glans penis
c. radiata
c. seborrheica
c. veneris
Zinn c.
coronad
coronal
c. epispadias
c. hypospadias
c. plane
c. pulp
c. section
c. suture
coronale
coronalis
coronaria
coronarism
coronaritis
coronary
c. angiography
c. arteriosclerosis
c. arteritis
c. artery
c. artery aneurysm
c. artery bypass
c. atherectomy
cafe c.
c. care unit (CCU)
c. cataract
c. endarterectomy
c. failure

c. groove
c. insufficiency
c. ligament of knee
c. ligament of liver
c. nodal rhythm
c. node
c. occlusion
c. ostial stenosis
c. perfusion pressure
c. plexus
c. sinus
c. sinus rhythm
c. steal
c. sulcus
c. tendon
c. thrombosis
c. valve
c. vein
coronary-prone behavior
Coronaviridae
Coronavirus
coronavirus
coroner
coronion
coronoid
c. fossa of humerus
c. process
c. process of the mandible
c. process of the ulna
coronoidectomy
corpora (*pl. of* corpus)
corporeal
corporin
corporis
corpse
corps ronds
corpulence, corpulency
corpulent
corpus, pl. **corpora**
c. adiposum
c. adiposum buccae
c. adiposum fossae ischioanalis
c. adiposum fossae ischiorectalis
c. adiposum infrapatellare
c. adiposum orbitae
c. albicans
c. amygdaloideum
c. amylaceum, pl. corpora amylacea
c. aorticum
c. arantii
corpora arenacea
atretic c. luteum
c. atreticum
corpora bigemina
c. callosum
c. candicans
corpora cavernosa recti
c. cavernosum clitoridis
c. cavernosum of clitoris
c. cavernosum conchae
c. cavernosum penis
c. cavernosum urethrae
c. ciliare
c. claviculae
c. clitoridis

C

corpus (*continued*)

c. coccygeum
c. costae
c. dentatum
c. epididymidis
c. epididymis
c. femoris
c. fibrosum
c. fibulae
c. fimbriatum
c. fornicis
c. gastricum
c. geniculatum externum
c. geniculatum internum
c. geniculatum laterale
c. geniculatum mediale
c. glandulae sudoriferae
c. hemorrhagicum
c. highmori, c. highmorianum
c. humeri
c. incudis
c. juxtarestiforme
c. linguae
corpora lutea cyst
c. luteum
c. luteum deficiency syndrome
c. luteum hematoma
c. luteum hormone unit
c. luteum spurium
c. luteum verum
c. luysi
c. mammae
c. mammillare
c. mandibulae
c. maxillae
c. medullare cerebelli
c. metacarpale
c. metatarsale
c. nuclei caudati
c. olivare
c. ossis femoris
c. ossis hyoidei
c. ossis ilii
c. ossis ischii
c. ossis metacarpalis
c. ossis pubis
c. ossis sphenoidalis
c. pampiniforme
c. pancreatis
c. papillare
corpora para-aortica
c. paraterminale
c. penis
c. phalangis
c. pineale
c. pontobulbare
corpora quadrigemina
c. quadrigeminum anterius
c. quadrigeminum posterius
c. radii
c. restiforme
c. spongiosum penis
c. spongiosum urethrae muliebris
c. sterni

c. striatum
c. tali
c. tibiae
c. trapezoideum
c. triticeum
c. ulnae
c. unguis
c. uteri
c. vertebrae
c. vesicae
c. vesicae biliaris
c. vesicae felleae
c. vitreum

corpuscle

amnionic c.
amylaceous c.
amyloid c.
articular c.
axile c.
axis c.
basal c.
Bizzozero c.
blood c.
bone c.
bridge c.
bulboid c.
calcareous c.
cement c.
chyle c.
colloid c.
colostrum c.
concentrated human red blood c.
corneal c.
Dogiel c.
Donné c.
dust c.
Eichhorst c.
exudation c.
genital c.
ghost c.
Gluge c.
Golgi c.
Golgi-Mazzoni c.
Hassall concentric c.'s
inflammatory c.
lamellated c.
lymph c., lymphoid c.
lymphatic c.
malpighian c.
Mazzoni c.
Meissner c.
Merkel c.
Mexican hat c.
milk c.
molluscum c.
Negri c.
Norris c.
oval c.
pacchionian c.
pacinian c.
pessary c.
phantom c.
plastic c.
Purkinje c.
pus c.

Rainey c.
red c.
renal c.
reticular c.
Ruffini c.
salivary c.
Schwalbe c.
shadow c.
splenic c.
tactile c.
taste c.
terminal nerve c.
third c.
thymic c.
touch c.
Toynbee c.
Traube c.
Tröltsch c.
Valentin c.
Vater c.
Vater-Pacini c.
Virchow c.
white c.
Zimmermann c.

corpuscular
 c. lymph
 c. radiation

corpusculum, pl. **corpuscula**
 corpuscula articularia
 corpuscula bulboidea
 corpuscula genitalia
 corpuscula lamellosa
 corpuscula nervosa terminalia
 c. renis, pl. corpuscula renis
 c. tactus, pl. corpuscula tactus

corpus highmorianum (var. of corpus highmori)

corralin yellow

corrected
 c. dextrocardia
 c. transposition of the great vessels

correction
 occlusal c.
 spontaneous c. of placenta previa

corrective emotional experience

correlation
 c. coefficient
 product-moment c.
 rank-difference c.

correlational method

correlative differentiation

Correra line

correspondence
 abnormal c.
 anomalous retinal c.
 dysharmonious retinal c.
 harmonious retinal c.

Corrigan
 C. disease
 C. pulse
 C. sign

corrigent

corrin

corrinoid

corrode

corrosion preparation

corrosive sublimate

corrugator
 c. cutis muscle of anus
 c. muscle
 c. supercilii muscle

cortex, pl. **cortices**
 adrenal c.
 agranular c.
 association c.
 auditory c.
 cerebellar c.
 c. cerebelli
 cerebral c.
 c. cerebri
 deep c.
 dysgranular c.
 fetal adrenal c.
 frontal c.
 c. glandulae suprarenalis
 granular c.
 c. of hair shaft
 heterotypic c.
 homotypic c.
 insular c.
 laminated c.
 c. of lens
 c. lentis
 c. of lymph node
 mastoid c.
 motor c.
 c. nodi lymphatici
 olfactory c.
 orbitofrontal c.
 ovarian c.
 c. ovarii
 c. of ovary
 parastriate c.
 peristriate c.
 piriform c.
 prefrontal c.
 premotor c.
 primary visual c.
 provisional c.
 renal c.
 c. renalis
 secondary sensory c.
 secondary visual c.
 sensory c.
 somatic sensory c.,
  somatosensory c.
 striate c.
 supplementary motor c.
 suprarenal c.
 c. of suprarenal gland
 temporal c.
 tertiary c.
 c. thymi
 c. of thymus
 visual c.

cortexolone

cortexone

Corti
 C. arch
 C. auditory tooth

C

Corti *(continued)*
    C. canal
    C. cell
    C. ganglion
    C. membrane
    C. organ
    C. pillar
    C. rod
    C. tunnel
cortical
    c. amygdaloid nucleus
    c. apraxia
    c. arch of kidney
    c. audiometry
    c. blindness
    c. bone
    c. cataract
    c. convexity
    c. deafness
    c. dysgenesis
    c. dysplasia
    c. epilepsy
    c. hormone
    c. implantation
    c. lobule of kidney
    c. osteitis
    c. part
    c. part of middle cerebral artery
    c. radiate artery
    c. sensibility
    c. substance
corticalization
corticalosteotomy
corticectomy
cortices (*pl. of* cortex)
corticifugal
corticipetal
corticis
corticoafferent
corticobasal degeneration
corticobulbar
    c. fiber
    c. tract
corticocerebellum
corticoefferent
corticofugal
corticoid
    17-OH-c. test
corticomedial
corticomesencephalic fiber
corticonuclear fiber
corticopontine
    c. fiber
    c. tract
corticoreticular fiber
corticorubral fiber
corticospinal
    c. fiber
    c. tract
corticosteroid
corticosteroid-binding
    c.-b. globulin (CBG)
    c.-b. protein
corticosteroid-induced glaucoma

corticosterone
corticothalamic fiber
corticotroph
corticotropic hormone
β-corticotropin
corticotropin-releasing
    c.-r. factor (CRF)
    c.-r. hormone (CRH)
corticotropin-zinc hydroxide
Corticoviridae
corticovirus
cortilymph
cortin
cortisol acetate
cortisone
corundum
Corvisart facies
corymbiform
corynebacteria (*pl. of* corynebacterium)
corynebacteriophage
    beta c.
Corynebacterium
    C. *acnes*
    C. *amycolatum*
    C. *diphtheriae*
    C. *equi*
    C. *glucuronolyticum*
    C. *haemolyticum*
    C. *hofmannii*
    C. *jeikeium*
    C. *matruchotii*
    C. *minutissimum*
    C. *parvum*
    C. *pseudodiphtheriticum*
    C. *striatum*
    C. *xerosis*
corynebacterium, pl. **corynebacteria**
coryneform bacteria
coryza
    allergic c.
Coryzavirus
cosmesis
cosmetic
    c. dermatitis
    c. surgery
cosmetics
cosmic ray
cosmid
cosmopolitan
costa, pl. **costae**
    c. cervicalis
    costae fluctuantes [XI–XII]
    costae fluitantes
    c. lumbalis
    c. prima [I]
    costae spuriae [VII–XII]
    costae verae [I–VII]
costal
    c. angle
    c. arch
    c. arch reflex
    c. cartilage
    c. chondritis
    c. facet
    c. fringe

c. groove
c. line of pleural reflection
c. margin
c. notch
c. part of diaphragm
c. part of parietal pleura
c. pit of transverse process
c. pleura
c. pleurisy
c. process
c. respiration
c. surface
c. surface of lung
c. surface of scapula
c. tuberosity
costalgia
costectomy
Costen syndrome
costicartilage
costiform
costimulatory molecule
costive
costiveness
costoaxillary vein
costocentral
costocervical
c. (arterial) trunk
c. artery
costochondral
c. joint
c. junction
c. syndrome
costochondritis
costoclavicular
c. ligament
c. line
c. syndrome
costocolic ligament
costocoracoid
costodiaphragmatic recess
costogenic
costoinferior
costomediastinal
c. recess
c. sinus
costopectoral reflex
costophrenic
c. angle
c. septal line
c. sulcus
costoscapular
costoscapularis
costosternal
costosternoplasty
costosuperior
costotome
costotomy
costotransverse
c. foramen
c. joint
c. ligament
costotransversectomy
costovertebral
c. angle
c. joint

costoxiphoid
c. angle
c. ligament
cosubstrate
cosyntropin
Cotard syndrome
cotarnine
cot death
COTe
cathodal opening tetanus
Côte-d'Ivoire virus
cotinine
cotranslational
cotransport
Cotte operation
cotton
absorbent c.
C. effect
purified c.
soluble gun c.
styptic c.
cotton-dust asthma
cotton-fiber embolism
cotton-mill fever
cottonpox
cotton-root bark
cottonseed oil
cotton-wool
c.-w. patch
c.-w. spot
Cotunnius
C. aqueduct
C. canal
C. liquid
C. space
cotyle
cotyledon
fetal c.
maternal c.
cotyledonary placenta
Cotylogonimus
cotyloid
c. cavity
c. joint
c. ligament
c. notch
cough
aneurysmal c.
brassy c.
c. fracture
habit c.
privet c.
reflex c.
c. reflex
weaver's c.
whooping c.
coulomb (C, Q)
coumaranone
coumaric anhydride
coumarin
Coumel tachycardia
coumetarol
Councilman
C. hyaline body
Councilmania

counseling
  genetic c.
  marital c.
  pastoral c.
  c. psychology
count
  Addis c.
  Arneth c.
  blood c.
  CD4/CD8 c.
  c. density
  epidermal ridge c.
  filament-nonfilament c.
  total cell c.
  viable cell c.
counter
  automated differential leukocyte c.
  electronic cell c.
  Geiger-Müller c.
  proportional c.
  scintillation c.
  c. transference
  well c.
  whole-body c.
counterbalancing
counterconditioning
countercurrent
  c. distribution
  c. mechanism
countercurrent exchanger
countercurrent multiplier
counterdie
counterextension
counterimmunoelectrophoresis
counterincision
counterinvestment
counterirritant
counterirritation
counteropening
counterphobic
counterpulsation
  intraaortic balloon c.
counterpuncture
countershock
counterstain
countertraction
countertransference
countertransport
counting chamber
coup
  c. de sabre
  c. injury of brain
couple
coupled
  c. beats
  c. pulse
  c. rhythm
coupling
  constant c.
  c. defect
  c. factor
  fixed c.
  c. interval
  c. phase
  variable c.

Cournand dip
Courvoisier
  C. gallbladder
  C. law
  C. sign
couvade
Couvelaire
Couvelaire uterus
couvercle
covalent modification
cove plane
cover
  c. glass
  c. test
coverage
coverings of spermatic cord
coverslip
covert sensitization
cover-uncover test
cow
  c. face
  c. kidney
  c. milk anemia
Cowden disease
Cowdry
  C. type A inclusion body
  C. type B inclusion body
CO_2-withdrawal seizure test
Cowling rule
cowl muscle
Cowper
  C. cyst
  C. gland
  C. ligament
cowperian
cowpox virus
coxa, pl. **coxae**
  c. adducta
  false c. vara
  c. magna
  c. plana
  c. valga
  c. vara
  c. vara luxans
coxal bone
coxalgia
Coxiella burnetii
coxitic scoliosis
coxitis
coxodynia
coxofemoral
coxotuberculosis
coxsackie encephalitis
coxsackievirus
c.p.
  chemically pure
CPAP
  continuous positive airway pressure
CPEO
  chronic progressive external
    ophthalmoplegia
C-peptide
CPK
  creatine phosphokinase

CPM
    continuous passive motion
cpm
    continuous passive motion
CPPD
    calcium pyrophosphate deposition disease
CPPV
    continuous positive pressure ventilation
CPR
    cardiopulmonary resuscitation
cps
    cycles per second
CR
    conditioned reflex
Cr
    creatinine
crab hand
Crabtree effect
crack
    c. cocaine
    lacquer c.
cracked heel
cracked-pot
    c.-p. resonance
    c.-p. sound
crackle
crackling
    c. jaw
    parchment c.
    c. rale
cradle cap
Crafoord clamp
Craigia
Cramer wire splint
cramp
    heat c.'s
    intermittent c.
    miner's c.
    musician's c.
    pianist's c.
    piano-player's c.
    seamstress's c.
    shaving c.
    stoker's c.
    tailor's c.
    typist's c.
    violinist's c.
    waiter's c.
    watchmaker's c.
    writer's c.
Crampton
    C. line
    C. muscle
    C. test
Crandall syndrome
crania (*pl. of* cranium)
craniad
cranial
    c. arachnoid mater
    c. arteritis
    c. base
    c. bone
    c. capacity
    c. cavity
    c. dura mater

    c. flexure
    c. fontanelle
    c. index
    c. nerve
    c. neuropore
    c. part of parasympathetic part of autonomic division of nervous system
    c. pia mater
    c. root of accessory nerve
    c. sinus
    c. suture
    c. synchondroses
    c. synovial joint
    c. vault
    c. vertebra
cranialis
craniamphitomy
Craniata
craniectomy
    linear c.
cranioaural
craniocardiac reflex
craniocarpotarsal
    c. dysplasia
    c. dystrophy
craniocele
craniocerebral
craniocervical part of peripheral autonomic plexuses and ganglia
cranioclasia, cranioclasis
cranioclast
craniocleidodysostosis
craniodiaphysial dysplasia
craniodidymus
craniofacial
    c. angle
    c. appliance
    c. axis
    c. dysjunction fracture
    c. dysostosis
    c. fixation
    c. surgery
    c. suspension wiring
craniofenestria
craniognomy
craniograph
craniography
craniolacunia
craniology
craniomalacia
    circumscribed c.
craniomeningocele
craniometaphysial dysplasia
craniometer
craniometric point
craniometry
craniopagus
    c. occipitalis
    c. parasiticus
craniopathy
    metabolic c.
craniopharyngeal
    c. canal
    c. duct

C

craniopharyngioma
  ameloblastomatous c.
  cystic papillomatous c.
craniophore
cranioplasty
craniopuncture
craniorrhachidian
craniorrhachischisis
craniosacral
  c. division of autonomic nervous
    system
  c. nervous system
cranioschisis
craniosclerosis
cranioscopy
craniospinal sensory ganglia
craniostenosis
craniostosis
craniosynostosis
craniotabes
craniotome
craniotomy
  attached c.
  detached c.
  osteoplastic c.
craniotonoscopy
craniotrypesis
craniotympanic
cranium, pl. **crania**
  bifid c.
  c. bifidum
  cerebral c.
  c. cerebrale
  c. viscerale, visceral c.
crapulent
crash cart
crassamentum
crater arc
crateriform
craterization
cravat bandage
craw-craw
crazing
C-reactive protein (CRP)
cream
  cleansing c.
  cold c.
  greaseless c.
  leukocyte c.
  lubricating c.
  c. of tartar
  vanishing c.
crease
  digital c.
  digital flexion c.
  ear lobe c.
  flexion c.
  palmar c.
  simian c.
  Sydney c.
  c. wound
creatinase
creatine
  c. kinase (CK)

  c. kinase isoenzyme
  c. phosphate
  c. phosphokinase (CPK)
creatinemia
creatininase
creatinine (Cr)
  c. clearance
  c. coefficient
creatinuria
creative thinking
Credé
  C. maneuver
  C. method
credentialing
creeping
  c. eruption
  c. thrombosis
creep recovery
cremaster
  c. muscle
cremasteric
  c. artery
  c. fascia
  c. reflex
cremnocele
cremnophobia
crena, pl. **crenae**
  c. analis
  c. ani
  c. clunium
  c. cordis
  c. interglutealis
crenate, crenated
crenation
crenocyte
crenocytosis
Crenosoma vulpis
creola body
creophagy, creophagism
creosol
creosote
crepitant rale
crepitation
crepitus
  articular c.
  bony c.
crescendo
  c. angina
  c. murmur
crescent
  articular c.
  c. cell
  Giannuzzi c.
  glomerular c.
  Heidenhain c.
  malarial c.
  myopic c.
  c. sign
  sublingual c.
crescentic lobule of the cerebellum
crescograph
m-**cresol**
cresolase
cresol red

CREST
  calcinosis, Raynaud phenomenon,
    esophageal motility disorder,
    sclerodactyly and telangiectasia
    CREST syndrome
crest
  acoustic c.
  alveolar c.
  c. of alveolar ridge
  ampullary c.
  ampullary c. (of semicircular duct)
  anterior lacrimal c.
  arched c.
  arcuate c.
  arcuate c. of arytenoid cartilage
  articular c.
  basal c. of cochlear duct
  basilar c. of cochlear duct
  c. of body of rib
  buccinator c.
  c. of cochlear opening
  conchal c.
  conchal c. of body of maxilla
  conchal c. of palatine bone
  deltoid c.
  dental c.
  ethmoidal c.
  ethmoidal c. of maxilla
  ethmoidal c. of palatine bone
  external occipital c.
  falciform c.
  c. of fenestrae cochleae
  frontal c.
  ganglionic c.
  gingival c.
  gluteal c.
  c. of greater tubercle
  c. of head of rib
  iliac c.
  incisor c.
  infratemporal c. of greater wing of
    sphenoid
  inguinal c.
  intermediate sacral c.
  internal occipital c.
  interosseous c.
  intertrochanteric c.
  interureteric c.
  lateral epicondylar c.
  lateral sacral c.
  lateral supracondylar c.
  c. of lesser tubercle
  marginal c. of tooth
  medial epicondylar c.
  medial c. of fibula
  medial supracondylar c.
  median sacral c.
  c.'s of nail bed
  c.'s of nail matrix
  nasal c.
  nasal c. of horizontal plate of
    palatine bone
  nasal c. of palatine process of
    maxilla
  c. of neck of rib

  neural c.
  obturator c.
  c. of palatine bone
  palatine c. of horizontal process of
    palatine bone
  c. of petrous part of temporal bone
  c. of petrous temporal bone
  posterior lacrimal c.
  pubic c.
  c. of round window
  sacral c.
  sagittal c.
  c. of scapular spine
  sphenoidal c.
  spiral c.
  spiral c. of cochlear duct
  c. of supinator muscle
  supinator c. of ulna
  supramastoid c.
  suprastyloid c. of radius
  supraventricular c.
  temporal c. of mandible
  terminal c.
  tibial c.
  transverse c.
  transverse c. of internal acoustic
    meatus
  triangular c.
  trigeminal c.
  trochanteric c.
  turbinated c.
  urethral c.
  urethral c. of female
  urethral c. of male
  vertical c. of internal acoustic
    meatus
  vestibular c.
  c. of vestibule
  vomerine c. of choana
cresta
cresyl
  c. blue, c. blue brilliant
  c. echt
  c. fast violet
  c. violet acetate
cresylate
Cresylecht violet stain
creta
cretin
cretinism
cretinistic
cretinoid
cretinous
Creutzfeldt-Jakob disease (CJD)
crevice
  gingival c.
crevicular
  c. epithelium
  c. fluid
CRF
  corticotropin-releasing factor
CRH
  corticotropin-releasing hormone
crib death
cribra (*pl. of* cribrum)

cribrate
cribration
cribriform
    c. area of the renal papilla
    c. fascia
    c. foramina
    c. hymen
    c. plate of ethmoid bone
cribrous lamina
cribrum, pl. **cribra**
Cricetinae
Cricetulus
Cricetus
cricoarytenoid
    c. articular capsule
    c. articulation
    c. joint
    c. ligament
cricoarytenoideus
cricoesophageal tendon
cricoid
    c. cartilage
    c. split operation
cricoidynia
cricopharyngeal
    c. achalasia
    c. ligament
    c. myotomy
    c. part of inferior constrictor
      muscle of pharynx
cricopharyngeus muscle
cricosantorinian ligament
cricothyroid
    c. artery
    c. articular capsule
    c. articulation
    c. branch of superior thyroid artery
    c. joint
    c. membrane
    c. muscle
cricothyroideus
cricothyroidotomy
cricothyrotomy
cricotomy
cricotracheal
    c. ligament
    c. membrane
cricovocal membrane
cri-du-chat syndrome, cri du chat
  syndrome
Crigler-Najjar
    C.-N. disease
    C.-N. syndrome
Crile clamp
Crimean-Congo
    C.-C. hemorrhagic fever
    C.-C. hemorrhagic fever virus
Crimean fever
criminal
    c. abortion
    c. anthropology
    c. hygiene
    c. insanity
    c. irresponsibility
    c. psychology

criminology
crines
crinin
crinogenic
crinophagy
crippled
crisis, pl. **crises**
    addisonian c.
    adolescent c.
    adrenal c.
    anaphylactoid c.
    blast c.
    blood c.
    Dietl c.
    febrile c.
    gastric c.
    glaucomatocyclitic c.
    hemolytic c.
    identity c.
    c. intervention
    laryngeal c.
    midlife c.
    myasthenic c.
    myelocytic c.
    ocular c.
    oculogyric c.
    otolithic c.
    salt-depletion c.
    sickle cell c.
    tabetic c.
    therapeutic c.
    thyroid c.
    thyrotoxic c.
    vasoocclusive c.
    visceral c.
crispation
crisscross heart
crista, pl. **cristae**
    c. ampullaris
    c. ampullaris (ductuum
      semicircularium)
    c. arcuata cartilaginis arytenoideae
    c. basalaris ductus cochlearis
    c. basilaris ductus cochlearis
    c. buccinatoria
    c. capitis costae
    c. choanalis vomeris
    c. colli costae
    c. conchalis
    c. conchalis corporis maxillae
    c. conchalis ossis palatini
    c. corporis costae
    cristae cutis
    c. dentalis
    c. dividens
    c. ethmoidalis
    c. ethmoidalis maxillae
    c. ethmoidalis ossis palatini
    c. fenestrae cochleae
    c. frontalis
    c. galli
    c. glutea
    c. helicis
    c. iliaca

c. infratemporalis alaris majoris ossis sphenoidalis
c. intertrochanterica
c. lacrimalis anterior
c. lacrimalis posterior
c. marginalis dentis
cristae matricis unguis
c. medialis fibulae
cristae of mitochondria
cristae mitochondriales
c. musculi supinatoris ulnae
c. nasalis
c. nasalis laminae horizontalis ossis palatini
c. nasalis processus palatini maxillae
c. obturatoria
c. occipitalis externa
c. occipitalis interna
c. palatina
c. palatina laminae horizontalis ossis palatini
c. phallica
c. pubica
c. quarta
c. sacralis
c. sacralis intermedia
c. sacralis lateralis
c. sacralis medialis
c. sacralis mediana
c. sphenoidalis
c. spiralis
c. spiralis ductus cochlearis
c. supracondylaris lateralis
c. supracondylaris medialis
c. supraepicondylaris lateralis
c. supraepicondylaris medialis
c. supramastoidea
c. suprastyloidea radii
c. supraventricularis
c. temporalis mandibulae
c. terminalis
c. terminalis atrii dextri
c. terminalis of right atrium
c. transversalis
c. transversa meatus acustici interni
c. triangularis
c. tuberculi majoris
c. tuberculi minoris
c. urethralis
c. urethralis femininae
c. urethralis masculinae
c. verticalis meatus acustici interni
c. vestibuli
criterion, pl. **criteria**
Amsel criteria
Hill criteria of evidence
Jones criteria
Spiegelberg criteria
criterion-related validity
Crithidia
crithidia
critical
c. angle
c. care unit

c. flicker fusion frequency
c. fusion frequency (CFF)
c. illness polyneuropathy
c. illumination
c. limit
c. micelle concentration (cmc)
c. organ
c. pathway
c. period
c. pH
c. point
c. pressure
c. rate
c. temperature
CRL
crown-rump length
CR lead
CRM
certified reference material
CRM
cross-reacting material
CRNA
certified registered nurse anesthetist
cRNA
complementary ribonucleic acid
CRO
cathode ray oscilloscope
crocodile
c. tears
c. tears syndrome
Crocq disease
crocus
Crohn disease
cromolyn sodium
Cronkhite-Canada syndrome
Crooke
C. granule
C. hyaline change
C. hyaline degeneration
Crookes glass
Crookes-Hittorf tube
Crosby capsule
cross
c. agglutination
back c.
c. circulation
double back c.
c. flap
hair c.
c. hybridization
c. infection
maltese c.
c. mating
Ranvier c.
c. section
test c.
c. tolerance
crossbite tooth
crossbreed
crossbreeding
cross-cultural psychiatry
cross-cut bur
cross-dressing
crossed
c. adductor jerk

C

crossed *(continued)*
    c. adductor reflex
    c. anesthesia
    c. aphasia
    c. cylinder
    c. diplopia
    c. embolism
    c. extension reflex
    c. eyes
    c. fixation
    c. hemianesthesia
    c. hemianopia
    c. hemiplegia
    c. immunoelectrophoresis
    c. knee jerk
    c. knee reflex
    c. laterality
    c. paralysis
    c. pyramidal tract
    c. reflex of pelvis
    c. renal ectopia
    c. spino-adductor reflex
    c. testicular ectopia
cross-eye
crossing-over, crossover
    somatic c.-o.
    unequal c.-o.
    uneven c.-o.
cross-level bias
cross-link
cross-linked
    c.-l. polymer
    c.-l. resin
cross-matching
crossover *(var. of* crossing-over)
cross-over study
cross-reacting
    c.-r. agglutinin
    c.-r. antibody
    c.-r. material (CRM)
cross-section
cross-sectional
    c.-s. echocardiography
    c.-s. method
    c.-s. study
cross-table lateral projection
cross-taper
crossway
    sensory c.
crotalaria poisoning
crotalid
Crotalidae
crotalin
crotalism
Crotalus
Crotalus
    C. antitoxin
    C. toxin
crotamiton
crotaphion
crotonase
croton oil
crotonyl-ACP reductase
crotoxin

crottle
croup
croup-associated (CA)
    c.-a. virus
croupous
    c. bronchitis
    c. laryngitis
    c. lymph
    c. membrane
croupy
Crouzon
    C. disease
    C. syndrome
crowding phenomenon
Crowe-Davis mouth gag
Crow-Fukase syndrome
crowing inspiration
crown
    anatomical c.
    artificial c.
    bell-shaped c.
    c. cavity
    ciliary c.
    clinical c.
    c. flask
    c. glass
    c. of head
    jacket c.
    c. pulp
    radiate c.
    c. of tooth
    c. tubercle
    c. of Venus
crown-heel length (CH, CHL)
crowning
crown-rump length (CRL)
CRP
    cAMP receptor protein
    C-reactive protein
CRT
    cathode ray tube
cruces (*pl. of* crux)
crucial
    c. anastomosis
    c. bandage
    c. ligament
cruciate
    c. anastomosis
    c. eminence
    c. ligament of the atlas
    c. ligament of knee
    c. ligament of leg
    c. muscle
crucible
cruciform
    c. eminence
    c. ligament of atlas
    c. loop
    c. part of fibrous digital sheath
    c. part of fibrous sheath
    c. pulley
crude
    c. calcium sulfide
    c. death rate

c. drug
c. urine
crufomate
crunch
cruor
crura (*pl. of* crus)
crural
c. arch
c. fascia
c. fossa
c. hernia
c. interosseous nerve
c. ring
c. septum
c. sheath
c. triangle
crureus
crus, pl. **crura**
ampullary c. of semicircular duct
anterior c. of stapes
c. anterius capsulae internae
c. anterius stapedis
crura anthelicis
crura antihelicis
c. of antihelix
c. of bony semicircular canal
c. breve incudis
c. cerebri
c. clitoridis
c. of clitoris
common c. of semicircular duct
c. corporis cavernosi penis
c. dextrum diaphragmatis
c. dextrum fasciculi atrioventricularis
c. fornicis
c. of fornix
c. helicis
c. of helix
c. inferius marginis falciformis
hiatus sapheni
lateral c.
c. laterale
c. laterale anuli inguinalis
superficialis
c. laterale cartilaginis alaris majoris
lateral c. of facial canal
lateral c. of horizontal part of the
facial canal
lateral c. of the major alar
cartilage of the nose
lateral c. of the superficial inguinal
ring
left c. of atrioventricular bundle
left c. of diaphragm
long c. of incus
c. longum incudis
medial c.
c. mediale
c. mediale anuli inguinalis
superficialis
c. mediale cartilaginis alaris majoris
medial c. of facial canal
medial c. of the horizontal part of
the facial canal

medial c. of major alar cartilage of
nose
medial c. of the superficial inguinal
ring
crura membranacea ampullaria
ductuum semicircularium
c. membranaceum commune
ductuum semicircularium
c. membranaceum simplex ductus
semicircularis
crura ossea canalium semicircularium
c. penis
c. of penis
posterior c. of stapes
c. posterius capsulae internae
c. posterius stapedis
right c. of atrioventricular bundle
right c. of diaphragm
short c. of incus
simple c. of semicircular duct
c. sinistrum diaphragmatis
c. sinistrum fasciculi
atrioventricularis
c. superius marginis falciformis
hiatus sapheni
crush
c. kidney
c. syndrome
crusotomy
crust
milk c.
crusta, pl. **crustae**
c. inflammatoria
c. lactea
c. phlogistica
Crustacea
crusted
c. ringworm
c. scabies
crutch
c. palsy
c. paralysis
Cruveilhier
C. fascia
C. fossa
C. joint
C. ligament
C. plexus
Cruveilhier-Baumgarten
C.-B. disease
C.-B. murmur
C.-B. sign
C.-B. syndrome
crux, pl. **cruces**
c. of heart
cruces pilorum
Cruz trypanosomiasis
cryalgesia
cryanesthesia
cryesthesia
cry for help
crymophilic
crymophylactic
cryoanesthesia
cryobiology

C

cryocautery
cryoconization
cryoextraction
cryoextractor
cryofibrinogen
cryofibrinogenemia
cryofluorane
cryofracture
cryogen
cryogenic
cryogenics
cryoglobulinemia
cryoglobulins
cryohydrate
cryohypophysectomy
cryolysis
cryometer
cryopallidectomy
cryopathy
cryopexy
cryophilic
cryophylactic
cryoprecipitate
cryoprecipitation
cryopreservation
cryoprobe
cryoprostatectomy
cryoprotein
cryopulvinectomy
cryoscope
cryoscopy
cryospasm
cryostat
cryosurgery
cryothalamectomy
cryotherapy
cryotolerant
crypt
    c. abscess
    anal c.
    dental c.
    enamel c.
    c. of Henle
    c. of iris
    c. of Lieberkühn
    c. of Lieberkühn of large intestine
    c. of Lieberkühn of small intestine
    lingual c.
    Morgagni c.
    synovial c.
    tonsillar c.
crypta, pl. cryptae
    cryptae tonsillares
    c. tonsillaris
cryptectomy
cryptenamine acetate
cryptenamine tannate
cryptic
cryptitis
cryptochrome
cryptococcoma
cryptococcosis
Cryptococcus neoformans
cryptocrystalline
Cryptocystis trichodectis

cryptodidymus
Cryptogamia
cryptogenic
    c. cirrhosis
    c. epilepsy
    c. fibrosing alveolitis
    c. infection
    c. pyemia
    c. septicemia
cryptolith
cryptomenorrhea
cryptophthalmus, cryptophthalmia
    c. syndrome
cryptopodia
cryptopyrrole
cryptorchidism
cryptorchid testis
cryptorchism
cryptoscope
cryptosporidiosis
Cryptosporidium parvum
Cryptostroma corticale
cryptotia
cryptoxanthin
cryptozoite
cryptozygous
crystal
    asthma c.
    blood c.
    Böttcher c.
    Charcot-Leyden c.
    Charcot-Neumann c.
    Charcot-Robin c.
    chiral c.
    chlorohemin c.
    clathrate c.
    ear c.
    Florence c.
    hematoidin c.
    hydrate c.
    knife-rest c.
    Leyden c.
    Lubarsch c.
    c. rash
    sperm c.
    spermin c.
    c. structure
    Teichmann c.
    thorn apple c.
    twin c.
    c. violet vaccine
    Virchow c.
    whetstone c.
crystallin
    gamma c.
crystalline
    c. capsule
    c. cataract
    c. digitalin
    c. insulin zinc suspension
    c. interface
    c. lens
crystallization
crystallized trypsin
crystallogram

crystallography
crystalloid
    Charcot-Böttcher c.
    Reinke c.
crystallophobia
crystalluria
crystal violet
Cs
    cesium
CSD
    catscratch disease
C section
CSF
    cerebrospinal fluid
CSI
    Calculus Surface Index
"C" sliding osteotomy
CT
    computed tomography
      dynamic CT
      helical CT
      CT number
      CT pelvimetry
      CT scan
      spiral CT
      CT unit
CTD
    cumulative trauma disorder
Ctenocephalides
CTL
CTP
    cytidine 5′-triphosphate
Cu
    copper
^{67}**Cu**
    copper-67
^{64}**Cu**
    copper-64
Cuban itch
cubeb
cube pessary
cubic
    c. centimeter (cc)
    c. niter
cubital
    c. anastomosis
    c. bone
    c. fossa
    c. joint
    c. lymph node
    c. nerve
    c. tunnel syndrome
cubitus, pl. **cubiti**
    c. valgus
    c. varus
cuboid, cuboidal
    c. articular surface of calcaneus
    c. bone
    c. carcinoma
    c. epithelium
cuboideonavicular
    c. joint
    c. ligament
cuboidodigital reflex
cudbear

cue
    response-produced c.
cued speech
cuff
    musculotendinous c.
    perivascular c.
    rotator c. of shoulder
    vaginal c.
cuffing
cuirass
    analgesic c.
    c. respirator
    tabetic c.
    c. ventilator
cul-de-sac, pl. **culs-de-sac**
    conjunctival c.-d.-s.
    Douglas c.-d.-s.
    greater c.-d.-s.
    Gruber c.-d.-s.
    lesser c.-d.-s.
    c.-d.-s. smear
culdocentesis
culdoplasty
culdoscope
culdoscopy
culdotomy
Culex
    C. nigripalpus
    C. pipiens
    C. quinquefasciatus
    C. restuans
    C. salinarius
    C. tarsalis
Culicidae
culicidal
culicide
culicifuge
Culicoides
    C. austeni
    C. furens
    C. milnei
Culiseta
    C. inornata
    C. melanura
Cullen sign
culmen, pl. **culmina**
Culp pyeloplasty
culs-de-sac (*pl. of* cul-de-sac)
cult
cultivated yeast
cultivation
cultural
    c. anthropology
    c. diversity
    c. shock
culture
    batch c.
    cell c.
    continuous c.
    discontinuous c.
    elective c.
    enrichment c.
    hanging-block c.
    Harada-Mori filter paper strip c.
    c. medium

C

culture *(continued)*
> mixed lymphocyte c.
> monoxenic c.
> needle c.
> neotype c.
> organ c.
> Petri dish c.
> plastic envelope c.
> pouch c.
> pure c.
> roll-tube c.
> sensitized c.
> shake c.
> slant c.
> slope c.
> smear c.
> stab c.
> stock c.
> streak c.
> tissue c.
> type c.
> xenic c.

Culver root
cum (c̄)
cumarin
cumetharol
cumethoxaethane
Cummer
> C. classification
> C. guideline

cUMP
> cyclic uridine 3,5-monophosphate

cumulative
> c. action
> c. dose
> c. effect
> C. Index Medicus
> c. trauma disorder (CTD)

cumulus, pl. **cumuli**
> c. oöphorus
> c. ovaricus

cuneate
> c. fasciculus
> c. funiculus
> c. nucleus
> c. tubercle

cunei (*pl. of* cuneus)
cuneiform
> c. bone
> c. cartilage
> c. cataract
> c. lobe
> c. nucleus
> c. part of vomer
> c. tubercle

cuneocerebellar
> c. fiber
> c. tract

cuneocuboid
> c. interosseous ligament
> c. joint
> c. ligament

cuneometatarsal
> c. interosseous ligament
> c. joint

cuneonavicular
> c. articulation
> c. joint
> c. ligament

cuneoscaphoid
cuneospinal fiber
cuneus, pl. **cunei**
cuniculus, pl. **cuniculi**
cunnilingus
Cunninghamella elegans
cunnus
cup
> c. biopsy forceps
> Diogenes c.
> dry c.
> eye c.
> glaucomatous c.
> ocular c.
> optic c.
> c. of palm
> perilimbal suction c.
> physiologic c.
> suction c.
> wet c.

Cupid's bow
cupola
cupped
cupping glass
cupric
> c. acetate
> c. acetate normal
> c. arsenite
> c. chloride
> cupric citrate
> c. sulfate

cupriuresis
cupula, pl. **cupulae**
> c. ampullaris
> ampullary c.
> c. of cochlea
> c. cochleae
> cochlear c.
> c. pleurae
> pleural c.

cupular
> c. blind sac
> c. cecum of the cochlear duct
> c. part of epitympanic recess

cupulate
cupuliform cataract
cupulogram
cupulolithiasis
curage
curare
> calabash c.
> pot c.
> tube c.

curariform
curarimimetic
curarine
curarization
curative dose (CD^{50})

curb tenotomy
curcumin
curd soap
curdy pus
cure
curettage
 dilation and c. (D & C)
 periapical c.
 subgingival c.
 suction c.
curette, curet
 Hartmann c.
curettement
curie (c, Ci)
curing
 dental c.
curium (Cm)
curlicue ureter
Curling ulcer
currant
 c. jelly clot
 c. jelly stool
 c. jelly thrombus
current
 action c.
 after-c.
 alternating c. (AC)
 anodal c.
 ascending c.
 axial c.
 centrifugal c.
 centripetal c.
 d'Arsonval c.
 demarcation c.
 descending c.
 direct c. (DC)
 electrotonic c.
 galvanic c.
 high-frequency c.
 c. of injury
 labile c.
 Tesla c.
Curschmann spiral
curse
 Ondine c.
curvatura, pl. curvaturae
 c. primaria columnae vertebralis
 curvaturae secondariae columnae
  vertebralis
 c. ventriculi major
 c. ventriculi minor
curvature
 c. aberration
 angular c.
 anterior c.
 backward c.
 gingival c.
 greater c. of stomach
 c. hyperopia
 lateral c.
 lesser c. of stomach
 c. myopia
 occlusal c.
 posterior c.
 Pott c.

 primary c. of vertebral column
 secondary c. of vertebral column
 spinal c.
curve
 active length-tension c.
 alignment c.
 anti-Monson c.
 area under the c. (AUC)
 Barnes c.
 buccal c.
 calibration c.
 Carus c.
 cephalic c.
 characteristic c.
 compensating c.
 distribution c.
 dose-response c.
 dye-dilution c.
 epidemic c.
 flow-volume c.
 force-velocity c.
 Frank-Starling c.
 frequency c.
 Friedman c.
 gaussian c.
 growth c.
 H and D c.
 Heidelberger c.
 Hunter and Driffield c.
 indicator-dilution c.
 intracardiac pressure c.
 isovolume pressure-flow c.
 labor c.
 logistic c.
 milled-in c.
 Monson c.
 muscle c.
 c. of occlusion
 passive length-tension c.
 Pleasure c.
 precipitation c.
 Price-Jones c.
 probability c.
 progress c.
 pulse c.
 receiver operating characteristic c.
 reverse c.
 ROC c.
 c. of Spee
 Starling c.
 strength-duration c.
 stress-strain c.
 tension c.
 Traube-Hering c.
 tuning c.
 volume-time c.
 von Spee c.
 whole-body titration c.
Curvularia
Cushing
 C. disease
 C. disease of the omentum
 C. effect
 C. phenomenon
 C. pituitary basophilism

Cushing *(continued)*
  C. response
  C. suture
  C. syndrome
  C. syndrome medicamentosus
cushingoid
cushion
  anal c.
  atrioventricular canal c.
  endocardial c.
  c. of epiglottis
  eustachian c.
  hemorrhoidal c.
  levator c.
  Passavant c.
  pharyngoesophageal c.
  sucking c.
cusp
  c. angle
  anterior c. of left atrioventricular
    valve
  anterior c. of mitral valve
  anterior c. of right atrioventricular
    valve
  anterior c. of tricuspid valve
  c. of Carabelli
  c. height
  posterior c. of left atrioventricular
    valve
  posterior c. of mitral valve
  posterior c. of right atrioventricular
    valve
  posterior c. of tricuspid valve
  semilunar c.
  septal c. of right atrioventricular
    valve
  septal c. of tricuspid valve
  talon c.
  c. of tooth
cuspad
cuspal interference
cuspid tooth
cuspis, pl. **cuspides**
  c. anterior valvae atrioventricularis
    dextrae
  c. anterior valvae atrioventricularis
    sinistrae
  c. anterior valvae mitralis
  c. anterior valvae tricuspidalis
  c. coronae
  c. dentis
  c. posterior valvae atrioventricularis
    dextrae
  c. posterior valvae atrioventricularis
    sinistrae
  c. posterior valvae mitralis
  c. posterior valvae tricuspidalis
  c. septalis valvae atrioventricularis
    dextrae
  c. septalis valvae tricuspidalis
cuspless tooth
cusum
cutaneomeningospinal angiomatosis
cutaneomucosal

cutaneomucouveal syndrome
cutaneous
  c. absorption
  c. albinism
  c. ancylostomiasis
  c. anthrax
  c. blastomycosis
  c. branch of anterior branch of
    obturator nerve
  c. branch of mixed nerve
  c. branch of obturator nerve
  c. cervical nerve
  c. diphtheria
  c. emphysema
  c. focal mucinosis
  c. gangrene
  c. gland
  c. graft versus host reaction
  c. hemorrhoid
  c. horn
  c. larva migrans
  c. layer of tympanic membrane
  c. leishmaniasis
  c. leishmaniasis granuloma
  c. loop ureterostomy
  c. lupus erythematosus
  c. meningioma
  c. muscle
  c. nerve
  c. pseudolymphoma
  c. pupil reflex
  c. reflex
  c. schistosomiasis japonica
  c. tuberculin test
  c. tuberculosis
  c. ureterostomy
  c. vasculitis
  c. vein
cutch
cutdown
Cuterebra
cuticle
  acquired c.
  acquired enamel c.
  dental c.
  enamel c.
  c. of hair
  c. of nail
  Nasmyth c.
  posteruption c.
  c. of root sheath
cuticula, pl. **cuticulae**
  c. 2
  c. dentis
  c. pili
  c. vaginae folliculi pili
cuticular drusen
cutin
cutis
  c. anserina
  c. laxa
  c. marmorata
  c. marmorata telangiectatica
    congenita
  c. plate

c. rhomboidalis nuchae
c. vera
c. verticis gyrata
cutization
cutpoint
cutting
c. edge
c. forceps
c. needle
c. tooth
cuttlefish disk
cuvet, cuvette
c. oximeter
Cuvier
C. duct
C. vein
CV
coefficient of variation
CVA
cerebrovascular accident
CVP
central venous pressure
CX
phosgene oxime
CxT
concentration × time
cyanalcohol
cyanamide
cyanate
cyanemia
cyanide
c. methemoglobin
c. poisoning
cyanide-nitroprusside test
cyanidenon
cyanidol
cyanmethemoglobin
Cyanobacteria
cyanobacterialike (CLB)
cyanobacteriumlike body
cyanochroic, cyanochrous
cyanocobalamin
radioactive c.
cyanogen chloride
cyanogenic glycoside
cyanohydrin
cyanophil, cyanophile
cyanophilous
Cyanophyceae
cyanopia
cyanopsia
cyanosed
cyanose tardive
cyanosis
compression c.
enterogenous c.
false c.
hereditary methemoglobinemic c.
late c.
c. retinae
shunt c.
tardive c.
toxic c.
cyanotic
c. asphyxia

c. atrophy
c. atrophy of the liver
c. induration
cyanuria
cyanuric acid
Cyathostoma bronchialis
Cyathostomum
cybernetics
cybrid
cyclamate
cyclamic acid
cyclamide
cyclandelate
cyclarthrodial
cyclarthrosis
cyclase
cycle
anovulatory c.
brain wave c.
carbon c.
carbon dioxide c.
cardiac c.
cell c.
chewing c.
citric acid c.
Cori c.
dicarboxylic acid c.
endogenous c.
erythrocytic c.
estrous c.
exoerythrocytic c.
exogenous c.
fatty acid oxidation c.
forced c.
futile c.
gamma-glutamyl c.
glycine-succinate c.
glyoxylic acid c.
gonadotrophic c.
hair c.
heterogonic life c.
homogonic life c.
Krebs-Henseleit c.
Krebs-Kornberg c.
Krebs ornithine c.
Krebs urea c.
c. length alternans
life c.
masticating c.
menstrual c.
mitotic c.
nitrogen c.
ornithine c.
ovarian c.
pentose phosphate c.
c.'s per second (cps)
reproductive c.
restored c.
returning c.
Ross c.
Shemin c.
substrate c.
succinic acid c.
tricarboxylic acid c.

C

cycle *(continued)*
    urea c.
    visual c.
cyclectomy
cyclencephaly, cyclencephalia
cycle-specific agent
cyclic
    c. adenylic acid
    c. albuminuria
    c. AMP
    c. compound
    c. esotropia
    c. GMP
    c. guanosine 3′,5′-monophosphate
    c. inosine 3,5-monophosphate (cIMP)
    c. neutropenia
    c. nucleotide
    c. peptide
    c. phosphate
    c. phosphoric acid
    c. strabismus
    c. uridine 3′,5′-monophosphate
    c. vomiting
3′,5′-cyclic AMP synthetase
cyclin D
cyclitis
    Fuchs heterochromic c.
    heterochromic c.
    plastic c.
    purulent c.
cyclizine
    cyclizine hydrochloride
    cyclizine lactate
cyclobenzaprine hydrochloride
cyclocephaly, cyclocephalia
cyclochoroiditis
cyclocryotherapy
cyclocumarol
cyclodestructive
cyclodialysis
cyclodiathermy
cycloduction
cycloguanil pamoate
cyclohexanesulfamic acid
cycloheximide
cyclohexylsulfamic acid
cycloid
cyclol
cyclonamine
cyclooxygenase
cyclopea
cyclopentamine hydrochloride
cyclopentane
cyclopenta[a]phenanthrene
cyclopenthiazide
cyclopentolate hydrochloride
cyclopeptide
cyclophenazine hydrochloride
cyclophorase
cyclophoria
cyclophosphamide
    c., doxorubicin (Adriamycin), vincristine, prednisone (CHOP)
    c., hexamethylmelamine, doxorubicin (Adriamycin), and cisplatin (CHAP)
cyclophotocoagulation
Cyclophyllidae
cyclopia
cyclopian eye
cycloplegia
cycloplegic
cyclopropane
cyclops
cycloserine
cyclosis
Cyclospora cayetanensis
cyclosporin A
cyclosporine
cyclothiazide
cyclothymia
cyclothymiac, cyclothymic
    c. personality
    c. personality disorder
cyclotomy
cyclotorsion
cyclotron
cyclotropia
cyclozoonosis
Cyd
    cytidine
cyesis
cyl.
    cylinder
cylinder (cyl.)
    Bence Jones c.
    crossed c.
    Külz c.
    c. retinoscopy
cylindraxis
cylindrical
    c. bronchiectasis
    c. epithelium
    c. joint
    c. lens
cylindroadenoma
cylindroid aneurysm
cylindroma
cylindromatous carcinoma
cylindruria
cyllosoma
cymarin
cymba conchae
cymbocephalic, cymbocephalous
cymbocephaly
cynanthropy
cynocephaly
cynodont
cynophobia
Cyon nerve
CYP
    cytochrome P450 enzyme
      CYP 1A2
      CYP 3A
      CYP 2C9
      CYP 2C19
      CYP 2D6
      CYP 2E1

cypridophobia
cyproheptadine hydrochloride
cyproterone acetate
Cys
   cysteine
cyst
   adventitious c.
   allantoic c.
   alveolar hydatid c.
   aneurysmal bone c.
   angioblastic c.
   apical periodontal c.
   apoplectic c.
   arachnoid c.
   Baker c.
   Bartholin c.
   bile c.
   blood c.
   blue dome c.
   bone c.
   botryoid odontogenic c.
   Boyer c.
   branchial c.
   branchial cleft c.
   bronchogenic c.
   bursal c.
   calcifying and keratinizing
     odontogenic c.
   calcifying odontogenic c.
   cerebellar c.
   chocolate c.
   choledochal c.
   chyle c.
   colloid c.
   compound c.
   corpora lutea c.
   Cowper c.
   daughter c.
   dentigerous c.
   dermoid c.
   dermoid c. of ovary
   distention c.
   duplication c.
   echinococcus c.
   endodermal c.
   endometrial c.
   endothelial c.
   enterogenous c.
   ependymal c.
   epidermal c.
   epidermoid c.
   epithelial c.
   eruption c.
   extravasation c.
   exudation c.
   false c.
   fissural c.
   follicular c.
   Gartner c.
   gas c.
   gingival c.
   globulomaxillary c.
   glomerular c.
   Gorlin c.
   granddaughter c.

   hemorrhagic c.
   hepatic c.
   heterotrophic oral gastrointestinal c.
   hydatid c.
   implantation c.
   incisive canal c.
   inclusion c.
   junctional c.
   keratinous c.
   Klestadt c.
   lacteal c.
   lateral periodontal c.
   leptomeningeal c.
   lymphoepithelial c.
   median anterior maxillary c.
   median palatal c.
   median raphe c. of the penis
   meibomian c.
   milk c.
   morgagnian c.
   mother c.
   mucous c.
   multilocular hydatid c., multiloculate
     hydatid c.
   myxoid c.
   nabothian c.
   nasoalveolar c.
   nasolabial c.
   nasopalatine duct c.
   necrotic c.
   neural c.
   neurenteric c.
   odontogenic c.
   oil c.
   omphalomesenteric c.
   omphalomesenteric duct c.
   oophoritic c.
   osseous hydatid c.
   ovarian c.
   paraphysial c.
   parasitic c.
   parent c.
   paroophoritic c.
   parvilocular c.
   pearl c.
   periapical c.
   phaeomycotic c.
   pilar c.
   piliferous c.
   pilonidal c.
   pineal c.
   posttraumatic leptomeningeal c.
   primordial c.
   proliferating tricholemmal c.
   proliferation c.
   proliferative c.
   protozoan c.
   pseudomucinous c.
   radicular c.
   Rathke cleft c.
   residual c.
   retention c.
   rete c. of ovary
   root end c.
   sanguineous c.

C

cyst *(continued)*
>   sebaceous c.
>   secretory c.
>   seminal vesical c.
>   sequestration c.
>   serous c.
>   simple bone c.
>   solitary bone c.
>   Stafne bone c.
>   static bone c.
>   sterile c.
>   sublingual c.
>   sudoriferous c.
>   suprasellar c.
>   surgical ciliated c.
>   synovial c.
>   Tarlov c.
>   tarry c.
>   tarsal c.
>   teratomatous c.
>   thyroglossal duct c.
>   thyrolingual c.
>   Tornwaldt c.
>   traumatic bone c.
>   trichilemmal c.
>   tubular c.
>   umbilical c.
>   unicameral bone c.
>   unilocular hydatid c.
>   urachal c.
>   urinary c.
>   utricular c.
>   vitellointestinal c.
>   wolffian c.

cystacanth
cystadenocarcinoma
cystadenoma
>   papillary c. lymphomatosum

cystalgia
cystamine
cystathionase
β-cystathionase
cystathionine
cystathionine beta-lyase
cystathionine beta-synthase
cystathionine gamma-lyase
cystathionine gamma-synthase
cystathioninuria
cysteamine
cystectomy
>   Bartholin c.
>   partial c.
>   radical c.
>   salvage c.
>   total c.
>   vulvovaginal c.

cysteic acid
cysteine (Cys)
>   c. desulfhydrase
>   c. hydrolase
>   c. sulfinic acid
>   c. synthase

cysteinyl

cystic
>   c. acne
>   c. adenomatoid malformation
>   c. artery
>   c. bronchiectasis
>   c. carcinoma
>   c. diathesis
>   c. disease of the breast
>   c. disease of renal medulla
>   c. duct
>   c. duct cholangiography
>   c. fibrosis
>   c. fibrosis of the pancreas
>   c. gall duct
>   c. goiter
>   c. hygroma
>   c. hyperplasia
>   c. hyperplasia of the breast
>   c. kidney
>   c. lung
>   c. lymphangiectasis
>   c. lymph node
>   c. medial necrosis
>   c. mole
>   c. node
>   c. papillomatous craniopharyngioma
>   c. polyp
>   c. vein

cysticerci (*pl. of* cysticercus)
cysticercoid
cysticercosis
Cysticercus
>   *C. bovis*
>   *C. cellulosae*
>   *C.* disease

cysticercus, pl. **cysticerci**
cystiform
cystine
>   c. bridge
>   c. calculus
>   c. desulfhydrase
>   half c.
>   c. lyase
>   c. storage disease

meso-**cystine**
cystinemia
cystinosis
cystinotic leukocyte
cystinuria
cystinyl
cystis
>   c. fellea
>   c. urinaria

cystistaxis
cystitis
>   bacterial c.
>   c. colli
>   c. cystica
>   emphysematous c.
>   eosinophilic c.
>   follicular c.
>   c. glandularis
>   hemorrhagic c.
>   incrusted c.

interstitial c.
viral c.
cystoadenoma
cystocarcinoma
cystocele
cystochromoscopy
cystoduodenal ligament
cystoduodenostomy
pancreatic c.
cystoenterocele
cystoenterostomy
cystoepiplocele
cystofibroma
cystogastrostomy
cystogram
voiding c.
cystography
antegrade c.
cystohepatic triangle
cystoid
c. macular edema
c. maculopathy
cystojejunostomy
cystolith
cystolithiasis
cystolithic
cystolitholapaxy
cystolithotomy
cystoma
cystometer
cystometrogram (CMG)
cystometrography
cystometry
cystomorphous
cystomyoma
cystomyxoadenoma
cystomyxoma
cystopanendoscopy
cystoparalysis
cystopexy
cystophotography
cystoplasty
cystoplegia
cystoprostatectomy
cystopyelitis
cystopyelonephritis
cystorrhaphy
cystorrhea
cystosarcoma phyllode
cystoscope
cystoscopic urography
cystoscopy
cystospasm
cystostomy
cystotome
cystotomy
suprapubic c.
cystoureteritis
cystoureterogram
cystoureterography
cystourethritis
cystourethrocele
cystourethrogram
micturating c.

retrograde c.
voiding c. (VCUG)
cystourethrography
cystourethroscope
Cystoviridae
cystyl-aminopeptidase
Cyt
cytosine
cytapheresis
cytarabine
cytase
cythemolytic icterus
cytidine (Cyd)
c. 5′-diphosphate (CDP)
c. diphosphate choline
c. diphosphocholine (CDP-choline)
c. diphosphoglyceride (CDP-glyceride)
c. diphosphosugar (CDP-sugar)
c. 5′-monophosphate (CMP)
c. phosphate
c. 5′-triphosphate (CTP)
cytidylic acid
cytisine
cytoanalyzer
cytoarchitectonics
cytoarchitectural
cytoarchitecture
cytobiology
cytobiotaxis
cytocentrum
cytochalasin
cytochemistry
cytochrome
c. aa_3
c. b
c. b_5
c. b_5 reductase
c. c
c. cd
c. c_3 hydrogenase
c. c oxidase
c. c reductase
c. c_2 reductase
c. oxidase (*Pseudomonas*)
c. P-450$_{SCC}$
c. P450 enzyme (CYP)
c. peroxidase
c. P-450 system
c. reductase
c. system
cytochylema
cytocidal
cytocide
cytoclasis
cytoclastic
cytoclesis
cytocrine secretion
cytocuprein
cytocyst
cytodiagnosis
cytodieresis
cytogene
cytogenesis
cytogeneticist

C

cytogenetic map
cytogenetics
cytogenic reproduction
cytogenous
cytoglucopenia
cytoid body
cytokeratin filament
cytokine network
cytokinesis
cytolemma
cytolipin
    c. H, K
cytologic
    c. examination
    c. filter preparation
    c. screening
    c. smear
    c. specimen
cytologist
cytology
    exfoliative c.
cytolysin
cytolysis
cytolysosome
cytolytic
cytomatrix
cytomegalic
    c. cell
    c. inclusion disease
Cytomegalovirus disease
cytomembrane
cytomere
cytometer
    image c.
cytometry
    Feulgen c.
    flow c.
cytomicrosome
cytomorphology
cytomorphosis
cytopathic effect
cytopathogenic virus
cytopathologic, cytopathological
cytopathologist
cytopathology
cytopathy
cytopempsis
cytopenia
cytophagic histiocytic panniculitis
cytophagy
cytophanere
cytopharynx
cytophil group
cytophilic antibody
cytophotometry
    flow c.
cytophylactic
cytophylaxis
cytophyletic
cytopipette
cytoplasm
    ground-glass c.

cytoplasmic
    c. bridge
    c. inclusion body
    c. inheritance
    c. matrix
cytoplasmon
cytoplast
cytopoiesis
cytopreparation
cytopyge
cytoreductive therapy
cytorycte, cytorrhycte
cytoscreener
cytoside
cytosine (Cyt)
    c. arabinoside (AraC)
    c. ribonucleoside
cytosis
cytoskeleton
cytosmear
cytosol
cytosolic
cytosome
cytostasis
cytostatic chemotherapy
cytostome
cytotactic
cytotaxis, cytotaxia
    negative c.
    positive c.
cytotechnologist
cytothesis
cytotonic enterotoxin
cytotoxic
    c. cell
    c. chemotherapy
    c. reaction
    c. T lymphocyte
cytotoxicity
    antibody-dependent cell-mediated c.
    (ADCC)
    lymphocyte-mediated c.
cytotoxin
    vero c.
cytotrophoblast
cytotrophoblastic
    c. cell
    c. shell
cytotropic
    c. antibody
    c. antibody test
cytotropism
cytozoic
cytozoon
cyturia
Czapek-Dox medium
Czapek solution agar
CZE
    capillary zone electrophoresis
Czerny-Lembert suture
Czerny suture

δ (*var. of* delta)
Δ (*var. of* delta)
D
dexter
D antigen
D cell
D enzyme
D loop
D wave
2,4-D
2,4-dichlorophenoxy acetic acid
d
dexter
D-
-*d*
D-3-hydroxybutyric acid dehydrogenase
DA
developmental age
Da
dalton
dA, dAdo
deoxyadenosine
Daae disease
DAB
3′3-diaminobenzidine
dacarbazine (DTIC)
Adriamycin, bleomycin, vinblastine, d. (ABVD)
dacryadenitis
dacryoadenitis
dacryoblennorrhea
dacryocele
dacryocyst
dacryocystalgia
dacryocystectomy
dacryocystitis
dacryocystocele
dacryocystogram
dacryocystorhinostomy
dacryocystotomy
dacryohemorrhea
dacryolith
Desmarres d.
Nocardia d.
dacryolithiasis
dacryon
dacryops
dacryopyorrhea
dacryorrhea
dacryostenosis
dactinomycin
dactyl
dactylalgia
Dactylaria
dactyli (*pl. of* dactylus)
dactylitis
blistering distal d.
sickle cell d.
dactylocampsis
dactylocampsodynia
dactylodynia
dactylogryposis

dactylology
dactylomegaly
dactyloscopy
dactylospasm
dactylus, pl. **dactyli**
dacuronium
dAdo (*var. of* dA)
Da Fano stain
DAG
diacylglycerol
dagga
DAH
disordered action of heart
dahlia
dahlin
dahllite
daily dose
daisy
Dakin
D. fluid
D. solution
Dakin-Carrel treatment
Dale-Feldberg law
Dalen-Fuchs nodule
Dale reaction
Dalrymple sign
dalton (Da)
Dalton-Henry law
daltonian
daltonism
Dalton law
DALYs
disability-adjusted life years
DAM
diacetylmonoxime
post dam
rubber dam
dam
damage
diffuse alveolar d.
Damalinia
dammar
dam methylase
dAMP
deoxyadenylic acid
damp
damping
Dam unit
Damus-Kaye-Stancel procedure
Damus-Stancel-Kaye anastomosis
Dana operation
danazol
dance
hilar d.
Saint Anthony d.
Saint John d.
Saint Vitus d.
D. sign
dancing chorea
dander
dandruff

D

Dandy
  d. fever
  d. operation
Dandy-Walker syndrome
Dane
  D. particle
  D. stain
Danforth sign
Danielssen-Boeck disease
Danielssen disease
DANS
  1-dimethylaminonaphthalene-5-sulfonic
  acid
dansyl (Dns, DNS)
danthron
dantrolene sodium
Danubian endemic familial nephropathy
Danysz phenomenon
DAPI
  4'6-diamidino-2-phenylindole-2HCl
  DAPI stain
DA pregnancy test
dapsone neuropathy
d'Arcet metal
Darier
  D. disease
  D. sign
dark
  d. adaptation
  d. cell
  d. reaction
dark-adapted eye
dark-field
  d.-f. condenser
  d.-f. illumination
  d.-f. microscope
dark-ground illumination
Darling disease
Darrow red
d'Arsonval
  d. current
  d. galvanometer
dartoic
  d. tissue
dartos
  d. fascia
  d. muliebris
  d. muscle
darwinian
  d. ear
  d. evolution
  d. reflex
  d. theory
  d. tubercle
Dasyprocta
data processing
date
  d. boil
  d. fever
datum plane
Datura
  d. metel
  d. stramonium
Datura poisoning
daturine

Daubenton
  D. angle
  D. line
  D. plane
daughter
  d. cell
  d. colony
  d. cyst
  DES (diethylstilbestrol) d.
  d. isotope
  d. star
daunomycin
daunorubicin
Davidoff cell
Davidson syringe
Daviel
  D. operation
  D. spoon
Davies disease
Davis
  D. battery model of transduction
  D. graft
  D. interlocking sound
dawn phenomenon
Dawson encephalitis
day
  d. blindness
  d. hospital
  d. residue
  d. sight
  D. test
dazzling glare
dB
  decibel
DBP
  vitamin dbinding protein
DC
  direct current
  Doctor of Chiropractic
D & C
  dilation and curettage
dCMP
  deoxycytidylic acid
DDA
  dideoxyadenosine
DDI
  dideoxyinosine
DDS
  Doctor of Dental Surgery
DDT
  dichlorodiphenyltrichloroethane
D & E
  dilation and evacuation
de
  de Clerambault syndrome
  de Lange syndrome
  De Morgan spot
  de Morsier syndrome
  De Musset sign
  de Pezzer catheter
  de Quervain disease
  de Quervain tenosynovitis
  de Quervain thyroiditis
  De Sanctis-Cacchione syndrome
  de Wecker scissors

deacidification
deactivation
deacylase
dead
 d. arm syndrome
 d. fetus syndrome
 d. finger
 d. nerve
 d. on arrival (DOA)
 d. pulp
 d. space
 d. tooth
 d. tract
dead-end host
dead-in-bed syndrome
deadly
 d. agaric
 d. nightshade
DEAE-cellulose
deaf
deafferentation
deafness
 central d.
 chondrodystrophy with
  sensorineural d. (OSMED)
 cortical d.
 hereditary d.
 lentigines (multiple),
  electrocardiographic abnormalities,
  ocular hypertelorism, pulmonary
  stenosis, abnormalities of genitalia,
  retardation of growth, and d.
  (LEOPARD)
 nerve d.
 neural d.
 postlingual d.
 prelingual d.
 sudden d.
 word d.
dealbation
dealcoholization
deallergize
deamidase
deamidation, deamidization
deamidize
deamidizing enzyme
deaminase
deaminating enzyme
deamination, deaminization
 oxidative d.
deaminize
Dean fluorosis index
deanol acetamidobenzoate
death
 black d.
 brain d.
 cerebral d.
 d. certificate
 cot d.
 crib d.
 crude d. rate
 direct maternal d.
 early neonatal d.
 fetal d.
 genetic d.

 indirect maternal d.
 infant d.
 d. instinct
 late neonatal d.
 local d.
 maternal d.
 neonatal d.
 perinatal d.
 programmed cell d.
 d. rate
 d. rattle
 somatic d.
 sudden d.
 systemic d.
 d. trance
Deaver
 D. incision
 D. method
DeBakey
 D. classification
 D. forceps
debanding
debilitant
debilitating
debility
debond
debouch
débouchement
debrancher deficiency
debranching
 d. deficiency limit dextrinosis
 d. enzyme
 d. factor
Debré phenomenon
Debré-Sémélaigne syndrome
débridement
debris
 particulate wear d.
debrisoquine sulfate
debt
 alactic oxygen d.
 lactacid oxygen d.
 oxygen d.
debulking operation
decagram
decalcification
decalcify
decalcifying
decaliter
decalvant
decameter
decamethonium bromide
decamine
n-**decane**
decannulation
n-**decanoic acid**
decanoin
decanormal
decant
decantation
decapacitation factor
decapeptide
decapitate
decapitation
decapsulation of kidney

decarbonization
decarboxylase
decarboxylated dopa
decarboxylation
    oxidative d.
decay
    d. constant
    free induction d. (FID)
    d. theory
decayed
    d., extracted, and filled tooth (def, DEF)
    d., missing, and filled surface (DMFS, dmfs)
    d., missing, and filled teeth (DMF, dmf)
deceleration
    early d.
    late d.
    variable d.
decentered lens
decentration
decerebrate
    d. rigidity
    d. state
decerebration
    bloodless d.
decerebrize
dechloridation
dechlorination
dechloruration
decholesterolization
decibel (dB)
decidua
    d. basalis
    d. capsularis
    ectopic d.
    d. menstrualis
    d. parietalis
    d. polyposa
    d. reflexa
    d. serotina
    d. spongiosa
    d. vera
decidual
    d. cast
    d. cell
    d. endometritis
    d. fissure
    d. reaction
deciduate placenta
deciduation
deciduitis
deciduoma
    Loeb d.
deciduous
    d. dentition
    d. membrane
    d. skin
    d. tooth
decigram
deciliter
decimeter
decimorgan
decinormal

decision
    d. analysis
    limiting d.
decision tree
declamping
    d. phenomenon
    d. shock
declinator
declive
declivis
decoction
décollement
decompensation
    corneal d.
decompose
decomposition of movement
decompression
    cardiac d.
    cerebral d.
    d. chamber
    d. disease
    explosive d.
    internal d.
    nerve d.
    d. operation
    optic nerve sheath d.
    orbital d.
    pericardial d.
    rapid d.
    d. sickness
    spinal d.
    suboccipital d.
    subtemporal d.
    trigeminal d.
decongestant
decongestive
decontamination
deconvolution
decorticate
    d. rigidity
    d. state
decortication
    cerebral d.
    reversible d.
decoy cell
decrement
decremental conduction
decrepitation
decrudescence
decubital gangrene
decubitus
    Andral d.
    d. film
    d. radiograph
    d. ulcer
    ventral d.
decurrent
decussate
decussatio, pl. **decussationes**
    d. brachii conjunctivi
    d. fibrarum nervorum trochlearium
    d. fontinalis
    d. lemnisci mediales
    d. motoria

d. pedunculorum cerebellarium superiorum
d. pyramidum
d. sensoria
decussationes tegmentales
d. tegmentalis anterior
d. tegmentalis posterior

decussation
anterior tegmental d.
d. of brachia conjunctiva
dorsal tegmental d.
d. of the fillet
Forel d.
fountain d.
Held d.
d. of medial lemniscus
Meynert d.
motor d.
optic d.
posterior tegmental d.
d. of pyramid
rubrospinal d.
sensory d. of medulla oblongata
d. of superior cerebellar peduncles
tectospinal d.
tegmental d.
d. of trochlear nerve fiber
ventral tegmental d.
Wernekinck d.

dedentition
dedifferentiation
dedolation
deduction
deefferentation
de-emetinized ipecacuanha
deep
d. abdominal reflex
d. anterior cervical lymph node
d. artery of arm
d. artery of clitoris
d. artery of penis
d. artery of thigh
d. artery of tongue
d. auricular artery
d. bite
d. brachial artery
d. branch
d. branch of the lateral plantar nerve
d. branch of the medial circumflex femoral artery
d. branch of the medial plantar artery
d. branch of radial nerve
d. branch of the superior gluteal artery
d. branch of the transverse cervical artery
d. branch of the ulnar nerve
d. cardiac plexus
d. cell
d. cerebral vein
d. cervical artery
d. cervical fascia
d. cervical vein

d. circumflex iliac artery
d. circumflex iliac vein
d. cortex
d. crural arch
d. dorsal sacrococcygeal ligament
d. dorsal vein of clitoris
d. dorsal vein of penis
d. epigastric artery
d. epigastric vein
d. facial vein
d. fascia
d. fascia of arm
d. fascia of forearm
d. fascia of leg
d. fascia of neck
d. fascia of penis
d. fascia of thigh
d. femoral vein
d. fibular nerve
d. flexor muscle of finger
d. gray layer of superior colliculus
d. head of flexor pollicis brevis
d. hypothermic arrest
d. infrapatellar bursa
d. inguinal lymph node
d. inguinal ring
d. lamina
d. lateral cervical lymph node
d. layer
d. layer of levator palpebrae superioris
d. layer of temporal fascia
d. lingual artery
d. lingual vein
d. lymph vessel
d. middle cerebral vein
d. muscle of back
d. origin
d. palmar (arterial) arch
d. palmar branch of ulnar artery
d. palmar venous arch
d. parotid lymph node
d. part of anterior compartment of forearm
d. part of external anal sphincter
d. part of flexor retinaculum
d. part of masseter
d. part of palpebral part of orbicularis oculi
d. part of parotid gland
d. part of posterior (flexor) compartment of leg
d. percussion
d. perineal fascia
d. perineal pouch
d. perineal space
d. peroneal nerve
d. petrosal nerve
d. plantar artery
d. plantar branch of dorsalis pedis artery
d. posterior sacrococcygeal ligament
d. punctate keratitis
d. scleritis
d. sensibility

D

deep *(continued)*
 d. temporal artery
 d. temporal nerve
 d. temporal vein
 d. tendon reflex (DTR)
 d. transitional gyrus
 d. transverse metacarpal ligament
 d. transverse metatarsal ligament
 d. transverse muscle of perineum
 d. transverse perineal muscle
 d. vein of clitoris
 d. vein of penis
 d. vein of thigh
 d. white layer of superior colliculus
de-epicardialization
deer-fly
 d.-f. disease
 d.-f. fever
Deetjen body
def, DEF
 decayed, extracted, and filled tooth
  def caries index
defatigation
defecate
defecation
defecography
defect
 aorticopulmonary septal d.
 aortic septal d.
 atrial septal d.
 atrial ventricular canal d.
 birth d.
 congenital ectodermal d.
 coupling d.
 Eisenmenger d.
 endocardial cushion d.
 fibrous cortical d.
 filling d.
 Gerbode d.
 iodide transport d.
 iodotyrosine deiodinase d.
 luteal phase d.
 metaphyseal fibrous cortical d.
 organification d.
 osteoporotic marrow d.
 postinfarction ventricular septal d.
 relative afferent pupillary d.
 salt-losing d.
 ventricular septal d.
defective
 d. bacteriophage
 d. interfering particle
 d. organism
 d. phage
 d. probacteriophage
 d. prophage
 d. virus
defemination
defense
 d. mechanism
 d. reflex
 screen d.
 ur-d.'s
defensin

defensive
 d. circle
 d. medicine
deferent
 d. canal
 d. duct
deferential
 d. artery
 d. plexus
deferentitis
deferoxamine mesylate
deferred shock
defervescence
defervescent stage
defibrillation
defibrillator
 external d.
defibrination
deficiency
 adult lactase d.
 alpha$_1$-antitrypsin d.
 d. anemia
 antitrypsin d.
 arch length d.
 arginosuccinate lyase d.
 arylsulfatase A d.
 arylsulfatase B d.
 beta-*d*-glucuronidase d.
 biotinidase d.
 carnitine d.
 debrancher d.
 d. disease
 familial high density lipoprotein d.
 fructokinase d.
 galactokinase d.
 glucose-6-phosphate dehydrogenase d.
 glucosephosphate isomerase d.
 glutathione synthetase d.
 11-hydroxylase d.
 21-hydroxylase d.
 hypoxanthine guanine
  phosphoribosyltransferase d.
 immune d.
 immunity d.
 immunologic d.
 LCAT d.
 leukocyte adhesion d. (LAD)
 long-chain 3-hydroxyacyl-CoA
  dehydrogenase d.
 long-chain/very long-chain acyl-CoA
  dehydrogenase d.
 luteal phase d.
 medium-chain acyl-CoA
  dehydrogenase d.
 mental d.
 muscle phosphorylase d.
 d. mutant
 phosphohexose isomerase d.
 placental sulfatase d.
 primary carnitine d.
 proximal femoral focal d. (PFFD)
 pseudocholinesterase d.
 pyruvate kinase d.
 riboflavin d.
 secondary antibody d.

short-chain acyl-CoA
  dehydrogenase d.
d. symptom
taste d.
deficit
base d.
oxygen d.
pulse d.
sleep d.
definition
definitive
d. callus
d. host
d. lysosome
d. method
d. prosthesis
deflection
intrinsic d.
intrinsicoid d.
deflective occlusal contact
deflexion
deflorescence
defluoridation
defluvium
defluxion
deformability
deformation
deforming
deformity
Åkerlund d.
Arnold-Chiari d.
bell clapper d.
boutonnière d.
contracture d.
Erlenmeyer flask d.
gunstock d.
Haglund d.
J-sella d.
keyhole d.
lobster-claw d.
Madelung d.
mermaid d.
parachute d.
reduction d.
silver-fork d.
Sprengel d.
swan-neck d.
torsional d.
whistling d.
Whitehead d.
defurfuration
deganglionate
degeneracy
degenerate
degeneratio
degeneration
adipose d.
adiposogenital d.
age-related macular d.
albuminous d.
amyloid d.
angiolithic d.
ascending d.
atheromatous d.
axon d.

axonal d.
ballooning d.
basophilic d.
calcareous d.
carneous d.
caseous d.
colloid d.
cone d.
corticobasal d.
Crooke hyaline d.
descending d.
disciform macular d.
ectatic marginal d. of cornea
elastoid d.
elastotic d.
familial pseudoinflammatory
  macular d.
fascicular d.
fatty d.
fibrinoid d.
fibrinous d.
fibrous d.
granular d.
granulovacuolar d.
gray d.
hepatolenticular d.
hyaline d.
hyaloideoretinal d.
hydropic d.
infantile neuronal d.
liquefaction d.
macular d.
Mönckeberg d.
mucinoid d.
mucoid medial d.
myelinic d.
myopic d.
myxoid d.
myxomatous d.
neurofibrillary d.
Nissl d.
olivopontocerebellar d.
parenchymatous d.
pellucid marginal corneal d.
primary neuronal d.
primary pigmentary d. of retina
primary progressive cerebellar d.
pseudotubular d.
red d.
reticular d.
retrograde d.
Salzmann nodular corneal d.
senile d.
snail track d.
Sorsby macular d.
spheroid d.
spongy d. of infancy
subacute combined d. of the spinal
  cord
tapetoretinal d.
Terrien marginal d.
transsynaptic d.
Türck d.
vacuolar d.
vitelliform d.

D

degeneration *(continued)*
    vitelliruptive d.
    wallerian d.
    waxy d.
    xerotic d.
    Zenker d.
degenerative
    d. arthritis
    d. chorea
    d. index
    d. inflammation
    d. joint disease
    d. myopia
degloving injury
deglut.
    deglutiatur
deglutiatur (deglut.)
deglutition
    d. apnea
    d. pneumonia
    d. reflex
    d. syncope
deglutitive
Degos
    D. disease
    D. syndrome
degradation
degranulation
degree
    d.'s of freedom (d.f.)
    d. of kindred
degustation
dehalogenase
Dehio test
dehiscence
    iris d.
    root d.
    wound d.
dehumanization
dehydrase
dehydratase
dehydrate
dehydrated alcohol
dehydration
    absolute d.
    d. fever
    relative d.
    voluntary d.
dehydroacetic acid
L-dehydroascorbic acid
dehydrobilirubin
dehydrocholate test
7-dehydrocholesterol
24-dehydrocholesterol
dehydrocholic acid
11-dehydrocorticosterone
dehydroemetine resinate
dehydroepiandrosterone (DHEA)
    sulfate salt of d. (DHEAS)
dehydro-3-epiandrosterone (DHEA)
dehydrogenase
    aerobic d.
    alpha-keto acid d.

    anaerobic d.
    Robison ester d.
dehydrogenate
dehydrogenation
dehydroisoandrosterone
dehydroretinaldehyde
dehydroretinoic acid
dehydroretinol
dehydrosugar
dehypnotize
deiminase
deinstitutionalization
deionization
deionized water
deiterospinal tract
Deiters
    D. cell
    D. nucleus
    D. terminal frame
déjà
    d. voulu
    d. vu
    d. vu phenomenon
dejecta
dejection
Dejerine
    D. disease
    D. hand phenomenon
    D. reflex
    D. sign
Dejerine-Klumpke
    D.-K. palsy
    D.-K. syndrome
Dejerine-Roussy syndrome
Dejerine-Sottas disease
Delafield hematoxylin
delamination
Delaney clause
delayed
    d. allergy
    d. coma after hypoxia
    d. conduction
    d. dentition
    d. eruption
    d. flap
    d. graft
    d. hypersensitivity
    d. puberty
    d. reaction
    d. reaction experiment
    d. reflex
    d. sensation
    d. shock
    d. suture
delayed-type hypersensitivity (DTH)
Delbet sign
Del Castillo syndrome
de-lead
deleterious
deletion
    chromosomal d.
    gene d.
    interstitial d.
    d. mutation
    nucleotide d.

point d.
terminal d.

Delhi
D. boil
D. sore

delicate
delimitation
delimiting keratotomy
deliquesce
deliquescence
deliquescent
delirious
delirium, pl. **deliria**
acute d.
alcohol withdrawal d.
anxious d.
d. cordis
posttraumatic d.
senile d.
toxic d.
d. tremens (DT)

delitescence
deliver
delivery
assisted cephalic d.
breech d.
forceps d.
high forceps d.
low forceps d.
midforceps d.
outlet forceps d.
perimortem d.
postmortem d.
premature d.
spontaneous cephalic d.

delle
dellen
delomorphous
delouse
delphian node
delphinine
Delphinium ajacis
delta, Δ, δ
d. agent
d. antigen
d. bilirubin
d. cell of anterior lobe of hypophysis
d. cell of pancreas
d. check
d. fiber
d. fornicis
Galton d.
d. granule
d. hepatitis
d. mesoscapulae
d. rhythm
d. virus
d. wave

delta-aminobutyric acid amino transferase
delta-aminolevulinate dehydratase
delta-aminolevulinate dehydratase porphyria
delta-aminolevulinic acid (ALA)

delta-aminolevulinic acid synthase
delta check
delta-hydroxylysine
deltoid
d. branch
d. crest
d. eminence
d. impression
d. ligament
d. muscle
d. region
d. tubercle
d. tuberosity

deltoideopectoral
d. triangle
d. trigone

deltopectoral
d. flap
d. triangle

delusion
d. of being controlled
d. of control
encapsulated d.
expansive d.
d. of grandeur
grandiose d.
d. of negation
nihilistic d.
organic d.
d. of passivity
d. of persecution
persecutory d.
d. of reference
somatic d.
systematized d.
unsystematized d.

delusional disorder
demand
biochemical oxygen d. (BOD)
d. pacemaker
d. pulse generator

demarcation
d. current
d. line of retina
d. potential

Demarquay sign
demasculinizing
dematiaceous fungi
deme
demecarium bromide
demeclocycline
demecolcine
demented
dementia
AIDS d.
Alzheimer d.
catatonic d.
dialysis d.
epileptic d.
hebephrenic d.
Lewy body d.
multiinfarct d.
paralytic d.
d. paralytica
posttraumatic d.

D

dementia *(continued)*
    d. praecox
    presenile d.
    d. presenilis
    primary d.
    primary senile d.
    secondary d.
    senile d.
    toxic d.
    vascular d.
demethylase
demethylation
demigauntlet bandage
demilune
    d. body
    Giannuzzi d.
    Heidenhain d.
    serous d.
demineralization
demipenniform
demodectic
    d. blepharitis
    d. mange
Demodex folliculorum
demography
    dynamic d.
Demoivre formula
demoniac
demonstration ophthalmoscope
demonstrator
demorphinization
demucosation
demulcent
demyelinated myelitis
demyelinating
    d. disease
    d. encephalopathy
    d. polyneuropathy
demyelination, demyelinization
denarcotize
denarcotized opium *(var. of* deodorized
  opium)
denatonium benzoate
denaturation temperature of DNA
denatured
    d. alcohol
    d. protein
dendriform keratitis
dendrite
    apical d.
dendritic
    d. calculus
    d. cataract
    d. cell
    d. corneal ulcer
    d. depolarization
    d. keratitis
    d. process
    d. spine
    d. thorn
dendrogram
dendroid
dendron
denervate

denervation
dengue
    hemorrhagic d.
    d. hemorrhagic fever
    d. shock syndrome
    d. virus
denial
denidation
Denis
    D. Browne pouch
    D. Browne splint
denitration
denitrification
denitrify
denitrogenation
Dennie line
Dennie-Morgan fold
denominator
Denonvilliers
    D. aponeurosis
    D. ligament
dens, pl. **dentes**
    dentes acustici
    d. angularis
    d. axis
    d. bicuspidus
    d. caninus
    d. cuspidatus
    d. deciduus
    d. in dente
    d. incisivus
    d. invaginatus
    d. lacteus
    d. molaris
    d. molaris tertius
    d. permanens
    d. premolaris
    d. sapientiae
    d. serotinus
    d. succedaneus
dense body
dense-deposit disease
densimeter
densitometer
densitometry
density
    bone d.
    buoyant d.
    count d.
    flux d.
    d. gradient
    d. gradient centrifugation
    incidence d.
    optic d. (OD)
    photon d.
    spin d.
    vapor d.
dental
    d. abscess
    d. anatomy
    d. anesthesia
    d. ankylosis
    d. apparatus
    d. arch
    d. articulation

d. biomechanics
d. biophysics
d. branch
d. bulb
d. calculus
d. canal
d. cap
d. caries
d. cast
d. cement
d. cord
d. crest
d. crypt
d. curing
d. cuticle
d. drill
d. dysfunction
d. engine
d. engineering
d. fiber
d. fistula
d. floss
d. follicle
d. forceps
d. formula
d. furnace
d. geriatrics
d. germ
d. granuloma
d. groove
d. hygienist
d. impaction
d. implant
d. index (DI)
d. jurisprudence
d. lamina
d. ledge
d. lever
d. lymph
d. material
d. neck
d. nerve
d. orthopedics
d. osteoma
d. papilla
d. pathology
d. plaque
d. polyp
d. process
d. prophylaxis
d. prosthesis
d. prosthetics
d. pulp
d. pump
d. ramus
d. ridge
d. sac
d. sealant
d. senescence
d. shelf
d. surgeon
d. syringe
d. tubercle
d. tubule

d. ulcer
d. wedge
dentalgia
dentary center
dentate
d. fascia
d. fissure
d. fracture
d. gyrus
d. ligament of spinal cord
d. line
d. nucleus of cerebellum
d. suture
dentatectomy
dentatorubral
d. cerebellar atrophy with polymyoclonus
d. fiber
dentatothalamic
d. fiber
d. tract
dentatum
dentes (*pl. of* dens)
dentia
d. praecox
d. tarda
denticle
denticulate, denticulated
d. hymen
d. ligament
dentiform
dentifrice
dentigerous cyst
dentilabial
dentilingual
dentin
d. bridge
d. dysplasia
d. globule
hereditary opalescent d.
hypersensitive d.
interglobular d.
irregular d.
irritation d.
opalescent d.
peritubular d.
primary d.
reparative d.
sclerotic d.
secondary d.
tertiary d.
transparent d.
vascular d.
dentinal
d. canal
d. fiber
d. fluid
d. papilla
d. pulp
d. sheath
d. tubule
dentinalgia
dentine
dentinocemental junction
dentinoenamel junction

D

dentinogenesis imperfecta
dentinoid
dentinoma
dentinum
dentiparous
dentist
dentistry
    community d.
    esthetic d.
    forensic d.
    legal d.
    Master of Science in D. (M.S.D.)
    operative d.
    pediatric d.
    preventive d.
    prosthetic d.
    public health d.
    restorative d.
dentition
    artificial d.
    deciduous d.
    delayed d.
    first d.
    mandibular d.
    maxillary d.
    natural d.
    primary d.
    retarded d.
    secondary d.
    succedaneous d.
dentoalveolar
    d. abscess
    d. joint
dentode
dentogingival lamina
dentoid
dentolegal
dentoliva
dentulous
denture
    bar joint d.
    d. basal surface
    d. base
    d. border
    d. brush
    d. characterization
    complete d.
    design d.
    d. edge
    d. esthetics
    fixed partial d.
    d. flange
    d. flask
    d. foundation
    d. foundation area
    d. foundation surface
    full d.
    d. hyperplasia
    immediate insertion d.
    implant d.
    d. impression surface
    interim d.
    d. occlusal surface
    overlay d.
    d. packing

    partial d.
    d. polished surface
    d. prognosis
    provisional d.
    removable partial d.
    d. retention
    d. service
    d. sore mouth
    d. space
    d. stability
    telescopic d.
    temporary d.
    transitional d.
    treatment d.
    trial d.
    wax model d.
denture-bearing area
denture-supporting
    d.-s. area
    d.-s. structure
denturist
Denucé ligament
denucleated
denudation
denude
denumerable character
Denver
    D. classification
    D. Developmental Screening Test
    D. shunt
Denys-Drash syndrome
Denys-Leclef phenomenon
deodorant
deodorize
deodorized opium
deodorizer
deontology
deorsumduction
deossification
deoxidation
deoxidize
deoxyadenosine (dA, dAdo)
deoxyadenosine methylase
5′-deoxyadenosylcobalamin
deoxyadenylic acid (dAMP)
deoxybarbiturate
deoxycholate
deoxycholic acid
deoxycoformycin
2-deoxycoformycin
deoxycorticosterone (DOC)
    d. acetate
    d. pivalate
deoxycortone
deoxycytidine
deoxycytidylic acid (dCMP)
deoxyepinephrine
2-deoxyglucose (dGlc)
deoxyguanosine
deoxyguanylic acid (dGMP)
deoxyhexose
deoxynucleoside
deoxynucleotide
deoxypentose
deoxyriboaldolase

deoxyribodipyrimidine photolyase
deoxyribonuclease (DNAse)
    acid d.
    d. I, II
    pancreatic d.
    d. S_1
    spleen d.
deoxyribonucleic acid (DNA)
deoxyribonucleoprotein (DNP, Dnp, DNR)
deoxyribonucleoside
deoxyribonucleotide
deoxyribose phosphate
deoxyribosephosphate aldolase
deoxyriboside
deoxyribosyl
deoxyribosyltransferase
deoxyribotide
deoxyribovirus
deoxy sugar
deoxythymidine (dT)
deoxythymidylic acid (dTMP)
deoxyuridine
deoxyuridine 5-triphosphate (dUTP)
deozonize
dependence
    anchorage d.
    substance d.
dependency
    pyridoxine d. with seizure
dependent
    d. beat
    d. drainage
    d. edema
    d. personality
    d. personality disorder
    d. variable
Dependovirus
depersonalization
    d. disorder
    d. syndrome
dephasing
dephosphorylation
depigmentation
depilate
depilation
depilatory
    chemical d.
depletion
    d. response
    salt d.
    water d.
depletional hyponatremia
depolarization
    alternating failure of response,
    mechanical, to electrical d.
    (AFORMED)
    dendritic d.
depolarize
depolarizing
    d. block
    d. relaxant
depolymerase
deposit
    brickdust d.

depot
    d. injection
    d. reaction
    d. therapy
depravation
depraved
depravity
deprenyl
depressant
depressed
    d. skull fracture
depression
    agitated d.
    anaclitic d.
    clinical d.
    endogenous d.
    exogenous d.
    involutional d.
    lingual salivary gland d.
    major d.
    nonreactive d.
    d. of optic disk
    pacchionian d.
    postdrive d.
    pterygoid d.
    reactive d.
    spreading d.
depressive
    d. neurosis
    d. psychosis
    d. reaction
    d. stupor
    d. syndrome
depressor
    d. anguli oris muscle
    d. fiber
    d. labii inferioris muscle
    d. muscle of epiglottis
    d. muscle of eyebrow
    d. muscle of lower lip
    d. muscle of septum
    d. nerve of Ludwig
    d. reflex
    d. septi nasi muscle
    d. supercilii muscle
    tongue d.
deprivation
    d. amblyopia
    d. dwarfism
    emotional d.
    sensory d.
depsipeptide
depth
    anesthetic d.
    d. compensation
    d. dose
    focal d.
    d. of focus
    d. perception
    d. psychology
    d. recording
deptropine citrate
depulization
depurant
depuration

D

depurative
dequalinium
    d. acetate
    d. chloride
deradelphus
derailment
deranencephaly, deranencephalia
derangement
derby hat fracture
Dercum disease
derealization
dereism
dereistic
derencephalia
derencephalocele
derencephaly
derepression
derivation
derivative
    d. chromosome
    piperidine d. (MPTP)
derived protein
dermabrader
dermabrasion
Dermacentor
    D. albopictus
    D. andersoni
    D. marginatus
    D. occidentalis
    D. reticulatus
    D. variabilis
Dermacoccus
dermad
dermal
    d. bone
    d. duct tumor
    d. fat graft
    d. leishmanoid
    d. papillae
    d. ridge
    d. sinus
Dermanyssus gallinae
dermatalgia
dermatan sulfate
dermatitis, pl. **dermatitides**
    actinic d.
    d. aestivalis
    allergic contact d.
    ancylostoma d.
    d. artefacta
    atopic d.
    berloque d., berlock d.
    blastomycetic d.
    d. blastomycotica
    bubble gum d.
    d. calorica
    caterpillar d.
    chemical d.
    d. combustionis
    contact d.
    contagious pustular d.
    cosmetic d.
    diaper d.
    d. exfoliativa infantum
    d. exfoliativa neonatorum

    exfoliative d.
    exudative discoid and lichenoid d.
    factitial d.
    d. gangrenosa infantum
    d. herpetiformis
    d. hiemalis
    infectious eczematoid d.
    irritant contact d.
    mango d.
    meadow grass d.
    d. medicamentosa
    nickel d.
    d. nodosa
    d. nodularis necrotica
    nummular d.
    papular d. of pregnancy
    d. pediculoides ventricosus
    primary irritant d.
    proliferative d.
    rat mite d.
    d. repens
    Rhus d.
    sandal strap d.
    schistosomal d.
    seborrheic d.
    d. seborrheica
    solar d.
    stasis d.
    subcorneal pustular d.
    traumatic d.
    d. vegetans
dermatitis-arthritis-tenosynovitis syndrome
dermatitis-causing caterpillar.
dermatoarthritis
    lipoid d.
Dermatobia
    D. cyaniventris
    D. hominis
dermatobiasis
dermatocellulitis
dermatochalasis
dermatoconiosis
dermatocyst
dermatodynia
dermatofibroma
dermatofibrosarcoma protuberans
    pigmented d. p.
dermatofibrosis lenticularis disseminata
dermatogenic torticollis
dermatoglyphics
dermatograph
dermatographism
dermatoid
dermatologic paste
dermatologist
dermatology
dermatolysis
dermatoma
dermatomal distribution
dermatome
dermatomegaly
dermatomere
dermatomic area
dermatomycosis pedis
dermatomyoma

dermatomyositis
dermatoneurosis
dermatonosology
dermatopathia pigmentosa reticularis
dermatopathic
    d. lymphadenitis
    d. lymphadenopathy
dermatopathology
dermatopathy
Dermatophagoides pteronyssinus
dermatophilosis
Dermatophilus congolensis
dermatophobia
dermatophylaxis
dermatophyte
dermatophytid
dermatophytosis
dermatopolyneuritis
dermatorrhagia
dermatorrhea
dermatorrhexis
dermatoscopy
dermatosis, pl. **dermatoses**
    acute febrile neutrophilic d.
    ashy d.
    Bowen precancerous d.
    chronic bullous d. of childhood
    dermolytic bullous d.
    digitate d.
    juvenile plantar d.
    lichenoid d.
    d. medicamentosa
    d. papulosa nigra
    pigmented purpuric lichenoid d.
    progressive pigmentary d.
    radiation d.
    subcorneal pustular d.
    transient acantholytic d. (TAD)
dermatotherapy
dermatothlasia
dermatotropic
dermatozoon
dermatozoonosis
dermatrophia, dermatrophy
dermenchysis
dermis
Dermobacter
dermoblast
dermocyma
dermoepidermal interface
dermoid
    d. cyst
    d. cyst of ovary
    inclusion d.
    d. system
    d. tumor
dermoidectomy
dermolysis
dermolytic bullous dermatosis
dermonecrotic
dermopathy
    diabetic dermopathy
dermophlebitis
dermoskeleton
dermostenosis

dermotoxin
dermotropic
dermotuberculin reaction
dermovascular
derodidymus
derotation
DES
    diethylstilbestrol
desamidize
desaturate
desaturation
Desault bandage
Descartes law
descemetitis
Descemet membrane
descemetocele
descendens
    d. cervicalis
    d. hypoglossi
descending
    d. anterior branch
    d. aorta
    d. artery of knee
    d. branch
    d. branch of anterior segmental
      artery of left and right lungs
    d. branch of hypoglossal nerve
    d. branch of lateral circumflex
      femoral artery
    d. branch of medial circumflex
      femoral artery
    d. branch of occipital artery
    d. branch of posterior segmental
      artery of left and right lungs
    d. branch of superficial cervical
      artery
    d. colon
    d. current
    d. degeneration
    d. genicular artery
    d. neuritis
    d. nucleus of the trigeminus
    d. palatine artery
    d. part of aorta
    d. part of duodenum
    d. part of facial canal
    d. part of iliofemoral ligament
    d. part of trapezius muscle
    d. posterior branch
    d. scapular artery
    d. tract of trigeminal nerve
descensus
    d. testis
    d. uteri
    d. ventriculi
descent
Deschamps needle
descriptive
    d. anatomy
    d. myology
    d. psychiatry
    d. statistics
DES (diethylstilbestrol) daughter
desensitization
    heterologous d.

D

desensitization *(continued)*
    homologous d.
    systematic d.
desensitize
desensitizing paste
deserpidine
desert
    d. fever
    d. sore
desetope
desferrioxamine mesylate
desflurane
deshydremia
desiccant
desiccate
desiccated
    d. liver
    d. pituitary
desiccation
desiccative
desiccator
    vacuum d.
design denture
desipramine hydrochloride
deslanoside
Desmarres
    D. dacryolith
    D. retractor
desmin
desmitis
desmo-
desmocranium
desmodentium
desmodontium
Desmodus
desmogenous
desmography
desmoid
    extra-abdominal d.
    d. tumor
desmolase
desmology
desmopathy
desmoplasia
desmoplastic
    d. cerebral astrocytoma
    d. fibroma
    d. malignant melanoma
    d. medulloblastoma
    d. small cell tumor
    d. trichoepithelioma
desmopressin acetate
desmosine
desmosome
desmosterol
desmoteric medicine
desonide
desoximetasone
desoxy-
desoxycorticosterone
desoxycortone
desoxy sugar
despeciated antitoxin
despeciation

D'Espine sign
despumation
desquamate
desquamation
    branny d.
desquamative
    d. inflammatory vaginitis
    d. interstitial pneumonia (DIP)
    d. pneumonia
desthiobiotin
destructive distillation
destrudo
desulfhydrases
desulfinase
Desulfotomaculum nigrificans
desulfurase
desynchronous
DET
    diethyltryptamine
det.
    detur
detachable balloon
detached
    d. cranial section
    d. craniotomy
    d. retina
detachment
    exudative retinal d.
    d. of retina
    retinal d.
    rhegmatogenous retinal d.
    vitreous d.
detection
detector
    d. coil
    solid-state d.
detergent
    anionic d.
    cationic d.
    zwitterionic d.
deterioration
    alcoholic d.
    senile d.
determinant
    allotypic d.
    antigenic d.
    disease d.
    genetic d.
    d. group
    idiotypic antigenic d.
    isoallotypic d.
    mathematical d.
determinate cleavage
determination
    cell d.
    sex d.
determinism
    psychic d.
detersive
detoxicate
detoxication
    ammonia d.
detoxification
detoxify
detrition

detritus
detrusor
    d. areflexia
    d. compliance
    d. hyperreflexia
    d. instability
    d. pressure
    d. sphincter dyssynergia
    d. stability
detrusorrhaphy
detumescence
detur (det.)
deturgescence
deutencephalon
deuteranomaly
deuteranope
deuteranopia
deuterio-
deuterium
    d. oxide
deuteromycetes
Deuteromycota
deuteron
deuteropathic
deuteropathy
deuteroplasm
deuteroporphyrin
deuterosome
deuterotocia
deuterotoky
deutogenic
deutomerite
deuton
deutonymph
deutoplasm
deutoplasmic
deutoplasmigenon
deutoplasmolysis
Deutschländer disease
DEV
    duck embryo origin vaccine
devascularization
develop
developer
development
    cognitive d.
    life-span d.
    psychosexual d.
developmental
    d. age (DA)
    d. anatomy
    d. anomaly
    d. disability
    d. groove
    d. hip dysplasia
    d. line
    d. psychology
Deventer pelvis
deviance
deviant
deviation
    axis d.
    conjugate d. of the eye
    dissociated horizontal d.
    dissociated vertical d.

    immune d.
    d. to the left
    left axis d.
    primary d.
    d. to the right
    right axis d.
    secondary d.
    sexual d.
    skew d.
    standard d.
deviational nystagmus
Devic disease
device
    central-bearing tracing d.
    contraceptive d.
    intrauterine d. (IUD)
    intrauterine contraceptive d. (IUCD)
    left-ventricular assist d.
    ventricular assist d.
devil grip
deviometer
devitalization
devitalize
devitalized tooth
devolution
Devonshire colic
Dewar flask
dew point
dexamethasone suppression test
dexamphetamine sodium phosphate
dexbrompheniramine maleate
dexchlorpheniramine maleate
dexiocardia
dexpanthenol
dexter (D, d)
dextrad
dextral
dextrality
dextran
    d. 40, 70, 75, 110
    acid d.
    animal d.
    blue d.
    d. sulfate
dextranase
dextransucrase
dextrase
dextriferron
dextrin
    acid d.
    d. 6-alpha-D-glucosidase
    d. dextranase
    d. 6-glucosyltransferase
    d. glycosyltransferase
    limit d.
    d. limit
    Schardinger d.
    d. transglycosylase
dextrinase
    limit d.
dextrin → dextran transglucosidase
dextrinogenic
dextrinosis
    debranching deficiency limit d.
dextrinuria

D

dextroamphetamine
> d. phosphate
> d. sulfate

dextrocardia
> corrected d.
> false d.
> isolated d.
> mirror image d.
> secondary d.
> type 1, 2, 3, 4 d.
> d. with situs inversus

dextrocardiogram
dextrocerebral
dextrocular
dextrocycloduction
dextroduction
dextrogastria
dextroglucose
dextrogram
dextrogyration
dextromanual
dextromethorphan hydrobromide
dextromoramide tartrate
dextropedal
dextroposition of the heart
dextropropoxyphene
> d. hydrochloride
> d. napsylate

dextrorotation
dextrorotatory
dextrose
dextrosinistral
dextrothyroxine sodium
dextrotorsion
dextrotropic
dextroversion of the heart
DF, df
> DF caries index

d.f.
> degrees of freedom

DFP
> diisopropyl fluorophosphate

dGlc
> 2-deoxyglucose

dGMP
> deoxyguanylic acid

DHAP
> dihydroxyacetone phosphate

Dharmendra antigen
DHEA
> dehydroepiandrosterone
> dehydro-3-epiandrosterone

DHEAS
> sulfate salt of dehydroepiandrosterone

d'Herelle phenomenon
DHF
> dihydrofolic acid

DHFR
> dihydrofolate reductase

D-homosteroid
D Hy
> Doctor of Hygiene

DI
> dental index

Di
> Di antigen
> Di Ferrante syndrome
> Di Guglielmo disease
> Di Guglielmo syndrome

diabetes
> adult-onset d.
> alimentary d.
> alloxan d.
> brittle d.
> bronze d.
> bronzed d.
> calcinuric d.
> chemical d.
> galactose d.
> gestational d.
> growth-onset d.
> d. innocens
> d. insipidus
> insulin-dependent d. mellitus (IDDM)
> insulinopenic d.
> d. intermittens
> juvenile d.
> juvenile-onset d.
> ketosis-prone d.
> ketosis-resistant d.
> latent d.
> lipoatrophic d.
> lipogenous d.
> maturity-onset d.
> maturity onset d. of youth
> d. mellitus
> metahypophysial d.
> Mosler d.
> nephrogenic d. insipidus
> non-insulin-dependent d. mellitus (NIDDM)
> pancreatic d.
> phlorizin d.
> phosphate d.
> piqûre d.
> pregnancy d.
> puncture d.
> renal d.
> starvation d.
> steroid d.
> steroidogenic d.
> subclinical d.
> thiazide d.
> type 1, 2 d.
> type 1 d. mellitus
> vasopressin-resistant d.

diabetic
> d. acidosis
> d. amyotrophy
> d. arthropathy
> d. cataract
> d. coma
> d. dermopathy
> d. diet
> d. fetopathy
> d. gangrene
> d. gingivitis
> d. glomerulosclerosis

d. lipemia
d. myelopathy
d. nephropathy
d. neuropathic cachexia
d. neuropathy
d. polyneuropathy
d. polyradiculopathy
d. puncture
d. retinitis
d. retinopathy
d. thoracic radiculopathy
diabetogenic factor
diabetogenous
diabetology
diacetal (*var. of* diacetyl)
diacetate
diacetemia
diacetonuria
diaceturia
diacetyl, diacetal
diacetylcholine
diacetylmonoxime (DAM)
diacetylmorphine
diacetyltannic acid
diachronic study
diacid
diaclasis, diaclasia
diacrinous
diacrisis
diacritic, diacritical
diactinic
diacylglycerol (DAG)
d. acyltransferase
d. lipase
diad
diadochocinesia
diadochokinesia, diadochokinesis
diadochokinetic
diagnose
diagnosis
antenatal d.
clinical d.
differential d.
d. by exclusion
laboratory d.
neonatal d.
pathologic d.
physical d.
prenatal d.
diagnosis-related group (DRG)
diagnostic
d. anesthesia
d. audiometry
d. cast
d. diphtheria toxin
DNA d.'s
d. radiology
d. sensitivity
d. specificity
D. and Statistical Manual of Mental Disorders (DSM)
d. ultrasound
diagnostician
diagonal
d. band

d. conjugate
d. conjugate diameter
d. section
diagonalis stria
diagram
Dieuaide d.
flow d.
Venn d.
diakinesis
dial
astigmatic d.
d. manometer
Dialister
diallyl
dialysance
dialysate
dialysis
continuous ambulatory peritoneal d. (CAPD)
d. dementia
d. disequilibrium syndrome
d. encephalopathy syndrome
equilibrium d.
extracorporeal d.
peritoneal d.
d. retinae
d. shunt
dialyze
dialyzer
diamagnetic
diamagnetism
di-amelia
diameter
anteroposterior d. of the pelvic inlet
biparietal d.
buccolingual d.
conjugate d. of pelvic inlet
conjugate d. of pelvic outlet
diagonal conjugate d.
external conjugate d.
d. obliqua
oblique d.
obstetric conjugate d.
occipitofrontal d.
occipitomental d.
posterior sagittal d.
suboccipitobregmatic d.
total end-diastolic d. (TEDD)
total end-systolic d. (TESD)
trachelobregmatic d.
d. transversa
transverse d.
zygomatic d.
diamide
diamidine
4′6-diamidino-2-phenylindole-2HCl (DAPI)
diamine oxidase
3′3-diaminobenzidine (DAB)
diamniotic
diamond
d. cutting instrument
d. disk
d. fuchsin
D. TYM medium

Diamond-Blackfan
> D.-B. anemia
> D.-B. syndrome

diamond-shaped murmur
diamthazole dihydrochloride
Diana complex
diandry, diandria
dianoetic
diapause
> embryonic d.

diapedesis
diaper
> d. dermatitis
> d. rash

diaphanography
diaphanoscope
diaphanoscopy
diaphemetric
diaphen hydrochloride
diaphorase
diaphoresis
diaphoretic
diaphragm
> aperture d.
> Bucky d.
> d. of mouth
> pelvic d.
> d. of pelvis
> d. pessary
> Potter-Bucky d.
> d. sellae
> sellar d.
> d. of sella turcica
> urogenital d.

diaphragma, pl. **diaphragmata**
> d. oris
> d. pelvis
> d. sellae
> d. urogenitale

diaphragmalgia
diaphragmatic
> d. constriction of esophagus
> d. flutter
> d. hernia
> d. ligament of the mesonephros
> d. myocardial infarction
> d. pacemaker
> d. part of parietal pleura
> d. peritonitis
> d. pleura
> d. pleurisy
> d. surface

diaphragmatocele
diaphragmodynia
diaphyseal
diaphysectomy
diaphysial
> d. center
> d. dysplasia

diaphysis, pl. **diaphyses**
diaphysitis
diapiresis
diaplacental
diaplexus
diapnoic, diapnotic

diapophysis
Diaptomus
diarrhea
> cachectic d.
> choleraic d.
> chronic bacillary d.
> Cochin China d.
> colliquative d.
> dientamoeba d.
> dysenteric d.
> fatty d.
> flagellate d.
> gastrogenous d.
> lienteric d.
> morning d.
> mucous d.
> nocturnal d.
> pancreatic d.
> d. pancreatica
> pancreatogenous d.
> serous d.
> summer d.
> toddler's d.
> traveler's d.
> tropical d.

diarrheal, diarrheic
diarrhetic
diarthric
diarthrodial
> d. cartilage
> d. joint

diarthrosis, pl. **diarthroses**
diarticular
diaschisis
diascope
diascopy
diastalsis
diastaltic
diastase
diastasis
> d. cordis
> d. recti

diastasuria
diastatic skull fracture
diastema, pl. **diastemata**
diastematocrania
diastematomyelia
diaster
diastereoisomer
diastole
> atrial d.
> electrical d.
> gastric d.
> late d.
> ventricular d.

diastolic
> d. afterpotential
> d. murmur
> d. pressure
> d. shock
> d. thrill

diastology
diastrophic
> d. dwarfism
> d. dysplasia

diastrophism
diataxia
    cerebral d.
diatela
diathermal
diathermancy
diathermanous
diathermic therapy
diathermocoagulation
diathermy
    medical d.
    short wave d.
    surgical d.
    ultrashortwave d.
diathesis
    contractural d.
    cystic d.
    gouty d.
    spasmophilic d.
diathetic
diatom
diatomaceous earth
diatomic
diatoric
diatrizoate
diazepam
diazine
diazinon
diazo
    d. reaction
    d. reagent
    d. stain for argentaffin granule
diazo-
diazonium salt
diazotize
diazoxide
dibasic
    d. acid
    d. amino acid
    d. ammonium phosphate
    d. calcium phosphate
    d. potassium phosphate
    d. sodium phosphate
dibenamine
dibenzepin hydrochloride
dibenzheptropine citrate
dibenzopyridine
dibenzothiazine
dibenzthione
Di blood group (*var. of* Diego blood group)
Dibothriocephalus latus
dibromopropamidine isethionate
dibromsalan
dibucaine
    d. hydrochloride
    d. number (DN)
dibutoline sulfate
dibutyl phthalate
DIC
    disseminated intravascular coagulation
dicacodyl
dicarboxylic acid cycle
dicelous
dicentric chromosome

dicephalous
dicephalus
    d. diauchenos
    d. dipus dibrachius
    d. dipus tetrabrachius
    d. dipus tribrachius
    d. dipygus
    d. monauchenos
dicheilia, dichilia
dicheiria, dichiria
Dichelobacter nodosus
dichilia (*var. of* dicheilia)
dichloramine-T
dichloride
dichlorisone
dichlorobenzene
dichlorodifluoromethane
p,p′-dichlorodiphenyl methyl carbinol (DMC)
dichlorodiphenyltrichloroethane (DDT)
di(2-chloroethyl)sulfide
dichloroformoxime
dichlorohydrin
2,6-dichloroindophenol
dichloroisopropyl alcohol
dichlorophen
dichlorophenarsine hydrochloride
2,6-dichlorophenol-indophenol
(2,4-dichlorophenoxy) acetic acid (2,4-D)
dichlorovos
dichlorphenamide
dichlorvos
dichorial, dichorionic
    d. diamnionic placenta
    d. twins
dichotic
dichotomous
dichotomy
dichroic
dichroism
    circular d. (CD)
dichromat
dichromate
dichromatic
dichromatism
dichromatopsia
dichromic
dichromophil, dichromophile
Dick
    D. method
    D. test
    D. test toxin
Dickens shunt
diclofenac
dicloxacillin sodium
DICOM
    Digital Imaging and Communications in Medicine
dicophane
dicoria
dicotyledon
dicrocoeliosis
Dicrocoelium
dicrotic
    d. notch

D

dicrotic *(continued)*
    d. pulse
    d. wave
dicrotism
dicto
    more d. (m. dict., mor. dict.)
dictyoma
dictyosome
dictyotene
dicumarol resistance
dicyclomine hydrochloride
dicysteine
didactic
    d. analysis
didactylism
didelphic
Didelphis
dideoxy
    d. procedure
    d. sequencing
dideoxyadenosine (DDA)
dideoxycytidine
dideoxyinosine (DDI)
DIDMOD
    Wolfram syndrome
didymus
in die
    ter in die (t.i.d.)
die
dieb. alt.
    diebus alternis
diebus alternis (dieb. alt.)
diecious
Diego blood group, Di blood group
diel
dieldrin
dielectrography
dielectrolysis
Diels hydrocarbon
diencephala (*pl. of* diencephalon)
diencephalic
    d. epilepsy
    d. syndrome of infancy
diencephalohypophysial
diencephalon, pl. **diencephala**
diener
dienestrol
dientamoeba diarrhea
Dientamoeba fragilis
dieresis
dieretic
in dies (in d.)
diesterase
diestrous
diestrus
diet
    acid-ash d.
    alkaline-ash d.
    balanced d.
    basal d.
    basic d.
    bland d.
    BRAT d.
    challenge d.

    clear liquid d.
    diabetic d.
    elimination d.
    full liquid d.
    Giordano-Giovannetti d.
    Giovannetti d.
    gluten-free d.
    gout d.
    high-calorie d.
    high-fat d.
    high-fiber d.
    Kempner d.
    ketogenic d.
    low-calorie d.
    low-fat d.
    low purine d.
    low residue d.
    low salt d.
    macrobiotic d.
    Meulengracht d.
    Minot-Murphy d.
    Ornish prevention d.
    Ornish reversal d.
    purine-free d.
    purine-restricted d.
    d. quality index
    rachitic d.
    reducing d.
    rice d.
    Schmidt d.
    Schmidt-Strassburger d.
    Sippy d.
    smooth d.
    soft d.
    subsistence d.
    Wilder d.
dietary
    d. amenorrhea
    d. fiber
Dieterle stain
dietetic
    d. albuminuria
    d. treatment
dietetics
diethadione
diethanolamine
diethazine
diethenoid fatty acid
diethyl
O-**diethylaminoethyl cellulose**
5,5-diethylbarbituric acid
diethylcarbamazine citrate
diethylenediamine
1,4-diethylene dioxide
diethylene glycol
diethylenetriamine pentaacetic acid (DTPA)
diethyl ether
diethylolamine
diethylpropion hydrochloride
diethylstilbestrol (DES)
diethyltoluamide
diethyltryptamine (DET)
dietician, dietitian
    registered d. (RD)

Dietl crisis
Dieuaide diagram
Dieulafoy
    D. erosion
    D. lesion
difarnesyl group
difenoxin
difenoxylic acid
difference
    alveolar-arterial oxygen d.
    arteriovenous carbon dioxide d.
    arteriovenous oxygen d.
    AV d.
    cation-anion d.
    individual d.
    light d.
    d. limen
    masking level d.
    standard error of d.
differential
    d. blood pressure
    d. diagnosis
    d. display
    d. gene expression
    d. growth
    d. manometer
    d. renal function test
    d. spinal anesthesia
    d. stain
    d. stethoscope
    d. thermometer
    threshold d.
    d. threshold
    d. ureteral catheterization test
    d. white blood count
differentiated
differentiation
    correlative d.
    echocardiographic d.
    invisible d.
    pressure pulse d.
diffluence
diffraction
diffraction grating
diffusate
diffuse
    d. abscess
    d. alveolar damage
    d. aneurysm
    d. angiokeratoma
    d. arterial ectasia
    d. choroiditis
    d. cutaneous leishmaniasis
    d. cutaneous mastocytosis
    d. deep keratitis
    d. esophageal spasm
    d. ganglion
    d. glomerulonephritis
    d. goiter
    d. hyperkeratosis of palms and soles
    d. idiopathic skeletal hyperostosis (DISH)
    d. infantile familial sclerosis
    d. Lewy body disease

    d. mastocytosis
    d. mesangial proliferation
    d. obstructive emphysema
    d. panbronchiolitis
    d. peritonitis
    d. small cleaved cell lymphoma
    d. unilateral subacute neuroretinitis (DUSN)
    d. waxy spleen
diffused
    d. psoriasis
    d. reflex
diffusible stimulant
diffusing
    d. capacity
    d. factor
diffusion
    d. anoxia
    d. coefficient
    d. constant
    facilitated d.
    gel d.
    d. hypoxia
    d. method
    passive d.
    d. respiration
    d. shell
diflorasone diacetate
diflucortolone
diflunisal
digametic
digastric
    d. branch of facial nerve
    d. fossa
    d. groove
    d. muscle
    d. notch
    d. triangle
digastricus
Digenea
digenesis
digenetic
DiGeorge syndrome
digest
digestant
digestion
    buccal d.
    duodenal d.
    gastric d.
    intercellular d.
    intestinal d.
    intracellular d.
    pancreatic d.
    peptic d.
    primary d.
    salivary d.
    secondary d.
digestive
    d. albuminuria
    d. apparatus
    d. enzyme
    d. fever
    d. glycosuria
    d. leukocytosis
    d. system

D

digestive *(continued)*
    d. tract
    d. tube
    d. vacuole
digit
    binary d.
    clubbed d.
    d. of foot
    primary d. of foot
digital
    d. collateral artery
    d. crease
    d. dilatation
    d. flexion crease
    d. fossa
    d. furrow
    d. gray scale
    d. hearing aid
    D. Imaging and Communications in Medicine (DICOM)
    d. joint
    d. plethysmograph
    d. pulp
    d. pulp of hand
    d. radiography (DR)
    d. reflex
    d. subtraction angiography (DSA)
    d. vein
    d. whorl
digitalin
    crystalline d.
Digitalis
digitalis
    d. tincture
    d. unit
digitalism
digitalization
digitate
    d. dermatosis
    d. impression
    d. wart
digitation
digitationes hippocampi
digiti (*pl. of* digitus)
digitin
digitonin reaction
digitoxigenin
digitoxin
digitoxose
ᴅ-digitoxose
digitus, pl. **digiti**
    d. anularis
    d. auricularis
    digiti hippocratici
    d. manus
    d. (manus) medius
    d. (manus) minimus
    d. (manus) primus
    d. (manus) quartus IV
    d. (manus) quintus [V]
    d. (manus) secundus [II]
    d. (manus) tertius [III]
    d. pedis
    d. (pedis) minimus [V]

    d. pedis primus I
    d. (pedis) quartus [IV]
    d. (pedis) quintus [V]
    d. (pedis) secundus [II]
    d. (pedis) tertius [III]
    d. valgus
    d. varus
diglossia
diglyceride lipase
diglycocoll hydroiodide-iodine
dignathus
digoxigenin
digoxin
digyny, digynia
diheterozygote
dihybrid
dihydralazine
dihydrate
dihydrazone
dihydric alcohol
dihydroascorbic acid
dihydrobiopterin reductase
dihydrocodeine tartrate
dihydrocodeinone
dihydrocortisone
dihydroergocornine
dihydroergocristine
dihydroergocryptine
dihydroergotamine
dihydroergotoxine mesylate
dihydrofolate
    dihydrofolate reductase (DHFR)
dihydrofolic acid (DHF)
7,8-dihydrofolic acid
dihydrogen phosphate
dihydrolipoamide *S*-acetyltransferase
dihydrolipoamide dehydrogenase
dihydrolipoic acid
dihydromorphinone hydrochloride
dihydro-orotase
dihydro-orotate
dihydropteridine reductase
dihydropteroic acid
dihydropyrimidine dehydrogenase
dihydrostreptomycin
dihydrotachysterol
dihydrotestosterone
dihydrouracil
dihydrouracil dehydrogenase
dihydrouridine (hU)
dihydroxyacetone
    d. phosphate (DHAP)
    d. phosphate acyltransferase
2,8-dihydroxyadenine
    -d. lithiasis
dihydroxyaluminum aminoacetate
dihydroxyaluminum sodium carbonate
1,25-dihydroxyergocalciferol
3,4-dihydroxyphenylalanine
diiodide
diiodohydroxyquin
diiodotyrosine (DIT)
diisopromine
diisopropyl fluorophosphate (DFP)
diisopropyl iminodiacetic acid (DISIDA)

2,6-diisopropyl phenol
2,3-diketo-L-gulonate
diketohydrindylidene-diketohydrindamine
diketone
diketopiperazine
dil.
    dilute
dilaceration
dilantin gingivitis
dilatancy
dilatation
    digital d.
dilatator
dilate
dilated
    d. cardiomyopathy
    d. pore
dilation
    d. and curettage (D & C)
    d. and evacuation (D & E)
    d. and extraction
    post-stenotic d.
    d. and suction
    d. thrombosis
    urethral d.
dilator
    Chevalier-Jackson d.
    Hanks d.
    Hegar d.
    hydrostatic d.
    d. iridis
    Kollmann d.
    d. muscle of ileocecal sphincter
    d. muscle of pylorus
    pneumatic d.
    Pratt d.
    d. of pupil
    d. pupillae muscle
    Walther d.
dildo, dildoe
dilemma
    masking d.
dileptic seizure
dill oil
diloxanide furoate
diltiazem hydrochloride
diluent
dilute (dil.)
    d. alcohol
    d. phosphoric acid
diluted
    d. acetic acid
    d. hydrochloric acid
dilutional hyponatremia
dilution anemia
dim.
    dimidius
dimazole dihydrochloride
dimazon
dimelia
dimenhydrinate
dimension
    buccolingual d.
    occlusal vertical d.
    rest vertical d.
    vertical d.
dimensional stability
dimer
    D-d.
    pyrimidine d.
    thymine d.
dimercaprol
dimercurion
dimeric
dimerous
D-dimer test
dimetacrine tartrate
dimethadione
dimethicone
dimethindene maleate
dimethisterone
dimethothiazine mesylate
dimethoxanate hydrochloride
dimethoxyamphetamine (DMA)
2,5-dimethoxy-4-methylamphetamine (DOM)
dimethylallylpyrophosphate
dimethylaminoazobenzene
1-dimethylaminonaphthalene-5-sulfonic acid (DANS)
dimethylarsinic acid
dimethylbenzene
5,6-dimethylbenzimidazole
dimethylcarbinol
dimethyl-1-carbomethoxy-1-propen-2-yl phosphate
dimethyl iminodiacetic acid (HIDA)
dimethyl ketone
dimethylmercury
dimethylphenol
dimethylphenylpiperazinium (DMPP)
dimethyl phthalate
dimethylpiperazine tartrate
dimethyl sulfate
dimethyl sulfoxide (DMSO)
N,N-dimethyltryptamine (DMT)
dimethyl *d*-tubocurarine
dimethyl tubocurarine chloride
dimethyl tubocurarine iodide
dimetria
dimidiate hermaphroditism
dimidius (dim.)
Dimmer keratitis
dimorphic anemia
dimorphism
    sexual d.
dimorphous leprosy
dimple
    coccygeal d.
    postanal d.
    d. sign
dimpling
dineric
dinitrocellulose
4,6-dinitro-*o*-cresol
dinitrogen monoxide
2,4-dinitrophenol (DNP, Dnp)
dinitrophenylhydrazine test
dinner pad

D

dinoflagellate toxin
Dinoflagellida
dinoprostone
dinoprost tromethamine
dinucleotide
    d. domain
    d. fold
Dioctophyma renale
dioctophymiasis
dioctyl
    d. calcium sulfosuccinate
    d. sodium sulfosuccinate
Diodon
diodone
diodoquin
Diogenes cup
diolamine
diopter
    prism d. (p.d.)
dioptric aberration
dioptrics
dioscin
diose
diosgenin
diotic
diovular twin
diovulatory
dioxane
dioxide
dioxin
dioxybenzone
dioxygenase
DIP
    desquamative interstitial pneumonia
    distal interphalangeal
        DIP joint
dip
    Cournand d.
    d. phenomenon
D.I. particle
dipeptidase
    methionyl d.
dipeptide
dipeptidyl
    d. carboxypeptidase
    d. peptidase
    d. transferase
Dipetalonema
    D. reconditum
    D. streptocerca
diphallus
diphasic
    d. complex
    d. milk fever
diphemanil methylsulfate
diphemethoxidine
diphenadione
diphenan
diphenhydramine hydrochloride
diphenidol
o-diphenolase
diphenol oxidase
diphenoxylate hydrochloride
diphenyl
diphenylchlorarsine

diphenylcyanoarsine
diphenylenimine
5,5-diphenylhydantoin
diphenylhydantoin gingivitis
diphenylmethane
    d. dye
    d. laxative
2,5-diphenyloxazole (PPO)
diphenylpyraline hydrochloride
diphosgene
diphosphatase
    inorganic d.
diphosphate
diphosphoglycerate (P$_2$Gri)
diphosphothiamin
diphtheria
    d. antitoxin
    d. antitoxin unit
    cutaneous d.
    false d.
    faucial d.
    laryngeal d.
    laryngotracheal d.
    d., tetanus, and acellular pertussis
        vaccine (DTaP)
    d. toxin
    d. toxoid, tetanus toxoid, and
        pertussis vaccine (DPT, DTP)
diphtherial, diphtheritic
    d. conjunctivitis
    d. enteritis
    d. membrane
    d. neuropathy
    d. paralysis
    d. ulcer
diphtheric
diphtheroid
diphtherotoxin
diphyllobothriasis
Diphyllobothrium
    D. cordatum
    D. dendriticum
    D. hians
    D. houghtoni
    D. latum
    D. linguloides
    D. mansoni
    D. mansonoides
    D. nihonkaiense
    D. orcini
    D. pacificum
    D. scoticum
diphyllobothrium anemia
diphyodont
dipiproverine
dipivefrin hydrochloride
diplacusis
    d. binauralis
    d. dysharmonica
    d. echoica
    d. monauralis
diplegia
    congenital facial d.
    facial d.
    infantile d.

distropin
disturbance
    emotional d.
    mental d.
disulfamide
disulfate
disulfide
    asymmetric d.
    d. bond
    d. bridge
    glutathione d. (GSSG)
    mixed d.
    symmetric d.
disulfiram
disuse atrophy
DIT
    diiodotyrosine
diterpene
dithiazanine iodide
dithiothreitol
dithranol
Dittrich
    D. plug
    D. stenosis
diuresis
    alcohol d.
    osmotic d.
    water d.
diuretic
    cardiac d.
    direct d.
    indirect d.
    loop d.
    mercurial d.
    osmotic d.
    potassium sparing d.
diurnal
    d. enuresis
    d. periodicity
    d. rhythm
divalence, divalency
divalent
divalproex sodium
divarication
divergence
    d. excess exotropia
    d. insufficiency
    d. insufficiency exotropia
    d. paresis
divergent
    d. evolution
    d. squint
    d. strabismus
diverging meniscus
diver's
    d. palsy
    d. paralysis
diversity
    cultural d.
divers' spectacles
diverticula (*pl. of* diverticulum)
diverticular
    d. disease
diverticulectomy
diverticulitis

diverticuloma
diverticulopexy
diverticulosis
diverticulum, pl. **diverticula**
    allantoenteric d.
    allantoic d.
    d. of ampulla of ductus deferens
    d. ampullae ductus deferentis
    caliceal d.
    cervical d.
    d. of colon
    colonic d.
    duodenal d.
    epiphrenic d.
    false d.
    Heister d.
    hypopharyngeal d.
    Kommerell d.
    laryngotracheal d.
    Meckel d.
    metanephric d.
    Nuck d.
    pancreatic d.
    Pertik d.
    pharyngoesophageal d.
    pituitary d.
    pulsion d.
    Rathke d.
    thyroid d., thyroglossal d.
    tracheobronchial d.
    traction d.
    true d.
    urethral d.
    ventricular d.
    vesical d.
    Zenker d.
divicine
divided
    d. dose
    d. spectacles
divide into equal parts (div. in p. aeg.)
diving
    d. goiter
    d. reflex
divisio
    d.'s anteriores plexus brachialis
    d. autonomica systematis nervosi
      peripherici
    d. lateralis dextra hepatis
    d. lateralis sinistra
    d. lateralis sinistra hepatis
    d. medialis dextra hepatis
    d. medialis sinistra hepatis
    d.'s posteriores plexus brachialis
division
    anterior primary d.
    anterior d. of (trunks of) brachial
      plexus
    autonomic d. of nervous system
    cleavage d.
    conjugate d.
    craniosacral d. of autonomic
      nervous system
    direct nuclear d.
    equatorial d.

D

division (*continued*)
indirect nuclear d.
lateral d. of left liver
left lateral d. of liver
left medial d. of liver
meiotic d.
mitotic d.
multiplicative d.
posterior d. of brachial plexus
posterior primary d.
reduction d.
Remak nuclear d.
right lateral d. of liver
right medial d. of liver
divisional block
div. in p. aeg.
divide into equal parts
divulse
divulsion
divulsor
Dix-Hallpike maneuver
dixyrazine
dizygotic
d. twins
dizziness
djenkolic acid
djenkol poisoning
dl-**narcotine**
DM
adamsite
DMA
dimethoxyamphetamine
DMARD
disease modifying antirheumatic drug
DMC
p,p-dichlorodiphenyl methyl carbinol
DMD
Doctor of Dental Medicine
DMF, dmf
decayed, missing, and filled teeth
DMFS, dmfs
decayed, missing, and filled surface
DMFS caries index
DMPP
dimethylphenylpiperazinium
DMSA
^{99m}Tc-dimercaptosuccinic acid
DMSO
dimethyl sulfoxide
DMT
n,n-dimethyltryptamine
DN
dibucaine number
DNA
deoxyribonucleic acid
A-DNA
antisense DNA
B-DNA
blunt-ended DNA
competitor DNA
complementary DNA (cDNA)
DNA diagnostics
extrachromosomal DNA
DNA fingerprinting

DNA gap
genomic DNA
DNA helix
DNA homology
DNA hybridization
junk DNA
DNA ligase
linker DNA
DNA marker
DNA nucleotidylexotransferase
palindromic DNA
DNA polymerase
DNA polymorphism
DNA profiling
recombinant DNA
repetitive DNA
satellite DNA
selfish DNA
sticky-ended DNA
DNA typing
DNA virus
Z-DNA
zero time-binding DNA
dnaG
primase
DNA-RNA hybrid
DNAse
deoxyribonuclease
DNP, Dnp
deoxyribonucleoprotein
2,4-dinitrophenol
DNR
deoxyribonucleoprotein
Dns, DNS
dansyl
DO
Doctor of Osteopathy
DOA
dead on arrival
dobutamine
DOC
deoxycorticosterone
d'Ocagne nomogram
docking protein
n-**docosanoic acid**
doctor (Dr.)
D. of Chiropractic (DC)
D. of Dental Medicine (DMD)
D. of Dental Surgery (DDS)
D. of Hygiene (D Hy)
D. of Osteopathy (DO)
D. of Pharmacy (Pharm. D.)
D. of Philosophy (PhD)
D. of Podiatric Medicine (DPM)
D. of Podiatry (DP)
D. of Public Health (DPH, DrPH)
D. of Surgery (ChD)
doctrine
Arrhenius d.
humoral d.
Monro d.
Monro-Kellie d.
docusate
d. calcium
d. sodium

dodecane
n-dodecanoic acid
dodecanoyl-CoA synthetase
dodecarbonium chloride
dodecyl
    d. gallate
    d. sulfate
Döderlein bacillus
Doerfler-Stewart test
dog
    d. disease
    d. distemper virus
    d. ear
    d. nose
    d. unit
Dogiel
    D. cell
    D. corpuscle
dogma
    central d.
dogmatic school
dogmatist
Döhle
    D. body
    D. inclusion
Doisy
dol
dolichocephalic, dolichocephalous
dolichocephaly, dolichocephalism
dolichocolon
dolichocranial
dolichoectatic artery
dolichofacial
dolichol phosphate
dolichopellic, dolichopelvic
    d. pelvis
dolichoprosopic, dolichoprosopous
dolichostenomelia
dolichouranic, dolichuranic
doll's eye sign
dolor capitis
dolorific
dolorimetry
dolorogenic zone
dolorology
DOM
    2,5-dimethoxy-4-methylamphetamine
domain
    dinucleotide d.
Dombrock blood group
dome
    d. cell
    d. of pleura
domiciliated
dominance
    cerebral d.
    false d.
    genetic d.
    d. hierarchy
    d. of traits
dominant
    d. character
    d. eye
    d. frequency
    d. gene

    d. hemisphere
    d. idea
    d. inheritance
    d. lethal trait
    d. optic atrophy
    d. trait
dominantly inherited Lévi disease
domiodol
domiphen bromide
domperidone
Donath-Landsteiner
    D.-L. cold autoantibody
    D.-L. phenomenon
Donders
    D. law
    D. pressure
Don Juanism
Donnan equilibrium
Donné corpuscle
Donohue
    D. disease
    D. syndrome
donor
    hydrogen d.
    d. insemination
    universal d.
do not resuscitate
Donovan body
Doose syndrome
dopa, DOPA, Dopa
    alpha methyl d.
    d. decarboxylase
    decarboxylated d.
    d. oxidase
    d. quinone
    d. reaction
L-dopa
dopamine
    d. beta-hydroxylase
    d. beta-monooxygenase
    d. hydrochloride
dopaminergic
dope
doping
Doppler
    D. color flow
    D. echocardiography
    D. effect
    D. phenomenon
    D. shift
    D. ultrasonography
Dor
    D. fundoplication
    D. procedure
doraphobia
Dorello canal
Dorendorf sign
Dorfman-Chanarin syndrome
dornase
    pancreatic d.
Dorno
doromania
dorsa (*pl. of* dorsum)
dorsabdominal
dorsad

D

dorsal

d. accessory olivary nucleus
d. artery of clitoris
d. artery of foot
d. artery of nose
d. artery of penis
d. branch
d. branch of first and second posterior intercostal artery
d. branch of the lumbar artery
d. branch of the posterior intercostal artery 3–11
d. branch of the posterior intercostal veins 4–11
d. branch of the subcostal artery
d. branch of the superior intercostal artery
d. branch of the ulnar nerve
d. calcaneocuboid ligament
d. callosal vein
d. carpal arterial arch
d. carpal branch of radial artery
d. carpal branch of ulnar artery
d. carpal ligament
d. carpal network
d. carpal tendinous sheath
d. carpometacarpal ligament
d. column of spinal cord
d. column stimulation
d. cuboideonavicular ligament
d. cuneocuboid ligament
d. cuneonavicular ligamens
d. digital artery
d. digital nerve
d. digital nerve of deep fibular nerve
d. digital nerve of foot
d. digital nerve of hand
d. digital nerve of superficial fibular nerve
d. digital nerve of ulnar nerve
d. digital vein of foot
d. digital vein of toes
d. fascia of foot
d. fascia of hand
d. flexure
d. funiculus
d. hood
d. hypothalamic area
d. hypothalamic region
d. intercuneiform ligament
d. intermediate sulcus
d. interosseous artery
d. interosseous nerve
d. interosseus of foot
d. interosseus of hand
d. lateral cutaneous nerve
d. lateral geniculate nucleus
d. lingual branch of lingual artery
d. lingual vein
d. longitudinal fasciculus
d. medial cutaneous nerve
d. median sulcus
d. mesocardium
d. mesogastrium

d. metacarpal artery
d. metacarpal ligament
d. metacarpal vein
d. metatarsal artery
d. metatarsal ligament
d. metatarsal vein
d. midbrain syndrome
d. motor nucleus of vagus
d. muscle
d. nasal artery
d. nerve of clitoris
d. nerve of penis
d. nerve of scapula
d. nerve of toes
d. nucleus
d. nucleus of thalamus
d. nucleus of trapezoid body
d. nucleus of vagus
d. pallidum
d. pancreas
d. pancreatic artery
d. part of intertransversarii laterales lumborum
d. part of pons
d. plate of neural tube
d. position
d. premammillary nucleus
d. primary ramus of spinal nerve
d. radiocarpal ligament
d. reflex
d. root ganglion
d. root of spinal nerve
d. sacrococcygeal muscle
d. sacrococcygeus muscle
d. sacroiliac ligament
d. scapular artery
d. scapular nerve
d. scapular vein
d. septal nucleus
d. spine
d. spinocerebellar tract
d. striatum
d. supraoptic commissure
d. surface
d. surface of digit
d. surface of sacrum
d. surface of scapula
d. talonavicular bone
d. tarsal ligament
d. tarsometatarsal ligament
d. tegmental decussation
d. thalamus
d. thoracic artery
d. thoracic nucleus
d. trigeminothalamic tract
d. tubercle of radius
d. vagal nucleus
d. vein of clitoris
d. vein of corpus callosum
d. vein of penis
d. venous arch of foot
d. venous network
d. vertebrae

dorsalis pedis artery
Dorset culture egg medium

dorsi
dorsiduct
dorsiflexion
dorsiflexor compartment of leg
dorsiscapular
dorsispinal vein
dorsocephalad
dorsolateral
    d. fasciculus
    d. nucleus
    d. plate of neural tube
    d. sulcus
    d. tract
dorsolumbar
dorsomedial
    d. hypothalamic nucleus
    d. nucleus
    d. nucleus of hypothalamus
dorsosacral position
dorsoventrad
dorsum, pl. **dorsa**
    d. ephippii
    d. of foot
    d. of foot reflex
    d. of hand
    d. linguae
    d. manus
    d. nasi
    d. of nose
    d. pedis
    d. pedis reflex
    d. of penis
    d. penis
    d. scapulae
    d. sellae
    d. of tongue
dosage
dose
    absorbed d.
    air d.
    bone marrow d.
    booster d.
    cumulative d.
    curative d. (CD^{50})
    daily d.
    depth d.
    divided d.
    effective d. (ED)
    epilation d.
    equianalgesic d.
    equivalent d.
    erythema d.
    exit d.
    exposure d.
    fractional d.
    gonad d.
    gonadal d.
    infecting d. (ID)
    initial d.
    integral d.
    L d.
    L^+ d.
    lethal d. (LD)
    Lf d.
    Lo d.

    loading d.
    Lr d.
    maintenance d.
    maximum permissible d. (MPD)
    maximum tolerated d.
    median effective dose (ED_{50})
    minimal infecting d. (MID)
    minimal lethal d. (MLD)
    minimal reacting d. (MRD)
    optimum d.
    preventive d.
    sensitizing d.
    shocking d.
    skin d.
    therapeutic d.
    tissue culture infectious d. ($TCID_{50}$)
    tolerance d.
dose-response
    d.-r. curve
    d.-r. relationship
dosimeter
dosimetry
    thermoluminescence d.
    x-ray d.
dot
    Gunn d.
    Horner-Trantas d.
    Maurer d.
    Mittendorf d.
    Schüffner d.
    Trantas d.
    Ziemann d.
dotage
dotted tongue
double
    d. antibody immunoassay
    d. antibody method
    d. antibody precipitation
    d. antibody sandwich assay
    d. aortic arch
    d. aortic stenosis
    d. back cross
    d. bind
    d. blind experiment
    d. blind study
    d. bond
    d. bubble sign
    d. chin
    d. compartment hydrocephalus
    d. concave lens
    d. congenital athetosis
    d. consciousness
    d. contrast enema
    d. convex lens
    d. displacement mechanism
    d. elevator palsy
    d. enterostomy
    d. flap amputation
    d. fracture
    d. (gel) diffusion precipitin test in one dimension
    d. (gel) diffusion precipitin test in two dimensions
    d. helix
    d. hemiplegia

D

double *(continued)*
    d. immunodiffusion
    d. inlet atrioventricular connection
    d. intussusception
    d. lip
    d. loop hernia
    d. membrane
    d. minute chromosome
    d. outlet right ventricle
    d. pedicle flap
    d. pleurisy
    d. pneumonia
    d. product
    d. protrusion
    d. quartan
    d. quotidian fever
    d. refraction
    d. ring sign
    d. salt
    d. stain
    d. tachycardia
    d. tertian
    d. tertian malaria
    d. track sign
    d. vision
double-channel catheter
double-masked experiment
double-mouthed uterus
double-point threshold
double-reciprocal plot
double-shock sound
double-strand break
double-stranded (ds)
doublet
        Wollaston d.
doubling time
doubly
        d. armed suture
        d. heterozygous
douche bath
doughnut pessary
Douglas
        D. abscess
        D. bag
        D. cul-de-sac
        D. fold
        D. line
        D. mechanism
        D. pouch
dousing bath
dovetail stress-broken abutment
dowager hump
dowel graft
downbeat nystagmus
Downey cell
downgrowth
        epithelial d.
down-regulation
Downs analysis
Down syndrome
downward drainage
downy hair
doxacurium chloride
doxapram hydrochloride

doxazocin
doxepin hydrochloride
doxophylline
doxorubicin
doxycycline
doxylamine succinate
Doyère eminence
Doyle operation
Doyne honeycomb choroidopathy
DP
        Doctor of Podiatry
DPH
        Doctor of Public Health
DPM
        Doctor of Podiatric Medicine
D-proline reductase
DPT
        diphtheria toxoid, tetanus toxoid, and
            pertussis vaccine
DR
        digital radiography
Dr.
        doctor
dr
        dram
Drabkin reagent
drachm
dracunculiasis, dracunculosis
Dracunculus
        D. lova
        D. medinensis
        D. oculi
        D. persarum
draft
drag
        solvent d.
dragée
Dragendorff
        D. reagent
        D. test
Dräger respirometer
drain
        cigarette d.
        Mikulicz d.
        Penrose d.
        stab d.
        sump d.
drainage
        capillary d.
        closed d.
        dependent d.
        downward d.
        infusion-aspiration d.
        open d.
        postural d.
        suction d.
        through d.
        tidal d.
        d. tube
        Wangensteen d.
drain-trap stomach
dram (dr)
drape
Draper law
draught

drawer
    d. sign
    d. test
draw-sheet
dream
    anxiety d.
    d. associations
    wet d.
dream-work
dreamy state
Drechslera
Dreifuss
drepanidium
drepanocyte
drepanocytic anemia
dresser
dressing
    adhesive absorbent d.
    antiseptic d.
    bolus d.
    dry d.
    fixed d.
    d. forceps
    Lister d.
    occlusive d.
    pressure d.
    tie-over d.
    water d.
    wet-to-dry d.
Dressler
    D. beat
    D. syndrome
Dreyer formula
DRG
    diagnosis-related group
dribble
dried
    d. alum
    d. ferrous sulfate
    d. human albumin
    d. human plasma protein fraction
    d. human serum
    d. yeast
drift
    antigenic d.
    genetic d.
    d. movement
    pure random d.
drifting
drifts
drill
    bur d.
    dental d.
drill-out
    cochlear d.-o.
Drinker respirator
drip
    alkaline milk d.
    intravenous d.
    Murphy d.
    d. phleboclysis
    postnasal d.
    d. transfusion
drive
    acquired d.

    exploratory d.
    learned d.
    meiotic d.
    physiologic d.
    primary d.
    secondary d.
driving
    photic d.
dromomania
dromostanolone propionate
dronabinol
drooping lily sign
drop
    d. attack
    enamel d.
    eye d.'s
    d. finger
    d. foot
    d. hand
    hanging d.
    d. heart
    knock-out d.'s
    nose d.'s
    stomach d.'s
droperidol
dropfoot
droplet
    d. infection
    d. nucleus
dropped beat
dropper
dropsical
dropsy
    abdominal d.
    cardiac d.
    epidemic d.
    famine d.
    nutritional d.
    d. of pericardium
drowning
    dry d.
    near d.
    secondary d.
drowsiness
DrPH
    Doctor of Public Health
drug
    d. abuse
    addictive d.
    d. allergy
    crude d.
    disease modifying antirheumatic d.
      (DMARD)
    d. eruption
    d. fever
    d. holiday
    d. interaction
    nonsteroidal antiinflammatory d.
      (NSAID)
    orphan d.
    d. pathogenesis
    psychedelic d.
    psychodysleptic d.
    psycholytic d.
    d. psychosis

D

drug *(continued)*
    psychotomimetic d.
    psychotropic d.
    recreational d.
    residue remaining after percolation
       of a d. (marc)
    d. resistance
    scheduled d.
    street d.
    d. tetanus
    d. utilization review
drug-fast
druggist
drug-induced
    d.-i. disease
    d.-i. hepatitis
    d.-i. lupus
drum
    d. membrane
Drummond sign
drumstick appendage
drunkenness
    sleep d.
drusen
    basal laminar d.
    basal linear d.
    cuticular d.
    exudative d.
    hard d.
    intrapapillary d.
    d. of the macula
    macular d.
    d. of the optic nerve head
    soft d.
    typical d.
dry
    d. abscess
    d. amputation
    d. beriberi
    d. bronchiectasis
    d. cup
    d. cutaneous leishmaniasis
    d. distillation
    d. dressing
    d. drowning
    d. eye syndrome
    d. gangrene
    d. hernia
    d. ice
    d. labor
    d. leprosy
    d. nurse
    d. pack
    d. pericarditis
    d. pleurisy
    d. rale
    d. socket
    d. synovitis
    d. vomiting
    d. weight
ds
    double-stranded
DSA
    digital subtraction angiography

DSM
    Diagnostic and Statistical Manual of
      Mental Disorders
D-S test
DT
    delirium tremens
dT
    deoxythymidine
DTaP
    diphtheria, tetanus, and acellular pertussis
      vaccine
DT-diaphorase
dTDP
    thymidine 5′-diphosphate
dTDP-sugar
DTH
    delayed-type hypersensitivity
dThd
    thymidine
DTIC
    dacarbazine
dTMP
    deoxythymidylic acid
DTP
    diphtheria toxoid, tetanus toxoid, and
      pertussis vaccine
DTPA
    diethylenetriamine pentaacetic acid
DTR
    deep tendon reflex
dTTP
    thymidine 5′-triphosphate
dual
    d. personality
    d. relationship
dual-cure resin
dualism
Duane syndrome
duarte dolare (dur. dolor.)
Dubin-Johnson syndrome
Dubois
    D. abscess
    D. disease
DuBois formula
duboisine
Du Bois-Reymond law
Duboscq colorimeter
Dubowitz score
Dubreuil-Chambardel syndrome
Duchenne
    D. disease
    D. dystrophy
    D. sign
Duchenne-Aran disease
Duchenne-Erb paralysis
duck
    d. embryo origin vaccine (DEV)
    d. hepatitis virus
    d. influenza virus
    d. plague virus
duckbill speculum
Duckworth phenomenon
Ducrey
    D. bacillus
    D. test

duct

aberrant d.
aberrant bile d.
accessory pancreatic d.
alveolar d.
amnionic d.
anal d.
arterial d.
Bartholin d.
Bellini d.
Bernard d.
bile d.
biliary d.
Blasius d.
Botallo d.
bucconeural d.
d. of bulbourethral gland
canalicular d.
d. carcinoma
carotid d.
cervical d.
choledoch d.
cochlear d.
common bile d.
common hepatic d.
craniopharyngeal d.
Cuvier d.
cystic d.
cystic gall d.
deferent d.
efferent d.
ejaculatory d.
endolymphatic d.
d. of epididymis
excretory d.
excretory d. of lacrimal gland
excretory d. of seminal gland
excretory d. of seminal vesicle
frontonasal d.
galactophorous d.
gall d.
Gartner d.
genital d.
guttural d.
hemithoracic d.
Hensen d.
hepatic d.
hepatocystic d.
Hoffmann d.
hypophysial d.
incisive d.
intercalated d.
interlobar d.
interlobular d.
intralobular d.
jugular d.
lactiferous d.
left d. of caudate lobe of liver
left hepatic d.
longitudinal d. of epoöphoron
Luschka d.
lymphatic d.
major sublingual d.
mamillary d.
mammary d.

mesonephric d.
metanephric d.
milk d.
minor sublingual d.
Müller d.
müllerian d.
nasal d.
nasolacrimal d.
nephric d.
omphalomesenteric d.
pancreatic d.
papillary d.
d. papilloma
paramesonephric d.
paraurethral d.
parotid d.
Pecquet d.
perilymphatic d.
pharyngobranchial d.
pronephric d.
prostatic d.
right d. of caudate lobe of liver
right hepatic d.
right lymphatic d.
Rivinus d.
saccular d.
salivary d.
Santorini d.
Schüller d.
secretory d.
semicircular d.
seminal d.
d. of Skene gland
spermatic d.
Steno d.
Stensen d.
striated d.
subclavian d.
submandibular d.
submaxillary d.
sudoriferous d.
sweat d.
d. of sweat gland
testicular d.
thoracic d.
thyroglossal d.
thyrolingual d.
umbilical d.
uniting d.
utricular d.
utriculosaccular d.
vitelline d.
vitellointestinal d.
Walther d.
Wharton d.
Wirsung d.
wolffian d.

ductal

d. aneurysm
d. carcinoma
d. hyperplasia

ductile
duction

forced d.
passive d.

D

ductless gland
ductular
ductule
    aberrant d.
    biliary d.
    efferent d. of testis
    excretory d. of lacrimal gland
    inferior aberrant d.
    interlobular d.
    prostatic d.
    superior aberrant d.
    transverse d. of epoöphoron
ductulus, pl. **ductuli**
    d. aberrans inferior
    d. aberrans superior
    ductuli aberrantes
    d. alveolaris
    ductuli biliferi
    ductuli efferentes testis
    ductuli excretorii glandulae
      lacrimalis
    ductuli interlobulares
    ductuli paroöphori
    ductuli prostatici
    ductuli transversi epoöphori
ductus, gen. and pl. **ductus**
    d. aberrantes
    d. arteriosus
    d. biliaris
    d. biliferi
    d. caroticus
    d. choledochus
    d. cochlearis
    d. cysticus
    d. deferens
    d. deferens vestigialis
    d. diverticulum
    d. dorsopancreaticus
    d. ejaculatorius
    d. endolymphaticus
    d. epididymidis
    d. excretorius
    d. excretorius glandulae vesiculosae
    d. excretorius vesiculae seminalis
    d. glandulae bulbourethralis
    d. hemithoracicus
    d. hepaticus communis
    d. hepaticus dexter
    d. hepaticus sinister
    d. incisivus
    d. lactiferi
    d. lingualis
    d. lobi caudati dexter hepatis
    d. lobi caudati sinister hepatis
    d. longitudinalis epoöphori
    d. lymphaticus dexter
    d. mesonephricus
    d. nasolacrimalis
    d. pancreaticus
    d. pancreaticus accessorius
    d. paramesonephricus
    d. paraurethrales
    d. parotideus
    patent d. arteriosus
    d. perilymphaticus

    d. pharyngobranchialis III
    d. pharyngobranchialis IV
    d. prostatici
    d. reuniens
    d. saccularis
    d. semicirculares
    d. semicircularis anterior
    d. semicircularis lateralis
    d. semicircularis posterior
    d. sublinguales minores
    d. sublingualis major
    d. submandibularis
    d. submaxillaris
    d. sudoriferus
    d. thoracicus
    d. thoracicus dexter
    d. thyroglossus
    d. utricularis
    d. utriculosaccularis
    d. venosus
    d. venosus arantii
Duddell membrane
Duffy
    D. antigen
    D. blood group
Duhring disease
Dührssen incision
Duke bleeding time test
Dukes
    D. classification
    D. disease
dulcin
dulcite, dulcitol, dulcose
dull
dullness, dulness
    shifting d.
Dulong-Petit law
dumbbell ganglioneuroma
dumb rabies
Dumdum fever
dummy consultand
Dumontpallier pessary
dumping syndrome
Duncan
    D. disease
    D. fold
    D. mechanism
    D. placenta
    D. syndrome
    D. ventricle
duocrinin
duodena (*pl. of* duodenum)
duodenal
    d. ampulla
    d. branch of anterior superior
      pancreaticoduodenal artery
    d. branch of posterior superior
      pancreaticoduodenal artery
    d. bulb
    d. cap
    d. digestion
    d. diverticulum
    d. fistula
    d. fossae
    d. gland

d. impression on liver
d. smear
d. sphincter
duodenectomy
duodenitis
duodenocholangitis
duodenocholecystostomy
duodenocholedochotomy
duodenocystostomy
duodenoenterostomy
duodenojejunal
d. angle
d. flexure
d. fold
d. fossa
d. hernia
d. junction
d. recess
d. sphincter
duodenojejunostomy
duodenolysis
duodenomesocolic fold
duodenorenal ligament
duodenorrhaphy
duodenoscopy
duodenostomy
duodenotomy
duodenum, pl. **duodena**
duovirus
duplex
d. Doppler scan
d. kidney
d. transmission
d. ultrasonography
d. uterus
duplication
d. of chromosome
d. cyst
gene d.
duplicitas
d. anterior
d. posterior
duplicity theory of vision
Dupré muscle
Dupuytren
D. amputation
D. canal
D. contracture
D. disease of the foot
D. fascia
D. fracture
D. hydrocele
D. sign
D. suture
D. tourniquet
duraencephalosynangiosis
dural
d. cavernous sinus fistula
d. part of filum terminale
d. sheath
d. sheath of optic nerve
d. venous sinus
dura mater
d. m. of brain
cranial d. m.

d. m. cranialis
d. m. encephali
spinal d. m.
d. m. of spinal cord
d. m. spinalis
duramatral
Duran-Reynals
D.-R. permeability factor
D.-R. spreading factor
duraplasty
duration
half amplitude pulse d.
pulse wave d.
Dürck node
dur. dolor.
duarte dolare
Duret
D. hemorrhage
D. lesion
Durham
D. rule
D. tube
Duroziez
D. disease
D. murmur
D. sign
DUSN
diffuse unilateral subacute neuroretinitis
dust
d. asthma
d. cell
d. corpuscle
dUTP
deoxyuridine 5-triphosphate
Dutton
D. disease
D. relapsing fever
Duvenhage virus
Duverney
D. fissure
D. gland
D. muscle
dwarf
hypophysial d.
hypothyroid d.
d. pelvis
pituitary d.
dwarfed enamel
dwarfism
achondroplastic d.
acromelic d.
acromesomelic d.
aortic d.
asexual d.
ateliotic d.
camptomelic d.
chondrodystrophic d.
deprivation d.
diastrophic d.
disproportionate d.
Fröhlich d.
Hunter-Thompson d.
hypothyroid d.
infantile d.
Laron-type d.

D

dwarfism (*continued*)
    lethal d.
    Lorain-Lévi d.
    mesomelic d.
    metatropic d.
    micromelic d.
    panhypopituitary d.
    phocomelic d.
    physiologic d.
    pituitary d.
    primordial d.
    proportionate d.
    psychosocial d.
    rhizomelic d.
    Robinow d.
    Seckel d.
    senile d.
    sexual d.
    Silver-Russell d.
    snub-nose d.
    thanatophoric d.
    true d.
Dwyer osteotomy
Dy
    dysprosium
dyad
dyadic
    d. psychotherapy
    d. symbiosis
dyclonine hydrochloride
dydrogesterone
dye
    acidic d.
    acridine d.
    azin d.
    azo d.
    azocarmine d.
    basic d.
    chlorotriazine d.
    diphenylmethane d.
    d. disappearance test
    d. exclusion test
    ketonimine d.
    natural d.
    nitro d.
    oxazin d.
    rosanilin d.
    salt d.
    synthetic d.
    thiazin d.
    triphenylmethane d.
    xanthene d.
dye-dilution curve
Dyggve-Melchior-Clausen syndrome
dynamic
    d. aorta
    d. compliance of lung
    d. computed tomography
    d. CT
    d. demography
    d. equilibrium
    d. force
    d. friction
    d. ileus

    d. murmur
    d. posturography
    d. psychiatry
    d. psychology
    d. psychotherapy
    d. refraction
    d. relation
    d. school
    d. splint
    d. viscosity
dynamics
    group d.
dynamogenesis
dynamogenic
dynamogeny
dynamograph
dynamometer
dynamoscope
dynamoscopy
dynatherm
dyne
dynein arm
dynorphin
dyphylline
dysacousia, dysacusia
dysacusis
dysadaptation
dysantigraphia
dysaphia
dysaphic
dysarteriotony
dysarthria
    ataxic d.
    hyperkinetic d.
    hypokinetic d.
    lower motor neuron d.
    rigid d.
    spastic d.
dysarthria–clumsy hand syndrome
dysarthric
dysarthrosis
dysautonomia
    familial d.
dysbarism
dysbasia
    d. angiosclerotica
    d. angiospastica
    d. lordotica progressiva
dysbetalipoproteinemia
dysbolism
dysbulia
dysbulic
dyscalculia
dyscephalia mandibulooculofacialis
dyscephaly
dyscheiral, dyschiral
dyscheiria, dyschiria
dyschezia
dyschiral (*var. of* dyscheiral)
dyschondrogenesis
dyschondroplasia with hemangioma
dyschondrosteosis
dyschroia, dyschroa
dyschromatopsia
dyschromatosis

dyschromia
dyscinesia
dysconjugate gaze
dyscontrol
dyscoria
dyscrasia
    blood d.
dyscrasic, dyscratic
dysdiadochokinesia, dysdiadochocinesia
dysdiadochokinesis
dysembryoplastic neuroepithelial tumor
dysemia
dysencephalia splanchnocystica
dysenteric
    d. algid malaria
    d. diarrhea
dysentery
    amebic d.
    d. antitoxin
    bacillary d.
    d. bacillus
    balantidial d.
    bilharzial d.
    fulminating d.
    helminthic d.
    malignant d.
    viral d.
dyserethism
dysergia
dysesthesia
dysfibrinogenemia
dysfunction
    constitutional hepatic d.
    dental d.
    minimal brain d.
    papillary muscle d.
    phagocyte d.
    placental d.
    psychosexual d.
    sexual d.
    sphincter of Oddi d.
    temporomandibular joint d. (TMD, TMJ)
dysfunctional uterine bleeding
dysgammaglobulinemia
dysgenesis
    cortical d.
    gonadal d.
    iridocorneal mesenchymal d.
    seminiferous tubule d.
    testicular d.
    XO gonadal d.
    XX gonadal d.
    XY gonadal d.
dysgenic
dysgerminoma
dysgeusia
dysgnathia
dysgnathic
dysgnosia
dysgonic
dysgranular cortex
dysgraphia
dysharmonious retinal correspondence
dyshematopoiesis

dyshematopoietic
dyshemopoiesis
dyshemopoietic anemia
dyshidria
dyshidrosis
dyshidrotic eczema
dysjunction
    Le Fort III craniofacial d.
dysjunctive nystagmus
dyskaryosis
dyskaryotic
dyskeratoma
    warty d.
dyskeratosis
    benign d.
    d. congenita
    intraepithelial d.
    isolated d. follicularis
dyskeratotic
dyskinesia
    biliary d.
    extrapyramidal d.
    lingual-facial-buccal d.
    d. syndrome
    tardive d.
    tracheobronchial d.
dyskinesis
    ciliary d.
dyskinetic
dyslexia
dyslexic
dyslogia
dysmasesis
dysmature
dysmaturity
dysmelia
dysmenorrhea
    functional d.
    mechanical d.
    membranous d.
    obstructive d.
    ovarian d.
    primary d.
    secondary d.
    spasmodic d.
    tubal d.
    ureteric d.
    uterine d.
    vaginal d.
dysmenorrheal membrane
dysmetria
    ocular d.
dysmnesic syndrome
dysmorphia
dysmorphism
dysmorphogenesis
dysmorphology
dysmorphophobia
dysmyelination
dysmyotonia
dysnystaxis
dysodontiasis
dysontogenesis
dysontogenetic
dysorexia

D

dysosmia
dysosteogenesis
dysostosis
    acrofacial d.
    cleidocranial d.
    clidocranial d.
    craniofacial d.
    mandibuloacral d.
    mandibulofacial d.
    metaphysial d.
    d. multiplex
    orodigitofacial d.
    otomandibular d.
    peripheral d.
dyspallia
dyspareunia
dyspepsia
    acid d.
    adhesion d.
    atonic d.
    fermentative d.
    flatulent d.
    functional d.
    nervous d.
    reflex d.
dyspeptic
dysphagia, dysphagy
    d. lusoria
    d. nervosa
    nervous d.
    sideropenic d.
    vallecular d.
dysphagocytosis
    congenital d.
dysphasia
dysphemia
dysphonia
    abductor spasmodic d.
    adductor spasmodic d.
    d. plicae ventricularis
    spasmodic d.
    spastic d.
    d. spastica
dysphoria
    late luteal phase d.
dysphrasia
dyspigmentation
dyspinealism
dyspituitarism
dysplasia
    anhidrotic ectodermal d.
    anterofacial d., anteroposterior
      facial d.
    anteroposterior d.
    asphyxiating thoracic d.
    branchiootorenal d.
    bronchopulmonary d.
    cemental d.
    cerebral d.
    cervical d.
    chondroectodermal d.
    cleidocranial d., clidocranial d.
    cochlear d.
    congenital ectodermal d.
    congenital hip d.

    cortical d.
    craniocarpotarsal d.
    craniodiaphysial d.
    craniometaphysial d.
    dentin d.
    developmental hip d.
    diaphysial d.
    diastrophic d.
    ectodermal d.
    enamel d.
    d. epiphysealis multiplex
    d. epiphysialis hemimelia
    d. epiphysialis punctata
    epithelial d.
    faciodigitogenital d.
    familial white folded d.
    fibromuscular d.
    fibrous d. of bone
    fibrous d. of jaw
    florid osseous d.
    hidrotic ectodermal d.
    hypohidrotic ectodermal d.
    mandibulofacial d.
    McKusick metaphyseal d.
    metaphysial d.
    Mondini d.
    monostotic fibrous d.
    mucoepithelial d.
    multiple epiphyseal d. (EDM)
    neuronal intestinal d.
    OAV d.
    oculoauriculovertebral d.
    oculodentodigital d.
    oculovertebral d.
    odontogenic d.
    ophthalmomandibulomelic d.
    otospondylomegaepiphyseal d.
    periapical cemental d.
    polyostotic fibrous d.
    pseudoachondroplastic
      spondyloepiphysial d.
    retinal d.
    septooptic d.
    skeletal d.
    spondyloepiphyseal d.
    spondyloepiphyseal d. congenita
      (SEDC)
    spondyloepiphyseal d. tarda
    ventriculoradial d.
dysplastic
    d. nevus
    d. nevus syndrome
dyspnea
    cardiac d.
    exertional d.
    expiratory d.
    functional d.
    nocturnal d.
    paroxysmal nocturnal d.
    Traube d.
dyspneic
dyspraxia
dysprosium (Dy)
dysproteinemia
dysproteinemic retinopathy

dysraphism, dysraphia
    spinal d.
dysrhythmia
    cardiac d.
    electroencephalographic d.
    esophageal d.
    paroxysmal cerebral d.
dyssomnia
dysspermatogenic sterility
dysspondylism
dysstasia
dysstatic
dyssyllabia
dyssynergia
    d. cerebellaris myoclonica
    detrusor sphincter d.
dystasia
dystelephalangy
dysthymia
dysthymic disorder
dysthyroid
    d. myopathy
    d. orbitopathy
dysthyroidal infantilism
dystocia
    arrest of active phase d.
    arrest of descent d.
    fetal d.
    maternal d.
    placental d.
    shoulder d.
dystonia
    d. lenticularis
    d. musculorum deformans
    torsion d.
dystonic
    d. reaction
    d. torticollis
dystopia
    pituitary d.
dystopic
dystrophia
    d. adiposogenitalis
    d. brevicollis
    d. myotonica
    d. unguium
dystrophic
    d. calcification
    d. calcinosis
dystrophin
dystrophy
    adiposogenital d.
    adult foveomacular retinal d.
    adult pseudohypertrophic muscular d.
    anterior corneal d.
    asphyxiating thoracic d.
    Becker muscular d.
    Becker-type tardive muscular d.
    central areolar choroidal d.
    central cloudy corneal d. of
      François

    central crystalline corneal d. of
      Snyder
    childhood muscular d.
    Cogan d.
    cone d.
    cone-rod retinal d.
    congenital hereditary endothelial d.
    corneal d.
    craniocarpotarsal d.
    Duchenne d.
    Emery-Dreifuss muscular d.
    facioscapulohumeral muscular d.
    Favre d.
    fingerprint d.
    fleck d. of cornea
    Fuchs endothelial d.
    gelatinous droplike corneal d.
    granular corneal d.
    Groenouw corneal d.
    gutter d. of cornea
    hereditary epithelial d.
    hypertrophic d.
    infantile neuroaxonal d.
    Landouzy-Dejerine d.
    lattice corneal d.
    Leyden-Möbius muscular d.
    limb-girdle muscular d.
    macular corneal d.
    macular retinal d.
    map-dot-fingerprint d.
    Meesman d.
    microcystic epithelial d.
    mucopolysaccharide keratin d.
    muscular d.
    myotonic d.
    neuroaxonal d.
    oculopharyngeal d.
    pattern retinal d.
    pelvofemoral muscular d.
    posterior polymorphous corneal d.
    pre-Descemet corneal d.
    progressive tapetochoroidal d.
    pseudohypertrophic muscular d.
    reflex sympathetic d. (RSD)
    Reis-Bücklers corneal d.
    ringlike corneal d.
    scapulohumeral muscular d.
    stromal corneal d.
    sympathetic reflex d.
    thoracic-pelvic-phalangeal d.
    twenty-nail d.
    vitelliform retinal d.
    vitreotapetoretinal d.
    vortex corneal d.
    vulvar d.
dystropin
dystropy
dysuria
dysuric
dysury
dysversion

D

ε (*var. of* epsilon)
E

extraction ratio
E rosette
E selectin

E_0^+

oxidation-reduction potential

E_1

estrone

E_2

estradiol

E

entgegen

E_a

energy of activation

e

elementary charge

EAC

EAC rosette
EAC rosette assay

Eadie-Hofstee plot
EAE

experimental allergic encephalitis

Eagle

E. basal medium
E. minimum essential medium
(MEM)

Eagle-Barrett syndrome
EAHF complex
Eales disease
ear

Aztec e.
bat e.
bladder e.
Blainville e.
e. bone
boxer's e.
Cagot e.
e. canal
cauliflower e.
e. crystal
darwinian e.
dog e.
external e.
glue e.
inner e.
internal e.
e. lobe
e. lobe crease
lop e.
middle e.
Morel e.
Mozart e.
e.'s, nose, and throat (ENT)
outstanding e.
protruding e.
scroll e.
Stahl e.
swimmer's e.
telephone e.
e. wax
Wildermuth e.

earache
eardrum
Earle

E. L fibrosarcoma
E. solution

early

e. deceleration
e. diastolic murmur
e. discharge
e. dumping syndrome
e. infantile autism
e. latent syphilis
e. neonatal death
e. posttraumatic epilepsy
e. reaction
e. receptor potential (ERP)
e. seizure

early-phase response
earpiece
earplug
earth

alkaline e.
diatomaceous e.
fuller's e.
rare e.
e. wax

earthy water
earwax
east

E. African sleeping sickness
E. African trypanosomiasis

eastern

e. equine encephalomyelitis (EEE)
e. equine encephalomyelitis virus

eating

e. disorder
e. epilepsy

Eaton agent
Eaton-Lambert syndrome
E.B., EB

elementary body

Ebbinghaus test
Eberth

E. bacillus
E. line
E. perithelium

Ebner

E. gland
E. reticulum

Ebola

E. hemorrhagic fever
E. virus
E. virus Côte-d'Ivoire
E. virus Reston
E. virus Sudan
E. virus Zaire

ebonation
ébranlement
Ebstein

E. anomaly
E. disease
E. sign

E

EBT
electron beam tomography
ebullism
ebur dentis
eburnation of dentin
eburneous
eburnitis
EBV
Epstein-Barr virus
EB virus
EC
Enzyme Commission of the International
Union of Biochemistry
E-cadherin
écarteur
ecaudate
ecboline
eccentric
e. amputation
e. fixation
e. hypertrophy
e. implantation
e. interocclusal record
e. occlusion
e. position
e. relation
eccentrochondroplasia
eccentropiesis
ecchondroma
ecchondrosis
ecchordosis physaliphora
ecchymoma
ecchymosis
bilateral medial orbital e.
Tardieu e.
ecchymotic
eccrine
e. acrospiroma
e. gland
e. poroma
e. spiradenoma
eccrinology
eccrisis
eccritic
eccyesis
ecdemic
ecdysial gland
ecdysiasm
ecdysis
ecdysist
ECF
extracellular fluid
ECF-A
eosinophil chemotactic factor of
anaphylaxis
ECFV
extracellular fluid volume
ECG
electrocardiogram
ECG trigger
ecgonine
ecgonine e.
Echidnophaga gallinacea
echinate
Echinochasmus

echinococciasis
echinococcosis
Echinococcus
E. granulosus
E. multilocularis
E. vogeli
echinococcus
e. cyst
e. disease
echinocyte
echinoderm
Echinodermata
Echinorhynchus
echinosis
Echinostoma
E. ilocanum
E. malayanum
echinostomiasis
echinulate
Echis
echo
atrial e.
e. beat
navigator e.
nodus sinuatrialis e.
NS e.
e. planar
e. reaction
e. speech
spin e.
echoacousia
echoaortography
echocardiogram
echocardiographic differentiation
echocardiography
contrast e.
cross-sectional e.
Doppler e.
M-mode e.
real-time e.
sector e.
stress e.
transesophageal e.
transthoracic e.
two-dimensional e.
echoencephalography
echo-free
echogenic
echogram
echographer
echographia
echography
echolalia
echolocation
echomotism
echopathy
echophony, echophonia
echophrasia
echopraxia
echoscope
echothiophate iodide
ECHO virus, echovirus
Echovirus 28
Ecker fissure
Eck fistula

eclabium
eclampsia
    puerperal e.
    superimposed e.
eclamptic
eclamptogenic
eclectic
eclecticism
eclipse
    e. blindness
    e. period
    e. phase
ECMO virus
ecoendocrinology
ECoG
    electrocorticography
ecologic
    e. chemistry
    e. study
ecological
    e. ectocrine
    e. fallacy
    e. system
ecology
    human e.
    landscape e.
econazole
economic
    e. coefficient
    e. triage
economy
ecospecies
ecosystem
    parasite-host e.
ecotaxis
ecotropic virus
écouvillon
ECP
    eosinophil cationic protein
ecphyma
ECS
    electrocerebral silence
ECSO virus
ecstasy
ecstatic
ecstrophe
ECT
    electroconvulsive therapy
ectad
ectal origin
ectasia, ectasis
    annuloaortic e.
    aortoannular e.
    e. cordis
    corneal e.
    diffuse arterial e.
    familial aortic e.
    hypostatic e.
    mammary duct e.
    scleral e.
    e. ventriculi paradoxa
ectatic
    e. aneurysm
    e. emphysema
    e. marginal degeneration of cornea

ectental
ectethmoid
ecthyma
    contagious e.
    e. gangrenosum
ectiris
ectoantigen
ectoblast
ectocardia
ectocervical smear
ectochoroidea
ectocornea
ectocrine
    ecological e.
ectocyst
ectoderm
    amnionic e.
    chorionic e.
    epithelial e.
    extraembryonic e.
    superficial e.
ectodermal
    e. cloaca
    e. dysplasia
ectodermatosis
ectodermic
ectodermosis
ectoentad
ectoental
ectoenzyme
ectoethmoid
ectogenic teratosis
ectogenous
ectohormone
ectomere
ectomerogony
ectomesenchyme
ectomorph
ectomorphic
ectopagus
ectoparasite
ectoparasiticide
ectoparasitism
ectoperitonitis
ectophyte
ectopia
    e. cloacae
    e. cordis
    crossed renal e.
    crossed testicular e.
    e. lentis
    e. lentis et pupillae
    e. maculae
    e. pupillae congenita
    e. renis
    e. testis
    testis e.
    thoracoabdominal e. cordis
    ureteral e.
    e. vesicae
ectopic
    e. ACTH syndrome
    e. beat
    e. decidua
    e. eyelash

E

ectopic *(continued)*
  e. hormone
  e. impulse
  e. pacemaker
  e. pinealoma
  e. pregnancy
  e. rhythm
  e. schistosomiasis
  e. tachycardia
  e. teratosis
  e. testis
  e. ureter
  e. ureterocele
ectoplacental cavity
ectoplasm
ectoplasmatic, ektoplasmic, ektoplastic
ectopy
ectoretina
ectosarc
ectoscopy
ectosteal
ectostosis
ectothrix
ectotoxin
ectotrophoblastic cavity
ectozoon
ectrocheiry, ectrochiry
ectrodactyly, ectrodactylia, ectrodactylism
ectrodactyly–ectodermal dysplasia–clefting
  syndrome
ectrogenic
ectrogeny
ectromelia virus
ectromelic
ectropion, ectropium
  atonic e.
  cicatricial e.
  flaccid e.
  paralytic e.
  spastic e.
  e. uveae
ectropody
ectrosyndactyly
ectylurea
ectype
ecuresis
eczema
  allergic e.
  atopic e.
  baker's e.
  chronic e.
  dyshidrotic e.
  e. erythematosum
  flexural e.
  hand e.
  e. herpeticum
  infantile e.
  e. intertrigo
  lichenoid e.
  nummular e.
  e. papulosum
  e. parasiticum
  e. pustulosum
  seborrheic e.

  stasis e.
  tropical e.
  e. tyloticum
  varicose e.
  e. verrucosum
  e. vesiculosum
  weeping e.
  winter e.
eczematization
eczematoid seborrhea
eczematous
ED
  effective dose
ED$_{50}$
  median effective dose
edathamil
EDC
  estimated date of confinement
eddy sound
edea
edema
  ambulatory e.
  angioneurotic e.
  Berlin e.
  blue e.
  brain e.
  brawny e.
  brown e.
  bullous e.
  bullous e. vesicae
  cachectic e.
  cardiac e.
  cerebral e.
  cystoid macular e.
  dependent e.
  gestational e.
  e. glottidis
  heat e.
  hereditary angioneurotic e. (HANE)
  hydremic e.
  infantile acute hemorrhagic e. of
    the skin
  inflammatory e.
  lymphatic e.
  marantic e.
  menstrual e.
  e. neonatorum
  nephrotic e.
  noninflammatory e.
  nonpitting e.
  nutritional e.
  periodic e.
  pitting e.
  premenstrual e.
  pulmonary e.
  salt e.
  solid e.
  Yangtze e.
edematization
edematous
edentate
edentulous
Eder-Pustow bougie
edestin
edetate calcium disodium

edetic acid
edge
    cutting e.
    denture e.
    e. enhancement
    incisal e.
    leading e.
    shearing e.
edge-to-edge
    e.-t.-e. bite
    e.-t.-e. occlusion
edgewise appliance
Edinger-Westphal nucleus
edisylate
Edlefsen reagent
EDM
    multiple epiphyseal dysplasia
Edman
    E. method
    E. reagent
EDRF
    endothelium-derived relaxing factor
Edridge-Green lamp
edrophonium chloride
EDS
    Ehlers-Danlos syndrome
EDSS
    expanded disability status scale
EDTA
    ethylenediaminetetraacetic acid
educational psychology
educt
edulcorant
edulcorate
Edwardsiella
Edwards syndrome
EEE
    eastern equine encephalomyelitis
    EEE virus
EEG
    electroencephalogram
    EEG activation
eel
    vinegar e.
EENT
    eye, ear, nose, and throat
effacement
effect
    abscopal e.
    additive e.
    after-e.
    Anrep e.
    Arias-Stella e.
    autokinetic e.
    Bernoulli e.
    Bohr e.
    Bowditch e.
    Circe e.
    clasp-knife e.
    Compton e.
    Cotton e.
    Crabtree e.
    cumulative e.
    Cushing e.
    cytopathic e.

    Doppler e.
    electrophonic e.
    experimenter e.
    Fahraeus-Lindqvist e.
    Fenn e.
    first-pass e.
    flash-lag e.
    founder e.
    gene dosage e.
    generation e.
    Haldane e.
    halo e.
    Hawthorne e.
    healthy worker e.
    hyperchromic e.
    hypochromic e.
    Mach e.
    e. modifier
    nuclear Overhauser e. (NOE)
    Orbeli e.
    oxygen e.
    Pasteur e.
    photechic e.
    photoelectric e.
    piezoelectric e.
    position e.
    Purkinje e.
    quantal e.
    Raman e.
    Rivero-Carvallo e.
    Russell e.
    second gas e.
    sigma e.
    Somogyi e.
    Staub-Traugott e.
    Stiles-Crawford e.
    synergistic e.
    Tyndall e.
    Venturi e.
    Wedensky e.
    Wolff-Chaikoff e.
    Zeeman e.
effective
    e. conjugate
    e. dose (ED)
    e. half-life
    e. osmotic pressure
    e. refractory period
    e. renal blood flow (ERBF)
    e. renal plasma flow (ERPF)
    e. stroke
    e. temperature
    e. temperature index
effectiveness
    relative biologic e.
effector cell
effemination
efferent
    e. duct
    e. ductule of testis
    e. fiber
    gamma e.
    e. glomerular arteriole
    e. lymphatic

E

efferent *(continued)*
    e. nerve
    e. vessel
effervesce
effervescent
    e. lithium citrate
    e. magnesium citrate
    e. magnesium sulfate
    e. potassium citrate
    e. salt
    e. sodium phosphate
efficacy
efficiency
    quantum e.
    visual e.
effleurage
effloresce
efflorescent
effluvium, pl. **effluvia**
    anagen e.
    telogen e.
effort
    distributed e.
effort-induced thrombosis
effuse
effusion
    complex pleural e.
    joint e.
    loculated pleural e.
    middle-ear e.
    parapneumonic e.
    pericardial e.
    pleural e.
    subpulmonic e.
eflornithine hydrochloride
EGD
    esophagogastroduodenoscopy
egesta
EGF
    epidermal growth factor
EGFR
    epidermal growth factor receptor
egg
    e. albumin
    e. cell
    centrolecithal e.
    e. cluster
    homolecithal e.
    isolecithal e.
    e. membrane
    microlecithal e.
    e. shell nail
    telolecithal e.
Egger line
Eggleston method
eggshell calcification
egg-white
    e.-w. injury
    e.-w. syndrome
eglandulous
Eglis gland
ego
    e. analysis
    e. ideal

    e. identity
    e. instincts
ego-alien
egobronchophony
egocentric
egocentricity
ego-dystonic homosexuality
ego-ideal
egomania
egophonic
egophony
ego-syntonic
egotropic
EGTA
    ethyleneglycotetraacetic acid
Egyptian
    E. hematuria
    E. ophthalmia
    E. splenomegaly
EHEC
    enterohemorrhagic escherichia coli
Ehlers-Danlos syndrome (EDS)
Ehrenritter ganglion
Ehret phenomenon
Ehrlich
    E. acid hematoxylin stain
    E. anemia
    E. aniline crystal violet stain
    E. benzaldehyde reaction
    E. diazo reaction
    E. diazo reagent
    E. inner body
    E. phenomenon
    E. postulate
    E. theory
    E. triacid stain
    E. triple stain
Ehrlichia
    E. canis
    E. chaffeensis
    E. equi
    E. phagocytophila
    E. risticii
    E. sennetsu
Ehrlichieae
ehrlichiosis
    human e.
    human granulocytic e. (HGE)
    human monocytic e. (HME)
Ehrlich-Türk line
Eichhorst
    E. corpuscle
    E. neuritis
Eicken method
***n*-eicosanoic acid**
eicosanoid
9-eicosenoic acid
eidetic image
EIEC
    enteroinvasive escherichia coli
eighth
    e. cranial nerve [CN VIII]
    e. nerve tumor
Eikenella corrodens
eikonometer

eiloid
Eimeriidae
Einarson gallocyanin-chrome alum stain
einstein
einsteinium (Es)
Einthoven
    E. equation
    E. law
    E. string galvanometer
    E. triangle
Eisenmenger
    E. complex
    E. defect
    E. disease
    E. syndrome
    E. tetralogy
eisodic
ejaculate
ejaculation
    premature e.
    retrograde e.
ejaculatory duct
ejecta
ejection
    e. click
    e. fraction
    e. murmur
    e. period
    e. sound
ejector
    saliva e.
EJP
    excitatory junction potential
Ejrup maneuver
Ekbom syndrome
EKG
    electrocardiogram
    EKG trigger
ekiri
ektoplasmic (*var. of* ectoplasmatic)
ektoplastic (*var. of* ectoplasmatic)
EKY
    electrokymogram
elaboration
    secondary e.
Elaeophora schneideri
elaidic acid
elaiopathia
E-LAM
    endothelial-leukocyte adhesion molecule
elapid
Elapidae
elastance
elastase
elastic
    e. artery
    e. bandage
    e. band fixation
    e. bougie
    e. cartilage
    e. cone
    e. fiber
    intermaxillary e.
    e. lamella
    e. laminae of artery

    e. layer of artery
    e. layer of cornea
    e. ligature
    e. limit
    e. membrane
    e. skin
    e. tissue
    vertical e.
elastica
elasticin
elasticity
    physical e. of muscle
    physiologic e. of muscle
    total e. of muscle
elastin
elastofibroma
elastoid degeneration
elastoidin
elastolysis
    generalized e.
elastoma
    juvenile e.
    Miescher e.
elastometer
elastomucin
elastorrhexis
elastosis
    e. colloidalis conglomerata
    e. dystrophica
    e. perforans serpiginosa
    solar e.
elastotic degeneration
elation
elaunin
Elaut triangle
elbow
    e. bone
    e. jerk
    e. joint
    little league e.
    Little Leaguer's e.
    miner's e.
    nursemaid's e.
    e. reflex
    tennis e.
elbowed
    e. bougie
    e. catheter
elder abuse
elder flowers
elderly primigravida
elective
    e. abortion
    e. culture
    e. mutism
Electra complex
electric
    e. anesthesia
    e. bath
    e. cardiac pacemaker
    e. cataract
    e. cautery
    e. chorea
    e. irritability
    e. retinopathy

E

electric *(continued)*
    e. shock
    e. sleep
electrical
    e. alternans
    e. alternation of heart
    e. axis
    e. diastole
    e. failure
    e. formula
    e. heart position
    e. systole
electroanalgesia
electroanalysis
electroanesthesia
electroaxonography
electrobioscopy
electrocardiogram (ECG, EKG)
    concordant changes e.
    discordant changes e.
    scalar e.
    unipolar e.
electrocardiograph
electrocardiographic
    e. complex
    e. wave
electrocardiography
    fetal e.
    precordial e.
electrocardiophonogram
electrocardiophonography
electrocauterization
electrocautery
electrocerebral inactivity
electrocerebral silence (ECS)
electrochemical gradient
electrocoagulation
electrocochleogram
electrocochleography
electrocontractility
electroconvulsive therapy (ECT)
electrocorticogram
electrocorticography (ECoG)
electrocute
electrocution
electrocystography
electrode
    active e.
    calomel e.
    carbon dioxide e.
    e. catheter ablation
    central terminal e.
    Clark e.
    dispersing e.
    exciting e.
    exploring e.
    glass e.
    hydrogen e.
    indifferent e.
    ion-selective e.
    e. knife
    localizing e.
    negative e.
    oxidation-reduction e.

    oxygen e.
    positive e.
    quinhydrone e.
    redox e.
    reference e.
    resectoscope e.
    rollerball e.
    Severinghaus e.
    silent e.
    therapeutic e.
electrodermal
electrodesiccation
electrodiagnosis
electrodiagnostic medicine
electrodialysis
electroencephalogram (EEG)
    flat e.
    isoelectric e.
electroencephalograph
electroencephalographic dysrhythmia
electroencephalography
electroendosmosis
electrofocusing
electrogastrogram
electrogastrograph
electrogastrography
electrogram
    His bundle e. (HBE, HB_eAg)
electrographic seizure
electrohemostasis
electrohydraulic shock wave lithotripsy
electrohysterograph
electroimmunodiffusion
electrokymogram (EKY)
electrokymograph
electrolysis
electrolyte
    amphoteric e.
    e. metabolism
electrolytic
electrolyze
electrolyzer
electromagnet
electromagnetic
    e. flowmeter
    e. induction
    e. radiation
    e. unit (emu)
electromassage
electromechanical
    e. dissociation
    e. systole
electromicturation
electromorph
electromotility
electromotive force (EMF)
electromuscular sensibility
electromyogram (EMG)
electromyograph
electromyography
    evoked e.
electron
    Auger e.
    e. beam
    e. beam tomography (EBT)

e. capture
conversion e.
emission e.
e. interferometer
e. interferometry
internal conversion e.
e. magneton
e. micrograph
e. microscope
e. microscopy
e. paramagnetic resonance (EPR)
positive e.
e. radiography
e. resonance absorption
e. spin resonance
e. transfer flavin
transition e.
e. transport particle (ETP)
valence e.

electronarcosis
electronegative element
electroneurography
electroneurolysis
electroneuromyography
electronic

e. cell counter
e. fetal monitor
e. number
e. pacemaker
e. pacemaker load

electron-transport

e.-t. chain
e.-t. system

electron-volt (eV)

one million e.-v.'s (Mev)

electronystagmography (ENG)
electrooculogram
electrooculography (EOG)
electroolfactogram
electroosmosis
electroparacentesis
electropherogram
electrophil, electrophile
electrophilic
electrophobia
electrophonic effect
electrophoresis

capillary zone e. (CZE)
carrier e.
disk e.
free e.
gel e.
isoenzyme e.
lipoprotein e.
polyacrylamide gel e. (PAGE)
pulsed-field gel e.
thin-layer e. (TLE)

electrophoretic
electrophoretogram
electrophrenic respiration
electrophysiology
electroporation
electropositive element
electropuncture
electroradiology

electroradiometer
electroretinogram (ERG)
electroretinography
electroscission
electroscope
electroshock therapy
electrosol
electrospectrography
electrospinogram
electrospinography
electrostatic

e. bond
e. unit (esu)

electrostenolysis
electrostethograph
electrostriction
electrosurgery
electrotaxis

negative e.
positive e.

electrothanasia
electrotherapeutic

e. bath
e. sleep
e. sleep therapy

electrotherapeutics, electrotherapy
electrotherm
electrotome
electrotomy
electrotonic

e. current
e. junction
e. synapse

electrotonus
electrotropism
electuary
eledoisin
eleidin
element

actinide e.
alkaline earth e.
amphoteric e.
anatomical e.
copia e.
electronegative e.
electropositive e.
extrachromosomal e.
extrachromosomal genetic e.
fold-back e.
labile e.
long interspersed e. (LINES)
morphologic e.
neutral e.
noble e.
P e.
picture e.
rare earth e.
short interspersed e. (SINES)
trace e.
transposable e.
volume e.

elementary

e. body (E.B., EB)
e. charge (e)

E

elementary *(continued)*
    e. granule
    e. particle
eleoma
eleometer
eleopathy
eleostearic acid
eleotherapy
elephant
    e. leg
    e. man's disease
elephantiasis
    congenital e.
    gingival e.
    e. neuromatosa
    e. scroti
    e. telangiectodes
    e. vulvae
elephantoid fever
elevation
    e. of levator palati
    tactile e.
elevator
    e. disease
    e. muscle of anus
    e. muscle of prostate
    e. muscle of rib
    e. muscle of scapula
    e. muscle of soft palate
    e. muscle of thyroid gland
    e. muscle of upper eyelid
    e. muscle of upper lip
    e. muscle of upper lip and wing
      of nose
    periosteal e.
    screw e.
eleventh cranial nerve [CN XI]
elfin
    e. facies
    e. facies syndrome
eliminant
elimination
    carbon dioxide e. ($\dot{V}_{CO2}$)
    e. diet
elinguation
elinin
ELISA
    enzyme-linked immunosorbent assay
elixir
    phenobarbital e.
Ellik evacuator
Elliot
    E. operation
    E. position
Elliott law
ellipsis
ellipsoid
ellipsoidal joint
elliptical
    e. amputation
    e. anastomosis
    e. recess of bony labyrinth
elliptocytary anemia
elliptocytosis

elliptocytotic anemia
Ellis-van Creveld syndrome
Ellsworth-Howard test
Eloesser
    E. flap
    E. procedure
elongation factor
Elschnig
    E. pearl
    E. spot
El Tor vibrio
eluant
eluate
eluent
elusive ulcer
elutant
elute
elution
    gradient e.
elutriate
elutriation
EMA
    epithelial membrane antigen
emaciation
emaculation
emanation
    actinium e.
    radium e.
    thorium e.
emanatorium
emancipation
emanon
emanotherapy
emarginate
emargination
emasculation
EMB
    eosin-methylene blue
Embadomonas
EMB agar
embalm
Embden ester
Embden-Meyerhof-Parnas pathway
Embden-Meyerhof pathway
embed
embedding agent
embelin
emboitement
embole
embolectomy
embolemia
emboli (*pl. of* embolus)
embolia
embolic
    e. abscess
    e. gangrene
    e. infarct
    e. pneumonia
emboliform nucleus
embolism
    air e.
    amnionic fluid e.
    atheromatous e.
    bland e.
    bone marrow e.

cellular e.
cholesterol e.
cotton-fiber e.
crossed e.
direct e.
fat e.
gas e.
hematogenous e.
infective e.
lymph e.
lymphogenous e.
miliary e.
multiple e.
obturating e.
oil e.
paradoxical e.
pulmonary e.
pyemic e.
retinal e.
retrograde e.
riding e.
saddle e.
straddling e.
tumor e.
venous e.
embolization
embolomycotic
embolotherapy
embolus, pl. **emboli**
catheter e.
emboly
embouchement
embrasure
buccal e.
gingival e.
incisal e.
labial e.
lingual e.
occlusal e.
embrocation
embryo
heterogametic e.
hexacanth e.
homogametic e.
oncosphere e.
presomite e.
previllous e.
e. transfer
embryoblast
embryocardia
embryogenesis
embryogenic, embryogenetic
embryogeny
embryoid
embryologist
embryology
embryoma
embryomorphous
embryonal
e. adenoma
e. area
e. carcinoma
e. inducer
e. leukemia
e. medulloepithelioma

e. rhabdomyosarcoma
e. tumor
e. tumor of ciliary body
embryonate
embryonic
e. anideus
e. area
e. axis
e. blastoderm
e. cataract
e. cell
e. circulation
e. diapause
e. disk
e. hemoglobin
e. membrane
e. shield
e. tumor
embryoniform
embryonization
embryonoid
embryony
embryopathic cataract
embryopathy
embryophore
embryoplastic
embryotomy
embryotoxicity
embryotoxon
anterior e.
posterior e.
embryotroph
embryotrophic
embryotrophy
EMC virus
emedullate
emeiocytosis
emergence
property e.
emergency
e. hormonal contraception
e. theory
emergent evolution
emerging virus
emery disk
Emery-Dreifuss muscular dystrophy
emesis basin
emetic
emetine
emetocathartic
emetogenic
emetogenicity
EMF
electromotive force
EMG
electromyogram
EMG biofeedback
EMG examination
EMG syndrome
emiction
emigration
eminence
abducens e.
arcuate e.
articular e. of temporal bone

E

eminence *(continued)*
    canine e.
    collateral e.
    e. of concha
    cruciate e.
    cruciform e.
    deltoid e.
    Doyère e.
    facial e.
    forebrain e.
    frontal e.
    genital e.
    hypobranchial e.
    hypoglossal e.
    hypothenar e.
    ileocecal e.
    iliopectineal e.
    iliopubic e.
    intercondylar e.
    maxillary e.
    medial e.
    median e.
    olivary e.
    omental e. of pancreas
    orbital e. of zygomatic bone
    parietal e.
    pyramidal e.
    radial e. of wrist
    restiform e.
    round e.
    e. of scapha
    thenar e.
    thyroid e.
    e. of triangular fossa of auricle
    ulnar e. of wrist
eminentia, pl. **eminentiae**
    e. abducentis
    e. arcuata
    e. articularis ossis temporalis
    e. carpi radialis
    e. carpi ulnaris
    e. collateralis
    e. conchae
    e. cruciformis
    e. facialis
    e. fossae triangularis auricularis
    e. frontalis
    e. hypoglossi
    e. hypothena'ris
    e. iliopubica
    e. intercondylaris
    e. intercondyloidea
    e. maxillae
    e. medialis
    e. mediana
    e. orbitalis (ossis zygomatici)
    e. parietalis
    e. pyramidalis
    e. restiformis
    e. scaphae
    e. symphysis
    e. teres
    e. thena'ris

    e. triangularis
    vagi e.
emiocytosis
EMI scan
emissarium
    e. condyloideum
    e. mastoideum
    e. occipitale
    e. parietale
emissary vein
emission
    characteristic e.
    continuous otoacoustic e.
    distortion-product otoacoustic e.
    e. electron
    evoked otoacoustic e.
    nocturnal e.
    otoacoustic e.
    transient evoked otoacoustic e.
emissivity
EMIT
    enzyme-multiplied immunoassay
    technique
Emmet
    E. needle
    E. operation
emmetropia
emmetropic
emmetropization
Emmonsia
    E. parva var. crescens
    E. parva var. parva
Emmonsiella capsulata
emodin
emollient
emotion
emotional
    e. age
    e. amenorrhea
    e. amnesia
    e. attitudes
    e. deprivation
    e. disease
    e. disorder
    e. disturbance
    e. leukocytosis
    e. overlay
    e. tone
emotiovascular
empasm, empasma
empathic index
empathize
empathy
    generative e.
emperipolesis
emphraxis
emphysema
    alveolar duct e.
    bullous e.
    centriacinar e.
    centrilobular e.
    compensating e.
    compensatory e.
    congenital lobar e.
    cutaneous e.

diffuse obstructive e.
ectatic e.
familial e.
gangrenous e.
generalized e.
increased markings e.
interlobular e.
interstitial e.
intestinal e.
irregular e.
mediastinal e.
panacinar e.
panlobular e.
paracicatricial e.
paraseptal e.
pulmonary e.
scar e.
senile e.
subcutaneous e.
subgaleal e.
surgical e.
unilateral lobar e.
emphysematous
e. cholecystitis
e. cystitis
e. gangrene
empiric
e. risk
e. treatment
empirical
e. formula
e. horopter
empiricism
emporiatrics
emprosthotonos
empty sella
empyectomy
empyema
e. benignum
e. of gallbladder
latent e.
loculated e.
mastoid e.
e. necessitatis
e. of the pericardium
pneumococcal e.
pulsating e.
streptococcal e.
e. tube
empyemic scoliosis
empyesis
empyocele
empyreuma
E-M syndrome
emu
electromagnetic unit
emulgent
emulsifier
emulsify
emulsifying wax
emulsin
emulsion colloid
emulsive
emulsoid
emuresis

emylcamate
enalaprilat
enalapril maleate
enamel
e. cap
e. cell
e. cleavage
e. cleaver
e. crypt
e. cuticle
e. drop
dwarfed e.
e. dysplasia
e. epithelium
e. fiber
e. fissure
e. germ
e. hypocalcification
e. hypoplasia
interrod e.
e. lamella
e. layer
e. ledge
e. membrane
mottled e.
nanoid e.
e. niche
e. nodule
e. organ
e. pearl
e. prism
e. projection
e. pulp
e. rod
e. rod inclination
e. rod sheath
e. tuft
e. wall
whorled e.
enamelins
enameloblast
enamelogenesis imperfecta
enameloma
enamelum
enanthal
enanthate
enanthem, enanthema
enantiomer
enantiomeric
enantiomerism
enantiomorph
enantiomorphic
enantiomorphism
enantiomorphous
enarthrodial joint
enarthrosis
en bloc
encainide hydrochloride
encapsulated delusion
encapsulation
encapsuled
encarditis
encelitis, enceliitis
encephala (*pl. of* encephalon)
encephalalgia

E

encéphale isolé
encephalemia
encephalic vesicle
encephalithogenic protein
encephalitic
encephalitis, pl. encephalitides
    acute hemorrhagic e.
    acute inclusion body e.
    acute necrotizing e.
    Australian X e.
    bacterial e.
    bunyavirus e.
    California e.
    coxsackie e.
    Dawson e.
    epidemic e.
    equine e.
    experimental allergic e. (EAE)
    Far East Russian e.
    e. hemorrhagica
    herpes e.
    herpes simplex e.
    hyperergic e.
    Ilhéus e.
    inclusion body e.
    Japanese B e.
    e. japonica
    lead e.
    e. lethargica
    Mengo e.
    Murray Valley e.
    necrotizing e.
    e. neonatorum
    e. periaxialis concentrica
    e. periaxialis diffusa
    postvaccinal e.
    Powassan e.
    purulent e.
    e. pyogenica
    rasmussen e.
    Russian autumn e.
    Russian spring-summer e., Eastern subtype
    Russian spring-summer e., Western subtype
    Russian tick-borne e.
    secondary e.
    subacute inclusion body e.
    e. subcorticalis chronica
    suppurative e.
    tick-borne e. (Central European subtype)
    tick-borne e. (Eastern subtype)
    van Bogaert e.
    varicella e.
    vernal e.
    e. virus
    woodcutter's e.
encephalitogen
encephalitogenic
Encephalitozoon
    E. cuniculi
    E. hellem
    E. intestinale
    E. intestinalis

encephalization
encephalocele
    basal e.
encephaloclastic microcephaly
encephalocraniocutaneous lipomatosis
encephalocystocele
encephaloduroarteriosynangiosis
encephalodynia
encephalodysplasia
encephalogram
encephalography
    gamma e.
encephaloid
encephalolith
encephalology
encephaloma
encephalomalacia
encephalomeningitis
encephalomeningocele
encephalomeningopathy
encephalomere
encephalometer
encephalomyelitis
    acute disseminated e.
    acute necrotizing hemorrhagic e.
    e. associated with carcinoma
    benign myalgic e.
    eastern equine e. (EEE)
    epidemic myalgic e.
    equine e.
    experimental allergic e.
    granulomatous e.
    herpes B e.
    mouse e.
    postvaccinal e.
    Venezuelan equine e. (VEE)
    viral e.
    virus e.
    western equine e. (WEE)
    zoster e.
encephalomyelocele
encephalomyeloneuropathy
encephalomyelonic axis
encephalomyelopathy
    carcinomatous e.
    epidemic myalgic e.
    necrotizing e.
    paracarcinomatous e.
    paraneoplastic e.
    subacute necrotizing e. (SNE)
encephalomyeloradiculitis
encephalomyeloradiculopathy
encephalomyocarditis virus
encephalon, pl. encephala
encephalopathia
encephalopathy
    bilirubin e.
    Binswanger e.
    bovine spongiform e. (BSE)
    demyelinating e.
    hepatic e.
    HIV e.
    hypernatremic e.
    hypertensive e.
    hypoxic-hypercarbic e.

hypoxic ischemic e.
lead e.
metabolic e.
necrotizing e.
palindromic e.
pancreatic e.
portal-systemic e.
progressive subcortical e.
pulmonary e.
recurrent e.
saturnine e.
severe postanoxic e.
spongiform e.
subacute spongiform e.
subcortical arteriosclerotic e.
thyrotoxic e.
traumatic progressive e.
Wernicke e.
Wernicke-Korsakoff e.
encephalopyosis
encephalorrhachidian
encephaloschisis
encephalosclerosis
encephaloscope
encephaloscopy
encephalosis
encephalospinal
encephalotome
encephalotomy
encephalotrigeminal
e. angiomatosis
e. vascular syndrome
enchondral
enchondroma
enchondromatosis
enchondromatous
enclave
encoding
encopresis
encounter group
encranial
encranius
encu method
encysted
e. calculus
e. pleurisy
encystment
end
acromial e. of clavicle
e. artery
e. bud
e. bulb
e. cell
distal e.
fixed e.
mobile e.
e. organ
e. oxidation
e. piece
e. plate
e. point
e. product
e. product inhibition
e. product repression

e. stage
sternal e. of clavicle
endadelphos
Endamoeba
endangiitis, endangeitis
e. obliterans
endaortitis
endarterectomy
carotid e.
coronary e.
endarteritis
bacterial e.
e. deformans
e. obliterans
obliterating e.
e. proliferans
proliferating e.
endaural incision
endbrain
end-brush
end-bulb
end-cutting bur
end-diastolic volume
endectocide
endemia
endemic
e. disease
e. funiculitis
e. goiter
e. hematuria
e. hemoptysis
e. hypertrophy
e. index
e. influenza
e. neuritis
e. nonbacterial infantile
gastroenteritis
e. paralytic vertigo
e. stability
e. syphilis
e. typhus
endemoepidemic
endergonic
endermic, endermatic
endermosis
end-feet
endgut
ending
annulospiral e.
caliciform e.
calyciform e.
epilemmal e.
flower-spray e.
free nerve e.
grape e.
hederiform e.
nerve e.
sole-plate e.
synaptic e.
Endo
E. agar
E. medium
endoabdominal fascia
endoamylase
endoaneurysmoplasty

E

endoaneurysmorrhaphy
endoangiitis
endo-aortitis
endoappendicitis
endoarteritis
endoauscultation
endobag
endobasion
endobiotic
endobronchial tube
endocardia (*pl. of* endocardium)
endocardial, endocardiac
    e. cushion
    e. cushion defect
    e. fibroelastosis
    e. fibrosis
    e. murmur
    e. sclerosis
endocardiography
endocarditic
endocarditis
    abacterial thrombotic e.
    acute bacterial e.
    atypical verrucous e.
    bacterial e.
    cachectic e.
    e. chordalis
    constrictive e.
    infectious e.
    infective e.
    isolated parietal e.
    Libman-Sacks e.
    Löffler parietal fibroplastic e.
    malignant e.
    marantic e.
    mural e.
    mycotic e.
    nonbacterial thrombotic e.
    nonbacterial verrucous e.
    polypous e.
    rheumatic e.
    septic e.
    subacute bacterial e. (SBE)
    terminal e.
    valvular e.
    vegetative e.
    verrucous e.
endocardium, pl. endocardia
endoceliac
endocervical
    e. sinus tumor
    e. smear
endocervicitis
endocervix
endochondral
    e. bone
    e. ossification
endocoagulation
endocochlear potential
endocolitis
endocranial
endocranium
endocrine
    e. exophthalmos
    e. gland

    e. hormone
    e. ophthalmopathy
    e. part of pancreas
    e. system
endocrinologist
endocrinology
endocrinoma
endocrinopathic
endocrinopathy
endocrinotherapy
endocyclic
endocyst
endocystitis
endocytosis
endoderm
endodermal
    e. canal
    e. cell
    e. cloaca
    e. cyst
    e. pouch
    e. sinus tumor
endodiascope
endodiascopy
endodontia
endodontic
    e. stabilizer
    e. treatment
endodontics
endodontist
endodontologist
endodontology
endodyocyte
endodyogeny
endoenteritis
endoenzyme
endoesophagitis
endofaradism
end-of-life care
endogalvanism
endogamy
endogastric
endogastritis
endogenic toxicosis
endogenote
endogenous
    e. creatinine clearance
    e. cycle
    e. depression
    e. fiber
    e. hyperglyceridemia
    e. infection
    e. pyrogen (EP)
endoglin
endognathion
endoherniotomy
endointoxication
endolaryngeal
endolemniscal nucleus
Endolimax
endolith
endolymph
endolympha
endolymphatic
    e. duct

e. hydrops
e. sac
e. sac surgery
e. shunt operation
e. space
endolymphic
endomembrane system
endomerogony
endometria (*pl. of* endometrium)
endometrial
e. ablation
e. canal
e. cyst
e. hyperplasia
e. implant
e. smear
e. stromal sarcoma
endometrioid
e. carcinoma
e. tumor
endometrioma
endometriosis
endometritis
decidual e.
e. dissecans
endometrium, pl. endometria
Swiss cheese e.
endometropic
endomitosis
endomorph
endomorphic
endomotorsonde
Endomycetales
endomyocardial
endomyocardial fibroelastosis
e. fibrosis
endomyocarditis
endomyometritis
endomysium
endoneurium
end-on mattress suture
endonuclease
micrococcal e.
nucleate e.
restriction e.
e. S_1 *Aspergillus*
e. *Serratia marcescens*
single-stranded nucleate e.
spleen e.
endonucleolus
endo-osseous implant
endoparasite
endopeduncular nucleus
endopelvic fascia
endopeptidase
endoperiarteritis
endopericardiac
endoperimyocarditis
endoperitonitis
endoperoxide
endophlebitis
endophthalmitis
granulomatous e.
e. ophthalmia nodosa
e. phacoanaphylactica

endophthalmodonesis
endophyte
endophytic
endoplasm
endoplasmic reticulum (ER)
endoplast
endoplastic
endopolygeny
endopolyploid
endopolyploidy
endorectal pull-through procedure
endoreduplication
endorphin
endorphinergic
endorrhachis
endosac
endosalpingiosis
endosalpingitis
endosalpinx
endosarc
endoscope
flexible e.
endoscopic
e. biopsy
e. retrograde cholangiopancreatography (ERCP)
endoscopist
endoscopy
peroral e.
virtual e.
endoskeleton
endosome
endosonography
endosonoscopy
endosperm
endospore
endosseous implant
endosteal implant
endosteitis, endostitis
endosteoma
endostethoscope
endosteum
endostitis (*var. of* endosteitis)
endostoma
endotendineum
endoteric bacterium
endothelia (*pl. of* endothelium)
endothelial
e. cell
e. cyst
e. leukocyte
e. myeloma
e. relaxing factor
endothelial-leukocyte adhesion molecule (E-LAM)
endothelin
endotheliochorial placenta
endotheliocyte
endothelio-endothelial placenta
endothelioid
endothelioma
endotheliosis
endothelium, pl. endothelia
e. of anterior chamber

E

endothelium *(continued)*
  e. camerae anterioris
  e. posterius corneae
endothelium-derived relaxing factor (EDRF)
endothermic
endothoracic fascia
endothrix
endotoxemia
endotoxic
endotoxicosis
endotoxin shock
endotracheal
  e. anesthesia
  e. intubation
  e. stylet
  e. tube
endourology
endovaccination
endovaginal ultrasonography
endovasculitis
  hemorrhagic e.
endovenous septum
endpiece
endplate, end-plate
  motor e.
end-point
  e.-p. measurement
  e.-p. nystagmus
endstage lung
end-systolic volume
end-tidal
  e.-t. sample
end-to-end
  e.-t.-e. anastomosis
  e.-t.-e. bite
  e.-t.-e. occlusion
endyma
E.N.E.
  ethylnorepinephrine
enediol
enema
  air contrast e.
  air contrast barium e.
  analeptic e.
  barium e.
  blind e.
  contrast e.
  double contrast e.
  flatus e.
  high e.
  Hypaque e.
  nutrient e.
  oil retention e.
  small bowel e.
  soapsuds e.
  turpentine e.
enemator
enemiasis
energetics
energy
  e. of activation (E_a)
  binding e.
  chemical e.

free e.
fusion e.
Gibbs e. of activation
Gibbs free e.
Helmholtz e.
internal e. (U)
kinetic e.
latent e.
e. metabolism
nuclear e.
nutritional e.
e. of position
potential e.
psychic e.
radiant e.
solar e.
e. subtraction
total e.
energy-rich
  e.-r. bond
  e.-r. phosphate
enflurane
ENG
  electronystagmography
engagement
engastrius
Engelmann
  E. basal knob
  E. disease
engine
  dental e.
  e. reamer
engineering
  biomedical e.
  dental e.
  genetic e.
Englisch sinus
English
  E. lock
  E. position
  E. sweating disease
englobe
englobement
engorged
engorgement
engram
engraphia
en grappe
enhancement
  acoustic e.
  contrast e.
  edge e.
  immunologic e.
  ring e.
enhancers
enkephalin
enkephalinergic
enlargement
  cervical e.
  cervical e. of spinal cord
  choroid e.
  gingival e.
  lumbosacral e.
  lumbosacral e. of spinal cord

tympanic e.
e. of the vestibular aqueduct
enol
enolase
neuron-specific e.
enolization
enol **pyruvate**
enophthalmia
enophthalmos
enorganic
enostosis
enoyl-ACP reductase (NADPH)
enoyl-CoA
e.-c. hydratase
e.-c. reductase
2-enoyl-CoA reductase
enoyl hydrase
enrichment culture
E.N.S.
ethylnorepinephrine
ensheathing callus
ensiform
e. cartilage
e. process
ensisternum cartilage
ensu method
ENT
ears, nose, and throat
entactin
entad
ental origin
entamebiasis
Entamoeba
E. *buccalis*
E. *chattoni*
E. *coli*
E. *dispar*
E. *gingivalis*
E. *hartmanni*
E. *histolytica*
E. *moshkovskii*
E. *polecki*
enteralgia
enteral hyperalimentation
enteramine
enterdynia
enterectasis
enterectomy
enterelcosis
enteric
e. coated tablet
e. cytopathogenic human orphan
virus
e. cytopathogenic monkey orphan
virus
e. cytopathogenic swine orphan
virus
e. fever
e. orphan viruses
e. plexus
e. tuberculosis
e. viruses
entericoid fever
enteritis
e. anaphylactica

chronic cicatrizing e.
diphtherial e.
granulomatous e.
human eosinophilic e.
mucomembranous e.
e. necroticans
phlegmonous e.
e. polyposa
pseudomembranous e.
regional e.
tuberculous e.
enteroanastomosis
enteroanthelone
Enterobacter
E. *aerogenes*
E. *cloacae*
E. *sakazakii*
Enterobacteriaceae
enterobacterium, pl. **enterobacteria**
enterobiasis
Enterobius **granuloma**
enterocele
partial e.
enterocentesis
enterocholecystostomy
enterocholecystotomy
enterochromaffin cell
enterocidal
enterocleisis
omental e.
enteroclysis
radiologic e.
enterococcemia
Enterococcus
E. *faecalis*
E. *faecium*
enterococcus, pl. **enterococci**
enterocolitis
antibiotic e.
necrotizing e.
pseudomembranous e.
regional e.
enterocolostomy
enterocutaneous fistula
enterocyst
enterocystocele
enterocystoma
enterocyte cobalamin malabsorption
Enterocytozoon
E. *bieneusi*
enterodynia
enteroendocrine cell
enteroenterostomy
enterogastric reflex
enterogastritis
enterogastrone
enterogenous
e. cyanosis
e. cyst
e. methemoglobinemia
enterograph
enterography
enterohemorrhagic *Escherichia coli*
(EHEC)
enterohepatic circulation

E

enterohepatitis
enterohepatocele
enteroidea
enteroinvasive *Escherichia coli* (EIEC)
enterokinase
enterokinesis
enterokinetic agent
enterolith
enterolithiasis
enterology
enterolysis
enteromegaly, enteromegalia
enteromenia
enteromerocele
enterometer
Enteromonas
enteromycosis
enteroparesis
enteropathic arthritis
enteropathogen
enteropathogenic *Escherichia coli*
enteropathy
    gluten e.
    protein-losing e.
enteropeptidase
enteropexy
enteroplegia
enteroproctia
enteroptosis, enteroptosia
enteroptotic
enterorenal
enterorrhagia
enterorrhaphy
enterorrhexis
enteroscope
enterosepsis
enterospasm
enterostasis
enterostenosis
enterostomy
    double e.
enterotome
enterotomy
enterotoxication
enterotoxigenic *Escherichia coli*
enterotoxin
    Clostridium perfringens e.
    cytotonic e.
    Escherichia coli e.
    staphylococcal e.
enterotoxism
enterotropic
enterovaginal fistula
enterovesical fistula
Enterovirus
enterozoic
enterozoon
entgegen (*E*)
enthalpy (*H*)
enthesitis
enthesopathic
enthesopathy
enthlasis
en thyrse
entire

entity
Entner-Douderoff pathway
ento-
entoblast
entocele
entochoroidea
entocone
entoconid
entocornea
entocranial
entocranium
entoderm
entodermal cell
entoectad
Entoloma sinuatum
entomion
entomology
entomophobia
Entomophthora
    E. coronata
Entomophthorales
entomophthoramycosis
    e. basidiobolae
    e. conidiobolae
Entomopoxvirus
entopic
entoplasm
entoptic pulse
entoretina
entorhinal area
entosarc
entozoal
entozoon, pl. entozoa
entrails
entrance block
entrapment neuropathy
entropion, entropium
    atonic e.
    cicatricial e.
    spastic e.
entropionize
entropy (*S*)
entry zone
entypy
enucleate
enucleation
enuresis
    diurnal e.
    nocturnal e.
envelope
    e. conformation
    corneocyte e.
    e. flap
    nuclear e.
    viral e.
envenomation
environment
environmental
    e. illness
    e. psychology
envy
    penis e.
enzootic
    e. encephalomyelitis virus
    e. stability

enzygotic twin
enzymatic synthesis
enzyme
  acetyl-activating e.
  acyl-activating e.
  adaptive e.
  allosteric e.
  amino acid activating e.
  e. analog
  angiotensin-converting e. (ACE)
  e. antagonist
  antitumor e.
  autolytic e.
  beta-carotene-cleavage e.
  branching e.
  citrate-cleavage e.
  cold-sensitive e.
  E. Commission of the International
    Union of Biochemistry (EC)
  condensing e.
  constitutive e.
  cooperative e.
  cytochrome P450 e. (CYP)
  D e.
  deamidizing e.
  deaminating e.
  debranching e.
  digestive e.
  disproportionating e.
  extracellular e.
  heat-stable e.
  hydrolyzing e.
  immobilized e.
  e. immunoassay
  induced e.
  inducible e.
  e. inhibition theory of narcosis
  e. interconversion
  intracellular e.
  e. isomerization
  e. kinetics
  Kornberg e.
  malate-condensing e.
  malic e.
  marker e.
  membrane e.
  methionine-activating e.
  new yellow e.
  old yellow e.
  overall catalytic rate of an e. (k_{cat})
  P e.
  pantoate-activating e.
  e. parameter
  phosphorylase-rupturing e. (PR
    enzyme)
  photoreactivating e.
  PR e.
    phosphorylase-rupturing enzyme
  Q e.
  R e.
  reducing e.
  e. regulation
  repair e.
  repressible e.
  e. repression

  respiratory e.
  restriction e.
  RNA e.
  Schardinger e.
  splitting e.
  T e.
  terminal addition e.
  thermostable e.
  thiol e.
  transferring e.
  Warburg old yellow e.
  Warburg respiratory e.
  yellow e.
enzyme-catalyzed ligation
**enzyme-linked immunosorbent assay
  (ELISA)**
**enzyme-multiplied immunoassay technique
  (EMIT)**
enzyme-substrate complex
enzymic
enzymologist
enzymology
enzymolysis
enzymopathy
EOG
  electrooculography
eosin
  e. B
  e. I bluish
  e. y
  e. yellowish
eosin-methylene
  eosin-methylene blue (EMB)
  eosin-methylene blue agar
eosinocyte
eosinopenia
eosinopenic reaction
eosinophil, eosinophile
  e. adenoma
  e. cationic protein (ECP)
  e. chemotactic factor of anaphylaxis
    (ECF-A)
  e. granule
eosinophilia
  simple pulmonary e.
  tropical e.
eosinophilia-myalgia syndrome
eosinophilic
  e. cellulitis
  e. cystitis
  e. endomyocardial disease
  e. fasciitis
  e. gastritis
  e. gastroenteritis
  e. granuloma
  e. leukemia
  e. leukocyte
  e. leukocytosis
  e. leukopenia
  e. meningitis
  e. meningoencephalitis
  e. pneumonia
  e. pneumonopathy
  e. pustular folliculitis
eosinophiluria

E

eosinotactic
eosinotaxis
eosophobia
EP
  endogenous pyrogen
epactal
  e. bone
  e. ossicle
epamniotic cavity
eparterial bronchus
epaxial
EPEC
  enteropathogenic escherichia coli
ependyma
ependymal
  e. cell
  e. cyst
  e. layer
  e. zone
ependymitis
ependymoblast
ependymoblastoma
ependymocyte
ependymoma
  myxopapillary e.
ephapse
ephaptic
ephebic
ephebology
ephedra
ephedrine
ephelis, pl. **ephelides**
ephemeral
  e. fever
  e. fever virus
ephilides
  nevi, atrial myxoma, myxoid
    neurofibromas, and e.
epiandrosterone
epibatidine
epiblast
epiblastic
epiblepharon
epiboly, epibole
epibranchial placode
epibulbar
epicanthal fold
epicanthus
  e. inversus
  e. palpebralis
  e. supraciliaris
  e. tarsalis
epicardia
epicardial
epicardium
epichordal
epicillin
epicomus
epicondylalgia externa
epicondyle
  lateral e. of femur
  lateral e. of humerus
  medial e. of femur
  medial e. of humerus
epicondyli (*pl. of* epicondylus)

epicondylian
epicondylic
epicondylitis
  lateral humeral e.
epicondylus, pl. **epicondyli**
  e. lateralis femoris
  e. lateralis humeri
  e. lateralis ossis femoris
  e. medialis femoris
  e. medialis humeri
  e. medialis ossis femoris
epicoracoid
epicranial
  e. aponeurosis
  e. muscle
epicranium
epicranius
  e. muscle
epicrisis
epicritic sensibility
epicystitis
epicyte
epidemic
  behavioral e.
  e. benign dry pleurisy
  e. cerebrospinal meningitis
  e. curve
  e. diaphragmatic pleurisy
  e. disease
  e. dropsy
  e. encephalitis
  e. exanthema
  e. gangrenous proctitis
  e. gastroenteritis virus
  e. hemoglobinuria
  e. hemorrhagic fever
  e. hepatitis
  e. hiccup
  e. hysteria
  e. keratoconjunctivitis
  e. keratoconjunctivitis virus
  e. myalgia
  e. myalgia virus
  e. myalgic encephalomyelitis
  e. myalgic encephalomyelopathy
  e. myositis
  e. nausea
  e. neuromyasthenia
  e. nonbacterial gastroenteritis
  e. parotiditis
  e. parotitis virus
  e. pleurodynia
  e. pleurodynia virus
  point e.
  e. polyarthritis
  e. roseola
  e. stomatitis
  e. transient diaphragmatic spasm
  e. typhus
  e. vertigo
  e. vomiting
epidemicity
epidemiography
epidemiological distribution
epidemiologic genetics

episode
>acute schizophrenic e.
>e. of care
>manic e.

episodic
>e. dyscontrol syndrome
>e. hypertension

episome
>resistance-transferring e.

epispadias
>balanitic e.
>coronal e.
>penile e.
>penopubic e.

epispinal
episplenitis
epistasis
epistasy
epistatic
epistaxis
>renal e.

epistemology
epistemophilia
epistenocardiac pericarditis
episternal bone
episternum
epistropheus
epitarsus
epitaxy
epitendineum
epitenon
17-epitestosterone
epithalamus
epithalaxia
epithelia (*pl. of* epithelium)
epithelial
>e. attachment
>e. attachment of Gottlieb
>e. body
>e. cancer
>e. cast
>e. choroid layer
>e. cyst
>e. downgrowth
>e. dysplasia
>e. ectoderm
>e. inlay
>e. lamina
>e. membrane antigen (EMA)
>e. migration
>e. myoepithelial carcinoma
>e. nest
>e. pearl
>e. plug
>e. reticular cell
>e. tissue

epithelialization
epitheliochorial placenta
epitheliocyte
epitheliofibril
epithelioglandular
epithelioid
>e. cell
>e. cell nevus

epitheliolytic
epithelioma
>e. adenoides cysticum
>basal cell e.
>Borst-Jadassohn type
> intraepidermal e.
>e. cuniculatum
>Malherbe calcifying e.
>malignant ciliary e.
>multiple self-healing squamous e.
>sebaceous e.

epitheliomatous
epitheliopathy
>acute multifocal placoid pigment e.

epitheliosis
epitheliotropic
epithelium, pl. **epithelia**
>anterior e. of cornea
>e. anterius corneae
>Barrett e.
>ciliated e.
>columnar e.
>crevicular e.
>cuboid e.
>cylindrical e.
>e. ductus semicircularis
>enamel e.
>external dental e.
>external enamel e.
>germinal e.
>gingival e.
>glandular e.
>inner dental e.
>inner enamel e.
>junctional e.
>laminated e.
>e. of lens
>e. lentis
>mesenchymal e.
>muscle e.
>olfactory e.
>pavement e.
>pigment e.
>pigment e. of optic retina
>pseudostratified e.
>reduced enamel e.
>respiratory e.
>e. of semicircular duct
>seminiferous e.
>simple squamous e.
>stratified e.
>stratified ciliated columnar e.
>stratified squamous e.
>sulcular e.
>surface e.
>transitional e.

epithelization
epithem
epithermal
>e. chemistry
>e. neutron

epithet
>specific e.

epithiazide

E

epitope
  e. for a monoclonal antibody
  shared e.
epitoxoid
epitrichial layer
epitrichium
epitrochlea
epitrochlear
epituberculosis
epituberculous infiltration
epitympanic
  e. recess
  e. space
epitympanum
epityphlitis
epizoa (*pl. of* epizoon)
epizoic commensalism
epizoology
epizoon, pl. **epizoa**
epizootic
epizootiology
épluchage
EPO
  exclusive provider organization
epoetin alfa
eponychia
eponychium
eponym
eponymic
epoophoron
epoprostenol
epornitic
epoxy resin
2,3-epoxysqualene
EPR
  electron paramagnetic resonance
EPS
  exophthalmos-producing substance
epsilon, ε
  e. wave
Epsom salt
EPSP
  excitatory postsynaptic potential
Epstein
  E. disease
  E. pearl
  E. sign
  E. symptom
Epstein-Barr virus (EBV)
epulis
  congenital e. of newborn
  e. fissuratum
  giant cell e.
  e. gravidarum
  pigmented e.
epuloid
Eq, eq
  equivalent
equal cleavage
equation
  alveolar gas e.
  Arrhenius e.
  Bohr e.
  chemical e.
  constant field e.

Einthoven e.
Gay-Lussac e.
GHK e.
Gibbs-Helmholtz e.
Goldman e.
Goldman-Hodgkin-Katz e.
Henderson-Hasselbalch e.
Henri-Michaelis-Menten e.
Hill e.
Hüfner e.
Lineweaver-Burk e.
Michaelis-Menten e.
Nernst e.
personal e.
rate e.
Rayleigh e.
Svedberg e.
van't Hoff e.
equator
  e. bulbi oculi
  e. of eyeball
  e. of lens
  e. lentis
equatorial
  e. cleavage
  e. division
  e. plane
  e. plate
  e. staphyloma
equianalgesic dose
equiaxial
equicaloric
equilenin
equilibration
equilibrium
  acid-base e.
  e. constant (K_{eq})
  e. dialysis
  Donnan e.
  dynamic e.
  genetic e.
  Gibbs-Donnan e.
  Hardy-Weinberg e.
  homeostatic e.
  nitrogenous e.
  nutritive e.
  physiologic e.
  radioactive e.
  random mating e.
  secular e.
  stable e.
  transient e.
  unstable e.
equilin
equimolar
equimolecular
equine
  e. encephalitis
  e. encephalomyelitis
  e. gait
  e. gonadotropin unit
  e. Morbillivirus
  e. rhinoviruses
equinovalgus
equinovarus

equiphasic complex
equitoxic
equivalence, equivalency
    e. point
    e. zone
equivalent (Eq, eq)
    combustion e.
    e. dose
    e. extract
    e. form reliability
    gold e.
    gram e.
    Joule e.
    lethal e.
    metabolic e. (MET)
    nitrogen e.
    e. power
    starch e.
    e. temperature
    toxic e.
    e. weight
equivocal symptom
ER
    endoplasmic reticulum
Er
    erbium
eradication
Eranko fluorescence stain
Erb
    E. disease
    E. palsy
    E. paralysis
Erb-Charcot disease
ERBF
    effective renal blood flow
erbium (Er)
ercalcidiol
ercalciol
ercalcitriol
ERCP
    endoscopic retrograde
      cholangiopancreatography
Erdheim
    E. disease
    E. tumor
Erdmann reagent
erectile tissue
erect illumination
erection
erector
    e. muscle of hair
    e. muscle of spine
    e. spinae
erector-spinal reflex
eremophobia
ereuthophobia
ERG
    electroretinogram
ergasia
ergasiophobia
ergasthenia
ergastoplasm
ergine
ergobasine
ergocalciferol

ergocornine
ergocristine
ergocryptine
ergodynamograph
ergoesthesiograph
ergogenic
ergograph
    Mosso e.
ergographic
ergolines
ergometer
ergometrine maleate
ergonomics
ergonovine maleate
ergosine
ergosterin
ergosterol
ergostetrine
ergot
    e. alkaloid
    e. alkaloid-associated heart disease
    corn e.
    e. poisoning
ergotamine
ergotaminine
ergothioneine
ergotism
ergotoxine
ergotropic
eriodictyon
erisophake
Erlenmeyer
    E. flask
    E. flask deformity
erode
erogenous zone
eros
erose
E-rosette test
erosion
    Dieulafoy e.
    recurrent corneal e.
erosive adenomatosis of nipple
erotic zoophilism
erotism, eroticism
    anal e.
erotization
erotogenesis
erotogenic zone (*var. of* erogenous zone)
erotomania
erotomanic disorder
erotopathic
erotopathy
erotophobia
ERP
    early receptor potential
ERPF
    effective renal plasma flow
erratic
erroneous projection
error
    alpha e.
    beta e.
    experimental e.
    e. of the first kind

E

error *(continued)*
    interobserver e.
    intraobserver e.
    residual e.
    e. of the second kind
    technical e.
    type I, II e.
error-prone
    e.-p. polymerase chain reaction
    e.-p. repair
ertacalciol
erubescence
erucic acid
eructation
eruption
    accelerated e.
    butterfly e.
    clinical e.
    continuous e.
    creeping e.
    e. cyst
    delayed e.
    drug e.
    feigned e.
    fixed drug e.
    iodine e.
    Kaposi varicelliform e.
    medicinal e.
    passive e.
    polymorphous light e.
    seabather's e.
    e. sequestrum
    serum e.
    surgical e.
eruptive
    e. fever
    e. phase
    e. stage
    e. xanthoma
ERV
    expiratory reserve volume
Erwinia **L-asparaginase**
erysipelas
    ambulatory e.
    e. internum
    e. migrans
    e. perstans faciei
    phlegmonous e.
    e. pustulosum
    surgical e.
    swine e.
    wandering e.
erysipeloid
Erysipelothrix
    E. insidiosa
    E. rhusiopathiae
erysipelotoxin
erythema
    e. ab igne
    acrodynic e.
    e. annulare
    e. annulare centrifugum
    e. annulare rheumaticum
    e. arthriticum epidemicum

    e. caloricum
    e. chronicum migrans
    e. circinatum
    cold e.
    e. dose
    e. dyschromicum perstans
    e. elevatum diutinum
    e. exfoliativa
    e. figuratum perstans
    e. gyratum
    e. induratum
    e. infectiosum
    e. intertrigo
    e. keratodes
    macular e.
    e. marginatum
    e. multiforme
    e. multiforme bullosum
    e. multiforme exudativum
    e. multiforme major
    necrolytic migratory e.
    e. neonatorum
    e. nodosum
    e. nodosum leprosum
    e. nodosum migrans
    e. nuchae
    e. palmare hereditarium
    e. papulatum
    e. paratrimma
    e. pernio
    e. perstans
    scarlatiniform e.
    e. scarlatinoides
    e. simplex
    e. solare
    symptomatic e.
    e. threshold
    e. toxicum
    e. toxicum neonatorum
    e. tuberculatum
erythematous
erythermalgia
erythralgia
erythrasma
erythredema
erythremia
    altitude e.
erythremic myelosis
erythristic
erythrite
erythritol
erythrityl tetranitrate
erythroblast
erythroblastemia
erythroblastic anemia
erythroblastopenia
    transient e. of childhood
erythroblastosis
    fetal e.
    e. fetalis
erythroblastotic
erythrocatalysis
erythrochromia
erythroclasis
erythroclastic

erythrocuprein
erythrocyanosis
erythrocyte
    e. adherence phenomenon
    e. adherence test
    e. fragility test
    e. indices
    e. maturation factor
    e. sedimentation rate (ESR)
erythrocythemia
erythrocytic
    e. cycle
    e. series
erythrocytoblast
erythrocytolysin
erythrocytolysis
erythrocytometer
erythrocytopenia
erythrocytopoiesis
erythrocytorrhexis
erythrocytoschisis
erythrocytosis
erythrocyturia
erythrodegenerative
erythroderma
    bullous congenital ichthyosiform e.
    congenital ichthyosiform e.
    e. desquamativum
    nonbullous congenital
      ichthyosiform e.
    e. psoriaticum
    Sézary e.
erythrodermatitis
erythrodextrin
erythrodontia
erythrodysesthesia syndrome
erythrogenesis imperfecta
erythrogenic toxin
erythrogonium, pl. erythrogonia
erythroid cell
erythroidin
erythrokeratodermia variabilis
erythrokinetics
erythroleukemia
erythroleukosis
erythrol tetranitrate
erythrolysin
erythrolysis
erythromelalgia
erythromelia
erythromycin
    e. estolate
    e. glucoheptonate
    e. propionate
    e. stearate
erythron
erythroneocytosis
erythronormoblastic anemia
erythropenia
erythrophagia
erythrophagocytosis
erythrophil
erythrophilic
erythrophore
erythroplakia

erythroplasia of Queyrat
erythropoiesis
erythropoietic
    e. hormone
    e. porphyria
    e. protoporphyria
erythropoietin
erythroprosopalgia
erythropsia
erythropyknosis
erythrorrhexis
erythrose 4-phosphate
erythrosin B
erythroxyline
erythrulose
erythruria
Es
    einsteinium
Esbach reagent
escape
    e. beat
    e. conditioning
    e. contraction
    e. impulse
    e. interval
    junctional e.
    e. phenomenon
    e. rhythm
    e. training
    ventricular e.
    e. ventricular contraction
escape-capture bigeminy
eschar
escharectomy
escharotic
escharotomy
Escherichia
    E. coli
    E. coli enterotoxin
    E. coli RNase I
    enterohemorrhagic *E. coli* (EHEC)
    enteroinvasive *E. coli* (EIEC)
    enteropathogenic *E. coli* (EPEC)
    enterotoxigenic *E. coli* (ETEC)
    E. freundii
escorcin, escorcinol
esculapian
esculent
esculin
eseridine
eserine
    e. aminoxide
    e. oxide
    e. salicylate
Esmarch
    E. bandage
    E. tourniquet
esmolol hydrochloride
esodeviation
esodic nerve
esophagalgia
esophageal
    e. achalasia
    e. artery
    e. atresia

E

esophageal *(continued)*
 e. branch
 e. branch of the inferior thyroid artery
 e. branch of the left gastric artery
 e. branch of the recurrent laryngeal nerve
 e. branch of the thoracic aorta
 e. branch of thoracic ganglia
 e. branch of the vagus nerve
 e. cardiogram
 e. constriction
 e. dysrhythmia
 e. gland
 e. hiatus
 e. impression on liver
 e. lead
 e. manometry
 e. mucosa
 e. opening
 e. plexus
 e. reflux
 e. smear
 e. spasm
 e. speech
 e. varix
 e. vein
 e. web
esophagectomy
 Ivor Lewis e.
 three-incision e.
 transhiatal e.
 transthoracic e.
esophagi (*pl. of* esophagus)
esophagism
esophagitis
 peptic e.
 reflux e.
esophagocardioplasty
esophagocele
esophagodynia
esophagoenterostomy
esophagogastrectomy
esophagogastric
 e. junction
 e. orifice
 e. vestibule
esophagogastroanastomosis
esophagogastroduodenoscopy (EGD)
esophagogastromyotomy
esophagogastroplasty
esophagogastrostomy
esophagogram
esophagography
esophagology
esophagomalacia
esophagomyotomy
esophagoplasty
esophagoplication
esophagoptosis, esophagoptosia
esophagosalivary reflex
esophagoscope
esophagoscopy
esophagospasm

esophagostenosis
esophagostomiasis
esophagostomy
esophagotomy
esophagram
esophagus, pl. **esophagi**
 Barrett e.
esophoria
esophoric
esotropia
 A-pattern e.
 basic e.
 consecutive e.
 cyclic e.
 mixed e.
 nonaccommodative e.
 nonrefractive accommodative e.
 refractive accommodative e.
 V-pattern e.
 X-pattern e.
esotropic
ESP
 extrasensory perception
espundia
esquinancea
ESR
 erythrocyte sedimentation rate
essence of rose
essential
 e. albuminuria
 e. amino acid
 e. anemia
 e. anisocoria
 e. bradycardia
 e. fatty acid
 e. fever
 e. food factor
 e. fructosuria
 e. hypertension
 e. nutrient
 e. oil
 e. pentosuria
 e. progressive atrophy of iris
 e. pruritus
 e. tachycardia
 e. telangiectasia
 e. thrombocytopenia
 e. tremor
Essick cell band
Essig splint
established cell line
estazolam
ester
 carboxylic acid e.
 Cori e.
 Embden e.
 Harden-Young e.
 Neuberg e.
 Robison e.
 Robison-Embden e.
 sugar e.
 thiol e.
esterase
 C1 e.
esterification

esterified estrogen
Estes operation
esthematology
esthesia
esthesic
esthesiodic system
esthesiogenesis
esthesiogenic
esthesiography
esthesiology
esthesiometer
esthesiometry
esthesioneuroblastoma
    olfactory e.
esthesioneurocytoma
esthesiophysiology
esthesioscopy
esthesodic
esthetic
    e. dentistry
    e. surgery
esthetics
    denture e.
estimate
    Kaplan-Meier e.
estimated date of confinement (EDC)
estimation
estimator
    least squares e.
    maximum likelihood e.
estival
estivation
estivoautumnal
Estlander flap
estradiol (E$_2$)
    e. benzoate
    e. benzoate unit
    e. cypionate
    e. dipropionate
    ethinyl e.
    ethynyl e.
    e. undecylate
    e. valerate
estragon oil
estramustine phosphate sodium
estrane
estratriene
estrin
estriol
estrodienol
estrogen
    catechol e.
    conjugated e.
    esterified e.
    e. receptor
    e. replacement therapy
estrogenic hormone
estrone (E$_1$)
    e. unit
estrous cycle
estrual
estrus
    postpartum e.
esu
    electrostatic unit

ESWL
    extracorporeal shock wave lithotripsy
esylate
Et
    ethyl
eta
etafedrine hydrochloride
etafenone
etamsylate
état
    e. criblé
    e. mamelonné
ETEC
    enterotoxigenic escherichia coli
ethacridine lactate
ethacrynate sodium
ethacrynic acid
ethadione
ethambutol hydrochloride
ethamivan
ethamoxytriphetol
ethamsylate
ethanal
ethane
ethanediamine
ethanoic acid
ethanol
ethanolamine
ethanolaminephosphotransferase
ethaverine hydrochloride
ethchlorvynol
ethenyl
ethenylbenzene
ethenylene
ether
    anesthetic e.
    glycol e.
    solvent e.
    xylostyptic e.
ethereal
    e. oil
    e. solution
    e. tincture
etherification
etherization
ethiazide
ethical
ethics
    medical e.
ethidene
ethidium bromide
ethindrone
ethinyl
    e. estradiol
    e. trichloride
ethinylestrenol
ethiodized oil
ethionamide
ethionine
ethisterone
ethmocranial
ethmofrontal
ethmoid
    e. air cell
    e. angle

E

ethmoid (*continued*)
    e. bone
    e. infundibulum
ethmoidal
    e. bulla
    e. cell
    e. crest
    e. crest of maxilla
    e. crest of palatine bone
    e. foramen
    e. groove
    e. infundibulum
    e. labyrinth
    e. notch
    e. process of inferior nasal concha
    e. sinus
    e. vein
ethmoidale
ethmoidal-lacrimal fistula
ethmoidectomy
ethmoiditis
ethmoidolacrimal suture
ethmoidomaxillary suture
ethmolacrimal
ethmomaxillary
ethmonasal
ethmopalatal
ethmosphenoid
ethmoturbinal
ethmovomerine plate
ethnic group
ethnocentrism
ethnology
ethnopharmacology
ethoheptazine citrate
ethohexadiol
ethologist
ethology
ethomoxane
ethopharmacology
ethopropazine hydrochloride
ethosuximide
ethotoin
ethotrimeprazine
ethoxazene hydrochloride
ethoxy
ethoxybutamoxane
ethoxyzolamide
ethyl (Et)
    e. alcohol
    e. aminobenzoate
    e. biscoumacetate
    e. butyrate
    e. carbamate
    e. chloride
    e. ether
    e. formate
    e. green
    e. oleate
    e. oxide
    e. salicylate
ethylate
ethylbenztropine
ethylcellulose

ethyldichloroarsine
ethylene
    ethylene dibromide
    e. glycol
    e. oxide
    e. tetrachloride
ethylenediamine
ethylenediaminetetraacetic acid (EDTA)
ethyleneglycotetraacetic acid (EGTA)
ethylestrenol
ethylidene
ethylidyne
ethylmorphine hydrochloride
ethylnorepinephrine (E.N.E., E.N.S.)
ethylpapaverine hydrochloride
ethylparaben
ethylphenylephrine hydrochloride
ethylstibamine
ethynodiol diacetate
ethynyl estradiol
etidocaine
etidronate disodium
etidronic acid
etilefrine hydrochloride
etiocholanolone
etiogenic
etiolated
etiolation
etiologic
etiology
etiopathic
etiopathology
etioporphyrin
etiotropic
etofamide
etomidate
etoposide
etorphine
etozolin
ETP
    electron transport particle
etretinate
etymemazine
"e"-type cholinesterase
Eu
    europium
euallele
Eubacteriales
Eubacterium
    E. aerofaciens
    E. combesi
    E. contortum
    E. crispatum
    E. filamentosum
    E. lentum
    E. limosum
    E. minutum
    E. moniliforme
    E. parvum
    E. poeciloides
    E. pseudotortuosum
    E. quartum
    E. quintum
    E. rectale

E. tenue
E. tortuosum
eubiotics
eucaine
eucalyptol
eucalyptus
e. gum
e. oil
eucapnia
Eucaryotae (*var. of* Eukaryotae)
eucaryote
eucaryotic
eucasin
eucatropine hydrochloride
Eucestoda
euchlorhydria
eucholia
euchromatic
euchromatin
euchromosome
Eucoleus
eucorticalism
eucrasia
eucupine
eudiaphoresis
eudipsia
Euflagellata
eugenic acid
eugenics
eugenism
eugenol
Euglena
E. gracilis
E. viridis
Euglenidae
euglobulin clot lysis time
euglycemia
euglycemic
eugnathia
eugnathic anomaly
eugnosia
eugonic
Eugregarinida
euhydration
Eukaryotae, Eucaryotae
eukaryote
eukaryotic
eukeratin
eukinesia
Eulenburg disease
eumelanin
eumelanosome
eumetria
eumorphism
eumycetes
eumycetoma
Eumycetozoea
eunuch
eunuchism
eunuchoid
e. gigantism
e. state
e. voice

eunuchoidism
hypergonadotropic e.
hypogonadotropic e.
euosmia
eupancreatism
euparal
Euparyphium
eupaverin
eupepsia
eupeptic
eupeptide bond
euphenics
Euphorbia pilulifera
euphoretic
euphoria
euphoriant
euplasia
euplastic lymph
euploid
euploidy
eupnea
eupraxia
euprocin hydrochloride
Euproctis
eurhythmia
European
E. bat Lyssavirus
E. snakeroot
E. tarantula
E. typhus
europium (Eu)
euroxenous parasite
euryblepharon
eurycephalic, eurycephalous
eurygnathic
eurygnathism
eurygnathous
euryon
euryopic
eurysomatic
euscope
Eusimulium
eustachian
e. catheter
e. cushion
e. tonsil
e. tube
e. tuber
e. valve
eustachitis
eusthenia
eustrongyloides
Eustrongylus
eusystole
eusystolic
eutectic
e. alloy
e. temperature
euthanasia
euthenics
eutherapeutic
Eutheria
euthermic
euthymia
euthymic

E

euthyroid
    e. hypometabolism
    e. sick syndrome
euthyroidism
euthyscope
euthyscopy
eutonic
eutrichosis
eutrophia
eutrophic
eutrophy
euvolia
eV
    electron-volt
evacuant
evacuate
evacuation
    dilation and e. (D & E)
evacuator
    Ellik e.
evagination
evaluation
    acute physiology and chronic
       health e. (APACHE)
evanescent
Evans
    E. blue
    E. forceps
    E. syndrome
evaporate
evaporation
evasion
    macular e.
event
    sentinel e.
eventration of the diaphragm
eversion
evert
evidence-based medicine
eviration
evisceration
evisceroneurotomy
evocation
evocator
evoked
    e. electromyography
    e. otoacoustic emission
    e. potential
    e. response
evolution
    biologic e.
    chemical e.
    coincidental e.
    concerted e.
    convergent e.
    darwinian e.
    divergent e.
    emergent e.
    organic e.
    saltatory e.
    spontaneous e.
evolutionary fitness
evulsion

Ewart
    E. procedure
    E. sign
Ewing
    E. sarcoma
    E. sign
    E. tumor
Ewingella
exacerbation
exaltation
examination
    cytologic e.
    direct wet mount e.
    EMG e.
    fecal e.
    ova and parasite e.
    Papanicolaou e.
    permanent stained smear e.
    physical e.
    postmortem e.
examiner
    medical e.
examining table
exanthem
exanthema
    Boston e.
    epidemic e.
    keratoid e.
    e. subitum
exanthematous
    e. disease
    e. fever
    e. typhus
exanthesis arthrosia
exanthrope
exanthropic
exarteritis
excalation
excavatio
    e. disci
    e. papillae
    e. rectouterina
    e. rectovesicalis
    e. vesicouterina
excavation
    atrophic e.
    glaucomatous e.
    e. of optic disk
    physiologic e.
excavator
    hatchet e.
    hoe e.
excementosis
excentric amputation
excess
    antibody e.
    antigen e.
    base e.
    convergence e.
    e. lactate
    negative base e.
exchange
    sister chromatid e.
    e. transfusion

exchanger
  anion e.
  cation e.
  countercurrent e.
  ion e.
excimer laser
excipient
excise
excision
  e. biopsy
  large loop e. of transformation zone of the cervix of the uterus (LLETZ)
  loop e.
  e. repair
excitability
  supranormal e.
excitable
  e. area
  e. gap
excitant
excitation
  anomalous atrioventricular e.
  e. spectrum
  e. wave
excitatory
  e. junction potential (EJP)
  e. postsynaptic potential (EPSP)
excited
  e. atom
  e. catatonia
  e. state
excitement
  catatonic e.
  manic e.
exciting
  e. cause
  e. electrode
  e. eye
excitoglandular
excitometabolic
excitomotor
excitomuscular
excitoreflex nerve
excitor nerve
excitosecretory
excitotoxic
excitotoxin
exclamation point hair
exclave
exclusion
  allelic e.
  e. of pupil
exclusive provider organization (EPO)
exconjugant
excoriate
excoriation
  neurotic e.
excrement
excrementitious
excrescence
  Lambl e.
excreta
excrete
excretion

excretory
  e. duct
  e. duct of lacrimal gland
  e. duct of seminal gland
  e. duct of seminal vesicle
  e. ductule of lacrimal gland
  e. gland
  e. urography
excursion
  lateral e.
  protrusive e.
  retrusive e.
excycloduction
excyclophoria
excyclotorsion
excyclotropia
excyclovergence
excystation
exduction
exemia
exencephalia
exencephalic
exencephalocele
exencephalous
exencephaly
exenteration
  anterior pelvic e.
  orbital e.
  pelvic e.
  posterior pelvic e.
  total pelvic e.
exenteritis
exercise
  e. imaging
  isometric e.
  isotonic e.
  Kegel e.'s
  e. radionuclide angiocardiography
  e. test
exercise-induced amenorrhea
exeresis
exergonic
exertional
  e. dyspnea
  e. rhabdomyolysis
exflagellation
exfoliation
  e. of lens
  e. syndrome
exfoliative
  e. cytology
  e. dermatitis
  e. gastritis
  e. psoriasis
exhalation
exhale
exhaustion
  heat e.
exhibitionism
exhibitionist
exhilarant
existential
  e. psychiatry
  e. psychology
  e. psychotherapy

E

exit
    e. block
    e. dose
exitus
Exner plexus
exo-1,4-alpha-D-glucosidase
exoamylase
exoantigen
exocardia
exoccipital bone
exocelomic membrane
exocrine
    e. gland
    e. pancreatic insufficiency
    e. part of pancreas
exocyclic
exocytosis
exodeviation
exodic nerve
exodontia
exodontist
exoenzyme
exoerythrocytic
    e. cycle
    e. stage
exogamy
exogastrula
exogenetic
exogenic toxicosis
exogenote
exogenous
    e. creatinine clearance
    e. cycle
    e. depression
    e. fiber
    e. hemochromatosis
    e. hyperglyceridemia
    e. ochronosis
    e. pigmentation
    e. pyrogens
exolever
exomphalos
exon shuffle
exonuclease
exopeptidase
Exophiala
    E. jeanselmei
    E. werneckii
exophoria
exophoric
exophthalmic
    e. goiter
    e. ophthalmoplegia
exophthalmometer
exophthalmos, exophthalmus
    endocrine e.
    malignant e.
exophthalmos-producing substance (EPS)
exophyte
exophytic
exoplasm
exoserosis
exoskeleton
exospore
exosporium

exostectomy
exostosectomy
exostosis, pl. **exostoses**
    e. bursata
    e. cartilaginea
    hereditary multiple exostoses
    ivory e.
    multiple e.
    solitary osteocartilaginous e.
    subungual e.
exoteric bacterium
exothermic
exotoxic
exotoxin
exotropia
    A-pattern e.
    basic e.
    divergence excess e.
    divergence insufficiency e.
    V-pattern e.
    X-pattern e.
expandable stent
expanded disability status scale (EDSS)
expansion
    e. arch
    clonal e.
    extensor e.
    extensor digital e.
    hygroscopic e.
    perceptual e.
    setting e.
    wax e.
expansive delusion
expansiveness
expectation of life
    e. o. l. at age *x*
    e. o. l. at birth
expected
expectorant
expectorate
expectoration
    prune-juice e.
experience
    corrective emotional e.
experiential aura
experiment
    Carr-Purcell e.
    control e.
    delayed reaction e.
    double blind e.
    double-masked e.
    factorial e.
    hertzian e.
    Mariotte e.
    pulse-chase e.
    Scheiner e.
experimental
    e. allergic encephalitis (EAE)
    e. allergic encephalomyelitis
    e. error
    e. group
    e. medicine
    e. method
    e. neurosis
    e. psychology

experimenter effect
expiration
expiratory
    e. center
    e. dyspnea
    e. reserve volume (ERV)
    e. resistance
    e. stridor
expire
expired gas
explant
explantation
exploration
exploratory drive
explorer
exploring
    e. electrode
    e. needle
explosion
explosive
    e. decompression
    e. speech
exponential
    e. distribution
    e. growth
expose
exposed pulp
exposure
    e. dose
    e. keratitis
express
expressed
    e. mustard oil
    e. skull fracture
expression
    differential gene e.
    gene e.
    integrated rate e.
    e. library
    e. vector
expressive aphasia
expressivity
expulsive pain
exquisite
exsanguinate
exsanguination transfusion
exsanguine
exsect
exsection
Exserohilum
exsiccant
exsiccate
exsiccated
    e. alum
    e. sodium sulfite
exsiccation fever
exsomatize
exsorption
exstrophy
    e. of the bladder
    cloacal e.
extemporaneous mixture
extend
extended
    e. clasp

    e. family
    e. family therapy
    e. insulin zinc suspension
    e. mediastinoscopy
    e. pyelotomy
    e. radical mastectomy
    e. thymectomy
extension
    e. bridge
    Buck e.
    e. form
    primer e.
    ridge e.
    skeletal e.
extensor
    e. aponeurosis
    e. carpi radialis brevis muscle
    e. carpi radialis longus muscle
    e. carpi ulnaris muscle
    e. compartment of arm
    e. compartment of forearm
    e. compartment of leg
    e. compartment of thigh
    e. digital expansion
    e. digiti minimi muscle
    e. digitorum brevis muscle
    e. digitorum brevis muscle of hand
    e. digitorum longus muscle
    e. digitorum muscle
    e. expansion
    e. hallucis brevis muscle
    e. hallucis longus muscle
    e. indicis muscle
    e. muscle
    e. muscle of finger
    e. muscle of little finger
    e. pollicis brevis muscle
    e. pollicis longus muscle
    e. retinaculum
exterior
exteriorize
extern
external
    e. absorption
    e. acoustic aperture
    e. acoustic foramen
    e. acoustic meatus
    e. acoustic pore
    e. anal sphincter
    e. aperture of cochlear canaliculus
    e. aperture of vestibular aqueduct
    e. arcuate fiber
    e. artery of nose
    e. auditory foramen
    e. auditory meatus
    e. auditory pore
    e. axis of eye
    e. base of skull
    e. branch of superior laryngeal nerve
    e. branch of trunk of accessory nerve
    e. canthus
    e. capsule
    e. cardiac massage

E

external *(continued)*
e. carotid artery
e. carotid nerve
e. carotid plexus
e. cephalic version
e. collateral ligament of wrist
e. conjugate
e. conjugate diameter
e. cuneate nucleus
e. defibrillator
e. dental epithelium
e. ear
e. enamel epithelium
e. exudative retinopathy
e. female genital organ
e. fistula
e. fixation
e. genitalia
e. hemorrhoid
e. hydrocephalus
e. iliac artery
e. iliac lymphatic plexus
e. iliac lymph node
e. iliac vein
e. inguinal ring
e. intercostal membrane
e. intercostal muscle
e. jugular vein
e. lip of iliac crest
e. male genital organ
e. malleolus
e. mammary artery
e. matrix
e. maxillary artery
e. maxillary plexus
e. medium
e. medullary lamina
e. meningitis
e. naris
e. nasal artery
e. nasal branch of infraorbital nerve
e. nasal vein
e. nose
e. nuclear layer of retina
e. oblique muscle
e. oblique reflex
e. oblique ridge
e. obturator muscle
e. occipital crest
e. occipital protuberance
e. opening
e. opening of cochlear canaliculus
e. opening of urethra
e. ophthalmopathy
e. ophthalmoplegia
e. os of uterus
e. ovular e.
e. pacemaker
e. palatine vein
e. phase
e. pillar cell
e. pin fixation
e. pin fixation, biphase
e. pterygoid muscle

e. pudendal vein
e. pyocephalus
e. respiration
e. respiratory nerve of Bell
e. root sheath
e. salivary gland
e. saphenous nerve
e. secretion
e. semilunar fibrocartilage
e. sheath of optic nerve
e. spermatic artery
e. spermatic fascia
e. spermatic nerve
e. sphincter muscle of anus
e. sphincterotomy
e. spiral sulcus
e. squint
e. surface
e. surface of cochlear duct
e. surface of cranial base
e. surface of frontal bone
e. surface of parietal bone
e. table of calvaria
e. traction
e. urethral orifice
e. urethral sphincter
e. urethral sphincter of female
e. urethral sphincter of male
e. urethrotomy
e. urinary meatus
e. wall of cochlear duct
externus
exteroceptive
exteroceptor
exterofective system
extinction
e. coefficient
specific e.
visual e.
extinguish
extirpation
Exton reagent
extorsion
extortor
extra-abdominal desmoid
extraamniotic pregnancy
extraanatomic bypass
extra-articular
extra-axial
extrabuccal
extrabulbar
extracaliceal
extracapsular
e. ankylosis
e. fracture
e. ligament
extracardiac murmur
extracarpal
extracellular
e. enzyme
e. fluid (ECF)
e. fluid volume (ECFV)
e. toxin
extrachorial pregnancy

extrachromosomal
    e. DNA
    e. element
    e. gene
    e. genetic element
    e. inheritance
extracoronal retainer
extracorporeal
    e. circulation
    e. dialysis
    e. photophoresis
    e. shock wave lithotripsy (ESWL)
extracorpuscular
extracranial
    e. arteritis
    e. ganglia
    e. pneumatocele
    e. pneumocele
extracranial-intracranial bypass
extract
    alcoholic e.
    allergenic e.
    allergic e.
    belladonna e.
    Büchner e.
    equivalent e.
    fluid e.
    hydroalcoholic e.
    liquid e.
    pollen e.
extractant
extracting forceps
extraction
    Baker pyridine e.
    breech e.
    e. coefficient
    partial breech e.
    podalic e.
    e. ratio (E)
    serial e.
    spontaneous breech e.
    total breech e.
extractive
extractor
    vacuum e.
extracystic
extradural
    e. anesthesia
    e. hematorrhachis
    e. hemorrhage
    e. space
    e. space
extraembryonic
    e. blastoderm
    e. celom
    e. ectoderm
    e. membrane
    e. mesoderm
extraepiphysial
extragenital
extraglomerular mesangium
extrahepatic
extraligamentous
extramalleolus
extramammary Paget disease

extramedullary
extramembranous pregnancy
extramitochondrial
extramural practice
extraneous
extranodal marginal zone lymphoma
extranuclear inheritance
extraocular
    e. muscle
    e. part of central retinal artery and vein
extraoral
    e. anchorage
    e. fracture appliance
extraovular
extrapapillary
extraparenchymal
extraperineal
extraperiosteal
extraperitoneal
    e. fascia
    e. space
extraphysiologic
extrapineal pinealoma
extraplacental
extrapleural pneumothorax
extraprostatic
extrapsychic
extrapulmonary
extrapyramidal
    e. cerebral palsy
    e. disease
    e. dyskinesia
    e. motor system
    e. motor system disease
    e. syndrome
extrasaccular hernia
extrasensory
    e. perception (ESP)
    e. thought transference
extraserous
extraskeletal chondroma
extrasomatic
extrasystole
    atrial e.
    atrioventricular e.
    auricular e.
    interpolated e.
    junctional e.
    return e.
    supraventricular e.
    ventricular e.
extratarsal
extrathyroidal hypermetabolism
extratracheal
extratubal
extrauterine pregnancy
extravaginal torsion
extravasate
extravasation cyst
extravascular fluid
extraventricular
extraversion
extravert
extravesical reimplantation

E

extravisual
extravital ultraviolet
extremal quotient
extreme capsule
in extremis
extremital
extremitas
    e. acromialis claviculae
    e. anterior splenica
    e. inferior
    e. inferior renis
    e. inferior testis
    e. posterior splenica
    e. sternalis claviculae
    e. superior
    e. superior renis
    e. superior testis
    e. tubaria ovarii
    e. uterina ovarii
extremity
    acromial e. of clavicle
    anterior e. of caudate nucleus
    anterior e. of spleen
    inferior e.
    inferior e. of kidney
    lower e.
    posterior e. of spleen
    sternal e. of clavicle
    superior e.
    superior e. of kidney
    tubal e. of ovary
    upper e.
    upper e. of fibula
    uterine e. of ovary
extrinsic
    e. allergic alveolitis
    e. asthma
    e. color
    e. factor
    e. incubation period
    e. motivation
    e. muscle
    e. muscle of eyeball
    e. protein
    e. sphincter
extrogastrulation
extroversion
extrovert
extrude
extruded tooth
extrusion of a tooth
extubate
extubation
exuberant
exudate
exudation
    e. cell
    e. corpuscle
    e. cyst
exudative
    e. bronchiolitis
    e. choroiditis
    e. discoid and lichenoid dermatitis
    e. drusen
    e. glomerulonephritis

    e. inflammation
    e. retinal detachment
    e. retinitis
    e. tuberculosis
    e. vitreoretinopathy
exude
exulcerans
exumbilication
ex vivo
eye
    amaurotic cat e.
    aphakic e.
    artificial e.
    e. bank
    black e.
    blear e.
    bleary e.
    e. capsule
    compound e.
    crossed e.'s
    e. cup
    cyclopian e.
    dark-adapted e.
    dominant e.
    e. drops
    e., ear, nose, and throat (EENT)
    epiphysial e.
    exciting e.
    fixing e.
    hare's e.
    e. lens
    light-adapted e.
    Listing reduced e.
    master e.
    e. ointment
    parietal e.
    phakic e.
    photopic e.
    pineal e.
    raccoon e.'s
    reduced e.
    e. reflex
    right e. (R.E.)
    schematic e.
    scotopic e.
    shipyard e.
    e. socket
    e. speculum
    squinting e.
    sympathizing e.
    e. tooth
    watery e.
    web e.
eyeball compression reflex
eyeball-heart reflex
eyebrow
eye-closure
    e.-c. pupil reaction
    e.-c. reflex
eye-ear plane
eyeglasses
eyegrounds
eyelash
    ectopic e.
    piebald e.

eyelid
    e. imbrication
    inferior e.
    lower e.
    superior e.
    third e.
    upper e.

eyepiece
eyespot
eyestone
eyestrain
eyewash

E

F

French scale
  F agent
  F pili
  F plasmid
  F thalassemia
  F wave

F

faraday
  f distribution
  f wave

FAAN

Fellow of the American Academy of
Nursing

FAB

French-American-British
  FAB classification

Fab

Fab fragment
Fab piece

fabella

Faber

F. anemia
F. syndrome

fabism

fabrication

Fabricius, Fabrizzi

Fabricius ship

Fabry disease

FACCP, Fellow of the American College of Chest Physicians

Fellow of the American College of Chest
Physicians

FACD

Fellow of the American College of
Dentists

face

bird f.
cow f.
dish f.
f. form
frog f.
hippocratic f.
masklike f.
moon f.
moon shaped f.
f. peel
f. presentation
f. region
superolateral f. of cerebral
hemisphere
f. validity

face-bow

adjustable axis f.-b.
f.-b. fork
kinematic f.-b.
f.-b. record

facelift

facet, facette

acromial f. of clavicle
articular f.

articular f. of head of fibula
articular f. of head of rib
articular f. of lateral malleolus
articular f. of medial malleolus
articular f. of radial head
articular f. of tubercle of rib
clavicular f.
clavicular articular f. of acromion
corneal f.
costal f.
fibular articular f. of tibia
inferior articular f. of atlas
inferior costal f.
f. joint
lateral malleolar f. of talus
Lenoir f.
locked f.
medial malleolar f. of talus
f. (of atlas) for dens
f. (on talus) for calcaneonavicular
part of bifurcate ligament
f. (on talus) for plantar
calcaneonavicular ligament
posterior articular f. of dens
f. rhizotomy
sternal f. of clavicle
superior articular f. of atlas
superior costal f.
superior f. of trochlear of talus
transverse costal f.

facetectomy

facial

f. angle
f. artery
f. aspect
f. axis
f. bone
f. canal
f. cleft
f. colliculus
f. diplegia
f. eminence
f. height
f. hemiatrophy
f. hemiatrophy of Romberg
f. hemiplegia
f. hillock
f. index
f. lymph node
f. motor nucleus
f. muscle
f. myokymia
f. nerve area
f. nerve [CN VII]
f. neuralgia
f. nucleus
f. palsy
f. paralysis
f. plane
f. plexus
f. profile

F

facial *(continued)*
- f. recess approach
- f. reflex
- f. root
- f. skeleton
- f. spasm
- f. surface of tooth
- f. tic
- f. triangle
- f. vein
- f. vision

facialis phenomenon

facies, pl. **facies**
- acromial articular f. of clavicle
- adenoid f.
- f. antebrachialis anterior
- f. antebrachialis posterior
- f. anterior
- f. anterior antebrachii
- f. anterior brachii
- f. anterior corneae
- f. anterior corporis maxillae
- f. anterior cruris
- f. anterior glandulae suprarenalis
- f. anterior iridis
- f. anterior lateralis corporis humeri
- f. anterior lentis
- f. anterior medialis corporis humeri
- f. anterior membri inferioris
- f. anterior palpebrarum
- f. anterior partis petrosae ossis temporalis
- f. anterior patellae
- f. anterior prostatae
- f. anterior radii
- f. anterior renis
- f. anterior ulnae
- f. anterior uteri
- f. anteroinferior corporis pancreatis
- f. anterolateralis cartilaginis arytenoideae
- f. anterolateralis corporis humeri
- f. anteromedialis corporis humeri
- f. anterosuperioris corporis pancreatis
- f. antonina
- aortic f.
- f. approximalis dentis
- f. articularis
- f. articularis acromialis claviculae
- f. articularis anterior dentis
- f. articularis arytenoidea cricoideae
- f. articularis calcanea tali
- f. articularis capitis costae
- f. articularis capitis fibulae
- f. articularis carpi radii
- f. articularis cartilaginis arytenoideae
- f. articularis clavicularis acromii
- f. articularis cuboidea ossis calcanei
- f. articularis fibularis tibiae
- f. articularis fossae mandibularis ossis temporalis
- f. articularis inferior atlantis
- f. articularis inferior tibiae
- f. articularis malleoli lateralis fibulae
- f. articularis malleoli medialis tibiae
- f. articularis navicularis tali
- f. articularis partis calcaneonavicularis ligamenti bifurcati tali
- f. articularis patellae
- f. articularis posterior dentis
- f. articularis sternalis claviculae
- f. articularis superior atlantis
- f. articularis superior tibiae
- f. articularis talaris anterior calcanei
- f. articularis talaris calcanei
- f. articularis talaris media calcanei
- f. articularis talaris posterior calcanei
- f. articularis thyroidea cricoideae
- f. articularis tuberculi costae
- f. auricularis ossis ilii
- f. auricularis ossis sacri
- f. bovina
- f. brachialis anterior
- f. brachialis posterior
- f. cerebralis
- cherubic f.
- f. colica splenis
- f. contactus dentis
- Corvisart f.
- f. costalis
- f. costalis pulmonis
- f. costalis scapulae
- f. cruralis anterior
- f. cruralis posterior
- f. cubitalis anterior
- f. cubitalis posterior
- f. diaphragmatica
- f. digitalis dorsalis (manus et pedis)
- f. digitalis palmaris
- f. digitalis plantaris
- f. digitalis ventralis
- f. distalis dentis
- f. dolorosa
- f. dorsalis
- f. dorsalis ossis sacri
- f. dorsalis scapulae
- elfin f.
- f. externa
- f. externa ossis frontalis
- f. externa ossis parietalis
- f. facialis dentis
- f. femoralis anterior
- f. femoralis posterior
- f. gastrica splenis
- f. glutea ossis ilii
- hippocratic f.
- f. hippocratica
- hound-dog f.
- Hutchinson f.
- f. inferior hemispherii cerebri
- f. inferior linguae
- f. inferior partis petrosae ossis temporalis
- f. inferolateralis prostatae

f. infratemporalis alaris majoris ossis sphenoidalis
f. infratemporalis corporis maxillae
f. interlobares pulmonis
f. interna
f. interna ossis frontalis
f. interna ossis parietalis
f. intestinalis uteri
f. lateralis
f. lateralis brachii
f. lateralis cruris
f. lateralis digiti manus
f. lateralis digiti pedis
f. lateralis fibulae
f. lateralis membri inferioris
f. lateralis ossis zygomatici
f. lateralis ovarii
f. lateralis testis
f. lateralis tibiae
leonine f.
f. ligamenti calcaneonavicularis plantaris tali
f. lingualis dentis
f. lunata acetabuli
f. malleolaris lateralis tali
f. malleolaris medialis tali
f. masticatoria
f. maxillaris alaris majoris ossis sphenoidalis
f. maxillaris ossis palatini
f. medialis
f. medialis cartilaginis arytenoideae
f. medialis digiti pedis
f. medialis fibulae
f. medialis hemispherii cerebri
f. medialis ovarii
f. medialis pulmonis
f. medialis testis
f. medialis tibiae
f. medialis ulnae
f. mediastinalis pulmonis
f. mesialis dentis
mitral f.
moon f.
myasthenic f.
myopathic f.
f. nasalis maxillae
f. nasalis ossis palatini
f. occlusalis dentis
f. orbitalis
f. palatina laminae horizontalis ossis palatini
f. palmares digitorum
f. pancreatica splenica
Parkinson f.
f. patellaris femoris
f. pelvica ossis sacri
f. poplitea femoris
f. posterior
f. posterior cartilaginis arytenoideae
f. posterior corneae
f. posterior corporis humeri
f. posterior cruris
f. posterior fibulae

f. posterior glandulae suprarenalis
f. posterior iridis
f. posterior lentis
f. posterior membri inferioris
f. posterior palpebrarum
f. posterior pancreatis
f. posterior partis petrosae ossis temporalis
f. posterior prostatae
f. posterior radii
f. posterior renis
f. posterior scapulae
f. posterior tibiae
f. posterior ulnae
Potter f.
f. pulmonales cordis dextra/sinistra
f. renalis glandulae suprarenalis
f. renalis lienis
f. renalis splenis
f. sacropelvina ossis ilii
f. scaphoidea
f. sternocostalis cordis
f. superior hemispherii cerebelli
f. superior tali
f. superolateralis hemispherii cerebri
f. symphysialis
f. temporalis
f. urethralis penis
f. vesicalis uteri
f. vestibularis dentis
f. visceralis hepatis
f. visceralis splenis

facilitated
f. diffusion
f. transport
facilitation
Wedensky f.
facing
faciodigitogenital dysplasia
faciolingual
facioplasty
facioplegia
facioscapulohumeral
f. atrophy
f. muscular dystrophy
FACNM
Fellow of the American College of Nuclear Medicine
FACNP
Fellow of the American College of Nuclear Physicians
FACOG
Fellow of the American College of Obstetricians and Gynecologists
FACP
Fellow of the American College of Physicians
FACR
Fellow of the American College of Radiology
FACS
Fellow of the American College of Surgeons
fluorescence-activated cell sorter

F

FACSM
  Fellow of the American College of Sports
  Medicine
F-actin
factitial dermatitis
factitious
  f. disorder
  f. illness by proxy
  f. melanin
  f. purpura
  f. urticaria
factor
  f. 3
  ABO f.
  accelerator f.
  acetate replacement f.
  adrenal weight f.
  adrenocorticotropic releasing f.
  angiogenesis f.
  animal protein f. (APF)
  antialopecia f.
  antianemic f.
  antiangiogenesis f.
  antiberiberi f.
  anti–black-tongue f.
  anticomplementary f.
  antidermatitis f.
  antihemophilic f. A, B
  antihemorrhagic f.
  antineuritic f.
  antinuclear f. (ANF)
  antipellagra f.
  antipernicious anemia f. (APA)
  antisterility f.
  atrial natriuretic f.
  f. B
  B_T f.
  bacteriocin f.
  B cell differentiating f.
  B cell differentiation/growth f.
  B cell stimulatory f. 2
  bifidus f.
  biotic f.
  Bittner milk f.
  branching f.
  C f.
  CAMP f.
  capillary permeability f.
  Castle intrinsic f.
  Christmas f.
  citrovorum f. (CF)
  clearing f.
  clotting f.
  coagulation f.
  cobra venom f.
  coenzyme f.
  colony-stimulating f.
  complement chemotactic f.
  complement f. I
  corticotropin-releasing f. (CRF)
  coupling f.
  f. D
  debranching f.
  decapacitation f.
  diabetogenic f.

  diffusing f.
  direct lytic f. of cobra venom
  Duran-Reynals permeability f.
  Duran-Reynals spreading f.
  elongation f.
  endothelial relaxing f.
  endothelium-derived relaxing f.
    (EDRF)
  eosinophil chemotactic f. of
    anaphylaxis (ECF-A)
  epidermal growth f. (EGF)
  erythrocyte maturation f.
  essential food f.
  extrinsic f.
  fermentation *Lactobacillus casei* f.
  fertility f.
  fibrin-stabilizing f.
  filtrate f.
  Fitzgerald f.
  Flaujeac f.
  Fletcher f.
  G f.
  glass f.
  glucose tolerance f.
  f. Gm
  gonadotropin-releasing f.
  granulocyte colony-stimulating f. (G-
    CSF)
  granulocyte-macrophage colony-
    stimulating f. (GM-CSF)
  growth f.
  growth hormone-releasing f. (GHRF,
    GH-RF)
  f. H
  Hageman f.
  HG f.
  histamine-releasing f.
  human antihemophilic f.
  hyperglycemic-glycogenolytic f.
    (HGF)
  f. I, II, IIa, III, IV, V, Va, Via,
    VII, VIII, VIII:C, VIIIR, IX, X,
    X for *Haemophilus*, XI, XII, XIII
  impact f.
  inhibition f.
  initiation f. (IF)
  insulinlike growth f. (IGF)
  intrinsic f.
  ischemia-modifying f.
  labile f.
  Lactobacillus bulgaricus f. (LBF)
  Lactobacillus casei f.
  Laki-Lorand f.
  LE f.
  lethal f.
  leukemia inhibitory f.
  leukocytosis-promoting f.
  leukopenic f.
  lipotropic f.
  liver filtrate f.
  liver *Lactobacillus casei* f.
  L-L f.
  luteinizing hormone/follicle-
    stimulating hormone-releasing f.
    (LH/FSH-RF)

luteinizing hormone-releasing f. (LH-RF, LRF)
lymph node permeability f. (LNPF)
macrophage-activating f. (MAF)
macrophage colony-stimulating f. (M-CSF)
maize f.
mammotropic f.
maturation f.
megakaryocyte growth and development f.
melanotropin-releasing f. (MRF)
mesodermal f.
migration-inhibitory f. (MIF)
milk f.
monocyte-derived neutrophil chemotactic f. (MDNCF)
mouse antialopecia f.
müllerian duct inhibitory f.
müllerian inhibiting f.
müllerian regression f.
multicolony-stimulating f. (multi-CSF)
myocardial depressant f. (MDF)
natural killer cell stimulating f.
nephritic f.
nerve growth f. (NGF)
neural f.
neutrophil-activating f.
neutrophil chemotactant f.
nuclear f.-kappa B
osteoclast activating f.
P f.
f. P
pellagra-preventing f. (p-p factor)
plasma labile f.
plasma thromboplastin f. (PTF)
plasma thromboplastin f. B
plasma f. X
plasmin prothrombins conversion f. (PPCF)
platelet f. 3
platelet-activating f.
platelet-aggregating f. (PAF)
platelet-derived growth f. (PDGF)
platelet tissue f.
p-p f.
    pellagra-preventing factor
predisposing f.
prolactin-inhibiting f.
properdin f. B, D
protein f.
pyruvate oxidation f.
quality f. (QF)
ρ f.
R f.
radiation weighting f.
releasing f. (RF)
resistance f.
resistance-inducing f. (RIF)
resistance-transfer f. (RTF)
Rh f.
Rhesus f.
rheumatoid f.
rho f.

risk f.
σ f.
S f.
secretor f.
sex f.
sigma f.
slow-reacting f. of anaphylaxis (SRF-A)
SLR f.
somatotropin release-inhibiting f. (SIF, SRIF)
somatotropin-releasing f. (SRF)
spreading f.
stable f.
stem cell f.
Streptococcus lactis R f.
stringent f.
Stuart f.
Stuart-Prower f.
sun protection f. (SPF)
T-cell growth f.
T-cell growth f.-1, -2
termination f.
testis-determining f. (TDF)
thymic lymphopoietic f.
thyroid-stimulating hormone-releasing f. (TSH-RF)
thyrotropin-releasing f. (TRF)
tissue weighting f.
transfer f.
transforming f.
transforming growth f. (TGF)
transforming growth f. α (TGFalpha)
transforming growth f. β (TGFbeta)
transmethylation f.
tumor angiogenic f. (TAF)
tumor necrosis f. (TNF)
tumor necrosis f.-alpha
tumor necrosis f.-beta
uncoupling f.
von Willebrand f.
W f.
Williams f.
ρ factor
σ factor
factorial
factorial experiment
facultative
    f. anaerobe
    f. heterochromatin
    f. hyperopia
    f. parasite
    f. saprophyte
faculty
FAD
    flavin adenine dinucleotide
Faden suture
fading time
Faget sign
Fahraeus-Lindqvist effect
Fahr disease
Fahrenheit scale
failure
    backward heart f.

F

failure *(continued)*
    cardiac f.
    congestive heart f.
    coronary f.
    electrical f.
    forward heart f.
    heart f.
    high output f.
    left-sided heart f.
    left ventricular f.
    low output f.
    pacemaker f.
    power f.
    premature ovarian f.
    pump f.
    pure autonomic f.
    renal f.
    respiratory f.
    right ventricular f.
    secondary f.
    f. to thrive
faint
faith healing
falcate
falces (*pl. of* falx)
falcial
falciform
    f. cartilage
    f. crest
    f. ligament
    f. ligament of liver
    f. lobe
    f. margin of saphenous opening
    f. process of sacrotuberous ligament
    f. retinal fold
falcine
falciparum
    f. fever
    f. malaria
falcula
falcular
fallacy
    ecological f.
fallen arch-
falling
    f. palate
    f. sickness
    f. of the womb
fallopian
    f. aqueduct
    f. arch
    f. canal
    f. hiatus
    f. ligament
    f. neuritis
    f. pregnancy
    f. tube
Fallot
    F. tetrad
    F. triad
false
    f. agglutination
    f. albuminuria
    f. anemia

    f. aneurysm
    f. angina
    f. ankylosis
    f. blepharoptosis
    f. branching
    f. cast
    f. chordae tendineae
    f. conjugate
    f. coxa vara
    f. cyanosis
    f. cyst
    f. dextrocardia
    f. diphtheria
    f. diverticulum
    f. dominance
    f. glottis
    f. hellebore
    f. hematuria
    f. hermaphroditism
    f. hypertrophy
    f. image
    f. joint
    f. knot
    f. knot of umbilical cord
    f. labor
    f. lumen
    f. macula
    f. membrane
    f. memory syndrome
    f. negative
    f.-negative reaction
    f. neuroma
    f. nucleolus
    f. pain
    f. paracusis
    f. pelvis
    f. positive
    f.-positive reaction
    f. pregnancy
    f. projection
    f. rib
    f. suture
    f. tendinous cord
    f. thirst
    f. vertebra
    f. vocal cord
    f. water
falsetto
falsification
    retrospective f.
falx, pl. **falces**
    f. aponeurotica
    cerebellar f.
    f. cerebelli
    cerebral f.
    f. cerebri
    inguinal f.
    f. inguinalis
    f. septi
familial
    f. adenomatous polyposis (FAP)
    f. aggregation
    f. aminoglycoside ototoxicity
    f. amyloid neuropathy
    f. amyloidosis

f. aortic ectasia
f. aortic ectasia syndrome
f. bipolar mood disorder
f. cancer
f. chylomicronemia syndrome
f. combined hyperlipemia
f. dysautonomia
f. emphysema
f. erythrophagocytic lymphohistiocytosis (FEL)
f. fat-induced hyperlipemia
f. glycinuria
f. goiter
f. hemophagocytic lymphohistiocytosis (FMLH)
f. high density lipoprotein deficiency
f. hyperbetalipoproteinemia
f. hyperbetalipoproteinemia and hyperprebetalipoproteinemia
f. hypercholesteremic xanthomatosis
f. hypercholesterolemia
f. hypercholesterolemia with hyperlipemia
f. hyperchylomicronemia
f. hyperchylomicronemia with hyperprebetalipoproteinemia
f. hyperlipoproteinemia
f. hyperprebetalipoproteinemia
f. hypertriglyceridemia
f. hypertrophic cardiomyopathy
f. hypobetalipoproteinemia
f. hypogonadotropic hypogonadism
f. hypoparathyroidism
f. hypophosphatemic rickets
f. hypoplastic anemia
f. juvenile nephrophthisis
f. lipoprotein lipase inhibitor
f. Mediterranean fever
f. microcytic anemia
f. multiple endocrine adenomatosis
f. nephrosis
f. neuroviscerolipidosis
f. nonhemolytic jaundice
f. paroxysmal polyserositis
f. paroxysmal rhabdomyolysis
f. partial lipodystrophy
f. periodic paralysis
f. polyposis coli
f. pseudoinflammatory macular degeneration
f. pseudoinflammatory maculopathy
f. pyridoxine-responsive anemia
f. recurrent polyserositis
f. screening
f. spinal muscular atrophy
f. tremor
f. white folded dysplasia
family
alu f.
alu-equivalent f.
cancer f.
extended f.
gene f.
f. medicine

nuclear f.
f. physician
f. practice
f. therapy
famine dropsy
famotidine
famotine hydrochloride
Fañanás cell
FANA test (*var. of* fluorescent antinuclear antibody test)
Fanconi
F. anemia
F. pancytopenia
F. syndrome
fang
fango
Fannia
fan sign
fantasy
FAP
familial adenomatous polyposis
FAPA syndrome
far
F. East hemorrhagic fever
F. East Russian encephalitis
f. point
f. point of convergence
f. sight
Farabeuf
F. amputation
F. triangle
farad
faraday (*F*)
F. constant
F. law
faradism
surging f.
faradization
faradocontractility
faradomuscular
faradopalpation
faradotherapy
far-and-near suture
Farber
F. disease
F. syndrome
farcy
fardel
farfara
farina
f. avenae
f. tritici
farinaceous
farmer's
f. lung
f. skin
farnesene alcohol
farnesol
farnesyl pyrophosphate
farnoquinone
Farnsworth-Munsell color test
Farrant mounting fluid
Farre line
Farr law
farsightedness

F

Fas
    F. ligand
    F. receptor
fascia, pl. **fasciae, fascias**
    f. abdominalis parietalis
    Abernethy f.
    f. adherens
    anal f.
    antebrachial f.
    f. antebrachii
    f. axillaris
    axillary f.
    bicipital f.
    brachial f.
    f. brachii
    broad f.
    f. buccopharyngea
    buccopharyngeal f.
    Buck f.
    f. bulbi
    Camper f.
    f. cervicalis
    f. cervicalis profunda
    f. cinerea
    clavipectoral f.
    f. clavipectoralis
    f. clitoridis
    f. of clitoris
    Colles f.
    Cooper f.
    cremasteric f.
    f. cremasterica
    cribriform f.
    f. cribrosa
    crural f.
    f. cruris
    Cruveilhier f.
    dartos f.
    deep f.
    deep f. of arm
    deep cervical f.
    deep f. of forearm
    deep f. of leg
    deep f. of neck
    deep f. of penis
    deep perineal f.
    deep f. of thigh
    f. dentata hippocampi
    dentate f.
    f. diaphragmatis pelvis inferior
    f. diaphragmatis urogenitalis inferior
    dorsal f. of foot
    dorsal f. of hand
    f. dorsalis manus
    f. dorsalis pedis
    Dupuytren f.
    endoabdominal f.
    f. endoabdominalis
    endopelvic f.
    f. endopelvina
    endothoracic f.
    f. endothoracica
    external spermatic f.
    f. of extraocular muscle
    extraperitoneal f.

    f. extraperitonealis
    f. of forearm
    Gallaudet f.
    Gerota f.
    Godman f.
    f. graft
    Hesselbach f.
    hypothenar f.
    iliac f.
    f. iliaca
    iliopectineal f.
    inferior f. of pelvic diaphragm
    inferior f. of urogenital diaphragm
    f. infraspinata
    infraspinatus f.
    infraspinous f.
    infundibuliform f.
    intercolumnar fasciae
    internal spermatic f.
    interosseous f.
    f. investiens
    f. investiens perinei superficialis
    investing f.
    lacrimal f.
    f. lata
    f. of leg
    lumbodorsal f.
    masseteric f.
    f. masseterica
    middle cervical f.
    muscular f.
    muscular f. of extraocular muscle
    f. muscularis musculorum bulbi
    f. musculi quadrati lumborum
    f. nuchae
    nuchal f.
    obturator f.
    f. obturatoria
    f. of obturator internus
    orbital fasciae
    fasciae orbitales
    palmar f.
    parietal abdominal f.
    parietal pelvic f.
    parotid f.
    f. parotidea
    parotideomasseteric f.
    f. parotideomasseterica
    pectoral f.
    f. pectoralis
    pelvic f.
    f. pelvica
    f. pelvis
    f. pelvis parietalis
    f. pelvis visceralis
    f. penis
    f. of penis
    f. penis profunda
    f. penis superficialis
    perineal f.
    f. perinei
    f. perinei superficialis
    perirenal f.
    pharyngobasilar f.
    f. pharyngobasilaris

phrenicopleural f.
f. phrenicopleuralis
plantar f.
popliteal f.
Porter f.
prececocolic f.
f. prececocolica
presacral f.
f. presacralis
pretracheal f.
prevertebral f.
f. profunda
f. prostatae
f. of prostate
rectosacral f.
f. rectosacralis
rectovesical f.
renal f.
f. renalis
Scarpa f.
semilunar f.
Sibson f.
f. spermatica externa
f. spermatica interna
subperitoneal f.
f. subperitonealis
subsartorial f.
superficial f.
superficial investing f. of perineum
f. superficialis
superficial f. of penis
superficial f. of perineum
superficial f. of scrotum
f. superior diaphragmatis pelvis
superior f. of pelvic diaphragm
temporal f.
f. temporalis
f. thoracolumbalis
thoracolumbar f.
Toldt f.
f. transversalis
transversalis f.
Treitz f.
triangular f.
f. triangularis abdominis
Tyrrell f.
umbilical f.
f. umbilicalis
umbilical prevesical f.
umbilicovesical f.
vastoadductor f.
visceral f.
visceral pelvic f.
Zuckerkandl f.

fascial

f. hernia
f. sheath of extraocular muscle
f. sheath of eyeball

fascicle

anterior f. of palatopharyngeus
  muscle
muscle f.
nerve f.
posterior f. of palatopharyngeus
  muscle

fascicular

f. block
f. degeneration
f. graft
f. keratitis
f. ophthalmoplegia
f. sarcoma
f. ulcer

fasciculata cell
fasciculate
fasciculation
fasciculus, fasciculi, pl. fasciculi

f. anterior musculi palatopharyngei
anterior f. proprius
anterior pyramidal f.
arcuate f.
f. atrioventricularis
Burdach f.
calcarine f.
central tegmental f.
f. circumolivaris pyramidis
f. corticospinalis anterior
f. corticospinalis lateralis
cuneate f.
f. cuneatus
dorsal longitudinal f.
dorsolateral f.
f. dorsolateralis
Flechsig fasciculi
Foville f.
fronto-occipital f.
gracile f.
f. gracilis
hooked f.
inferior longitudinal f.
inferior occipitofrontal f.
interfascicular f.
f. interfascicularis
intersegmental fasciculi
f. lateralis plexus brachialis
lateral f. proprius
lateral pyramidal f.
lenticular f.
f. lenticularis
Lissauer f.
fasciculi longitudinales ligamenti
  cruciformis atlantis
fasciculi longitudinales pontis
f. longitudinalis inferior
f. longitudinalis medialis
f. longitudinalis posterior
f. longitudinalis superior
longitudinal pontine fasciculi
macular f.
f. macularis
mammillotegmental f.
f. mammillotegmentalis
mammillothalamic f.
f. mammillothalamicus
marginal f.
f. marginalis
f. medialis plexus brachialis
f. medialis telencephali
medial longitudinal f.
f. of Meynert

F

fasciculus *(continued)*
    oblique pontine f.
    f. obliquus pontis
    occipitofrontal f.
    f. occipitofrontalis
    f. occipitofrontalis inferior
    f. occipitofrontalis superior
    oval f.
    f. pedunculomammillaris
    pedunculomammillary f.
    perpendicular f.
    f. posterior musculi palatopharyngei
    f. posterior plexus brachialis
    posterior f. proprius
    proper fasciculi
    fasciculi proprii
    f. proprius anterior
    f. proprius lateralis
    f. pyramidalis anterior
    f. pyramidalis lateralis
    retroflex f.
    f. retroflexus
    f. rotundus
    round f.
    rubroreticular fasciculi
    fasciculi rubroreticulares
    semilunar f.
    f. semilunaris
    septomarginal f.
    f. septomarginalis
    slender f.
    f. solitarius
    solitary f.
    subcallosal f.
    f. subcallosus for superior
       occipitofrontal fasciculus
    subthalamic f.
    f. subthalamicus
    superior longitudinal f.
    superior occipitofrontal f.
    thalamic f.
    f. thalamicus
    f. thalamomammillaris
    transverse fasciculi
    fasciculi transversi
    unciform f.
    uncinate f.
    uncinate f. of cerebellum
    uncinate f. of Russell
    f. uncinatus
    f. uncinatus cerebelli
    wedge-shaped f.
fasciectomy
fasciitis
    eosinophilic f.
    group A streptococcal necrotizing f.
    necrotizing f.
    nodular f.
    parosteal f.
    plantar f.
    proliferative f.
    pseudosarcomatous f.
fasciodesis

Fasciola
    f. cinerea
    f. gigantica
    f. hepatica
fasciolar gyrus
fascioliasis
fasciolid
fasciolopsiasis
Fasciolopsis
    f. buski
    f. rathouisi
fasciorrhaphy
fasciotomy
fascitis
fast
    f. component of nystagmus
    f. green FCF
    f. smear
fastidious organism
fastigatum
fastigial nucleus
fastigiobulbar
    f. fiber
    f. tract
fastigiospinal
    f. fiber
    f. tract
fastigium
fasting hypoglycemia
fastness
fast-neutron radiation therapy
fat
    f. body
    f. body of cheek
    f. body of ischioanal fossa
    f. body of ischiorectal fossa
    f. body of orbit
    brown f.
    f. cell
    f. embolism
    f. graft
    f. hernia
    f. indigestion
    f. metabolism
    multilocular f.
    f. necrosis
    neutral f.
    f. pad
    f. pad of ischioanal fossa
    paranephric f.
    retrobulbar f.
    saturated f.
    f. solvent
    split f.
    f. tide
    unilocular f.
    unsaturated f.
    white f.
fatal
fatality rate
fate
    f. map
    prospective f.
father complex
fatigability

fatigable
fatigue
    auditory f.
    battle f.
    f. fever
    f. fracture
    functional vocal f.
    f. strength
fat-pad
    Bichat f.-p.
    buccal f.-p.
    Imlach f.-p.
    infrapatellar f.-p.
    ischiorectal f.-p.
fat-soluble vitamin
fat-storing cell
fatty
    f. acid
    f. acid–binding protein
    f. acid oxidation cycle
    f. alcohol
    f. appendix of colon
    f. ascites
    f. atrophy
    f. cast
    f. change
    f. cirrhosis
    f. degeneration
    f. diarrhea
    f. fold of pleura
    f. heart
    f. hernia
    f. infiltration
    f. kidney
    f. layer of subcutaneous tissue
    f. layer of subcutaneous tissue of abdomen
    f. layer of superficial fascia
    f. liver
    f. metamorphosis
    f. oil
    f. phanerosis
    f. renal capsule
    f. series
    f. stool
    f. tissue
fatty acid
    ω-3 fatty acids
    activated fatty acid
    diethenoid fatty acid
    essential fatty acid
    omega-3 fatty acids
    saturated fatty acid
    fatty acid synthase complex
    fatty acid thiokinase
    unesterified free fatty acid (FFA, UFA)
    unsaturated fatty acid
fauces
faucial
    f. branch of lingual nerve
    f. diphtheria
    f. paralysis
    f. reflex
    f. tonsil

faulty union
fauna
faun tail nevus
faveolate
faveolus, pl. **faveoli**
favic chandelier
favid
FA virus
favism
Favre-Durand-Nicholas disease
Favre dystrophy
Favre-Racouchot
    F.-R. disease
    F.-R. syndrome
favus
Fazio-Londe disease
Fc
    Fc fragment
    Fc piece
    Fc receptor
FCAP
    Fellow of the College of American Pathologists
FCCP
    Fellow of the College of Chest Physicians
Fd
    ferredoxin
FDA
    Food and Drug Administration of the United States Department of Health and Human Services
FDNB
    fluoro-2,4-dinitrobenzene
FDP
    fibrin/fibrinogen degradation product
Fe
    iron
^{59}Fe
    iron-59
^{52}Fe
    iron-52
^{55}Fe
    iron-55
fear
feature
febricant
febricula
febrifacient
febriferous
febrific
febrifugal
febrifuge
febrile
    f. albuminuria
    f. convulsion
    f. crisis
    f. psychosis
    f. seizure
    f. urine
    f. urticaria
febris
    f. melitensis
    f. undulans
fecal
    f. abscess

F

fecal *(continued)*
    f. concentration
    f. examination
    f. fistula
    f. impaction
    f. incontinence
    f. tumor
    f. vomiting
fecalith
fecaloid
fecaloma
fecaluria
feces
Fechner-Weber law
feculent
fecund
fecundate
fecundation
fecundity
feedback
    f. activation
    auditory f.
    f. inhibition
    negative f.
    positive f.
    f. system
    tubuloglomerular f.
feed-forward activation
feeding
    f. center
    fictitious f.
    forced f.
    forcible f.
    gastric f.
    nasal f.
    sham f.
    f. tube
fee-for-service insurance
feeling tone
Feer disease
FEF
    forced expiratory flow
Fehling
    F. reagent
    F. solution
feigned eruption
Feiss line
FEL
    familial erythrophagocytic lymphohistiocytosis
felbamate
Felidae
feline
fellatio
Fellow
    F. of the American Academy of Nursing (FAAN)
    F. of the American College of Chest Physicians (*var. of* FACCP) (FACCP, Fellow of the American College of Chest Physicians)
    F. of the American College of Dentists (FACD)

    F. of the American College of Nuclear Medicine (FACNM)
    F. of the American College of Nuclear Physicians (FACNP)
    F. of the American College of Obstetricians and Gynecologists (FACOG)
    F. of the American College of Physicians (FACP)
    F. of the American College of Radiology (FACR)
    F. of the American College of Sports Medicine (FACSM)
    F. of the American College of Surgeons (FACS)
    F. of the College of American Pathologists (FCAP)
    F. of the College of Chest Physicians (FCCP)
    F. of the Faculty of Radiologists (United Kingdom) (FFR)
    F. of the Royal College of Physicians (Canada) (FRCP(C))
    F. of the Royal College of Physicians (Edinburgh) (FRCP(E), FRCP(Edin))
    F. of the Royal College of Physicians (Ireland) (FRCP(I))
    F. of the Royal College of Physicians (of England) (FRCP)
    F. of the Royal College of Surgeons (Canada) (FRCS(C))
    F. of the Royal College of Surgeons (Edinburgh) (FRCS(E), FRCS(Edin))
    F. of the Royal College of Surgeons (Ireland) (FRCS(I))
    F. of the Royal College of Surgeons (of England) (FRCS)
    F. of the Royal Society (FRS)
    F. of the Royal Society (Canada) (FRSC)
fellow
felodipine
felon
feltwork
Felty syndrome
felypressin
female
    f. catheter
    f. circumcision
    f. external genitalia
    genetic f.
    f. gonad
    f. hermaphroditism
    f. homosexuality
    f. internal genitalia
    f. pattern alopecia
    f. prostate
    f. pseudohermaphroditism
    f. sterility
    f. urethra
    XO f.
    XXX f.
femininity complex

feminization
    testicular f.
femora (*pl. of* femur) (*pl. of* femoral)
femoral, pl. **femora**
    f. arch
    f. branch of genitofemoral nerve
    f. canal
    f. fossa
    f. hernia
    f. muscle
    f. nerve
    f. nutrient artery
    f. opening
    f. plexus
    f. reflex
    f. region
    f. ring
    f. septum
    f. sheath
    f. triangle
    f. vein
femoris
femoroabdominal reflex
femorocele
femoropatellar joint
femoropopliteal
    f. bypass
    f. occlusive disease
femorotibial
femur, pl. **femora**
fenbufen
fencamine
fenclofenac
fenclonine
fenestra, fenestrae, pl. **fenestrae**
    f. of the cochlea
    f. cochleae
    f. nov-ovalis
    f. ovalis
    f. rotunda
    f. of the vestibule
    f. vestibuli
fenestrated
    f. capillary
    f. membrane
    f. sheath
fenestration
    f. operation
    optic nerve sheath f.
    tracheal f.
fenethylline hydrochloride
fenfluramine hydrochloride
Fenn effect
fennel
fenoprofen calcium
fenoterol
fenpipramide
fentanyl citrate
fenticlor
Fenton reaction
fenugreek
Fenwick-Hunner ulcer
feral
Ferguson reflex
Fergusson incision

ferment
fermentable
fermentation
    acetic f.
    acetous f.
    alcoholic f.
    amylic f.
    lactic acid f.
    f. *Lactobacillus casei* factor
fermentative dyspepsia
fermenter
fermium
Fernandez reaction
Fernbach flask
ferning
fern test
Ferrata cell
ferredoxin (Fd)
Ferrein
    F. canal
    F. cord
    F. foramen
    F. ligament
    F. pyramid
    F. tube
    F. vasa aberrantia
ferri-
ferric
    f. alum
    f. and ammonium acetate solution
    f. ammonium citrate
    f. ammonium citrate, green
    f. ammonium sulfate
    f. chloride
    f. chloride reaction of epinephrine
    f. chloride test
    f. fructose
    f. glycerophosphate
    f. hydroxide
    f. oxide
    f. sulfate
ferric phosphate
    soluble f. p.
ferricyanide
ferricytochrome
ferriheme chloride
ferrihemoglobin
ferriporphyrin
    f. chloride
ferriprotoporphyrin
ferritin
ferrochelatase
ferrocholinate
ferrocyanide
ferrocytochrome
ferroheme
ferrokinetics
ferroporphyrin
ferroprotein
ferroprotoporphyrin
ferrosoferric
ferrotherapy
ferrous
    f. citrate
    f. fumarate

F

ferrous *(continued)*
 f. gluconate
 f. lactate
 f. succinate
ferrous sulfate
 dried f. s.
ferrugination
ferruginous body
ferrule
Ferry line
Ferry-Porter law
fertile period
fertility
 f. agent
 f. factor
 f. ratio
 f. vitamin
fertilization
 f. membrane
 in vitro f. (IVF)
 in vivo f.
fertilized ovum
fertilizin
Ferula
fervescence
FESS
 functional endoscopic sinus surgery
fester
festinant
festinating gait
festination
festoon
 gingival f.
festooning
FET
 forced expiratory time
fetal
 f. adrenal cortex
 f. alcohol syndrome
 f. aspiration syndrome
 f. attitude
 f. bradycardia
 f. circulation
 f. cotyledon
 f. death
 f. death rate
 f. distress
 f. dystocia
 f. electrocardiography
 f. erythroblastosis
 f. face syndrome
 f. fracture
 f. gigantism
 f. growth restriction
 f. habitus
 f. heart rate
 f. hemoglobin
 f. hydantoin syndrome
 f. hydrops
 f. inclusion
 f. membrane
 f. movement
 f. ovoid
 f. placenta

 f. reticularis
 f. scalp stimulation
 f. souffle
 f. tachycardia
 f. trimethadione syndrome
 f. warfarin syndrome
 f. zone
fetalism
fetation
feticide
fetid
fetish
fetishism
fetoglobulin
fetography
fetology
fetomaternal transfusion
fetometry
fetopathy
 diabetic f.
fetoplacental anasarca
fetoprotein
 α f.
α-fetoprotein
β-fetoprotein
β-fetoprotein
γ-fetoprotein
γ-fetoprotein
fetor
 f. hepaticus
 f. oris
fetoscope
fetoscopy
fetuin
fetus, pl. **fetuses**
 f. in fetu
 harlequin f.
 impacted f.
 f. papyraceus
 f. sanguinolentis
Feulgen
 F. cytometry
 F. reaction
 F. stain
FEV
 forced expiratory volume
fever
 absorption f.
 acclimating f.
 Aden f.
 aestivoautumnal f.
 African hemorrhagic f.
 African tick f.
 African tick-bite f.
 algid pernicious f.
 ardent f.
 Argentinean hemorrhagic f.
 artificial f.
 aseptic f.
 Assam f.
 Australian Q f.
 autumn f.
 benign tertian f.
 bilious remittent f.
 black f.

blackwater f.
f. blister
blue f.
Bolivian hemorrhagic f.
bouquet f.
boutonneuse f.
brass founder's f.
Brazilian hemorrhagic f.
Brazilian purpuric f.
Brazilian spotted f.
breakbone f.
Bunyamwera f.
Burdwan f.
Bwamba f.
cachectic f.
camp f.
canicola f.
catarrhal f.
cat-bite f.
catheter f.
catscratch f.
Central European tick-borne f.
cerebrospinal f.
Charcot intermittent f.
childbed f.
Colorado tick f.
Congolian red f.
continued f.
cotton-mill f.
Crimean f.
Crimean-Congo hemorrhagic f.
dandy f.
date f.
deer-fly f.
dehydration f.
dengue hemorrhagic f.
desert f.
digestive f.
diphasic milk f.
double quotidian f.
drug f.
Dumdum f.
Dutton relapsing f.
Ebola hemorrhagic f.
elephantoid f.
enteric f.
entericoid f.
ephemeral f.
epidemic hemorrhagic f.
epimastical f.
eruptive f.
essential f.
exanthematous f.
exsiccation f.
falciparum f.
familial Mediterranean f.
Far East hemorrhagic f.
fatigue f.
field f.
five-day f.
Flinders Island spotted f.
flood f.
food f.
Fort Bragg f.
foundryman's f.

Gambian f.
glandular f.
Haverhill f.
hay f.
hematuric bilious f.
hemoglobinuric f.
hemorrhagic f.
hemorrhagic f. with renal syndrome
hepatic intermittent f.
herpetic f.
hospital f.
icterohemorrhagic f.
Ilhéus f.
inanition f.
induced f.
intermittent malarial f.
inundation f.
island f.
jail f.
Japanese river f.
Japanese spotted f.
jungle f.
jungle yellow f.
Katayama f.
kedani f.
Kenya f.
Kew Gardens f.
Kinkiang f.
Korean hemorrhagic f.
Lassa f.
Lassa hemorrhagic f.
laurel f.
malarial f.
malignant tertian f.
Malta f.
Manchurian hemorrhagic f.
Marseilles f.
marsh f.
Mediterranean erythematous f.
Mediterranean exanthematous f.
Mediterranean spotted f.
meningotyphoid f.
metal fume f.
Mexican spotted f.
miliary f.
milk f.
mill f.
miniature scarlet f.
monoleptic f.
Mossman f.
mud f.
mumu f.
nanukayami f.
nine mile f.
nodal f.
North Queensland tick f.
Omsk hemorrhagic f.
o'nyong-nyong f.
Oropouche f.
Oroya f.
Pahvant Valley f.
paludal f.
pappataci f.
paratyphoid f.
parenteric f.

F

357

fever *(continued)*
    parrot f.
    Pel-Ebstein f.
    periodic f.
    Persian relapsing f.
    pharyngoconjunctival f.
    Philippine hemorrhagic f.
    phlebotomus f.
    pinta f.
    polka f.
    polyleptic f.
    polymer fume f.
    pretibial f.
    protein f.
    puerperal f.
    Pym f.
    pyogenic f.
    Q f.
    quartan f.
    quintan f.
    quotidian f.
    rabbit f.
    rat-bite f.
    recrudescent typhus f.
    recurrent f.
    red f.
    red f. of the Congo
    relapsing f.
    remittent malarial f.
    rheumatic f.
    rice-field f.
    Rift Valley f.
    Rocky Mountain spotted f.
    Roman f.
    Ross River f.
    sakushu f.
    Salinem f.
    salt f.
    sandfly f.
    San Joaquin Valley f.
    São Paulo f.
    scarlet f.
    Schamberg f.
    Sennetsu f.
    septic f.
    seven-day f.
    shin bone f.
    ship f.
    shoddy f.
    simian hemorrhagic f.
    Sindbis f.
    slime f.
    slow f.
    smelter's f.
    snail f.
    solar f.
    Songo f.
    South African tick-bite f.
    spirillum f.
    spotted f.
    steroid f.
    symptomatic f.
    syphilitic f.
    tertian f.

    therapeutic f.
    f. therapy
    thermic f.
    thirst f.
    three-day f.
    Tobia f.
    traumatic f.
    trench f.
    trypanosome f.
    tsutsugamushi f.
    typhoid f.
    undifferentiated type f.
    undulant f.
    undulating f.
    f. of unknown origin (FUO)
    urethral f.
    urinary f.
    urticarial f.
    uveoparotid f.
    Uzbekistan hemorrhagic f.
    valley f.
    Venezuelan hemorrhagic f.
    viral hemorrhagic f.
    vivax f.
    Wesselsbron f.
    West African f.
    West Nile f.
    wound f.
    Yangtze Valley f.
    yellow f.
    Zika f.
    zinc fume f.
feverish urine
FF
    filtration fraction
FFA
    unesterified free fatty acid
FFP
    fresh frozen plasma
FFR
    Fellow of the Faculty of Radiologists
    (United Kingdom)
ff waves *(var. of* f wave)
FGAR
    n-formylglycinamide ribotide
FH₄
    tetrahydrofolic acid
fiat (ft.)
fiber
    A f.
    accelerator f.
    adrenergic f.
    afferent f.
    alpha f.
    anastomosing f.
    anastomotic f.
    anterior external arcuate f.
    arcuate f.
    arcuate f. of cerebrum
    argyrophilic f.
    association f.
    astral f.
    augmentor f.
    autonomic nerve f.
    B f.

Bergmann f.
beta f.
bulbar corticonuclear f.
C f.
cerebellohypothalamic f.
cerebelloolivary f.
cerebellospinal f.
cholinergic f.
chromatic f.
circular f.
climbing f.
collagen f.
collagenous f.
commissural f.
cone f.
corticobulbar f.
corticomesencephalic f.
corticonuclear f.
corticopontine f.
corticoreticular f.
corticorubral f.
corticospinal f.
corticothalamic f.
cuneocerebellar f.
cuneospinal f.
decussation of trochlear nerve f.
delta f.
dental f.
dentatorubral f.
dentatothalamic f.
dentinal f.
depressor f.
dietary f.
efferent f.
elastic f.
enamel f.
endogenous f.
exogenous f.
external arcuate f.
fastigiobulbar f.
fastigiospinal f.
frontopontine f.
gamma f.
Gerdy f.
gracilespinal f.
Gratiolet f.
gray f.
hypothalamocerebellar f.
hypothalamospinal f.
inhibitory f.
inner cone f.
intercolumnar f.
intercrural f. of superficial ring
internal arcuate f.
intrafusal f.
intrathalamic f.
intrinsic f.
James f.
kinetochore f.
Korff f.
Kühne f.
f. of lens
long association f.
longitudinal pontine f.
Mahaim f.

medullated nerve f.
meridional f. of ciliary muscle
mesencephalic corticonuclear f.
mossy f.
motor f.
Müller f.
myelinated nerve f.
Nélaton f.
nerve f.
nodoventricular f.
nonmedullated f.
nuclear bag f.
nuclear chain f.
nucleocortical f.
oblique f. of muscular layer of
  stomach
occipitopontine f.
occipitotectal f.
olivocochlear f.
olivospinal f.
osteocollagenous f.
osteogenic f.
outer cone f.
parietopontine f.
pectinate f.
perforating f.
periodontal ligament f.
periventricular f.
pilomotor f.
polar f.
pontine corticonuclear f.
pontocerebellar f.
postcommissural f.
posterior external arcuate f.
postganglionic f.
postganglionic nerve f.
precollagenous f.
precommissural f.
preganglionic nerve f.
pressor f.
pretectoolivary f.
projection f.
Prussak f.
Purkinje f.
pyramidal f.
raphespinal f.
red f.
Reissner f.
Remak f.
reticular f.
Retzius f.
rod f.
Rosenthal f.
rubroolivary f.
Sappey f.
Sharpey f.
short association f.
skeletal muscle f.
somatic nerve f.
spindle f.
spinocuneate f.
spinogracile f.
spinohypothalamic f.
spinomesencephalic f.
spinoolivary f.

F

fiber *(continued)*
  spinoperiaqueductal f.
  spinoreticular f.
  spinotectal f.
  stress f.
  striatonigral f.
  strionigral f.
  sudomotor f.
  sustentacular f. of retina
  T f.
  tautomeric f.
  tectoolivary f.
  tectopontine f.
  tectoreticular f.
  temporopontine f.
  thalamocortical f.
  Tomes f.
  transseptal f.
  transverse pontine
  unmyelinated f.
  vasomotor f.
  visceral motor f.
  Weitbrecht f.
  white f.
  yellow f.
  zonular f.
fiberoptic gastroscope
fiberoptics
fiberscope
fibra, pl. **fibrae**
  fibrae arcuatae cerebri
  fibrae arcuatae externae
  fibrae arcuatae externae anteriores
  fibrae arcuatae externae posteriores
  fibrae arcuatae internae
  fibrae associationes breves
  fibrae associationes longae
  fibrae cerebelloolivares
  fibrae circulares
  fibrae corticomesencephalicae
  fibrae corticonucleares
  fibrae corticonucleares bulbi
  fibrae corticonucleares mesencephali
  fibrae corticonucleares pontis
  fibrae corticopontinae
  fibrae corticoreticulares
  fibrae corticorubrales
  fibrae corticospinales
  fibrae cuneocerebellares
  fibrae cuneospinales
  fibrae dentatorubrales
  fibrae frontopontinae
  fibrae gracilispinales
  fibrae hypothalamospinales
  fibrae intercrurales anuli inguinalis
    superficialis
  fibrae intrathalamicae
  fibrae lentis
  fibrae meridionales muscularis
    ciliaris
  fibrae obliquae tunicae muscularis
  fibrae occipitopontinae
  fibrae occipitotectales
  fibrae olivospinales

  fibrae parietopontinae
  fibrae periventriculares
  fibrae pontis longitudinales
  fibrae pontis transversae
  fibrae pontocerebellares
  fibrae postcommissurales
  fibrae precommissurales
  fibrae pretectoolivares
  fibrae pyramidales
  fibrae rubroolivares
  fibrae spinocuneatae
  fibrae spinograciles
  fibrae spinohypothalamicae
  fibrae spinomesencephalicae
  fibrae spinoolivares
  fibrae spinoperiaqueductales
  fibrae spinoreticulares
  fibrae spinotectales
  fibrae tectoolivares
  fibrae tectopontinae
  fibrae tectoreticulares
  fibrae temporopontinae
  fibrae zonulares
fibrates
fibre
fibremia
fibric acid
fibril
  anchoring f.
  collagen f.
  muscular f.
  subpellicular f.
  unit f.
fibrilla, pl. **fibrillae**
fibrillar, fibrillary
  f. astrocyte
  f. astrocytoma
  f. baskets
  f. chorea
  f. contraction
  f. myoclonia
  f. neuroma
  f. wave
fibrillate
fibrillated
fibrillation
  atrial f.
  auricular f.
  f. threshold
  ventricular f.
fibrillatory wave
fibrillin
fibrilloflutter
fibrillogenesis
fibrin
  f. calculus
  f. thrombus
fibrinase
fibrin/fibrinogen degradation product
  (FDP)
fibrinocellular
fibrinogen
  human f.
fibrinogenase
fibrinogenemia

fibrinogenesis
fibrinogen-fibrin conversion syndrome
fibrinogenic
fibrinogenolysis
fibrinogenopenia
fibrinoid
    f. degeneration
    f. necrosis
fibrinokinase
fibrinolysin
    streptococcal f.
fibrinolysis
fibrinolysokinase
fibrinolytic purpura
fibrinopeptide
fibrinopurulent inflammation
fibrinoscopy
fibrinous
    f. adhesion
    f. bronchitis
    f. cast
    f. cataract
    f. degeneration
    f. inflammation
    f. iritis
    f. lymph
    f. pericarditis
    f. pleurisy
fibrin-stabilizing factor
fibrinuria
fibroadenoma
    giant f.
    intracanalicular f.
    pericanalicular f.
fibroadipose
fibroareolar
fibroblastic
fibroblast interferon
fibrocartilage
    basilar f.
    circumferential f.
    external semilunar f.
    interarticular f.
    internal semilunar f. of knee joint
    interpubic f.
    semilunar f.
    stratiform f.
fibrocartilaginous ring of tympanic
  membrane
fibrocartilago
    f. basalis
    f. interarticularis
    f. interpubica
    f. intervertebralis
fibrocaseous peritonitis
fibrocellular
fibrochondritis
fibrochondroma
fibrocongestive
fibrocystic
    f. condition of the breast
    f. disease of the pancreas
fibrocyte
fibrodysplasia ossificans progressiva
fibroelastic membrane of larynx

fibroelastosis
    endocardial f.
    endomyocardial f.
fibroepithelial polyp
fibroepithelioma
fibrofatty
fibrofolliculoma
fibrogenesis
fibrogliosis
fibrohyaline tissue
fibroid
    f. cataract
    f. inflammation
    f. lung
    f. tumor
fibroidectomy
fibroin
fibrolamellar liver cell carcinoma
fibroleiomyoma
fibrolipoma
fibroma
    ameloblastic f.
    aponeurotic f.
    cementoossifying f.
    central ossifying f.
    chondromyxoid f.
    concentric f.
    desmoplastic f.
    giant cell f.
    irritation f.
    f. molle
    f. molle gravidarum
    f. myxomatodes
    nonossifying f.
    nonosteogenic f.
    odontogenic f.
    peripheral ossifying f.
    periungual f.
    rabbit f.
    recurring digital f. of childhood
    Shope f.
    telangiectatic f.
fibromatoid
fibromatosis
    abdominal f.
    aggressive infantile f.
    f. colli
    congenital generalized f.
    gingival f.
    infantile digital f.
    juvenile hyalin f.
    juvenile palmo-plantar f.
    palmar f.
    penile f.
    plantar f.
fibromatous
fibromectomy
fibrometer
fibromuscular
    f. dysplasia
    f. hyperplasia
fibromusculocartilagenous layer of
  bronchi
fibromyalgia syndrome
fibromyectomy

F

fibromyoma
fibromyositis
fibromyxoma
fibronectin
    large, external transformation-
      sensitive f. (LETS)
    plasma f.
fibroneuroma
fibroosteoma
fibropapilloma
fibroplasia
    retrolental f.
fibroplastic
fibroplate
fibropolypus
fibroreticulate
fibrosa
    pericardium f.
fibrosarcoma
    ameloblastic f.
    Earle L f.
    infantile f.
fibrose
fibroserous
fibrosing
    f. adenomatosis
    f. adenosis
    f. alveolitis
    f. colonopathy
    f. mediastinitis
fibrosis
    African endomyocardial f.
    congenital f. of the extraocular
      muscles
    cystic f.
    cystic f. of the pancreas
    endocardial f.
    endomyocardial f.
    idiopathic interstitial f.
    idiopathic pulmonary f. (IPF)
    interstitial pulmonary f.
    leptomeningeal f.
    mediastinal f.
    nodular subepidermal f.
    oral submucous f.
    pericentral f.
    perimuscular f.
    pipestem f.
    replacement f.
    retroperitoneal f.
    subadventitial f.
    Symmers clay pipestem f.
fibrositic headache
fibrositis
    cervical f.
fibrothorax
fibrotic ophthalmoplegia
fibrous
    f. adhesion
    f. ankylosis
    f. appendix of liver
    f. articular capsule
    f. astrocyte
    f. bacterial virus-
    f. capsule

    f. capsule of kidney
    f. capsule of liver
    f. capsule of parotid gland
    f. capsule of spleen
    f. capsule of thyroid gland
    f. cavernitis
    f. cortical defect
    f. degeneration
    f. digital sheath of foot
    f. digital sheath of hand
    f. digital sheath of toes
    f. dysplasia of bone
    f. dysplasia of jaw
    f. goiter
    f. hamartoma of infancy
    f. histiocytoma
    f. joint
    f. layer
    f. layer of eyeball
    f. layer of joint capsule
    f. layer in or on deep aspect of
      fatty layer of subcutaneous tissue
    f. mediastinitis
    f. membrane of joint capsule
    f. pericarditis
    f. pericardium
    f. pneumonia
    f. polyp
    f. protein
    f. ring
    f. ring of intervertebral disk
    f. sheath
    f. sheath of digits of hand
    f. skeleton of heart
    f. tendon sheath
    f. tissue
    f. trigone
    f. tubercle
    f. tunic of corpus spongiosum
    f. tunic of eye
    f. union
    f. xanthoma
fibroxanthoma
    atypical f.
fibula
fibular
    f. artery
    f. articular facet of tibia
    f. articular surface of tibia
    f. collateral ligament
    f. collateral ligament of ankle
    f. compartment of leg
    f. lymph node
    f. margin of foot
    f. node
    f. notch
    f. nutrient artery
    f. (peroneal) border of foot
    f. tarsal tendinous sheath
    f. trochlea of calcaneus
    f. vein
fibularis
    f. brevis muscle
    f. longus muscle
    f. tertius muscle

fibulocalcaneal
ficain
ficin
Fick
>   F. law of diffusion
>   F. method
>   F. principle
Ficoll-Hypaque technique
fictitious feeding
FID
>   free induction decay
Fiedler myocarditis
field
>   auditory f.
>   f. block
>   f. block anesthesia
>   Broca f.
>   f. carcinogenesis
>   Cohnheim f.
>   f. of consciousness
>   f. emission tube
>   f. fever
>   f. of fixation
>   f. of Forel
>   free f.
>   f. gradient
>   H f.
>   individuation f.
>   involved f.
>   f. lens
>   magnetic f.
>   microscopic f.
>   nerve f.
>   prerubral f.
>   F. rapid stain
>   sound f.
>   f. survey
>   tegmental f. of Forel
>   visual f.
>   Wernicke f.
Fielding membrane
field-vole
Fiessinger-Leroy-Reiter syndrome
fièvre
>   fièvre boutonneuse
fifth
>   f. cranial nerve [CN V]
>   f. digit syndrome
>   f. disease
>   f. finger
>   f. ventricle
fig
fight or flight reaction
FIGLU
>   formiminoglutamic acid
figuratus
figure
>   authority f.
>   flame f.
>   fortification f.
>   mitotic f.
>   myelin f.
>   f.-of-eight abnormality
>   f.-of-eight bandage

>   f.-of-eight suture
>   Purkinje f.
figure and ground
fila (*pl. of* filum)
filaceous
filaggrin
filamen, filamin
filament, pl. **filamenta**
>   actin f.
>   axial f.
>   cytokeratin f.
>   intermediate f.
>   keratin f.
>   myosin f.
>   parabasal f.
>   pial f.
>   f. polymorphonuclear leukocyte
>   root f.
>   spermatic f.
>   thick f.
>   thin f.
>   Z f.
filamenta (*pl. of* filament) (*pl. of* filamentum)
filamentary
>   f. keratitis
>   f. keratopathy
filament-nonfilament count
filamentous
>   f. bacterial virus-
>   f. bacteriophage
>   f. colony
filamentum, pl. **filamenta**
filamin (*var. of* filamen)
filar
>   f. mass
>   f. micrometer
>   f. substance
Filaria
filaria, pl. **filariae**
filarial
>   f. arthritis
>   f. funiculitis
>   f. hydrocele
>   f. periodicity
>   f. synovitis
filariasis
>   bancroftian f.
>   Brug f.
>   periodic f.
filaricidal
filaricide
filariform larva
Filariicae
Filarioidea
Filatov
>   F. disease
>   F. flap
Filatov-Dukes disease
Filatov-Gillies flap
file
>   Hedström f.
>   periodontal f.
>   root canal f.
filial generation

F

filiform
- f. adnatum
- f. bougie
- f. nucleus
- f. papilla
- f. pulse
- f. wart

filioparental

fillet
- lateral f.
- f. layer
- medial f.

filling
- f. defect
- f. internal urethral orifice

film
- absorbable gelatin f.
- bitewing f.
- decubitus f.
- horizontal beam f.
- latitude f.
- panoramic x-ray f.
- plain f.
- precorneal f.
- right or left lateral decubitus f.
- scout f.
- f. speed
- spot f.
- tear f.
- wide-latitude f.

film changer
- rapid f. c.
- serial f. c.

filmless radiography

filopodium, pl. **filopodia**

filopressure

filovaricosis

Filoviridae

Filovirus

filter
- bandpass f.
- Berkefeld f.
- bird's nest f.
- Greenfield f.
- high-pass f.
- low-pass f.
- nitinol f.
- f. paper
- vena cava f.
- venocaval f.

filtering
- f. bleb
- f. cicatrix
- f. operation

filtrable
- f. virus

filtrate
- f. factor
- f. nitrogen

filtration
- f. angle
- f. coefficient
- f. fraction (FF)
- gel f.

filtrum
- Merkel f. ventriculi
- f. ventriculi

filum, pl. **fila**
- f. durae matris spinalis
- fila olfactoria
- olfactory fila
- radicular f.
- fila radicularia
- f. of spinal dura mater
- terminal f.
- f. terminale
- f. terminale externum
- f. terminale internum

fimbria, pl. **fimbriae**
- f. hippocampi
- f. of hippocampus
- ovarian f.
- f. ovarica
- fimbriae tubae uterinae
- fimbriae of uterine tube

fimbriate

fimbriated fold of inferior surface of tongue

fimbriectomy

fimbrin

fimbriocele

fimbriodentate sulcus

fimbrioplasty

final
- f. host
- f. impression

finasteride

Finckh test

finding

fine
- f. needle biopsy
- f. structure
- f. tremor

fineness

finger
- f. agnosia
- baseball f.
- blubber f.
- clubbed f.
- dead f.
- drop f.
- fifth f.
- first f.
- fourth f.
- hammer f.
- hippocratic f.
- index f.
- jerk f.
- little f.
- lock f.
- mallet f.
- middle f.
- f. percussion
- f. phenomenon
- ring f.
- sausage f.
- seal f.

second f.
snap f.
spade f.
f. spelling
spider f.
spring f.
stuck f.
third f.
trigger f.
waxy f.
webbed f.
whale f.
white f.
zinc f.
fingernail
finger-nose test
fingerprint
f. dystrophy
Galton system of classification of f.'s
genetic f.
finger-thumb reflex
finger-to-finger test
finishing bur
Finkelstein test
Fink-Heimer stain
Finney
F. operation
F. pyloroplasty
fire ant
firedamp
first
f. aid
f. arch syndrome
f. cervical vertebra
f. cranial nerve [CN I]
f. cuneiform bone
f. dentition
f. duodenal sphincter
f. finger
f. heart sound (S_1)
f. messenger
f. molar
f. parallel pelvic plane
f. part of duodenum
f. permanent molar
f. rank symptom (FRS)
f. rib [I]
f. and second posterior intercostal artery
f. stage
f. temporal convolution
f. visceral cleft
first-degree
f.-d. AV block
f.-d. burn
f.-d. prolapse
first-order reaction
first-pass
f.-p. effect
f.-p. metabolism
first-set rejection
Fischer
F. projection
F. projection formula

F. projection formula of sugar
F. sign
F. symptom
fish
f. berry
f. eye disease
f. poison
f. skin
f. tapeworm anemia
Fishberg concentration test
Fisher
F. exact test
F. syndrome
Fishman-Lerner unit
fish-mouth
f.-m. meatus
f.-m. mitral stenosis
fish-tank granuloma
fission
binary f.
bud f.
multiple f.
f. product
simple f.
fissiparity
fissiparous
fissula ante fenestram
fissura, pl. **fissurae**
f. antitragohelicina
f. calcarina
fissurae cerebelli
f. cerebri lateralis
f. choroidea
f. collateralis
f. dentata
f. hippocampi
f. horizontalis
f. horizontalis pulmonis dextri
f. intersemilunaris
f. intraculminalis
f. ligamenti teretis hepatis
f. ligamenti venosi
f. longitudinalis cerebri
f. mediana anterior medullae oblongatae
f. mediana anterior medullae spinalis
f. obliqua pulmonis
f. orbitalis inferior
f. orbitalis superior
f. parietooccipitalis
f. petrooccipitalis
f. petrosquamosa
f. petrotympanica
f. posterior superior
f. posterolateralis
f. precentralis
f. preculminalis
f. prepyramidalis
f. prima cerebelli
f. pterygoidea
f. pterygomaxillaris
f. pterygopalatina
f. pudendi
f. secunda cerebelli

F

fissura *(continued)*
  f. sphenopetrosa
  f. transversa cerebelli
  f. transversa cerebri
  f. tympanomastoidea
  f. tympanosquamosa
fissural cyst
fissuration
fissure
  abdominal f.
  Ammon f.
  anal f.
  ansoparamedian f.
  anterior median f. of medulla
    oblongata
  anterior median f. of spinal cord
  antitragohelicine f.
  ape f.
  auricular f.
  azygos f.
  Bichat f.
  branchial f.
  Broca f.
  f. bur
  calcarine f.
  callosomarginal f.
  f. caries
  caudal transverse f.
  cerebellar f.
  cerebral f.
  choroid f.
  choroidal f.
  Clevenger f.
  collateral f.
  decidual f.
  dentate f.
  Duverney f.
  Ecker f.
  enamel f.
  glaserian f.
  great horizontal f.
  great longitudinal f.
  Henle f.
  hippocampal f.
  horizontal f. of right lung
  horizontal f. [TA] of cerebellum
  inferior accessory f.
  inferior orbital f.
  intersemilunar f.
  intraculminate f.
  lateral cerebral f.
  left sagittal f.
  f. for ligamentum teres
  f. for ligamentum venosum
  linguogingival f.
  f. of liver
  longitudinal cerebral f.
  lunate f.
  f. of lung
  major f.
  minor f.
  oblique f.
  oblique f. of lung
  optic f.

  oral f.
  palpebral f.
  Pansch f.
  paracentral f.
  parietooccipital f.
  petrooccipital f.
  petrosphenoidal f.
  petrosquamous f.
  petrotympanic f.
  portal f.
  postcentral f.
  posterior median f. of the medulla
    oblongata
  posterior median f. of spinal cord
  posterior superior f.
  posterolateral f.
  posthippocampal f.
  postlingual f.
  postlunate f.
  postpyramidal f.
  postrhinal f.
  precentral f.
  preculminate f.
  prenodular f.
  prepyramidal f.
  primary f. of cerebellum
  pterygoid f.
  pterygomaxillary f.
  rhinal f.
  right sagittal f.
  f. of Rolando
  f. for round ligament of liver
  Santorini f.
  f. sealant
  secondary f. of cerebellum
  f. sign
  simian f.
  sphenoidal f.
  sphenomaxillary f.
  sphenopetrosal f.
  squamotympanic f.
  superior orbital f.
  superior temporal f.
  sylvian f.
  f. of Sylvius
  transverse f. of cerebellum
  transverse cerebral f.
  transverse f. of the right lung
  tympanomastoid f.
  tympanosquamous f.
  umbilical f.
  f. of venous ligament
  vestibular f. of cochlea
  zygal f.
fissured
  f. fracture
  f. tongue
fistula, pl. **fistulae**, **fistulas**
  abdominal f.
  amphibolic f.
  amphibolous f.
  anal f.
  arteriovenous f.
  f. auris congenita
  biliary f.

f. bimucosa
blind f.
BP f.
branchial f.
Brescia-Cimino f.
bronchobiliary f.
bronchocavitary f.
bronchoesophageal f.
bronchopleural f.
bronchopleural-cutaneous f.
carotid-cavernous f.
cholecystoduodenal f.
chyle f.
coccygeal f.
colocutaneous f.
coloileal f.
colonic f.
colovaginal f.
colovesical f.
complete f.
congenital pulmonary
  arteriovenous f.
dental f.
duodenal f.
dural cavernous sinus f.
Eck f.
enterocutaneous f.
enterovaginal f.
enterovesical f.
ethmoidal-lacrimal f.
external f.
fecal f.
gastric f.
gastrocolic f.
gastrocutaneous f.
gastroduodenal f.
gastrointestinal f.
genitourinary f.
gingival f.
hepatic f.
hepatopleural f.
horseshoe f.
H-type tracheoesophageal f.
incomplete f.
internal lacrimal f.
intestinal f.
f. knife
labyrinthine f.
lacrimal f.
f. lacrimalis
lacteal f.
lymphatic f.
mammary f.
Mann-Bollman f.
metroperitoneal f.
oroantral f.
orofacial f.
oronasal f.
parietal f.
perilymphatic f.
perineovaginal f.
pilonidal f.
pulmonary f.
rectolabial f.
rectourethral f.

rectovaginal f.
rectovesical f.
rectovestibular f.
rectovulvar f.
reverse Eck f.
salivary f.
sigmoidovesical f.
spermatic f.
T-E f.
f. test
Thiry f.
Thiry-Vella f.
thoracic f.
tracheobiliary fistula
tracheoesophageal f.
umbilical f.
urachal f.
ureterocutaneous f.
ureterovaginal f.
urethrocutaneous f.
urethrovaginal f.
urinary f.
urogenital f.
uteroperitoneal f.
Vella f.
vesical f.
vesicocolic f.
vesicocutaneous f.
vesicointestinal f.
vesicouterine f.
vesicovaginal f.
vesicovaginorectal f.
vitelline f.

fistulation
fistulatome
fistulectomy
fistuloenterostomy
fistulotomy
fistulous
fit
  induced f.
  uncinate f.
FITC
  fluorescein isothiocyanate
fitness
  clinical f.
  evolutionary f.
  genetic f.
  physical f.
FIT test
  fusion-inferred threshold test
Fitzgerald factor
Fitz-Hugh and Curtis syndrome
five-day fever
five-year survival rate
fixation
  ammonia f.
  bifoveal f.
  binocular f.
  circumalveolar f.
  circummandibular f.
  circumzygomatic f.
  complement f.
  craniofacial f.
  crossed f.

F

fixation *(continued)*
    f. disparity
    eccentric f.
    elastic band f.
    external f.
    external pin f.
    external pin f., biphase
    freudian f.
    genetic f.
    intermaxillary f.
    internal f.
    intraosseous f.
    mandibulomaxillary f.
    maxillomandibular f.
    nasomandibular f.
    nitrogen f.
    f. nystagmus
    f. reaction
    f. suppression
fixational ocular movement
fixative
    acetone f.
    AFA f.
    alcohol-glycerin f.
    Altmann f.
    Bouin f.
    Carnoy f.
    Champy f.
    Flemming f.
    formaldehyde f.
    formol-calcium f.
    formol-Müller f.
    formol-saline f.
    formol-Zenker f.
    glutaraldehyde f.
    Golgi osmiobichromate f.
    Helly f.
    Hermann f.
    Kaiserling f.
    Luft potassium permanganate f.
    Marchi f.
    methanol f.
    Müller f.
    neutral buffered formalin f.
    Newcomer f.
    Orth f.
    osmic acid f.
    Park-Williams f.
    picroformol f.
    PVA f.
    Regaud f.
    SAF f.
    Schaudinn f.
    single vial f.
    Thoma f.
    Zenker f.
fixator muscle
fixed
    f. alkali
    f. alkaloid
    f. bridge
    f. contracture
    f. coupling
    f. dressing

    f. drug eruption
    f. end
    f. idea
    f. macrophage
    f. oil
    f. partial denture
    f. pupil
    f. rate pulse generator
    f. torticollis
    f. virus
fixed-interval reinforcement schedule
fixed-rate pacemaker
fixed-ratio reinforcement schedule
fixing eye
flaccid
    f. ectropion
    f. membrane
    f. paralysis
    f. part of tympanic membrane
flaccidity
Flack node
flagella (*pl. of* flagellum)
flagellar
    f. agglutinin
    f. antigen
Flagellata
flagellate
    collared f.
    f. diarrhea
flagellated
flagellation
flagellin
flagellosis
flagellum, pl. **flagella**
flag sign
flail
    f. chest
    f. joint
flame
    f. arc
    f. cell
    f. emission spectrophotometry
    f. figure
    f. nevus
    f. photometer
    f. spot
flammable anesthetic
flange
    buccal f.
    f. contour
    denture f.
    labial f.
    lingual f.
flank
    f. bone
    f. incision
    f. position
flap
    Abbe f.
    advancement f.
    f. amputation
    arterial f.
    axial pattern f.
    bipedicle f.
    bone f.

buried f.
Byars f.
composite f.
compound f.
cross f.
delayed f.
deltopectoral f.
direct f.
distant f.
double pedicle f.
Eloesser f.
envelope f.
Estlander f.
Filatov f.
Filatov-Gillies f.
free f.
free bone f.
full-thickness f.
gingival f.
hinged f.
Indian f.
interpolated f.
island f.
Italian f.
jump f.
lined f.
liver f.
local f.
mucoperichondrial f.
mucoperiosteal f.
musculocutaneous f.
myocutaneous f.
myodermal f.
neurovascular f.
omental f.
f. operation
osteoplastic bone f.
pedicle f.
pericoronal f.
pharyngeal f.
random pattern f.
rotation f.
skin f.
subcutaneous f.
tubed f.
tubed pedicle f.
V-Y f.
flapless amputation
flapping tremor
flare
aqueous f.
flash
f. blindness
f. burn
f. dispersal
hot f.
f. keratoconjunctivitis
f. method
f. point
flashback
flashing pain syndrome
flash-lag effect
flask
casting f.
f. closure

crown f.
denture f.
Dewar f.
Erlenmeyer f.
Fernbach f.
Florence f.
hatching f.
injection f.
refractory f.
vacuum f.
volumetric f.
flasking
flat
f. affect
f. bone
f. chest
f. condyloma
f. electroencephalogram
f. muscle
f. pelvis
f. plate
f. top wave
f. wart
Flatau law
flatfoot
flatulence
flatulent dyspepsia
flatus
f. enema
f. vaginalis
flatworm
Flaujeac factor
flavedo
flavianic acid
flavin
f. adenine dinucleotide (FAD)
electron transfer f.
f. mononucleotide (FMN)
f. nucleotide
Flaviviridae
Flavivirus
Flavobacterium
F. aquatile
F. breve
F. meningisepticum
F. piscicida
flavoenzyme
flavokinase
flavone
flavonoid
flavonol
flavoprotein
flavor
flavoxate hydrochloride
flavus
flax-dresser's disease
flaxseed oil
flea
flea-bitten kidney
flea-borne typhus
flecainide acetate
Flechsig
F. area
F. fasciculi

F

Flechsig *(continued)*
    F. ground bundle
    F. tract
fleck
    f. dystrophy of cornea
    f. retina of Kandori
flecked
    f. retina
    f. retina syndrome
Flegel disease
Fleischer
    F. ring
    F. vortex
Fleischer-Strümpell ring
Fleischmann bursa
Fleischner line
Fleisch pneumotachograph
Fleitmann test
Flemming
    F. fixative
    F. triple stain
Flesch formula
flesh
    f. fly
    goose f.
    proud f.
fleshflies
fleshy
    f. mole
    f. polyp
Fletcher factor
flex
flexibilitas cerea
flexible
    f. collodion
    f. endoscope
    f. hysteroscope
fleximeter
flexion
    f. crease
    palmar f.
    plantar f.
flexion-extension injury
Flexner bacillus
flexor
    f. accessorius muscle
    f. carpi radialis muscle
    f. carpi ulnaris muscle
    f. compartment of arm
    f. compartment of forearm
    f. compartment of leg
    f. compartment of thigh
    f. digiti minimi brevis muscle of foot
    f. digiti minimi brevis muscle of hand
    f. digitorum brevis muscle
    f. digitorum longus muscle
    f. digitorum profundus muscle
    f. digitorum superficialis muscle
    f. hallucis brevis muscle
    f. hallucis longus muscle
    f. muscle
    f. pollicis brevis muscle

    f. pollicis longus muscle
    f. reflex
    f. retinaculum
    f. retinaculum of forearm
    f. retinaculum of lower limb
flexura, pl. **flexurae**
    f. anorectalis
    f. colica splenica
    f. coli dextra
    f. coli hepatis
    f. coli sinistra
    f. duodeni inferior
    f. duodeni superior
    f. duodenojejunalis
    f. perinealis (canalis ani)
    f. sacralis recti
    f. sigmoidea
flexural
    f. eczema
    f. psoriasis
flexure
    anorectal f.
    basicranial f.
    caudal f.
    cephalic f.
    cerebral f.
    cervical f.
    cranial f.
    dorsal f.
    duodenojejunal f.
    hepatic f.
    inferior duodenal f.
    left colic f.
    lumbar f.
    mesencephalic f.
    perineal f. of anal canal
    perineal f. of rectum
    pontine f.
    right colic f.
    sacral f.
    sacral f. of rectum
    sigmoid f.
    splenic f.
    superior duodenal f.
    telencephalic f.
    transverse rhombencephalic f.
flick
flicker
    f. fusion
    f. fusion frequency technique
    f. movement
    f. perimetry
    f. photometer
Flieringa ring
flight
    f. blindness
    f. or fight response
    f. of idea
    f. into disease
    f. into health
    f. nurse
Flinders Island spotted fever
flint
    F. arcade
    f. disease

f. glass
F. murmur
flip angle
flitter
flittering scotoma
floater
floating
f. cartilage
f. kidney
f. organ
f. patella
f. rib
f. spleen
f. villus
floc
floccillation
floccose
flocculable
floccular fossa
flocculate
flocculation
limes f. (Lf)
f. reaction
f. test
floccule
flocculence
flocculent
flocculonodular lobe
flocculus, pl. **flocculi**
accessory f.
flood
f. fever
flooding
Flood ligament
floor
f. of orbit
f. plate
f. of tympanic cavity
floppy valve syndrome
flora
florantyrone
Florence
F. crystal
F. flask
Florey unit
florid
f. oral papillomatosis
f. osseous dysplasia
floriform cataract
Florschütz formula
floss
dental f.
f. silk
flotation
f. constant (S$_f$)
f. method
Flourens theory
floury cornea
flow
Bingham f.
blood f. (Q̇)
cerebral blood f. (CBF)
f. cytometry
f. cytophotometry
f. diagram

Doppler color f.
effective renal blood f. (ERBF)
effective renal plasma f. (ERPF)
forced expiratory f. (FEF)
gas f. (V̇)
gene f.
laminar f.
newtonian f.
peak expiratory f.
renal blood f. (RBF)
renal plasma f. (RPF)
shear f.
f. void
flower
f. of antimony
f. basket of Bochdalek
f. of benzoin
f. bone
f. dental index
f. of sulfur
f. of zinc
flower-spray
f.-s. ending
f.-s. organ of Ruffini
flowing hyperostosis
flowmeter
electromagnetic f.
flow-over vaporizer
flow-volume
f.-v. curve
f.-v. loop study
floxacillin
floxuridine
flu
fluanisone
flucrylate
fluctuance
fluctuate
fluctuation
flucytosine
fludrocortisone acetate
fluence
fluency
fluent aphasia
flufenamic acid
fluid
allantoic f.
amnionic f.
Brodie f.
bronchoalveolar f.
Callison f.
cerebrospinal f. (CSF)
crevicular f.
Dakin f.
dentinal f.
extracellular f. (ECF)
f. extract
extravascular f.
Farrant mounting f.
gingival f.
infranatant f.
interstitial f.
intracellular f. (ICF)
intraocular f.
f. mosaic model

F

fluid *(continued)*
    newtonian f.
    non-newtonian f.
    pleural f.
    prostatic f.
    pseudoplastic f.
    Rees-Ecker f.
    f. retinopexy
    Scarpa f.
    seminal f.
    sulcular f.
    supernatant f.
    synovial f.
    thixotropic f.
    tissue f.
    transcellular f.
    ventricular f.
    f. wave
fluidextract
fluidglycerates
fluidism
fluidity
fluidounce
fluidrachm
fluke
flumazenil
flumen, pl. **flumina**
    flumina pilorum
flumethasone
flumethiazide
flumina (*pl. of* flumen)
flunarizine
flunisolide
flunitrazepam
fluocinolone acetonide
fluocinonide
fluocortolone
    f. caproate
    f. hexanoate
    f. pivalate
fluorapatite
9*H*-fluorene
fluorescamine
fluoresce, fluorescing
fluorescein
    f. angiography
    f. instillation test
    f. isothiocyanate (FITC)
    f. sodium
    f. string test
fluorescence
    f. microscope
    f. microscopy
    f. plus Giemsa stain
    f. quenching
    f. in situ hybridization
    f. spectrum
fluorescence-activated cell sorter (FACS)
fluorescent
    f. antibody
    f. antibody technique
    f. antinuclear antibody test
    f. screen
    f. in situ hybridization

    f. stain
    f. treponemal antibody-absorption
      test (FTA-ABS test)
fluorescin
fluorescing (*var. of* fluoresce)
fluoridated tooth
fluoridation
fluoride number
fluoridization
fluorine
fluorochrome
fluorochroming
fluorocyte
fluorodeoxyuridine (FUDR)
fluoro-2,4-dinitrobenzene (FDNB)
fluorography
fluorometer
fluorometholone
fluorometry
fluorophotometry
fluoroquinolone
fluororoentgenography
fluoroscope
fluoroscopic
fluoroscopy
    video f.
fluorosis
    chronic endemic f.
fluorouracil
fluosol-DA
fluoxetine hydrochloride
fluoxymesterone
flupentixol
fluperolone acetate
fluphenazine
    f. enanthate
    f. hydrochloride
fluprednisolone
flurandrenolide
flurazepam hydrochloride
flurbiprofen
flurogestone acetate
flurothyl
fluroxene
Flury
    F. strain rabies virus
    F. strain vaccine
flush
    carcinoid f.
    hectic f.
    histamine f.
    hot f.
    malar f.
    f. technique
flutamide
flutter
    atrial f.
    auricular f.
    diaphragmatic f.
    impure f.
    ocular f.
    ventricular f.
flutter-fibrillation
    f.-f. wave
flux (*J*)

f. density
luminous f.
net f.
f. ratio
unidirectional f.
fluxionary hyperemia
fly
f. agaric
f. blister
flesh f.
heel f.
louse f.
mangrove f.
Russian f.
Spanish f.
warble f.
flying spot microscope
Flynn-Aird syndrome
Flynn phenomenon
Fm
FMD
foot-and-mouth disease
FMD virus
fMet
n-formylmethionine
fMet-tRNA
formylmethionyl-tRNA
FMLH
familial hemophagocytic
lymphohistiocytosis
FMN
flavin mononucleotide
FMR1
FNA
fine needle aspiration biopsy
foam
f. cell
human fibrin f.
f. stability test
foamy
f. agent
f. virus-
focal
f. acrohyperkeratosis
f. amyloidosis
f. appendicitis
f. condensing osteitis
f. depth
f. dermal hypoplasia
f. distance
f. embolic glomerulonephritis
f. epilepsy
f. epithelial hyperplasia
f. illumination
f. infection
f. interval
f. lymphocytic thyroiditis
f. metastatic disease
f. motor seizure
f. necrosis
f. nephritis
f. point
f. reaction
f. sclerosing glomerulopathy
f. segmental glomerulosclerosis

f. spot
f. spot size
focimeter
focus, pl. **foci**
conjugate foci
depth of f.
Ghon f.
natural f. of infection
principal f.
real f.
virtual f.
focused grid
fodrin
Fogarty
F. clamp
F. embolectomy catheter
fogging retinoscopy
fogo selvagem
foil
Foix-Alajouanine
F.-A. myelitis
F.-A. syndrome
Foix-Cavany-Marie syndrome
folate
fold
adipose f. of the pleura
alar f. of intrapatellar synovial fold
amnionic f.
ampullary f. of uterine tube
anterior axillary f.
aryepiglottic f.
arytenoepiglottidean f.
axillary f.
caval f.
cecal f.
f. of chorda tympani
ciliary f.
circular f.'s of small intestine
Dennie-Morgan f.
dinucleotide f.
Douglas f.
Duncan f.
duodenojejunal f.
duodenomesocolic f.
epicanthal f.
epigastric f.
epiglottic f.
falciform retinal f.
fatty f. of pleura
fimbriated f. of inferior surface of
tongue
gastric f.
gastropancreatic f.
genital f.
giant gastric f.
glossopalatine f.
gluteal f.
Guérin f.
Hasner f.
head f.
Houston f.
ileocecal f.
incudal f.
inferior duodenal f.
infrapatellar synovial f.

F

fold *(continued)*
  inguinal aponeurotic f.
  interarytenoid f.
  interdigital f.
  interureteric f.
  f. of iris
  Kerckring f.
  Kohlrausch f.
  labioscrotal f.
  lacrimal f.
  f. of laryngeal nerve
  lateral f.
  lateral glossoepiglottic f.
  lateral nasal f.
  lateral umbilical f.
  f. of left vena cava
  longitudinal f. of duodenum
  malar f.
  mallear f.
  mammary f.
  Marshall vestigial f.
  medial canthic f.
  medial nasal f.
  medial umbilical f.
  median glossoepiglottic f.
  median umbilical f.
  medullary f.
  mesonephric f.
  middle glossoepiglottic f.
  middle transverse rectal f.
  middle umbilical f.
  mongolian f.
  mucobuccal f.
  mucosal f. of gallbladder
  nail f.
  nasojugal f.
  Nélaton f.
  neural f.
  opercular f.
  palmate f. of cervical canal
  palpebronasal f.
  paraduodenal f.
  pharyngoepiglottic f.
  pleuropericardial f.
  pleuroperitoneal f.
  posterior axillary f.
  presplenic f.
  rectal f.
  rectouterine f.
  rectovesical f.
  retinal f.
  retroauricular f.
  retrotarsal f.
  Rindfleisch f.
  sacrogenital f.
  sacrouterine f.
  sacrovaginal f.
  sacrovesical f.
  salpingopalatine f.
  salpingopharyngeal f.
  Schultze f.
  semilunar f.
  semilunar f. of colon
  semilunar conjunctival f.

  spiral f. of cystic duct
  stapedial f.
  f. of stapes
  sublingual f.
  superior duodenal f.
  f. of superior laryngeal nerve
  synovial f.
  tail f.
  tarsal f.
  transverse palatine f.
  transverse f. of rectum
  transverse vesical f.
  Treves f.
  triangular f.
  urachal f.
  ureteric f.
  urorectal f.
  f. of uterine tube
  uterovesical f.
  vascular f. of the cecum
  Vater f.
  ventricular f.
  vestibular f.
  vestigial f.
  vocal f.
foldable intraocular lens
fold-back element
folded-lung syndrome
folding fracture
Foley
  F. catheter
  F. Y-plasty pyeloplasty
folia *(pl. of* folium)
foliaceous
foliar
foliate
  f. papillae
  f. papillitis
folic
  f. acid
  f. acid antagonists
  f. acid conjugate
  f. acid deficiency anemia
folie
  f. à deux
  f. du doute
  f. du pourquoi
  f. gémellaire
Folin
  F. reaction
  F. reagent
  F. test
folinate
folinic acid
Folin-Looney test
foliose
folium, pl. **folia**
  folia cerebelli
  folia of cerebellum
  folia linguae
  f. of vermis
  f. vermis
folk medicine
follian process

follicle
> aggregated lymphatic f.'s of small intestine
> aggregated lymphatic f.'s of vermiform appendix
> anovular ovarian f.
> antral f.
> atretic ovarian f.
> dental f.
> gastric f.
> graafian f.
> growing ovarian f.
> hair f.
> intestinal f.
> Lieberkühn f.
> lingual f.
> luteinized unruptured f.
> lymphatic f.'s of larynx
> lymphatic f.'s of rectum
> mature ovarian f.
> Montgomery f.
> multilaminar primary f.
> nabothian f.
> ovarian f.
> polyovular ovarian f.
> primary ovarian f.
> primordial ovarian f.
> sebaceous f.
> secondary ovarian f.
> solitary f.
> solitary lymphatic f.
> splenic lymph f.
> f. of thyroid gland
> unilaminar primary f.
> vesicular f.
> vesicular ovarian f.

follicle-stimulating
> f.-s. hormone (FSH)
> f.-s. principle

follicular
> f. abscess
> f. adenoma
> f. antrum
> f. carcinoma
> f. conjunctivitis
> f. cyst
> f. cystitis
> f. epithelial cell
> f. gland
> f. goiter
> f. hormone
> f. impetigo
> f. iritis
> f. lymphoma
> f. mucinosis
> f. ovarian cell
> f. papule
> f. predominantly large cell lymphoma
> f. predominantly small cleaved cell lymphoma
> f. stigma
> f. trachoma
> f. urethritis
> f. vulvitis

folliculi (*pl. of* folliculus)
folliculin
folliculin hydrate
folliculitis
> f. abscedens et suffodiens
> f. barbae
> f. decalvans
> eosinophilic pustular f.
> f. keloidalis
> f. nares perforans
> perforating f.
> f. ulerythematosa reticulata

folliculoma
folliculosis
folliculus, pl. **folliculi**
> folliculi glandulae thyroideae
> folliculi linguales
> folliculi lymphatici aggregati
> folliculi lymphatici aggregati appendicis vermiformis
> folliculi lymphatici gastrici
> folliculi lymphatici laryngei
> folliculi lymphatici lienales
> folliculi lymphatici recti
> folliculi lymphatici solitarii
> f. lymphaticus
> f. ovaricus primarius
> f. ovaricus vesiculosus
> f. pili

Folling disease
Folli process
follistatin
follitropin
following bougie
follow-up study
Foltz valvule
fomentation
fomes, pl. **fomites**
fomite
fonazine mesylate
Fonio solution
Fonsecaea
Fontan
> F. operation
> F. procedure

Fontana
> F. canal
> F. space
> F. stain

Fontana-Masson silver stain
fontanelle, fontanel
> anterior f.
> anterolateral f.
> bregmatic f.
> Casser f.
> cranial f.
> frontal f.
> Gerdy f.
> mastoid f.
> occipital f.
> posterior f.
> posterolateral f.
> sagittal f.
> sphenoidal f.

fonticulus, pl. **fonticuli**

F

fonticulus *(continued)*
>   f. anterior
>   f. anterolateralis
>   fonticuli cranii
>   f. mastoideus
>   f. posterior
>   f. posterolateralis
>   f. sphenoidalis

food
>   f. asthma
>   f. ball
>   f. fever
>   f. impaction
>   f. poisoning

Food and Drug Administration of the United States Department of Health and Human Services (FDA)

foot
>   athlete's f.
>   f. bone
>   claw f.
>   club f.
>   contracted f.
>   drop f.
>   f. of hippocampus
>   immersion f.
>   Madura f.
>   Morand f.
>   mossy f.
>   f. plate
>   f. plugger
>   f. presentation
>   f. process
>   f.'s reticulin impregnation stain
>   sandal f.
>   spastic flat f.
>   trench f.
>   f. yaws

foot-and-mouth
>   f.-a.-m. disease (FMD)
>   f.-a.-m. disease virus
>   f.-a.-m. disease virus vaccines

footcandle
footdrop
footling presentation
footplate, foot-plate
foot-pound
foot-poundal
foot-pound-second
>   f.-p.-s. system (FPS, fps)
>   f.-p.-s. unit

footprinting
forage
foramen, pl. **foramina**
>   foramina alveolaria corporis maxillae
>   alveolar foramina of maxilla
>   anterior condyloid f.
>   anterior palatine f.
>   aortic f.
>   apical dental f.
>   apical f. of tooth
>   f. apicis dentis
>   arachnoid f.
>   f. of Arnold

blind f. of frontal bone
blind f. of the tongue
Bochdalek f.
f. of Bochdalek hernia
Botallo f.
f. caecum medullae oblongatae
f. caecum posterius
carotid f.
cecal f. of frontal bone
cecal f. of the tongue
f. cecum of frontal bone
f. cecum linguae
f. cecum ossis frontalis
f. cecum of tongue
conjugate f.
f. costotransversarium
costotransverse f.
cribriform foramina
foramina cribrosa
f. diaphragmatis sellae
epiploic f.
f. epiploicum
ethmoidal f.
f. ethmoidale (anterior et posterior)
external acoustic f.
external auditory f.
Ferrein f.
frontal f.
f. frontale
great f.
greater palatine f.
Huschke f.
Hyrtl f.
incisive f.
f. incisivum
incisor f.
inferior dental f.
infraorbital f.
f. infraorbitale
interatrial f. primum
interatrial f. secundum
f. intermesocolica transversa
internal acoustic f.
internal auditory f.
interventricular f.
f. interventriculare
intervertebral f.
f. intervertebrale
f. ischiadicum (anterior et posterior)
f. ischiadicum majus et minor
jugular f.
f. jugulare
f. of Key-Retzius
lacerated f.
f. lacerum
f. lacerum anterius
f. lacerum medium
f. lacerum posterius
Lannelongue foramina
f. lateralis ventriculi quarti
lesser palatine foramina
f. of Luschka
f. of Magendie
f. magnum
malar f.

f. mandibulae
mandibular f.
mastoid f.
f. mastoideum
mental f.
f. mentale
Monro f.
Morgagni f.
nasal f.
foramina nervosa
f. nutricium
nutrient f.
obturator f.
f. obturatum
olfactory f.
omental f.
f. omentale
optic f.
f. opticum
oval f.
f. ovale
f. ovale cordis
f. ovale of heart
oval f. of heart
foramina palatina minora
f. palatinum majus
foramina papillaria renis
papillary foramina of kidney
parietal f.
f. parietale
petrosal f.
f. petrosum
posterior condyloid f.
posterior palatine foramina
postglenoid f.
primary interatrial f.
f. processus transversi
f. quadratum
f. recessus superioris bursae
  omentalis
f. of Retzius
root f.
f. rotundum
round f.
sacral foramina
f. sacrale
foramina sacralia anterior et
  posterior
foramina sacralia dorsalia
foramina sacralia pelvica
Scarpa foramina
sciatic f.
secondary interatrial f.
f. of sellar diaphragm
singular f.
f. singulare
foramina of the smallest veins of
  heart
sphenoidal emissary f.
sphenopalatine f.
f. sphenopalatinum
sphenotic f.
f. spinosum
Stensen f.
stylomastoid f.

f. stylomastoideum
f. subseptale
f. of superior recess of omental
  bursa
supraorbital f.
f. supraorbitale
thebesian foramina
thyroid f.
f. thyroideum
f. transversarium
transverse f.
f. of transverse process
f. of vena cava
vena caval f.
f. venae cavae
foramina of the venae minimae
foramina venarum minimarum cordis
f. venosum
venous f.
vertebral f.
f. vertebrale
vertebroarterial f.
f. vertebroarteriale
Vesalius f.
Vicq d'Azyr f.
Vieussens foramina
Weitbrecht f.
f. of Winslow
zygomaticofacial f.
f. zygomaticofaciale
zygomatico-orbital f.
f. zygomatico-orbitale
zygomaticotemporal f.
f. zygomaticotemporale
foraminal
f. herniation
f. lymph node
f. node
Foraminifera
foraminiferous
foraminotomy
foraminulum, pl. **foraminula**
Forbes-Albright syndrome
Forbes disease
force
animal f.
chewing f.
dynamic f.
electromotive f. (EMF)
G f.
f. of mastication
masticatory f.
nervous f.
occlusal f.
psychic f.
reciprocal f.'s
reserve f.
van der Waals f.'s
vital f.
forced
f. alimentation
f. beat
f. cycle
f. duction
f. expiratory flow (FEF)

F

forced *(continued)*
    f. expiratory time (FET)
    f. expiratory volume (FEV)
    f. feeding
    f. grasping reflex
    f. respiration
    f. spirometry
    f. vital capacity (FVC)
force platform
forceps
    Adson f.
    alligator f.
    Allis f.
    f. anterior
    Arruga f.
    arterial f.
    axis-traction f.
    Barton f.
    bayonet f.
    bone f.
    Brown-Adson f.
    bulldog f.
    bullet f.
    capsule f.
    Chamberlen f.
    clamp f.
    clip f.
    cup biopsy f.
    cutting f.
    DeBakey f.
    f. delivery
    dental f.
    dressing f.
    Evans f.
    extracting f.
    frontal f.
    f. frontalis
    Graefe f.
    hemostatic f.
    jeweller f.
    Kjelland f.
    Lahey f.
    Laplace f.
    Levret f.
    lion-jaw bone-holding f.
    Löwenberg f.
    magic f.
    Magill f.
    major f.
    f. major
    minor f.
    f. minor
    mosquito f.
    mouse-tooth f.
    needle f.
    nonfenestrated f.
    obstetric f.
    occipital f.
    f. occipitalis
    O'Hara f.
    Piper f.
    f. posterior
    Randall stone f.
    rubber dam clamp f.

    Simpson f.
    speculum f.
    Tarnier f.
    tenaculum f.
    thumb f.
    tubular f.
    Tucker-McLean f.
    tying f.
    vulsella f.
    vulsellum f.
    Willett f.
force-velocity curve
Forchheimer sign
forcipate
forcipressure
Fordyce
    F. angiokeratoma
    F. disease
    F. granule
    F. spot
forearm
forebrain
    f. eminence
    f. prominence
    f. vesicle
foreconscious
forefinger
foregut
forehead
    olympian f.
foreign
    f. body
    f. body giant cell
    f. body granuloma
    f. body salpingitis
    f. body tumorigenesis
    f. protein
    f. protein therapy
    f. serum
foreign-body appendicitis
forekidney
Forel decussation
forelock
    white f.
foremilk
forensic
    f. dentistry
    f. medicine
    f. odontology
    f. psychiatry
    f. psychology
foreplay
forepleasure
forequarter amputation
foreskin of penis
Forestier disease
forestomach
forewaters
forgetting
fork
    bite f.
    face-bow f.
    tuning f.
form
    accolé f.

appliqué f.
arch f.
boat f.
cavity preparation f.
chair f.
convenience f.
extension f.
face f.
half-chair f.
involution f.
L f.
occlusal f.
outline f.
posterior tooth f.
replicative f.
resistance f.
retention f.
sickle f.
skew f.
tooth f.
twist f.
wave f.
wax f.
-form
Formad kidney
formaldehyde
active f.
f. fixative
**formalin-ether sedimentation
concentration**
**formalin-ethyl acetate sedimentation
concentration**
formalinize
formalin pigment
formal operation
formamidase
**5-formamidoimidazole-4-carboximide
ribotide**
formant
formate
active f.
formatio, pl. **formationes**
f. hippocampalis
f. reticularis
formation
concept f.
personality f.
reaction f.
reticular f.
rouleau f.
symptom f.
formative cell
formazan
formboard
formed visual hallucination
forme fruste, pl. **formes frustes**
formic
f. acid
f. aldehyde
formication
formiminoglutamic acid (FIGLU)
***N*-formiminotetrahydrofolate**
formin
formocresol
formol-calcium fixative

formol-gel test
formol-Müller fixative
formol-saline fixative
formol titration
formol-Zenker fixative
formosulfathiazole
formula, pl. **formulas, formulae**
Arneth f.
Bazett f.
Bernhardt f.
Black f.
Broca f.
chemical f.
Christison f.
constitutional f.
Demoivre f.
dental f.
Dreyer f.
DuBois f.
electrical f.
empirical f.
Fischer projection f.
Flesch f.
Florschütz f.
Gorlin f.
graphic f.
Hamilton-Stewart f.
Häser f.
Haworth perspective and
conformational formulas
Jellinek f.
Ledermann f.
Long f.
Mall f.
Meeh f.
Meeh-Dubois f.
molecular f.
official f.
Pignet f.
Poisson-Pearson f.
Ranke f.
rational f.
Reuss f.
Runeberg f.
spatial f.
stereochemical f.
structural f.
Toronto f. for pulmonary artery
banding
Trapp f.
Trapp-Häser f.
Van Slyke f.
vertebral f.
formulary
hospital f.
formyl
active f.
formyl-methionyl-f.
formylase
***N*-formylglycinamide ribotide (FGAR)**
***N*-formylkynurenine**
***N*-formylmethionine (fMet)**
formylmethionyl-tRNA (fMet-tRNA)
N^{10}-formyltetrahydrofolate
fornicate gyrus

F

fornication
fornix, pl. **fornices**
    f. conjunctivae
    f. conjunctivae inferior
    f. conjunctivae superior
    conjunctival f.
    f. gastricus
    f. of lacrimal sac
    pharyngeal f.
    f. pharyngis
    f. sacci lacrimalis
    f. of stomach
    transverse f.
    f. uteri
    f. vaginae
    vaginal f.
Forsius-Eriksson albinism
forskolin
Forssman
    F. antibody
    F. antigen
    F. antigen-antibody reaction
    F. hapten
Förster uveitis
Fort Bragg fever
fortification
    f. figure
    f. spectrum
fortified
    f. milk
    f. vitamin D milk
forward
    f. conduction
    f. heart failure
foscarnet
Fosdick-Hansen-Epple test
Foshay test
fossa, pl. **fossae**
    acetabular f.
    f. acetabuli
    adipose f.
    amygdaloid f.
    anconal f.
    anterior cranial f.
    f. anthelicis
    f. of anthelix
    f. antihelica
    articular f. of temporal bone
    f. axillaris
    axillary f.
    Bichat f.
    Biesiadecki f.
    Broesike f.
    f. canina
    canine f.
    f. carotica
    cerebellar f.
    f. cerebellaris
    Claudius f.
    condylar f.
    f. condylaris
    f. coronoidea humeri
    coronoid f. of humerus
    f. cranii anterior
    f. cranii media

    f. cranii posterior
    crural f.
    Cruveilhier f.
    cubital f.
    f. cubitalis
    digastric f.
    f. digastrica
    digital f.
    f. ductus venosi
    f. of ductus venosus
    duodenal fossae
    duodenojejunal f.
    epigastric f.
    f. epigastrica
    femoral f.
    floccular f.
    f. for gallbladder
    gallbladder f.
    Gerdy hyoid f.
    f. glandulae lacrimalis
    glenoid f.
    greater supraclavicular f.
    Gruber-Landzert f.
    f. of helix
    hyaloid f.
    f. hyaloidea
    hypophysial f.
    f. hypophysialis
    iliac f.
    f. iliaca
    iliacosubfascial f.
    f. iliacosubfascialis
    iliopectineal f.
    f. incisiva
    incisive f.
    incudal f.
    f. incudis
    f. of incus
    inferior duodenal f.
    infraclavicular f.
    f. infraclavicularis
    infraduodenal f.
    f. infraspinata
    infraspinous f.
    infratemporal f.
    f. infratemporalis
    inguinal f.
    f. inguinalis lateralis
    f. inguinalis medialis
    f. innominata
    innominate f.
    intercondylar f.
    f. intercondylaris
    intercondylic f.
    f. intermesocolica transversa
    interpeduncular f.
    f. interpeduncularis
    intrabulbar f.
    ischioanal f.
    f. ischioanalis
    ischiorectal f.
    f. ischiorectalis
    Jobert de Lamballe f.
    Jonnesco f.
    jugular f.

f. jugularis
lacrimal f.
f. for lacrimal gland
f. for lacrimal sac
Landzert f.
lateral f. of brain
lateral cerebral f.
lateral inguinal f.
f. lateralis cerebri
f. of lateral malleolus
lenticular f.
lesser supraclavicular f.
little f. of the cochlear window
little f. of the oval (vestibular)
   window
Malgaigne f.
f. malleoli fibulae
f. malleoli lateralis
mandibular f.
f. mandibularis
mastoid f.
f. mastoidea
medial inguinal f.
Merkel f.
mesentericoparietal f.
middle cranial f.
Mohrenheim f.
Morgagni f.
mylohyoid f.
f. navicularis auriculae
f. navicularis auris
f. navicularis Cruveilhier
f. navicularis urethrae
f. navicularis vestibulae vaginae
navicular f. of urethra
f. olecrani
olecranon f.
oval f.
f. ovalis
f. of oval window
ovarian f.
f. ovarica
paraduodenal f.
parajejunal f.
f. parajejunalis
pararectal f.
f. pararectalis
paravesical f.
f. paravesicalis
patellar f. of vitreous
peritoneal fossae
petrosal f.
piriform f.
pituitary f.
f. poplitea
popliteal f.
posterior cranial f.
f. provesicalis
pterygoid f.
f. pterygoidea
pterygomaxillary f.
f. pterygopalatina
pterygopalatine f.
radial f. of humerus
f. radialis humeri

retroduodenal f.
retromandibular f.
f. retromandibularis
retromolar f.
f. retromolaris
rhomboid f.
f. rhomboidea
Rosenmüller f.
f. of round window
f. sacci lacrimalis
scaphoid f.
f. scaphoidea
f. scaphoidea ossis sphenoidalis
scaphoid f. of sphenoid bone
f. scarpae major
sigmoid f.
sphenomaxillary f.
f. subarcuata
subarcuate f.
subcecal f.
subinguinal f.
sublingual f.
submandibular f.
f. submandibularis
submaxillary f.
subscapular f.
f. subscapularis
superior duodenal f.
f. supraclavicularis major
f. supraclavicularis minor
supramastoid f.
f. supraspinata
supraspinous f.
supratonsillar f.
f. supratonsillaris
supravesical f.
f. supravesicalis
f. of Sylvius
temporal f.
f. temporalis
f. terminalis urethrae
tonsillar f.
f. tonsillaris
transverse intermesocolic f.
Treitz f.
triangular f. of auricle
f. triangularis auriculae
trochanteric f.
f. trochanterica
trochlear f.
f. trochlearis
umbilical f.
Velpeau f.
f. venae cavae
f. venae umbilicalis
f. venosa
vermian f.
f. vesicae biliaris
f. vesicae felleae
vestibular f.
f. of vestibule of vagina
f. vestibuli vaginae
Waldeyer fossae
zygomatic f.

F

fossette
fossula, pl. **fossulae**
    f. fenestrae cochleae
    f. fenestrae vestibuli
    f. petrosa
    petrosal f.
    f. post fenestram
    f. rotunda
    tonsillar fossulae
    fossulae tonsillarum (palatini et
      pharyngealis)
fossulate
Foster
    F. frame
    F. Kennedy syndrome
Fothergill
    F. disease
    F. neuralgia
    F. operation
    F. sign
Fouchet
    F. reagent
    F. stain
foulage
foundation
    denture f.
founder
    f. effect
    f. principle
foundryman's fever
fountain
    f. decussation
    f. syringe
fourchette
Four Corners virus
four-headed muscle
Fourier
    F. analysis
    F. transfer
    F. transform
Fourneau
    F. 710
    F. 933
Fournier
    F. disease
    F. gangrene
four-tailed bandage
fourth
    f. cranial nerve [CN IV]
    f. disease
    f. finger
    f. heart sound (S_4)
    f. lumbar nerve [L4]
    f. parallel pelvic plane
    f. toe [IV]
    f. turbinated bone
    f. ventricle
fovea, pl. **foveae**
    f. anterior
    anterior f.
    f. articularis capitis radii
    f. articularis inferior atlantis
    f. articularis superior atlantis
    f. capitis femoris
    f. cardiaca

    f. centralis maculae luteae
    central retinal f.
    f. costalis inferior
    f. costalis processus transversi
    f. costalis superior
    f. dentis atlantis
    f. elliptica
    f. ethmoidalis
    f. of the femoral head
    f. femoralis
    f. hemielliptica
    f. hemispherica
    inferior f.
    f. inferior
    f. inguinalis interna
    f. for ligament of head of femur
    Morgagni f.
    f. oblonga cartilaginis arytenoideae
    oblong f. of arytenoid cartilage
    pterygoid f.
    f. pterygoidea
    f. of radial head
    f. spherica
    f. sublingualis
    f. submandibularis
    f. submaxillaris
    superior f.
    f. superior
    f. supravesicalis
    triangular f. of arytenoid cartilage
    f. triangularis cartilaginis
      arytenoideae
    trochlear f.
    f. trochlearis
foveate
foveated
    f. chest
foveation
foveola, pl. **foveolae**
    f. coccygea
    coccygeal f.
    f. gastrica
    granular foveolae
    foveolae granulares
    f. ocularis
    f. papillaris
    f. of retina
    f. retinae
    f. suprameatalis
    f. suprameatica
foveolar
    f. cell of stomach
foveolate
Foville
    F. fasciculus
    F. syndrome
Fowler position
fowl typhoid
Fox-Fordyce disease
foxglove
FPLC
    fast protein liquid chromatography
FPS, fps
    foot-pound-second system
      FPS unit

Fr
 francium
FRACP
fractals
fraction
 amorphous f. of adrenal cortex
 blood plasma f.'s
 f. collector
 dried human plasma protein f.
 ejection f.
 filtration f. (FF)
 human antihemophilic f.
 human plasma protein f.
 mole f.
 radionuclide ejection f.
 recombination f.
 regurgitant f.
fractional
 f. distillation
 f. dose
 f. epidural anesthesia
 f. spinal anesthesia
 f. sterilization
fractionation
fracture
 apophysial f.
 articular f.
 avulsion f.
 Barton f.
 basal skull f.
 f. bed
 bending f.
 Bennett f.
 bimalleolar f.
 birth f.
 f. blister
 blowout f.
 boxer's f.
 capillary f.
 Chance f.
 clay shoveler's f.
 closed skull f.
 Colles f.
 comminuted skull f.
 complex f.
 compound skull f.
 f. by contrecoup
 cough f.
 craniofacial dysjunction f.
 dentate f.
 depressed skull f.
 derby hat f.
 diastatic skull f.
 direct f.
 dishpan f.
 dislocation f.
 f. dislocation
 double f.
 Dupuytren f.
 epiphysial f.
 expressed skull f.
 extracapsular f.
 fatigue f.
 fetal f.
 fissured f.

folding f.
freeze f.
Galeazzi f.
Gosselin f.
greenstick f.
growing f.
Guérin f.
gutter f.
hairline f.
hangman's f.
horizontal f.
impacted f.
incomplete f.
indirect f.
intertrochanteric f.
intraarticular f.
intracapsular f.
intrauterine f.
Le Fort I, II, III f.
linear f.
linear skull f.
longitudinal f.
march f.
Monteggia f.
multiple f.
neurogenic f.
oblique f.
occult f.
open skull f.
parry f.
pathologic f.
pertrochanteric f.
pilon f.
ping-pong f.
pond f.
Pott f.
pyramidal f.
segmental f.
Shepherd f.
silver-fork f.
simple skull f.
Skillern f.
skull f.
Smith f.
spiral f.
splintered f.
spontaneous f.
sprain f.
stable f.
stellate skull f.
strain f.
stress f.
subcapital f.
subperiosteal f.
supracondylar f.
toddler's f.
torsion f.
torus f.
transcervical f.
transcondylar f.
transverse facial f.
trimalleolar f.
tripod f.
unstable f.
ununited f.

F

Fraenkel pneumococcus
fragile
> f. site
> f. X chromosome
> f. X syndrome

fragilitas
> f. crinium
> f. sanguinis

fragility
> f. of the blood
> capillary f.
> osmotic f.
> f. test

fragilocyte
fragilocytosis
fragment
> acentric f.
> Brimacombe f.
> butterfly f.
> Fab f.
> Fc f.
> Klenow f.
> Okazaki f.
> one-carbon f.
> f. reaction
> two-carbon f.

fragmentation of the myocardium
fragment length polymorphism (*var. of*
> restriction length polymorphism)

fraise
Fraley syndrome
frambesia tropica
frambesiform
frambesioma
frame
> Balkan f.
> Bradford f.
> Deiters terminal f.
> Foster f.
> occluding f.
> Stryker f.
> trial f.
> Whitman f.

frameshift
> f. mutagen
> f. mutation

framework region
Framingham Heart Study
Franceschetti-Jadassohn syndrome
Franceschetti syndrome
Francisella
> *F. tularensis*

francium (Fr)
Francke needle
frangula
frangulic acid
frangulin
frank breech presentation
Frankenhäuser ganglion
Frankfort
> F. horizontal plane
> F. plane

Frankfort-mandibular incisor angle
frankincense

Franklin
> F. disease
> F. spectacles

franklinic taste
Frank-Starling curve
Fräntzel murmur
Fraser-Lendrum stain for fibrin
Fraser syndrome
fraternal twins
Fraunhofer line
Frazier needle
Frazier-Spiller operation
FRC
> functional residual capacity

FRCP
> Fellow of the Royal College of Physicians
> (of England)

FRCP(C)
> Fellow of the Royal College of Physicians
> (Canada)

FRCP(E), FRCP(Edin)
> Fellow of the Royal College of Physicians
> (Edinburgh)

FRCP(I)
> Fellow of the Royal College of Physicians
> (Ireland)

FRCS
> Fellow of the Royal College of Surgeons
> (of England)

FRCS(C)
> Fellow of the Royal College of Surgeons
> (Canada)

FRCS(E), FRCS(Edin)
> Fellow of the Royal College of Surgeons
> (Edinburgh)

FRCS(I)
> Fellow of the Royal College of Surgeons
> (Ireland)

freckle
> Hutchinson f.
> iris f.'s
> melanotic f.

Fredet-Ramstedt operation
free
> f. association
> f. bone flap
> f. border
> f. border of nail
> f. border of ovary
> f. electrophoresis
> f. energy
> f. field
> f. flap
> f. gingiva
> f. graft
> f. induction decay (FID)
> f. macrophage
> f. mandibular movement
> f. margin
> f. margin of eyelid
> f. nerve ending
> f. part of lower limb
> f. part of upper limb
> f. radical
> f. tenia

f. thyroxine index (FTI)
f. villus
f. water
f. water clearance
free-floating anxiety
free-hand knife
Freeman-Sheldon syndrome
freeway space
freeze-drying
freeze fracture
freezing
gastric f.
f. point
Freiberg
F. disease
F. infarction
Frei-Hoffmann reaction
Frei test
Frejka pillow splint
frémissement cattaire
fremitus
bronchial f.
hydatid f.
pericardial f.
pleural f.
rhonchal f.
subjective f.
tactile f.
tussive f.
vocal f.
frena (*pl. of* frenum)
frenal
French
F. chalk
F. scale (F)
French-American-British (FAB)
French-American-British classification
frenectomy
frenoplasty
frenotomy
frenulum, pl. **frenula**
cerebellar f.
f. cerebelli
f. clitoridis
f. of clitoris
f. epiglottidis
f. of foreskin
f. of Giacomini
f. of ileal orifice
f. of ileocecal valve
f. of labia minora
f. labii inferioris
f. labii superioris
f. labiorum minorum
f. labiorum pudendi
f. linguae
lingual f.
f. of lower lip
f. of M'Dowel
f. of Morgagni
f. ostii ilealis
f. of prepuce
f. preputii
f. preputii clitoridis
f. of pudendal lips

f. pudendi
f. of superior medullary velum
synovial frenula
f. of tongue
f. of upper lip
f. valvae ileocecalis
f. veli medullaris superioris
frenum, pl. **frena, frenums**
Morgagni f.
synovial frena
frenzy
frequency
best f.
characteristic f.
critical flicker fusion f.
critical fusion f. (CFF)
f. curve
f. distribution
f. domain
dominant f.
f. encoding
fundamental f.
gene f.
Larmor f.
f. of micturition
mutational f.
nearest neighbor f.
resonant f.
respiratory f.
f. spectrum
Frerichs theory
freshening
fresh frozen plasma (FFP)
Fresnel
F. lens
F. prism
fressreflex
fretting
fretum, pl. **freta**
freudian
f. fixation
f. psychoanalysis
f. slip
Freud theory
Freund
F. anomaly
F. complete adjuvant
F. incomplete adjuvant
F. operation
Frey
F. hair
F. syndrome
FRF
FRH
follitropin-releasing hormone
friable
fricative
friction
dynamic f.
f. murmur
f. rub
f. sound
starting f.
static f.
frictional attachment

F

Friderichsen-Waterhouse syndrome
Friedländer
    F. bacillus
    F. bacillus pneumonia
    F. stain for capsule
Friedman curve
Friedreich
    F. ataxia
    F. phenomenon
    F. sign
Friend
    F. disease
    F. leukemia virus
    F. virus
fright reaction
frigid
frigidity
frigorific
frigorism
fringe
    costal f.
    synovial f.
frit
Froehde reagent
frog
    f. face
    f. leg position
frog-leg lateral projection
Fröhlich
    F. dwarfism
    F. syndrome
Frohn reagent
Froin syndrome
frôlement
Froment sign
frons
front
frontad
frontal
    f. angle of parietal bone
    f. area
    f. artery
    f. aspect
    f. belly of occipitofrontalis muscle
    f. bone
    f. border
    f. border of parietal bone
    f. border of sphenoid bone
    f. branch of middle meningeal artery
    f. branch of superficial temporal artery
    f. cortex
    f. crest
    f. eminence
    f. fontanelle
    f. foramen
    f. forceps
    f. groove
    f. horn
    f. lobe
    f. lobe of cerebrum
    f. lobe epilepsy
    f. margin
    f. margin of sphenoid

    f. nerve
    f. notch
    f. part of corpus callosum
    f. plane
    f. plate
    f. pole
    f. pole of cerebrum
    f. process of maxilla
    f. process of zygomatic bone
    f. region of head
    f. section
    f. sinus
    f. sinus aperture
    f. squama
    f. suture
    f. triangle
    f. tuber
    f. vein
frontalis muscle
frontoanterior position
frontoethmoidal suture
frontolacrimal suture
frontomalar
frontomaxillary suture
frontonasal
    f. duct
    f. process
    f. prominence
    f. suture
fronto-occipital fasciculus
fronto-orbital area
frontoparietal
frontopolar artery
frontopontine
    f. fiber
    f. tract
frontoposterior position
frontosphenoidal process
frontotemporale
frontotemporal tract
frontotransverse position
frontozygomatic suture
front-tap
    f.-t. contraction
    f.-t. reflex
Froriep ganglion
frost
    f. itch
    F. suture
    urea f.
    uremic f.
frostbite
frosted
    f. branch angiitis
    f. heart
frottage
frotteur
frozen
    f. pelvis
    f. section
    f. shoulder
FRS
    Fellow of the Royal Society
    first rank symptom

FRSC
Fellow of the Royal Society (Canada)
Fru
fructan
fructo
fructofuranose
fructokinase deficiency
fructolysis
fructosan
fructose
f.-bisphosphatase
f. 1,6-bisphosphate
f. 2,6-bisphosphate
f.-bisphosphate aldolase
f.-diphosphate aldolase
f. malabsorption
f. 1-phosphate
f. 6-phosphate
fructosemia
fructoside
fructosuria
benign f.
essential f.
fructosyl
fruiting body
fruit sugar
frusemide
frustration-aggression hypothesis
frustration tolerance
FSH
follicle-stimulating hormone
FSH-RH
ft.
fiat
FTA-ABS
fluorescent treponemal antibody
absorption
F.-A. test
fluorescent treponemal antibody-
absorption test
FTI
free thyroxine index
Fuc
fucose
Fuchs
F. adenoma
F. black spot
F. coloboma
F. endothelial dystrophy
F. heterochromic cyclitis
F. spur
F. stoma
F. syndrome
F. uveitis
fuchsin
acid f.
aldehyde f.
aniline f.
basic f.
f. body
carbol f.
diamond f.
fuchsinophil
f. cell

f. granule
f. reaction
fuchsinophilia
fuchsinophilic
fucose (Fuc)
fucosidosis
FUDR
fluorodeoxyuridine
fugacity
-fugal
-fuge
fugitive
f. swelling
f. wart
fugue
fugu poison
fugutoxin
fulcrum, pl. **fulcra, fulcrums**
f. line
fulgurant
fulgurating migraine
fulguration
direct f.
indirect f.
full
f. breech presentation
f. denture
f. liquid diet
fuller's earth
full-thickness
f.-t. burn
f.-t. flap
f.-t. graft
fulminant
f. hepatitis
f. hyperpyrexia
fulminating
f. dysentery
f. smallpox
fumarase
fumarate
f. hydratase
f. reductase (NADH)
fumaric
f. acid
f. acidemia
f. aminase
f. hydrogenase
fumarylacetoacetate hydrolase
fumigant
fumigate
fumigation
fuming
f. nitric acid
f. sulfuric acid
functio laesa
function
allomeric f.
arousal f.
atrial transport f.
f. corrector
discriminant f.
isomeric f.
line spread f. (LSF)
modulation transfer f. (MTF)

F

functional
    f. albuminuria
    f. anatomy
    f. aphasia
    f. apoplexy
    f. asplenia
    f. autonomy
    f. blindness
    f. cardiovascular disease
    f. castration
    f. chew-in record
    f. congestion
    f. contracture
    f. disease
    f. disorder
    f. dysmenorrhea
    f. dyspepsia
    f. dyspnea
    f. endoscopic sinus surgery (FESS)
    f. genomics
    f. group
    f. hearing impairment
    f. hypertrophy
    f. illness
    f. jaw orthopedics
    f. mandibular movement
    f. murmur
    f. neck dissection
    f. neurosurgery
    f. occlusal harmony
    f. occlusion
    f. orthodontic therapy
    f. pathology
    f. pleiotropy
    f. prepubertal castration syndrome
    f. psychosis
    f. refractory period
    f. residual air
    f. residual capacity (FRC)
    f. sphincter
    f. splint
    f. stricture
    f. terminal innervation ratio
    f. visual loss
    f. vocal fatigue
functionalism
fundament
fundamental
    f. frequency
    f. tone
fundectomy
fundi (*pl. of* fundus)
fundic gland
fundiform
    f. ligament of clitoris
    f. ligament of foot
    f. ligament of penis
fundoplication
    Belsey f.
    Collis-Belsey f.
    Collis-Nissen f.
    Dor f.
    Nissen f.
    Toupet f.
fundus, pl. **fundi**
    f. albipunctatus
    f. of bladder
    f. diabeticus
    f. flavimaculatus
    f. of gallbladder
    f. gastricus
    f. of internal acoustic meatus
    f. of internal auditory meatus
    leopard f.
    f. meatus acustici interni
    mosaic f.
    f. oculi
    f. polycythemicus
    f. reflex
    salt-and-pepper f.
    f. of stomach
    tessellated f.
    f. tigré
    tigroid f.
    f. tympani
    f. of urinary bladder
    f. uteri
    f. of uterus
    f. ventriculi
    f. vesicae biliaris
    f. vesicae felleae
    f. vesicae urinariae
funduscope
funduscopy
fundusectomy
fungal
fungate
fungemia
fungi (*pl. of* fungus)
fungicidal
fungicide
fungicidin
fungiform papillae
fungilliform
fungistat
fungistatic
fungitoxic
fungitoxicity
fungoid
fungous
fungus, pl. **fungi**
    f. ball
    f. cerebri
    dematiaceous fungi
    imperfect f.
    fungi imperfecti
    perfect f.
    ray f.
    thrush f.
    umbilical f.
    yeast f.
funicle
funic souffle
funicular
    f. f.
    f. graft
    f. hydrocele
    f. myelitis
    f. myelosis

f. part of ductus deferens
f. process
funiculitis
    endemic f.
    filarial f.
funiculus, pl. funiculi
    anterior f.
    f. anterior
    cuneate f.
    dorsal f.
    f. dorsalis
    f. gracilis
    lateral f.
    f. lateralis
    lateral f. of spinal cord
    funiculi medullae spinalis
    f. posterior
    posterior f.
    f. separans
    f. solitarius
    f. spermaticus
    f. teres
    f. umbilicalis
    ventral f.
funiform
funipuncture
funis
funisitis
funnel
    f. breast
    Büchner f.
    f. chest
    Martegiani f.
    pial f.
    f. plot
funnel-shaped pelvis
funny bone
FUO
    fever of unknown origin
fur
fura-2
furaltadone
furan
furanose
furazolidone
furcal nerve
furcation
furcula
furfur, pl. furfures
furfuraceous
furfural
furfures (*pl. of* furfur)
furfurol reaction
furfuryl alcohol
furious rabies
furnace
    dental f.
    muffle f.
furnacemen's cataract
furosemide
furred tongue
furrow
    digital f.

genital f.
gluteal f.
mentolabial f.
primitive f.
skin f.'s
furuncle
furunculosis
furunculus, pl. furunculi
Fusarium
fuseau
fused
    f. kidney
    f. silver nitrate
    f. teeth
fusel oil
fusible metal
fusidate sodium
fusidic acid
fusiform
    f. aneurysm
    f. cataract
    f. cell of cerebral cortex
    f. gyrus
    f. layer
    f. muscle
Fusiformis
fusimotor
fusin
fusing point
fusion
    f. area
    f. beat
    bone block f.
    cell f.
    centric f.
    f. energy
    flicker f.
    nuclear f.
    spinal f.
    spine f.
    splenogonadal f.
    f. temperature (wire method)
    vertebral f.
fusional movement
fusion-inferred threshold test (FIT test)
Fusobacterium
    F. mortiferum
    F. necrophorum
    F. nucleatum
fusocellular
fusospirochetal
    f. disease
    f. gingivitis
    f. stomatitis
fustic
fustigation
futile cycle
FVC
    forced vital capacity
Fy
    Fy antigen
    Fy blood group

F

γ (*var. of* gamma)
G
  gauss
    G acid
    G antigen
    G cell
    G factor
    G force
    G protein
    G syndrome
    G unit of streptomycin
G1
  gap 1
G2
  gap 2
g
  gram
Ga
  gallium
⁶⁷Ga
⁶⁸Ga
GABA
  gamma-aminobutyric acid
    GABA pathway
Gaboon ulcer
G-actin
GAD
  glutamate decarboxylase
Gaddum and Schild test
gadfly
gadodiamide
gadoleic acid
gadolinium (Gd)
gadopentetate
gadoteridol
Gaenslen sign
Gaffky
    G. scale
    G. table
GAG
  glycosaminoglycan
    Crowe-Davis mouth G.
gag
    g. reflex
gage
gain
    primary g.
    secondary g.
    time-compensated g.
    time compensation g. (TCG)
    time-varied g. (TVG)
Gairdner disease
Gaisböck syndrome
gait
    antalgic g.
    g. apraxia
    ataxic g.
    calcaneal g.
    cerebellar g.
    Charcot g.
    circumduction g.
    equine g.

  festinating g.
  gluteus maximus g.
  gluteus medius g.
  helicopod g.
  hemiplegic g.
  high-steppage g.
  hysterical g.
  scissor g.
  spastic g.
  steppage g.
  toppling g.
  Trendelenburg g.
  waddling g.
Gal
  galactose
galact- (*var. of* galacto-)
galactacrasia
galactagogue
galactan
galactic
galactidrosis
galactitol
galacto-, galact-
galactoblast
galactocele
galactogen
galactokinase
    g. deficiency
    g. deficiency galactosemia
galactometer
galactophagous
galactophore
galactophoritis
galactophorous
    g. canal
    g. duct
galactopoiesis
galactopoietic hormone
galactopyranose
galactorrhea
galactosamine
galactosaminoglycan
galactosan
galactoscope
galactose (Gal)
    g. cataract
    g. diabetes
    g. tolerance test
galactosemia
    epimerase deficiency g.
    galactokinase deficiency g.
    transferase deficiency g.
galactose-1-phosphate uridylyltransferase
galactose-6-sulfatase
galactose-6-sulfurase
β-galactosidase
galactoside
galactosis
galactosuria
galactosyl
galactosylceramide lipoidosis
galactotherapy

G

galacturonan
D-galacturonic acid
galangal
galanthamine
Galant reflex
Galassi pupillary phenomenon
galea aponeurotica
Galeati gland
galeatomy
Galeazzi fracture
Galen
> G. anastomosis
> G. nerve

galena
galenic
galenical
galla
gallamine triethiodide
Gallaudet fascia
Gallavardin phenomenon
gallbladder
> Courvoisier g.
> g. fossa
> porcelain g.
> sandpaper g.
> strawberry g.

gall duct
Gallego differentiating solution
gallein
gallic acid
Gallie transplant
Galliformes
gallinaceous
gallium (Ga)
gallium-67, -68
gallocyanin, gallocyanine
gallon
gallop
> atrial g.
> presystolic g.
> protodiastolic g.
> g. rhythm
> S_7 g.
> g. sound
> summation g. (S_7)
> systolic g.

gallstone
> g. colic
> g. ileus
> opacifying g.
> silent g.

Gallus
gallus adenolike virus
GALT
> gut-associated lymphoid tissue

Galton
> G. delta
> G. law
> G. system of classification of fingerprints
> G. whistle

galtonian
> g. genetics
> g. inheritance
> g. trait

Galtonian-Fisher genetics
galvanic
> g. current
> g. nystagmus
> g. skin reaction
> g. skin reflex
> g. skin response (GSR)
> g. threshold

galvanism
galvanization
galvanocaustic snare
galvanocautery
galvanocontractility
galvanofaradization
galvanometer
> d'Arsonval g.
> Einthoven string g.

galvanomuscular
galvanopalpation
galvanoscope
galvanosurgery
galvanotaxis
galvanotherapy
galvanotonus
galvanotropism
GAL virus
gamabufagin
gamabufogenin
gamabufotalin
Gambian
> G. fever
> G. trypanosomiasis

gambir
game
> language g.
> model g.
> g. theory

gamekeeper's thumb
gametangium
gamete
> g. intrafallopian transfer (GIFT)
> joint g.

gametic nucleus
gameto
gametocide
gametocyst
gametocyte
gametogenesis
gametogonia
gametogony
gametoid
gametokinetic hormone
gametophagia
Gamgee tissue
gamic
gamma, γ
> g. angle
> g. benzene hexachloride (GBH)
> g. camera
> g. cell of pancreas
> g. crystallin
> g. efferent
> g. encephalography
> g. fiber
> g.-glutamyl carboxylase

g.-glutamyl cycle
g.-glutamylcysteine
g.-glutamyl hydrolase
g.-glutamyltransferase
g.-glutamyl transpeptidase
g. knife
g. loop
g. motor neuron
g. motor system
g. radiation
g. ray
gamma-aminobutyric acid (γ-Abu, GABA)
gamma-amylase
gammacism
gamma-cystathionase
gamma-glutamate (glutamate γ-) carboxypeptidase
gammagram
gamma-heavy-chain disease
Gammaherpesvirinae
gamma-hydroxybutyrate (GHB)
gamma-iodopropyleneglycol
gamma-T
gamma-tocopherol
gammopathy
    benign monoclonal g.
    biclonal g.
    monoclonal g.
    monoclonal g. of undetermined significance
    monoclonal g. of unknown significance (MGUS)
    polyclonal g.
Gamna disease
Gamna-Favre body
Gamna-Gandy
    G.-G. body
    G.-G. nodule
gamogenesis
gamogony
gamont
gamophagia
gamophobia
ganciclovir
Gandy-Gamna body
Gandy-Nanta disease
ganga
ganglia (*pl. of* ganglion)
ganglial
gangliate, gangliated
    g. cord
    g. nerve
gangliform
gangliitis
ganglioblast
gangliocyte
gangliocytoma
ganglioform
ganglioglioma
gangliolysis
    percutaneous radiofrequency g.
ganglioma
ganglion, pl. ganglia
    aberrant g.

acousticofacial g.
Acrel g.
Andersch g.
aorticorenal ganglia
ganglia aorticorenalia
Arnold g.
auditory g.
Auerbach ganglia
auricular g.
autonomic ganglia
ganglia of autonomic plexuses
basal ganglia
Bezold g.
Bochdalek g.
Bock g.
Böttcher g.
cardiac ganglia
ganglia cardiaca
carotid g.
celiac ganglia
g. cell
g. cell of dorsal spinal root
g. cell of retina
g. cervicale inferius
g. cervicale medium
g. cervicale superius
cervicothoracic g.
g. cervicothoracicum
chain ganglia
g. ciliare
ciliary g.
coccygeal g.
cochlear g.
g. cochleare
ganglia coeliaca
Corti g.
ganglia craniospinalia sensoria
craniospinal sensory ganglia
diffuse g.
dorsal root g.
Ehrenritter g.
extracranial ganglia
g. extracraniale
g. of facial nerve
Frankenhäuser g.
Froriep g.
gasserian g.
geniculate g.
g. geniculatum
g. geniculi
Gudden g.
g. habenulae
hypogastric ganglia
g. impar
inferior cervical g.
inferior g. of glossopharyngeal nerve
inferior mesenteric g.
inferior g. of vagus nerve
g. inferius nervi glossopharyngei
g. inferius nervi vagi
intercrural g.
ganglia intermedia
intermediate ganglia
g. of intermediate nerve

G

ganglion *(continued)*
  interpeduncular g.
  intervertebral g.
  intracranial g.
  g. isthmi
  jugular g.
  Laumonier g.
  Lee g.
  lenticular g.
  Lobstein g.
  Ludwig g.
  ganglia lumbalia
  lumbar ganglia
  Meckel g.
  g. mesentericum inferius
  g. mesentericum superius
  middle cervical g.
  nasal g.
  nerve g.
  g. of nervus intermedius
  neural g.
  nodose g.
  otic g.
  g. oticum
  parasympathetic ganglia
  ganglia parasympathetica
  paravertebral ganglia
  pelvic ganglia
  ganglia pelvica
  periosteal g.
  petrosal g.
  petrous g.
  phrenic g.
  ganglia phrenica
  ganglia plexuum autonomicorum
  prevertebral ganglia
  pterygopalatine g.
  g. pterygopalatinum
  Remak ganglia
  renal ganglia
  ganglia renalia
  Ribes g.
  g. ridge
  sacral ganglia
  ganglia sacralia
  Scarpa g.
  Schacher g.
  semilunar g.
  g. sensorium nervi spinalis
  sensory g.
  Soemmerring g.
  solar ganglia
  sphenopalatine g.
  spinal g.
  g. spinale
  spiral g. of cochlea
  spiral cochlear g.
  g. spirale cochleae
  stellate g.
  g. stellatum
  sublingual g.
  g. sublinguale
  submandibular g.
  g. submandibulare

  submaxillary g.
  superior cervical g.
  superior g. of glossopharyngeal
    nerve
  superior mesenteric g.
  superior g. of vagus nerve
  g. superius nervi glossopharyngei
  g. superius nervi vagi
  sympathetic ganglia
  g. of sympathetic trunk
  terminal g.
  g. terminale
  thoracic ganglia
  ganglia thoracica
  thoracic splanchnic g.
  g. thoracicum splanchnicum
  trigeminal g.
  g. trigeminale
  Troisier g.
  ganglia trunci sympathici
  g. of trunk of vagus
  tympanic g.
  g. tympanicum
  Valentin g.
  vertebral g.
  g. vertebrale
  vestibular g.
  g. vestibulare
  Vieussens ganglia
  Walther g.
  Wrisberg ganglia
ganglionated
ganglionectomy
ganglioneuroblastoma
ganglioneuroma
  central g.
  dumbbell g.
ganglioneuromatosis
ganglionic
  g. blockade
  g. blocking agent
  g. branch of internal carotid artery
  g. branch of lingual nerve
  g. branch of lingual nerve to
    sublingual ganglion
  g. branch of lingual nerve to
    submandibular ganglion
  g. branch of maxillary nerve
  g. branch of maxillary nerve to
    pterygopalatine ganglion
  g. cell layer of retina
  g. chain
  g. crest
  g. layer
  g. layer of cerebellar cortex
  g. layer of cerebral cortex
  g. layer of optic nerve
  g. motor neuron
  g. saliva
ganglionitis
ganglionostomy
ganglioplegic
gangliosialidosis
ganglioside lipidosis

gangliosidosis
G_{M2} g.
G_{M1} g.
generalized g.
infantile G_{M2} g.
infantile, generalized G_{M1} g.
Type 1 G_{M1} g.
gangosa
gangrene
arteriosclerotic g.
cold g.
cutaneous g.
decubital g.
diabetic g.
disseminated cutaneous g.
dry g.
embolic g.
emphysematous g.
Fournier g.
gas g.
hemorrhagic g.
hospital g.
hot g.
Meleney g.
moist g.
presenile spontaneous g.
pressure g.
progressive bacterial synergistic g.
senile g.
spontaneous g. of newborn
static g.
symmetrical g.
thrombotic g.
trophic g.
venous g.
wet g.
white g.
gangrenous
g. appendicitis
g. cellulitis
g. emphysema
g. pharyngitis
g. pneumonia
g. rhinitis
g. stomatitis
ganoblast
Ganser
G. commissure
G. syndrome
Gant clamp
gantry
Gantzer
G. accessory bundle
G. muscle
Ganzfeld stimulation
gap
g. 1 (G1)
g. 2 (G2)
air-bone g.
anion g.
g. arthroplasty
auscultatory g.
Bochdalek g.
chromosomal g.
DNA g.

excitable g.
interocclusal g.
g. junction
g. phenomenon
silent g.
gap₂
g. period
g. phase
gap₀
g. period
g. phase
gap₁
g. period
g. phase
garapata disease
Gardner-Diamond syndrome
Gardnerella
Gardnerella vaginalis
Gardnerella **vaginitis**
Gardner syndrome
gargantuan mastitis
gargle
Gariel pessary
Garland triangle
garlic oil
garment
antishock g.
pneumatic antishock g.
Garré
G. disease
G. osteomyelitis
Gartner
G. canal
G. cyst
G. duct
Gärtner
G. method
G. tonometer
G. vein phenomenon
GAS
group A streptococci
gas
g. abscess
alveolar g.
anesthetic g.
arterial blood g. (ABG)
g. bacillus
blood g.'s
carbonic acid g.
g. cautery
g. chromatography
g. constant
g. cyst
g. embolism
expired g.
g. flow (V)
g. gangrene
g. gangrene antitoxin
hemolytic g.
ideal alveolar g.
inert g.
inspired g.
laughing g.
marsh g.
mixed expired g.

G

gas *(continued)*
 mustard g. (HD)
 noble g.
 g. peritonitis
 g. retinopexy
 sewer g.
 sneezing g.
 suffocating g.
 tear g.
 g. thermometer
 vesicating g.
 vomiting g.
 water g.
gaseous
 g. mediastinography
 g. pulse
Gaskell
 G. bridge
 G. clamp
gas-liquid chromatography (GLC)
gasometer
gasometric
gasometry
gasserian ganglion
gassing
gaster
Gasterophilidae
gastralgia
gastral mesoderm
gastrea theory
gastrectasis
gastrectomy
 Hofmeister g.
 Pólya g.
gastric
 g. algid malaria
 g. analysis
 g. area
 g. artery
 g. branch of anterior vagal trunk
 g. branch of posterior vagal trunk
 g. bypass
 g. calculus
 g. canal
 g. cardia
 g. colic
 g. crisis
 g. diastole
 g. digestion
 g. feeding
 g. fistula
 g. fold
 g. follicle
 g. freezing
 g. gland
 g. hemorrhage
 g. hypersecretion
 g. impression on liver
 g. impression on spleen
 g. indigestion
 g. inhibitory peptide (GIP)
 g. inhibitory polypeptide (GIP)
 g. juice
 g. lymphoid nodule

 g. mucin
 g. mucosa
 g. nervous plexus
 g. neurasthenia
 g. pit
 g. plexus of autonomic system
 g. rugae
 g. smear
 g. stapling
 g. surface of spleen
 g. tetany
 g. ulcer
 g. vein
 g. volvulus
gastricsin
gastricus
gastrin
gastrinoma
gastritis
 alkaline reflux g.
 atrophic g.
 bile g.
 catarrhal g.
 g. cystica polyposa
 eosinophilic g.
 exfoliative g.
 hypertrophic g.
 interstitial g.
 polypous g.
 pseudomembranous g.
 sclerotic g.
gastroacephalus
gastroalbumorrhea
gastroamorphus
gastroanastomosis
gastroatonia
gastroblennorrhea
gastrocardiac syndrome
gastrocele
gastrochronorrhea
gastrocnemius muscle
gastrocolic
 g. fistula
 g. ligament
 g. omentum
 g. reflex
gastrocolitis
gastrocoloptosis
gastrocolostomy
gastrocutaneous fistula
gastrocystoplasty
gastrodialysis
gastrodiaphragmatic ligament
Gastrodiscoides hominis
Gastrodiscus hominis
gastroduodenal
 g. artery
 g. fistula
 g. lymph node
 g. orifice
gastroduodenitis
gastroduodenoscopy
gastroduodenostomy
gastrodynia
gastroenteric

gastroenteritis
    acute infectious nonbacterial g.
    endemic nonbacterial infantile g.
    eosinophilic g.
    epidemic nonbacterial g.
    infantile g.
    viral g.
    g. virus type A, B
gastroenteroanastomosis
gastroenterocolitis
gastroenterocolostomy
gastroenterologist
gastroenterology
gastroenteropathy
gastroenteroplasty
gastroenteroptosis
gastroenterostomy
gastroenterotomy
gastroepiploic
    g. artery
    g. vein
gastroesophageal
    • g. hernia
    g. reflux disease (GERD)
    g. vestibule
gastroesophagitis
gastroesophagostomy
gastrogastrostomy
gastrogavage
gastrogenic
gastrogenous diarrhea
Gastrografin swallow
gastrograph
gastrohepatic omentum
gastrohydrorrhea
gastroileac reflex
gastroileitis
gastroileostomy
gastrointestinal (GI)
    g. autonomic nerve tumor
    g. fistula
    g. hormone
    g. stromal tumor
    g. tract
gastrojejunal loop obstruction syndrome
gastrojejunocolic
gastrojejunostomy
gastrokinesograph
gastrolavage
gastrolienal ligament
gastrolith
gastrolithiasis
gastrologist
gastrology
gastrolysis
gastromalacia
gastromegaly
gastromelus
gastromyxorrhea
gastronesteostomy
gastroomental artery
gastropagus
gastropancreatic fold
gastroparalysis
gastroparasitus

gastroparesis diabeticorum
gastropathic
gastropathy
    hypertrophic hypersecretory g.
gastropexy
Gastrophilidae
gastrophrenic ligament
gastroplasty
    Collis g.
    vertical banded g.
gastroplication
gastropneumonic
gastropod
Gastropoda
gastroptosis
gastroptyxis
gastropulmonary
gastropyloric
gastrorrhagia
gastrorrhaphy
gastrorrhea
gastrorrhexis
gastroschisis
gastroscope
    fiberoptic g.
gastroscopic
gastroscopy
gastrospasm
gastrosplenic
    g. ligament
    g. omentum
gastrostaxis
gastrostenosis
gastrostogavage
gastrostolavage
gastrostomy
    percutaneous endoscopic g.
gastrothoracopagus
gastrotome
gastrotomy
gastrotonometer
gastrotonometry
gastrotoxic
gastrotoxin
gastrotropic
gastroxia
gastroxynsis
gastrula
gastrulation
Gatch bed
gate
gate-control
    g.-c. hypothesis
    g.-c. theory
gated radionuclide angiocardiography
gatekeeper
gating
    cardiac g.
    g. mechanism
    respiratory g.
Gaucher
    G. cell
    G. disease
gauge
    bite g.

G

gauge *(continued)*
>Boley g.
>catheter g.
>g. pressure
>strain g.
>undercut g.

gaultheria oil
gaultherin
gauntlet bandage
gauss (G)
>G. sign

gaussian
>g. curve
>g. distribution

gauze bandage
gavage
Gavard muscle
gay
>g. bowel syndrome
>g. gland

Gay-Lussac
>G.-L. equation
>G.-L. law

gaze
>conjugate g.
>dysconjugate g.
>g. paretic nystagmus

G-banding
>G.-b. stain

GBG
>gonadal steroid-binding globulin

GBH
>gamma benzene hexachloride

GB virus
GC
>guanosine and cytosine
>GC content

G-CSF
>granulocyte colony-stimulating factor

Gd
>gadolinium

GDP
>guanosine 5′-diphosphate

GDPmannose phosphorylase
Ge
>germanium
>Ge antigen

Gedoelstia
gedoelstiosis
Geigel reflex
Geiger-Müller
>G.-M. counter
>G.-M. tube

gel
>colloidal g.
>g. diffusion
>g. diffusion precipitin test
>g. diffusion precipitin test in one
>dimension
>g. diffusion precipitin test in two
>dimensions
>g. diffusion reaction
>g. electrophoresis
>g. filtration

>g. filtration chromatography
>pharmacopeial g.
>g. structure

gelastic seizure
gelate
gelatin
>glycerinated g.
>Irish moss g.
>g. sugar
>vegetable g.
>zinc g.

gelatinase
gelatiniferous
gelatinization
gelatinize
gelatinoid
gelatinous
>g. ascites
>g. bone marrow
>g. droplike corneal dystrophy
>g. infiltration
>g. nucleus
>g. polyp
>g. scleritis
>g. substance
>g. tissue
>g. varix

gelation
gelatum
Gélineau syndrome
Gell
>G. and Coombs Classification
>G. and Coombs reaction

Gellé test
gelosis
gelsemine
gelsolin
Gély suture
gem-
Gemella
>*G. morbillorum*

gemellology
gemellus
gemfibrozil
geminate
geminated tooth
gemination
geminous
gemistocyte
gemistocytic
>g. astrocyte
>g. astrocytoma
>g. cell
>g. reaction

gemistocytoma
gemma
gemmation
gemmule
>Hoboken g.'s

gena
genal gland
gender
>g. dysphoria syndrome
>g. identity

g. identity disorder
g. role

gene

g. activation
allelic g.
autosomal g.
BRCA1 g.
BRCA2 g.
C g.
codominant g.
control g.
g. deletion
dominant g.
g. dosage compensation
g. dosage effect
g. duplication
g. expression
extrachromosomal g.
g. family
g. flow
g. frequency
H g.
histocompatibility g.
holandric g.
homeotic g.'s
housekeeping g.'s
immune response g.'s
jumping g.
lethal g.
g. library
g. mapping
microophthalmia transcription
   factor g.'s
mimic g.'s
mitochondrial g.
modifier g.
g. mosaicism
mutant g.
operator g.
pleiotropic g.
polyphenic g.
g. pool
P53 tumor suppressor g.
g. regulation
regulator g.
repressor g.
SOS g.'s
g. splicing
split g.
structural g.
g. therapy
transfer g.'s
transforming g.
tumor suppressor g.
V g.
X-linked g.
Y-linked g.
Z g.

genealogy
genera (*pl. of* genus)
general

g. adaptation reaction
g. adaptation syndrome
g. anatomy
g. anesthesia
g. anesthetic
g. bloodletting
g. duty nurse
g. fertility rate
g. hospital
g. immunity
g. paresis
g. peritonitis
g. physiology
g. practice
g. sensation
g. somatic afferent column
g. somatic efferent column
g. stimulant
g. transduction
g. visceral afferent column
g. visceral efferent column

generalist
generalization

stimulus g.

generalized

g. anaphylaxis
g. anxiety disorder
g. chondromalacia
g. cortical hyperostosis
g. elastolysis
g. emphysema
g. epidermolytic hyperkeratosis
g. eruptive histiocytoma
g. gangliosidosis
g. glycogenosis
g. lentiginosis
g. myokymia
g. paralysis
g. plane xanthomatosis
g. pustular psoriasis of Zambusch
g. Shwartzman phenomenon
g. tetanus
g. tonic-clonic epilepsy
g. tonic-clonic seizure
g. tuberculosis
g. vaccinia
g. xanthelasma

generalized seizure
generate
generated occlusal path
generation

asexual g.
g. effect
filial g.
nonsexual g.
parental g. (P_1)
sexual g.
skipped g.
spontaneous g.
virgin g.

generational
generative empathy
generator

aerosol g.
asynchronous pulse g.
atrial synchronous pulse g.
atrial triggered pulse g.
demand pulse g.
fixed rate pulse g.

G

generator *(continued)*
    g. potential
    pulse g.
    radionuclide g.
    standby pulse g.
    ventricular inhibited pulse g.
    ventricular synchronous pulse g.
    ventricular triggered pulse g.
    x-ray g.
generic
    g. name
    g. substitution
genesial
genesiology
genesis
genetic
    g. amplification
    g. association
    g. burden
    g. carrier
    g. code
    g. colonization
    g. compound
    g. counseling
    g. death
    g. determinant
    g. disequilibrium
    g. dominance
    g. drift
    g. engineering
    g. epidemiology
    g. equilibrium
    g. female
    g. fingerprint
    g. fitness
    g. fixation
    g. heterogeneity
    g. homeostasis
    g. human male
    g. isolate
    g. lethal
    g. linkage
    g. load
    g. locus
    g. map
    g. marker
    g. material
    g. model
    g. penetrance
    g. polymorphism
    g. psychology
    g. recombination
    g. testing
geneticist
genetics
    behavioral g.
    biochemical g.
    classical g.
    clinical g.
    epidemiologic g.
    galtonian g.
    Galtonian-Fisher g.
    human g.
    mathematical g.

    medical g.
    mendelian g.
    microbial g.
    modern g.
    molecular g.
    multilocal g.
    population g.
    quantitative g.
    reverse g.
    somatic cell g.
    statistical g.
    transplantation g.
genetotrophic
Geneva
    G. Convention
    G. lens G.
Gengou phenomenon
genial
    g. tubercle
genicula (*pl. of* geniculum)
genicular
    g. anastomosis
    g. artery
    g. vein
geniculate
    g. body
    g. ganglion
    g. neuralgia
    g. otalgia
    g. zoster
geniculated
geniculatus lateralis nucleus
geniculocalcarine
    g. radiation
    g. tract
geniculum, pl. **genicula**
    g. canalis facialis
    g. of facial canal
    g. of facial nerve
    g. nervus facialis
genioglossal muscle
genioglossus muscle
geniohyoideus
geniohyoid muscle
genion
genioplasty
genital
    g. ambiguity
    g. branch of genitofemoral nerve
    g. branch of iliohypogastric nerve
    g. cord
    g. corpuscle
    g. duct
    g. eminence
    g. fold
    g. furrow
    g. gland
    g. herpes
    g. ligament
    g. organ
    g. phase
    g. primacy
    g. primordium
    g. ridge
    g. stage

g. swelling
g. system
g. tract
g. tubercle
g. wart
genitalia
ambiguous g.
ambiguous external g.
external g.
female external g.
female internal g.
indifferent g.
male external g.
male internal g.
genitality
genitals
genitocrural nerve
genitofemoral nerve
genitoinguinal ligament
genitourinary (GU)
g. apparatus
g. fistula
g. surgeon
g. system
genius epidemicus
Gennari
G. band
G. stria
genoblast
genocopy
genodermatology
genodermatosis
genome
genomic
g. clone
g. DNA
g. imprinting
g. library
genomics
functional g.
genospecies
genote
genotoxic
genotype
ZZ g.
genotypic
genotypical
gentamicin
gentian, gentian root
g. aniline water
g. violet
gentianophil, gentianophile
gentianophilous
gentianophobic
gentiobiase
gentiobiose
gentisic acid
genu, pl. **genua**
g. capsulae internae
g. corporis callosi
g. of corpus callosum
g. of facial canal
g. of facial nerve
g. of internal capsule
g. nervi facialis

g. recurvatum
g. valgum
g. varum
genual
genucubital position
genupectoral position
genus, pl. **genera**
genyantrum
geode
geographic
g. choroidopathy
g. information system
g. keratitis
g. retinal atrophy
g. stippling of nail
g. tongue
geographic stippling of nail, geographic stippling of nail
geomedicine
geometric
g. isomer
g. isomerism
g. mean
g. sense
geopathology
geophagia
geophilic
Geophilus
geotaxis
geotrichosis
Geotrichum
geotropism
gephyrin
gephyrophobia
gepirone
geraniol
geranylgeranyl pyrophosphate
geranyl pyrophosphate
geratology
Gerbich antigen
Gerbode defect
GERD
gastroesophageal reflux disease
Gerdy
G. fiber
G. fontanelle
G. hyoid fossa
G. interatrial loop
G. ligament
G. tubercle
Gerhardt
G. reaction
G. test for acetoacetic acid
G. test for urobilin in the urine
Gerhardt-Mitchell disease
geriatric
g. medicine
g. therapy
geriatrics
dental g.
Gerlach
G. annular tendon
G. tonsil
G. valve
G. valvula

G

Gerlier disease
germ
- g. cell
- dental g.
- g. disk
- enamel g.
- g. layer
- g. layer theory
- g. line
- g. membrane
- g. nucleus
- reserve tooth g.
- tooth g.
- g. tube
- g. tube test
- wheat g.

German
- G. measles
- G. measles virus

germanium (Ge)
germicidal
germicide
germinal
- g. membrane
- g. aplasia
- g. area
- g. cell
- g. center of Flemming
- g. cord
- g. disk
- g. epithelium
- g. localization
- g. mosaicism
- g. pole
- g. rod
- g. streak
- g. vesicle

germinative
- g. layer
- g. layer of nail

germine
germinoma
Germiston virus
geroderma
gerodontics, gerodontology
geromarasmus
gerontal
gerontine
gerontologist
gerontology
gerontophilia
gerontophobia
gerontotherapeutics
gerontotherapy
gerontoxon
Gerota
- G. capsule
- G. fascia
- G. method

Gerstmann-Sträussler-Scheinker syndrome
Gerstmann syndrome
gestagen
gestagenic
gestalt
- g. phenomenon
- g. psychology
- g. theory
- g. therapy

gestaltism
gestation
gestational
- g. age
- g. diabetes
- g. edema
- g. hypertension
- g. proteinuria
- g. ring
- g. sac
- g. trophoblastic disease

gestin
gestosis, pl. **gestoses**
gesture
- suicide g.

Gey solution
GFR
- glomerular filtration rate

G$_{M1}$ gangliosidosis
G$_{M2}$ gangliosidosis
GH
- growth hormone

ghatti gum
GHB
- gamma-hydroxybutyrate

ghee
GHK equation
Ghon
- G. complex
- G. focus
- G. primary lesion
- G. tubercle

ghost
- g. cell
- g. cell glaucoma
- g. corpuscle
- g. tooth

ghoul hand
GHRF, GH-RF
- growth hormone-releasing factor

GHRH, GH-RH
- growth hormone-releasing hormone

GHz
- gigahertz

GI
- gastrointestinal
- Gingival Index

Giannuzzi
- G. crescent
- G. demilune

Gianotti-Crosti syndrome
giant
- g. axonal neuropathy
- g. cell
- g. cell aortitis
- g. cell arteritis
- g. cell carcinoma
- g. cell carcinoma of thyroid gland
- g. cell epulis
- g. cell fibroma
- g. cell glioblastoma multiforme
- g. cell granuloma

g. cell hepatitis
g. cell hyaline angiopathy
g. cell monstrocellular sarcoma of Zülch
g. cell myeloma
g. cell myocarditis
g. cell pneumonia
g. cell sarcoma
g. cell thyroiditis
g. cell tumor of bone
g. cell tumor of tendon sheath
g. chromosome
g. colon
g. condyloma
g. fibroadenoma
g. follicular lymphoblastoma
g. follicular thyroiditis
g. gastric fold
g. hives
g. hypertrophy of gastric mucosa
g. melanosome
g. osteoid osteoma
g. papillary conjunctivitis
g. pigmented nevus
g. urticaria

giantism
Giardia

G. intestinalis
G. lamblia

giardiasis
gibberellic acid
gibberellin
gibbon
gibbous
Gibb phase rule
Gibbs

G. energy of activation
G. free energy
G. theorem

Gibbs-Donnan equilibrium
Gibbs-Helmholtz equation
gibbus
Gibney

G. boot
G. fixation bandage

Gibson

G. bandage
G. murmur

Giemsa

G. chromosome banding stain

Gierke

G. cell
G. disease
G. respiratory bundle

Gifford reflex
GIFT

gamete intrafallopian transfer

gigahertz (GHz)
gigantiform cementoma
gigantism

acromegalic g.
cerebral g.
eunuchoid g.
fetal g.

pituitary g.
primordial g.

gigantocellular

g. glioma
g. nucleus of medulla oblongata

gigantomastia
Gigantorhynchus
Gigli saw
GIH

growth hormone-inhibiting hormone

Gila monster
Gilbert

G. disease
G. syndrome

gilbert
Gilchrist disease
gill

g. arch skeleton
g. cleft

Gilles

G. de la Tourette disease
G. de la Tourette syndrome

Gillespie syndrome
Gillette suspensory ligament
Gilliam operation
Gillies operation
Gillmore needle
Gilmer wiring
Gil-Vernet operation
Gimbernat ligament
ginger

Chinese g.
Indian g.
g. oleoresin
g. paralysis
wild g.

gingili oil
gingiva, pl. **gingivae**

alveolar g.
attached g.
buccal g.
free g.
labial g.
lingual g.
septal g.

gingival

g. abrasion
g. abscess
g. atrophy
g. clamp
g. cleft
g. contour
g. crest
g. crevice
g. curvature
g. cyst
g. elephantiasis
g. embrasure
g. enlargement
g. epithelium
g. festoon
g. fibromatosis
g. fistula
g. flap
g. fluid

G

gingival *(continued)*
    g. groove
    g. hyperplasia
    G. Index (GI)
    g. margin
    g. massage
    g. mucosa
    g. papilla
    g. pocket
    g. proliferation
    g. recession
    g. repositioning
    g. resorption
    g. retraction
    g. septum
    g. space
    g. sulcus
    g. tissue
    g. trough
    g. zone
Gingival-Periodontal Index (GPI)
gingivectomy
gingivitis
    acute necrotizing ulcerative g. (ANUG)
    atypical g.
    chronic desquamative g.
    diabetic g.
    dilantin g.
    diphenylhydantoin g.
    fusospirochetal g.
    hormonal g.
    hyperplastic g.
    leukemic hyperplastic g.
    marginal g.
    necrotizing ulcerative g. (NUG)
    plasma cell g.
    pregnancy g.
    proliferative g.
    suppurative g.
    ulceromembranous g.
gingivoaxial
gingivobuccal
    g. groove
    g. sulcus
gingivodental ligament
gingivoglossitis
gingivolabial
    g. groove
    g. sulcus
gingivolingual
    g. groove
    g. sulcus
gingivolinguoaxial
gingivoosseous
gingivoplasty
gingivosis
gingivostomatitis
    primary herpetic g.
ginglyform
ginglymoarthrodial
ginglymoid joint

ginglymus
    helicoid g.
    lateral g.
Ginkgo biloba
ginseng
Giordano-Giovannetti diet
Giovannetti diet
GIP
    gastric inhibitory peptide
    gastric inhibitory polypeptide
Girard reagent
girdle
    g. anesthesia
    Hitzig g.
    Neptune g.
    g. pain
    pectoral g.
    pelvic g.
    g. sensation
    shoulder g.
    thoracic g.
    white limbal g. of Vogt
Girdlestone procedure
gitalin
Gitelman syndrome
githagism
gitogenin
gitonin
gitoxigenin
gitoxin
gitter cell
gitterzelle
Gla
    4-carboxyglutamic acid
glabella
glabellad
glabrous
    g. skin
glacial
    g. acetic acid
    g. phosphoric acid
gladiate
gladiolus
glairy mucus
glancing wound
gland
    accessory g.
    accessory lacrimal g.
    accessory parotid g.
    accessory suprarenal g.
    accessory thyroid g.
    acid g.
    acinotubular g.
    acinous g.
    admaxillary g.
    adrenal g.
    aggregate g.
    agminate g.
    Albarran g.
    albuminous g.
    alveolar g.
    anal g.
    anterior lingual g.
    apical g.
    apocrine g.

apocrine sweat g.
areolar g.
arteriococcygeal g.
arytenoid g.
Aselli g.
g. of auditory tube
axillary g.
axillary sweat g.
Bartholin g.
basal g.
Bauhin g.
Baumgarten g.
biliary g.
g. of biliary mucosa
Blandin g.
Bowman g.
brachial g.
bronchial g.
Bruch g.
Brunner g.
buccal g.
bulbourethral g.
cardiac g.
cardiac g. of esophagus
cardiac g. of stomach
ceruminous g.
cervical g.
cervical g. of uterus
Ciaccio g.
ciliary g.
circumanal g.
coccygeal g.
coil g.
g. of (common) bile duct
compound g.
conjunctival g.
convoluted g.
Cowper g.
cutaneous g.
ductless g.
duodenal g.
Duverney g.
Ebner g.
eccrine g.
ecdysial g.
Eglis g.
endocrine g.
esophageal g.
g. of eustachian tube
excretory g.
exocrine g.
external salivary g.
g. of the female urethra
follicular g.
fundic g.
Galeati g.
gastric g.
gay g.
genal g.
genital g.
Gley g.
glomiform g.
greater vestibular g.
Guérin g.
hemal g.

hematopoietic g.
hemolymph g.
Henle g.
hibernating g.
holocrine g.
internal salivary g.
g. of internal secretion
interscapular g.
interstitial g.
intestinal g.
intraepithelial g.
jugular g.
Knoll g.
Krause g.
labial g.
lacrimal g.
lactiferous g.
g. of large intestine
laryngeal g.
lesser vestibular g.
Lieberkühn g.
Littré g.
Luschka g.
Luschka cystic g.
lymph g.
major salivary g.
g. of the male urethra
malpighian g.
mammary g.
marrow-lymph g.
master g.
maxillary g.
meibomian g.
merocrine g.
Méry g.
mesenteric g.
milk g.
minor salivary g.
mixed g.
molar g.
Moll g.
Montgomery g.
g. of mouth
mucilaginous g.
muciparous g.
mucous g.
mucous g. of auditory tube
nasal g.
Nuhn g.
odoriferous g.
oil g.
olfactory g.
oxyntic g.
pacchionian g.
palatine g.
palpebral g.
parathyroid g.
paraurethral g.
parotid g.
pectoral g.
peptic g.
peritracheal g.
perspiratory g.
Peyer g.
pharyngeal g.

G

gland (*continued*)
  Philip g.
  pileous g.
  pineal g.
  pituitary g.
  Poirier g.
  prehyoid g.
  preputial g.
  prostate g.
  prothoracic g.
  pyloric g.
  racemose g.
  Rivinus g.
  Rosenmüller g.
  saccular g.
  salivary g.
  sebaceous g.
  seminal g.
  sentinel g.
  seromucous g.
  serous g.
  Serres g.
  sexual g.
  Skene g.
  g. of small intestine
  solitary g.
  sublingual g.
  submandibular g.
  submaxillary g.
  sudoriferous g.
  suprahyoid g.
  suprarenal g.
  Suzanne g.
  sweat g.
  target g.
  tarsal g.
  Terson g.
  Theile g.
  thoracic g.
  thymus g.
  thyroid g.
  Tiedemann g.
  tracheal g.
  trachoma g.
  tubal g. of pharyngotympanic tube
  tubular g.
  tubuloacinar g.
  tubuloalveolar g.
  tympanic g.
  Tyson g.
  unicellular g.
  urethral g.
  uterine g.
  vaginal g.
  vascular g.
  ventral g.
  vesical g.
  vestibular g.
  vulvovaginal g.
  Waldeyer g.
  Wasmann g.
  Weber g.
  Wepfer g.
  Wölfler g.

  Wolfring g.
  Zeis g.
glanders
glandes (*pl. of* glans)
glandilemma
glandula, pl. **glandulae**
  glandulae areolares
  g. atrabiliaris
  g. basilaris
  glandulae bronchiales
  glandulae buccales
  g. bulbourethralis
  glandulae ceruminosae
  glandulae cervicales uteri
  glandulae ciliares
  glandulae circumanales
  glandulae conjunctivales
  glandulae cutis
  glandulae ductus biliaris
  glandulae ductus choledochi
  glandulae duodenales
  glandulae endocrinae
  glandulae esophageae
  glandulae gastricae
  glandulae glomiformes
  glandulae intestinales
  glandulae intestini crassi
  glandulae intestini tenuis
  glandulae labiales
  glandulae lacrimales accessoriae
  g. lacrimalis
  glandulae laryngeae
  g. lingualis anterior
  g. mammaria
  glandulae molares
  g. mucosa
  glandulae mucosae biliosae
  glandulae nasales
  glandulae olfactoriae
  glandulae oris
  glandulae palatinae
  g. parathyroidea
  g. parotidea
  g. parotidea accessoria
  g. parotis
  g. parotis accessoria
  glandulae pharyngeales
  g. pinealis
  g. pituitaria
  glandulae preputiales
  g. prostatica
  glandulae pyloricae
  g. salivaria
  glandulae salivariae majores
  glandulae salivariae minores
  glandulae sebaceae
  g. seminalis
  g. seromucosa
  g. serosa
  glandulae sine ductibus
  g. sublingualis
  g. submandibularis
  glandulae sudoriferae
  glandulae suprarenales accessoriae
  g. suprarenalis

glandulae tarsales
g. thyroidea
g. thyroidea accessoria
glandulae thyroideae accessoriae
glandulae tracheales
glandulae tubariae
glandulae urethrales femininae
glandulae urethrales masculinae
glandulae uterinae
g. vesiculosa
glandulae vestibulares minores
g. vestibularis major
glandular
g. branch
g. branch of facial artery
g. branch of inferior thyroid artery
g. branch of submandibular
  ganglion
g. cancer
g. carcinoma
g. epithelium
g. fever
g. lobe of hypophysis
g. mastitis
g. plague
g. substance of prostate
g. system
g. tularemia
glandule
glandulopreputial lamella
glandulous
glans, pl. **glandes**
g. clitoridis
g. of clitoris
g. penis
glanular hypospadias
Glanzmann
G. disease
G. thrombasthenia
glaphenine
glare
blinding g.
dazzling g.
peripheral g.
specular g.
veiling g.
glarometer
glaserian
g. artery
g. fissure
Glasgow
G. coma scale
G. sign
glass, pl. **glasses**
g. bead sterilizer
g. body
cover g.
Crookes g.
crown g.
cupping g.
g. electrode
g. factor
flint g.
g. ionomer cement
object g.

quartz g.
g. ray
soluble g.
vita g.
water g.
Wood g.
glassworker's cataract
glassy membrane
Glauber salt
glaucine
glaucoma
absolute g.
acute g.
alpha-chymotrypsin-induced g.
angle-closure g.
aphakic g.
chronic g.
closed-angle g.
combined g.
compensated g.
congenital g.
corticosteroid-induced g.
g. fulminans
ghost cell g.
hemorrhagic g.
hypersecretion g.
low-tension g.
malignant g.
narrow-angle g.
neovascular g.
normal-tension g.
open-angle g.
phacogenic g.
phacolytic g.
phacomorphic g.
pigmentary g.
pseudoexfoliative g.
pupillary block g.
secondary g.
simple g., g. simplex
glaucomatocyclitic crisis
glaucomatous
g. cataract
g. cup
g. excavation
g. halo
g. nerve-fiber bundle scotoma
g. ring
glaucosuria
GLC
gas-liquid chromatography
Gleason
G. score
G. tumor grade
gleet
Glenn
G. operation
G. shunt
Glenner-Lillie stain for pituitary
glenohumeral
g. articulation
g. joint
g. ligament
glenoid
g. cavity

G

glenoid *(continued)*
    g. cavity of scapula
    g. fossa
    g. labrum of scapula
    g. ligament
    g. surface
glenoidal lip
Gley gland
glia cell
gliacyte
gliadin
glial
    g. fibrillary acidic protein
    g. limiting membrane
gliclazide
glide
    mandibular g.
glidewire
gliding
    g. joint
    g. occlusion
glioblast
glioblastoma multiforme
    giant cell g. m.
glioblastosis cerebri
glioma
    brainstem g.
    gigantocellular g.
    mixed g.
    nasal g.
    g. of optic chiasm
    optic nerve g.
    g. of the spinal cord
    telangiectatic g.
    g. telangiectodes
gliomatosis cerebri
gliomatous
gliomyxoma
glioneuroma
gliosarcoma
gliosis
    isomorphous g.
    piloid g.
    g. uteri
GLIP
    glucagonlike insulinotropic peptide
glipizide
Glisson
    G. capsule
    G. cirrhosis
    G. sphincter
glissonitis
glitazones
glitter cell
Gln
    glutamine
    glutamyl
global
    g. aphasia
    g. burden of disease
    g. paralysis
    g. warming

globe
    g. of eye
    pale g.
globi (*pl. of* globus)
globin
    g. insulin
    g. zinc insulin
Globocephalus
globoid
    g. cell
    g. cell leukodystrophy
globoside
globosus nucleus
globotriaosylceramide
globular
    g. heart
    g. leukocyte
    g. process
    g. protein
    g. sputum
    g. thrombus
globule
    dentin g.
    Morgagni g.'s
    polar g.
globuliferous
globulin
    accelerator g. (AcG)
    antihemophilic g. (AHG)
    antihemophilic g. A, B
    antihuman g.
    antilymphocyte g. (ALG)
    $beta_{1C}$ g.
    chickenpox immune g. (human)
    corticosteroid-binding g. (CBG)
    gonadal steroid-binding g. (GBG)
    human gamma g.
    immune serum g.
    measles immune g. (human)
    pertussis immune g.
    plasma accelerator g.
    poliomyelitis immune g. (human)
    rabies immune g.
    $RH_o(D)$ immune g.
    serum accelerator g.
    sex hormone-binding g. (SHBG)
    sex steroid-binding g.
    specific immune g. (human)
    testosterone-estrogen-binding g.
    tetanus immune g.
    thyroxine-binding g. (TBG)
    zoster immune g.
globulinuria
globulomaxillary cyst
globulus
globus, pl. **globi**
    g. hystericus
    g. major
    g. minor
    g. pallidus
glomal
glomangioma
glomangiosis
    pulmonary g.
glome

glomectomy
glomera (*pl. of* glomus)
glomerular
    g. capsule
    g. crescent
    g. cyst
    g. filtration rate (GFR)
    g. layer of olfactory bulb
    g. nephritis
    g. sclerosis
glomerule
glomeruli (*pl. of* glomerulus)
glomerulitis
glomerulonephritis
    acute crescentic g.
    acute hemorrhagic g.
    acute poststreptococcal g.
    anti-basement membrane g.
    Berger focal g.
    chronic g.
    diffuse g.
    exudative g.
    focal embolic g.
    hypocomplementemic g.
    immune complex g.
    lobular g.
    local g.
    membranoproliferative g.
    membranous g.
    mesangial proliferative g.
    mesangiocapillary g.
    proliferative g.
    rapidly progressive g.
    segmental g.
    subacute g.
glomerulopathy
    focal sclerosing g.
glomerulosa cell
glomerulosclerosis
    diabetic g.
    focal segmental g.
    intercapillary g.
glomerulose
glomerulus, pl. **glomeruli**
    juxtamedullary g.
    malpighian g.
    g. of mesonephros
    olfactory g.
    g. of pronephros
glomiform gland
glomus, pl. **glomera**
    aortic glomera
    glomera aortica
    g. aorticum
    g. body
    g. caroticum
    choroid g.
    g. choroideum
    g. coccygeum
    intravagal g.
    g. intravagale
    jugular g.
    g. jugulare
    g. jugulare tumor
    g. pulmonale

    pulmonary g.
    g. tympanicum tumor
glossa
glossagra
glossal
glossalgia
glossectomy
Glossina
    G. *morsitans*
    G. *pallidipes*
    G. *palpalis*
glossitis
    g. areata exfoliativa
    atrophic g.
    benign migratory g.
    g. desiccans
    Hunter g.
    median rhomboid g.
    Moeller g.
glossocele
glossocinesthetic
glossodontotropism
glossodynamometer
glossodynia
glossodyniotropism
glossoepiglottic, glossoepiglottidean
    g. ligament
glossograph
glossohyal
glossokinesthetic
glossolabiolaryngeal paralysis
glossolabiopharyngeal paralysis
glossolalia
glossology
glossoncus
glossopalatine
    g. arch
    g. fold
glossopalatinus
glossopalatolabial paralysis
glossopathy
glossopharyngeal
    g. breathing
    g. nerve [CN IX]
    g. neuralgia
    g. part of superior pharyngeal
      constrictor
    g. tic
glossopharyngeolabial paralysis
glossopharyngeus
glossoplasty
glossoplegia
glossoptosis
glossopyrosis
glossorrhaphy
glossospasm
glossosteresis
glossotomy
glossotrichia
glossy skin
glottal
glottalization
glottic
glottidospasm
glottis, pl. **glottides**

G

glottis *(continued)*
    false g.
    g. respiratoria
    g. spuria
    true g.
    g. vera
    g. vocalis
glottitis
glottology
glove anesthesia
gloved-finger sign
glover
    G. phenomenon
    g. suture
GLP-1
    glucagonlike peptide
Glp
    5-oxoproline
Glu
    glutamic acid
    glutamyl
glucagon
    gut g.
glucagonlike
    g. insulinotropic peptide (GLIP)
    g. peptide (GLP-1)
glucagonoma syndrome
glucal
glucan
4-α-D-glucanotransferase
gluceptate
gluciphore
glucoamylase
glucoascorbic acid
glucocerebroside
glucocorticoid
glucocorticotrophic
glucocyamine
glucofuranose
glucogenesis
glucogenic
glucoinvertase
glucokinase
glucokinetic
glucolipid
glucolysis
gluconeogenesis
gluconic acid
gluconolactonase
glucopenia
glucoplastic
glucoprotein
glucopyranose
glucosamine
glucosaminoglycan
glucosan
glucose
    g. oxidase method
    g. oxidase paper strip test
    g. 6-phosphate
    g. tolerance factor
    g. tolerance test
    g. transport maximum

D-glucose
    activated glucose
    glucose dehydrogenase
    liquid glucose
    glucose oxidase
    glucose oxyhydrase
    glucose phosphomutase
glucose-6-phosphate dehydrogenase deficiency
D-glucose 1,6-bisphosphate
glucose-dependent insulinotropic polypeptide
glucose-6-phosphatase
    g.-p. hepatorenal glycogenosis
D-glucose 1-phosphate
D-glucose 6-phosphate
glucose-6-phosphate dehydrogenase
glucose-phosphate isomerase
glucosephosphate isomerase deficiency
glucose-1-phosphate kinase
glucose-1-phosphate phosphodismutase
glucose-6-phosphate translocase
glucose-1-phosphate uridylyltransferase
glucosidase inhibitor
glucosidases
glucoside
glucosinolates
glucosone
glucosulfone sodium
glucosuria
glucosyl
glucosylceramide
glucosyltransferase
glucuronate
glucurone
glucuronic acid
glucuronide
D-glucuronolactone
glucuronoside
glucuronosyltransferase
glue ear
glue-sniffing
Gluge corpuscle
glusulase
glutaconic acid
glutamate
    g. acetyltransferase
    g. decarboxylase (GAD)
    g. dehydrogenases
    g. formiminotransferase
    g. gamma-semialdehyde
    g. synthase
glutamic acid (Glu)
    g. a. dehydrogenases
    g. a. hydrochloride
glutamic-aspartic transaminase
glutamic-oxaloacetic transaminase (GOT)
glutamic-pyruvic transaminase (GPT)
glutaminase
glutaminate
glutamine (Gln)
    g. aminotransferase
    g. synthetase
    g. transaminase
glutaminyl

glutamoyl
glutamyl (Gln, Glu, Glx)
γ-glutamylcysteine
 γ-glutamylcysteine synthetase
glutaral
glutaraldehyde fixative
glutaric acid
glutaryl-CoA
 glutaryl-CoA dehydrogenase
 glutaryl-CoA synthetase
glutathione (GSH)
 oxidized g.
 g. peroxidase
 reduced g.
 g. reductase
 g. synthetase
 g. synthetase deficiency
 g. *S*-transferase
glutathionuria
gluteal
 g. cleft
 g. crest
 g. fold
 g. furrow
 g. hernia
 g. line
 g. lymph node
 g. reflex
 g. region
 g. ridge
 g. surface of ilium
 g. tuberosity
 g. vein
glutelin
gluten
 g. ataxia
 g. casein
 g. enteropathy
gluten-free diet
glutenin
gluteofemoral bursa
gluteoinguinal
glutethimide
gluteus
 g. maximus gait
 g. maximus muscle
 g. medius bursae
 g. medius gait
 g. medius muscle
 g. minimus bursa
 g. minimus muscle
glutinoid
glutinous
glutitis
Glx
 glutamyl
Gly
 glycine
glyburide
glycal
glycan
glycanohydrolases
glycate
glycation
glycemia

glycemic index
glyceraldehyde
glyceraldehyde 3-phosphate
glyceric
 g. acid
 g. aldehyde
D-glyceric aciduria
L-glyceric aciduria
glyceridase
glyceride
 mixed g.'s
glycerin
 g. jelly
 g. suppository
glycerinated
 g. gelatin
 g. tincture
glycerite
 starch g.
 tannic acid g.
glycerogelatin
glycerokinase
glycerol
 g. dehydration test
 iodinated g.
 g. kinase
 g. phosphate
glycerol-3-phosphate acyltransferase
glycerol-3-phosphate dehydrogenase (NAD⁺)
glycerone
glycerophosphate shuttle
glycerophosphocholine
glycerophosphoric acid
glycerophosphorylcholine
glycerulose
glyceryl
 g. alcohol
 g. borate
 g. guaiacolate
 g. iodide
 g. monostearate
 g. triacetate
 g. tributyrate
 g. tricaprate
 g. trinitrate
glycinamide ribonucleotide
glycinate
glycine (Gly)
 g. acyltransferase
 g. amidinotransferase
 g. betaine
 g. cleavage complex
 g. dehydrogenases
 g. synthase
 g. transamidinase
glycineamide ribonucleotide
glycine-succinate cycle
glycinin
glycinium
glycinuria
 familial g.
glyco-
glycobiarsol
glycocalyx

G

glycocholate sodium
glycocholic acid
glycoconjugate
glycocorticoid
glycocyamine
glycogelatin
glycogen
  g. cardiomegaly
  g. granule
  g. phosphorylase
  g. starch synthase
  g. synthase
glycogenase
glycogenesis
glycogenetic
glycogenic
  g. acanthosis
  g. cardiomegaly
glycogenolysis
glycogenosis
  brancher deficiency g.
  generalized g.
  glucose-6-phosphatase hepatorenal g.
  hepatophosphorylase deficiency g.
  myophosphorylase deficiency g.
  type 1, 2, 3, 4, 5, 6, 7 g.
D-glycogenous
glycogen-storage disease
glycogeusia
glycoglycinuria
glycohistochemistry
  lectin glycohistochemistry
glycolaldehyde
  active g.
glycolaldehydetransferase
glycolate
glycol ether
glycoleucine
glycolic
  g. acid
  g. aciduria
glycolipid lipidosis
glycolyl
glycolylurea
glycolysis
glycolytic
glyconeogenesis
glyconic acids
glycopenia
glycopeptide
Glycophagus
glycophilia
glycophorin
glycoprotein
  alpha$_1$-acid g.
glycoptyalism
glycopyrrolate
glycorrhachia
glycorrhea
glycosaminoglycan (GAG)
glycosecretory
glycosialia
glycosialorrhea
glycosidase

glycoside
  cardiac g.
  cyanogenic g.
N-glycoside
glycosidic
glycosphingolipid
glycostatic
glycosuria
  alimentary g.
  benign g.
  digestive g.
  nondiabetic g.
  nonhyperglycemic g.
  normoglycemic g.
  orthoglycemic g.
  pathologic g.
  phloridzin g.
  phlorizin g.
  renal g.
glycosylated hemoglobin
glycosylation
glycosyl compound
glycosyltransferase
glycotropic
glycuresis
glycuronate
glycuronic acid
glycuronidase
glycuronide
glycuronuria
glycyclamide
glycyl
glycyrrhiza
glyoxal
glyoxalase
glyoxylate transacetylase
glyoxyldiureide
glyoxylic acid cycle
Gm
  Gm allotype
  Gm antigen
gm
  gram
GM-CSF (granulocyte-macrophage colony-
  stimulating factor)
  granulocyte-macrophage colony-
    stimulating factor
Gmelin test
GMP
  guanylic acid
    cyclic GMP
  GMP reductase
    guanylic acid reductase
  GMP synthetase
    guanylic acid synthetase
GMS
  Gomori methenamine-silver stain
gnashing
gnat
gnathic index
gnathion
gnathocephalus
gnathodynamics
gnathodynamometer
gnathography

gnathological
gnathology
gnathoschisis
gnathostatics
Gnathostoma
    G. *doloresi*
    G. *hispidum*
    G. *nipponicum*
    G. *siamense*
    G. *spinigerum*
gnathostomiasis
gnoscopine
gnosia
gnotobiology
gnotobiota
gnotobiote
gnotobiotic
GnRH
    gonadotropin-releasing hormone
goal
goatpox virus
goat's milk anemia
goblet cell
Godélier law
Godman fascia
Godwin tumor
Goeckerman treatment
Goethe bone
Gofman test
Goggia sign
goggle
    plethysmographic g.
goiter
    aberrant g.
    acute g.
    adenomatous g.
    Basedow g.
    cabbage g.
    colloid g.
    cystic g.
    diffuse g.
    diving g.
    endemic g.
    exophthalmic g.
    familial g.
    fibrous g.
    follicular g.
    lingual g.
    microfollicular g.
    multinodular g.
    nontoxic g.
    nontoxic nodular g. (NTNG)
    parenchymatous g.
    simple g.
    substernal g.
    suffocative g.
    thoracic g.
    toxic g.
    wandering g.
goitrogen
goitrogenic
goitrous
gold (Au)
    g. alloy
    g. casting

    cohesive g.
    colloidal radioactive g.
    g. equivalent
    g. foil
    g. inlay
    mat g.
    noncohesive g.
    g. number
    powdered g.
    g. sodium thiomalate
    g. sodium thiosulfate
    g. sol test
    g. standard
    g. thioglucose
Goldblatt
    G. hypertension
    G. kidney
Goldenhar syndrome
golden seal
Goldflam disease
Goldie-Coldman hypothesis
Goldman equation
Goldman-Fox knife
Goldman-Hodgkin-Katz equation
Goldmann
    G. applanation tonometer
    G. perimeter
Goldmann-Favre syndrome
gold-myokymia syndrome
Goldscheider test
Goldstein toe sign
golfer's skin
golf-hole ureteral orifice
Golgi
    G. apparatus
    G. body
    G. cell
    G. complex
    G. corpuscle
    G. epithelial cell
    G. internal reticulum
    G. osmiobichromate fixative
    G. stain
    G. tendon organ
    G. type I, II neuron
    G. zone
Golgi-Mazzoni corpuscle
golgiokinesis
Goll column
Goltz syndrome
Gombault triangle
gomenol
gomitoli
gommelin
Gomori
    G. aldehyde fuchsin stain
    G. chrome alum hematoxylin-
      phloxine stain
    G. methenamine-silver stain (GMS)
    G. nonspecific acid phosphatase
      stain
    G. nonspecific alkaline phosphatase
      stain
    G. one-step trichrome stain
    G. silver impregnation stain

G

Gomori-Jones periodic acid-methenamine-silver stain
Gompertz
    G. hypothesis
    G. law
gompholic joint
gomphosis
gonad
    g. dose
    female g.
    indifferent g.
    male g.
    g. nucleus
    streak g.
gonadal
    g. agenesis
    g. aplasia
    g. cord
    g. dose
    g. dysgenesis
    gonadal g.
    g. hormone
    g. ridge
    g. steroid-binding globulin (GBG)
    g. streak
gonadectomy
gonado-
gonadoblastoma
gonadocrin
gonadoliberin
gonadopathy
gonadorelin hydrochloride
gonadotroph
gonadotrophic cycle
gonadotrophin
gonadotropic hormone
gonadotropin
    anterior pituitary g.
    beta-human chorionic g.
    chorionic g. (CG)
    human chorionic g. (HCG)
    human menopausal g. (HMG)
    placenta g.
gonadotropin-producing adenoma
gonadotropin-releasing
    g.-r. factor
    g.-r. hormone (GnRH, GRH)
gonaduct
gonalgia
gonane
gonarthritis
gonecyst
Gongylonema
    g. *pulchrum*
gongylonemiasis
gonia (*pl. of* gonion)
gonio-
goniocraniometry
goniodysgenesis
goniometer
gonion, pl. **gonia**
goniopuncture
gonioscope
gonioscopy
goniosynechia

goniotomy
gonochorism
gonocide
gonococcal
    g. arthritis
    g. conjunctivitis
    g. stomatitis
gonococcemia
gonococci (*pl. of* gonococcus)
gonococcic
gonococcicide
gonococcus, pl. **gonococci**
gonocyte
gonohemia
gonoopsonin
gonophage
gonophore
gonorrhea
gonorrheal
    g. arthritis
    g. conjunctivitis
    g. ophthalmia
    g. rheumatism
    g. salpingitis
    g. urethritis
gonosome
gonotoxemia
gonotoxin
gonotyl
Gonyaulax catanella
gonycampsis
good
    G. antigen
    g. object
Goodell sign
Goodenough draw-a-man test
goodness
    g. of fit
    g. of fit test
Goodpasture
    G. stain
    G. syndrome
Goormaghtigh cell
gooseflesh
Gopalan syndrome
Gordius
Gordon
    G. reflex
    G. sign
    G. and Sweet stain
    G. symptom
Gordona
gorget
    probe g.
Gorham
    G. disease
    G. syndrome
Goriaew rule
Gorlin
    G. cyst
    G. formula
    G. sign
    G. syndrome
Gorlin-Chaudhry-Moss syndrome
gorondou

goserelin
Gosselin fracture
gossypol
gossypose
GOT
　glutamic-oxaloacetic transaminase
gothic
　G. arch
　G. arch tracing
　G. palate
Göthlin test
gouge
Gougerot and Blum disease
Gougerot-Carteaud syndrome
Gougerot-Sjögren disease
Gould suture
Gouley catheter
goundou
gout
　abarticular g.
　articular g.
　calcium g.
　g. diet
　idiopathic g.
　interval g.
　latent g.
　lead g.
　masked g.
　primary g.
　retrocedent g.
　saturnine g.
　secondary g.
　tophaceous g.
gouty
　g. arthritis
　g. diathesis
　g. pearl
　g. tophus
　g. urine
government hospital
Gowers
　G. column
　G. contraction
　G. disease
　G. syndrome
　G. tract
Gower sign
GPI
　Gingival-Periodontal Index
GPT
　glutamic-pyruvic transaminase
gr
　grain
graafian follicle
gracile
　g. fasciculus
　g. habitus
　g. lobule
　g. nucleus
　g. tubercle
gracilespinal fiber
gracilis
　g. muscle
　g. syndrome

grad.
　gradatim
gradatim (grad.)
grade
　Gleason tumor g.
　Heath-Edwards g.'s
　g. I, II, III, IV astrocytoma
Gradenigo syndrome
gradient
　atrioventricular g.
　concentration g.
　density g.
　electrochemical g.
　g. elution
　g. encoding
　field g.
　magnetic field g.
　mitral g.
　systolic g.
　ventricular g.
gradient-recalled acquisition in the steady state (GRASS)
graduated
　g. compress
　g. pipette
　g. tenotomy
graduate nurse
Graefe
　G. forceps
　G. knife
　G. operation
　G. sign
Graefenberg ring
Graffi virus
graft
　allogenic g.
　animal g.
　autogeneic g.
　autologous g.
　autoplastic g.
　bone g.
　chorioallantoic g.
　composite g.
　corneal g.
　Davis g.
　delayed g.
　dermal fat g.
　dowel g.
　fascia g.
　fascicular g.
　fat g.
　free g.
　full-thickness g.
　funicular g.
　H g.
　heterologous g.
　heteroplastic g.
　heterotopic g.
　homologous g.
　homoplastic g.
　inlay g.
　isogeneic g.
　isologous g.
　isoplastic g.
　Krause g.

G

graft *(continued)*
    Krause-Wolfe g.
    mesh g.
    mucosal g.
    nerve g.
    Ollier g.
    Ollier-Thiersch g.
    onlay g.
    orthotopic g.
    osteoperiosteal g.
    partial-thickness g.
    pedicle g.
    periosteal g.
    pinch g.
    porcine g.
    primary skin g.
    punch g.
    Reverdin g.
    skin g.
    sleeve g.
    split-skin g.
    split-thickness g.
    Stent g.
    syngeneic g.
    tendon g.
    Thiersch g.
    g. versus host (GVH)
    g. versus host disease
    g. versus host reaction (GVHR)
    Wolfe g.
    Wolfe-Krause g.
    xenogeneic g.
    zooplastic g.
grafting
Graham
    G. law
    G. Steell murmur
Graham-Cole test
Grahamella
grain (gr)
    g. alcohol
    g. itch
gram (g, gm)
    g. calorie
    g. equivalent
    G. iodine
    G. stain
gram-atomic weight
gram-centimeter
Gram-chromotrope stain
gramicidin
gram-ion
gram-meter
gram-molecular weight
gram-molecule
Gram-negative
Gram-positive
grana (*pl. of* granum)
granatum
grand
    g. mal
    g. mal epilepsy
    g. mal seizure
    g. multipara

granddaughter cyst
grandiose
    g. delusion
    g. type of paranoid disorder
Granger
    G. line
    G. projection
Granit loop
granny knot
Gr antigen
granular
    g. cast
    g. cell myoblastoma
    g. cell tumor
    g. conjunctivitis
    g. corneal dystrophy
    g. cortex
    g. degeneration
    g. endoplasmic reticulum
    g. foveolae
    g. kidney
    g. layer
    g. layer of cerebellar cortex
    g. layer of cerebellum
    g. layer of cerebral cortex
    g. layer of epidermis
    g. layer of a vesicular ovarian
      follicle
    g. leukocyte
    g. lid
    g. ophthalmia
    g. pit
    g. pneumonocytes
    g. trachoma
    g. urethritis
granulated opium
granulatio, pl. **granulationes**
    granulationes arachnoideae
granulation
    arachnoid g.
    arachnoidal g.
    pacchionian g.
    g. tissue
granule
    acidophil g.
    acrosomal g.
    alpha g.
    Altmann g.
    amphophil g.
    argentaffin g.
    azurophil g.
    basal g.
    basophil g.
    Bensley specific g.
    beta g.
    Birbeck g.
    Bollinger g.
    g. cell
    g. cell of connective tissue
    chromatic g.
    chromophil g.
    chromophobe g.
    cone g.
    Crooke g.
    delta g.

elementary g.
eosinophil g.
Fordyce g.
fuchsinophil g.
glycogen g.
iodophil g.
juxtaglomerular g.
kappa g.
keratohyalin g.
lamellar g.
Langerhans g.
Langley g.
membrane-coating g.
metachromatic g.
mucinogen g.
Neusser g.
neutrophil g.
Nissl g.
oxyphil g.
Palade g.
proacrosomal g.
prosecretion g.
rod g.
Schüffner g.
secretory g.
seminal g.
specific g.
volutin g.
Zimmermann g.
zymogen g.

granuloblast
granulocyte
g. colony-stimulating factor (G-CSF)
immature g.
granulocyte-macrophage colony-stimulating factor (GM-CSF)
GM-CSF
granulocytic
g. leukemia
g. sarcoma
g. series
granulocytopenia
granulocytopoiesis
granulocytopoietic
granulocytosis
granuloma
actinic g.
amebic g.
g. annulare
apical g.
beryllium g.
bilharzial g.
Capillaria g.
cholesterol g.
coccidioidal g.
cutaneous leishmaniasis g.
dental g.
Enterobius g.
eosinophilic g.
g. faciale
fish-tank g.
foreign body g.
g. gangrenescens
giant cell g.
g. gravidarum

infectious g.
g. inguinale
laryngeal g.
lethal midline g.
lipoid g.
lipophagic g.
lymphatic filariasis g.
Majocchi g.'s
malignant g.
Miescher g.
g. multiforme
ocular larva migrans g.
oily g.
paracoccidioidal g.
Paragonimus g.
periapical g.
pulse g.
pyogenic g.
g. pyogenicum
reparative g.
reparative giant cell g.
root end g.
sarcoidal g.
schistosome g.
sea urchin g.
silica g.
silicotic g.
swimming pool g.
trichinosis g.
g. tropicum
umbilical g.
g. venereum
zirconium g.
granulomatosis
allergic g.
lipid g., g. granulomatosis
lymphomatoid g.
g. siderotica
Wegener g.
granulomatous
g. arteritis
g. colitis
g. disease
g. encephalomyelitis
g. endophthalmitis
g. enteritis
g. inflammation
g. mastitis
g. nocardiosis
g. rosacea
granulomere
granulopenia
granuloplasm
granuloplastic
granulopoiesis
granulopoietic
granulosa
g. cell
g. cell tumor
g. lutein cell
granulosis rubra nasi
granulovacuolar degeneration
granum, pl. **grana**
granzyme

G

grape
  g. ending
  g. sugar
graph
graphanesthesia
graphesthesia
graphic
  g. aphasia
  g. formula
graphite
grapho-
graphology
graphomania
graphomotor aphasia
graphopathology
graphophobia
graphospasm
grasp
  palm g.
  pen g.
  g. reflex
grasping reflex
GRASS
  gradient-recalled acquisition in the steady
  state
grass bacillus
Grasset
  G. law
  G. phenomenon
  G. sign
Grasset-Gaussel phenomenon
Gratiolet
  G. fiber
  G. radiation
grattage
gratuitous inducer
gravel
Graves
  G. disease
  G. ophthalmopathy
  G. optic neuropathy
  G. orbitopathy
grave wax
gravida
  g. I, II
gravidic
gravidism
graviditas
  g. examnialis
  g. exochorialis
gravidity
gravid uterus
gravimeter
gravimetric
gravireceptor
gravitation abscess
gravitational
  g. ulcer
  g. units
gravity
  g. concentration
  specific g. (sp. gr.)
  zero g.

Grawitz
  G. basophilia
  G. tumor
gray (Gy)
  g. baby syndrome
  g. cataract
  g. column
  g. commissure
  g. degeneration
  g. fiber
  g. hepatization
  g. induration
  g. infiltration
  g. layer of superior colliculus
  g. literature
  g. matter
  g. rami communicantes
  g. scale
  g. substance
  g. syndrome
  g. tuber
  g. tubercle
  g. wing
gray-scale ultrasonography
greaseless cream
great
  g. adductor muscle
  g. alveolar cell
  g. anastomotic artery
  g. auricular nerve
  g. cardiac vein
  g. cerebral vein
  g. cerebral vein of Galen
  g. foramen
  g. horizontal fissure
  g. longitudinal fissure
  g. radicular artery
  g. saphenous vein
  g. sciatic nerve
  g. segmental medullary artery
  g. superior pancreatic artery
  g. toe I
  g. vein of Galen
greater
  g. alar cartilage
  g. arterial circle of iris
  g. circulation
  g. cul-de-sac
  g. curvature of stomach
  g. horn of hyoid bone
  g. multangular bone
  g. occipital nerve
  g. omentum
  g. palatine artery
  g. palatine canal
  g. palatine foramen
  g. palatine groove
  g. palatine nerve
  g. pancreatic artery
  g. pectoral muscle
  g. pelvis
  g. peritoneal cavity
  g. petrosal nerve
  g. posterior rectus muscle of head
  g. psoas muscle

g. rhomboid muscle
g. ring of iris
g. sciatic notch
g. splanchnic nerve
g. superficial petrosal nerve
g. supraclavicular fossa
g. trochanter
g. tubercle
g. tuberosity of humerus
g. tympanic spine
g. vestibular gland
g. wing of sphenoid bone
g. zygomatic muscle
greatest length
great-toe reflex
green

g. hemoglobin
g. monkey virus
g. pus
Scheele g.
g. soap
g. soap tincture
g. sputum
g. stain
g. tobacco sickness
g. tooth
g. vision
Greenfield filter
greenstick fracture
gregaloid
Gregarina
gregarine
Gregarinia
gregarinosis
Greig

G. cephalopolysyndactyly syndrome
G. syndrome
grenz

g. ray
g. zone
gression
Greville bath
grey

g. matter
G. Turner sign
GRH

gonadotropin-releasing hormone
grid

Amsler g.
focused g.
g. ratio
Wetzel g.
Gridley

G. stain
G. stain for fungi
grief
Griesinger

G. disease
G. sign
grindelia
grinding

selective g.
g. surface
grinding-in

grip

devil g.
grippe
griseofulvin
griseus
Grisonella ratellina
gristle
Gritti operation
Gritti-Stokes amputation
Grocco

G. sign
G. triangle
grocer's itch
Grocott-Gomori methenamine-silver stain
Groenouw corneal dystrophy
groin
Grönblad-Strandberg syndrome
groove

alveolobuccal g.
alveololabial g.
alveololingual g.
ampullary g.
anterior auricular g.
anterior intermediate g.
anterior interventricular g.
anterolateral g.
anteromedian g.
g. for arch of aorta
arterial g.
atrioventricular g.
g. for auditory tube
auriculoventricular g.
bicipital g.
branchial g.
carotid g.
carpal g.
cavernous g.
chiasmatic g.
coronary g.
costal g.
g. of crus of helix
dental g.
g. for the descending aorta
developmental g.
digastric g.
ethmoidal g.
g. of first rib for subclavian artery
frontal g.'s
gingival g.
gingivobuccal g.
gingivolabial g.
gingivolingual g.
greater palatine g.
g. for greater petrosal nerve
Harrison g.
inferior petrosal g.
g. for inferior petrosal sinus
g. for inferior venae cava
infraorbital g.
interosseous g.
interosseous g. of calcaneus
interosseous g. of talus
intertubercular g.
interventricular g.
lacrimal g.

G

groove *(continued)*
 laryngotracheal g.
 lateral bicipital g.
 g. of lesser petrosal nerve
 linguogingival g.
 Lucas g.
 g. of lung for subclavian artery
 major g.
 malleolar g.
 mastoid g.
 medial bicipital g.
 median g. of tongue
 medullary g.
 middle meningeal artery g.
 g. for middle temporal artery
 minor g.
 musculospiral g.
 mylohyoid g.
 g. of nail matrix
 nasolabial g.
 nasopalatine g.
 nasopharyngeal g.
 neural g.
 obturator g.
 occipital g.
 olfactory g.
 olfactory g. of nasal cavity
 optic g.
 palatine g.
 palatovaginal g.
 paraglenoid g.
 pharyngeal g.
 pharyngotympanic g.
 pontomedullary g.
 popliteal g.
 g. for popliteus
 posterior auricular g.
 posterior intermediate g.
 posterior interventricular g.
 posterolateral g.
 preauricular g.
 primary labial g.
 primitive g.
 g. of promontory of labyrinthine
  wall of tympanic cavity
 g. of pterygoid hamulus
 g. for pterygoid hamulus
 pterygopalatine g.
 pulmonary g.
 radial g.
 g. for radial nerve
 retention g.
 rhombic g.
 sagittal g.
 Sibson g.
 sigmoid g.
 g. for sigmoid sinus
 g. sign
 skin g.
 g. for spinal nerve
 spiral g.
 subclavian g.
 g. for subclavian vein
 g. for subclavius

 subcostal g.
 g. for superior petrosal sinus
 g. for superior sagittal sinus
 g. for superior vena cava
 supplemental g.
 supra-acetabular g.
 g. for tendon of fibularis longus
 g. for tendon of flexor hallucis
  longus
 g. for tendon of peroneus longus
 g. for tibialis posterior tendon
 tracheobronchial g.
 transverse anthelicine g.
 transverse nasal g.
 g. for transverse sinus
 tympanic g.
 g. for ulnar nerve
 urethral g.
 venous g.
 vertebral g.
 g. for vertebral artery
 vomeral g.
 vomerine g.
 vomerovaginal g.
grooved tongue
gross
 g. anatomy
 g. hematuria
 g. lesion
 G. leukemia virus
 g. reproduction rate
ground
 g. bundle
 g. itch
 g. itch anemia
 g. lamella
 g. state
 g. substance
ground-glass
 g.-g. cytoplasm
 g.-g. pattern
group
 ABO blood g.
 g. agglutination
 g. agglutinin
 aluminum g.
 g. antigen
 g. A streptococcal necrotizing
  fasciitis
 g. A streptococci (GAS)
 blood g.
 g. B streptococci
 calcium g.
 CDE blood g.
 characterizing g.
 connective tissue g.
 control g.
 cytophil g.
 determinant g.
 diagnosis-related g. (DRG)
 Duffy blood g.
 g. dynamics
 encounter g.
 experimental g.
 functional g.

HACEK g.
g. hospital
g. immunity
linkage g.
matched g.'s
g. practice
prosthetic g.
g. psychotherapy
g. reaction
sensitivity training g.
symptom g.
T g.
    training group
g. test
therapeutic g.
training g. (T group)
g. transfer
g. translocation
Grover disease
growing
g. fracture
g. ovarian follicle
g. pain
growth
accretionary g.
appositional g.
g. arrest line
auxetic g.
bacterial g.
g. curve
differential g.
exponential g.
g. factor
g. hormone (GH)
g. hormone-inhibiting hormone
  (GIH)
g. hormone–producing adenoma
g. hormone-releasing factor (GHRF,
  GH-RF)
g. hormone-releasing hormone
  (GHRH, GH-RH)
interstitial g.
intussusceptive g.
g. medium
multiplicative g.
new g.
g. plate
g. rate
g. rate of population
g. regulator
growth-onset diabetes
grub
Gruber
G. cul-de-sac
G. method
G. reaction
Gruber-Landzert fossa
Gruber-Widal reaction
gruel
grumous
Grunert spur
Grunstein-Hogness assay
Grynfeltt triangle
gryochrome
gryposis penis

GSH
glutathione
GSR
galvanic skin response
GSSG
glutathione disulfide
G-strophanthin
gt.
gutta
g-tolerance
GTP
guanosine 5′-triphosphate
  G. binding protein
gtt.
gutta
GU
genitourinary
Gua
guanine
guaiac
g. gum
g. test
guaiacin
guaiacol
g. glyceryl ether
g. phosphate
guaifenesin
Guama virus
guanabenz acetate
guanacline sulfate
guanadrel sulfate
Guanarito virus
guanase
guanazolo
guanethidine sulfate
guanfacine
guanidine
guanidinium
guanidinoacetate
guanidinoacetate *N*-methyltransferase
guanine (Gua)
g. aminase
g. cell
g. deaminase
g. deoxyribonucleotide
g. ribonucleotide
guanochlor sulfate
guanosine (Guo)
cyclic g. 3′,5′-monophosphate
  (cGMP)
g. 5′-diphosphate (GDP)
g. 5′-monophosphate
g. 5′-triphosphate (GTP)
guanosine and cytosine (GC)
guanosine 5′-triphosphate (GTP)
GTP cyclohydrolase
guanoxan sulfate
guanylate cyclase
guanyl cyclase
guanylic acid (GMP)
g. a. reductase (GMP reductase,
  GMP reductase)
g. a. synthetase (GMP synthetase,
  GMP synthetase)
guanyloribonuclease

G

guanylyl
>g. cyclase

guarana

guaranine

guarding
>abdominal g.
>involuntary g.
>voluntary g.

guar gum

Guarnieri body

Guaroa virus

gubernacular
>g. canal
>g. cord

gubernaculum
>g. dentis
>Hunter g.
>g. testis

Gubler
>G. line
>G. paralysis
>G. syndrome

Gudden
>G. commissure
>G. ganglion
>G. tegmental nucleus

Guedel airway

Guéneau de Mussy point

Guérin
>G. fold
>G. fracture
>G. gland
>G. sinus
>G. valve

guidance
>condylar g.
>incisal g.

guide
>anterior g.
>catheter g.
>condylar g.
>incisal g.
>mold g.
>g. plane

guided tissue regeneration

guideline
>clasp g.
>clinical practice g.'s
>Cummer g.
>practice g.'s

guidewire

Guillain-Barré
>G.-B. reflex
>G.-B. syndrome

guillotine amputation

guinea green B

guinea pig

Guldberg-Waage law

Gulf War syndrome

gullet

Gullstrand slitlamp

L-gulonic acid

L-gulonolactone

L-gulono-γ-lactone

L-gulonolactone
>L-gulonolactone oxidase

gulose

gum
>g. arabic
>Bassora g.
>g. benjamin
>g. benzoin
>British g.
>g. contour
>eucalyptus g.
>ghatti g.
>guaiac g.
>guar g.
>Indian g.
>karaya g.
>g. lancet
>g. line
>locust g.
>g. opium
>red g.
>g. resection
>g. resin
>senegal g.
>starch g.
>sterculia g.
>wheat g.

gumboil

gumma, pl. **gummata, gummas**

gummatous
>g. abscess
>g. ulcer

Gumprecht shadow

Gunn
>G. crossing sign
>G. dot
>G. phenomenon
>G. pupil
>G. syndrome

Günning reaction

Gunning splint

gunshot wound

gunstock deformity

Günzberg
>G. reagent
>G. test

Günz ligament

Guo
>guanosine

gurgling rale

gurney

gusher
>perilymphatic g.

Gussenbauer suture

gustation

gustatory
>g. agnosia
>g. anesthesia
>g. aura
>g. bud
>g. cell
>g. hallucination
>g. hyperesthesia
>g. hyperhidrosis
>g. lemniscus

g. nucleus
g. organ
g. pore
g. rhinorrhea
g. sweating syndrome
gustatory-sudorific reflex
gustducin
gut
blind g.
g. glucagon
postanal g.
postcloacal g.
preoral g.
primitive g.
gut-associated lymphoid tissue (GALT)
Guthrie
G. muscle
G. test
gutta, pl. **guttae (gt., gtt.)**
g. serena
gutta-percha
g.-p. cone
g.-p. point
g.-p. spreader
guttat.
guttatim
guttate
guttatim (guttat.)
gutter
g. dystrophy of cornea
g. fracture
paracolic g.
paravertebral g.
g. wound
Guttman scale
guttural
g. duct
g. pulse
g. rale
gutturotetany
Gutzeit test
Guyon
G. amputation
G. canal
G. isthmus
G. sign
G. tunnel syndrome
GVH
graft versus host
GVH disease
GVHR
graft versus host reaction
Gy
gray
gym-**diol**
Gymnamoebida
gymnastics
Swedish g.
Gymnoascaceae
Gymnodinium
G. breve
Gymnophalloides seoi
gymnophobia
gymnothecium

GYN
gynecology
gynandrism
gynandroblastoma
gynandroid
gynandromorphism
gynandromorphous
gynatresia
gynecic
gynecogenic
gynecoid
g. obesity
g. pelvis
gynecologic
gynecologist
gynecology (GYN)
obstetrics and g.
gynecomania
gynecomastia
refeeding g.
gynecophoric canal
gynephobia
gyniatrics
gyniatry
gynocardia oil
gynogenesis
gynopathy
gynoplasty
gypsum
gyrase
gyrate atrophy of choroid and retina
gyration
gyrectomy
gyrencephalic
gyri (*pl. of* gyrus)
gyrochrome cell
gyromagnetic ratio
Gyromitra esculenta
gyrose
gyrospasm
gyrus, pl. **gyri**
angular g.
g. angularis
annectent g.
anterior central g.
anterior paracentral g.
anterior piriform g.
anterior transverse temporal g.
ascending frontal g.
ascending parietal g.
gyri breves insulae
callosal g.
central gyri
cerebral gyri
gyri cerebri
cingulate g.
g. cinguli
deep transitional g.
dentate g.
g. dentatus
fasciolar g.
g. fasciolaris
fornicate g.
g. fornicatus
g. frontalis inferior

G

gyrus *(continued)*
    g. frontalis medialis
    g. frontalis medius
    g. frontalis superior
    fusiform g.
    g. fusiformis
    Heschl gyri
    hippocampal g.
    inferior frontal g.
    inferior occipital g.
    inferior parietal g.
    inferior temporal g.
    gyri insulae
    insular gyri
    interlocking gyri
    lateral occipitotemporal g.
    lateral olfactory g.
    lingual g.
    g. lingualis
    long g. of insula
    g. longus insulae
    marginal g.
    medial frontal g.
    medial occipitotemporal g.
    medial olfactory g.
    middle frontal g.
    middle temporal g.
    occipital g.
    g. occipitotemporalis lateralis
    g. occipitotemporalis medialis
    g. olfactorius lateralis
    g. olfactorius medialis
    orbital gyri
    gyri orbitales
    g. paracentralis anterior
    g. paracentralis posterior

    parahippocampal g.
    g. parahippocampalis
    paraterminal g.
    g. paraterminalis
    postcentral g.
    g. postcentralis
    posterior central g.
    posterior paracentral g.
    posterior transverse temporal g.
    precentral g.
    g. precentralis
    prepiriform g.
    g. rectus
    Retzius g.
    short gyri of insula
    splenial g.
    straight g.
    subcallosal g.
    g. subcallosus
    superior frontal g.
    superior occipital g.
    superior parietal g.
    superior temporal g.
    supracallosal g.
    supramarginal g.
    g. supramarginalis
    gyri temporales transversi
    g. temporalis inferior
    g. temporalis medius
    g. temporalis superior
    g. temporalis transversus anterior
    g. temporalis transversus posterior
    transitional g.
    transverse temporal gyri
    uncinate g.

H
    henry
    heroin
    hydrogen
        H agglutinin
        H antigen
        H band
        H colony
        H and D curve
        H disk
        H field
        H gene
        H graft
        H ray
        H reflex
        H shunt
        H substance

H-2
        H-2 antigen
        H-2 complex

H⁺
    hydrogen ion

³H
    hydrogen-3

²H
    hydrogen-2

¹H
    hydrogen-1

H
    enthalpy

h
    hecto-

hν
    photon

h
    Planck constant

HAA
    hepatitis-associated antigen

Haase rule
habena, pl. **habenae**
habenal
habenula, pl. **habenulae**
    h. of cecum
    Haller h.
    habenulae perforatae
    pineal h.
    Scarpa h.
    h. urethralis
habenular
    h. commissure
    h. nucleus
    h. sulcus
    h. trigone
habenulointerpeduncular tract
Haber syndrome
Haber-Weiss reaction
habit
    h. chorea
    h. cough
    h. scoliosis
    h. spasm
    h. tic

habitual abortion
habituation
habitus
    fetal h.
    gracile h.
Habronema
    H. majus
    H. megastoma
    H. microstoma
    H. muscae
HACEK group
hacking
Hadrurus
Haeckel
    H. gastrea theory
    H. law
Haemadipsa ceylonica
Haemamoeba
Haemaphysalis
    H. cinnabarina
    H. concinna
    H. leachi
    H. spinigera
Haematopinus
Haemococcidium
Haemodipsus ventricosus
Haemogregarina
Haemonchus
Haemophilus
    H. actinomycetemcomitans
    H. aegyptius
    H. aphrophilus
    H. ducreyi
    H. haemolyticus
    H. influenzae
    H. influenzae type B
    H. influenzae type B vaccine
    nontypeable *H. influenzae*
    H. parahaemolyticus
    H. parainfluenzae
    H. paratropicalis
    H. segnis
Haemoproteus
Haemosporina
Haff disease
Haffkine vaccine
Hafnia
hafnium (Hf)
hafussi bath
Hagedorn needle
Hageman factor
hagiotherapy
Haglund
    H. deformity
    H. disease
HA1, HA2 virus
hahnemannian
Hahn oxine reagent
Haidinger brush
Hailey-Hailey disease
hair
    auditory h.

H

hair *(continued)*
　　axillary h.
　　bamboo h.
　　bayonet h.
　　beaded h.
　　h. bulb
　　burrowing h.
　　h. cast
　　h. cell
　　club h.
　　h. cross
　　h. cycle
　　h. disk
　　downy h.
　　exclamation point h.
　　h. follicle
　　Frey h.'s
　　h. of head
　　ingrown h.
　　kinky h.
　　lanugo h.
　　moniliform h.
　　nettling h.
　　h. papilla
　　primary h.
　　pubic h.
　　ringed h.
　　h. root
　　scalp h.
　　Schridde cancer h.
　　h. shaft
　　spun glass h.
　　stellate h.
　　h. stream
　　taste h.
　　terminal h.
　　h. of tragus
　　h. transplant
　　twisted h.
　　vellus h.
　　h. of vestibule of nose
　　h. whorls
　　woolly h.
HAIR-AN syndrome
hairline fracture
hairpin
　　h. loop
　　h. vessels
hairworm
hairy
　　h. cell
　　h. cell leukemia
　　h. heart
　　h. leukoplakia
　　h. mole
　　h. tongue
halation
halazone
Halberstaedter-Prowazek body
Haldane
　　H. apparatus
　　H. effect
　　H. relationship

　　H. transformation
　　H. tube
Haldane-Priestley sample
Hale colloidal iron stain
Hales piesimeter
half
　　h. amplitude pulse duration
　　h. axial view
　　h. cystine
　　h. and half nail
　　h. hapten
half-axial projection
half-chair form
half-glass spectacles
half-hapten
half-life
　　biologic h.-l.
　　effective h.-l.
　　physical h.-l.
half-moon
　　red h.-m.
half-time
half-value (HV)
half-value layer (HVL)
halibut liver oil
halide
haliphagia
halisteresis
halisteretic
halitosis
halitus
hallachrome
Hallé point
Haller
　　H. ansa
　　H. anulus
　　H. arch
　　H. cell
　　H. circle
　　H. cones
　　H. habenula
　　H. insula
　　H. line
　　H. plexus
　　H. rete
　　H. tripod
　　H. tunica vasculosa
　　H. unguis
　　H. vas aberrans
　　H. vascular tissue
Hallermann-Streiff-François syndrome
Hallermann-Streiff syndrome
Hallervorden-Spatz
　　H.-S. disease
　　H.-S. syndrome
Hallervorden syndrome
hallex, pl. **hallices**
Hallgren syndrome
Hallopeau disease
hallucal
halluces (*pl. of* hallux)
hallucination
　　auditory h.
　　command h.
　　formed visual h.

gustatory h.
haptic h.
hypnagogic h.
hypnopompic h.
kinesthesia h.
lilliputian h.
mood-congruent h.
mood-incongruent h.
olfactory h.
stump h.
tactile h.
unformed visual h.
hallucinatory neuralgia
hallucinogen
hallucinogenesis
hallucinogenic
hallucinosis
organic h.
hallus
hallux, pl. **halluces**
h. dolorosus
h. extensus
h. flexus
h. malleus
h. rigidus
h. valgus
h. varus
halo
anemic h.
h. cast
h. effect
glaucomatous h.
h. nevus
senile h.
h. sign
h. sign of hydrops
h. traction
h. vision
haloalkylamines
halogen
h. acne
h. atom (X)
halogenation
halogenoderma
Halogeton
halometer
halophil
halophilic
halosteresis
halothane-ether azeotrope
halothane hepatitis
Halstead-Reitan battery
Halsted
H. law
H. operation
H. suture
Halteridium
halzoun
ham
H. test
HAMA
human antimouse antibody
hamamelis
hamartia
hamartoblastoma

hamartochondromatosis
hamartoma
fibrous h. of infancy
pulmonary h.
hamartomatous
hamartophobia
hamate bone
hamatum
Hamburger phenomenon
Hamilton
H. anxiety rating scale
H. depression rating scale
Hamilton-Stewart
H.-S. formula
H.-S. method
Hamman
H. disease
H. murmur
H. sign
H. syndrome
Hamman-Rich syndrome
Hammarsten reagent
hammer
h. finger
h. nose
h. toe
Hammerschlag method
hammock
h. bandage
h. ligament
Hammond disease
Hampton
H. hump
H. line
H. maneuver
H. technique
hamster
hamstring
lateral h.
medial h.
h. muscle
h. tendon
hamular
h. notch
h. process of lacrimal bone
h. process of sphenoid bone
hamulus, pl. **hamuli**
h. cochleae
lacrimal h.
h. lacrimalis
h. laminae spiralis
h. ossis hamati
pterygoid h.
h. pterygoideus
h. of spiral lamina
Hancock amputation
hand
accoucheur h.
ape h.
claw h.
cleft h.
club h.
crab h.
dorsum of h.
drop h.

H

hand (*continued*)
  h. eczema
  ghoul h.
  Marinesco succulent h.
  monkey h.
  obstetric h.
  opera-glass h.
  h. ratio
  simian h.
  skeleton h.
  spade h.
  split h.
  trident h.
  writing h.
hand-and-foot syndrome
handedness
hand-foot-and-mouth
  h.-f.-a.-m. disease
  h.-f.-a.-m. disease virus
hand-foot syndrome
handicap
handpiece
Hand-Schüller-Christian disease
handshapes
HANE
  hereditary angioneurotic edema
Hanes plot
hanging
  h. drop
  h. septum
hanging-block culture
hangman's fracture
hangnail
Hanhart syndrome
Hanks
  H. dilators
  H. solution
Hannover canal
Hanot cirrhosis
Hansemann macrophage
Hansen
  H. bacillus
  H. disease
Hantaan virus
Hantavirus
hantavirus pulmonary syndrome
hapalonychia
haphalgesia
haphazard sampling
haphephobia
haplo-
haplodont
haploid set
haplology
haploprotein
haploscope
  mirror h.
haploscopic vision
Haplosporidia
haplotype
happy puppet syndrome
Hapsburg
  H. jaw
  H. lip

hapten
  conjugated h.
  Forssman h.
  half h.
  h. inhibition of precipitation
haptic hallucination
haptodysphoria
haptoglobin (HP)
haptometer
Har
  homoarginine
Harada
  H. disease
  H. syndrome
Harada-Ito procedure
Harada-Mori filter paper strip culture
hard
  h. cataract
  h. chancre
  h. corn
  h. drusen
  h. palate
  h. papilloma
  h. paraffin
  h. pulse
  h. ray
  h. soap
  h. sore
  h. tissue
  h. tubercle
  h. ulcer
  h. water
hardened pelvis
hardening
Harden-Young ester
hardiness
Harding-Passey melanoma
hardness
  indentation h.
  h. scale
hardware
Hardy-Rand-Ritter test
Hardy-Weinberg
  H.-W. equilibrium
  H.-W. law
harelip
hare's eye
harlequin
  h. fetus
  h. ichthyosis
  h. reaction
harmaline
harmidine
harmine
harmonia
harmonic
  h. mean
  h. suture
harmonious retinal correspondence
harmony
  functional occlusal h.
  occlusal h.
harpaxophobia
harpoon
Harrington-Flocks test

Harris
  H. hematoxylin
  H. line
  H. migraine
  H. and Ray test
  H. syndrome
Harrison groove
Harris and Ray test
Hartel technique
Hartmann
  H. curette
  H. operation
  H. pouch
  H. solution
Hartmannella
Hartman solution
Hartnup
  H. disease
  H. syndrome
hartshorn
harvest bug
harvester ant
hasamiyami
Häser formula
Hashimoto
  H. disease
  H. struma
  H. thyroiditis
hashish
Hasner fold
Hassall
  H. body
  H. concentric corpuscle
Hassall-Henle body
Hasson
  H. cannula
  H. trocar
hatchet excavator
hatching flask
Haudek niche
haustorium, pl. **haustoria**
haustra (*pl. of* haustrum)
haustral
haustrations of colon
haustrum, pl. **haustra**
  haustra coli
  haustra of colon
haustus
HAV
  hepatitis A virus
Haverhill fever
Haverhillia multiformis
haversian
  h. canal
  h. lamella
  h. space
  h. system
Hawkins impingement sign
Hawley
  H. appliance
  H. retainer
Haworth
  H. conformational formulas of cyclic sugar

H. perspective and conformational formulas
H. perspective formulas of cyclic sugar
H. projection
Hawthorne effect
hay
  h. asthma
  h. bacillus
  h. fever
Hayem
  H. hematoblast
  H. solution
Hayem-Widal syndrome
Hayflick limit
Haygarth node
hazard rate
hazelwort
Hb
  hemoglobin
Hb$_{Chesapeake}$
  hemoglobin Chesapeake
HB$_c$Ab
  hepatitis B core antigen
HB$_s$Ab
  hepatitis B surface antigen
HB$_e$Ab
  hepatitis B e antigen
HB$_c$Ag
  hepatitis B core antigen
HbCO
  carboxyhemoglobin
HBE, HB$_e$Ag
  His bundle electrogram
HBe
  hepatitis B e antigen
HbO$_2$
  oxyhemoglobin
Hb S
  sickle cell hemoglobin
HBV
  hepatitis B virus
HCC
  25-hydroxycholecalciferol
HCFA
  Health Care Financing Administration
HCG
  human chorionic gonadotropin
HCS
  human chorionic somatomammotropic hormone
Hct
  hematocrit
HCV
  hepatitis C virus
Hcy
  homocysteine
HD
  mustard gas
h.d.
  hora decubitus
HDCV
  human diploid cell vaccine
HDL
  high density lipoprotein

H

HDV
> hepatitis delta virus

He
> helium

³He
> helium-3

⁴He
> helium-4

head
> h. area
> h. botflies
> bulldog h.
> h. cap
> h. of caudate nucleus
> h. cavity
> clavicular h. of pectoralis major muscle
> h. cold
> deep h. of flexor pollicis brevis
> h. of epididymis
> h. of femur
> h. of fibula
> h. fold
> hourglass h.
> humeral h.
> humeroulnar h. of flexor digitorum superficialis muscle
> h. of humerus
> h. kidney
> lateral h.
> h. line
> little h. of humerus
> long h.
> h. of malleus
> h. of mandible
> medial h.
> Medusa h.
> h. of metacarpal
> h. of metatarsal
> h. mirror
> h. nurse
> oblique h.
> optic nerve h.
> h. of pancreas
> h. of phalanx (of hand or foot)
> h. presentation
> h. process
> h. of radius
> h. of rib
> saddle h.
> short h.
> short h. of biceps brachii
> short h. of biceps femoris
> h. of stapes
> sternocostal h. of pectoralis major muscle
> superficial h. of flexor pollicis brevis
> h. of talus
> h. of thigh bone
> transverse h.
> h. tremor
> h. of ulna
> ulnar h.
> h. zone

headache
> benign exertional h.
> bilious h.
> blind h.
> cluster h.
> coital h.
> fibrositic h.
> histaminic h.
> Horton h.
> ice pick h.
> idiopathic stabbing h.
> migraine h.
> muscle contraction h.
> nodular h.
> organic h.
> posttraumatic h.
> reflex h.
> sick h.
> spinal h.
> symptomatic h.
> tension h.
> tension-type h.
> thunderclap h.
> vacuum h.
> vascular h.

head-bobbing doll syndrome
head-dropping test
headgear
headgut
head-nodding
head-tilt
heal
healed
> h. tuberculosis
> h. ulcer

healer
healing
> faith h.
> h. by first intention
> h. by second intention
> h. by third intention

health
> h. behavior
> behavioral h.
> h. care
> H. Care Financing Administration (HCFA)
> h. center
> Doctor of Public H. (DPH, DrPH)
> h. education
> h. indicator
> h. information system
> h. maintenance organization
> mental h.
> h. promotion
> h. psychology
> public h.
> H. Resources and Services Administration (HRSA)
> h. risk assessment (h.r.a.)
> h. status index

healthy worker effect
Heaney operation
He antigen
hear

hearing
- color h.
- h. instrument
- h. level
- normal h.
- h. protectors

hearing aid
- behind-the-ear h. a.
- completely in the canal h. a. (CIC)
- digital h. a.
- in-the-canal h. a.
- in-the-ear h. a.

hearing impairment, hearing loss
- acoustic trauma h. i.
- Alexander h. i.
- boilermaker's hearing loss
- conductive h. i.
- functional h. i.
- hereditary h. i.
- high-frequency h. i.
- hysterical h. i.
- industrial hearing loss
- low-tone hearing loss
- mixed h. i.
- Mondini h. i.
- neural h. i.
- noise-induced h. i.
- occupational hearing loss
- organic h. i.
- perceptive h. i.
- psychogenic h. i.
- retrocochlear h. i.
- Scheibe h. i.
- sensorineural h. i.
- sensory h. i.

heart
- h. antigen
- armor h.
- armored h.
- h. arrest
- artificial h.
- athlete's h.
- athletic h.
- h. attack
- h. beat
- beer h.
- beriberi h.
- h. block
- bony h.
- h. chamber remodeling
- chaotic h.
- crisscross h.
- disordered action of h. (DAH)
- drop h.
- h. failure
- h. failure cell
- fatty h.
- frosted h.
- globular h.
- hairy h.
- Holmes h.
- horizontal h.
- h. hormone
- hyperthyroid h.
- hypoplastic h.

- icing h.
- intermediate h.
- Jarvik artificial h.
- h. knife
- h. law
- left h.
- h. massage
- mechanical h.
- movable h.
- myxedema h.
- ox h.
- parchment h.
- pendulous h.
- h. position
- pulmonary h.
- h. rate
- h. rate turbulence
- right h.
- round h.
- sabot h.
- h. sac
- semihorizontal h.
- semivertical h.
- h. sound
- stone h.
- h. stroke
- systemic h.
- h. tamponade
- three-chambered h.
- tiger h.
- tobacco h.
- h. tones
- h. transplantation
- univentricular h.
- h. valve prosthesis
- venous h.
- vertical h.
- wooden-shoe h.

heartbeat

heartburn

heart-lung
- h.-l. machine
- h.-l. preparation
- h.-l. transplantation

heart-shaped
- h.-s. pelvis
- h.-s. uterus

heartworm

heat
- h. apoplexy
- atomic h.
- h. capacity
- h. coagulation test
- h. of combustion
- h. of compression
- conductive h.
- convective h.
- conversive h.
- h. cramps
- h. of crystallization
- h. of dissociation
- h. edema
- h. of evaporation
- h. exhaustion
- h. of formation

H

heat *(continued)*
    h. hyperpyrexia
    initial h.
    innate h.
    h. instability test
    h. lamp
    latent h.
    molecular h.
    prickly h.
    h. prostration
    radiant h.
    h. rash
    h. rigor
    sensible h.
    h. shock protein (hsp)
    h. of solution
    specific h.
    h. stroke
    h. treatment
    h. urticaria
    h. of vaporization
heat-curing resin
Heath-Edwards grades
heat-labile
heat-rigor point
heat-stable enzyme
heatstroke
heavy
    h. chain
    h. chain disease
    h. hydrogen
    h. liquid petrolatum
    h. metal
    h. metal neuropathy
    h. nitrogen
    h. oxygen
    h. water
Hebeloma
hebephrenia
hebephrenic
    h. dementia
    h. schizophrenia
Heberden
    H. angina
    H. node
hebetic
hebetude
hebiatrics
Hebra prurigo
hecateromeric
hecatomeral, hecatomeric
Hecht pneumonia
Heck disease
hectic flush
hecto- (h)
hectogram
hectoliter
hedeoma
hederiform ending
hedonophobia
Hedström file
heel
    black h.
    h. bone

    cracked h.
    h. fly
    h. jar
    h. pad
    painful h.
    prominent h.
    h. region
    h. spur
    h. tap
    h. tendon
heel-tap
    h.-t. reaction
    h.-t. test
heel-to-knee-to-toe test
heel-to-shin test
Heerfordt disease
Hegar
    H. dilator
    H. sign
Hegglin
    H. anomaly
    H. syndrome
Hehner
    H. number
    H. value
Heidelberger curve
Heidenhain
    H. azan stain
    H. crescent
    H. demilune
    H. iron hematoxylin stain
    H. law
    H. pouch
height
    anterior facial h. (AFH)
    h. of contour
    cusp h.
    facial h.
    nasal h.
    orbital h.
    h. vertigo
height-length index
Heilbronner thigh
Heim-Kreysig sign
Heimlich maneuver
Heineke-Mikulicz pyloroplasty
Heinz
    H. body
    H. body anemia
    H. body test
Heinz-Ehrlich body
Heister
    H. diverticulum
    H. valve
HeLa cell
helcomenia
held
    H. bundle
    H. decussation
helianthine
helical
    h. computed tomography
    h. CT
helices *(pl. of* helix)

helicine
>h. artery of penis
>h. artery of the uterus

helicis
>h. major muscle
>h. minor muscle

Helicobacter
>*H. cinaedi*
>*H. fennelliae*
>*H. heilmannii*
>*H. pylori*

helicoid
>h. choroidopathy
>h. ginglymus

helicopod gait
helicopodia
helicotrema
Helie bundle
heliencephalitis
helioaerotherapy
heliopathy
heliophobia
heliosis
heliotaxis
heliotropism
Heliozoea
helium (He)
>h. speech

helium-3 (^{3}He)
helium-4 (^{4}He)
helix, pl. helices
>3_{10} h.
>3.6_{13} h.
>alpha h.
>collagen h.
>DNA h.
>double h.
>Pauling-Corey h.
>pi h.
>triple h.
>twin h.
>Watson-Crick h.

hellebore
>false h.

helleborin
helleborism
helleborus
Heller
>H. myotomy
>H. operation
>H. plexus

Hellin law
HELLP syndrome
Helly fixative
helmet cell
Helmholtz
>H. axis ligament
>H. energy
>H. theory of accommodation
>H. theory of color vision
>H. theory of hearing

Helmholtz-Gibbs theory
helminth
helminthagogue
helminthemesis
helminthiasis
helminthic dysentery
helminthism
helminthoid
helminthology
helminthoma
helminthophobia
Helminthosporium
helmintic
Heloderma
helper
>h. cell
>h. virus

Helvella esculenta
Helweg bundle
Helweg-Larssen syndrome
hemachrome
hemacytometer
hemacytozoon
hemadostenosis
hemadsorption
>h. virus test
>h. virus type 1, 2

hemafacient
hemagglutinating cold autoantibody
hemagglutination
>h. inhibition
>passive h.
>reverse passive h.
>h. test
>viral h.

hemagglutinin
hemagogic
hemal
>h. arch
>h. gland
>h. node
>h. spine

hemalum
hemamebiasis
hemanalysis
hemangiectasis, hemangiectasia
hemangiectatic hypertrophy
hemangioblast
hemangioblastoma
hemangioendothelioblastoma
hemangioendothelioma tuberosum multiplex
hemangiofibroma
>juvenile h.

hemangioma
>capillary h.
>capillary h. of infancy
>cavernous h.
>lobular capillary h.
>racemose h.
>sclerosing h.
>senile h.
>spider h.
>strawberry h.
>verrucous h.

hemangiomatosis
hemangiopericytoma
hemangiosarcoma
hemapheic

H

hemaphein
hemapheism
hemarthrosis
hemastrontium
hemat-
hematachometer
hematapostema
hematein
    Baker acid h.
hematemesis
hematencephalon
hematherapy
hematherm
hemathermal
hemathermous
hemathorax
hematic
hematid
hematidrosis
hematimeter
hematin
    h. chloride
    reduced h.
hematinemia
hematinic principle
hematobilia
hematobium
hematoblast
    Hayem h.
hematocele
    pelvic h.
    pudendal h.
hematocephaly
hematochezia
hematochlorin
hematochyluria
hematocolpometra
hematocolpos
hematocrit (Hct)
hematocryal
hematocyst
hematocystis
hematocyte
hematocytoblast
hematocytolysis
hematocytometer
hematocytozoon
hematodyscrasia
hematodystrophy
hematogenesis
hematogenetic calculus
hematogenous, hematogenic
    h. abscess
    h. embolism
    h. jaundice
    h. metastasis
    h. osteitis
    h. pigment
hematohistioblast
hematohiston
hematoidin crystal
hematologist
hematology
hematolymphangioma
hematolysis

hematolytic
hematoma
    communicating h.
    corpus luteum h.
    epidural h.
    intracranial h.
    intramural h.
    pulsatile h.
    subdural h.
hematometra
hematometry
hematomphalocele
hematomyelia
hematomyelopore
hematonic
hematopathology
hematopathy
hematopenia
hematophagia
hematophagous
hematophagus
hematoplastic
hematopoiesis
hematopoietic
    h. gland
    h. system
hematopoietin
hematoporphyria
hematoporphyrin
hematoporphyrinemia
hematoporphyrinuria
hematopsia
hematorrhachis
    h. externa
    extradural h.
    h. interna
    subdural h.
hematosalpinx
hematosepsis
hematosin
hematosis
hematospectroscope
hematospectroscopy
hematospermatocele
hematospermia
hematostatic
hematostaxis
hematosteon
hematothermal
hematotoxic (*var. of* hemotoxic)
hematotoxin
hematotropic
hematotympanum
hematoxic (*var. of* hemotoxic)
hematoxin
hematoxylin
    h. body
    Boehmer h.
    Delafield h.
    h. and eosin stain
    Harris h.
    iron h.
    phosphotungstic acid h. (PTAH)
hematoxylin-malachite green-basic fuchsin
  stain

hematoxylin-phloxine B stain
hematoxyphil body
hematozoic
hematozoon
hematuria
    Egyptian h.
    endemic h.
    false h.
    gross h.
    initial h.
    microscopic h.
    painful h.
    painless h.
    renal h.
    terminal h.
    total h.
    urethral h.
    vesical h.
hematuric bilious fever
heme
    h. a, c
hemeralopia
hemeranopia
hemerythrins
hemiacardius
hemiacetal
hemiacrosomia
hemiageusia
hemiageustia
hemialgia
hemianalgesia
hemianencephaly
hemianesthesia
    alternate h.
    crossed h.
hemianopia
    absolute h.
    altitudinal h.
    binasal h.
    bitemporal h.
    complete h.
    congruous h.
    crossed h.
    heteronymous h.
    homonymous h.
    incomplete h.
    incongruous h.
    pseudo-h.
    quadrantic h.
    unilateral h.
    unilocular h.
hemianopic
    h. scotoma
    h. spectacles
hemianopsia
hemianosmia
hemiaplasia
hemiapraxia
hemiarthroplasty
hemiasynergia
hemiataxia
hemiathetosis
hemiatrophy
    facial h.

    facial h. of Romberg
    lingual h.
hemiazygos vein
hemiballism
hemiballismus
hemiblock
hemibody radiation
hemic
    h. calculus
    h. distomiasis
    h. murmur
hemicardia
    h. dextra
    h. sinistra
hemicellulose
hemicentrum
hemicephalalgia
hemicephalia
hemicerebrum
hemicholinium
Hemichorda
Hemichordata
hemichorea
hemicolectomy
hemicorporectomy
hemicrania
hemicraniectomy
hemicraniosis
hemicraniotomy
hemidesmosomes
hemidiaphoresis
hemidrosis
hemidysesthesia
hemidystrophy
hemiectromelia
hemifacial spasm
hemigastrectomy
hemigeusia
hemiglossal
hemiglossectomy
hemiglossitis
hemignathia
hemihepatectomy
hemihidrosis
hemihydranencephaly
hemihypalgesia
hemihyperesthesia
hemihyperhidrosis
hemihypertonia
hemihypertrophy
hemihypesthesia
hemihypoesthesia
hemihypotonia
hemikaryon
hemiketal
hemilaminectomy
hemilaryngectomy
hemilateral chorea
hemilesion
hemilingual
hemimacroglossia
hemimandibulectomy
hemimelia
hemimetabolous
hemin

H

435

hemiopalgia
hemipagus
hemipancreatectomy
hemiparesis
hemipelvectomy
hemiplegia
    alternating h.
    contralateral h.
    crossed h.
    double h.
    facial h.
    infantile h.
    spastic h.
hemiplegic
    h. amyotrophy
    h. gait
    h. migraine
Hemiptera
hemisection
hemisensory
hemiseptum
hemispasm
hemisphere
    h. of bulb of penis
    h. of cerebellum
    h. of cerebellum [HII–HX]
    cerebral h.
    dominant h.
hemispherectomy
hemisphericum
    h. cerebelli [HII–HX]
hemispherium
    h. bulbi urethrae
    h. cerebelli [HII–HX]
    h. cerebri
Hemispora
hemistrumectomy
hemisubstance
hemisulfur mustard
hemisyndrome
hemiterpene
hemithermoanesthesia
hemithoracic duct
hemithorax
hemitremor
hemitruncus
hemivertebra
hemizona assay
hemizygosity
hemizygote
hemizygotic
hemizygous
hemlock
hemoagglutination
hemoagglutinin
hemoantitoxin
hemobilia
hemoblast
    lymphoid h. of Pappenheim
hemoblastosis
hemocatharsis
hemocatheresis
hemocatheretic
Hemoccult test
hemocele

hemocholecystitis
hemochorial placenta
hemochromatosis
    exogenous h.
    primary h.
    secondary h.
hemochrome
hemochromogen
hemoclasis, hemoclasia
hemoclastic reaction
hemoconcentration
hemoconia
hemoconiosis
hemocryoscopy
hemocuprein
hemocyanin
hemocyte
hemocytoblast
hemocytocatheresis
hemocytolysis
hemocytometer
hemocytometry
hemocytotripsis
hemocytozoon
hemodiagnosis
hemodialysis
hemodialyzer
    ultrafiltration h.
hemodiastase
hemodilution
hemodynamic
hemodynamics
hemodyscrasia
hemodystrophy
hemoendothelial placenta
hemofiltration
hemoflagellate
hemofuscin
hemogenesis
hemogenic
hemoglobin (Hb)
    h. A
    h. A_2
    h. A_{Ic}
    aberrant h.
    h. anti-Lepore
    h. Bart
    bile pigment h.
    h. C
    h. $C_{Georgetown}$
    h. C_{Harlem}
    carbon monoxide h.
    h. C, H disease
    h. Chesapeake ($Hb_{Chesapeake}$)
    h. Constant Spring
    h. D_{Punjab}
    h. E
    embryonic h.
    h. F
    fetal h.
    h. F (hereditary persistence of)
    glycosylated h.
    h. Gower-1, -2
    green h.
    h. H

h. I
h. J$_{Capetown}$
h. Kansas
h. Lepore
h. M
mean corpuscular h. (MCH)
muscle h.
oxygenated h.
h. Portland
h. Rainier
reduced h.
h. S
sickle cell h. (Hb S)
unstable h.'s
variant h.
h. Yakima
hemoglobinemia
paroxysmal nocturnal h.
puerperal h.
hemoglobinocholia
hemoglobinolysis
hemoglobinopathy
hemoglobinopepsia
hemoglobinophilic
hemoglobinuria
epidemic h.
intermittent h.
malarial h.
march h.
paroxysmal cold h.
paroxysmal nocturnal h.
postparturient h.
toxic h.
hemoglobinuric
h. fever
h. nephrosis
hemogram
hemohistioblast
hemolamella
hemolipase
hemolith
hemology
hemolymph
h. gland
h. node
hemolysate
hemolysin
alpha h.
bacterial h.
beta h.
cold h.
heterophil h.
immune h.
natural h.
specific h.
h. unit
warm-cold h.
hemolysinogen
hemolysis
alpha' h.
beta h.
biologic h.
conditioned h.
gamma h.
immune h.

phenylhydrazine h.
venom h.
viridans h.
hemolytic
h. anemia
h. anemia of newborn
h. crisis
h. disease of newborn
h. gas
h. jaundice
h. plaque assay
h. splenomegaly
h. streptococci
h. uremic syndrome
hemolytic unit (*var. of* hemolysin unit)
hemolyzation
hemolyze
hemomediastinum
hemometra
hemometry
hemopathology
hemopathy
hemoperfusion
hemopericardium
hemoperitoneum
hemopexin
hemophagia
hemophagocytosis
hemophil
hemophilia
h. A, B, C
classic h.
hemophiliac
hemophilic
h. arthritis
h. joint
hemophilosis
hemophobia
hemophoresis
hemophthalmia
hemophthisis
hemoplastic
hemoplasty
hemopneumopericardium
hemopneumothorax
hemopoiesis
hemopoietic tissue
hemopoietin
hemoporphyrin
hemoprecipitin
hemoprotein
hemoptysis
endemic h.
parasitic h.
hemopyelectasis
hemorepellant
hemorheology
hemorrhage
brainstem h.
cerebral h.
concealed h.
Duret h.
extradural h.
gastric h.
intermediate h.

H

hemorrhage *(continued)*
  internal h.
  intracerebral h.
  intracranial h.
  intrapartum h.
  intraventricular h.
  nasal h.
  parenchymatous h.
  h. per rhexis
  petechial h.
  pontine h.
  postpartum h.
  primary h.
  punctate h.
  renal h.
  secondary h.
  serous h.
  splinter h.
  subarachnoid h.
  subdural h.
  subgaleal h.
  syringomyelic h.
hemorrhagic
  h. anemia
  h. ascites
  h. bronchitis
  h. colitis
  h. cyst
  h. cystitis
  h. dengue
  h. disease of the newborn
  h. endovasculitis
  h. fever
  h. fever with renal syndrome
  h. gangrene
  h. glaucoma
  h. infarct
  h. iritis
  h. measles
  h. nephritis
  h. pachymeningitis
  h. pericarditis
  h. plague
  h. pleurisy
  h. rickets
  h. scurvy
  h. shock
  h. smallpox
hemorrhagin
hemorrhoid
  cutaneous h.
  external h.
  internal h.
hemorrhoidal
  h. cushion
  h. nerve
  h. plexus
  h. vein
  h. zone
hemorrhoidectomy
hemosalpinx
hemosialemesis
hemosiderin

hemosiderosis
  idiopathic pulmonary h.
  nutritional h.
hemospermia
  h. spuria
  h. vera
hemosporidium
hemosporine
hemostasia
hemostasis
hemostat
hemostatic
  h. collodion
  h. forceps
hemostyptic
hemosuccus pancreaticus
hemotachogram
hemotachometer
hemotherapy
hemothorax
hemotoxic, hematotoxic, hematoxic
hemotoxin
  cobra h.
hemotroph, hemotrophe
hemotropic
hemotympanum
hemozoic
hemozoon
HEMPAS
  hereditary erythroblastic multinuclearity
    associated with positive acidified serum
HEMPAS cell
henbane
hen-cluck stertor
Henderson-Hasselbalch equation
Hendersonula toruloidea
Hendra virus
Henke space
Henle
  H. ampulla
  H. ansa
  crypt of H.
  H. fenestrated elastic membrane
  H. fiber layer
  H. fissure
  H. gland
  H. layer
  H. loop
  H. nervous layer
  H. reaction
  H. sheath
  H. spine
  H. tubules
  H. warts
henna
Hennebert sign
Henoch
  H. chorea
  H. purpura
Henoch-Schönlein
  H.-S. purpura
  H.-S. syndrome
henpuye
Henri-Michaelis-Menten equation
henry (H)

Henry-Gauer response
Henry law
Hensen
    H. canal
    H. cell
    H. disk
    H. duct
    H. knot
    H. line
    H. node
    H. stripe
Hensing ligament
Hepadnaviridae
hepar
    h. lobatum
heparan
    h. *N*-sulfatase
    h. sulfate
heparin
    h. complement
    h. eliminase
    h. lyase
    h. sodium
    h. unit
heparinase
heparinemia
heparinic acid
heparinize
heparitin sulfate
hepat-
hepatatrophia, hepatatrophy
hepatectomy
hepatic
    h. adenoma
    h. amebiasis
    h. artery
    h. artery proper
    h. branch of anterior vagal trunk
    h. branch of vagus nerve
    h. capsulitis
    h. colic
    h. coma
    h. cord
    h. cyst
    h. duct
    h. encephalopathy
    h. fistula
    h. flexure
    h. infantilism
    h. insufficiency
    h. intermittent fever
    h. laminae
    h. lobule
    h. lymph node
    h. plexus
    h. porphyria
    h. portal system
    h. portal vein
    h. prominence
    h. segment
    h. steatosis
    h. triad
    h. vein
hepaticodochotomy
hepaticoduodenostomy

hepaticoenterostomy
hepaticogastrostomy
hepaticolithotomy
hepaticolithotripsy
hepaticopulmonary
hepaticostomy
hepaticotomy
hepatin
hepatis
hepatitic
hepatitis
    h. A
    acute parenchymatous h.
    anicteric h.
    anicteric virus h.
    h. A virus (HAV)
    h. B
    h. B core antigen (HB$_c$Ab, HB$_c$Ag)
    h. B e antigen (HB$_e$Ab, HBe)
    h. B surface antigen (HB$_s$Ab)
    h. B vaccine
    h. B virus (HBV)
    h. C
    cholangiolitic h.
    cholestatic h.
    chronic active h.
    chronic interstitial h.
    chronic persistent h.
    chronic persisting h.
    h. C virus (HCV)
    h. D
    delta h.
    h. delta virus (HDV)
    drug-induced h.
    h. D virus
    h. E
    epidemic h.
    h. E virus (HEV)
    h. externa
    h. F
    fulminant h.
    h. G
    giant cell h.
    h. G virus (HGV)
    halothane h.
    infectious h. (IH)
    long incubation h.
    lupoid h.
    MS-1 h.
    NANB h.
    NANBNC h.
        non-A, non-B, non-C hepatitis
    neonatal h.
    non–A-E h.
    non-A, non-B h.
    non-A, non-B, non-C h. (NANBNC
      hepatitis)
    peliosis h.
    plasma cell h.
    serum h. (SH)
    short incubation h.
    subacute h.
    suppurative h.
    transfusion h.
    viral h.

H

hepatitis *(continued)*
    viral h. type A, B, C, D, E
    virus h.
    virus A, B, C h.
hepatitis-associated antigen (HAA)
hepatization
    gray h.
    red h.
    yellow h.
hepatoblastoma
hepatocarcinoma
hepatocele
hepatocellular
    h. adenoma
    h. carcinoma
    h. jaundice
hepatocholangioenterostomy
hepatocholangiojejunostomy
hepatocholangiostomy
hepatocholangitis
hepatocolic ligament
hepatocuprein
hepatocystic duct
Hepatocystis
hepatocyte
hepatoduodenal ligament
hepatoduodenostomy
hepatodysentery
hepatoenteric recess
hepatoerythropoietic porphyria
hepatoesophageal ligament
hepatofugal
hepatogastric ligament
hepatogenic, hepatogenous
    h. jaundice
    h. pigment
hepatography
hepatohemia
hepatoid
hepatojugular
    h. reflex
    h. reflux
hepatojugularometer
hepatolenticular degeneration
hepatolienography
hepatolienomegaly
hepatolith
hepatolithectomy
hepatolithiasis
hepatologist
hepatology
hepatolysin
hepatoma
    malignant h.
hepatomalacia
hepatomegaly
hepatomelanosis
hepatomphalocele
hepatomphalos
hepatonecrosis
hepatonephric syndrome
hepatonephromegaly

hepatopancreatic
    h. ampulla
    h. sphincter
hepatopathic
hepatopathy
hepatoperitonitis
hepatopetal
hepatopexy
hepatophosphorylase deficiency glycogenosis
hepatophyma
hepatopleural fistula
hepatopneumonic
hepatoportal
hepatoptosis
hepatopulmonary
hepatorenal
    h. ligament
    h. pouch
    h. recess of subhepatic space
    h. syndrome
hepatorrhagia
hepatorrhaphy
hepatorrhexis
hepatoscopy
hepatosplenitis
hepatosplenography
hepatosplenomegaly
hepatosplenopathy
hepatostomy
hepatotherapy
hepatotomy
hepatotoxemia
hepatotoxic
hepatotoxicity
hepatotoxin
Hepatozoon
HEPES
heptachlor
heptad
heptanal
heptapeptide
heptose
heptulose
D-*altro*-2-**heptulose**
D-*manno*-**heptulose**
n-**heptylpenicillin**
HEP vaccine (*var. of* high-egg-passage vaccine)
herald patch
herbivorous
herd
    h. immunity
    h. instinct
hereditary
    h. amyloidosis
    h. angioedema
    h. angioneurotic edema (HANE)
    h. benign telangiectasia
    h. cerebellar ataxia
    h. chorea
    h. clubbing
    h. coproporphyria
    h. deafness
    h. deforming chondrodystrophy

h. epithelial dystrophy
h. erythroblastic multinuclearity associated with positive acidified serum (HEMPAS)
h. folate malabsorption
h. fructose intolerance
h. hearing impairment
h. hemorrhagic telangiectasia
h. hemorrhagic thrombasthenia
h. hypersegmentation of neutrophils
h. hyperthyroidism
h. hypertrophic neuropathy
h. hypophosphatemic rickets
h. lymphedema
h. methemoglobinemia
h. methemoglobinemic cyanosis
h. multiple exostoses
h. multiple trichoepithelioma
h. myokymia
h. nephritis
h. nonpolyposis colorectal cancer
h. opalescent dentin
h. photomyoclonus
h. progressive arthroophthalmopathy
h. pyropoikilocytosis
h. renal hypouricuria
h. sensory radicular neuropathy
h. spherocytosis
h. spinal ataxia
h. syphilis
heredity
heredofamilial tremor
heredopathia atactica polyneuritiformis
heredotaxia
Herellea
Hering
H. sinus nerve
H. test
H. theory of color vision
Hering-Breuer reflex
heritability
h. in the broad sense
h. in the narrow sense
heritage
Herlitz syndrome
Hermann fixative
Hermansky-Pudlak syndrome
hermaphrodism
hermaphrodite
hermaphroditism
adrenal h.
bilateral h.
dimidiate h.
false h.
female h.
lateral h.
male h.
transverse h.
true h.
unilateral h.
hermetic
hernia
abdominal h.
Barth h.
Béclard h.

bilocular femoral h.
h. of the broad ligament of the uterus
cecal h.
cerebral h.
Cloquet h.
complete h.
concealed h.
congenital diaphragmatic h.
Cooper h.
crural h.
diaphragmatic h.
direct inguinal h.
double loop h.
dry h.
duodenojejunal h.
h. en bissac
epigastric h.
extrasaccular h.
fascial h.
fat h.
fatty h.
femoral h.
foramen of Bochdalek h.
gastroesophageal h.
gluteal h.
Hesselbach h.
Hey h.
hiatal h.
hiatus h.
Holthouse h.
iliacosubfascial h.
incarcerated h.
incisional h.
indirect inguinal h.
infantile h.
inguinal h.
inguinocrural h.
inguinofemoral h.
inguinolabial h.
inguinoscrotal h.
inguinosuperficial h.
internal h.
intersigmoid h.
interstitial h.
intraepiploic h.
intrailiac h.
intrapelvic h.
irreducible h.
ischiatic h.
h. knife
Krönlein h.
labial h.
lateral ventral h.
Laugier h.
levator h.
Littré h.
lumbar h.
Malgaigne h.
meningeal h.
mesenteric h.
Morgagni foramen h.
obturator h.
orbital h.
pannicular h.

H

hernia *(continued)*
    pantaloon h.
    paraduodenal h.
    paraesophageal h.
    parahiatal h.
    paraperitoneal h.
    parasaccular h.
    parasternal h.
    parietal h.
    perineal h.
    Petit h.
    posterior vaginal h.
    properitoneal inguinal h.
    pudendal h.
    reducible h.
    retrograde h.
    retroperitoneal h.
    retropubic h.
    retrosternal h.
    Richter h.
    Rokitansky h.
    sciatic h.
    scrotal h.
    sliding esophageal hiatal h.
    slipped h.
    spigelian h.
    strangulated h.
    synovial h.
    Treitz h.
    umbilical h.
    h. uteri inguinale
    Velpeau h.
    ventral h.
    vesicle h.
    vitreous h.
    "w" h.
hernial
    h. aneurysm
    h. sac
herniated disk
herniation
    caudal transtentorial h.
    cingulate h.
    contained disk h.
    disk h.
    foraminal h.
    noncontained disk h.
    rostral transtentorial h.
    sphenoidal h.
    subfalcial h.
    tonsillar h.
    transtentorial h.
    uncal h.
hernioenterotomy
herniography
hernioid
herniolaparotomy
herniopuncture
herniorrhaphy
    Bassini h.
herniotome
    Cooper h.
herniotomy
    Petit h.

heroic
heroin (H)
    h. overdose syndrome
Herophilus
herpangina
herpes
    h. B encephalomyelitis
    h. catarrhalis
    h. corneae
    h. digitalis
    h. encephalitis
    h. facialis
    h. febrilis
    h. generalisatus
    h. genitalis
    h. gestationis
    h. gladiatorum
    h. labialis
    neonatal h.
    h. progenitalis
    h. simplex
    h. simplex encephalitis
    h. simplex virus (HSV)
    traumatic h.
    h. whitlow
    h. zoster
    h. zoster ophthalmicus
    h. zoster oticus
    h. zoster varicellosus
    h. zoster virus
Herpesviridae
herpesvirus
    cercopithecrine h.
    human h. (HHV)
    human h. 1, 2, 3, 4, 5, 6, 7, 8
    h. saimiri
    suid h.
herpetic
    h. fever
    h. keratitis
    h. keratoconjunctivitis
    h. meningoencephalitis
    h. ulcer
    h. whitlow
herpetiform aphthae
herpetologist
herpetology
Herpetomonas
Herpetoviridae
herpetovirus
Herring
    H. body
    H. law
herring-worm disease
Herrmann syndrome
hersage
Hers disease
Hershberg test
Hertwig sheath
hertz (Hz)
hertzian experiment
Herxheimer reaction
herz hormone
herzstoss
Heschl gyri

hesitancy
hesitant
hesperidin
Hess
    H. law
    H. screen
Hesselbach
    H. fascia
    H. hernia
    H. ligament
    H. triangle
hetastarch
heteradelphus
heteralius
heteraxial
heterecious
heterecism
heteresthesia
heteroagglutinin
heteroallele
heteroantibody
heteroantiserum
heteroatom
heteroblastic
heterocellular
heterocentric
heterocephalus
heterocheiral
heterochromatic
heterochromatin
    constitutive h.
    facultative h.
    satellite-rich h.
heterochromia
    atrophic h.
    binocular h.
    h. iridis
    h. of iris
    monocular h.
    simple h.
    sympathetic h.
heterochromic
    h. cyclitis
    h. uveitis
heterochromous
heterochron
heterochronia
heterochronic
heterochronous
heterocladic
heterocrine
heterocrisis
heterocyclic compound
heterocytotropic antibody
heterodetic peptide
heterodisperse
heterodont
Heterodoxus spiniger
heterodromous
heteroduplex
heterodymus
heteroeroticism
heterogametic embryo
heterogamous
heterogamy

heterogeneic antigen
heterogeneity
    genetic h.
heterogeneous
    h. nuclear RNA
    h. nucleation
    h. radiation
    h. system
heterogenesis
heterogenic
    h. antibody
    h. antigen
    h. parasite
heterogenote
heterogenous
    h. keratoplasty
    h. vaccine
heteroglycan
heterogonic life cycle
heterograft
heterokaryon
heterokaryotic
heterokeratoplasty
heterokinesia
heterokinesis
heterolateral
heterolipid
heteroliteral
heterologous
    h. antiserum
    h. desensitization
    h. graft
    h. insemination
    h. protein
    h. serotype
    h. stimulus
    h. tumor
    h. twins
heterology
heterolysin
heterolysis
heterolytic
heteromastigote
heteromeral
heteromeric
    h. cell
    h. peptide
heteromerous
heterometabolous metamorphosis
heterometaplasia
heterometric autoregulation
heterometropia
heteromorphism
heteromorphosis
heteromorphous
heteronomous psychotherapy
heteronomy
heteronuclear
heteronymous
    h. diplopia
    h. hemianopia
    h. image
    h. parallax
heteropagus
heteropathy

H

heterophagy
heterophil
  h. antibody
  h. antigen
  h. hemolysin
heterophonia
heterophoria
heterophthalmus
heterophthongia
Heterophyes
  H. brevicaeca
  H. heterophyes
  H. katsuradai
heterophyiasis
heterophyid
Heterophyidae
heterophyidiasis
heteroplasia
heteroplastic graft
heteroplastid
heteroploid
heteroploidy
heteropolar bond
heteropolysaccharide
heteroproteose
heteropyknosis
  negative h.
  positive h.
heteropyknotic chromatin
heteroreceptor
heterosaccharide
heteroscedasticity
heterosexual
heterosexuality
heteroside
heterosis
heterosmia
heterosome
heterospecific
heterosuggestion
heterotaxia
  cardiac h.
heterotaxic
heterotaxis, heterotaxy
heterothallic
heterotherm
heterothermic
heterotic
heterotonia
heterotopia maculae
heterotopic
  h. bone
  h. graft
  h. pregnancy
  h. stimulus
heterotopous
heterotransplantation
heterotrichosis
heterotroph
heterotrophic oral gastrointestinal cyst
heterotropia, heterotropy
heterotropic pregnancy
heterotype mitosis
heterotypical chromosome
heterotypic cortex

heterovaccine therapy
heteroxanthine
heteroxenous parasite
heterozoic
heterozygosity
heterozygote
  compound h.
  manifesting h.
heterozygous
  doubly h.
Heubner
  H. arteritis
  H. artery
Heuser membrane
HEV
  hepatitis E virus
hexacanth embryo
hexachlorocyclohexane
hexachlorophane
hexachlorophene
hexacosanoic acid
hexacosanol
hexacosyl
hexad
hexadactyly
hexadecanoic acid
1-hexadecanol
hexafluorenium bromide
hexamer
hexameric
hexametazime (HMPAO)
hexamethylpropyleneamine oxime
hexamidine isethionate
hexamine
hexane
hexanoate
n-hexanoic acid
hexanoyl
hexapeptide
hexaploidy
Hexapoda
hexaxial reference system
hexazonium salt
hexestrol
hexitol
hexokinase method
hexon antigen
hexone base
hexonic acid
hexosamine
hexosaminidase
  h. A, B
hexosans
hexose
  h. monophosphate pathway
  h. monophosphate shunt
hexosebisphosphatase
hexose phosphatase
hexosephosphate isomerase
hexose-1-phosphate uridylyltransferase
hexulose
hexuronic acid
hexyl
hexylresorcinol

Hey
>H. amputation
>H. hernia
>H. ligament

Heyer-Pudenz valve

Hf
>hafnium

HFR strain

Hg
>mercury

HGE
>human granulocytic ehrlichiosis

HGF
>hyperglycemic-glycogenolytic factor

HG factor

HGH
>human growth hormone

HGPRT
>hypoxanthine guanine
>phosphoribosyltransferase

HGSIL
>high-grade squamous intraepithelial lesion

HGV
>hepatitis G virus

HHV
>human herpesvirus

hiatal hernia

hiatus
>adductor h.
>h. adductorius
>aortic h.
>h. aorticus
>Breschet h.
>h. canalis facialis
>h. canalis nervi petrosi majoris
>h. canalis nervi petrosi minoris
>esophageal h.
>h. esophageus
>h. ethmoidalis
>h. of facial canal
>fallopian h.
>h. for greater petrosal nerve
>h. for lesser petrosal nerve
>h. maxillaris
>maxillary h.
>pleuropericardial h.
>pleuroperitoneal h.
>sacral h.
>h. sacralis
>saphenous h.
>h. saphenus
>scalene h.
>Scarpa h.
>semilunar h.
>h. semilunaris
>h. subarcuatus
>h. tendineus
>h. totalis sacralis

hibernating
>h. gland
>h. myocardium

hibernation

hibernoma
>interscapular h.

Hib vaccine

hiccup
>epidemic h.

Hickman catheter

HIDA
>dimethyl iminodiacetic acid

hidden
>h. border of nail
>h. nail skin
>h. part
>h. part of duodenum

hidradenitis
>neutrophilic eccrine h.
>h. suppurativa

hidradenoma
>clear cell h.
>nodular h.
>papillary h.
>h. papilliferum

hidroa

hidrocystoma
>apocrine h.

hidromeiosis

hidropoiesis

hidroschesis

hidrosis

hidrotic ectodermal dysplasia

hierarchy
>dominance h.
>Maslow h.
>response h.
>h. of terms

hierophobia

hierotherapy

high
>h. altitude chamber
>h. convex
>h. dose tolerance
>h. endothelial postcapillary venules
>h. enema
>h. energy phosphate bond
>h. forceps delivery
>h. lip line
>h. lithotomy
>h. molecular weight kininogen
>h. osmolar contrast agent (HOCA)
>h. osmolar contrast medium
>(HOCM)
>h. output failure
>h. pressure oxygen
>h. spinal anesthesia
>h. wine

high-calorie diet

high-dose-rate brachytherapy

high-egg-passage vaccine

high-energy
>h.-e. compound
>h.-e. phosphate

higher
>h. order conditioning
>h. order pregnancy

highest
>h. concha
>h. intercostal artery
>h. intercostal vein
>h. nuchal line

H

445

highest *(continued)*
    h. thoracic artery
    h. turbinated bone
high-fat diet
high-fiber diet
high-frequency
    h.-f. current
    h.-f. hearing impairment
    h.-f. transduction
    h.-f. ventilation
high-grade squamous intraepithelial lesion (HGSIL, HSIL)
high-kV technique
Highmore body
high-pass filter
high-performance liquid chromatography
high-pressure liquid chromatography (HPLC)
high-quality filter paper
high-resolution
    h.-r. banding
    h.-r. computed tomography (HRCT)
high-steppage gait
Higoumenakia sign
hila (*pl. of* hilum)
hilar
    h. cell tumor of ovary
    h. dance
    h. lymph node
    h. shadow
hilitis
hill
    H. coefficient
    H. constant
    H. criteria of evidence
    H. equation
    H. operation
    H. phenomenon
    H. plot
    H. reaction
    H. sign
Hillis-Müller maneuver
hillock
    axon h.
    facial h.
    seminal h.
Hill-Sachs lesion
Hilton
    H. law
    H. method
    H. sac
    H. white line
hilum, pl. **hila**
    h. of dentate nucleus
    h. of inferior olivary nucleus
    h. of kidney
    h. lienis
    h. of lung
    h. of lymph node
    h. nodi lymphatici
    h. nuclei dentati
    h. nuclei olivaris inferioris
    h. ovarii
    h. of ovary

    h. pulmonis
    h. renalis
    h. of spleen
    splenic h.
    h. splenicum
hilus cell
himantosis
hindbrain vesicle
hindgut
hind kidney
hindquarter amputation
hindwater
Hines-Brown test
hinge
    h. axis
    h. joint
    h. movement
    h. position
    h. region
hinge-bow
hinged flap
Hinman syndrome
Hinton test
hip
    h. bone
    h. joint
    h. phenomenon
    snapping h.
hipberries
hip-flexion phenomenon
Hippelates
Hippel disease
Hippobosca
hippocampal
    h. commissure
    h. convolution
    h. fissure
    h. gyrus
    h. sclerosis
    h. sulcus
hippocampus
    h. major
    major h.
    h. minor
    minor h.
hippocratic
    h. face
    h. facies
    h. finger
    h. nails
    H. Oath
    h. school
    h. succussion
    h. succussion sound
hippocratism
hippurate
hippuria
hippuric acid
hippuricase
hippus
    respiratory h.
hircismus
hircus, pl. **hirci**

Hirschberg
>H. method
>H. test

Hirschfeld canal
Hirsch-Peiffer stain
Hirschsprung disease
hirsute
hirsuties
hirsutism
>constitutional h.
>idiopathic h.

hirtellous
hirudicide
hirudin
Hirudinea
hirudiniasis
hirudinization
Hirudo
His
>H. band
>H. bundle
>H. bundle electrogram (HBE, HB$_e$Ag)
>H. copula
>H. line
>H. perivascular space
>H. spindle

Hiss stain
Histalog test
histaminase
histamine
>h. flush
>h. liberators
>h. phosphate
>h. shock
>h. test

histamine-fast
histaminemia
histamine-releasing factor
histaminic
>h. cephalalgia
>h. headache

histaminuria
histangic
His-Tawara system
histidase
histidinal
histidinase
histidine
>h. ammonia-lyase
>h. deaminase
>h. decarboxylase

histidinemia
histidino
histidinol
histidinuria
histidyl
histioblast
histiocyte
>cardiac h.
>sea-blue h.

histiocytic lymphoma
histiocytoma
>fibrous h.

>generalized eruptive h.
>malignant fibrous h.

histiocytosis
>Langerhans cell h.
>lipid h.
>malignant h.
>nodular non-X h.
>nonlipid h.
>sinus h. with massive lymphadenopathy
>h. X
>h. Y

histiogenic
histioid
histioma
histionic
histoangic
histoblast
histochemistry
histocompatibility
>h. antigen
>h. complex
>h. gene
>h. testing

histocyte
histocytosis
histodifferentiation
histofluorescence
histogenesis
histogenetic
histogenous
histogeny
histogram
histoid
>h. leprosy
>h. neoplasm
>h. tumor

histoincompatibility
histologic
>h. accommodation
>h. internal os of uterus

histologist
histology
>pathologic h.

histolysis
histoma
histometaplastic
histomorphometry
histone base
histonectomy
histoneurology
histonomy
histonuria
histopathogenesis
histopathology
histophysiology
Histoplasma capsulatum
histoplasmin
histoplasmin-latex test
histoplasmoma
histoplasmosis
>acute h.
>African h.
>chronic mediastinal h.

H

histoplasmosis *(continued)*
    disseminated h.
    presumed ocular h.
historadiography
historrhexis
histotome
histotomy
histotope
histotoxic anoxia
histotroph
histotrophic
histotropic
histozoic
histozyme
histrionic personality disorder
hitchhiker thumb
Hitzig girdle
HIV
    human immunodeficiency virus
        HIV encephalopathy
        HIV wasting syndrome
HIV-1
    human immunodeficiency virus-1
HIV-2
    human immunodeficiency virus-2
hives
    giant h.
hK3
    human glandular kallikrein 3
HL-7
    Health Level-7
HLA
    human leukocyte antigen
        HLA complex
        HLA typing
HL-A antigen
HMB-45 antibody
HME
    human monocytic ehrlichiosis
HMG
    human menopausal gonadotropin
        HMG-CoA
            beta-hydroxy-beta-methylglutaryl-CoA
        HMG CoA-reductase inhibitors
HMO
    hypothetical mean organism
HMPAO
    hexametazime
HMS
    hypothetical mean strain
HN2
    nitrogen mustard
hnRNA
    heterogeneous nuclear rna
Ho
    Ho antigen
Hoagland sign
hoarhound *(var. of* horehound)
hoarse
hoarseness
hobnail
    h. cell

    h. liver
    h. tongue
Hoboken
    H. gemmule
    H. nodule
    H. valve
HOCA
    high osmolar contrast agent
Hoche
    H. bundle
    H. tract
HOCM
    high osmolar contrast medium
Hodge pessary
Hodgkin
    H. disease
    H. lymphoma
Hodgkin-Key murmur
Hodgson disease
hodoneuromere
hodophobia
hoe
    h. excavator
    h. scaler
HOECHST 33258
hof
Hofbauer cell
Hoffa operation
Hoffmann
    H. duct
    H. muscular atrophy
    H. phenomenon
    H. reflex
    H. sign
Hoffman violet
Hofmann bacillus
Hofmeister
    H. gastrectomy
    H. operation
    H. series
Hofmeister-Pólya anastomosis
hog
    h. cholera vaccines
    h. cholera virus
Hogben number
Hogness box
holandric
    h. gene
    h. inheritance
holarthritic
holarthritis
Holden line
hole in retina
holiday
    h. heart syndrome
    h. syndrome
holism
holistic
    h. medicine
    h. psychology
Hollander test
Hollenhorst plaque
Holliday
    H. junction
    H. structure

Holl ligament
hollow
    h. back
    h. bone
    Sebileau h.
Holmes
    H. heart
    H. stain
Holmes-Adie
    H.-A. pupil
    H.-A. syndrome
Holmes-Rahe questionnaire
Holmgrén-Golgi canal
Holmgren wool test
holmium
holoacardius
    h. acephalus
    h. amorphus
holo-ACP synthase
holoacrania
holoanencephaly
holoblastic cleavage
holocarboxylase synthetase
holocephalic
holocord
holocrine gland
holodiastolic
holoendemic disease
holoenzyme
hologastroschisis
hologram
holography
hologynic inheritance
holomastigote
holometabolous metamorphosis
holomiantic (infection)
holomorphosis
holophytic
holoprosencephaly
holoprotein
holorachischisis
holoside
holosystolic murmur
holotelencephaly
holothurins
holotrichous
holozoic
Holter monitor
Holthouse hernia
Holt-Oram syndrome
Holzknecht unit
homalocephalous
Homalomyia
homaluria
Homans sign
homatropine
homaxial
home
    h. health nurse
    h. lobe
    h. monitor
homeobox
homeodomain
homeometric autoregulation
homeomorphous

homeopath
homeopathic
homeopathist
homeopathy
homeoplasia
homeoplastic
homeorrhesis
homeosis
homeostasis
    Bernard-Cannon h.
    genetic h.
    Lerner h.
    ontogenic h.
    physiologic h.
    waddingtonian h.
homeostatic
    h. equilibrium
    h. lag
homeotherapeutic
homeotherapy, homeotherapeutics
homeotherm
homeothermal
homeothermic
homeotic gene
homeotypical
homergy
Homer-Wright rosette
homicidal
homicide
homidium bromide
homigrade scale
hominal physiology
homing value
Hominidae
Hominoidea
Homo
    H. sapiens
homoarginine (Har)
homobiotin
homoblastic
homocarnosine
homocarnosinosis
homocentric
homochronous
homocitrullinuria
homocladic
homocyclic compound
homocysteine (Hcy)
homocystine
homocystinemia
homocystinuria
homocytotropic antibody
homodetic peptide
homodont
homodromous
homoeo-
homoerotism, homoeroticism
homogametic embryo
homogamy
homogenate
homogeneous
    h. immersion
    h. nucleation
    h. radiation
    h. system

H

homogenesis
homogenization
homogenize
homogenous keratoplasty
homogentisate 1,2-dioxygenase
homogentisic acid oxidase
homogeny
homoglycan
homogonic life cycle
homograft reaction
homoioplasia
homoiothermal
homokaryon
homokaryotic
homokeratoplasty
homolateral
homolecithal egg
homolipids
homolog, homologue
homologous
    h. antigen
    h. antiserum
    h. chromosome
    h. desensitization
    h. graft
    h. insemination
    h. protein
    h. recombination
    h. series
    h. serotype
    h. serum jaundice
    h. stimulus
    h. tumor
homology
    h. of chains
    DNA h.
    h. of strands
homolysin
homolysis
homomeric peptide
homomorphic
homonomous
homonomy
homonuclear
homonymous
    h. diplopia
    h. hemianopia
    h. image
    h. parallax
homophenes
homophil
homophobia
    internalized h.
homoplastic graft
homopolymer
homoproline
homoprotocatechuic acid
homorganic
homosalate
homoscedasticity
homoserine
    h. deaminase
    h. dehydratase
    h. lactone

homosexuality
    ego-dystonic h.
    female h.
    latent h.
    male h.
    overt h.
    unconscious h.
homosexual panic
homosteroid
4-homosulfanilamide
homothallic
homothermal
homotonic
homotopic
homotransplantation
homotropic
homotype
homotypic, homotypical
    h. cortex
homovanillic acid (HVA)
homovanillic acid test
homozoic
homozygosity, homozygosis
homozygote
homozygous
    h. achondroplasia
    h. by descent
homunculus
Honduras bark
honey (mel)
    h. urine
honeycomb
    h. lung
    h. macula
    h. pattern
    h. ringworm
Hong Kong influenza
honk
    systolic h.
hood
    dorsal h.
hooded prepuce
hook
    calvarial h.
    h. of hamate
    palate h.
    sliding h.
    h. of spiral lamina
    squint h.
    tracheotomy h.
hookean behavior
hooked
    h. bone
    h. bundle of Russell
    h. fasciculus
Hooke law
hooklet
hook-shaped cataract
hookworm
    h. anemia
    h. disease
Hoover sign
Hopkins rod-lens telescope
Hoplopsyllus anomalus

Hopmann
  H. papilloma
  H. polyp
hops
hora decubitus (h.d., hor. decub.)
hora somni (hor. som., h.s.)
hor. decub.
  hora decubitus
hordenine
hordeolum
  h. externum
  h. internum
  h. meibomianum
horehound, hoarhound
horizontal
  h. atrophy
  h. beam film
  h. cell of Cajal
  h. cell of retina
  h. fissure of right lung
  h. fissure [TA] of cerebellum
  h. fracture
  h. growth phase
  h. heart
  h. laryngectomy
  h. osteotomy
  h. overlap
  h. part of duodenum
  h. part of facial canal
  h. plane
  h. plate of palatine bone
  h. resorption
  h. transmission
  h. vertigo
horizontalis
hormesis
hormion
hormogonal
hormonal gingivitis
hormone
  adipokinetic h.
  adrenal androgen-stimulating h. (AASH)
  adrenocortical h.
  adrenocorticotropic h. (ACTH)
  adrenomedullary h.
  adrenotropic h.
  androgenic h.
  antidiuretic h. (ADH)
  anti-müllerian h.
  cardiac h.
  chorionic gonadotropic h.
  chorionic "growth h.-prolactin" (CGP)
  cortical h.
  corticotropic h.
  corticotropin-releasing h. (CRH)
  ectopic h.
  endocrine h.
  erythropoietic h.
  estrogenic h.
  follicle-stimulating h. (FSH)
  follicular h.
  follitropin-releasing h. (FRH)
  galactopoietic h.

  gametokinetic h.
  gastrointestinal h.
  gonadal h.
  gonadotropic h.
  gonadotropin-releasing h. (GnRH, GRH)
  growth h. (GH)
  growth h.-inhibiting h. (GIH)
  growth h.-releasing h. (GHRH, GH-RH)
  heart h.
  herz h.
  human chorionic somatomammotropic h. (HCS)
  human growth h. (HGH)
  hypophysiotropic h.
  inappropriate h.
  interstitial cell-stimulating h. (ICSH)
  lactation h.
  lactogenic h.
  lipid-mobilizing h.
  lipotropic h. (LPH)
  local h.
  luteinizing h. (LH)
  luteinizing hormone-releasing h. (LH-RH, LRH)
  mammotropic h.
  melanocyte-stimulating h. (MSH)
  melanotropin release-inhibiting h. (MIH)
  melanotropin-releasing h. (MRH)
  neurohypophysial h.
  ovarian hormone
  pancreatic hyperglycemic h.
  parathyroid h. (PTH)
  pituitary gonadotropic h.
  pituitary growth h.
  placental growth h.
  pregnancy h.
  progestational h.
  proparathyroid h.
  releasing h. (RH)
  h. replacement therapy (HRT)
  salivary gland h.
  sex h.
  somatotropic h. (STH)
  somatotropin release-inhibiting h. (SIH)
  somatotropin-releasing h. (SRH)
  steroid h.
  sympathetic h.
  thyroid-stimulating h. (TSH)
  thyrotropic h.
  thyrotropin-releasing h. (TRH)
  tissue h.
  trophic h.
  tropic h.
  vertebrate h.
hormonogenesis
hormonogenic
hormonopoiesis
hormonopoietic
hormonoprivia
hormonotherapy

H

horn
  Ammon h.
  anterior h.
  cicatricial h.
  coccygeal h.
  cutaneous h.
  frontal h.
  greater h. of hyoid bone
  h.'s of hyoid bone
  iliac h.
  inferior h.
  inferior h. of falciform margin of
    saphenous opening
  inferior h. of lateral ventricle
  inferior h. of thyroid cartilage
  lateral h.
  lesser h. of hyoid
  occipital h.
  posterior h.
  pulp h.
  sacral h.
  h.'s of saphenous opening
  sebaceous h.
  superior h. of falciform margin of
    saphenous opening
  superior h. of thyroid cartilage
  temporal h.
  h.'s of thyroid cartilage
  uterine h.
  h. of uterus
  ventral h.
  warty h.
Horner
  H. muscle
  H. pupil
  H. syndrome
  H. tooth
Horner-Trantas dot
horny
  h. cell
  h. layer of epidermis
  h. layer of nail
horopter
  empirical h.
horripilation
horror
  h. autotoxicus
  h. fusionis
horsefly
horsepower
horsepox virus
horseradish peroxidase
horseshoe
  h. fistula
  h. kidney
  h. placenta
Horsley bone wax
hor. som.
  hora somni
Hortega
  H. cell
  H. neuroglia stain
Horton
  H. arteritis

  H. cephalalgia
  H. headache
hospice
hospital
  base h.
  camp h.
  closed h.
  day h.
  h. fever
  h. formulary
  h. gangrene
  general h.
  government h.
  group h.
  maternity h.
  mental h.
  municipal h.
  night h.
  h. nurse
  open h.
  philanthropic h.
  private h.
  proprietary h.
  public h.
  h. record
  special h.
  state h.
  teaching h.
  Veterans Administration h.
  voluntary h.
  weekend h.
hospital-acquired pneumonia
hospital-based physician
hospitalist
hospitalization
host
  accidental h.
  amplifier h.
  h. cell
  dead-end h.
  definitive h.
  final h.
  intermediary h.
  intermediate h.
  paratenic h.
  reservoir h.
  secondary h.
  transport h.
hostile behavior
hot
  h. abscess
  h. flash
  h. flush
  h. gangrene
  h. nodule
  h. pack
  h. salt sterilizer
  h. snare
  h. spot
Hottentot tea
hound-dog facies
Hounsfield
  H. number
  H. unit

hour
> microliters of STPD of CO_2 given off per milligram of tissue per h. (Q_{CO2})

hourglass
> h. contraction
> h. head
> h. murmur
> h. pattern
> h. stomach
> h. vertebrae

house
> halfway h.
> h. officer
> h. staff

housefly
housekeeping gene
housemaid's knee
Houssay
> H. animal
> H. phenomenon
> H. syndrome

Houston
> H. fold
> H. muscle

Houston-Harris syndrome
Howard test
Howell-Jolly body
Howell unit
Howship lacunae
Hoyer
> H. anastomoses
> H. canal

HP
> haptoglobin

HPL
> human placental lactogen

HPLC
> high-pressure liquid chromatography

HPV
> human papillomavirus

H₂Q
> ubiquinol

h.r.a.
> health risk assessment

HR conduction time
HRCT
> high-resolution computed tomography

HRSA
> Health Resources and Services Administration

HRT
> hormone replacement therapy

Hruby lens
h.s.
> hora somni

H-shape vertebrae
HSIL
> high-grade squamous intraepithelial lesion

hsp
> heat shock protein

HSV
> herpes simplex virus

5-HT
> 5-hydroxytryptamine

Ht
> total hyperopia

HTLV
> human T-cell lymphoma/leukemia virus

HTLV-I, -II, -III
H-type
> H-t. tracheoesophageal fistula

hU
> dihydrouridine

Hu antigen
Hubbard tank
Hubrecht protochordal knot
Hückel rule
Hucker-Conn stain
Hudson-Stähli line
hue
Hueck ligament
Hueter maneuver
Hüfner equation
Hughes-Stovin syndrome
Huguier
> H. canal
> H. circle
> H. sinus

Huhner test
Hull triad
hum
> venous h.

human
> h. alpha₁-protease inhibitor
> h. antihemophilic factor
> h. antihemophilic fraction
> h. antimouse antibody (HAMA)
> h. babesiosis
> h. botfly
> h. botfly myiasis
> h. chorionic gonadotropin (HCG)
> h. chorionic somatomammotropic hormone (HCS)
> h. chorionic somatomammotropin
> h. communication
> h. diploid cell rabies vaccine
> h. diploid cell vaccine (HDCV)
> h. ecology
> h. ehrlichiosis
> h. eosinophilic enteritis
> h. fibrin foam
> h. fibrinogen
> h. gamma globulin
> h. genetics
> H. Genome Initiative
> H. Genome Project
> h. glandular kallikrein 3 (hK3)
> h. granulocytic ehrlichiosis (HGE)
> h. herpesvirus 1, 2, 3, 4, 5, 6, 7, 8
> h. immunodeficiency virus (HIV)
> h. immunodeficiency virus-2 (HIV-2)
> h. insulin
> h. leukocyte antigen (HLA)
> h. measles immune serum
> h. menopausal gonadotropin (HMG)
> h. monocytic ehrlichiosis (HME)
> h. normal immunoglobulin
> h. papillomavirus (HPV)

H

human (*continued*)
 h. pertussis immune serum
 h. placental lactogen (HPL)
 h. plasma protein fraction
 h. scarlet fever immune serum
 h. serum jaundice
 h. T-cell lymphoma/leukemia virus (HTLV)
 h. T-cell lymphotropic virus
 h. thrombin
 h. T lymphotrophic virus
humanistic psychology
humectant
humectation
humeral
 h. artery
 h. articulation
 h. axillary lymph node
 h. head
 h. nutrient artery
humeri (*pl. of* humerus)
humeroradial
 h. articulation
 h. joint
humeroscapular
humeroulnar
 h. head of flexor digitorum superficialis muscle
 h. joint
humerus, pl. **humeri**
humidity
 absolute h.
 relative h.
humin
Hummelsheim
 H. operation
 H. procedure
humor
 aqueous h.
 h. aquosus
 Morgagni h.
 ocular h.
 peccant h.
 vitreous h.
 h. vitreus
humoral
 h. doctrine
 h. hypercalcemia of benignancy
 h. immunity
 h. pathology
 h. regulator
 h. theory
humoralism, humorism
hump
 buffalo h.
 dowager h.
 Hampton h.
humpback
Humphry ligament
humulin
humulus
hunchback
hunger
 affect h.

 h. contractions
 narcotic h.
 h. pain
 h. swelling
Hung method
Hunner ulcer
Hunt
 H. neuralgia
 H. paradoxic phenomenon
 H. syndrome
hunter
 H. canal
 H. and Driffield curve
 H. glossitis
 H. gubernaculum
 H. ligament
 H. line
 H. membrane
 H. operation
 H. syndrome
Hunter-Schreger
 H.-S. bands
 H.-S. line
Hunter-Thompson dwarfism
hunting
 h. reaction
Huntington
 H. chorea
 H. disease
Hurler
 H. disease
 H. syndrome
Hurler-Scheie syndrome
Hurst
 H. bougie
 H. disease
Hürthle
 H. cell
 H. cell adenoma
 H. cell carcinoma
Huschke
 H. auditory tooth
 H. cartilage
 H. foramen
 H. valve
Hutchinson
 H. crescentic notch
 H. facies
 H. freckle
 H. incisor
 H. mask
 H. patch
 H. pupil
 H. tooth
 H. triad
Hutchinson-Gilford
 H.-G. disease
 H.-G. syndrome
Hutchison syndrome
Huxley
 H. layer
 H. membrane
 H. sheath

Huygens
  H. ocular
  H. principle
HV
  half-value
  HV conduction time
  HV interval
HVA
  homovanillic acid
  HVA test
HVL
  half-value layer
hyalin
  alcoholic h.
hyaline
  h. body
  h. body of pituitary
  h. cartilage
  h. cast
  h. degeneration
  h. leukocyte
  h. membrane
  h. membrane disease of the
    newborn
  h. membrane syndrome
  h. thrombus
  h. tubercle
hyalinization
hyalinosis
  h. cutis et mucosae
  systemic h.
hyalinuria
hyalitis
  suppurative h.
hyalobiuronic acid
hyalocapsular ligament
hyalocyte
hyalogen
hyalohyphomycosis
hyaloid
  h. artery
  h. body
  h. canal
  h. fossa
  h. membrane
hyaloideoretinal degeneration
hyalomere
Hyalomma
  H. anatolicum
  H. anatolicum anatolicum
  H. marginatum
  H. variegatum
hyalophagia
hyalophobia
hyaloplasm
  nuclear h.
hyaloserositis
hyalosis
  asteroid h.
  punctate h.
hyalosome
hyalurate
hyaluronate lyase

hyaluronic
  h. acid
  h. lyase
hyaluronidase
hyaluronoglucosaminidase
hyaluronoglucuronidase
H-Y antigen
hybaroxia
hybenzate
hybrid
  DNA-RNA h.
  h. prosthesis
  SV40-adenovirus h.
hybridism
hybridization
  cell h.
  cross h.
  DNA h.
  fluorescence in situ h.
  fluorescent in situ h.
  nucleic acid h.
  overlap h.
  in situ h.
  in situ nucleic acid h.
  somatic cell h.
hybridoma
hyclate
hydantoin
hydantoinate
hydatid
  h. cyst
  h. disease
  h. fremitus
  Morgagni h.
  nonpedunculated h.
  pedunculated h.
  h. polyp
  h. pregnancy
  h. rash
  h. resonance
  h. sand
  sessile h.
  stalked h.
  h. thrill
hydatidiform mole
hydatidocele
hydatidosis
hydatidostomy
Hydatigera taeniaeformis
hydatoid
hydnocarpus oil
hydracetin
hydradenitis
hydradenoma
hydragogue
hydralazine
  h. hydrochloride
  h. syndrome
hydrallostane
hydramitrazine tartrate
hydramnios
hydranencephaly
hydrargyria
hydrargyrum
hydrarthrodial

H

hydrarthrosis
    intermittent h.
hydrase
hydrastine
hydrastinine
hydrastis
hydratase
hydrate
    h. crystal
    h. microcrystal theory of anesthesia
hydrated alumina
hydration
    absolute h.
hydraulic conductivity
hydrazide
hydrazine yellow
hydrazinolysis
hydrazone
hydremic edema
hydrencephalocele
hydrencephalomeningocele
hydrencephalus
hydriatric
hydric
hydride ion
hydrindantin
hydroa
    h. aestivale
    h. puerorum
    h. vacciniforme
hydroadipsia
hydroalcoholic
    h. extract
    h. tincture
hydroappendix
hydrobilirubin
hydrobromate
hydrobromic acid
hydrocalycosis
hydrocarbon
    Diels h.
    saturated h.
hydrocele
    cervical h.
    h. colli
    communicating h.
    congenital h.
    cord h.
    Dupuytren h.
    h. feminae
    filarial h.
    funicular h.
    noncommunicating h.
    Nuck h.
    h. spinalis
hydrocelectomy
hydrocephalic
hydrocephalocele
hydrocephaloid
hydrocephalus
    communicating h.
    congenital h.
    double compartment h.
    external h.
    h. ex vacuo

    internal h.
    noncommunicating h.
    normal pressure h.
    obstructive h.
    occult h.
    otitic h.
    postmeningitic h.
    posttraumatic h.
    primary h.
    secondary h.
    thrombotic h.
    toxic h.
hydrocephaly
hydrochloric acid
    diluted h. a.
hydrochloride
hydrochlorothiazide
hydrocholecystis
hydrocholeresis
hydrocholeretic
hydrocodone
hydrocolloid
    irreversible h.
    reversible h.
hydrocolpocele
hydrocortamate hydrochloride
hydrocortisone
    h. acetate
    h. cyclopentylpropionate
    h. cypionate
    h. hydrogen succinate
    h. sodium phosphate
    h. sodium succinate
hydrocotarnine
hydrocyanic acid
hydrocyanism
hydrocyst
hydrocystoma
hydrodipsia
hydrodipsomania
hydrodiuresis
hydrodynamics
hydroelectric bath
hydroencephalocele
hydrofluoric acid
hydrogel
hydrogen (H)
    h. acceptor
    activated h.
    arseniureted h.
    h. bond
    h. bromide
    h. carrier
    h. chloride
    h. cyanide
    h. dehydrogenase
    h. dioxide
    h. donor
    h. electrode
    h. exponent
    heavy h.
    h. ion (H^+)
    h. number
    h. peroxide
    h. phosphide

phosphureted h.
h. pump
h. sulfide
sulfureted h.
h. transport
hydrogen-1 (^{1}H)
hydrogen-2 (^{2}H)
hydrogen-3 (^{3}H)
hydrogenase
hydrogenation
hydrogenlyase
hydrokinetic
hydrokinetics
hydrolabile
hydrolability
hydrolase
cysteine h.
serine h.
hydrolymph
hydrolysate
hydrolysis
hydrolytic cleavage
hydrolyze
hydrolyzing enzyme
hydroma
hydromassage
hydromeningocele
hydrometer
hydrometra
hydrometric
hydrometrocolpos
hydrometry
hydromicrocephaly
hydromorphone hydrochloride
hydromphalus
hydromyelia
hydromyelocele
hydronephrosis
hydronephrotic
hydronium ion
hydroparasalpinx
hydropathic
hydropathy
hydropenia
hydropenic
hydropericardium
hydroperitoneum, hydroperitonia
hydroperoxidases
hydroperoxide
hydrophil, hydrophile
h. colloid
hydrophilia
hydrophilic
h. colloid
h. ointment
h. petrolatum
hydrophilous
hydrophobia
hydrophobic
h. bond
h. colloid
h. interaction
hydrophthalmia, hydrophthalmos,
hydrophthalmus
Hydrophyidae

hydropic degeneration
hydropneumatosis
hydropneumopericardium
hydropneumoperitoneum
hydropneumothorax
hydroposia
hydrops
endolymphatic h.
fetal h.
h. fetalis
h. folliculi
h. of gallbladder
immune fetal h.
nonimmune fetal h.
h. ovarii
h. pericardii
h. tubae
h. tubae profluens
hydropyonephrosis
hydroquinol
hydroquinone
hydrorchis
hydrorheostat
hydrorrhea
h. gravidae
h. gravidarum
hydrosalpinx
intermittent h.
hydrosarca
hydrosarcocele
hydrosol
hydrosphygmograph
hydrostat
hydrostatic
h. dilator
h. pressure
hydrosudopathy
hydrosudotherapy
hydrosyringomyelia
hydrotaxis
hydrotherapeutic
hydrotherapeutics
hydrotherapy
hydrothermal
hydrothionemia
hydrothionuria
hydrothorax
chylous h.
hydrotomy
hydrotropism
negative h.
positive h.
hydrotubation
hydroureter
hydroureteronephrosis
hydrous wool fat
hydrovarium
hydroxamic acids
hydroxide
hydroxocobalamin
hydroxocobemine
hydroxyacetic acid
hydroxy acid
3-hydroxyacyl-CoA dehydrogenase
hydroxyacylglutathione hydrolase

H

3-hydroxyanthranilic acid
hydroxyapatite
    amorphous h.
    poorly crystalline h.
3-hydroxybutanoic acid
4-hydroxybutyrate
3-hydroxybutyric acid dehydrogenase
4-hydroxybutyric aciduria
hydroxycarbamide
hydroxychloroquine sulfate
25-hydroxycholecalciferol (HCC)
hydroxychroman
hydroxychromene
17-hydroxycorticosteroid test
hydroxyephedrine
25-hydroxyergocalciferol
hydroxyfatty acid
3-hydroxyglutaric acid
hydroxyhemin
3-L-hydroxykynurenine
hydroxykynureninuria
hydroxyl
hydroxylamine reductase
hydroxylamino
hydroxylapatite
11-hydroxylase deficiency
21-hydroxylase deficiency
17-hydroxylase deficiency syndrome
hydroxylases
hydroxylation
hydroxylysine (Hyl)
5-hydroxylysine (5Hyl)
p-hydroxymercuribenzoate
β-hydroxy-β-methylglutaryl-CoA
    β-hydroxy-β-methylglutaryl- lyase
    β-hydroxy-β-methylglutaryl- reductase
    β-hydroxy-β-methylglutaryl- synthase
3-hydroxy-3-methylglutaryl-CoA
hydroxynervone
hydroxynervonic acid
p-hydroxyphenylacetate
p-hydroxyphenyllactate
p-hydroxyphenylpyruvate
hydroxyphenyluria
17α-hydroxyprogesterone
21-hydroxyprogesterone
3-hydroxyproline (3Hyp)
4-hydroxyproline (4Hyp)
    4-h. oxidase
hydroxyprolinemia
15-hydroxyprostaglandin dehydrogenase
6-hydroxypurine
3-hydroxy-2-pyrrolidinecarboxylic acid
8-hydroxyquinoline
hydroxystilbamidine isethionate
hydroxytoluic acid
5-hydroxytryptamine (5-HT)
    -h. antagonist
hydroxytryptophan decarboxylase
3-hydroxytyramine
hydroxyurea
hydroxyzine
Hydrozoa
hygieiology
hygieist

hygiene
    criminal h.
    Doctor of H. (D Hy)
    industrial h.
    mental h.
    oral h.
hygienic laboratory coefficient
hygienist
    dental h.
hygric acid
hygroma
    h. axillare
    cervical h.
    h. colli cysticum
    cystic h.
    subdural h.
hygrometer
hygrometry
hygrophobia
hygroscopic expansion
hygrostomia
Hyl
    hydroxylysine
5Hyl
    5-hydroxylysine
hyla
hylephobia
hymen
    h. bifenestratus
    h. biforis
    cribriform h.
    denticulate h.
    imperforate h.
    infundibuliform h.
    h. sculptatus
    septate h.
    h. subseptus
    vertical h.
hymenal caruncula
hymenectomy
hymenitis
hymenoid
hymenolepiasis
hymenolepidid
Hymenolepididae
Hymenolepis
    H. diminuta
    H. lanceolata
    H. nana
    H. nana, var. *fraterna*
hymenology
Hymenoptera
hymenorrhaphy
hymenotomy
hyobranchial cleft
hyoepiglottic ligament
hyoepiglottidean
hyoglossal
    h. membrane
    h. muscle
hyoglossus muscle
hyoid
    h. apparatus
    h. arch
    h. bone

hyomandibular cleft
hyopharyngeus
hyoscine hydrobromide
dl-**hyoscyamine**
hyoscyamine sulfate
hyoscyamus
hyothyroid
Hyp
    hypoxanthine
3Hyp
    3-hydroxyproline
4Hyp
    4-hydroxyproline
hypacusia
hypacusis
hypalbuminemia
hypalgesia
hypalgesic, hypalgetic
hypamnion
hypanakinesia, hypanakinesis
Hypaque
    H. enema
    H. swallow
hyparterial bronchus
hypaxial
hypazoturia
hypencephalon
hypengyophobia
hyperabduction syndrome
hyperacidity
hyperactive child syndrome
hyperactivity
hyperacusis
hyperacute
    h. purulent conjunctivitis
    h. rejection
hyperadenosis
hyperadiposis, hyperadiposity
hyperadrenalcorticalism
hyperadrenocorticalism
hyperalaninemia
hyperaldosteronism
hyperalgesia
hyperalgesic, hyperalgetic
hyperalimentation
    enteral h.
    parenteral h.
hyperallantoinuria
hyperalphalipoproteinemia
hyperaminoaciduria
hyperammonemia
hyperamylasemia
hyperanacinesia, hyperanacinesis
hyperanakinesia, hyperanakinesis
hyperaphia
hyperaphic
hyperargininemia
hyperbaric
    h. chamber
    h. medicine
    h. oxygen
    h. oxygenation
    h. oxygen therapy
    h. spinal anesthesia
hyperbarism

hyperbasic aminoaciduria
hyper-beta-alaninemia
hyper-beta-aminoisobutyric aciduria
hyperbetalipoproteinemia
    familial h.
    familial h. and
      hyperprebetalipoproteinemia
hyperbilirubinemia
    neonatal h.
hyperbrachycephaly
hypercalcemia
    humoral h. of benignancy
    idiopathic h. of infant
hypercalcemic
    h. sarcoidosis
    h. uremia
hypercalcinuria
hypercalciuria
hypercalcuria
hypercapnia
hypercapnic acidosis
hypercarbia
hypercardia
hypercatabolic
hypercatabolism
hypercatharsis
hypercathexis
hypercementosis
hyperchloremia
hyperchloremic acidosis
hyperchlorhydria
hyperchloruria
hypercholesteremia
hypercholesterinemia
hypercholesterolemia
    familial h.
    familial h. with hyperlipemia
hypercholesterolia
hypercholia
hyperchromaffinism
hyperchromasia
hyperchromatic macrocythemia
hyperchromatism
hyperchromia
    macrocytic h.
hyperchromic effect
hyperchylia
hyperchylomicronemia
    familial h.
    familial h. with
      hyperprebetalipoproteinemia
hypercinesis, hypercinesia
hypercoagulability
hypercoagulable
hypercorticoidism
hypercortisolism
hypercryalgesia
hypercryesthesia
hypercupremia
hypercyanotic angina
hypercyesis, hypercyesia
hypercythemia
hypercytochromia
hypercytosis
hyperdicrotic

H

hyperdicrotism
hyperdiploid
hyperdipsia
hyperdistention
hyperechoic
hyperekplexia
hyperemesis
    h. gravidarum
    h. lactentium
hyperemetic
hyperemia
    active h.
    arterial h.
    Bier h.
    collateral h.
    fluxionary h.
    passive h.
    peristatic h.
    reactive h.
    venous h.
hyperemic
hyperencephaly
hyperendemic disease
hypereosinophilia
hypereosinophilic syndrome
hyperergia
hyperergic encephalitis
hypererythrocythemia
hyperesophoria
hyperesthesia
    auditory h.
    cervical h.
    gustatory h.
    muscular h.
    h. olfactoria
    olfactory h.
    h. optica
    tactile h.
hyperesthetic
hypereuryprosopic
hyperexophoria
hyperextension
hyperextension-hyperflexion injury
hyperferremia
hyperfibrinogenemia
hyperfibrinolysis
hyperflexion
hyperfractionated radiation
hyperfructosemia
hyperfunctional occlusion
hypergalactosis
hypergammaglobulinemia
hyperganglionosis
hypergenesis
hypergenetic
hypergenic teratosis
hypergenitalism
hypergeusia
hypergia
hypergic
hyperglandular
hyperglobulia, hyperglobulism
hyperglobulinemia
hyperglobulinemic purpura
hyperglobulism (*var. of* hyperglobulia)

hyperglycemia
    ketotic h.
    nonketotic h.
    posthypoglycemic h.
hyperglycemic-glycogenolytic factor (HGF)
hyperglyceridemia
    endogenous h.
    exogenous h.
hyperglycinemia
    ketotic h.
    nonketotic h.
hyperglycinuria
hyperglycogenolysis
hyperglycorrhachia
hyperglycosemia
hyperglycosuria
hyperglyoxylemia
hypergnosis
hypergonadism
hypergonadotropic
    h. eunuchoidism
    h. hypogonadism
hypergranulosis
hyperguanidinemia
hypergynecosmia
hyperhedonia, hyperhedonism
hyperhemoglobinemia
hyperheparinemia
hyperhidrosis
    gustatory h.
hyperhydration
hyperhydrochloria
hyperhydrochloridia
hyperhydropexy, hyperhydropexis
hyperhydroxyprolinemia
hyper-IgM syndrome
hyperimidodipeptiduria
hyperimmune serum
hyperimmunity
hyperimmunization
hyperimmunoglobulin E syndrome
hyperindicanemia
hyperinfection
hyperinflation
hyperinosemia
hyperinosis
hyperinsulinemia
hyperinsulinism
    alimentary h.
hyperinvolution
hyperisotonic
hyperkalemia
hyperkalemic periodic paralysis
hyperkaliemia
hyperkaluresis
hyperkeratinization
hyperkeratosis
    h. congenita
    diffuse h. of palms and soles
    epidermolytic h.
    h. follicularis et parafollicularis
    generalized epidermolytic h.
    h. lenticularis perstans
hyperketonemia
hyperketonuria

hyperkinemia
hyperkinesis, hyperkinesia
hyperkinetic
    h. dysarthria
    h. heart syndrome
    h. syndrome
hyperlactation
hyperleukocytosis
hyperlexia
hyperlipemia
    carbohydrate-induced h.
    combined fat- and carbohydrate-
      induced h.
    familial combined h.
    familial fat-induced h.
    idiopathic h.
    mixed h.
hyperlipidemia
    mixed h.
    mixed hyperlipoproteinemia familial,
      type 5 h.
hyperlipoidemia
hyperlipoproteinemia
    acquired h.
    familial h.
    lipoprotein(a) h.
    type I, II, III, IV, V familial h.
hyperliposis
hyperlithuria
hyperlogia
hyperlordosis
hyperlucent lung
hyperlysinemia
hyperlysinuria
hypermagnesemia
hypermastia
hypermature cataract
hypermenorrhea
hypermetabolism
    extrathyroidal h.
hypermetamorphosis
hypermethioninemia
hypermetria
hypermetrope
hypermetropia
    index h.
hypermnesia
hypermobility
hypermorph
hypermotor seizure
hypermyotrophy
hypernatremia
hypernatremic encephalopathy
hyperneocytosis
hypernephroid
hypernoia
hypernomic
hypernutrition
hyperoncotic
hyperonychia
hyperope
hyperopia
    absolute h.
    axial h.
    curvature h.

    facultative h.
    latent h.
    manifest h.
    total h. (Ht)
hyperopic astigmatism
hyperorality
hyperorexia
hyperornithinemia
hyperornithinemia-hyperammonemia-
    hypercitrullinuria syndrome
hyperorthocytosis
hyperosmia
hyperosmolality
hyperosmolar (hyperglycemic) nonketotic
    coma
hyperosmolarity
hyperosmotic
hyperosteoidosis
hyperostosis
    ankylosing h.
    h. corticalis deformans
    diffuse idiopathic skeletal h. (DISH)
    flowing h.
    h. frontalis interna
    generalized cortical h.
    infantile cortical h.
    streak h.
hyperostotic spondylosis
hyperovarianism
hyperoxaluria
    primary h. and oxalosis
hyperoxia
hyperoxidation
hyperpancreatism
hyperparasite
hyperparasitism
hyperparathyroidism
    primary h.
    secondary h.
hyperparotidism
hyperpathia
hyperpepsia
hyperpepsinia
hyperperistalsis
hyperphagia
hyperphalangism
hyperphenylalaninemia
    malignant h.
    non-PKU h.
hyperphonesis
hyperphonia
hyperphoria
hyperphosphatasemia
hyperphosphatasia
hyperphosphatemia
hyperphosphaturia
hyperphrenia
hyperpiesis, hyperpiesia
hyperpietic
hyperpigmentation
hyperpipecolatemia
hyperpipecolic acidemia
hyperpituitarism
hyperplasia
    adenomatous h.

H

461

hyperplasia *(continued)*
    angiofollicular mediastinal lymph node h.
    angiolymphoid h. with eosinophilia
    atypical endometrial h.
    atypical melanocytic h.
    basal cell h.
    benign giant lymph node h.
    benign prostatic h.
    cementum h.
    complex endometrial h.
    congenital adrenal h.
    congenital virilizing adrenal h.
    cystic h.
    cystic h. of the breast
    denture h.
    ductal h.
    endometrial h.
    fibromuscular h.
    focal epithelial h.
    gingival h.
    inflammatory fibrous h.
    inflammatory papillary h.
    intravascular papillary endothelial h.
    neuronal h.
    nodular h. of prostate
    nodular regenerative h.
    pseudocarcinomatous h.
    pseudoepitheliomatous h.
    senile sebaceous h.
    simple endometrial h.
    squamous cell h.
    verrucous h.
hyperplastic
    h. arteriosclerosis
    h. gingivitis
    h. inflammation
    h. osteoarthritis
    h. polyp
    h. pulpitis
hyperpnea
hyperpolarization
hyperpotassemia
hyperprebetalipoproteinemia
    familial h.
hyperprochoresis
hyperproinsulinemia
hyperprolactinemia
hyperprolactinemic amenorrhea
hyperprolinemia
hyperproteinemia
hyperproteosis
hyperpyretic
hyperpyrexia
    fulminant h.
    heat h.
    malignant h.
hyperpyrexial
hyperreactive malarious splenomegaly
hyperreflexia
    detrusor h.
hyperreflexic bladder
hyperresonance
hypersalemia

hypersaline
hypersalivation
hypersarcosinemia
hypersecretion
    gastric h.
    h. glaucoma
hypersegmentation
    hereditary h. of neutrophils
hypersegmented neutrophil
hypersensitive
    h. dentin
    h. xiphoid syndrome
hypersensitivity
    h. angiitis
    contact h.
    delayed h.
    delayed-type h. (DTH)
    immediate h.
    h. pneumonitis
    h. reaction
    tuberculin-type h.
    h. vasculitis
hypersensitization
hyperserotonemia
hyperskeocytosis
hypersomatotropism
hypersomnia
hypersonic
hypersphyxia
hypersplenism
hypersteatosis
hypersthenia
hypersthenic
hypersthenuria
hypersusceptibility
hypersystole
hypersystolic
hypertelorism
    Bixler type h.
    canthal h.
    ocular h.
hypertensin
hypertensinogen
hypertension
    accelerated h.
    adrenal h.
    benign h.
    borderline h.
    episodic h.
    essential h.
    gestational h.
    Goldblatt h.
    idiopathic h.
    labile h.
    malignant h.
    pale h.
    paroxysmal h.
    portal h.
    postpartum h.
    pregnancy-induced h.
    primary h.
    pulmonary h.
    renal h.
    renovascular h.

secondary h.
systemic venous h.
hypertensive
h. arteriopathy
h. arteriosclerosis
h. encephalopathy
h. retinopathy
h. upper esophageal sphincter
hypertensor
hypertestoidism
hyperthecosis
stromal h.
hyperthelia
hyperthermalgesia
hyperthermia
malignant h.
hyperthermoesthesia
hyperthrombinemia
hyperthymia
hyperthymic
hyperthymism
hyperthymization
hyperthyrea
hyperthyroid heart
hyperthyroidism
hereditary h.
iodine-induced h.
masked h.
ophthalmic h.
primary h.
secondary h.
hyperthyroxinemia
hypertonia
h. polycythemica
sympathetic h.
hypertonic bladder
hypertonicity
hypertrichiasis
hypertrichophrydia
hypertrichosis
h. lanuginosa
nevoid h.
h. partialis
h. universalis
hypertriglyceridemia
familial h.
hypertroph
hypertrophia
hypertrophic
h. arthritis
h. cardiomyopathy
h. cervical pachymeningitis
h. dystrophy
h. gastritis
h. hypersecretory gastropathy
h. interstitial neuropathy
h. pulmonary osteoarthropathy
h. pulpitis
h. pyloric stenosis
h. rhinitis
h. rosacea
h. scar
hypertrophy
adaptive h.

benign prostatic h.
compensatory h.
compensatory h. of the heart
complementary h.
concentric h.
eccentric h.
endemic h.
false h.
functional h.
giant h. of gastric mucosa
hemangiectatic h.
lipomatous h.
numerical h.
physiologic h.
quantitative h.
simple h.
simulated h.
true h.
vicarious h.
hypertropia
hypertyrosinemia
hyperuracil thyminuria
hyperuricemia
hyperuricemic
hyperuricuria
hypervaccination
hypervalinemia
hypervariable region
hypervascular
hyperventilation
h. syndrome
h. test
h. tetany
hyperviscosity syndrome
hypervitaminosis
hypervolemia
hypervolemic
hypervolia
hypesthesia
olfactory h.
hypha, pl. **hyphae**
racquet h.
spiral hyphae
hyphedonia
hyphema
hyphemia
intertropical h.
tropical h.
Hyphomyces destruens
Hyphomycetes
hyphomycosis
hypnagogic
h. hallucination
h. image
hypnoanalysis
hypnoanalytic
hypnocatharsis
hypnocyst
hypnogenesis
hypnogenic, hypnogenous
h. spot
hypnoidal
hypnoid state
hypnophobia

H

hypnopompic
  h. hallucination
  h. image
hypnosis
  lethargic h.
  major h.
  minor h.
hypnotherapy
hypnotic
  h. psychotherapy
  h. relationship
  h. sleep
  h. state
  h. suggestion
hypnotism
hypnotist
hypnotize
hypnozoite
hypoacidity
hypoacusis
hypoadenia
hypoadrenalism
hypoalbuminemia
hypoaldosteronism
  hyporeninemic h.
  isolated h.
  selective h.
hypoaldosteronuria
hypoalgesia
hypoalimentation
hypoazoturia
hypobaria
hypobaric spinal anesthesia
hypobarism
hypobaropathy
hypobetalipoproteinemia
  familial h.
  h. with apo B-37
hypoblast
hypoblastic
hypobranchial eminence
hypobromite
hypobromous acid
hypocalcemia
hypocalcemic cataract
hypocalcification
  enamel h.
hypocapnia
hypocarbia
hypocelom
hypochloremia
hypochloremic
hypochlorhydria
hypochlorite
hypochlorous acid
hypochloruria
hypocholesteremia
hypocholesterinemia
hypocholesterolemia
hypocholia
hypochondria (*pl. of* hypochondrium)
hypochondriacal
  h. melancholia
  h. neurosis
hypochondriac region

hypochondrial reflex
hypochondriasis
hypochondrium, pl. **hypochondria**
hypochondroplasia
hypochordal
hypochromasia
hypochromatic
hypochromatism
hypochromia
hypochromic
  h. effect
  h. microcytic anemia
hypochrosis
hypochylia
hypocinesis, hypocinesia
hypocitraturia
hypocomplementemia
hypocomplementemic
  h. glomerulonephritis
  h. vasculitis
hypocone
hypoconid
hypoconule
hypoconulid
hypocorticoidism
hypocupremia
hypocycloidal tomography
hypocystotomy
hypocythemia
hypocytosis
hypodactyly, hypodactylia, hypodactylism
hypoderm
Hypoderma
hypodermatoclysis
hypodermatomy
hypodermatosis
hypodermic
  h. injection
  h. needle
  h. syringe
  h. tablet
hypodermis
hypodermoclysis
hypodiploid
hypodipsia
hypodontia
hypodynamia cordis
hypodynamic
hypoeccrisis
hypoeccritic
hypoechoic
hypoeosinophilia
hypoesophoria
hypoesthesia
hypoexophoria
hypoferremia
hypoferric anemia
hypofibrinogenemia
hypofractionated radiation
hypofrontality
hypofunction
hypogalactia
hypogalactous
hypogammaglobinemia

hypogammaglobulinemia
    acquired h.
    primary h.
    secondary h.
    transient h. of infancy
    X-linked h., X-linked infantile h.
    X-linked h. with growth hormone
      deficiency
hypoganglionosis
hypogastric
    h. artery
    h. ganglia
    h. nerve
    h. reflex
    h. vein
hypogastrium
hypogastrocele
hypogastropagus
hypogastroschisis
hypogenesis
    polar h.
hypogenetic
hypogenitalism
hypogeusia
hypoglobulia
hypoglossal
    h. canal
    h. eminence
    h. nerve [CN XII]
    h. nucleus
    h. trigone
hypoglossis
hypoglossus
hypoglottis
hypoglycemia
    fasting h.
    ketotic h.
    leucine h.
    leucine-induced h.
    leucine-sensitive h.
    mixed h.
    neonatal h.
hypoglycemic coma
hypoglycogenolysis
hypoglycorrhachia
hypognathous
hypognathus
hypogonadism
    familial hypogonadotropic h.
    hypergonadotropic h.
    hypogonadotropic h.
    male h.
    primary h.
    secondary h.
    h. with anosmia
hypogonadotropic
    h. eunuchoidism
    h. hypogonadism
hypogranulocytosis
hypohepatia
hypohidrosis
hypohidrotic ectodermal dysplasia
hypohydremia
hypohydrochloria
hypoisotonic

hypokalemia
hypokalemic
    h. nephropathy
    h. periodic paralysis
hypokinemia
hypokinesis, hypokinesia
hypokinetic dysarthria
hypoleukemia
hypoleydigism
hypolipoproteinemia
hypoliposis
hypologia
hypolymphemia
hypomagnesemia
hypomania
hypomastia
hypomelancholia
hypomelanosis of Ito
hypomelia
hypomenorrhea
hypomere
hypometabolic
    h. state
    h. syndrome
hypometabolism
    euthyroid h.
hypometria
hypomnesia
hypomorph
hypomotility
hypomotor seizure
hypomyelination, hypomyelinogenesis
hypomyotonia
hypomyxia
hyponatremia
    depletional h.
    dilutional h.
hyponeocytosis
hyponoia
hyponychial
hyponychium
hyponychon
hypooncotic
hypoorthocytosis
hypoovarianism
hypopancreatism
hypopancreorrhea
hypoparathyroidism
    familial h.
    h. syndrome
hypoparathyroid tetany
hypopepsia
hypoperistalsis
hypophalangism
hypopharyngeal diverticulum
hypopharynx
hypophonesis
hypophonia
hypophoria
hypophosphatasemia
hypophosphatasia
    adult h.
    childhood h.
    congenital h.
hypophosphatemia

H

hypophosphaturia
hypophosphorous acid
hypophrasia
hypophyseal
    h. cachexia
    h. pouch
hypophysectomize
hypophysectomy
hypophyseoportal system
hypophyseoprivic
hypophyseotropic
hypophysial
    h. amenorrhea
    h. cachexia
    h. duct
    h. dwarf
    h. fossa
    h. infantilism
    h. portal circulation
    h. portal system
    h. syndrome
hypophysin
hypophysioportal system
hypophysioprivic
hypophysiosphenoidal syndrome
hypophysiotropic hormone
hypophysis
    h. cerebri
    pharyngeal h.
    h. sicca
hypophysitis
    lymphocytic h.
    lymphoid h.
hypopiesis
    orthostatic h.
hypopigmentation
hypopituitarism
hypoplasia
    cartilage-hair h.
    enamel h.
    focal dermal h.
    optic nerve h.
    renal h.
    h. of right ventricle
    right ventricular h.
    thymic h.
hypoplastic
    h. anemia
    h. fetal chondrodystrophy
    h. heart
    h. left heart syndrome
hypopnea
hypoposia
hypopotassemia
hypoproaccelerinemia
hypoproconvertinemia
hypoproteinemia
hypoproteinosis
hypoprothrombinemia
hypoptyalism
hypopyon
    recurrent h.
    h. ulcer
hyporeflexia
hyporeninemia

hyporeninemic hypoaldosteronism
hyporiboflavinosis
hyposalivation
hyposcheotomy
hyposcleral
hyposensitivity
hyposensitization
hyposkeocytosis
hyposmia
hyposmosis
hyposmotic
hyposomatotropism
hyposomia
hyposomniac
hypospadiac
hypospadias
    balanic h.
    coronal h.
    glanular h.
    penile h.
    penoscrotal h.
    perineal h.
    scrotal h.
    subcoronal h.
hyposphygmia
hyposplenism
hypostasis
    postmortem h.
    pulmonary h.
hypostatic
    h. abscess
    h. congestion
    h. ectasia
    h. pneumonia
hyposthenuria
hypostome
hypostomia
hypostosis
hyposupradrenalism
hyposystole
hypotelorism
hypotension
    arterial h.
    controlled h.
    idiopathic orthostatic h.
    induced h.
    intracranial h.
    orthostatic h.
    postural h.
hypotensive anesthesia
hypotensor
hypothalamic
    h. amenorrhea
    h. infundibulum
    h. obesity
    h. obesity with hypogonadism
    h. sulcus
hypothalamocerebellar fiber
hypothalamohypophysial
    h. portal circulation
    h. portal system
    h. tract
hypothalamospinal fiber
hypothalamus

hypothenar
   h. eminence
   h. fascia
   h. prominence
hypothermal
hypothermia
   accidental h.
   moderate h.
   profound h.
   regional h.
   total body h.
hypothermic anesthesia
hypothesis
   adapter h.
   alternative h.
   autocrine h.
   Avogadro h.
   bayesian h.
   frustration-aggression h.
   gate-control h.
   Goldie-Coldman h.
   Gompertz h.
   insular h.
   Knudsen h.
   Lyon h.
   Makeham h.
   Michaelis-Menten h.
   mnemic h.
   monoamine h.
   Neyman-Pearson statistical h.
   Norton-Simon h.
   null h.
   sequence h.
   sliding filament h.
   Starling h.
   upregulation/downregulation h.
   wobble h.
   zwitter h.
hypothetical
   h. mean organism (HMO)
   h. mean strain (HMS)
hypothrombinemia
hypothromboplastinemia
hypothymia
hypothymic
hypothymism
hypothyroid
   h. dwarf
   h. dwarfism
   h. infantilism
hypothyroidism
   congenital h.
   infantile h.
   secondary h.
hypothyroxinemia
hypotonia
   benign congenital h.
hypotonic
hypotonicity
hypotonus, hypotony
hypotrichiasis
hypotrichosis
hypotropia
hypotympanotomy
hypotympanum

hypouresis
hypouricemia
hypouricuria
   hereditary renal h.
hypovarianism
hypoventilation coma
hypovitaminosis
hypovolemia
hypovolemic shock
hypovolia
hypoxanthine (Hyp)
   h. guanine phosphoribosyltransferase (HGPRT)
   h. guanine phosphoribosyltransferase deficiency
   h. oxidase
   h. phosphoribosyltransferase
hypoxanthinosine
hypoxemia test
hypoxia
   anemic h.
   diffusion h.
   hypoxic h.
   ischemic h.
   oxygen affinity h.
   stagnant h.
   h. warning system
hypoxic
   h. hypoxia
   h. ischemic encephalopathy
   h. nephrosis
hypoxic-hypercarbic encephalopathy
hypsarhythmia, hypsarrhythmia
hypsi-, hypso-
hypsibrachycephalic
hypsicephaly
hypsiconchous
hypsiloid
   h. angle
   h. cartilage
   h. ligament
hypsistaphylia
hypsistenocephalic
hypso- (*var. of* hypsi-)
hypsocephaly
hypsochromic
hypsodont
hypurgia
Hyrtl
   H. anastomosis
   H. epitympanic recess
   H. foramen
   H. loop
   H. sphincter
hysteralgia
hysteratresia
hysterectomy
   abdominal h.
   abdominovaginal h.
   cesarean h.
   laparoscopic-assisted vaginal h. (LAVH)
   modified radical h.
   Porro h.
   radical h.

H

hysterectomy *(continued)*
    subtotal h.
    supracervical h.
    vaginal h.
hysteresis
    static h.
hysteria
    anxiety h.
    conversion h.
    dissociative h.
    epidemic h.
    mass h.
hysterical, hysteric
    h. amblyopia
    h. anesthesia
    h. aphonia
    h. ataxia
    h. blindness
    h. chorea
    h. convulsion
    h. gait
    h. hearing impairment
    h. joint
    h. neurosis
    h. paralysis
    h. personality
    h. personality disorder
    h. polydipsia
    h. pregnancy
    h. psychosis
    h. syncope
    h. torticollis
    h. tremor
    h. vertigo
hysterics
hysterocatalepsy
hysterocele
hysterocleisis
hysterocolposcope

hysterocystopexy
hysterodynia
hysterogenic, hysterogenous
hysterogram
hysterograph
hysterography
hysteroid convulsion
hysterolysis
hysterometer
hysteromyomectomy
hysteromyotomy
hystero-oophorectomy
hysteropathy
hysteropexy
    abdominal h.
hysteroplasty
hysterorrhaphy
hysterosalpingectomy
hysterosalpingography
hysterosalpingo-oophorectomy
hysterosalpingostomy
hysteroscope
    contact h.
    flexible h.
hysteroscopy
hysterospasm
hysterosystole
hysterothermometry
hysterotomy
    abdominal h.
    vaginal h.
hysterotrachelectomy
hysterotracheloplasty
hysterotrachelorrhaphy
hysterotrachelotomy
hysterotubography
Hz
    hertz

ι (*var. of* iota)

I

I antigen
I band
I cell
I disk
I pili
I region

^{123}I

iodine-123

^{125}I

iodine-125

^{127}I

iodine-127

^{131}I

iodine-131

^{132}I

iodine-132

-ia

IAHS

infection-associated hemophagocytic syndrome

IANC

International Anatomical Nomenclature Committee

IAP

intermittent acute porphyria

iatraliptic
iatraliptics
iatric
iatrochemical
iatrochemist
iatrochemistry
iatrogenic

i. pneumothorax
i. transmission

iatrology
iatromathematical school
iatromechanical
iatrophysical
iatrophysicist
iatrophysics
iatrotechnique

IBC

iron-binding capacity

ibogaine
ibotenic acid
ibuprofen
ICAM-1

intercellular adhesion molecule-1

ICAO standard atmosphere
iccosomes
ICD, ICDA

International Classification of Diseases

ice

i. pack
i. pick headache

Iceland

I. disease
I. moss

I-cell disease

ICF

intracellular fluid

ichor
ichoremia
ichoroid
ichorous pus
ichorrhea
ichorrhemia
ICHPPC

International Classification of Health Problems in Primary Care

ichthammol
ichthyism
ichthyismus

i. exanthematicus
i. hystrix

ichthyoacanthotoxism
ichthyocolla
ichthyohemotoxin
ichthyohemotoxism
ichthyoid
ichthyootoxin
ichthyophagous
ichthyophobia
ichthyosarcotoxin
ichthyosarcotoxism
ichthyosis

acquired i.
i. congenita
i. congenita neonatorum
i. corneae
i. fetalis
i. follicularis
harlequin i.
i. hystrix
lamellar i.
i. linearis circumflexa
nacreous i.
i. palmaris et plantaris
i. scutulata
i. simplex
i. vulgaris
X-linked i.

ichthyotic
ichthyotoxicology
ichthyotoxicon
ichthyotoxin
ichthyotoxism
ICIDH

International Classification of Impairments, Disabilities and Handicaps

icing heart
iconic sign
icosahedral
***n*-icosanoic acid**
ICP

intracranial pressure

ICRP

International Commission on Radiological Protection

ICSH

interstitial cell-stimulating hormone

ictal
icteric
icteroanemia
icterogenic
icterohematuric
icterohemoglobinuria
icterohemorrhagic fever
icteroid
icterus
    acquired hemolytic i.
    benign familial i.
    cholestatic hepatosis i. gravidarum
    chronic familial i.
    congenital hemolytic i.
    cythemolytic i.
    i. gravis
    infectious i.
    i. melas
    i. neonatorum
    physiologic i.
    i. praecox
ictometer
ictus
    i. cordis
    i. epilepticus
    i. paralyticus
    i. solis
ICU
    intensive care unit
        ICU psychosis
ID
    infecting dose
IDA
    iminodiacetate
IDDM
    insulin-dependent diabetes mellitus
idea
    autochthonous i.
    compulsive i.
    dominant i.
    fixed i.
    flight of i.'s
    overvalued i.
    i. of reference
ideal
    i. alveolar gas
    ego i.
ideation
ideational
idée fixe
identical twins
identification
    projective i.
    synthetic sentence i.
identity
    i. crisis
    i. disorder
    ego i.
    gender i.
    i. matrix
    sense of i.
ideokinetic apraxia
ideology
ideomotion

ideomotor
    i. apraxia
ideophobia
idioagglutinin
idiodynamic control
idiogenesis
idioglossia
idioglottic
idiogram
idiographic approach
idioheteroagglutinin
idioheterolysin
idiohypnotism
idioisoagglutinin
idioisolysin
idiojunctional rhythm
idiolalia
idiolysin
idiomuscular contraction
idionodal rhythm
idiopathetic
idiopathic
    i. aldosteronism
    i. bilateral vestibulopathy
    i. bone cavity
    i. bradycardia
    i. cardiomyopathy
    i. disease
    i. epilepsy
    i. fibrous mediastinitis
    i. fibrous retroperitonitis
    i. gout
    i. hirsutism
    i. hypercalcemia of infant
    i. hypercalcemic sclerosis of infant
    i. hyperlipemia
    i. hypertension
    i. hypertrophic osteoarthropathy
    i. hypertrophic subaortic stenosis
    i. infantilism
    i. interstitial fibrosis
    i. megacolon
    i. myocarditis
    i. neuralgia
    i. orthostatic hypotension
    i. paroxysmal rhabdomyolysis
    i. proctitis
    i. pulmonary fibrosis (IPF)
    i. pulmonary hemosiderosis
    i. roseola
    i. stabbing headache
    i. subglottic stenosis
    i. thrombocytopenic purpura (ITP)
idiopathy
idiophrenic
idiopsychologic
idioreflex
idiosome
idiosyncrasy
idiosyncratic sensitivity
idiotope
    set of i.'s
idiot-prodigy
idiotrophic
idiotropic

idiot-savant
idiotype autoantibody
idiotypic
>   i. antibody
>   i. antigenic determinant

idioventricular
>   i. kick
>   i. rhythm

iditol
IDL
>   intermediate density lipoprotein

idose
idoxuridine (IDU)
IDP
>   inosine 5′-diphosphate

id reaction
IDU
>   idoxuridine

iduronate sulfatase
iduronic acid
IEP
>   isoelectric point

IF
>   initiation factor

IFN
>   interferon

IFN-alpha
>   interferon alpha

IFN-beta
>   interferon beta

IFN-gamma
>   interferon gamma

Ig
>   immunoglobulin

IgA
>   immunoglobulin A
>   IgA nephropathy

IgD
>   immunoglobulin D

IgE
>   immunoglobulin E

IGF
>   insulinlike growth factor

IgG
>   immunoglobulin G

IgM
>   immunoglobulin M
>   IgM nephropathy

ignatia
ignipedites
ignipuncture
ignotine
IH
>   infectious hepatitis

IJP
>   inhibitory junction potential

ikota
IL-1
>   interleukin-1

IL-2
>   interleukin-2

IL-3
>   interleukin-3

IL-4
>   interleukin-4

IL-5
>   interleukin-5

IL-6
>   interleukin-6

IL-7
>   interleukin-7

IL-8
>   interleukin-8

IL-9
>   interleukin-9

IL-10
>   interleukin-10

IL-11
>   interleukin-11

IL-12
>   interleukin-12

IL-13
>   interleukin-13

IL-14
>   interleukin-14

IL-15
>   interleukin-15

IL-16
>   interleukin-16

IL-17
>   interleukin-17

IL-18
>   interleukin-18

ILA
>   insulinlike activity

ileac
ileadelphus
ileal
>   i. artery
>   i. bladder
>   i. conduit
>   i. intussusception
>   i. orifice
>   i. papilla
>   i. sphincter
>   i. ureter
>   i. vein

ileectomy
ileitis
>   backwash i.
>   distal i., regional i.
>   terminal i.

ileoanal pouch
ileocecal
>   i. eminence
>   i. fold
>   i. intussusception
>   i. junction
>   i. opening
>   i. orifice
>   i. valve

ileocecocolic sphincter
ileocecocystoplasty
ileocecostomy
ileocecum
ileocolic
>   i. artery
>   i. intussusception
>   i. lymph node

ileocolic *(continued)*
    i. valve
    i. vein
ileocolitis
ileocolonic
ileocolostomy
ileocystoplasty
ileoentectropy
ileoileostomy
ileojejunitis
ileopexy
ileoproctostomy
ileorectostomy
ileorrhaphy
ileosigmoidostomy
ileostomy
    Brooke i.
    Kock i.
ileotomy
ileotransversostomy
ileum duplex
ileus
    adynamic i.
    dynamic i.
    gallstone i.
    mechanical i.
    meconium i.
    occlusive i.
    paralytic i.
    spastic i.
    i. subparta
    terminal i.
    verminous i.
Ilhéus
    I. encephalitis
    I. fever
    I. virus
ilia (*pl. of* ilium)
iliac
    i. artery
    i. bone
    i. branch of iliolumbar artery
    i. bursa
    i. colon
    i. crest
    i. fascia
    i. fossa
    i. horn
    i. muscle
    i. plexus
    i. region
    i. roll
    i. spine
    i. steal
    i. tubercle
    i. tuberosity
    i. vein
iliacosubfascial
    i. fossa
    i. hernia
iliacus
    i. branch of iliolumbar artery
    i. minor muscle
    i. muscle

iliadelphus
iliococcygeal
    i. muscle
    i. raphe
iliococcygeus muscle
iliocolotomy
iliocostalis
    i. cervicis muscle
    i. lumborum muscle
    i. muscle
    i. thoracis muscle
iliocostal muscle
iliofemoral ligament
iliofemoroplasty
iliohypogastric nerve
ilioinguinal nerve
iliolumbar
    i. artery
    i. ligament
    i. vein
iliopagus
iliopectineal
    i. arch
    i. bursa
    i. eminence
    i. fascia
    i. fossa
    i. ligament
    i. line
iliopelvic sphincter
iliopsoas muscle
iliopubic
    i. eminence
    i. tract
iliosacral
iliosciatic notch
iliospinal
iliothoracopagus
iliotibial
    i. band
    i. band friction syndrome
    i. band syndrome
    i. tract
iliotrochanteric ligament
ilioxiphopagus
ilium, pl. **ilia**
Ilizarov technique
illegal abortion
illicium
illinition
illness
    environmental i.
    factitious i. by proxy
    functional i.
    manic-depressive i.
    mass sociogenic i.
    mental i.
    nonspecific building-related i.
    severity of i.
    specific building-related i.
illumination
    axial i.
    central i.
    contact i.
    critical i.

dark-field i.
dark-ground i.
direct i.
erect i.
focal i.
Köhler i.
lateral i.
oblique i.
vertical i.
illuminism
illusion
i. of doubles
i. of movement
oculogravic i.
oculogyral i.
optic i.
illusional
Ilosvay reagent
IM
internal medicine
intramuscular
ima
image
accidental i.
i. amplifier
body i.
catatropic i.
i. cytometer
direct i.
eidetic i.
false i.
heteronymous i.
homonymous i.'s
hypnagogic i.
hypnopompic i.
i. intensifier
inverted i.
magnitude i.
mental i.
mirror i.
motor i.
negative i.
optic i.
phase i.
Purkinje i.'s
Purkinje-Sanson i.'s
real i.
retinal i.
Sanson i.'s
sensory i.
specular i.
tactile i.
unequal retinal i.
virtual i.
visual i.
imagery
imaginal
imaging
blood pool i.
i. department
exercise i.
magnetic resonance i. (MRI)
NMR i.
nuclear magnetic resonance i.
pharmacologic stress i.

through transfer i.
transfer i.
imago, pl. **imagines**
imbalance
autonomic i.
occlusal i.
sex chromosome i.
sympathetic i.
vasomotor i.
imbecile
imbed
imbibition
imbricate, imbricated
imbrication
eyelid i.
i. line of von Ebner
Imerslünd-Grasbeck syndrome
imidazole alkaloids
4-imidazolone-5-propionate
imidazolyl
imide
imidodipeptidase
imidodipeptiduria
imidole
iminazolyl
imino acid
iminocarbonyl
iminodiacetate (IDA)
iminodipeptidase
iminoglycinuria
iminohydrolases
iminostilbenes
imipenem
imipramine hydrochloride
imiquimod
IML
intermediolateral cell column of spinal
cord
Imlach fat-pad
immature
i. cataract
i. granulocyte
i. neutrophil
immediate
i. allergy
i. amputation
i. auscultation
i. hypersensitivity
i. hypersensitivity reaction
i. insertion denture
i. percussion
i. posttraumatic automatism
i. posttraumatic convulsion
immedicable
immersion
i. bath
i. foot
homogeneous i.
i. lens
i. microscopy
i. objective
oil i.
water i.
immiscible
immission

immittance
immobilization
immobilize
immobilized enzyme
immobilizing antibody
immortalization
immotile cilia syndrome
immovable
    i. bandage
    i. joint
immune
    i. adherence
    i. adherence phenomenon
    i. adhesion test
    i. adsorption
    i. agglutination
    i. agglutinin
    i. complex
    i. complex disease
    i. complex disorder
    i. complex glomerulonephritis
    i. complex nephritis
    i. deficiency
    i. deviation
    i. electron microscopy
    i. fetal hydrops
    i. hemolysin
    i. hemolysis
    i. inflammation
    i. interferon
    i. opsonin
    i. paralysis
    i. precipitation
    i. protein
    i. reaction
    i. response
    i. response gene
    i. serum
    i. serum globulin
    i. suppression
    i. surveillance
    i. system
    i. thrombocytopenia
    i. thrombocytopenic purpura
immunifacient
immunity
    acquired i.
    active i.
    adoptive i.
    antiviral i.
    artificial active i.
    artificial passive i.
    bacteriophage i.
    cell-mediated i. (CMI)
    cellular i.
    concomitant i.
    i. deficiency
    general i.
    group i.
    herd i.
    humoral i.
    infection i.
    innate i.
    local i.
    maternal i.

    natural i.
    passive i.
    relative i.
    specific i.
    specific active i.
    specific passive i.
    stress i.
immunization
    active i.
    passive i.
immunize
immunoadjuvant
immunoagglutination
immunoassay
    double antibody i.
    enzyme i.
    enzyme-multiplied i. technique
    (EMIT)
    solid phase i.
    thin-layer i.
immunobiology
immunoblast
immunoblastic
    i. lymphadenopathy
    i. lymphoma
    i. sarcoma
immunoblot, immunoblotting
immunochemical assay
immunochemistry
immunocompetence
immunocompetent
immunocomplex
immunocompromised
immunoconglutinin
immunocyte
immunocytoadherence
immunocytochemistry
immunodeficiency
    cellular i. with abnormal
      immunoglobulin synthesis
    combined i.
    common variable i.
    phagocytic dysfunction i.
    phagocytic dysfunction disorders i.
    secondary i.
    severe combined i. (SCID)
    i. syndrome
    i. with elevated IgM
    i. with hypoparathyroidism
immunodeficient
immunodepressant
immunodepressor
immunodiagnosis
immunodiffusion
    double i.
    radial i. (RID)
    single i.
immunoelectrophoresis
    crossed i.
    rocket i.
    two-dimensional i.
immunoenhancement
immunoenhancer
immunoferritin

I

immunofluorescence
    direct i.
    indirect i.
    i. method
    i. microscopy
immunofluorescent stain
immunogen
immunogenetics
immunogenic
immunogenicity
immunoglobulin (Ig)
    i. A (IgA)
    anti-D i.
    chickenpox i.
    i. D (IgD)
    i. domains
    i. E (IgE)
    i. G (IgG)
    i. G subclass deficiency
    human normal i.
    i. M (IgM)
    measles i.
    monoclonal i.
    pertussis i.
    poliomyelitis i.
    rabies i.
    Rh_o(D) i.
    secretory i.
    secretory i. A
    selective i. A deficiency
    tetanus i.
    thyroid-stimulating i.'s (TSI)
immunohematology
immunohistochemistry
immunolocalization
immunologic
    i. competence
    i. deficiency
    i. enhancement
    i. high dose tolerance
    i. mechanism
    i. paralysis
    i. pregnancy test
immunologically
    i. activated cell
    i. competent cell
    i. privileged site
immunological surveillance
immunologist
immunology
immunomodulatory
immunopathology
immunoperoxidase technique
immunophilin
immunopotentiation
immunopotentiator
immunoprecipitation
immunoproliferative
    i. disorder
    i. small intestinal disease
immunoradiometric assay
immunoreaction
immunoreactive insulin
immunoselection
immunosorbent

immunosuppressant
immunosuppression
immunosuppressive
immunosurveillance
immunosympathectomy
immunotherapy
    adoptive i.
    biologic i.
immunotolerance
immunotransfusion
IMP
    inosine 5′-monophosphate
impact
    i. factor
    i. resistance
impacted
    i. fetus
    i. fracture
    i. tooth
impaction
    dental i.
    fecal i.
    food i.
    mucus i.
impaired glucose tolerance
impairment
    mental i.
IMP-aspartate ligase
impatent
impedance
    acoustic i.
    i. angle
    i. matching
    i. method
    i. plethysmography
imperative conception
imperception
imperfect
    i. fungus
    i. stage
    i. state
imperforate
    i. anus
    i. hymen
imperforation
impermeable junction
impermeant
impersistence
    motor i.
impervious
impetiginization
impetiginous cheilitis
impetigo
    Bockhart i.
    i. bullosa
    bullous i. of newborn
    i. circinata
    i. contagiosa
    i. contagiosa bullosa
    follicular i.
    i. herpetiformis
    i. neonatorum
    i. vulgaris
impetus

impingement
>i. sign
>i. syndrome
>i. test

implant
>carcinomatous i.
>cochlear i.
>dental i.
>i. denture
>i. denture substructure
>i. denture superstructure
>endometrial i.
>endo-osseous i.
>endosseous i.
>endosteal i.
>inflatable i.
>intracorneal i.
>intraocular i.
>magnetic i.
>orbital i.
>penile i.
>pin i.
>post i.
>root-form i.
>silicone i.
>submucosal i.
>subperiosteal i.
>supraperiosteal i.
>testicular i.
>threaded i.
>triplant i.

implantation
>central i.
>circumferential i.
>collagen i.
>i. cone
>cortical i.
>i. cyst
>eccentric i.
>interstitial i.
>nerve i.
>pellet i.
>periosteal i.
>subcutaneous i.
>superficial i.
>i. theory of the production of endometriosis

implanted suture
implosion
implosive therapy
impotence, impotency
>psychic i.
>vasculogenic i.

impregnate
impregnation
impressio, pl. **impressiones**
>i. aortica pulmonis sinistri
>i. cardiaca faciei diaphragmaticae hepatis
>i. cardiaca pulmonis
>i. colica hepatis
>impressiones digitatae
>i. duodenalis hepatis
>i. esophagea hepatis
>i. gastrica hepatis

impressiones gyrorum
>i. ligamenti costoclavicularis
>i. petrosa pallii
>i. renalis hepatis
>i. suprarenalis hepatis
>i. trigeminalis

impression
>aortic i. of left lung
>i. area
>basilar i.
>cardiac i. of diaphragmatic surface of liver
>cardiac i. on lung
>i. of cerebral gyri
>colic i. on liver
>colic i. of spleen
>complete denture i.
>i. compound
>i. for costoclavicular ligament
>deltoid i.
>digitate i.
>direct bone i.
>duodenal i. on liver
>esophageal i. on liver
>i.'s of esophagus
>final i.
>gastric i. on liver
>gastric i. on spleen
>i. material
>mental i.
>partial denture i.
>petrosal i. of the pallium
>preliminary i.
>primary i.
>renal i. on liver
>renal i. of spleen
>rhomboid i.
>sectional i.
>suprarenal i. on liver
>i. tray
>trigeminal i.

impressive aphasia
imprinting
>genomic i.

impromidine
impulse
>apex i.
>cardiac i.
>i. control disorder
>ectopic i.
>escape i.
>irresistible i.
>morbid i.
>right parasternal i.

impulsion
impulsive obsession
impure flutter
imus
IMV
>intermittent mandatory ventilation

IMViC
^{113m}In
>indium-113m

^{111}In
>indium-111

in
> inulin
>> in situ hybridization
>> in situ nucleic acid hybridization

in
>> *in vitro* fertilization
>> *in vivo* fertilization

in-
inaction
inactivate
inactivated
> i. poliovirus vaccine (IPV)
> i. serum

inactivation
> insertional i.
> X i.

inactive
> i. mutant
> i. repressor
> i. tuberculosis

inadequate
> i. personality
> i. stimulus

inanimate
inanition fever
inapparent infection
inappetence
inappropriate
> i. affect
> i. hormone

inarticulate
inassimilable
inattention
> selective i.
> sensory i.
> visual i.

inborn
> i. error of metabolism
> i. lysosomal disease
> i. reflex

inbred
inbreeding
incarcerated
> i. hernia
> i. placenta

incarceration symptom
incarial bone
incarnant
incarnative
incasement theory
incendiarism
incentive
inception rate
incertae sedis
incest barrier
incestuous
incidence
> i. density
> i. rate

incident
> i. angle
> i. point
> i. ray

incidental
> i. learning
> i. parasite

incidentaloma
incipient caries
incisal
> i. edge
> i. embrasure
> i. guidance
> i. guide
> i. guide angle
> i. margin
> i. path
> i. point
> i. rest
> i. surface

incise
incised wound
incision
> i. biopsy
> bucket-handle i.
> celiotomy i.
> chevron i.
> clamshell i.
> collar i.
> Deaver i.
> Dührssen i.
> endaural i.
> Fergusson i.
> flank i.
> Kocher i.
> lumbotomy i.
> McBurney i.
> midline i.
> paramedian i.
> Pfannenstiel i.
> postauricular i.
> transmeatal i.
> transverse abdominal i.

incisional hernia
incisive
> i. bone
> i. canal
> i. canal cyst
> i. duct
> i. foramen
> i. fossa
> i. papilla
> i. suture

incisor
> i. canal
> central i.
> i. crest
> i. foramen
> Hutchinson i.'s
> lateral i.
> second i.
> i. tooth

incisura, pl. incisurae
> i. acetabuli
> i. angularis
> i. anterior auriculae
> i. anterior auris
> i. apicis cordis
> i. cardiaca

incisura *(continued)*
   i. cardiaca pulmonis sinistri
   i. cartilaginis meatus acustici
   i. cerebelli anterior
   i. cerebelli posterior
   i. clavicularis
   incisurae costales
   i. ethmoidalis
   i. fibularis
   i. frontalis
   i. interarytenoidea
   i. intertragica
   i. ischiadica major
   i. ischiadica minor
   i. jugularis ossis occipitalis
   i. jugularis ossis temporalis
   i. jugularis sternalis
   i. lacrimalis
   i. ligamenti teretis hepatis
   i. mandibulae
   i. mastoidea
   i. nasalis
   i. pancreatis
   i. parietalis
   i. preoccipitalis
   i. pterygoidea
   i. radialis
   i. rivini
   i. santorini
   i. scapulae
   i. semilunaris ulnae
   i. sphenopalatina
   i. supraorbitalis
   i. tentorii
   i. of tentorium
   i. terminalis auricularis
   i. terminalis auris
   i. thyroidea inferior
   i. thyroidea superior
   i. tragica
   i. trochlearis
   i. tympanica
   i. ulnaris
   i. umbilicalis
   i. vertebralis
incisure
   angular i.
   Lanterman i.'s
   Rivinus i.
   Santorini i.'s
   Schmidt-Lanterman i.
   tympanic i.
inclinatio, pl. **inclinationes**
   i. pelvis
inclination
   condylar guidance i.
   enamel rod i.
   lateral condylar i.
   pelvic i.
   i. of pelvis
inclinometer
inclusion
   i. blennorrhea
   i. body

   i. body disease
   i. body encephalitis
   cell i.'s
   i. cell
   i. cell disease
   i. compound
   i. conjunctivitis
   i. conjunctivitis virus
   i. cyst
   i. dermoid
   Döhle i.
   fetal i.
   leukocyte i.'s
incoherent
incomitant strabismus
incompatibility
   physiologic i.
   Rh antigen i.
   therapeutic i.
incompatible blood transfusion reaction
incompetence, incompetency
   aortic i.
   cardiac i.
   cardiac valvular i.
   mitral i.
   muscular i.
   pulmonary i.
   pulmonic i.
   pyloric i.
   relative i.
   tricuspid i.
   valvular i.
incompetent cervical os
incomplete
   i. abortion
   i. achromatopsia
   i. agglutinin
   i. alexia
   i. antibody
   i. antigen
   i. ascertainment
   i. atrioventricular block
   i. atrioventricular dissociation
   i. AV dissociation
   i. cleavage
   i. conjoined twin
   i. disinfectant
   i. fistula
   i. foot presentation
   i. fracture
   i. hemianopia
   i. knee presentation
   i. metamorphosis
   i. neurofibromatosis
   i. tetanus
incongruent nystagmus
incongruous hemianopia
inconstant
incontinence
   fecal i.
   i. of feces
   i. of milk
   overflow i.
   paradoxical i.
   passive i.

i. of pigment
reflex i.
stress urinary i. (SUI)
urge i.
urgency i.
urinary exertional i.
i. of urine
incontinent
incontinentia
    i. pigmenti
    i. pigmenti achromians
incoordination
incorporation
increase
    absolute cell i.
    base i. at low levels
    treble i. at low levels
increased markings emphysema
increment
incremental
    i. line
    i. line of von Ebner
incretin
incretion
incrustation
incrusted cystitis
incubation period
incubative stage
incubator
incubatory carrier
incubus
incudal
    i. fold
    i. fossa
incudectomy
incudes (*pl. of* incus)
incudiform uterus
incudomalleal
incudomalleolar
    i. articulation
    i. joint
incudostapedial
    i. articulation
    i. joint
incurable
incurvation
incus, pl. **incudes**
incycloduction
incyclophoria
incyclotropia
in d.
    in dies
indanedione derivative
indanediones
indeciduate
indenization
indentation hardness
independence
    causal i.
    stochastic i.
independent
    i. assortment
    i. practice association (IPA)
    i. variable

indeterminate
    i. cleavage
    i. leprosy
index, pl. **indices, indexes**
    absorbancy i.
    alveolar i.
    i. ametropia
    amnionic fluid i.
    anesthetic i.
    antitryptic i.
    apnea-hypopnea i.
    Arneth i.
    auricular i.
    Ayala i.
    basilar i.
    Bödecker i.
    body mass i.
    buffer i.
    cardiac i.
    i. case
    centromeric i.
    cephalic i.
    cephaloorbital i.
    cerebral i.
    cerebrospinal i.
    chemotherapeutic i.
    chest i.
    cranial i.
    Cumulative I. Medicus
    Dean fluorosis i.
    def caries i.
    degenerative i.
    dental i. (DI)
    DF caries i.
    diet quality i.
    DMFS caries i.
    effective temperature i.
    empathic i.
    endemic i.
    erythrocyte indices
    i. extensor muscle
    facial i.
    i. finger
    Flower dental i.
    free thyroxine i. (FTI)
    glycemic i.
    gnathic i.
    health status i.
    height-length i.
    i. hypermetropia
    i. index
    international sensitivity i. (ISI)
    iron i.
    karyopyknotic i.
    length-breadth i.
    length-height i.
    leukopenic i.
    maturation i.
    metacarpal i.
    mitotic i.
    molar absorbancy i.
    i. myopia
    nasal i.
    nucleoplasmic i.
    obesity i.

index *(continued)*
    opsonic i.
    orbital i.
    orbitonasal i.
    palatal i.
    palatine i.
    palatomaxillary i.
    Pearl i.
    pelvic i.
    Periodontal Disease I. (PDI)
    phagocytic i.
    Pirquet i.
    Plaque I.
    PMA i.
    ponderal i.
    pressure-volume i.
    pulsatility i.
    refractive i. *(n)*
    Robinson i.
    Röhrer i.
    root caries i.
    sacral i.
    saturation i.
    Schilling i.
    shock i.
    short increment sensitivity i.
    small increment sensitivity i.
    spiro-i.
    splenic i.
    staphyloopsonic i.
    stroke work i.
    superior facial i.
    therapeutic i.
    thoracic i.
    tibiofemoral i.
    total facial i.
    transversovertical i.
    tuberculoopsonic i.
    ultraviolet i.
    uricolytic i.
    vertical i.
    vital i.
    Volpe-Manhold i. (V-MI)
    volume i.
    zygomaticoauricular i.
indexical sign
India ink capsule stain
Indian
    I. flap
    I. ginger
    I. gum
    I. podophyllum
    I. podophyllum resin
    I. sickness
    I. tick typhus
indican
    metabolic i.
    plant i.
indicanidrosis
indicant
indicanuria
indication
    causal i.
    off-label i.

    specific i.
    symptomatic i.
indicator
    alizarin i.
    clinical i.
    i. dilution method
    health i.
    oxidation-reduction i.
    redox i.
    i. system
    i. yellow
indicator-dilution curve
indices (*pl. of* index)
indicis
Indiella
indifference to pain syndrome
indifferent
    i. cell
    i. electrode
    i. genitalia
    i. gonad
    i. neutrotaxis
    i. oxide
    i. tissue
    i. water
indigenous
indigestion
    acid i.
    fat i.
    gastric i.
    nervous i.
indigo
    i. blue
    i. carmine
indigotin
indigouria, indiguria
indirect
    i. agglutination
    i. assay
    i. calorimetry
    i. Coombs test
    i. diuretic
    i. fluorescent antibody test
    i. fracture
    i. fulguration
    i. hemagglutination test
    i. immunofluorescence
    i. inguinal hernia
    i. laryngoscopy
    i. lead
    i. maternal death
    i. method for making inlays
    i. nuclear division
    i. ophthalmoscope
    i. ophthalmoscopy
    i. ovular transmigration
    i. oxidase
    i. pulp capping
    i. pupillary reaction
    i. ray
    i. reacting bilirubin
    i. retainer
    i. retention
    i. technique

i. transfusion
i. vision
indisposition
indium
indium-111 (^{111}In)
i. chloride
i. trichloride
indium-113m (^{113m}In)
individual
i. difference
i. psychology
i. therapy
i. thromboxane (TX)
i. tolerance
individuation field
indocyanine green
i. g. angiography
indocybin
indolaceturia
indolamine
indolent
i. bubo
i. ulcer
indole test
indolic acid
indologenous
indoluria
indolyl
indomethacin
indophenolase
indophenol method
indophenol oxidase
indoramin
indoxyl
indoxyluria
induce
induced
i. abortion
i. apnea
i. enzyme
i. fever
i. fit
i. fit model
i. hypotension
i. malaria
i. mutation
i. phagocytosis
i. psychotic disorder
i. radioactivity
i. sensitivity
i. symptom
i. trance
inducer
i. cell
embryonal i.
gratuitous i.
inducible enzyme
inductance
induction
i. chemotherapy
electromagnetic i.
lysogenic i.
i. period
spinal i.
inductive resistance

inductor
inductorium
inductotherm
inductothermy
indulin
indulinophil, indulinophile
indurated
induration
brown i. of the lung
cyanotic i.
gray i.
pigment i. of the lung
plastic i.
red i.
indurative myocarditis
indusium, pl. **indusia**
i. griseum
industrial
i. disease
i. hearing loss
i. hygiene
i. methylated spirit
i. psychiatry
i. psychology
indwelling catheter
inebriant
inebriation
inebriety
Inermicapsifer
Inermicapsifer madagascariensis
inert gas
inertia
magnetic i.
primary uterine i.
psychic i.
secondary uterine i.
i. time
true uterine i.
uterine i.
inevitable abortion
infancy
infant
i. death
i. Hercules
liveborn i.
i. mortality rate
postmature i.
postterm i.
preterm i.
stillborn i.
term i.
infanticide
infantile
i. acropustulosis
i. acute hemorrhagic edema of the skin
i. autism
i. beriberi
i. cataract
i. celiac disease
i. colic
i. convulsion
i. cortical hyperostosis
i. digital fibromatosis
i. diplegia

infantile *(continued)*
    i. dwarfism
    i. eczema
    i. fibrosarcoma
    i. gastroenteritis
    i. gastroenteritis virus
    i., generalized G_{M1} gangliosidosis
    i. G_{M2} gangliosidosis
    i. hemiplegia
    i. hernia
    i. hypothyroidism
    i. leishmaniasis
    i. myofibromatosis
    i. myxedema
    i. neuroaxonal dystrophy
    i. neuronal degeneration
    i. osteomalacia
    i. pellagra
    i. progressive spinal muscular atrophy
    i. purulent conjunctivitis
    i. scurvy
    i. sexuality
    i. spasm
    i. spastic paraplegia
    i. tetany
infantilism
    Brissaud i.
    dysthyroidal i.
    hepatic i.
    hypophysial i.
    hypothyroid i.
    idiopathic i.
    Lorain-Lévi i.
    myxedematous i.
    pancreatic i.
    pituitary i.
    proportionate i.
    renal i.
    sexual i.
    static i.
    tubal i.
    universal i.
infarct
    anemic i.
    bland i.
    bone i.
    Brewer i.'s
    embolic i.
    hemorrhagic i.
    pale i.
    red i.
    Roesler-Dressler i.
    septic i.
    thrombotic i.
    uric acid i.
    white i.
    Zahn i.
infarction
    anterior myocardial i.
    anteroinferior myocardial i.
    anterolateral myocardial i.
    anteroseptal myocardial i.
    apical i.

    cardiac i.
    diaphragmatic myocardial i.
    Freiberg i.
    inferior myocardial i.
    inferolateral myocardial i.
    lateral myocardial i.
    myocardial i. (MI)
    nontransmural myocardial i. (NTMI)
    posterior myocardial i.
    silent myocardial i.
    subendocardial myocardial i.
    thrombolysis in myocardial i. (TIMI)
    through-and-through myocardial i.
    transmural myocardial i.
    watershed i.
infect
infected abortion
infection
    agonal i.
    airborne i.
    apical i.
    i. calculus
    i. control nurse
    cross i.
    cryptogenic i.
    disseminated gonococcal i.
    droplet i.
    endogenous i.
    focal i.
    holomiantic (i.)
    i. immunity
    inapparent i.
    latent i.
    mass i.
    mixed i.
    pyogenic i.
    Salinem i.
    scalp i.
    secondary i.
    terminal i.
    i. transmission parameter
    urinary tract i. (UTI)
    vector-borne i.
    Vincent i.
    zoonotic i.
infection-associated hemophagocytic syndrome (IAHS)
infection-exhaustion psychosis
infection-immunity
infectiosity
infectious
    i. anemia
    i. crystalline keratopathy
    i. disease
    i. ectromelia virus
    i. eczematoid dermatitis
    i. endocarditis
    i. granuloma
    i. hepatitis (IH)
    i. hepatitis virus
    i. icterus
    i. jaundice
    i. mononucleosis
    i. myositis

I

i. nucleic acid
i. papilloma virus
i. plasmid
i. polyneuritis
i. porcine encephalomyelitis virus
i. wart
infectiousness
infective
i. disease
i. embolism
i. endocarditis
i. jaundice
i. thrombus
infectivity
infecundity
inference
inferential statistic
inferior
i. aberrant ductule
i. accessory fissure
i. alveolar artery
i. alveolar nerve
i. anal nerve
i. anastomotic vein
i. angle of scapula
i. articular facet of atlas
i. articular pit of atlas
i. articular process
i. articular surface of atlas
i. articular surface of tibia
i. basal vein
i. belly of omohyoid muscle
i. border
i. border of body of pancreas
i. border of liver
i. border of lung
i. border of pancreas
i. border of spleen
i. branch
i. branch of oculomotor nerve
i. branch of pubic bone
i. branch of superior gluteal artery
i. branch of transverse cervical
   nerve
i. calcaneonavicular ligament
i. cardiac vein
i. carotid triangle
i. cerebellar peduncle
i. cerebral surface
i. cerebral vein
i. cervical cardiac branch of vagus
   nerve
i. cervical cardiac nerve
i. cervical ganglion
i. choroid vein
i. clunial nerve
i. colliculus
i. constrictor muscle of pharynx
i. costal facet
i. costal pit
i. dental arch
i. dental artery
i. dental branch of inferior dental
   plexus
i. dental canal

i. dental foramen
i. dental nerve
i. dental plexus
i. dental rami
i. duodenal flexure
i. duodenal fold
i. duodenal fossa
i. duodenal recess
i. epigastric artery
i. epigastric lymph node
i. epigastric vein
i. esophageal constriction
i. esophageal sphincter
i. extensor retinaculum
i. extremity
i. extremity of kidney
i. eyelid
i. fascia of pelvic diaphragm
i. fascia of urogenital diaphragm
i. fibular retinaculum
i. fovea
i. frontal convolution
i. frontal gyrus
i. frontal sulcus
i. ganglion of glossopharyngeal
   nerve
i. ganglion of vagus nerve
i. gemellus muscle
i. gingival branch of inferior dental
   plexus
i. gluteal artery
i. gluteal nerve
i. gluteal vein
i. hemiazygos vein
i. hemorrhoidal artery
i. hemorrhoidal nerve
i. hemorrhoidal plexus
i. hemorrhoidal vein
i. horn
i. horn of falciform margin of
   saphenous opening
i. horn of lateral ventricle
i. horn of thyroid cartilage
i. hypogastric plexus
i. hypophysial artery
i. ileocecal recess
i. internal parietal artery
i. labial artery
i. labial branch of facial artery
i. labial branch of mental nerve
i. labial vein
i. laryngeal artery
i. laryngeal cavity
i. laryngeal nerve
i. laryngeal vein
i. laryngotomy
i. lateral brachial cutaneous nerve
i. lateral cutaneous nerve of arm
i. lateral genicular artery
i. ligament of epididymis
i. limb
i. limb of ansa cervicalis
i. lingual muscle
i. lingular artery

inferior *(continued)*

i. lingular branch of lingular branch of left pulmonary artery
i. lingular segment [S V]
i. lobar artery
i. lobe of (left/right) lung
i. longitudinal fasciculus
i. longitudinal muscle of tongue
i. longitudinal sinus
i. lumbar triangle
i. macular arteriole
i. macular venule
i. margin
i. maxillary nerve
i. medial genicular artery
i. mediastinum
i. medullary velum
i. member
i. mesenteric artery
i. mesenteric ganglion
i. mesenteric lymph node
i. mesenteric plexus
i. mesenteric vein
i. myocardial infarction
i. nasal arteriole of retina
i. nasal colliculus
i. nasal concha
i. nasal retinal venule
i. nasal venule of retina
i. nuchal line
i. oblique muscle
i. oblique muscle of head
i. occipital gyrus
i. occipital triangle
i. occipitofrontal fasciculus
i. olivary complex
i. olivary nucleus
i. olive
i. omental recess
i. ophthalmic vein
i. orbital fissure
i. palpebral (arterial) arch
i. palpebral vein
i. pancreatic artery
i. pancreaticoduodenal artery
i. parietal gyrus
i. parietal lobule
i. part
i. part of duodenum
i. part of lingular vein
i. part of trapezius muscle
i. part of vestibular ganglion
i. part of vestibulocochlear nerve
i. pelvic aperture
i. peroneal retinaculum
i. petrosal groove
i. petrosal sinus
i. petrosal sulcus
i. phrenic artery
i. phrenic lymph node
i. phrenic vein
i. pole
i. pole of kidney
i. pole of testis

i. polioencephalitis
i. posterior serratus muscle
i. pubic ligament
i. pubic ramus
i. quadrigeminal brachium
i. radioulnar joint
i. recess of omental bursa
i. rectal artery
i. rectal nerve
i. rectal plexus
i. rectal vein
i. rectus muscle
i. renal segment
i. retinaculum of extensor muscle
i. root of ansa cervicalis
i. sagittal sinus
i. salivary nucleus
i. salivatory nucleus
i. segment
i. segmental artery of kidney
i. semilunar lobule
i. strait
i. subtendinous bursa of biceps femoris
i. and superior lobar artery
i. suprarenal artery
i. surface of cerebellar hemisphere
i. surface of petrous part of temporal bone
i. surface of tongue
i. tarsal muscle
i. tarsus
i. temporal convolution
i. temporal gyrus
i. temporal line of parietal bone
i. temporal retinal arteriole
i. temporal retinal venule
i. temporal sulcus
i. temporal venule of retina
i. thalamic peduncle
i. thalamic radiation
i. thalamostriate vein
i. thoracic aperture
i. thyroid artery
i. thyroid notch
i. thyroid plexus
i. thyroid tubercle
i. thyroid vein
i. tibiofibular joint
i. tracheobronchial lymph node
i. transverse scapular ligament
i. triangle sign
i. trunk of brachial plexus
i. turbinated bone
i. tympanic artery
i. ulnar collateral artery
i. vein of cerebellar hemisphere
i. vein of vermis
i. vena cava (IVC)
i. ventricular vein
i. vesical artery
i. vesical venous plexus
i. vestibular area
i. vestibular nucleus

i. wall of orbit
i. wall of tympanic cavity
inferiority complex
inferolateral
i. margin
i. margin of cerebral hemisphere
i. myocardial infarction
i. surface of prostate
inferomedial margin of cerebral hemisphere
infertile male syndrome
infertility
infest
infestation
infibulation
infiltrate
Assmann tuberculous i.
infraclavicular i.
infiltration
adipose i.
i. anesthesia
calcareous i.
cellular i.
epituberculous i.
fatty i.
gelatinous i.
gray i.
lipomatous i.
paraneural i.
perineural i.
infinite distance
infinity
infirm
infirmary
infirmity
inflamed ulcer
inflammable
inflammation
active i.
acute i.
adhesive i.
allergic i.
alterative i.
atrophic i.
catarrhal i.
chronic active i.
degenerative i.
exudative i.
fibrinopurulent i.
fibrinous i.
fibroid i.
granulomatous i.
hyperplastic i.
immune i.
interstitial i.
necrotic i.
necrotizing i.
productive i.
proliferative i.
pseudomembranous i.
purulent i.
sclerosing i.
serofibrinous i.
serous i.

subacute i.
suppurative i.
inflammatory
i. carcinoma
i. corpuscle
i. edema
i. fibrous hyperplasia
i. linear verrucous epidermal nevus
i. lymph
i. macrophage
i. papillary hyperplasia
i. polyp
i. pseudotumor
i. rheumatism
inflatable
i. implant
i. splint
inflation
inflator
inflection, inflexion
influenza
i. A, B, C
Asian i.
i. bacillus
endemic i.
Hong Kong i.
i. nostras
i. pneumonia
Russian i.
Spanish i.
swine i.
i. virus
i. virus vaccine
influenzal virus pneumonia
infold
informatics
information
i. system
i. theory
informational RNA
informed consent
informofer
informosomes
infraauricular
i. deep parotid lymph node
i. subfascial parotid lymph node
infraaxillary
infrabony pocket
infrabulge
infracardiac bursa
infracerebral
infraclavicular
i. fossa
i. infiltrate
i. part of brachial plexus
i. triangle
infraclinoid aneurysm
infraclusion
infracortical
infracostal line
infracotyloid
infracristal
infraction
infradentale
infradian

infradiaphragmatic
infraduction
infraduodenal fossa
infraglenoid
    i. tubercle
    i. tuberosity
infraglottic
    i. cavity
    i. space
infragranular layer
infrahepatic
infrahyoid
    i. branch of superior thyroid artery
    i. bursa
    i. muscle
infralobar part of posterior vein
inframamillary
inframammary region
inframandibular
inframarginal
inframaxillary
infranatant fluid
infraocclusion
infraorbital
    i. artery
    i. canal
    i. foramen
    i. groove
    i. margin
    i. nerve
    i. region
    i. suture
infraorbitomeatal plane
infrapalpebral sulcus
infrapatellar
    i. branch of saphenous nerve
    i. fat body
    i. fat pad
    i. synovial fold
infrapsychic
infrared (IR)
    i. cataract
    i. light
    i. microscope
    i. ray
    i. spectroscopy
    i. spectrum
    i. thermography
infrascapular
    i. artery
    i. region
infrasegmental
    i. part
    i. vein
infrasonic
infraspinatus
    i. bursa
    i. fascia
    i. muscle
infraspinous
    i. fascia
    i. fossa
infrasplenic
infrasternal angle
infrasubspecific

infratemporal
    i. approach
    i. crest of greater wing of
      sphenoid
    i. fossa
    i. surface of (body of) maxilla
    i. surface of greater wing of
      sphenoid
infrathoracic
infratonsillar
infratrochlear nerve
infraumbilical
infraversion
infriction
infundibula (*pl. of* infundibulum)
infundibular
    i. part
    i. recess
    i. stalk
    i. stem
    i. stenosis
infundibulectomy
infundibuliform
    i. fascia
    i. hymen
    i. sheath
infundibulin
infundibuloma
infundibulo-ovarian ligament
infundibulopelvic ligament
infundibulum, pl. infundibula
    ethmoid i.
    ethmoidal i.
    i. ethmoidale
    i. of gallbladder
    i. hypophysis
    i. hypothalami
    hypothalamic i.
    i. of lung
    i. of pituitary gland
    i. of right ventricle
    i. tubae uterinae
    i. of uterine tube
    i. vesicae biliaris
    i. vesicae felleae
infusible
infusion
infusion-aspiration drainage
Infusoria
infusorian
Ingelfinger rule
ingesta
ingestion
ingestive
Ingrassia process
ingravescent
ingrowing toenail
ingrown
    i. hair
    i. nail
inguen
inguinal
    i. aponeurotic fold
    i. branch of deep external pudendal
      artery

i. canal
i. crest
i. falx
i. fossa
i. hernia
i. ligament
i. ligament of the kidney
i. lymphatic plexus
i. part of ductus deferens
i. region
i. triangle
i. trigone
inguinocrural hernia
inguinodynia
inguinolabial hernia
inguinoperitoneal
inguinoscrotal hernia
inguinosuperficial hernia
INH
isonicotinic acid hydrazide
inhalant
inhalation
i. analgesia
i. anesthesia
i. anesthetic
solvent i.
i. therapy
inhale
inhaler
metered-dose i.
inherent
inheritance
alternative i.
blending i.
codominant i.
collateral i.
cytoplasmic i.
dominant i.
extrachromosomal i.
extranuclear i.
galtonian i.
holandric i.
hologynic i.
maternal i.
mendelian i.
mosaic i.
multifactorial i.
polygenic i.
recessive i.
sex-influenced i.
sex-limited i.
sex-linked i.
X-linked i.
Y-linked i.
inherited
i. albumin variants
i. character
inhibin
inhibit
inhibitine
inhibiting antibody
inhibition
allogenic i.
central i.
competitive i.

contact i.
end product i.
i. factor
feedback i.
hapten i. of precipitation
hemagglutination i.
noncompetitive i.
potassium i.
proactive i.
product i.
reciprocal i.
reflex i.
residual i.
retroactive i.
selective i.
substrate i.
uncompetitive i.
Wedensky i.
inhibitor
alpha-glucosidase i.
5alpha-reductase i.
$alpha_1$-trypsin i.
angiotensin-converting enzyme i.
(ACEI)
aromatase i.
beta-lactamase i.'s
Bowman-Birk i.
carbonate dehydratase i.
carbonic anhydrase i.
C1 esterase i.
cholinesterase i.
familial lipoprotein lipase i.
glucosidase i.'s
HMG CoA-reductase i.'s
human $alpha_1$-protease i.
lipoprotein-associated coagulation i.
(LACI)
mechanism-based i.
monoamine oxidase i. (MAOI)
ovulation i.
protease i.
proton pump i.
residual i.
respiratory i.
selective norepinephrine reuptake i.
selective serotonin reuptake i.
serine protease i.
serotonin norepinephrine reuptake i.
suicide i.
trypsin i.
uncompetitive i.
inhibitory
i. fiber
i. junction potential (IJP)
i. nerve
i. obsession
i. postsynaptic potential (IPSP)
iniac
iniad
inial
iniencephaly
inion
iniopagus
iniops

initial
    i. contact
    i. dose
    i. heat
    i. hematuria
    i. rate
    i. velocity
initiating
    i. agent
    i. codon
initiation
    i. codon
    i. factor (IF)
    i. tRNA
initis
inject
injectable
injected
injection
    adrenal cortex i.
    collagen i.
    depot i.
    i. flask
    hypodermic i.
    insulin i.
    intracytoplasmic sperm i.
    intrathecal i.
    intraventricular i.
    jet i.
    lactated Ringer i.
    i. mass
    i. molding
    Regular insulin i.
    Ringer i.
    selective i.
    sensitizing i.
    test i.
    Z-tract i.
injector
    jet i.
    power i.
injure
injury
    blast i.
    brachial plexus i.
    closed head i.
    contrecoup i. of brain
    coup i. of brain
    current of i.
    degloving i.
    egg-white i.
    flexion-extension i.
    hyperextension-hyperflexion i.
    i. of intervertebral disk
    open head i.
    pneumatic tire i.
    i. potential
    reperfusion i.
    steering wheel i.
    whiplash i.
inkblot test
inlay
    epithelial i.
    gold i.
    i. graft

    porcelain i.
    i. wax
inlet
    laryngeal i.
    i. of larynx
    pelvic i.
    thoracic i.
innate
    i. heat
    i. immunity
    i. reflex
inner
    i. border of iris
    i. cell mass
    i. cone fiber
    i. dental epithelium
    i. ear
    i. enamel epithelium
    i. layer of eyeball
    i. limiting layer
    i. lip of iliac crest
    i. malleolus
    i. membrane
    i. nuclear layer
    i. plexiform layer
    i. sheath of optic nerve
    i. spiral sulcus
    i. stripe of renal medulla
    i. table of skull
    i. zone of renal medulla
innermost intercostal muscle
innervation
    i. apraxia
    reciprocal i.
innidiation
innocent
    i. bystander cell
    i. murmur
    i. tumor
innocuous
innominatal
innominate
    i. artery
    i. bone
    i. cardiac vein
    i. fossa
    i. substance
innoxious
INO
    internuclear ophthalmoplegia
Ino
ino
inoculability
inoculable
inoculate
inoculation
    stress i.
inoculum
Inocybe
inopectic
inoperable
inopexia
inorganic
    i. acid
    i. catalyst

i. chemistry
i. compound
i. dental cement
i. diphosphatase
i. murmur
i. orthophosphate
i. phosphate (Pi)
i. pyrophosphatase (PP$_i$)
inosamine
inoscopy
inose
inosemia
inosinate
inosine
cyclic i. 3,5-monophosphate (cIMP)
i. 5′-diphosphate (IDP)
i. 5′-monophosphate (IMP)
i. pranobex
i. 5′-triphosphate
inosine 5′-monophosphate (IMP)
IMP dehydrogenase
inosine 5′-triphosphate
inosinic acid
inosinicase
inosinyl
inosite
inositide
inositol
i. niacinate
i. 1,3,4,5-tetraphosphate
i. 1,4,5-trisphosphate (IP$_3$)
meso-**inositol**
myo-**inositol**
inosituria
inosuria
inotropic
i. agent
negatively i.
positively i.
Inoviridae
inquest
inquiline parasite
INR
international normalized ratio
insalubrious
insane
insanitary
insanity
criminal i.
i. defense
inscription
tendinous i.
inscriptio tendinea
Insecta
insectarium
insecticide
insectifuge
Insectivora
insectivorous
insect virus
insecurity
insemination
artificial i.
donor i.
heterologous i.

homologous i.
intrauterine i. (IUI)
insenescence
insensible
i. perspiration
i. thirst
insert
insertion
parasol i.
i. sequence
velamentous i.
insertional
i. inactivation
i. mutagenesis
insheathed
insidious
insight learning
insolation
insoluble soap
insomnia
conditioned i.
subjective i.
insomniac
insorption
inspection
visual i. with acetic acid
inspersion
inspiration
crowing i.
inspiratory
i. capacity
i. center
i. reserve volume (IRV)
i. stridor
inspire
inspired gas
inspirometer
inspissate
inspissated
i. bile syndrome
i. cerumen
inspissation
inspissator
instability
detrusor i.
spinal i.
instantaneous
i. electrical axis
i. vector
instar
instep
instillation
instillator
instinct
aggressive i.
death i.
ego i.'s
herd i.
life i.
sexual i.
social i.
instinctive, instinctual
institutional review board (IRB)
instructive theory

instrument
 diamond cutting i.
 hearing i.
 Krueger i. stop
 plugging i.
 purse-string i.
 Sabouraud-Noiré i.
 stereotactic i.
 test handle i.
instrumental
 i. amusia
 i. conditioning
instrumentarium
instrumentation
insuccation
insudate
insufficiency
 accommodative i.
 acute adrenocortical i.
 adrenocortical i.
 aortic i.
 cardiac i.
 chronic adrenocortical i.
 convergence i.
 coronary i.
 divergence i.
 exocrine pancreatic i.
 hepatic i.
 latent adrenocortical i.
 mitral i.
 muscular i.
 myocardial i.
 parathyroid i.
 partial adrenocortical i.
 primary adrenocortical i.
 pulmonary i.
 pyloric i.
 renal i.
 respiratory i.
 secondary adrenocortical i.
 thyroid i.
 tricuspid i.
 uterine i.
 valvular i.
 velopharyngeal i.
 venous i.
insufflate
insufflation
 i. anesthesia
 perirenal i.
 peritoneal i.
insufflator
insula, pl. **insulae**
 Haller i.
insular
 i. area
 i. artery
 i. cortex
 i. gyri
 i. hypothesis
 i. lobe
 i. part
 i. part of middle cerebral artery
 i. sclerosis
 i. vein

insulate
insulation
insulator
insulin
 i. antagonist
 biphasic i.
 i. coma therapy
 i. coma treatment
 globin i.
 globin zinc i.
 human i.
 i. hypoglycemia test
 immunoreactive i.
 i. injection
 isophane i.
 lente i.
 i. lipoatrophy
 i. lipodystrophy
 lispro i.
 NPH i.
 protamine zinc i.
 i. receptor substrate-1 (IRS-1)
 Regular i.
 i. resistance
 semilente i.
 i. shock
 i. shock treatment
 ultralente i.
 i. unit
 i. zinc suspension
insulin-dependent diabetes mellitus (IDDM)
insulinemia
insulinlike
 i. activity (ILA)
 i. growth factor (IGF)
insulinogenesis
insulinogenic, insulogenic
insulinoma
insulinopenic diabetes
insulitis
insulogenic (*var. of* insulinogenic)
insult
insurance
 fee-for-service i.
insusceptibility
int. cib.
 inter cibos
integral
 i. dose
 i. protein
integrated rate expression
integration
 personality i.
integrins
integrity
 marginal i. of amalgam
integument
integumentary system
integumentum commune
intellectual aura
intellectualization
intelligence
 abstract i.
 artificial i.

measured i.
mechanical i.
i. quotient (IQ)
social i.
i. test
intemperance
intensification chemotherapy
intensifying screen
intensity
luminous i.
performance i.
radiant i.
i. of sound
intensive
i. care
i. care unit (ICU)
i. psychotherapy
intention
i. spasm
i. tremor
intentional replantation
intention-to-treat analysis
interacinar
interacinous
interaction
apolar i.
drug i.
hydrophobic i.
i. process analysis
interalveolar
i. pore
i. septum
i. space
interannular segment
interarch distance
interarticular
i. fibrocartilage
i. joint
interarytenoid
i. fold
i. notch
interasteric
interatrial
i. block
i. conduction time
i. foramen primum
i. foramen secundum
i. septum
interaural attenuation
interauricular arc
interbody
intercadence
intercadent
intercalary
i. neuron
i. staphyloma
intercalated
i. disk
i. duct
i. nucleus
intercalation
intercanalicular
intercapillary
i. cell
i. glomerulosclerosis

intercapitular vein
intercarotid, intercarotic
i. body
i. nerve
intercarpal
i. joint
i. ligament
intercartilaginous
i. part of glottic opening
i. part of rima glottidis
intercavernous sinus
intercellular
i. adhesion molecule-1 (CD 54, ICAM-1)
i. bridge
i. canaliculus
i. cement
i. digestion
i. junction
i. lymph
intercentral
interceptive occlusal contact
intercerebral
interchondral
i. articulation
i. joint
inter cibos (int. cib.)
intercilium
interclavicular
i. ligament
i. notch
interclinoid ligament
intercoccygeal
intercolumnar
i. fasciae
i. fiber
i. tubercle
intercondylar, intercondyloid
i. eminence
i. fossa
i. line of femur
i. notch
i. tubercle
interconversion
enzyme i.
intercornual ligament
intercostal
i. anesthesia
i. artery
i. ligament
i. lymph node
i. membrane
i. nerve
i. neuralgia
i. space
i. vein
intercostobrachial nerve
intercostohumeralis
intercostohumeral nerve
intercourse
sexual i.
intercricothyrotomy
intercrine
intercristal
intercross

intercrural
  i. fiber of superficial ring
  i. ganglion
intercuneiform
  i. joint
  i. ligament
intercurrent disease
intercuspal position
intercuspation
intercusping
intercutaneomucous
interdeferential
interdental
  i. canal
  i. caries
  i. papilla
  i. septum
  i. splint
interdentium
interdigit
interdigital fold
interdigitating reticulum cell
interdigitation
interdisciplinary
interectopic interval
interface
  crystalline i.
  dermoepidermal i.
  metal i.
  structural i.
interfacial
  i. canal
  i. surface tension
interfascial space
interfascicular fasciculus
interfemoral
interference
  bacterial i.
  i. beat
  cuspal i.
  i. dissociation
  i. microscope
interferometer
  electron i.
interferometry
  electron i.
interferon (IFN)
  i. alfa 2b
  i. alpha (IFN-alpha)
  antigen i.
  i. beta (IFN-beta)
  i. beta 1b
  fibroblast i.
  i. gamma (IFN-gamma)
  immune i.
  leukocyte i.
  i.-omega
  i.-tau
  trophoblast i.
  type I, II i.
interferon-beta2
interfibrillar
interfibrous
interfilamentous
interfoveolar ligament

interfrontal
interganglionic branch of sympathetic trunk
intergemmal
intergenal
intergenic
  i. complementation
  i. suppression
interglobular
  i. dentin
  i. space
  i. space of Owen
intergluteal cleft
intergonial
intergyral
interhemicerebral
interictal
interiliac lymph node
interim denture
interior
interischiadic
interjudge reliability
interkinesis
interlamellar
interlaminar jelly
interleukin
  recombinant human i.-11 (rhIL-11)
interleukin-1 (IL-1)
interleukin-2 (IL-2)
interleukin-3 (IL-3)
interleukin-4 (IL-4)
interleukin-5 (IL-5)
interleukin-6 (IL-6)
interleukin-7 (IL-7)
interleukin-8 (IL-8)
interleukin-9 (IL-9)
interleukin-10 (IL-10)
interleukin-11 (IL-11)
interleukin-12 (IL-12)
interleukin-13 (IL-13)
interleukin-14 (IL-14)
interleukin-15 (IL-15)
interleukin-16 (IL-16)
interleukin-17 (IL-17)
interleukin-18 (IL-18)
interlobar
  i. artery
  i. artery of kidney
  i. duct
  i. surface of lung
  i. vein of kidney
interlobitis
interlobular
  i. artery
  i. artery of kidney
  i. artery of liver
  i. duct
  i. ductule
  i. emphysema
  i. pleurisy
  i. septum
  i. vein of kidney
  i. vein of liver
interlocal additivity
interlocking gyri

intermalleolar
intermammary
intermammillary
intermarriage
intermaxilla
intermaxillary
    i. anchorage
    i. bone
    i. elastic
    i. fixation
    i. relation
    i. segment
    i. suture
    i. traction
intermediary
    i. metabolism
    i. movement
    i. nerve
    i. system
intermediate
    i. abutment
    i. acoustic stria
    i. amputation
    i. antebrachial vein
    i. atrial branch of left coronary artery
    i. atrial branch of right coronary artery
    i. basilic vein
    i. body of Flemming
    i. branch of hepatic artery proper
    i. bronchus
    i. cephalic vein
    i. cervical septum
    i. column
    i. cubital vein
    i. cuneiform bone
    i. density lipoprotein (IDL)
    i. disk
    i. dorsal cutaneous nerve
    i. filament
    i. ganglia
    i. great muscle
    i. heart
    i. hemorrhage
    i. hepatic vein
    i. host
    i. hypothalamic area
    i. hypothalamic region
    i. junction
    i. lacunar lymph node
    i. lacunar node
    i. lamella
    i. laryngeal cavity
    i. layer
    i. line of iliac crest
    i. lumbar lymph node
    i. mass
    i. mesoderm
    i. nerve
    i. part
    i. part of adenohypophysis
    i. part of male urethra
    i. part of vestibular bulb
    i. ray

    replicative i.
    i. sacral crest
    i. supraclavicular nerve
    i. temporal artery
    i. temporal branch of lateral occipital artery
    i. trait
    i. uveitis
    i. variable
    i. vastus muscle
    i. vein of forearm
    i. white layer of superior colliculus
    i. zone
    i. zone of iliac crest
intermedin
intermediolateral
    i. cell column of spinal cord (IML)
    i. nucleus
intermediomedial
    i. frontal branch of callosomarginal artery
    i. nucleus
intermedius
intermembrane space
intermembranous
    i. part of glottic opening
    i. part of rima glottidis
intermeningeal
intermenstrual pain
intermesenteric
    i. arterial anastomoses
    i. plexus
intermetacarpal joint
intermetameric
intermetatarsal
    i. articulation
    i. joint
intermetatarseum
intermission
intermit
intermittence
intermittent
    i. acute porphyria (IAP)
    i. albuminuria
    i. arthralgia
    i. claudication
    i. cramp
    i. explosive disorder
    i. hemoglobinuria
    i. hydrarthrosis
    i. hydrosalpinx
    i. malaria
    i. malarial fever
    i. mandatory ventilation (IMV)
    i. positive pressure breathing (IPPB)
    i. positive pressure ventilation (IPPV)
    i. pulse
    i. reinforcement schedule
    i. self-obturation
    i. sterilization
intermuscular
    i. gluteal bursa
    i. septum

intern
internal
    i. acoustic foramen
    i. acoustic meatus
    i. acoustic opening
    i. acoustic pore
    i. adhesive pericarditis
    i. anal sphincter
    i. arcuate fiber
    i. attachment
    i. auditory artery
    i. auditory foramen
    i. auditory meatus
    i. auditory vein
    i. axis of eye
    i. base of skull
    i. branch of superior laryngeal nerve
    i. branch of trunk of accessory nerve
    i. canthus
    i. capsule
    i. capsule syndrome
    i. carotid artery
    i. carotid nerve
    i. carotid venous plexus
    i. cephalic version
    i. cerebral vein
    i. collateral ligament of the wrist
    i. conjugate
    i. conversion electron
    i. decompression
    i. ear
    i. energy (U)
    i. female genital organ
    i. fixation
    i. hemorrhage
    i. hemorrhoid
    i. hernia
    i. hydrocephalus
    i. iliac artery
    i. iliac lymph node
    i. iliac vein
    i. inguinal ring
    i. intercostal membrane
    i. intercostal muscle
    i. jugular vein
    i. lacrimal fistula
    i. limiting membrane
    i. lip of iliac crest
    i. male genital organ
    i. malleolus
    i. mammary artery
    i. mammary plexus
    i. maxillary artery
    i. maxillary plexus
    i. medicine (IM)
    i. medullary lamina
    i. meningitis
    i. naris
    i. nasal branch
    i. nostril
    i. oblique muscle
    i. obturator muscle
    i. occipital crest

    i. occipital protuberance
    i. ophthalmopathy
    i. ophthalmoplegia
    i. ovular transmigration
    i. phase
    i. pillar cell
    i. podalic version
    i. pterygoid muscle
    i. pudendal artery
    i. pudendal vein
    i. pyocephalus
    i. ramus of accessory nerve
    i. representation
    i. resorption
    i. respiration
    i. root sheath
    i. salivary gland
    i. saphenous nerve
    i. semilunar fibrocartilage of knee joint
    i. sheath of optic nerve
    i. spermatic artery
    i. spermatic fascia
    i. sphincter muscle of anus
    i. spiral sulcus
    i. squint
    i. surface
    i. surface of cranial base
    i. surface of frontal bone
    i. surface of parietal bone
    i. table of calvaria
    i. thoracic artery
    i. thoracic lymphatic plexus
    i. thoracic vein
    i. traction
    i. urethral opening
    i. urethral orifice
    i. urethral sphincter
    i. urethrotomy
internalization
internalized homophobia
internarial
internasal suture
international
    I. Classification of Diseases (ICD, ICDA)
    I. Classification of Health Problems in Primary Care (ICHPPC)
    I. Committee of the Red Cross
    I. Labour Organization Classification
    i. normalized ratio (INR)
    i. sensitivity index (ISI)
    i. unit (IU)
International Anatomical Nomenclature Committee (IANC)
International Classification of Impairments, Disabilities and Handicaps (ICIDH)
International Commission on Radiological Protection (ICRP)
International Union of Biochemistry (IUB)
International Union of Pure and Applied Chemistry (IUPAC)
interne

internet addiction disorder
interneuromeric cleft
interneurons
internist
internodal segment
internode
internuclear ophthalmoplegia (INO)
internuncial neuron
internus
interobserver error
interocclusal
    i. clearance
    i. distance
    i. gap
    i. record
    i. rest space
interoceptive
interoceptor
interofective system
interolivary
interorbital
interosseal
interosseous
    i. border
    i. border of fibula
    i. border of radius
    i. border of tibia
    i. border of ulna
    i. bursa of elbow
    i. cartilage
    i. crest
    i. cubital bursa
    i. cuneocuboid ligament
    i. cuneometatarsal ligament
    i. fascia
    i. groove
    i. groove of calcaneus
    i. groove of talus
    i. margin
    i. membrane of forearm
    i. membrane of leg
    i. metacarpal ligament
    i. metacarpal space
    i. metatarsal ligament
    i. metatarsal space
    i. muscle
    i. nerve of leg
    palmar i.'s
    i. sacroiliac ligament
    i. talocalcaneal ligament
    i. tibiofibular ligament
interosseus, pl. interossei
    dorsal i. of foot
    dorsal i. of hand
interpalpebral zone
interpapillary ridge
interparietal
    i. bone
    i. sulcus
    i. suture
interparoxysmal
interpectoral lymph node
interpediculate
interpeduncular
    i. cistern

    i. fossa
    i. ganglion
    i. nucleus
interpersonal conflict
interphalangeal
    i. articulation
    distal i. (DIP)
    i. joint of foot
    i. joint of hand
    proximal i. (PIP)
interphase
interphyletic
interplant
interplanting
interpleural space
interpolated
    i. extrasystole
    i. flap
interposition arthroplasty
interpositospinal tract
interpositus nucleus
interpretation
interproximal
    i. papilla
    i. space
    i. surface of tooth
interpubic
    i. disk
    i. fibrocartilage
interpulmonary septum
interpupillary
interradial
interradicular
    i. alveoloplasty
    i. septa of maxilla and mandible
    i. space
interrater reliability
interrenal
interridge distance
interrod enamel
interrupted
    i. respiration
    i. suture
interscalene triangle
interscapular
    i. gland
    i. hibernoma
    i. reflex
interscapulothoracic amputation
interscapulum
intersciatic
intersectio
    i. tendinea
    i.'s tendineae musculi recti
      abdominis
intersection
    tendinous i.
    tendinous i.'s of rectus abdominis
intersegmental
    i. fasciculi
    i. part of pulmonary vein
    i. vein
intersemilunar fissure
interseptal
interseptovalvular space

interseptum
intersexual
intersexuality
intersheath space of optic nerve
intersigmoid
    i. hernia
    i. recess
interspace
interspinal
    i. line
    i. muscle
    i. plane
interspinales
    i. cervicis muscle
    i. lumborum muscle
    i. muscle
    i. thoracis muscle
interspinalis
interspinous
    i. ligament
    i. plane
intersternebral joint
interstice
interstitial
    i. absorption
    i. amygdaloid nucleus
    i. brachytherapy
    i. cell
    i. cell-stimulating hormone (ICSH)
    i. cell tumor of testis
    i. cystitis
    i. deletion
    i. disease
    i. emphysema
    i. fluid
    i. gastritis
    i. gland
    i. growth
    i. hernia
    i. implantation
    i. inflammation
    i. keratitis
    i. lamella
    i. mastitis
    i. myositis
    i. nephritis
    i. neuritis
    i. nucleus
    i. nucleus of anterior hypothalamus
    i. nucleus of Cajal
    i. nucleus of medial longitudinal
      fasciculus
    i. pattern
    i. plasma cell pneumonia
    i. pregnancy
    i. pulmonary fibrosis
    i. therapy
    i. tissue
interstitiospinal tract
interstitium
intertarsal
    i. articulation
    i. joint
intertendinous connection of extensor
  digitorum

interthalamic adhesion
intertragic notch
intertransversalis
intertransversarii muscle
intertransverse
    i. ligament
    i. muscle
intertriginous
intertrigo
intertrochanteric
    i. crest
    i. fracture
    i. line
intertropical hyphemia
intertubercular
    i. groove
    i. line
    i. plane
    i. sulcus
    i. tendon sheath
intertubular zone
interureteral
interureteric
    i. crest
    i. fold
intervaginal subarachnoid space of optic
  nerve
interval
    a-c i.
    AH i.
    AN i.
    atrioventricular i.
    auriculoventricular i.
    AV i.
    BH i.
    calibration i.
    cardioarterial i., c-a i.
    cardioarterial i.
    confidence i.
    coupling i.
    escape i.
    focal i.
    i. gout
    HV i.
    interectopic i.
    isovolumic i.
    lucid i.
    i. operation
    PA i.
    PJ i.
    P-P i.
    PQ i.
    PR i.
    QR i.
    QRB i.
    QRS i.
    QS_2 i.
    QT i.
    R-R i.
    i. scale
    serial i.
    sphygmic i.
    Sturm i.
    systolic time i.
intervascular

intervening
    i. sequence
    i. variable
intervenous tubercle
intervention
    crisis i.
interventional
    i. angiography
    i. radiology
interventricular
    i. foramen
    i. groove
    i. septal branch of left/right coronary artery
    i. septum
intervertebral
    i. cartilage
    i. disk
    i. foramen
    i. ganglion
    i. notch
    i. symphysis
    i. vein
interview
    Zarit burden i.
intervillous
    i. lacuna
    i. space
interzonal mesenchyme
intestina (*pl. of* intestinum)
intestinal
    i. anastomosis
    i. angina
    i. anthrax
    i. arterial arcade
    i. artery
    i. atresia
    i. calculus
    i. capillariasis
    i. cecum
    i. digestion
    i. emphysema
    i. fistula
    i. follicle
    i. gland
    i. intoxication
    i. juice
    i. lymphangiectasis
    i. (lymphatic) trunks
    i. metaplasia
    i. myiasis
    i. pseudoobstruction
    i. rotation
    i. sand
    i. schistosomiasis
    i. sepsis
    i. stasis
    i. steatorrhea
    i. surface of uterus
    i. villi
intestine
    large i.
    small i.
intestinotoxin
intestinum, pl. **intestina**

    i. cecum
    i. crassum
    i. ileum
    i. jejunum
    i. rectum
    i. tenue
    i. tenue mesenteriale
in-the-canal hearing aid
in-the-ear hearing aid
intima
intimal
intimitis
    proliferative i.
intoe
intolerance
    hereditary fructose i.
    lactose i.
    lysinuric protein i.
intorsion
intortor
intoxation
intoxicant
intoxication
    acid i.
    anaphylactic i.
    citrate i.
    intestinal i.
    septic i.
    water i.
intraabdominal
intraacinous
intraadenoidal
intraalveolar septa
intraaortic
    i. balloon
    i. balloon counterpulsation
    i. balloon pump
intraarterial
intraarticular
    i. cartilage
    i. fracture
    i. ligament of costal head
    i. ligament of head of rib
    i. sternocostal ligament
intraatrial
    i. block
    i. conduction
    i. conduction time
intraaural
intraauricular
intrabony pocket
intrabronchial
intrabuccal
intrabulbar fossa
intracanalicular fibroadenoma
intracapsular
    i. ankylosis
    i. fracture
    i. ligament
    i. temporomandibular joint arthroplasty
intracardiac
    i. catheter
    i. lead
    i. pressure curve

intracarpal
intracartilaginous
intracatheter
intracavernous
    i. aneurysm
    i. plexus
intracavitary
intracelial
intracellular
    i. canaliculus
    i. digestion
    i. enzyme
    i. fluid (ICF)
    i. toxin
    i. water
intracerebellar
intracerebral hemorrhage
intracerebroventricular
intracervical
intracisternal
intracolic
intracordal
intracorneal implant
intracoronal retainer
intracorporeal
intracorpuscular
intracostal
intracranial
    i. aneurysm
    i. cavity
    i. ganglion
    i. granulomatous arteritis
    i. hematoma
    i. hemorrhage
    i. hypotension
    i. part of optic nerve
    i. part of vertebral artery
    i. pneumatocele
    i. pneumocele
    i. pressure (ICP)
intracrine
intractable
    i. epilepsy
    i. pain
intraculminate fissure
intracutaneous reaction
intracystic papilloma
intracytoplasmic sperm injection
intrad
intradermal
    i. nevus
    i. reaction
    i. test
intraduct
intraductal
    i. carcinoma
    i. papilloma
intradural
intraembryonic mesoderm
intraepidermal
    i. bulla
    i. carcinoma
intraepiphysial
intraepiploic hernia

intraepithelial
    i. carcinoma
    i. dyskeratosis
    i. gland
intrafaradization
intrafascicular
intrafebrile
intrafilar
intrafusal fiber
intragalvanization
intragastric
intragemmal
intragenal
intragenic
    i. complementation
    i. suppression
intraglandular
    i. deep parotid lymph node
    i. parotid lymph node
intraglobular
intragracile sulcus
intragyral
intrahepatic cholestasis of pregnancy
intrahyoid
intrailiac hernia
intrajugular process
intralaminar
    i. nuclei of thalamus
    i. part of intralocular part of optic
      nerve
intralaryngeal
intralesional therapy
intraligamentary pregnancy
intraligamentous
intralobar
    i. part of the posterior vein
intralobular duct
intralocal additivity
intralocular
intraluminal
intramaxillary anchorage
intramedullary
    i. anesthesia
    i. reamer
    i. tractotomy
    i. transfusion
intramembranous ossification
intrameningeal
intramitochondrial
intramolecular
intramural
    i. hematoma
    i. part of male urethra
    i. practice
    i. pregnancy
intramuscular (IM)
intramyocardial
intramyometrial
intranasal anesthesia
intranatal
intraneural
in-transit metastasis
intranuclear
intraobserver error

intraocular
    i. fluid
    i. implant
    i. neuritis
    i. part of optic nerve
    i. pressure
intraoral
    i. anchorage
    i. anesthesia
    i. antrostomy
    i. fracture appliance
intraorbital
intraosseous
    i. anesthesia
    i. fixation
intraosteal
intraovarian
intraovular
intrapapillary drusen
intraparietal
    i. sulcus
    i. sulcus of Turner
intraparotid plexus of facial nerve
intrapartum
    i. hemorrhage
    i. period
intrapelvic hernia
intrapericardiac, intrapericardial
intraperitoneal (IP)
    i. pregnancy
intrapersonal conflict
intrapial
intrapleural
intrapontine
intraprostatic
intraprotoplasmic
intrapsychic
intrapulmonary
    i. blood vessel
    i. lymph node
intrapyretic
intrarectal
intrarenal
    i. artery
    i. reflux
intraretinal space
intrarrhachidian
intrascrotal
intrasegmental
    i. bronchus
    i. part of pulmonary vein
    i. vein
intraseptal alveoloplasty
intraspinal anesthesia
intrasplenic
intrastromal
intrasynovial
intratarsal
intratendinous
    i. bursa of elbow
    i. olecranon bursa
intrathalamic fiber
intrathecal injection
intrathoracic
intrathyroid cartilage

intratonsillar
intratracheal
    i. anesthesia
    i. intubation
    i. tube
intratubal
intratubular
intratympanic
intrauterine
    i. amputation
    i. contraceptive device (IUCD)
    i. device (IUD)
    i. fracture
    i. growth retardation
    i. insemination (IUI)
    i. pneumonia
    i. transfusion
intravagal glomus
intravaginal torsion
intravascular
    i. ligature
    i. lymph
    i. papillary endothelial hyperplasia
intravenous (I.V.)
    i. anesthetic
    i. bolus
    i. cholangiography
    i. drip
    i. narcosis
    i. pyelography (IVP)
    i. regional anesthesia
    i. urogram (IVU)
    i. urography
intraventricular (IV, I-V)
    i. block (IVB)
    i. conduction
    i. hemorrhage
    i. injection
intravesical
intravital
    i. stain
    i. ultraviolet
intra vitam
    during life
intravitelline
intravitreous
intrinsic
    i. asthma
    i. color
    i. deflection
    i. factor
    i. fiber
    i. motivation
    i. muscle
    i. muscle of foot
    i. protein
    i. reflex
    i. sphincter
    i. sympathomimetic activity (ISA)
intrinsicoid deflection
introducer
introflection
introgastric
introitus
    i. canalis

introitus *(continued)*
 i. of facial canal
 vaginal i.
introject
introjection
intromission
intromittent organ
intron
introspection
introspective method
introsusception
introversion
introvert
intubate
intubation
 altercursive i.
 aqueductal i.
 blind nasotracheal i.
 endotracheal i.
 intratracheal i.
 nasotracheal i.
 orotracheal i.
 tracheal i.
intubator
intuitive stage
intumesce
intumescence
 tympanic i.
intumescent cataract
intumescentia
 i. cervicalis
 i. ganglioformis
 i. lumbosacralis
 i. tympanica
intussusception
 colic i.
 double i.
 ileal i.
 ileocecal i.
 ileocolic i.
 jejunogastric i.
 retrograde i.
intussusceptive growth
intussusceptum
intussuscipiens
inulase
inulin (in)
 i. clearance
inulinase
inulol
inunction
inundation fever
InV
 InV allotypes
 InV group antigen
invaccination
invaginate planula
invagination
 basilar i.
invaginator
invalid
invalidism
invasin
invasion

invasive
 i. carcinoma
 i. mole
 i. pituitary adenoma
inventory
 Millon clinical multiaxial i. (MCMI)
 Minnesota Multiphasic Personality I. (MMPI)
 personality i.
invermination
inverse
 i. anaphylaxis
 i. ocular bobbing
 i. square law
 i. symmetry
 i. syntropy
inversed jaw-winking syndrome
inverse-ratio ventilation
inversion
 i. of chromosome
 paracentric i.
 pericentric i.
 i. recovery
 i. of the uterus
 visceral i.
invertase
Invertebrata
invertebrate
inverted
 i. cone bur
 i. follicular keratosis
 i. image
 i. papilloma
 i. pelvis
 i. radial reflex
 i. repeat
invertin
invertor
invert sugar
investigatory reflex
investing
 i. cartilage
 i. fascia
 i. layer
 i. layer of cervical fascia
 i. tissues
 vacuum i.
investment
 i. cast
 refractory i.
inveterate
inviscation
invisible
 i. differentiation
 i. light
 i. spectrum
involucre
involucrin
involucrum
involuntary
 i. guarding
 i. muscle
 i. nervous system
involution
 i. form

senile i.
i. of the uterus
involutional
i. depression
i. melancholia
involved field
iobenzamic acid
iocetamic acid
iodamide
Iodamoeba
Iodamoeba bütschlii
iodate reaction of epinephrine
iodic
i. acid
iodide
i. acne
i. peroxidase
sodium i. iodine-131
i. transport defect
iodimetry
iodinase
iodinate
iodinated
i. casein
i. glycerol
i. ^{131}I human serum albumin
i. ^{125}I serum albumin
iodine
butanol-extractable i. (BEI)
i. eruption
Gram i.
i. number
protein-bound i. (PBI)
radioactive i.
i. reaction of epinephrine
i. stain
tamed i.
i. test
i. tincture
i. value
iodine-123 (^{123}I)
iodine-125 (^{125}I)
iodine-127 (^{127}I)
iodine-131 (^{131}I)
iodine-132 (^{132}I)
iodine-fast
iodine-induced hyperthyroidism
iodinophil
iodinophilous
iodipamide
methylglucamine i.
iodism
iodixanol
iodize
iodized
i. collodion
i. oil
iodoacetamide
iodoalphionic acid
iodocasein
iodochlorhydroxyquin
iodochlorol
iododerma
iodoform
iodoglobulin

iodogorgoic acid
iodohippurate sodium
iodomethamate sodium
iodometric
iodometry
iodopanoic acid
iodophendylate
iodophil granule
iodophilia
iodophor
iodophthalein
3-iodo-1,2-propanediol
iodopropylidene glycerol
iodoprotein
iodopsin
iodopyracet
iodoquinol
iodotherapy
iodothyronins
iodotyrosine
i. deiodase
i. deiodinase defect
iodoxamate meglumine
ioduria
ioglycamic acid
iohexol
iometer
ion
aquo-i.
i. channel
i. channel disorder
dipolar i.'s
i. exchange
i. exchange chromatography
i. exchanger
gram-i.
hydride i.
hydrogen i. (H$^+$)
hydronium i.
oxonium i.
i. pump
sulfonium i.
ion-exchange resin
ionic
i. medication
i. strength
ionium
ionization chamber
ionize
ionized atom
ionizing radiation
ionogram
ionone
ionopherogram
ionophore
ionophoresis
ionophoretic
ion-selective electrode
iontophoresis
iontophoretic
iontotherapy
iopamidol
iopanoic acid
iopentol
iophendylate

iophenoic acid
iophenoxic acid
iophobia
iopromide
iota, ι
iotacism
iothalamic acid
iothiouracil sodium
iotrol
iotrolan
ioversol
ioxaglate
ioxilan
ioxithalamate
IP
> intraperitoneal

IP$_3$
> inositol 1,4,5-trisphosphate

IPA
> independent practice association

ipecac
> powdered i.
> i. syrup

ipecacuanha
> de-emetinized i.
> prepared i.

IPF
> idiopathic pulmonary fibrosis

ipodate
ipomea resin
Ipomoea
> *Ipomoea rubrocoerulea* var. *praecox*
> *Ipomoea versicolor*

IPPB
> intermittent positive pressure breathing

IPPV
> intermittent positive pressure ventilation

ipratropium
iproniazid
iproveratril
iPrSGal
> isopropylthiogalactoside

Ips
> pipsyl

ipsefact
ipsilateral reflex
IPSP
> inhibitory postsynaptic potential

IPTG
> isopropylthiogalactoside

IPV
> inactivated poliovirus vaccine

IQ
> intelligence quotient

IR
> infrared

Ir
> iridium

IRB
> institutional review board

iridal
iridectomy
> buttonhole i.
> optic i.
> peripheral i.

> sector i.
> stenopeic i.
> therapeutic i.

iridencleisis
irideremia
irides (*pl. of* iris)
iridescent virus
iridesis
iridial
> i. part of retina

iridin
iridium (Ir)
iridoavulsion
iridocele
iridochoroiditis
iridocoloboma
iridocorneal
> i. angle
> i. endothelial syndrome
> i. mesenchymal dysgenesis
> i. syndrome

iridocyclectomy
iridocyclitis septica
iridocyclochoroiditis
iridocystectomy
iridodiagnosis
iridodialysis
iridodilator
iridodonesis
iridokinetic
iridology
iridomalacia
iridomesodialysis
iridomotor
iridoparalysis
iridopathy
iridoplegia
> complete i.
> reflex i.
> sympathetic i.

iridoptosis
iridopupillary lamina
iridorrhexis
iridoschisis
iridosclerotomy
iridotomy
> laser i.

Iridoviridae
Iridovirus
irigenin
IRI/G ratio
iris, pl. irides
> i. bicolor
> i. bombé
> crypt of i.
> i. dehiscence
> i. freckle
> i. frill
> i. pit
> plateau i.
> i. spatula
> tremulous i.

Irish
> I. moss
> I. moss gelatin

irisin
iris-nevus syndrome
iritic
iritis
  fibrinous i.
  follicular i.
  i. glaucomatosa
  hemorrhagic i.
  nodular i.
  plastic i.
  quiet i.
  serous i.
  sympathetic i.
iron (Fe)
  i. albuminate
  albuminized i.
  i. alum
  i. deficiency anemia
  i. filing
  i. hematoxylin
  i. index
  i. line
  i. lung
  i. protoporphyrin
  i. pyrite
  i. sulfate
iron-52 (^{52}Fe)
iron-55 (^{55}Fe)
iron-59 (^{59}Fe)
iron-binding capacity (IBC)
iron-dextran complex
iron-storage disease
iron-sulfur protein
irradiate
irradiated vitamin D milk
irradiation
irrational
irreducible hernia
irregular
  i. astigmatism
  i. bone
  i. dentin
  i. emphysema
  i. nystagmus
  i. pulse
irresistible impulse
irrespirable
irresponsibility
  criminal i.
irresuscitable
irreversible
  i. colloid
  i. hydrocolloid
  i. pulpitis
  i. reaction
  i. shock
irrigate
irrigation
irrigator
irritability
  electric i.
  myotatic i.
irritable
  i. breast
  i. colon

irritant
  i. contact dermatitis
  primary i.
irritation
  i. cell
  i. dentin
  i. fibroma
irritative
irrumation
irruption
irruptive
IRS-1
  insulin receptor substrate-1
IRV
  inspiratory reserve volume
Irvine-Gass syndrome
ISA
  intrinsic sympathomimetic activity
Isaac-Merton syndrome
Isaac syndrome
Isamine blue
isauxesis
ischemia
  myocardial i.
  postural i.
  i. retinae
  silent i.
ischemia-modifying factor
ischemic
  i. contracture of the left ventricle
  i. hypoxia
  i. lumbago
  i. mitral regurgitation
  i. muscular atrophy
  i. necrosis
  i. optic neuropathy
ischesis
ischia (*pl. of* ischium)
ischiadic
  i. plexus
  i. spine
ischiadicus
ischial
  i. bone
  i. bursa
  i. bursitis
  i. ramus
  i. spine
  i. tuberosity
ischialgia
ischiatic
  i. hernia
  i. notch
ischioanal fossa
ischiobulbar
ischiocapsular ligament
ischiocavernosus
ischiocavernous muscle
ischiocele
ischiococcygeal
ischiococcygeus
ischiodynia
ischiofemoral ligament
ischiofibular
ischiomelus

ischionitis
ischiopagus
ischioperineal
ischiopubic ramus
ischiorectal
>   i. abscess
>   i. fat-pad
>   i. fossa

ischiosacral
ischiothoracopagus
ischiotibial
ischiovaginal
ischiovertebral
ischium, pl. **ischia**
ischochymia
ischuretic
ischuria
isethionate
isethionic acid
Ishihara test
ISI
>   international sensitivity index

isinglass
island
>   blood i.
>   bone i.
>   i. of Calleja
>   i. disease
>   epimyoepithelial i.
>   i. fever
>   i. flap
>   Langerhans i.
>   pancreatic i.
>   i. of Reil

islet
>   blood i.
>   i. cell
>   i. cell tumor
>   i.'s of Langerhans
>   pancreatic i.'s
>   i. tissue

isoacceptor tRNA
isoagglutination
isoagglutinin
isoagglutinogen
isoallele
isoallotypic determinant
isoalloxazine
isoaminile
isoamyl
isoamylase
isoandrosterone
isoantibody
isoantigen
isobar
isobaric spinal anesthesia
isobornyl thiocyanoacetate
isobutane
isobuteine
isobutyl
>   i. alcohol
>   i. nitrite

isobutyric acid
isocapnia
isocellular

isochoric
isochromatic
isochromatophil
isochromic anemia
isochromosome
isochronia
isochronous
isochroous
isocitrase
isocitrate
>   i. dehydrogenase
>   i. lyase

isocitric acid dehydrogenase
isocitritase
isocline
isoconazole
isocoria
isocortex
isocyanate
isocyanic acid
isocyanide
isocyclic compound
isocytolysin
isodactylism
isodemographic map
isodense
isodesmosine
isodiphasic complex
isodose
isodulcit
isodynamic law
isodynamogenic
isoelectric
>   i. electroencephalogram
>   i. focusing
>   i. line
>   i. period
>   i. point (IEP, pI)
>   i. zone

isoenergetic
isoenzyme
>   creatine kinase i.
>   i. electrophoresis

isoerythrolysis
>   neonatal i.

isofluorphate
isoflurane
isogamete
isogamy
isogeneic, isogenic
>   i. graft
>   i. strain

isogenous
>   i. chondrocyte
>   i. nest

isogentiobiose
isoglutamine
isognathous
isograft
isohemagglutination
isohemagglutinin
isohemolysin
isohemolysis
isohydric
isohydruria

isoimmune neonatal thrombocytopenia
isoimmunization
isoionic point
isolate

    genetic i.
    mating i.

isolated

    i. abutment
    i. dextrocardia
    i. dyskeratosis follicularis
    i. explosive disorder
    i. hypoaldosteronism
    i. parietal endocarditis
    i. proteinuria

isolation
isolecithal

    i. egg
    i. ovum

isoleucine
isoleucyl
isoleukoagglutinin
isologous graft
isolysin
isolysis
isolytic
isomaltase
isomaltose
isomastigote
isomer

    geometric i.

isomerase
isomeric

    i. function
    i. transition

isomerism

    geometric i.
    optic i.
    stereochemical i.
    structural i.

isomerization

    enzyme i.

isomerous
isomethadone
isometheptene
isometric

    i. chart
    i. contraction
    i. contraction period
    i. exercise
    i. period of cardiac cycle
    i. relaxation
    i. relaxation period
    i. ruler
    i. traction

isometropia
isomorphic response
isomorphism
isomorphous gliosis
isonaphthol
isoncotic
isoniazid

    i. neuropathy
    i. polyneuropathy

isonicotinic acid
isonicotinic acid hydrazide (INH)

isonitrile
isonitrosoacetone
isoosmotic
isopathy
isopentenylpyrophosphate
isopentyl
isopeptide bond
isoperistaltic anastomosis
isophagy
isophane insulin
isoplassonts
isoplastic graft
isopleth
isopotential
isoprecipitin
isoprenaline

    i. hydrochloride
    i. sulfate

isoprene rule
isoprenoid
isoprenylation
isopropanol precipitation test
isoprophenamine hydrochloride
isopropyl

    i. alcohol
    i. myristate

isopropylarterenol hydrochloride
isopropylcarbinol
isopropylthiogalactoside (iPrSGal, IPTG)
isoproterenol

    i. hydrochloride
    i. sulfate

isopter
isopycnic zone
isopyknic
isopyrocalciferol
isoquinoline
isorhythmic dissociation
isoriboflavin
isorrhea
isosbestic point
isoschizomer
isosensitize
isoserum treatment
isosexual
isosmotic
isosorbide dinitrate
Isospora

    I. belli
    I. bigemina
    I. canis
    I. felis
    I. rivolta
    I. suis

isosporiasis
isostere
isostery
isosthenuria
isosuccinic acid
isosulfan blue
isothermal
isothiocyanate
isothipendyl
isotone
isotonia

isotonic
>i. coefficient
>i. contraction
>i. exercise
>i. traction

isotonicity
isotope
>i. clearance
>daughter i.
>radioactive i.
>stable i.

isotopic
isotransplantation
isotretinoin
isotropic, isotropous
>i. disk
>i. lipid

isotype
isotypic
isovaleric
>i. acid
>i. acidemia

isovaleryl-CoA
>isovaleryl-CoA dehydrogenase

isovalerylcoenzyme A
isovalthine
isovolume pressure-flow curve
isovolumetric relaxation
isovolumic
>i. interval
>i. period
>i. relaxation

isoxsuprine hydrochloride
isozyme
issue
>nature-nurture i.

isthmectomy
isthmi (*pl. of* isthmus)
isthmic, isthmian
isthmoparalysis
isthmoplegia
isthmus, pl. **isthmi, isthmuses**
>i. of aorta
>i. aortae
>aortic i.
>i. of auditory tube
>i. of cartilage of ear
>i. cartilaginis auricularis
>i. cartilaginis auris
>i. of cartilaginous auricle
>i. of cingulate gyrus
>i. of eustachian tube
>i. of external acoustic meatus
>i. of fauces
>i. faucium
>i. glandulae thyroideae
>Guyon i.
>i. gyri cinguli
>i. of gyrus fornicatus
>i. of His
>Krönig i.
>i. of limbic lobe
>i. meatus acustici externi
>oropharyngeal i.
>pharyngeal i.

>i. pharyngis
>i. pharyngonasalis
>i. of pharyngotympanic tube
>i. of pharynx
>pleural i.
>i. prostatae
>i. of prostate
>i. rhombencephali
>rhombencephalic i.
>i. of thyroid gland
>i. tubae auditivae
>i. tubae auditoriae
>i. tubae uterinae
>i. uteri
>i. of uterine tube
>i. of uterus
>Vieussens i.

itaconic acid
Itai-Itai disease
Italian flap
itch
>azo i.
>baker's i.
>barber's i.
>bath i.
>copra i.
>Cuban i.
>frost i.
>grain i.
>grocer's i.
>ground i.
>kabure i.
>Norway i.
>poultryman's i.
>rice i.
>Saint Ignatius i.
>straw i.
>straw-bed i.
>summer i.
>swimmer's i.
>water i.
>winter i.

itching
iter
>i. chordae anterius
>i. chordae posterius
>i. dentis
>i. dentium
>i. a tertio ad quartum ventriculum

iteral
Ito
>I. cell
>I. nevus

ITO method
ITP
>idiopathic thrombocytopenic purpura

itramin tosylate
IU
>international unit

IUB
>International Union of Biochemistry

IUCD
>intrauterine contraceptive device

IUD
>intrauterine device

IUI
> intrauterine insemination

IUPAC
> International Union of Pure and Applied
> Chemistry

^{131}**I uptake test**

I-V
> intraventricular

IV
> intraventricular
> > IV block

I.V.
> intravenous

IVB
> intraventricular block

IVC
> inferior vena cava

Ivemark syndrome

ivermectin

IVF
> in vitro fertilization

IVF-ET

Ivor Lewis esophagectomy

ivory
> i. exostosis

> i. membrane
> i. vertebra

IVP
> intravenous pyelography

IVU
> intravenous urogram

Ivy
> I. bleeding time test
> I. loop wiring

Ixodes
> *I. cookei*
> *I. dammini*
> *I. pacificus*
> *I. persulcatus*
> *I. redikorzevi*
> *I. ricinus*
> *I. scapularis*
> *I. spinipalpis*

ixodiasis

ixodic

ixodid

Ixodidae

Ixodoidea

J
J chain
J point

J
flux
Jaboulay
J. amputation
J. pyloroplasty
Jaccoud
J. arthritis
J. arthropathy
jacket
j. crown
Minerva j.
jackscrew
Jackson
J. law
J. membrane
J. rule
J. sign
J. veil
jacksonian
j. epilepsy
j. seizure
Jacobaeus operation
Jacobson
J. anastomosis
J. canal
J. cartilage
J. nerve
J. organ
J. plexus
J. reflex
Jacquart facial angle
Jacquemet recess
Jacquemin test
Jacques plexus
Jadassohn-Lewandowski syndrome
Jadassohn nevus
Jadassohn-Pellizzari anetoderma
Jaeger test types
Jaffe
J. reaction
J. test
Jaffe-Lichtenstein disease
Jahnke syndrome
jail fever
jake paralysis
jalap resin
Jamaican vomiting sickness
James
J. fiber
J. tract
Jamestown
J. Canyon virus
J. weed
Janet test
Janeway lesion
janiceps
j. asymmetrus
j. parasiticus
Jansen operation

Jansky-Bielschowsky disease
Jansky classification
Janus green B
Japanese
J. B encephalitis
J. B encephalitis virus
J. river fever
J. schistosomiasis
J. spotted fever
Japan wax
jar
heel j.
jargon aphasia
Jarisch-Herxheimer reaction
Jarman score
Jarvik artificial heart
Jatene procedure
Jatropha
J. curcas
J. glandulifera
J. urens
jaundice
acholuric j.
anhepatic j.
anhepatogenous j.
choleric j.
cholestatic j.
chronic acholuric j.
chronic familial j.
chronic idiopathic j.
congenital hemolytic j.
familial nonhemolytic j.
hematogenous j.
hemolytic j.
hepatocellular j.
hepatogenic j.
homologous serum j.
human serum j.
infectious j.
infective j.
leptospiral j.
malignant j.
mechanical j.
neonatal j.
j. of the newborn
nonobstructive j.
nuclear j.
obstructive j.
painless j.
physiologic j.
postarsphenamine j.
recurrent j. of pregnancy
regurgitation j.
retention j.
j. root
Schmorl j.
spherocytic j.
spirochetal j.
toxemic j.
jaw
j. bone
crackling j.

jaw *(continued)*
    Hapsburg j.
    jaw winking
    j. jerk
    j. joint
    lock-j.
    lower j.
    lumpy j.
    parrot j.
    j. reflex
    j. repositioning
    j. separation
    j. skeleton
    upper j.
Jaworski body
jaw-winking
    j.-w. phenomenon
    j.-w. syndrome
jaw-working reflex
JC virus
jealous type of paranoid disorder
Jeanselme nodule
Jeghers-Peutz syndrome
jejunal
    j. artery
    j. and ileal vein
jejunectomy
jejunitis
jejunocolostomy
jejunogastric intussusception
jejunoileal
    j. bypass
    j. shunt
jejunoileitis
jejunoileostomy
jejunojejunostomy
jejunoplasty
jejunostomy
jejunotomy
jejunum
Jellinek formula
jelly
    box j.
    cardiac j.
    interlaminar j.
    Wharton j.
jellyfish
Jena Nomina Anatomica (JNA)
Jendrassik maneuver
Jenner-Kay unit
Jenner stain
Jensen
    J. disease
    J. sarcoma
Jericho boil
jerk
    ankle j.
    chin j.
    crossed adductor j.
    crossed knee j.
    elbow j.
    j. finger
    jaw j.

    knee j.
    supinator j.
jerks
jerky
    j. nystagmus
    j. respiration
Jerne
    J. plaque assay
    J. technique
Jervell and Lange-Nielsen syndrome
Jesuits bark
Jesuit tea
jet
    j. ejector pump
    j. injection
    j. injector
    j. lag
    j. nebulizer
Jeune syndrome
jeweller forceps
Jewett
    J. sound
    J. and Strong staging
j-g complex
jigger
jimson weed
Jk
    Jk antigen
    Jk blood group
JNA
    Jena Nomina Anatomica
Jobbins antigen
Jobert
    J. de Lamballe fossa
    J. de Lamballe suture
Job syndrome
Jocasta complex
Jod-Basedow
Jod-Basedow phenomenon
Joffroy
    J. reflex
    J. sign
Johanson-Blizzard syndrome
johnin
Johnson method
joint
    acromioclavicular j.
    ankle j.
    anterior intraoccipital j.
    arthrodial j.
    atlantoaxial j.
    atlantooccipital j.
    j. of auditory ossicles
    ball and socket j.
    biaxial j.
    bicondylar j.
    bilocular j.
    j. branch
    Budin obstetrical j.
    calcaneocuboid j.
    capitular j.
    j. capsule
    carpal j.
    carpometacarpal j.
    carpometacarpal j. of thumb

cartilaginous j.
Charcot j.
Chopart j.
Clutton j.
coccygeal j.
cochlear j.
J. Commission on Accreditation of
  Healthcare Organizations
complex j.
composite j.
compound j.
condylar j.
costochondral j.
costotransverse j.
costovertebral j.
cotyloid j.
cranial synovial j.
cricoarytenoid j.
cricothyroid j.
Cruveilhier j.
cubital j.
cuboideonavicular j.
cuneocuboid j.
cuneometatarsal j.
cuneonavicular j.
cylindrical j.
dentoalveolar j.
diarthrodial j.
digital j.
DIP j.
distal interphalangeal j.
distal radioulnar j.
distal tibiofibular j.
j. of ear bone
j. effusion
elbow j.
ellipsoidal j.
enarthrodial j.
facet j.
false j.
femoropatellar j.
fibrous j.
flail j.
j. of foot
j. of free inferior limb
j. of free superior limb
J. gamete
ginglymoid j.
glenohumeral j.
gliding j.
gompholic j.
j. of hand
j. of head of rib
hemophilic j.
hinge j.
hip j.
humeroradial j.
humeroulnar j.
hysterical j.
immovable j.
incudomalleolar j.
incudostapedial j.
j. of inferior limb girdle
inferior radioulnar j.
inferior tibiofibular j.

interarticular j.
intercarpal j.
interchondral j.
intercuneiform j.
intermetacarpal j.
intermetatarsal j.
interphalangeal j. of foot
interphalangeal j. of hand
intersternebral j.
intertarsal j.
jaw j.
knee j.
lateral atlantoaxial j.
lateral atlantoepistrophic j.
Lisfranc j.
lumbosacral j.
Luschka j.
mandibular j.
manubriosternal j.
median atlantoaxial j.
metacarpophalangeal j.
metatarsophalangeal j.
j. mice
midcarpal j.
middle atlantoepistrophic j.
middle carpal j.
middle radioulnar j.
midtarsal j.
mortise j.
movable j.
MP j.
multiaxial j.
neurocentral j.
neuropathic j.
j. oil
j. of pectoral girdle
peg-and-socket j.
j. of pelvic girdle
petrooccipital j.
phalangeal j.
PIP j.
pisiform j.
pisotriquetral j.
pivot j.
plane j.
polyaxial j.
posterior intraoccipital j.
j. probability
proximal interphalangeal j.
proximal radioulnar j.
proximal tibiofibular j.
radiocarpal j.
rotary j.
rotatory j.
sacrococcygeal j.
sacroiliac j.
saddle j.
schindyletic j.
screw j.
secondary cartilaginous j.
j. sense
shoulder j.
simple j.
socket j.
sphenooccipital j.

joint (*continued*)
    spheroid j.
    spiral j.
    sternal j.
    sternoclavicular j.
    sternocostal j.
    stress-broken j.
    subtalar j.
    j. of superior limb girdle
    superior radioulnar j.
    superior tibiofibular j.
    suture j.
    synarthrodial j.
    synchondrodial j.
    syndesmodial j.
    syndesmotic j.
    synovial j.
    synovial j. of free lower limb
    synovial j. of free upper limb
    synovial j. of thorax
    talocalcaneal j.
    talocalcaneonavicular j.
    talocrural j.
    talonavicular j.
    tarsal j.
    tarsometatarsal j.
    temporomandibular j.
    thigh j.
    tibiofibular j.
    transverse tarsal j.
    trochoid j.
    uncovertebral j.
    uniaxial j.
    unilocular j.
    wedge-and-groove j.
    wrist j.
    xiphisternal j.
    zygapophysial j.
jojoba oil
Jolles test
Jolly
    J. body
    J. reaction
Jones
    J. criteria
    J. I, II test
    J. test
    J. transfer
Jonesia dentrificans
Jonnesco fossa
Joubert syndrome
joule
    J. equivalent
Js antigen
J-sella deformity
Judet view
Judkins technique
juga (*pl. of* jugum)
jugal
    j. bone
    j. ligament
    j. point
jugale
jugomaxillary

jugular
    j. bulb
    j. duct
    j. foramen
    j. foramen syndrome
    j. fossa
    j. ganglion
    j. gland
    j. glomus
    j. lymphatic plexus
    j. lymphatic trunk
    j. nerve
    j. notch of occipital bone
    j. notch of petrous part of
      temporal bone
    j. notch of sternum
    j. process of occipital bone
    j. pulse
    j. sinus
    j. tubercle of occipital bone
    j. vein
    j. venous arch
    j. wall of middle ear
jugulodigastric
    j. lymph node
    j. node
juguloomohyoid
    j. lymph node
    j. node
jugulum
jugum, pl. **juga**
    juga alveolaria
    juga cerebralia
    j. sphenoidale
juice
    appetite j.
    gastric j.
    intestinal j.
    pancreatic j.
jumper
    j. disease
    j. disease of Maine
jump flap
jumping
    j. the bite
    j. Frenchmen of Maine disease
    j. gene
junctio anorectalis
junction
    adhering j.'s
    amelodental j.
    amelodentinal j.
    amnioembryonic j.
    anorectal j.
    AV j.
    cardioesophageal j.
    cementodentinal j.
    cementoenamel j.
    choledochoduodenal j.
    communicating j.
    corneoscleral j.
    costochondral j.
    dentinocemental j.
    dentinoenamel j.
    duodenojejunal j.

electrotonic j.
esophagogastric j.
gap j.
Holliday j.
ileocecal j.
impermeable j.
intercellular j.'s
intermediate j.
j. of lips
manubriosternal j.
mucocutaneous j.
muscle-tendon j.
myoneural j.
neuroectodermal j.
neuromuscular j.
neurosomatic j.
j. nevus
rectosigmoid j.
right splicing j.
sacrococcygeal j.
sclerocorneal j.
squamocolumnar j.
ST j.
sternomanubrial j.
tight j.
tympanostapedial j.
ureteropelvic j. (UPJ)
ureterovesical j.
junctional
j. complex
j. cyst
j. epithelium
j. escape
j. extrasystole
j. rhythm
j. tachycardia
junctura, pl. **juncturae**
j. cartilaginea
j. fibrosa
j. lumbosacralis
juncturae membri inferioris liberi
juncturae membri superioris
juncturae membri superioris liberi
juncturae ossium
j. sacrococcygea
j. synovialis
juncturae tendinum
juncturae zygapophysiales
juncture
jungian psychoanalysis
jungle
j. fever
j. yellow fever
Jüngling disease
Jung muscle
Junin virus
juniper
j. berry oil
j. tar
junk DNA
jurisprudence
dental j.
medical j.

Jurkat cell
justice
justo
j. major
j. minor
juvenile
j. absence epilepsy
j. angiofibroma
j. arrhythmia
j. carcinoma
j. cataract
j. cell
j. cerebellar astrocytoma
j. chorea
j. chronic arthritis
j. cirrhosis
j. delinquent
j. diabetes
j. elastoma
j. hemangiofibroma
j. hyalin fibromatosis
j. kyphosis
j. myoclonic epilepsy
j. neutrophil
j.-onset diabetes
j. osteomalacia
j. osteoporosis
j. palmo-plantar fibromatosis
j. papillomatosis
j. pattern
j. pelvis
j. periodontitis
j. plantar dermatosis
j. polyp
j. retinoschisis
j. rheumatoid arthritis
j. spinal muscular atrophy
j. xanthogranuloma
juxtaarticular nodule
juxtacolic artery
juxtacortical
j. chondroma
j. osteogenic sarcoma
juxtacrine
juxtaepiphysial
juxtaesophageal lymph node
juxtaglomerular
j. apparatus
j. body
j. cell
j. cell tumor
j. complex
j. granule
juxtaintestinal mesenteric lymph node
juxtallocortex
juxtamedullary glomerulus
juxtaphrenic peak
juxtaposition
juxtapupillary choroiditis
juxtarestiform body

J

κ (*var. of* kappa)

K
- kalium
- kelvin
- lysine
- lysyl
- potassium

K
- K antigen
- K capture
- K cell
- K complex
- K region
- K shell
- K virus

^{43}**K**
- potassium-43

^{39}**K**
- potassium-39

^{40}**K**
- potassium-40

^{42}**K**
- potassium-42

K
- dissociation constant

K_a
- dissociation constant of an acid

K_b
- dissociation constant of a base

K_d
- dissociation constant

K_{eq}
- equilibrium constant

K_i
- dissociation constant of an inhibitor

K_m
- Michaelis constant

K_w
- autoprotolysis constant of water
- dissociation constant of water

k
- kilo

k
- rate constant

k_{cat}
- overall catalytic rate of an enzyme

kabure itch
Kaffir pox
kafindo
kainate receptor
kainic acid
kairomones
Kaiserling fixative
kak-, kako-
kal-, kali-
kala azar
kalemia
kali- (*var. of* kal-)
kaliopenia
kaliopenic
kalium (K)
kaliuresis

kaliuretic
kallidin
- k. 9, 10
- k. I, II

kallikrein
- human glandular k. 3 (hK3)
- k. system

Kallmann syndrome
kaluresis
kaluretic
kang cancer
kangri
- k. burn carcinoma
- k. cancer

Kanner syndrome
kanyemba
kaodzera
kaolin
kaolinosis
Kaplan-Meier
- K.-M. analysis
- K.-M. estimate

Kaposi
- K. sarcoma
- K. varicelliform eruption

kappa, κ
- k. angle
- k. granule
- k. particles

kappacism
K:A ratio
karaya gum
Karman cannula
Karmen unit
Karnofsky scale
Kartagener
- K. syndrome
- K. triad

karyochrome cell
karyoclasis
karyocyte
karyogamic
karyogamy
karyogenesis
karyogenic
karyogonad
karyogram
karyology
karyolymph
karyolysis
karyolytic
karyomere
karyomicrosome
karyomitome
karyomorphism
karyon
karyophage
karyoplasm
karyoplasmolysis
karyoplast
karyoplastin
karyopyknosis

K

karyopyknotic index
karyorrhexis
karyosome
karyostasis
karyotheca
karyotype
karyozoic
Kasabach-Merritt syndrome
Kasai operation
Kashin-Bek disease
Kasokero virus
Kasten
    K. fluorescent Feulgen stain
    K. fluorescent PAS stain
    K. fluorescent Schiff reagents
Kast syndrome
kat
    katal
kata-
katal (kat)
katathermometer
Katayama
    K. disease
    K. fever
    K. syndrome
    K. test
kathexis
kava
Kawasaki
    K. disease
    K. syndrome
Kayser-Fleischer ring
Kazanjian operation
kb
    kilobase
K blood group
kc
    kilocycle
kcal
    kilocalorie
Kearns-Sayre syndrome
Keating-Hart method
kedani fever
keel
keeled chest
Keen operation
Kegel exercises
Kehr sign
Keith
    K. bundle
    K. and Flack node
    K. node
kelectome
Kelev strain rabies virus
Kell blood group
Keller bunionectomy
Keller-Madlener operation
Kelly
    K. clamp
    K. operation
    K. rectal speculum
keloid
    acne k.
keloidosis

kelosomia
kelvin (K)
Kelvin scale
Kempner diet
Kendall
    K. compound
    K. substance
Kennedy
    K. classification
    K. disease
    K. syndrome
Kenny-Caffey syndrome
Kenny treatment
Kent bundle
Kent-His bundle
Kenya fever
kephalin
Kerandel sign
kerasin
keratan sulfate
keratectasia
keratectomy
    automated lamellar k.
    photorefractive k. (PRK)
    phototherapeutic k. (PTK)
keratein
keratic precipitate
keratin
    k. filament
    k. pearl
keratinases
keratinization
keratinized cell
keratinocyte
keratinophilic
keratinosome
keratinous cyst
keratitis
    actinic k.
    deep punctate k.
    dendriform k.
    dendritic k.
    diffuse deep k.
    Dimmer k.
    disciform k.
    k. disciformis
    exposure k.
    fascicular k.
    filamentary k.
    k. filamentosa
    geographic k.
    herpetic k.
    interstitial k.
    lagophthalmic k.
    k. linearis migrans
    marginal k.
    metaherpetic k.
    mycotic k.
    necrotizing k.
    neuroparalytic k.
    neurotrophic k.
    k. nummularis
    phlyctenular k.
    pneumococcal/suppurative k.
    polymorphic superficial k.

k. profunda
k. punctata
punctate k.
sclerosing k.
scrofulous k.
serpiginous k.
k. sicca
superficial linear k.
superficial punctate k.
trachomatous k.
vascular k.
vesicular k.
xerotic k.
keratoacanthoma
keratoangioma
keratocele
keratoconjunctivitis
atopic k.
epidemic k.
flash k.
herpetic k.
microsporidian k.
k. sicca
superior limbic k.
ultraviolet k.
vernal k.
virus k.
keratoconus
circumscribed posterior k.
keratocricoid
keratocyst
odontogenic k.
keratocyte
keratoderma
k. blennorrhagica
k. blennorrhagicum
lymphedematous k.
mutilating k.
k. palmaris et plantaris
palmoplantar k.
k. plantare sulcatum
punctate k.
senile k.
k. symmetrica
type III punctate palmoplantar k.
keratodermatitis
keratoectasia
keratoelastoidosis marginalis
keratoepithelioplasty
keratogenesis
keratogenetic
keratogenous membrane
keratoglobus
keratography
keratohyal
keratohyalin granule
keratoid exanthema
keratoleptynsis
keratoleukoma
keratolysis
k. exfoliativa
pitted k.
k. plantare sulcatum
keratolytic

keratoma
k. disseminatum
k. hereditarium mutilans
k. plantare sulcatum
senile k.
keratomalacia
keratome
keratometer
keratometry
keratomileusis
laser-assisted in situ k. (LASIK)
keratomycosis
keratonosis
keratopachyderma
keratopathia guttata
keratopathy
band-shaped k.
bullous k.
chronic actinic k.
climatic droplike k.
filamentary k.
infectious crystalline k.
Labrador k.
lipid k.
neuroparalytic k.
striate k.
vesicular k.
keratophakia
keratophakic keratoplasty
keratoplasia
keratoplasty
allopathic k.
autogenous k.
epikeratophakic k.
heterogenous k.
homogenous k.
keratophakic k.
lamellar k., layered k.
nonpenetrating k.
optic k.
penetrating k.
perforating k.
refractive k.
tectonic k.
total k.
keratoprosthesis
keratorefractive surgery
keratorhexis
keratorus
keratoscleritis
keratoscope
keratoscopy
keratosis
actinic k.
arsenical k.
k. blennorrhagica
k. follicularis
inverted follicular k.
k. labialis
lichenoid k.
lichen planus-like k.
k. obturans
k. palmaris et plantaris
k. pilaris
k. pilaris atrophicans faciei

K

keratosis *(continued)*
    k. punctata
    seborrheic k.
    senile k.
    solar k.
    tar k.
keratosulfate
keratotome
keratotomy
    delimiting k.
    radial k.
    refractive k.
keraunophobia
Kerckring
    K. center
    K. fold
    K. ossicle
    K. valve
kerion
Kerley
    K. A, B, C line
kernel
kernicterus
Kernig sign
Kernohan notch
kern-plasma relation theory
kerosene
Kestenbaum
    K. number
    K. procedure
    K. sign
ketal
ketamine
ketanserin
ketene
ketimine
3-ketoacid-CoA transferase
ketoacidemia
ketoacidosis
ketoaciduria
    branched chain k.
3-ketoacyl-CoA thiolase
2-ketoadipic acid
    2-k. a. dehydrogenase complex
2-ketoadipic acidemia
ketoconazole
ketogenesis
ketogenic
    k. corticoids test
    k. diet
    17-k. steroid assay test
ketogenic-antiketogenic ratio (K:A ratio)
α-ketoglutarate
    α-ketoglutarate dehydrogenase
ketoheptose
ketohexose
ketohydroxyestrin
ketol
ketole group
ketolytic
ketone
    k. alcohol
    k. body
ketone-aldehyde mutase

ketonemia
ketonic
ketonimine dye
ketonization
ketonuria
    branched chain k.
ketopantoic acid
ketopentose
ketorolac
ketose-1-phosphate aldolase
ketose reductase
ketosis
    bovine k.
ketosis-prone diabetes
ketosis-resistant diabetes
17-ketosteroids (17-KS)
ketosuccinic acid
ketosuria
ketotetrose
ketotic
    k. hyperglycemia
    k. hyperglycinemia
    k. hypoglycemia
ketotriose
Kety-Schmidt method
keV
    kiloelectron volts
Kew Gardens fever
Key
    k. attachment
    k. ridge
    k. vein
keyhole
    k. deformity
    k. pupil
keyway attachment
kg
    kilogram
khat
khellin
KHN
    Knoop hardness number
kick
    atrial k.
    idioventricular k.
Kidd blood group
kidney
    amyloid k.
    Armanni-Ebstein k.
    arteriolosclerotic k.
    arteriosclerotic k.
    artificial k.
    Ask-Upmark k.
    atrophic k.
    k. basin
    cake k.
    k. carbuncle
    contracted k.
    cow k.
    crush k.
    cystic k.
    disk k.
    duplex k.
    fatty k.
    flea-bitten k.

floating k.
Formad k.
fused k.
Goldblatt k.
granular k.
head k.
hind k.
horseshoe k.
k. lobe
medullary sponge k.
middle k.
mortar k.
movable k.
pancake k.
pelvic k.
polycystic k.
primordial k.
putty k.
pyelonephritic k.
Rose-Bradford k.
sclerotic k.
sigmoid k.
supernumerary k.
thoracic k.
k.'s, ureters, bladder (KUB)
wandering k.
waxy k.
Kiel classification
Kienböck
    K. disease
    K. dislocation
    K. unit (X)
Kiernan space
Kiesselbach area
Kikuchi disease
Kilham rat virus
Kiliani-Fischer
    K.-F. reaction
    K.-F. synthesis
Kilian line
killer
    k. cell
    natural k. (NK)
Killian
    K. bundle
    K. operation
    K. triangle
kilo (k)
kilobase (kb)
kilocalorie (kcal)
kilocycle (kc)
kilogram (kg)
kilogram-meter
kilohertz
kilohm
kilojoule
kilovolt (kv)
    k. peak (kVp)
kilovoltage
    peak k. (pkV)
kilovoltmeter
Ki-1+ lymphoma
Kimmelstiel-Wilson
    K.-W. disease
    K.-W. syndrome

Kimura disease
kin-
kinanesthesia
kinase
    k. II
kindling
kindred
    degree of k.
kinematic
    k. face-bow
    k. viscosity
kinematics
kinemometer
kineplastic amputation
kinesi-
kinesia
kinesiatrics
kinesics
kinesimeter
kinesin
kinesiology
kinesiometer
kinesipathist
kinesis
kinesitherapy
kinesophobia
kinesthesia hallucination
kinesthesiometer
kinesthesis
kinesthetic
    k. aura
    k. sense
kinetic
    k. analyzer
    k. ataxia
    k. energy
    k. measurement
    k. perimetry
    k. strabismus
    k. system
    k. tremor
kinetics
    chemical k.
    enzyme k.
kinetocardiogram
kinetocardiograph
kinetochore fiber
kinetochores
kinetogenic
kinetoplasm
kinetoplast
kinetoscope
kinetosome
King-Armstrong unit
kingdom
Kingella
    Kingella indologenes
    Kingella kingae
king's evil
Kingsley splint
King unit
kinic acid
kinin 9

K

kininogen
> high molecular weight k.
> low molecular weight k.

kininogenase
kininogenin
kink
> Lane k.

kinked aorta
Kinkiang fever
kinky hair
kino-
kinocentrum
kinocilium
kinomometer
kinoplasm
kinoplasmic
kinship
Kinyoun stain
kion
Kirk amputation
Kirkland knife
Kirschner
> K. apparatus
> K. wire

Kisch reflex
kissing puncta
Kitasato bacillus
Kjeldahl
> K. apparatus
> K. method

Kjelland forceps
Kjer optic atrophy
Klatskin tumor
Klebsiella
> *K. mobilis*
> *K. oxytoca*
> *K. ozaenae*
> *K. pneumoniae*
> *K. pneumoniae* subsp. *ozaenae*
> *K. rhinoscleromatis*

Klebs-Loeffler bacillus
kleeblattschädel
Kleihauer stain
Kleine-Levin syndrome
Klein-Gumprecht shadow nuclei
Klenow fragment
kleptomania
kleptomaniac
kleptophobia
Klestadt cyst
Klinefelter syndrome
Klinger-Ludwig acid-thionin stain for sex chromatin
Klippel-Feil syndrome
Klippel-Trenaunay-Weber syndrome
Klumpke
> K. palsy
> K. paralysis

Klüver-Barrera Luxol fast blue stain
Klüver-Bucy syndrome
Kluyvera
Km
> K. allotypes
> K. antigen

Knapp
> K. streak
> K. stria

knee
> Brodie k.
> k. disarticulation amputation
> housemaid's k.
> k. jerk
> k. joint
> locked k.
> k. presentation
> k. reflex
> runner's k.
> Wilbrand k.

knee-ankle-foot orthosis
kneecap
knee-chest position
knee-elbow position
knee-jerk reflex
Knemidokoptes
KNF model
> Koshland-Némethy-Filmer model

Kniest syndrome
knife, pl. **knives**
> amputation k.
> Beer k.
> cartilage k.
> cautery k.
> chemical k.
> electrode k.
> fistula k.
> free-hand k.
> gamma k.
> Goldman-Fox k.
> Graefe k.
> hernia k.
> Kirkland k.
> lenticular k.
> Liston knife
> Merrifield k.
> k. needle
> valvotomy k.

knife-rest crystal
knismogenic
knitting
knives (*pl. of* knife)
knob
> aortic k.
> Engelmann basal k.
> malarial k.

knock
> pericardial k.

knock-knee
knock-out
> k.-o. drops

knockout mouse
Knoll gland
Knoop
> K. hardness number (KHN)
> K. hardness test
> K. theory

knot
> false k.
> granny k.
> Hensen k.

Hubrecht protochordal k.
laparoscopic k.
net k.
primitive k.
protochordal k.
square k.
surgeon's k.
syncytial k.
true k.
true k. of umbilical cord
vital k.
Knott technique
knuckle
aortic k.
cervical aortic k.
k. pad
k. sign
Knudsen hypothesis
Kobberling-Dunnigan syndrome
Kobelt tubules
Kober test
Köbner phenomenon
Koch
K. bacillus
K. law
K. node
K. old tuberculin
K. phenomenon
K. postulates
K. triangle
Kocher
K. clamp
K. incision
K. sign
Kocher-Debré-Sémélaigne syndrome
Koch-Weeks bacillus
Kock
K. ileostomy
K. pouch
Koenig syndrome
Koerber-Salus-Elschnig syndrome
Koerte-Ballance operation
Koettstorfer number
Köhler
K. disease
K. illumination
Kohlmeier-Degos syndrome
Kohlrausch
K. fold
K. muscle
Kohn pore
Kohnstamm phenomenon
koilocyte
koilocytosis
koilonychia
koilosternia
Kojewnikoff epilepsy
kojic acid
kok disease
kokoi venom
Kokoskin stain
kola
Kölliker
K. layer
K. reticulum

Kollmann dilator
Kolmer test
kolp-
kolytic
Kommerell diverticulum
Kondoleon operation
koniocortex
Konno procedure
Konno-Rastan procedure
konzo
Koongol viruses
Koplik spot
kopophobia
kopro-
Korean
K. hemorrhagic fever
K. hemorrhagic fever virus
Korff fiber
Kornberg enzyme
koro
koronion
Korotkoff
K. sound
K. test
Korsakoff
K. psychosis
K. syndrome
Koshland-Némethy-Filmer model (KNF model)
Kossa stain
Kostmann syndrome
Kr
krypton
Krabbe disease
krait
Kraske operation
kraurosis vulvae
Krause
K. bone
K. end bulb
K. gland
K. graft
K. ligament
K. respiratory bundle
K. valve
Krause-Wolfe graft
krebiozen
Krebs
K.-Henseleit cycle
K.-Kornberg cycle
K. ornithine cycle
K.-Ringer solution
K. urea cycle
Kretschmann space
Kreysig sign
kriging
Krimsky test
kringle
Krogh spirometer
Kronecker stain
Krönig
K. isthmus
K. step

K

Krönlein
> K. hernia
> K. operation

Krueger instrument stop

Krukenberg
> K. amputation
> K. spindle
> K. tumor
> K. vein

Kruse brush

krypton (Kr)
> k. laser

17-KS
> 17-ketosteroids

KTP laser

KUB
> kidneys, ureters, bladder

kubisagari

Kufs disease

Kugel anastomotic artery

Kugelberg-Welander disease

Kühne
> K. fiber
> K. methylene blue
> K. phenomenon
> K. plate
> K. spindle

Kuhnt space

Kulchitsky cell

Külz cylinder

Küntscher nail

Kupffer cell

kurchi bark

Kürsteiner canal

kurtosis

Kurtzke multiple sclerosis disability scale

kuru

Kurzrok-Ratner test

Kuskokwim syndrome

Kussmaul
> K. coma

> K. disease
> K. respiration
> K. sign

Kussmaul-Kien respiration

kv
> kilovolt

Kveim
> K. antigen
> K. test

Kveim-Siltzbach
> K.-S. antigen
> K.-S. test

kVp
> kilovolt peak

kwashiorkor
> marasmic k.

Kyasanur
> K. Forest disease
> K. Forest disease virus

kymogram

kymograph

kymography

kymoscope

kynurenic acid

kynureninase

kynurenine
> k. formamidase
> k. 3-hydroxylase
> k. 3-monooxygenase

kyphos

kyphoscoliosis

kyphoscoliotic pelvis

kyphosis
> juvenile k.
> sacral k.
> k. sacralis TA]
> thoracic k.
> k. thoracica

kyphotic pelvis

Kyrle disease

Λ
    lambda
λ *(var. of* lambda)
L
    limes
L
    L chain
    L dose
    L form
    L selectin
    L shell
    L unit of streptomycin
L
    linking number
μl
    microliter
l
    length
    liquid
    liter
l-
    levarotatory
L-
La
    lanthanum
Laband syndrome
Labbé
    L. triangle
    L. vein
label (Sig.)
labeled
    l. atom
    l. thyroxine
la belle indifférence
labetalol hydrochloride
labia *(pl. of* labium)
labial
    l. arch
    l. bar
    l. branch of mental nerve
    l. commissure
    l. embrasure
    l. flange
    l. gingiva
    l. gland
    l. hernia
    l. occlusion
    l. part of orbicularis oris muscle
    l. splint
    l. sulcus
    l. swelling
    l. tubercle
    l. vein
    l. vestibule
labialism
labially
labile
    l. affect
    l. current
    l. element
    l. factor

    l. hypertension
    l. pulse
lability
labiocervical
labioclination
labiodental sulcus
labiogingival lamina
labioglossolaryngeal
labioglossopharyngeal
labiograph
labiolingual
    l. appliance
    l. plane
labiomental
labionasal
labiopalatine
labioplacement
labioplasty
labioscrotal
    l. fold
    l. swelling
labioversion
labitome
labium, pl. **labia**
    l. anterius ostii uteri
    l. externum cristae iliacae
    l. inferius oris
    l. internum cristae iliacae
    l. laterale lineae asperae
    l. limbi tympanicum laminae spiralis ossei
    l. limbi tympanicum limbi spiralis ossei
    l. limbi vestibulare laminae spiralis ossei
    l. limbi vestibulare limbi spiralis ossei
    labia majora
    l. majus
    l. majus pudendi
    l. mediale lineae asperae
    labia minora
    l. minus
    l. minus pudendi
    labia oris
    l. posterius ostii uteri
    l. superius oris
    tympanic l. of limbus of spiral lamina
    l. urethrae
    labia uteri
    vestibular l. of limbus of spiral lamina
    l. vocale
    labia vocalia
labor
    active l.
    l. curve
    dry l.
    false l.
    first stage l.
    missed l.

L

labor *(continued)*
l. pain
placental stage l.
precipitate l.
premature l.
second stage l.
third stage l.
trial of l. after cesarean section
laboratorian
laboratory
l. diagnosis
personal growth l.
labored respiration
labra (*pl. of* labrum)
Labrador keratopathy
labrale
l. inferius
l. superius
labrocyte
labrum, pl. **labra**
acetabular l.
l. acetabulare
articular l.
l. articulare
l. glenoidale scapulae
glenoid l. of scapula
labyrinth
bony l.
cochlear l.
ethmoidal l.
Ludwig l.
membranous l.
osseous l.
renal l.
Santorini l.
vestibular l.
labyrinthectomy
labyrinthine
l. apoplexy
l. artery
l. fistula
l. nystagmus
l. placenta
l. reflex
l. righting reflex
l. torticollis
l. vein
l. wall of middle ear
l. wall of tympanic cavity
labyrinthitis
labyrinthotomy
labyrinthus
l. cochlearis
l. ethmoidalis
l. membranaceus
l. osseus
l. vestibularis
lac
L. operon
l. sulfuris
l. vaccinum
lacca
laccase
lacerable

lacerated foramen
laceration
brain l.
scalp l.
through-and-through laceration
vaginal l.
lacertus
l. cordis
l. fibrosus
l. of lateral rectus muscle
l. medius
l. musculi recti lateralis
Lachman test
lachrymal
LACI
lipoprotein-associated coagulation inhibitor
laciniae tubae
laciniate ligament
lacis cell
lacquer crack
lacrimal
l. apparatus
l. artery
l. bay
l. bone
l. border of maxilla
l. calculus
l. canaliculus
l. caruncle
l. fascia
l. fistula
l. fold
l. fossa
l. gland
l. groove
l. hamulus
l. lake
l. margin of maxilla
l. nerve
l. notch
l. opening
l. papilla
l. part of orbicularis oculi muscle
l. pathway
l. process of inferior nasal concha
l. punctum
l. reflex
l. sac
l. vein
lacrimation
lacrimator
lacrimatory
lacrimoconchal suture
lacrimogustatory reflex
lacrimomaxillary suture
lacrimotomy
La Crosse virus
lactacidemia
lactacidosis
lactacid oxygen debt
lactalbumin
lactam, lactim
lactamase

lactase
l. persistence
l. restriction
lactate
l. dehydrogenase (LDH)
l. dehydrogenase virus
excess l.
l. 2-mono-oxygenase
Ringer l.
lactated
l. Ringer injection
l. Ringer solution
lactating adenoma
lactation
l. amenorrhea
l. hormone
lactational mastitis
lacteal
central l.
l. cyst
l. fistula
l. vessel
lactenin
lactescent
lactic
l. acid
l. acid bacillus
l. acid dehydrogenase
l. acidemia
l. acid fermentation
l. acidosis
l. acid oxidative decarboxylase
lactiferous
l. ampulla
l. duct
l. gland
l. sinus
lactifugal
lactifuge
lactigenous
lactim (*var. of* lactam)
lactimorbus
lactinated
Lactobacillaceae
lactobacillary milk
lactobacilli (*pl. of* lactobacillus)
lactobacillic acid
Lactobacillus
L. acidophilus
L. brevis
L. buchneri
L. bulgaricus
L. Bulgaricus factor
L. casei
L. casei factor
L. catenaformis
L. crispatus
L. curvatus
L. delbrueckii
L. fermentum
L. jensenii
L. plantarum
L. salivarius
L. trichodes
lactobacillus, pl. **lactobacilli**

lactobezoar
lactobutyrometer
lactocele
lactochrome
lactocrit
lactodensimeter
lactoferrin
lactoflavin
lactogen
human placental l. (HPL)
placental l. (PL)
lactogenesis
lactogenic hormone
lactoglobulin
lactometer
lactonase
lactone
lactoperoxidase
lactophenol cotton blue stain
lactoprotein
lactorrhea
lactoscope
lactose
l. intolerance
l. synthase
lactosuria
lactotherapy
lactotrophic
lactotropin
lactovegetarian
lactoylglutathione lyase
lactulose
lacuna, pl. **lacunae**
cartilage l.
cerebral l.
l. cerebri
Howship lacunae
intervillous l.
lateral lacunae
lacunae laterales
lateral lacunae of superior sagittal
sinus
lateral venous lacunae
l. magna
Morgagni l.
muscular l.
l. musculorum
l. musculorum retroinguinalis
osseous l.
pharyngeal l.
l. pharyngis
resorption lacunae
trophoblastic l.
urethral l.
l. urethralis, pl. lacunae urethrales
vascular l.
l. vasorum
l. vasorum retroinguinalis
lacunar
l. amnesia
l. ligament
l. state
l. tonsillitis
lacunar-molecular layer

L

lacunule
lacus, pl. **lacus**
 l. lacrimalis
 l. seminalis
LAD
 leukocyte adhesion deficiency
Ladd
 L. band
 L. operation
ladder splint
Ladd-Franklin theory
Lady Windemere's syndrome
Laelaps echidninus
Laënnec
 L. cirrhosis
 L. pearl
laetrile
Lafora
 L. body
 L. body disease
lag
 anaphase l.
 homeostatic l.
 l. phase
lagena, pl. **lagenae**
lagging
lagomorph
Lagomorpha
lagophthalmic keratitis
lagophthalmos
Lahey forceps
Lahore sore
Laimer-Haeckerman area
LAK
 lymphokine activated killer cell
lake
 capillary l.
 lacrimal l.
 lateral l.'s
 seminal l.
 subchorial l.
 venous l.'s
Laki-Lorand factor
laky blood
laliatry
laliophobia
Lallemand body
lalling
Lallouette pyramid
lalochezia
lalognosis
laloplegia
lamarckian theory
Lamaze method
LAMB
 lentigines, atrial myxoma, mucocutaneous
 myxomas, and blue nevi
 LAMB syndrome
Lam B
lambda, λ (Λ)
 L. phage
lambdacism
lambdoid
 l. border of occipital bone

 l. margin of occipital bone
 l. suture
Lambert
 L. law
 L. syndrome
Lambert-Eaton syndrome
Lambl excrescence
Lamblia intestinalis
lambliasis
lambo lambo
Lambrinudi operation
lamella
 annulate l.'s
 articular l.
 l. of bone
 circumferential l.
 concentric l.
 cornoid l.
 elastic l.
 enamel l.
 glandulopreputial l.
 ground l.
 haversian l.
 intermediate l.
 interstitial l.
 triangular l.
 tympanic l.
 l. tympanica (laminae spiralis ossei)
 l. vestibularis (laminae spiralis
  ossei)
 vestibular l. (of osseous spiral
  lamina)
 vitreous l.
lamellar
 l. bone
 l. cataract
 l. granule
 l. ichthyosis
 l. keratoplasty
lamellate, lamellated
 l. corpuscle
lamellipodium
lamina, pl. **laminae**
 l. affixa
 l. alaris
 alar l. of neural tube
 laminae albae cerebelli
 l. anterior fasciae thoracolumbalis
 anterior limiting l.
 l. anterior vaginae musculi recti
  abdominis
 l. arcus vertebrae
 basal l.
 basal l. of choroid
 basal l. of ciliary body
 basal l. of cochlear duct
 l. basalis
 l. basalis choroideae
 l. basalis corporis ciliaris
 basal l. of neural tube
 basal l. of semicircular duct
 basement l.
 basilar l.
 l. basilaris cochleae
 l. basilaris corporis ciliaris

l. basilaris ductus cochlearis
boundary l.
capillary l. of choroid
l. cartilaginis cricoideae
l. cartilaginis thyroideae
l. choriocapillaris
l. choroidea
l. choroidea epithelialis
l. choroidocapillaris
l. cinerea
l. cribrosa ossis ethmoidalis
l. cribrosa of sclera
l. cribrosa sclerae
cribrous l.
l. of cricoid cartilage
deep l.
l. densa
dental l.
l. dentata
dentogingival l.
l. dorsalis
l. dura
l. elastica anterior
l. elastica posterior
elastic laminae of artery
l. epiphysialis
episcleral l.
l. episcleralis
epithelial l.
l. epithelialis
l. externa calvaria
l. externa cranii
external medullary l.
l. fibrocartilaginea interpubica
l. fibroreticularis
l. fusca of sclera
l. fusca sclerae
hepatic laminae
l. horizontalis ossis palatini
l. interna calvariae
l. interna cranii
internal medullary l.
l. interna ossium cranii
iridopupillary l.
labiogingival l.
lateral l. of cartilage of
  pharyngotympanic auditory tube
l. lateralis cartilaginis tubae
  auditivae
l. lateralis cartilaginis tubae
  auditoriae
l. lateralis processus pterygoidei
lateral medullary l. of lentiform
  nucleus
l. of lens
l. limitans anterior
l. limitans anterior corneae
l. limitans posterior corneae
l. lucida
medial l. of cartilage of
  pharyngotympanic auditory tube
l. medialis cartilaginis tubae
  auditivae
l. medialis cartilaginis tubae
  auditoriae

l. medialis processus pterygoidei
medial medullary l. of lentiform
  nucleus
laminae medullares cerebelli
laminae medullares thalami
l. medullaris lateralis
l. medullaris lateralis nuclei
  lentiformis
l. medullaris medialis
l. medullaris medialis nuclei
  lentiformis
medullary laminae of thalamus
l. membranacea cartilaginis tubae
  auditivae
l. membranacea cartilaginis tubae
  auditoriae
membranous l. of cartilage of
  pharyngotympanic auditory plate
l. of mesencephalic tectum
l. modioli cochleae
l. of modiolus of cochlea
l. molecularis corticis cerebri
l. muscularis mucosae
nuclear l.
orbital l. of ethmoid bone
l. orbitalis ossis ethmoidalis
osseous spiral l.
l. papyracea
l. parietalis
l. parietalis pericardii serosi
l. parietalis tunicae vaginalis testis
periclaustral l.
l. perpendicularis
l. perpendicularis ossis ethmoidalis
l. perpendicularis ossis palatini
posterior limiting l. of cornea
l. posterior vaginae musculi recti
  abdominis
l. pretrachealis fasciae cervicalis
l. prevertebralis fasciae cervicalis
primary dental l.
l. profunda
l. profunda fasciae temporalis
l. profunda fasciae thoracolumbalis
l. profunda musculi levatoris
  palpebrae superioris
l. propria
l. propria mucosae
pterygoid l.
l. quadrigemina
quadrigeminal l.
l. rara
reticular l.
retrorectal l. of endopelvic fascia
retrorectal l. of hypogastric sheath
l. retrorectalis fasciae endopelvicae
l. of Rexed
rostral l.
l. rostralis
secondary spiral l.
l. septi pellucidi
l. of septum pellucidum
spinal l.
l. spinalis II
l. spiralis ossea

L

lamina *(continued)*
  l. spiralis secundaria
  successional l.
  superficial l.
  l. superficialis
  l. superficialis fasciae cervicalis
  l. superficialis fasciae temporalis
  l. superficialis musculi levatoris
    palpebrae superioris
  suprachoroid l. of sclera
  l. supraneuroporica
  l. tecti
  l. terminalis
  l. terminalis of cerebrum
  l. of thyroid cartilage
  tragal l.
  l. tragi
  l. of tragus
  vascular l. of choroid
  l. vasculosa choroideae
  l. ventralis
  l. of vertebral arch
  l. visceralis
  l. visceralis pericardii
  l. visceralis tunicae vaginalis testis
  l. vitrea
laminagram
laminagraph
laminagraphy, laminography
laminar
  l. cortical necrosis
  l. cortical sclerosis
  l. flow
laminaria
laminarin sulfate
laminated
  l. clot
  l. cortex
  l. epithelial plug
  l. epithelium
  l. thrombus
lamination
laminectomy
laminin receptor
laminitis
laminography *(var. of* laminagraphy*)*
laminotomy
lamins
lamotrigine
lamp
  annealing l.
  Edridge-Green l.
  heat l.
  mercury vapor l.
  mignon l.
  slit l.
  spirit l.
  tungsten arc l.
  ultraviolet l.
  Wood l.
lampbrush chromosome
lana
Lan antigen

lanatoside
  l. A, B, C, D
Lancaster red green test
lance
Lancefield classification
lancet
  gum l.
  spring l.
  thumb l.
lancinating
Lancisi sign
Landau-Kleffner syndrome
Landolfi sign
Landouzy-Dejerine dystrophy
Landouzy-Grasset law
Landry
  L. paralysis
  L. syndrome
Landry-Guillain-Barré syndrome
landscape ecology
Landschutz tumor
land scurvy
Landsteiner-Donath test
Landström muscle
Landzert fossa
Lane
  L. band
  L. disease
  L. kink
Lange
  L. solution
  L. test
Langenbeck triangle
Langendorff method
Langer
  L. arch
  L. line
  L. muscle
Langerhans
  L. cell
  L. cell histiocytosis
  L. granule
  L. island
Langer-Saldino syndrome
Langhans
  L. cell
  L. layer
  L. stria
Langhans-type giant cell
Langley granule
Langmuir trough
language
  American Sign L. (ASL)
  body l.
  l. game
  l. zone
laniary
lankamycin
Lannelongue
  L. foramina
  L. ligament
lanolin
  anhydrous l.
lanosterol

Lanterman
    L. incisures
    L. segment
lanthanic
lanthanides
lanthanum (La)
    l. nitrate
lanthionine
lanugo hair
Lanz line
LAO
    left anterior oblique projection
LAP
    leukocyte alkaline phosphatase
laparocele
laparoendoscopic
laparogastroscopy
laparomyositis
laparorrhaphy
laparosalpingo-oophorectomy
laparoscope
laparoscopic
    l. cannula
    l. cholecystotomy
    l. knot
    l. nephrectomy
    l. surgery
    l. uterosacral nerve ablation
laparoscopically assisted surgery
laparoscopic-assisted vaginal hysterectomy (LAVH)
laparoscopy
    closed l.
    open l.
laparotomy pad
Lapicque law
lapinization
lapinized
Laplace
    L. forceps
    L. law
L-AP₄ receptor
Laquer stain for alcoholic hyalin
larch turpentine
lard
    benzoinated l.
lardaceous
    l. liver
    l. spleen
large
    l. bowel
    l. calorie (C, Cal)
    l. cell carcinoma
    l. cell lymphoma
    l., external transformation-sensitive fibronectin (LETS)
    l. interarch distance
    l. intestine
    l. muscle of helix
    l. pelvis
    l. pudendal lip
    l. saphenous vein
larkspur
Larmor frequency
Laron-type dwarfism

Laroyenne operation
Larrey cleft
Larsen syndrome
larva, pl. **larvae**
    l. currens
    filariform l.
    rhabditiform l.
larvaceous
larval
    l. conjunctivitis
    l. plague
larva migrans
    cutaneous l. m.
    ocular l. m.
    spiruroid l. m.
    visceral l. m.
larvate
larvicidal
larvicide
larviparous
larviphagic
laryngeal
    l. aditus
    l. aperture
    l. atresia
    l. bursa
    l. cavity
    l. chorea
    l. crisis
    l. diphtheria
    l. epilepsy
    l. gland
    l. granuloma
    l. inlet
    l. lymphoid nodule
    l. mask
    l. mucosa
    l. papillomatosis
    l. part of pharynx
    l. pharynx
    l. polyp
    l. pouch
    l. prominence
    l. reflex
    l. saccule
    l. sinus
    l. stenosis
    l. stridor
    l. syncope
    l. tonsils
    l. vein
    l. ventricle
    l. vertigo
    l. web
laryngectomee
laryngectomy
    horizontal l.
    partial l.
    supraglottic l.
larynges (*pl. of* larynx)
laryngismus stridulus
laryngitic
laryngitis
    chronic posterior l.
    chronic subglottic l.

L

laryngitis *(continued)*
    croupous l.
    membranous l.
    l. sicca
    spasmodic l.
    l. stridulosa
laryngocele
laryngofissure
laryngograph
laryngography
laryngology
laryngomalacia
laryngoparalysis
laryngopharyngeal branch of superior cervical ganglion
laryngopharyngectomy
laryngopharyngeus
laryngopharyngitis
laryngopharynx
laryngophthisis
laryngoplasty
laryngoplegia
laryngoptosis
laryngoscope
laryngoscopic
laryngoscopist
laryngoscopy
    direct l.
    indirect l.
    suspension l.
    transnasal fiberoptic l.
laryngospasm
laryngospastic reflex
laryngostenosis
laryngostomy
laryngostroboscope
laryngotomy
    inferior l.
    median l.
    superior l.
laryngotracheal
    l. diphtheria
    l. diverticulum
    l. groove
laryngotracheitis
laryngotracheobronchitis
laryngotracheoesophageal cleft
laryngotracheoplasty
larynx, pl. **larynges**
    Cooper-Rand artificial l.
lase
Lasègue
    L. sign
    L. syndrome
laser
    argon l.
    continuous wave l.
    l. corepraxy
    excimer l.
    l. iridotomy
    krypton l.
    KTP l.
    l. microscope
    Nd:YAG l.

    l. photocoagulator
    l. plume
    pulsed l.
    pulsed dye l. (PDL)
    pumped l.
    Q-switched l.
    quasi-continuous wave l.
    l. trabeculoplasty (LTP)
laser-assisted in situ keratomileusis (LASIK)
lasering
Lash
    L. casein hydrolysate-serum medium
    L. operation
lash
LASIK
    laser-assisted in situ keratomileusis
Lasiohelea
Lassa
    L. fever
    L. hemorrhagic fever
    L. virus
lassitude
latah
Latarget
    L. nerve
    L. vein
late
    l. apical systolic murmur
    l. auditory-evoked response
    l. benign syphilis
    l. cyanosis
    l. deceleration
    l. diastole
    l. diastolic murmur
    l. dumping syndrome
    l. latent syphilis
    l. luteal phase dysphoria
    l. luteal phase dysphoric disorder
    l. neonatal death
    l. reaction
    l. replicating chromosome
    l. rickets
    l. seizure
    l. systole
latebra
latency
    l. period
    l. phase
latent
    l. adrenocortical insufficiency
    l. allergy
    l. carcinoma
    l. carrier
    l. content
    l. diabetes
    l. empyema
    l. energy
    l. gout
    l. heat
    l. homosexuality
    l. hyperopia
    l. infection
    l. learning
    l. membrane protein (LMP)

l. microbism
l. nystagmus
l. period
l. rat virus
l. reflex
l. scarlatina
l. schizophrenia
l. stage
l. syphilis
l. typhoid
l. zone

late-phase response
latera (*pl. of* latus)
laterad
lateral

l. abdominal/pectoral cutaneous branch of intercostal nerve
l. aberrant thyroid carcinoma
l. aberration
l. alveolar abscess
l. ampullar nerve
l. amygdaloid nucleus
l. angle of eye
l. angle of scapula
l. angle of uterus
l. antebrachial cutaneous nerve
l. anterior thoracic nerve
l. aperture of fourth ventricle
l. arcuate ligament
l. aspect
l. atlantoaxial joint
l. atlantoepistrophic joint
l. atrial branch of left coronary artery
l. atrial branch of right coronary artery
l. atrial vein
l. axillary lymph node
l. basal branch
l. basal segmental artery
l. basal segment [S IX]
l. bicipital groove
l. border
l. border of foot
l. border of forearm
l. border of humerus
l. border of kidney
l. border of nail
l. border of scapula
l. branch
l. branch of artery of tuber cinereum
l. branch of pontine artery
l. branch of posterior ramus of spinal nerve
l. bronchopulmonary segment S IV
l. calcaneal branch of sural nerve
l. canal
l. canthus
l. cartilage of nose
l. cartilaginous plate
l. central palmar space
l. cerebellomedullary cistern
l. cerebral fissure
l. cerebral fossa

l. cervical nucleus
l. cervical region
l. circumflex artery of thigh
l. circumflex femoral artery
l. circumflex femoral vein
l. collateral ligament of ankle
l. column
l. column of spinal cord
l. compartment of leg
l. condylar inclination
l. condyle
l. condyle of femur
l. condyle of tibia
l. cord of brachial plexus
l. corticospinal tract
l. costal branch of internal thoracic artery
l. costotransverse ligament
l. cricoarytenoid muscle
l. crus
l. crus of facial canal
l. crus of horizontal part of the facial canal
l. crus of the major alar cartilage of the nose
l. crus of the superficial inguinal ring
l. cuneate nucleus
l. cuneiform bone
l. curvature
l. cutaneous branch
l. cutaneous branch of intercostal nerve
l. cutaneous branch of ventral primary ramus of thoracic spinal nerve
l. cutaneous nerve of calf
l. cutaneous nerve of forearm
l. cutaneous nerve of thigh
l. decubitus radiograph
l. direct vein
l. division of left liver
l. dorsal cutaneous nerve
l. dorsal nucleus
l. epicondylar crest
l. epicondylar ridge
l. epicondyle of femur
l. epicondyle of humerus
l. excursion
l. fasciculus proprius
l. femoral circumflex artery
l. femoral cutaneous nerve
l. femoral tuberosity
l. fillet
l. fold
l. fossa of brain
l. frontobasal artery
l. funiculus
l. funiculus of spinal cord
l. geniculate body
l. geniculate nucleus
l. ginglymus
l. glossoepiglottic fold
l. great muscle
l. ground bundle

L

lateral (*continued*)

l. habenular nucleus
l. hamstring
l. head
l. hermaphroditism
l. horn
l. humeral epicondylitis
l. hypothalamic area
l. hypothalamic region
l. illumination
l. incisor
l. inferior genicular artery
l. inferior hepatic area
l. inguinal fossa
l. interocclusal record
l. jugular lymph node
l. lacunae
l. lacunae of superior sagittal sinus
l. lacunar lymph node
l. lacunar node
l. lake
l. lamina of cartilage of pharyngotympanic auditory tube
l. lemniscus
l. ligament of ankle
l. ligament of bladder
l. ligament of elbow
l. ligament of knee
l. ligament of malleus
l. ligament of temporomandibular joint
l. ligament of wrist
l. limb
l. lingual swelling
l. lip of linea aspera
l. lithotomy
l. longitudinal arch of foot
l. longitudinal stria
l. lumbar intertransversarii muscle
l. lumbar intertransverse muscle
l. lumbocostal arch
l. malleolar artery
l. malleolar branch of fibular peroneal artery
l. malleolar facet of talus
l. malleolar ligament
l. malleolar network
l. malleolar subcutaneous bursa
l. malleolar surface of talus
l. malleolus
l. malleolus bursa
l. mammary branch
l. mammary branch of lateral cutaneous branch of intercostal nerve
l. mammary branch of lateral cutaneous branch of thoracic spinal nerve
l. mammary branch of lateral thoracic artery
l. margin
l. mass of atlas
l. mass of ethmoid bone
l. and medial palpebral artery

l. and medial parietal artery
l. and medial posterior choroidal branch of posterior cerebral artery
l. medullary branch of intracranial part of vertebral artery
l. medullary lamina of lentiform nucleus
l. medullary syndrome
l. meniscus
l. mesoderm
l. midpalmar space
l. movement
l. myocardial infarction
l. nasal artery
l. nasal branch of anterior ethmoidal nerve
l. nasal branch of facial artery
l. nasal fold
l. nasal process
l. nasal prominence
l. nucleus
l. nucleus of mammillary body
l. nucleus of medulla oblongata
l. nucleus of thalamus
l. nucleus of trapezoid body
l. oblique radiograph
l. occipital artery
l. occipital sulcus
l. occipitotemporal gyrus
l. occlusion
l. olfactory gyrus
l. orbitofrontal artery
l. palpebral commissure
l. palpebral ligament
l. palpebral raphe
l. parabrachial nucleus
l. part of longitudinal arch of foot
l. part of middle lobe vein
l. part of occipital bone
l. part of posterior cervical intertransversarii muscle
l. part of posterior compartment of forearm
l. part of sacrum
l. part of vaginal fornix
l. patellar retinaculum
l. pectoral nerve
l. pelvic wall triangle
l. pericardial lymph node
l. pericuneate nucleus
l. periodontal abscess
l. periodontal cyst
l. pharyngeal space
l. plantar artery
l. plantar nerve
l. plate
l. plate of cartilaginous auditory tube
l. plate mesoderm
l. plate of pterygoid process
l. pole
l. posterior cervical intertransversarii muscle
l. posterior nucleus
l. preoptic nucleus

l. process of calcaneal tuberosity
l. process of malleus
l. process of septal nasal cartilage
l. process of talus
l. projection
l. proprius bundle
l. pterygoid muscle
l. pterygoid plate
l. puboprostatic ligament
l. pyramidal fasciculus
l. pyramidal tract
l. ramus radiograph
l. raphespinal tract
l. recess of fourth ventricle
l. rectus muscle
l. rectus muscle of the head
l. recumbent position
l. region of abdominal region
l. region of neck
l. reticular nucleus
l. reticulospinal tract
l. root of median nerve
l. root of optic tract
l. sacral artery
l. sacral branch of median sacral artery
l. sacral crest
l. sacral vein
l. sacrococcygeal ligament
l. segment
l. segmental artery
l. semicircular canal
l. septal nucleus
l. sinus
l. skull radiograph
l. spinal sclerosis
l. spinothalamic tract
l. splanchnic artery
l. striate artery
l. sulcus
l. superior genicular artery
l. superior hepatic area
l. superior olivary nucleus
l. supraclavicular nerve
l. supracondylar crest
l. supracondylar ridge
l. supraepicondylar ridge
l. sural cutaneous nerve
l. surface
l. surface of arm
l. surface of fibula
l. surface of finger
l. surface of leg
l. surface of lower limb
l. surface of ovary
l. surface of testis
l. surface of tibia
l. surface of toe
l. surface of zygomatic bone
l. talocalcaneal ligament
l. tarsal artery
l. tarsal strip procedure
l. temporomandibular ligament
l. thalamic peduncle
l. thoracic artery

l. thoracic region
l. thoracic vein
l. thyrohyoid ligament
l. tuberal nuclei
l. tubercle
l. umbilical fold
l. umbilical ligament
l. vaginal wall smear
l. vastus muscle
l. vein of lateral ventricle
l. venous lacunae
l. ventral hernia
l. ventricle
l. vertigo
l. vestibular nucleus
l. vestibulospinal tract
l. wall of middle ear
l. wall of orbit
l. wall of tympanic cavity
l. zone

lateralis
laterality
    crossed l.
lateralization
lateriflexion
latero-
lateroabdominal
laterodeviation
lateroduction
lateroflexion
lateroposition
lateropulsion
laterotorsion
laterotrusion
lateroversion
latex
    l. agglutination test
    l. fixation test
lathe
lathyrism
lathyrogen
Latin square
latissimus dorsi muscle
latitude film
Latrodectus
    Latrodectus mactans
LATS
    long-acting thyroid stimulator
lattice corneal dystrophy
latticed layer
latus, pl. **latera**
Latzko cesarean section
laudable pus
laudanine
laudanosine
laudanum
laughing gas
laughter reflex
Laugier hernia
Laumonier ganglion
Launois-Bensaude syndrome
Launois-Cléret syndrome
laurel fever
Laurence-Moon syndrome
Laurer canal

L

lauric acid
Lauth
 L. canal
 L. ligament
 L. violet
LAV
 lymphadenopathy-associated virus
lavage
 antral l.
 bronchoalveolar l. (BAL)
Lavdovsky nucleoid
Laverania
laveur
LAVH
 laparoscopic-assisted vaginal hysterectomy
law
 Alexander l.
 all or none l.
 Ångström l.
 Arndt l.
 Arrhenius l.
 l.'s of association
 l. of average localization
 Avogadro l.
 Baer l.
 Baruch l.
 Beer l.
 Beer-Lambert l.
 Behring l.
 Bell l.
 Bell-Magendie l.
 Bernoulli l.
 Berthollet l.
 l. of biogenesis
 biogenetic l.
 Blagden l.
 Bowditch l.
 Boyle l.
 Broadbent l.
 Bunsen-Roscoe l.
 Charles l.
 l. of constant numbers in ovulation
 l. of contiguity
 l. of contrary innervation
 Coppet l.
 Courvoisier l.
 Dale-Feldberg l.
 Dalton l.
 Dalton-Henry l.
 l. of definite proportions
 l. of denervation
 Descartes l.
 Donders l.
 Draper l.
 Du Bois-Reymond l.
 Dulong-Petit l.
 Einthoven l.
 Elliott l.
 l. of excitation
 Faraday l.
 Farr l.
 Fechner-Weber l.
 Ferry-Porter l.
 Fick l. of diffusion
 Flatau l.

 Galton l.
 Gay-Lussac l.
 Godélier l.
 Gompertz l.
 Graham l.
 Grasset l.
 l. of gravitation
 Guldberg-Waage l.
 Haeckel l.
 Halsted l.
 Hardy-Weinberg l.
 l. of the heart
 Heidenhain l.
 Hellin l.
 Henry l.
 Herring l.
 Hess l.
 Hilton l.
 Hooke l.
 l. of independent assortment
 l. of intestine
 inverse square l.
 isodynamic l.
 Jackson l.
 Koch l.
 Lambert l.
 Landouzy-Grasset l.
 Lapicque l.
 Laplace l.
 Le Chatelier l.
 Listing l.
 Louis l.
 Magendie l.
 Marey l.
 Marfan l.
 Mariotte l.
 mass l.
 l. of mass action
 Meltzer l.
 Mendeléeff l.
 Mendel first l.
 Mendel second l.
 l. of the minimum
 Müller l.
 l. of multiple proportions
 Nasse l.
 Neumann l.
 Newton l.
 Nysten l.
 Ochoa l.
 Ohm l.
 l. of partial pressure
 Pascal l.
 periodic l.
 Pflüger l.
 Plateau-Talbot l.
 Poiseuille l.
 l. of polar excitation
 l. of priority
 Profeta l.
 Proust l.
 Raoult l.
 l. of recapitulation
 l. of reciprocal proportions
 reciprocity l.

l. of referred pain
l. of refraction
l. of regression to mean
Ribot l. of memory
Ricco l.
Roscoe-Bunsen l.
Rosenbach l.
Rubner l.'s of growth
Schütz l.
second l. of thermodynamics
l. of segregation
Sherrington l.
l. of similars
Snell l.
Spallanzani l.
l. of specific nerve energies
Starling l.
Stokes l.
Tait l.
Thoma l.
van't Hoff l.
Vogel l.
wallerian l.
Weber l.
Weber-Fechner l.
Weigert l.
Williston l.
Wolff l.

Lawrence-Seip syndrome
lawrencium (Lr, Lw)
laxation
laxative
diphenylmethane l.

layer
ameloblastic l.
anterior elastic l.
anterior limiting l. of cornea
anterior l. of rectus sheath
anterior l. of thoracolumbar fascia
bacillary l.
basal cell l.
basal l. of choroid
basal l. of ciliary body
l. of Bechterew
blastodermic l.
Bowman l.
brown l.
cambium l.
l. of cerebellar cortex
l. of cerebral cortex
cerebral l. of retina
Chievitz l.
choriocapillary l.
choroid capillary l.
circular l. of detrusor muscle of
urinary bladder
circular l. of muscle coat of small
intestine
circular l. of muscular coat
circular l. of muscular tunics
circular l. of tympanic membrane
claustral l.
clear l. of epidermis
columnar l.
conjunctival l. of bulb

conjunctival l. of eyelid
corneal l. of epidermis
cornified l. of nail
cutaneous l. of tympanic membrane
deep l.
deep gray l. of superior colliculus
deep l. of levator palpebrae
superioris
deep l. of temporal fascia
deep white l. of superior colliculus
l. of dentate gyrus
elastic l. of artery
elastic l. of cornea
enamel l.
ependymal l.
episcleral l. of fibrous layer of
eyeball
epithelial choroid l.
epitrichial l.
external nuclear l. of retina
fatty l. of subcutaneous tissue
fatty l. of subcutaneous tissue of
abdomen
fatty l. of superficial fascia
fibromusculocartilagenous l. of
bronchi
fibrous l.
fibrous l. of eyeball
fibrous l. of joint capsule
fibrous l. in or on deep aspect of
fatty layer of subcutaneous tissue
fillet l.
fusiform l.
ganglionic l.
ganglionic cell l. of retina
ganglionic l. of cerebellar cortex
ganglionic l. of cerebral cortex
ganglionic l. of optic nerve
germ l.
germinative l.
germinative l. of nail
glomerular l. of olfactory bulb
granular l.
granular l. of cerebellar cortex
granular l. of cerebellum
granular l. of cerebral cortex
granular l. of epidermis
granular l. of a vesicular ovarian
follicle
gray l. of superior colliculus
half-value l. (HVL)
Henle l.
Henle fiber l.
Henle nervous l.
l. of hippocampus
horny l. of epidermis
horny l. of nail
Huxley l.
infragranular l.
inner l. of eyeball
inner limiting layer
inner nuclear l.
l. of inner and outer segment
inner plexiform l.
intermediate l.

L

layer *(continued)*

intermediate white l. of superior colliculus
investing l.
investing l. of cervical fascia
Kölliker l.
lacunar-molecular l.
Langhans l.
latticed l.
limiting l. of cornea
longitudinal l. of muscle coat of small intestine
longitudinal l. of muscular coat
longitudinal l. of muscular tunics
long pitch helicoidal l.
malpighian l.
mantle l.
marginal l.
medullary l. of thalamus
membranous l.
membranous l. of subcutaneous tissue of abdomen
membranous l. of superficial fascia
membranous l. of superficial fascia of perineum
meningeal l. of dura mater
Meynert l.
middle gray l. of superior colliculus
molecular l.
molecular l. of cerebellar cortex
molecular l. of cerebellum
molecular l. of cerebral cortex
molecular l. of olfactory bulb
molecular l. of retina
multiform l.
multiform l. of cerebral cortex
muscle l.
muscular l.
muscular l. of bronchi
muscular l. of colon
muscular l. of ductus deferens
muscular l. of esophagus
muscular l. of female urethra
muscular l. of gallbladder
muscular l. of intermediate part of male urethra
muscular l. of large intestine
muscular l. of male urethra
muscular l. of mucosa
muscular l. of pharynx
muscular l. of prostatic urethra
muscular l. of rectum
muscular l. of renal pelvis
muscular l. of seminal gland
muscular l. of small intestine
muscular l. of spongy male urethra
muscular l. of stomach
muscular l. of trachea
muscular l. of ureter
muscular l. of urinary bladder
muscular l. of uterine tube
muscular l. of vagina
l. of nerve fiber
neural l. of optic part of retina

neuroepithelial l. of retina
Nitabuch l.
nuclear l. of retina
odontoblastic l.
optic l.
orbital l. of ethmoid bone
oriens l.
osteogenic l.
outer limiting l.
outer nuclear l.
outer plexiform l.
palisade l.
papillary l.
parietal l.
parietal l. of leptomeninges
parietal l. of serous pericardium
parietal l. of tunica vaginalis of testis
perforated l. of sclera
periosteal l. of dura mater
pigmented l. of ciliary body
pigmented l. of iris
pigmented l. of retina
piriform neuron l.
l. of piriform neurons
plasma l.
plexiform l.
plexiform l. of cerebral cortex
plexiform l. of retina
polymorphous l.
posterior elastic l.
posterior limiting l. of cornea
posterior l. of rectus sheath
pretracheal l. of cervical fascia
prevertebral l. of cervical fascia
prickle cell l.
Purkinje cell l.
pyramidal l.
pyramidal cell l.
radiant l.
radiate l. of tympanic membrane
Rauber l.
reticular l. of corium
l. of retina
l. of rods and cones
rostral l.
Sattler elastic l.
serous l. of peritoneum
short pitch helicoidal l.
l. of skin
sluggish l.
somatic l.
spindle-celled l.
spinous l.
splanchnic l.
spongy l. of female urethra
spongy l. of vagina
still l.
subendocardial l.
subendothelial l.
subpapillary l.
subserous l.
superficial l.
superficial l. of deep cervical fascia

superficial gray l. of superior
  colliculus
superficial l. of the levator
  palpebrae superioris
superficial l. of temporal fascia
suprachoroid l.
Tomes granular l.
vascular l.
vascular l. of choroid coat of eye
vascular l. of eyeball
vascular l. of testis
ventricular l.
visceral l.
visceral l. of serous pericardium
visceral l. of tunica vaginalis of
  testis
Waldeyer zonal l.
Weil basal l.
zonular l.
layered keratoplasty (*var. of* lamellar
  keratoplasty)
lazaret
lb
  pound
LBF
  lactobacillus bulgaricus factor
LCAT
  lecithin-cholesterol acyltransferase
    LCAT deficiency
L-chain
    L.-c. disease
    L.-c. myeloma
LCM virus
l-cone
  long-wavelength-sensitive cone
LD
  lethal dose
L-D body
LDH
  lactate dehydrogenase
    LDH agent
LDL
  low density lipoprotein
LDL receptor disorder
LE, L.E.
  lupus erythematosus
Le
    Le antigen
    Le Bel–van't Hoff rule
    Le Blood Group
    Le body
    Le cell
    Le cell test
    Le Chatelier
    Le Chatelier law
    Le Chatelier principle
    Le factor
    Le Fort amputation
    Le Fort III craniofacial dysjunction
    Le Fort I, II, III fracture
    Le Fort osteotomy
    Le Fort sound
    Le phenomenon
leaching
lead (Pb)

ABC l.
l. acetate
l. anemia
augmented l.
bipolar l.
black l.
l. carbonate
CB l.
CF l.
chest l.
l. chromate
CL l.
l. colic
CR l.
direct l.
electrocardiographic l. (aVF, aVL,
  aVR)
l. encephalitis
l. encephalopathy
esophageal l.
l. gout
l. hydroxide stain
indirect l.
intracardiac l.
limb l.
l. line
l. monoxide
l. neuropathy
l. oxide (yellow)
l. palsy
l. paralysis
l. poisoning
precordial l.
red l.
red oxide of l.
semidirect l.
standard limb l.
l. stomatitis
l. sulfide
l. tetraethyl
l. tetroxide
unipolar l.
V l.
white l.
leader sequence
leading
    l. ancestor
    l. edge
lead-pipe
    l.-p. colon
    l.-p. rigidity
leaflet
League of Red Cross Societies
leak point pressure
leapfrog position
Lear complex
learned
    l. drive
    l. helplessness
learning
    l. disability
    incidental l.
    insight l.
    latent l.
    passive l.

L

learning *(continued)*
    rote l.
    l. set
    state-dependent l.
    l. theory
least
    l. confusion circle
    l. splanchnic nerve
    l. squares
    l. squares estimator
leather-bottle stomach
Leber
    L. hereditary optic atrophy
    L. idiopathic stellate neuroretinitis
    L. idiopathic stellate retinopathy
    L. plexus
lecithal
lecithin
    l. acyltransferase
    l.-cholesterol l.
lecithinase
    l. A, B, C, D
lecithin-cholesterol acyltransferase (LCAT)
lecithin/sphingomyelin ratio (L/S ratio)
lecithoblast
lecithoprotein
Leclercia
LeCompte
    L. maneuver
    L. operation
lectin
    l. glycohistochemistry
    mitogenic l.
    l. pathway molecule
Ledermann formula
ledge
    dental l.
    enamel l.
leech
leeching
Leede-Rumpel phenomenon
Lee ganglion
LEEP
    loop electrocautery excision procedure
Leeuwenhoek canal
leeway space
Lee-White method
left
    l. anterior descending artery
    l. anterior lateral hepatic segment [III]
    l. atrioventricular orifice
    l. atrioventricular valve
    l. atrium of heart
    l. auricle
    l. auricular appendage
    l. axis deviation
    l. branch
    l. branch of hepatic artery proper
    l. bundle of atrioventricular bundle
    l. colic artery
    l. colic flexure
    l. colic lymph node

l. colic vein
l. coronary artery
l. coronary vein
l. crus of atrioventricular bundle
l. crus of diaphragm
l. duct of caudate lobe of liver
l. fibrous trigone (of heart)
l.-footed
l. frontoanterior position (LFA)
l. frontoposterior position (LFP)
l. frontotransverse position (LFT)
l. gastric artery
l. gastric lymph node
l. gastric vein
l. gastroepiploic artery
l. gastroepiploic lymph node
l. gastroepiploic vein
l. gastroomental artery
l. gastroomental lymph node
l. gastroomental vein
l.-handed
l. heart
l. heart bypass
l. hepatic artery
l. hepatic duct
l. hepatic vein
l. inferior pulmonary vein
l. lateral division of liver
l. liver
l. lobe
l. lobe of liver
l. lumbar lymph node
l. main bronchus
l. marginal artery
l. medial division of liver
l. medial hepatic segment [IV]
l. mentoanterior position (LMA)
l. mentoposterior position (LMP)
l. mentotransverse position (LMT)
l. occipitoanterior position (LOA)
l. occipitoposterior position (LOP)
l. ovarian vein
l. part of liver
l. posterior lateral hepatic segment III
l. pulmonary artery
l. and right brachiocephalic veins
l. sacroanterior position (LSA)
l. sacroposterior position (LSP)
l. sacrotransverse position (LST)
l. sagittal fissure
l. superior intercostal vein
l. superior pulmonary vein
l. suprarenal vein
l. testicular vein
l. triangular ligament of liver
l. umbilical vein
l. upper quadrant of lung (LUQ)
l. ventricle
l. ventricular assist device
l. ventricular ejection time (LVET)
l. ventricular failure
l. ventricular myomectomy
l. ventricular volume reduction surgery

left-sided
    l.-s. appendicitis
    l.-s. heart failure
left-sidedness
    bilateral l.-s.
left-to-right shunt
leg
    l. of antihelix
    elephant l.
    l. phenomenon
    restless l.'s
    rider's l.
    tennis l.
legal
    l. blindness
    l. dentistry
    l. medicine
    l. psychiatry
    L. test
Legendre sign
Legg-Calvé-Perthes disease
Legg disease
Legg-Perthes disease
Legionella
    L. bozemanii
    L. dumoffii
    L. feeleii
    L. gormanii
    L. longbeachae
    L. micdadei
    L. pneumophila
    L. wadsworthii
legionellosis
Legionnaires disease
legumin
leguminivorous
Leigh disease
Leiner disease
leio-
leiomyofibroma
leiomyoma
    l. cutis
    parasitic l.
    vascular l.
leiomyomatosis peritonealis disseminata
leiomyomectomy
leiomyosarcoma
leiotrichous
leipo-
Leipzig yellow
Leishman
    L. chrome cell
    L. stain
Leishman-Donovan body
Leishmania
    L. aethiopica
    L. braziliensis
    L. braziliensis braziliensis
    L. braziliensis guyanensis
    L. braziliensis panamensis
    L. donovani
    L. donovani archibaldi
    L. donovani chagasi
    L. donovani donovani
    L. donovani infantum

    L. furunculosa
    L. major
    L. mexicana
    L. mexicana amazonensis
    L. mexicana garnhami
    L. mexicana mexicana
    L. mexicana pifanoi
    L. mexicana venezuelensis
    L. peruviana
    L. pifanoi
    L. tropica
    L. tropica major
    L. tropica mexicana
leishmania, pl. **leishmaniae**
leishmaniasis
    acute cutaneous l.
    American l.
    l. americana
    anergic l.
    anthroponotic cutaneous l.
    canine l.
    chronic cutaneous l.
    cutaneous l.
    diffuse cutaneous l.
    disseminated cutaneous l.
    dry cutaneous l.
    infantile l.
    lupoid l.
    mucocutaneous l.
    nasopharyngeal l.
    New World l.
    Old World l.
    pseudolepromatous l.
    l. recidivans
    rural cutaneous l.
    l. tegumentaria diffusa
    urban cutaneous l.
    visceral l.
    wet cutaneous l.
    zoonotic cutaneous l.
leishmanin test
leishmaniosis
leishmanoid
    dermal l.
    post-kala azar dermal l.
Leiter International Performance Scale
Lejeune syndrome
Lembert suture
lemic
Leminorella
lemmoblast
lemmocyte
lemniscal trigone
lemniscus, pl. **lemnisci**
    acoustic l.
    auditory l.
    gustatory l.
    lateral l.
    l. lateralis
    medial l.
    l. medialis
    spinal l.
    l. spinalis
    trigeminal l.
    l. trigeminalis

L

lemon
  l. sign
  l. yellow
Lendrum phloxine-tartrazine stain
Lenègre
  L. disease
  L. syndrome
length (l)
  arch l.
  available arch l.
  crown-heel l. (CH, CHL)
  crown-rump l. (CRL)
  greatest l.
  required arch l.
  resting l.
  spinal l. (SL)
length-breadth index
lengthening reaction
length-height index
Lenhossék process
lenitive
Lennert
  L. classification
  L. lymphoma
Lennox-Gastaut syndrome
Lennox syndrome
Lenoir facet
lens
  achromatic l.
  acoustic l.
  aplanatic l.
  apochromatic l.
  aspheric l.
  astigmatic l.
  bandage contact l.
  biconcave l.
  biconvex l.
  bifocal l.
  l. capsule
  cataract l.
  l. clock
  compound l.
  concave l.
  concavoconcave l.
  concavoconvex l.
  contact l.
  convex l.
  convexoconcave l.
  convexoconvex l.
  corneal l.
  crystalline l.
  cylindrical l.
  decentered l.
  dislocation of l.
  double concave l.
  double convex l.
  eye l.
  field l.
  foldable intraocular l.
  Fresnel l.
  Hruby l.
  immersion l.
  lighthouse l.
  meniscus l.
  minus l.

  multifocal l.
  ocular l.
  omnifocal l.
  orthoscopic l.
  periscopic l.
  photochromic l.
  l. pit
  l. placode
  planoconcave l.
  planoconvex l.
  plus l.
  safety l.
  slab-off l.
  spherical l. (S)
  spherocylindrical l.
  l. star
  l. suture
  toric l.
  trial l.
  trifocal l.
  l. vesicle
lensectomy
lens-induced uveitis
lensometer
lensopathy
lente insulin
lenticonus
lenticula
lenticular
  l. ansa
  l. apophysis
  l. astigmatism
  l. bone
  l. capsule
  l. colony
  l. fasciculus
  l. fossa
  l. ganglion
  l. knife
  l. loop
  l. nucleus
  l. papillae
  l. process of incus
  l. progressive disease
  l. vesicle
lenticuli (*pl. of* lenticulus)
lenticulooptic
lenticulopapular
lenticulostriate
  l. artery
lenticulothalamic
lenticulus, pl. **lenticuli**
lentiform bone
lentigines (*pl. of* lentigo)
lentiginosis
  centrofacial l.
  generalized l.
lentiglobus
lentigo, pl. **lentigines**
  lentigines, atrial myxoma,
    mucocutaneous myxomas, and blue
    nevi (LAMB)
  l. maligna
  lentigines (multiple),
    electrocardiographic abnormalities,

ocular hypertelorism, pulmonary stenosis, abnormalities of genitalia, retardation of growth, and deafness (LEOPARD)
senile l.
l. simplex
solar l.
Lentivirinae
lentivirus
lentogenic
lentula
leonine facies
leontiasis ossea
LEOPARD
lentigines (multiple), electrocardiographic abnormalities, ocular hypertelorism, pulmonary stenosis, abnormalities of genitalia, retardation of growth, and deafness
L. fundus
L. retina
L. syndrome
leopard's bane
Leopold maneuver
Lepehne-Pickworth stain
leper
lepidic
Lepidoptera
Lepore thalassemia
Leporipoxvirus
lepothrix
lepra cell
leprechaunism
leprid
leproma
lepromatous leprosy
lepromin
l. reaction
l. test
leprosarium
leprosery
leprostatic
leprosy
anesthetic l.
l. bacillus
borderline l.
dimorphous l.
dry l.
histoid l.
indeterminate l.
lepromatous l.
Lucio l.
macular l.
mutilating l.
nodular l.
smooth l.
trophoneurotic l.
tuberculoid l.
leprotic
leprous neuropathy
leptandra
leptin
leptocephalous
leptocephaly
leptochromatic

leptocyte
leptocytosis
leptodactylous
leptomeningeal
l. carcinoma
l. carcinomatosis
l. cyst
l. fibrosis
l. space
leptomeninges
leptomeningitis
basilar l.
leptomere
leptomonad
Leptomonas
leptonema
leptophonia
leptophonic
leptopodia
leptoprosopia
leptoprosopic
leptorrhine
leptoscope
leptosomatic
Leptospira
L. interrogans
leptospiral jaundice
leptospire
leptospirosis
anicteric l.
l. icterohemorrhagica
leptospiruria
leptotene
leptothricosis
Leptothrix
Leptotrichia
L. buccalis
Leptotrombidium
L. akamushi
LEP vaccine (*var. of* low-egg-passage vaccine)
lergotrile
Leri
L. pleonosteosis
L. sign
Leriche
L. operation
L. syndrome
Leri-Weill
L.-W. disease
L.-W. syndrome
Lermoyez syndrome
Lerner homeostasis
LES
lower esophageal sphincter
lesbian
lesbianism
Lesch-Nyhan syndrome
Leser-Trélat sign
lesion
Baehr-Lohlein l.
Bankart l.
benign lymphoepithelial l.
Bracht-Wächter l.
caviar l.

L

lesion *(continued)*
    coin l. of lung
    Dieulafoy l.
    Duret l.
    Ghon primary l.
    gross l.
    high-grade squamous
      intraepithelial l. (HGSIL, HSIL)
    Hill-Sachs l.
    Janeway l.
    Lohlein-Baehr l.
    lower motor neuron l.
    low-grade squamous intraepithelial l.
      (LGSIL, LSIL)
    Mallory-Weiss l.
    precancerous l.
    radial sclerosing l.
    ring-wall l.
    supranuclear l.
    upper motor neuron l.
    wire-loop l.

lesser
    l. alar cartilage
    l. arterial circle of iris
    l. circulation
    l. cul-de-sac
    l. curvature of stomach
    l. horn of hyoid
    l. internal cutaneous nerve
    l. multangular bone
    l. occipital nerve
    l. omentum
    l. palatine artery
    l. palatine canal
    l. palatine foramina
    l. palatine nerve
    l. pancreas
    l. pelvis
    l. peritoneal cavity
    l. peritoneal sac
    l. petrosal nerve
    l. rhomboid muscle
    l. ring of iris
    l. sciatic notch
    l. splanchnic nerve
    l. superficial petrosal nerve
    l. supraclavicular fossa
    l. triangle
    l. trochanter
    l. tubercle
    l. tuberosity of humerus
    l. tympanic spine
    l. vestibular gland
    l. wing of sphenoid bone
    l. zygomatic muscle
Lesshaft triangle
LET
    linear energy transfer
let-down reflex
lethal
    clinical l.
    l. coefficient
    l. dose (LD)
    l. dwarfism

    l. equivalent
    l. factor
    l. gene
    genetic l.
    l. midline granuloma
    l. mutation
lethality rate
lethargic hypnosis
lethargy
LETS
    large, external transformation-sensitive
    fibronectin
letter blindness
Letterer-Siwe disease
leucin
leucine
    l. aminopeptidase
    l. dehydrogenase
    l. hypoglycemia
    l. zipper
leucine-induced hypoglycemia
leucine-sensitive hypoglycemia
leucinosis
leucinuria
leucoharmine
leucoline
leucomethylene blue
Leuconostoc
    L. mesenteroides
leuco patent blue
leucovorin calcium
Leudet tinnitus
leuenkephalin
leukanemia
leukapheresis
leukemia
    acute lymphocytic leukemia (ALL)
    acute promyelocytic l.
    adult T-cell l. (ATL)
    aleukemic l.
    basophilic l.
    basophilocytic l.
    chronic granulocytic l.
    chronic myelocytic l.
    chronic myelogenous l. (CML)
    chronic myeloid l.
    l. cutis
    embryonal l.
    eosinophilic l.
    eosinophilocytic l.
    granulocytic l.
    hairy cell l.
    l. inhibitory factor
    leukemic l.
    leukopenic l.
    lymphatic l.
    lymphoblastic l.
    lymphocytic l.
    lymphoid l.
    mast cell l.
    mature cell l.
    megakaryocytic l.
    meningeal l.
    micromyeloblastic l.
    mixed l.

mixed cell l.
monocytic l.
murine l.
myeloblastic l.
myelocytic l.
myelogenic l.
myeloid l.
myelomonocytic l.
Naegeli type of monocytic l.
natural killer cell l.
neutrophilic l.
plasma cell l.
polymorphocytic l.
Rieder cell l.
Schilling type of monocytic l.
splenic l.
stem cell l.
subleukemic l.

leukemic
l. hyperplastic gingivitis
l. leukemia
l. myelosis
l. reticulosis
l. retinitis
l. retinopathy
leukemid
leukemogen
leukemogenesis
leukemogenic
leukemoid reaction
lymphocytic l. r.
monocytic l. r.
myelocytic l. r.
plasmocytic l. r.
leukemoid reaction
leukin
leukoagglutinin
leukobilin
leukoblast
leukoblastosis
leukochloroma
leukocidin
leukocoria, leukokoria
leukocytactic
leukocytal
leukocytaxia, leukocytaxis
leukocyte
acidophilic l.
l. adherence assay test
l. adhesion deficiency (LAD)
agranular l.
l. bactericidal assay test
basophilic l.
l. common antigen
l. cream
cystinotic l.
endothelial l.
eosinophilic l.
filament polymorphonuclear l.
globular l.
granular l.
hyaline l.
l. inclusion
l. interferon
mast l.

motile l.
multinuclear l.
neutrophilic l.
nonfilament polymorphonuclear l.
nongranular l.
nonmotile l.
oxyphilic l.
polymorphonuclear l.
polynuclear l.
segmented l.
transitional l.
Türk l.
leukocythemia
leukocytic
l. pyrogens
l. sarcoma
leukocytoblast
leukocytoclasis
leukocytoclastic vasculitis
leukocytogenesis
leukocytoid
leukocytolysin
leukocytolysis
leukocytolytic
leukocytoma
leukocytometer
leukocytopenia
leukocytoplania
leukocytopoiesis
leukocytosis
absolute l.
agonal l.
basophilic l.
digestive l.
distribution l.
emotional l.
eosinophilic l.
lymphocytic l.
monocytic l.
neutrophilic l.
l. of the newborn
physiologic l.
relative l.
terminal l.
leukocytosis-promoting factor
leukocytotactic
leukocytotaxia
negative l.
positive l.
leukocytotoxin
leukocyturia
leukoderma
acquired l.
l. acquisitum centrifugum
l. colli
syphilitic l.
leukodermatous
leukodontia
leukodystrophia cerebri progressiva
leukodystrophy
adrenal l.
globoid cell l.
metachromatic l.
l. with diffuse Rosenthal fiber
formation

L

leukoencephalitis
    acute epidemic l.
    acute hemorrhagic l.
    acute necrotizing hemorrhagic l.
    sclerosing l.
    subacute sclerosing l.
leukoencephalopathy
    progressive multifocal l. (PML)
leukoerythroblastic anemia
leukoerythroblastosis
leukokinetic
leukokinetics
leukokoria (*var. of* leukocoria)
leukokraurosis
leukolysin
leukolysis
leukolytic
leukoma
    adherent l.
leukomatous
leukomyelitis
    necrotizing hemorrhagic l.
leukomyelopathy
leukon
leukonecrosis
leukonychia
leukopathia
leukopedesis
leukopenia
    basophilic l.
    eosinophilic l.
    lymphocytic l.
    monocytic l.
    neutrophilic l.
leukopenic
    l. factor
    l. index
    l. leukemia
    l. myelosis
leukoplakia
    hairy l.
    l. vulvae
leukopoiesis
leukopoietic
leukoprotease
leukoriboflavin
leukorrhagia
leukorrhea
    menstrual l.
leukorrheal
leukotactic
leukotaxia
leukotaxine
leukotaxis
leukotome
leukotomy
    prefrontal l.
    transorbital l.
leukotoxin
leukotrichia
leukotriene receptor antagonist
leukotrienes (LT)
    peptidyl l.
Leukovirus
LEU M1

leupeptin
leuprolide acetate
leurocristine
Lev
    L. disease
    L. syndrome
Levaditi stain
levallorphan tartrate
levamisole
levan
levansucrase
levarotatory (*l-*)
levarterenol bitartrate
levator
    l. anguli oris muscle
    l. ani muscle
    l. cushion
    l. hernia
    l. labii superioris alaeque nasi
      muscle
    l. labii superioris muscle
    l. muscle of thyroid gland
    l. palati muscle
    l. palpebrae superioris muscle
    l. prostatae muscle
    l. scapulae muscle
    l. swelling
    l. veli palatini muscle
levatores
    l. costarum brevis muscle
    l. costarum longi muscle
    l. costarum muscle
Levay antigen
LeVeen shunt
level
    acoustic reference l.
    l. of aspiration
    background l.
    Clark l.
    Health L.-7 (HL-7)
    hearing l.
    loudness discomfort l.
    most comfortable l.
    saturation sound pressure l. (SSPL)
    sensation l.
    sensory acuity l.
    sound pressure l. (SPL)
    uncomfortable l.
    window l.
level-dependent frequency response
lever
    dental l.
leverage
Levey-Jennings chart
Levinea
    L. amalonatica
    L. diversus
    L. malonatica
Levin tube
levitation
Leviviridae
levoatriocardinal vein
levobunolol hydrochloride
levocardia
levocardiogram

levocarnitine
levoclination
levocycleduction
levocycloduction
levodopa
levoduction
levoform
levoglucose
levogram
levogyrate, levogyrous
levonordefrin
levophacetoperane
levophobia
levopropoxyphene napsylate
levorotation
levorotatory
levorphanol tartrate
levotorsion
levoversion
Levret forceps
levulan
levulic acid
levulin
levulinate
levulinic acid
levulosan
levulose
levulosemia
levulosuria
Lewis
    L. acid
    L. base
    L. Blood Group
lewisite
Lewy
    L. body
    L. body dementia
lexical
Leyden
    L. ataxia
    L. crystal
    L. neuritis
Leyden-Möbius muscular dystrophy
Leydig
    L. cell
    L. cell tumor
leydigarche
Lf
    limes flocculation
LFA
    left frontoanterior position
    lymphocyte function associated antigen
LFP
    left frontoposterior position
LFT
    left frontotransverse position
LGSIL
    low-grade squamous intraepithelial lesion
LH
    luteinizing hormone
Lhermitte sign
LH/FSH-RF
    luteinizing hormone/follicle-stimulating
      hormone-releasing factor

LH-RF
    luteinizing hormone-releasing factor
LH-RH
    luteinizing hormone-releasing hormone
Li
    lithium
liberator
    histamine l.'s
liberins
liberomotor
libidinization
libidinous
libido
    object l.
    l. theory
Libman-Sacks
    L.-S. endocarditis
    L.-S. syndrome
Liborius method
library
    cDNA l.
    genomic l.
    l. screening
lice (*pl. of* louse)
licensed
    l. practical nurse (LPN)
    l. vocational nurse (LVN)
Licentiate
    L. of the Royal College of
      Physicians (Edinburgh) (LRCP(E))
    L. of the Royal College of
      Physicians (Ireland) (LRCP(I))
    L. of the Royal College of
      Physicians (of England) (LRCP)
    L. of the Royal College of
      Surgeons (Edinburgh) (LRCS(E))
    L. of the Royal College of
      Surgeons (Ireland) (LRCS(I))
    L. of the Royal College of
      Surgeons (of England) (LRCS)
    L. of the Royal Faculty of
      Physicians and Surgeons (LRFPS)
lichen
    l. amyloidosis
    l. myxedematosus
    l. nitidus
    l. nuchae
    l. obtusus
    oral erosive l. planus
    l. planopilaris
    l. planus
    l. planus annularis
    l. planus follicularis
    l. planus hypertrophicus
    l. planus-like keratosis
    l. planus verrucosus
    l. ruber moniliformis
    l. sclerosus et atrophicus
    l. scrofulosorum
    l. simplex chronicus
    l. spinulosus
    l. striatus
    l. tropicus
lichenification
lichenin

L

lichenoid
    l. amyloidosis
    l. dermatosis
    l. eczema
    l. keratosis
licorice
lid
    l. crutch spectacles
    granular l.'s
    lower l.
    l. reflex
    upper l.
lid-closure reaction
Liddell-Sherrington reflex
lidocaine hydrochloride
lidoflazine
lie
    l. detector
    longitudinal l.
    oblique l.
    transverse l.
    unstable l.
Lieberkühn
    crypt of L.
    crypt of L. of large intestine
    crypt of L. of small intestine
    L. follicle
    L. gland
Liebermann-Burchard
    L.-B. reaction
    L.-B. test
Liebermeister rule
Liebig theory
lien
    l. accessorius
    l. mobilis
    l. succenturiatus
lienal artery
lienculus
lienectomy
lienomedullary
lienomyelogenous
lienopancreatic
lienophrenic ligament
lienorenal ligament
lienteric diarrhea
lientery
lienunculus
Liesegang ring
Lieutaud
    L. body
    L. triangle
    L. trigone
    L. uvula
life
    l. cycle
    during l. (intra vitam)
    l. event
    half-l.
    l. instinct
    postnatal l.
    prenatal l.
    quality of l.
    sexual l.
    l. stress

    l. table
    vegetative l.
life-belt cataract
lifespan
life-span development
lifestyle
Li-Fraumeni cancer syndrome
ligament
    accessory plantar l.
    accessory volar l.
    acromioclavicular l.
    alar l.
    alveolodental l.
    anococcygeal l.
    anterior costotransverse l.
    anterior cruciate l.
    anterior l. of fibular head
    anterior l. of Helmholtz
    anterior longitudinal l.
    anterior l. of malleus
    anterior meniscofemoral l.
    anterior sacrococcygeal l.
    anterior sacroiliac l.
    anterior sacrosciatic l.
    anterior sternoclavicular l.
    anterior talofibular l.
    anterior talotibial l.
    anterior tibiofibular l.
    anterior tibiotalar l.
    anular l.
    anular l. of radius
    anular l. of stapes
    anular l. of trachea
    apical l. of dens
    Arantius l.
    arcuate popliteal l.
    arcuate pubic l.
    arterial l.
    l. of auditory ossicle
    l. of auricle
    auricular l.
    axis l. of malleus
    Bardinet l.
    Barkow l.
    Bellini l.
    Berry l.
    Bertin l.
    Bichat l.
    bifurcate l.
    bifurcated l.
    Bigelow l.
    Botallo l.
    Bourgery l.
    broad l. of the uterus
    Brodie l.
    Burns l.
    calcaneocuboid l.
    calcaneofibular l.
    calcaneonavicular l.
    calcaneotibial l.
    Caldani l.
    Campbell l.
    Camper l.
    capsular l.
    cardinal l.

caroticoclinoid l.
carpometacarpal l. dorsal and palmar
caudal l.
ceratocricoid l.
cervical l. of uterus
check l.'s of eyeball, medial and lateral
check l.'s of medial and lateral rectus muscles
check l. of odontoid
chondroxiphoid l.
ciliary l.
Civinini l.
Clado l.
coccygeal l.
collateral l.
Colles l.
conoid l.
Cooper l.
coracoacromial l.
coracoclavicular l.
coracohumeral l.
corniculopharyngeal l.
coronary l. of knee
coronary l. of liver
costoclavicular l.
costocolic l.
costotransverse l.
costoxiphoid l.
cotyloid l.
Cowper l.
cricoarytenoid l.
cricopharyngeal l.
cricosantorinian l.
cricotracheal l.
crucial l.
cruciate l. of the atlas
cruciate l. of knee
cruciate l. of leg
cruciform l. of atlas
Cruveilhier l.
cuboideonavicular l.
cuneocuboid l.
cuneocuboid interosseous l.
cuneometatarsal interosseous l.
cuneonavicular l.
cystoduodenal l.
deep dorsal sacrococcygeal l.
deep posterior sacrococcygeal l.
deep transverse metacarpal l.
deep transverse metatarsal l.
deltoid l.
Denonvilliers l.
dentate l. of spinal cord
denticulate l.
Denucé l.
diaphragmatic l. of the mesonephros
dorsal calcaneocuboid l.
dorsal carpal l.
dorsal carpometacarpal l.
dorsal cuboideonavicular l.
dorsal cuneocuboid l.
dorsal cuneonavicular l.
dorsal intercuneiform l.

dorsal metacarpal l.
dorsal metatarsal l.
dorsal radiocarpal l.
dorsal sacroiliac l.
dorsal tarsal l.
dorsal tarsometatarsal l.
duodenorenal l.
l.'s of epididymis (inferior and superior)
epihyal l.
external collateral l. of wrist
extracapsular l.
falciform l.
falciform l. of liver
fallopian l.
Ferrein l.
fibular collateral l.
fibular collateral l. of ankle
Flood l.
fundiform l. of clitoris
fundiform l. of foot
fundiform l. of penis
gastrocolic l.
gastrodiaphragmatic l.
gastrolienal l.
gastrophrenic l.
gastrosplenic l.
genital l.
genitoinguinal l.
Gerdy l.
Gillette suspensory l.
Gimbernat l.
gingivodental l.
glenohumeral l.
glenoid l.
glossoepiglottic l.
Günz l.
hammock l.
l. of head of femur
Helmholtz axis l.
Hensing l.
hepatocolic l.
hepatoduodenal l.
hepatoesophageal l.
hepatogastric l.
hepatorenal l.
Hesselbach l.
Hey ligament
Holl l.
Hueck l.
Humphry l.
Hunter l.
hyalocapsular l.
hyoepiglottic l.
hypsiloid l.
iliofemoral l.
iliolumbar l.
iliopectineal l.
iliotrochanteric l.
inferior calcaneonavicular l.
inferior l. of epididymis
inferior pubic l.
inferior transverse scapular l.
infundibulo-ovarian l.
infundibulopelvic l.

L

ligament *(continued)*
  inguinal l.
  inguinal l. of the kidney
  intercarpal l.
  interclavicular l.
  interclinoid l.
  intercornual l.
  intercostal l.
  intercuneiform l.
  interfoveolar l.
  internal collateral l. of the wrist
  interosseous cuneocuboid l.
  interosseous cuneometatarsal l.
  interosseous metacarpal l.
  interosseous metatarsal l.
  interosseous sacroiliac l.
  interosseous talocalcaneal l.
  interosseous tibiofibular l.
  interspinous l.
  intertransverse l.
  intraarticular l. of costal head
  intraarticular l. of head of rib
  intraarticular sternocostal l.
  intracapsular l.
  ischiocapsular l.
  ischiofemoral l.
  jugal l.
  Krause l.
  laciniate l.
  lacunar l.
  Lannelongue l.
  lateral l. of ankle
  lateral arcuate l.
  lateral l. of bladder
  lateral collateral l. of ankle
  lateral costotransverse l.
  lateral l. of elbow
  lateral l. of knee
  lateral malleolar l.
  lateral l. of malleus
  lateral palpebral l.
  lateral puboprostatic l.
  lateral sacrococcygeal l.
  lateral talocalcaneal l.
  lateral temporomandibular l.
  lateral l. of temporomandibular joint
  lateral thyrohyoid l.
  lateral umbilical l.
  lateral l. of wrist
  Lauth l.
  l. of left superior vena cava
  left triangular l. of liver
  l. of left vena cava
  lienophrenic l.
  lienorenal l.
  Lisfranc l.
  Lockwood l.
  longitudinal l.
  long plantar l.
  lumbocostal l.
  Luschka l.
  Mackenrodt l.
  l. of malleus
  Mauchart l.

  Meckel l.
  medial l. of ankle joint
  medial arcuate l.
  medial canthal l.
  medial collateral l. of elbow
  medial l. of knee
  medial palpebral l.
  medial puboprostatic l.
  medial talocalcaneal l.
  medial l. of talocrural joint
  medial l. of temporomandibular joint
  medial umbilical l.
  medial l. of wrist
  median arcuate l.
  median cricothyroid l.
  median thyrohyoid l.
  median umbilical l.
  meniscofemoral l.
  metatarsal interosseous l.
  middle costotransverse l.
  middle umbilical l.
  nuchal l.
  oblique l. of elbow joint
  oblique popliteal l.
  occipitoaxial l.
  orbicular l.
  orbicular l. of radius
  ovarian l.
  l. of ovary
  palmar l.
  palmar carpal l.
  palmar carpometacarpal l.
  palmar l. of interphalangeal joint of hand
  palmar metacarpal l.
  palmar l. of metacarpophalangeal joint
  palmar radiocarpal l.
  palmar ulnocarpal l.
  patellar l.
  pectinate l. of iridocorneal angle
  pectinate l. of iris
  pectineal l.
  peridental l.
  periodontal l.
  phrenicocolic l.
  phrenicolienal l.
  phrenicosplenic l.
  phrenogastric l.
  pisohamate l.
  pisometacarpal l.
  pisouniform l.
  pisouncinate l.
  plantar l.
  plantar calcaneocuboid l.
  plantar calcaneonavicular l.
  plantar cuboideonavicular l.
  plantar cuneocuboid l.
  plantar cuneonavicular l.
  plantar l. of interphalangeal joint of foot
  plantar metatarsal l.
  plantar l. of metatarsophalangeal joint

plantar tarsal l.
plantar tarsometatarsal l.
posterior costotransverse l.
posterior cricoarytenoid l.
posterior cruciate l.
posterior l. of fibular head
posterior l. of head of fibula
posterior l. of incus
posterior l. of knee
posterior longitudinal l.
posterior meniscofemoral l.
posterior occipitoaxial l.
posterior sacroiliac l.
posterior sacrosciatic l.
posterior sternoclavicular l.
posterior talocalcaneal l.
posterior talofibular l.
posterior talotibial l.
posterior tibiofibular l.
posterior tibiotalar l.
Poupart l.
proper l. of ovary
pterygomandibular l.
pterygospinal l.
pterygospinous l.
pubocapsular l.
pubofemoral l.
puboprostatic l.
pubovesical l.
pulmonary l.
quadrate l.
radial collateral l.
radial collateral l. of elbow joint
radial collateral l. of wrist joint
radiate l.
radiate carpal l.
radiate l. of head of rib
radiate sternocostal l.
radiate l. of wrist
reflected inguinal l.
reflex l.
Retzius l.
rhomboid l.
right triangular l. of liver
ring l.
round l. of elbow joint
round l. of femur
round l. of liver
round l. of uterus
sacrodural l.
sacrospinous l.
sacrotuberous l.
serous l.
sheath l.
Simonart l.
skin l.
Soemmerring l.
sphenomandibular l.
spinoglenoid l.
spiral l. of cochlea
spiral l. of cochlear duct
splenorenal l.
spring l.
Stanley cervical l.
stellate l.

sternoclavicular l.
sternopericardial l.
stylohyoid l.
stylomandibular l.
stylomaxillary l.
superficial dorsal sacrococcygeal l.
superficial posterior
  sacrococcygeal l.
superficial transverse metacarpal l.
superficial transverse metatarsal l.
superior costotransverse l.
superior l. of epididymis
superior l. of incus
superior l. of malleus
superior pubic l.
superior transverse scapular l.
suprascapular l.
supraspinous l.
suspensory l. of axilla
suspensory l. of breast
suspensory l. of clitoris
suspensory l. of Cooper
suspensory l. of duodenum
suspensory l. of esophagus
suspensory l. of eyeball
suspensory l. of gonad
suspensory l. of lens
suspensory l. of ovary
suspensory l. of penis
suspensory l. of testis
suspensory l. of thyroid gland
sutural l.
synovial l.
talocalcaneal l.
talocalcaneal interosseous l.
talonavicular l.
tarsal l.
tarsal interosseous l.
tarsometatarsal l.
temporomandibular l.
Teutleben l.
Thompson l.
thyroepiglottic l.
tibial collateral l.
tibial collateral l. of ankle joint
tibiocalcaneal l.
tibiofibular l.
tibionavicular l.
transverse acetabular l.
transverse l. of acetabulum
transverse atlantal l.
transverse l. of the atlas
transverse carpal l.
transverse cervical l.
transverse crural l.
transverse l. of elbow
transverse genicular l.
transverse humeral l.
transverse l. of knee
transverse l. of leg
transverse metacarpal l.
transverse metatarsal l.
transverse l. of pelvis
transverse perineal l.
transverse l. of perineum

L

ligament (*continued*)
transverse tibiofibular l.
trapezoid l.
Treitz l.
triangular l.
triangular l. of liver
ulnar collateral l.
ulnar collateral l. of elbow joint
ulnar collateral l. of wrist joint
urachal l.
uterovesical l.
Valsalva l.
venous l.
ventral sacrococcygeal l.
ventral sacroiliac l.
ventricular l.
vertebropelvic l.
vesicoumbilical l.
vesicouterine l.
vestibular l.
vocal l.
volar carpal l.
Weitbrecht l.
Winslow l.
Wrisberg l.
yellow l.
Y-shaped l.
Zaglas l.
Zinn l.
ligamenta (*pl. of* ligamentum)
ligamentopexis
ligamentous
ligamentum, pl. **ligamenta**
l. acromioclaviculare
l. anococcygeum
l. anulare
l. anulare bulbi
l. anulare digitorum
l. anulare radii
l. anulare stapedis
ligamenta anularia trachealia
l. apicis dentis
l. arcuatum laterale
l. arcuatum mediale
l. arcuatum medianum
l. arcuatum pubis
l. arteriosum
ligamenta auricularia
l. bifurcatum
l. calcaneocuboideum
l. calcaneocuboideum plantare
l. calcaneofibulare
l. calcaneonaviculare
l. calcaneonaviculare plantare
l. calcaneotibiale
l. capitis costae intraarticulare
l. capitis costae radiatum
l. capitis femoris
l. capitis fibulae anterius
l. capitis fibulae posterius
ligamenta capitulorum transversa
l. capsulare
l. cardinale
l. carpi dorsale

l. carpi radiatum
l. carpi transversum
l. carpi volare
ligamenta carpometacarpalia dorsalia
ligamenta carpometacarpalia
(dorsalia/palmaria)
ligamenta carpometacarpalia palmaria
l. caudale
l. ceratocricoideum
l. collaterale, pl. ligamenta collateralia
l. collaterale carpi radiale
articulationis radiocarpalis
l. collaterale carpi ulnare
l. collaterale carpi ulnare
articulationis radiocarpalis
l. collaterale fibulare
l. collaterale laterale
l. collaterale mediale
l. collaterale radiale articulationis
cubiti
l. collaterale tibiale
l. collaterale ulnare articulationis
cubiti
ligamenta collateralia (*pl. of* l.
collaterale)
l. colli costae
l. conoideum
l. coracoacromiale
l. coracoclaviculare
l. coracohumerale
l. corniculopharyngeum
l. coronarium hepatis
l. costoclaviculare
l. costotransversarium
l. costotransversarium anterius
l. costotransversarium laterale
l. costotransversarium posterius
l. costotransversarium superius
l. costoxiphoideum
l. cotyloideum
l. cricoarytenoideum posterius
l. cricopharyngeum
l. cricotracheale
ligamenta cruciata digitorum
ligamenta cruciata genus
l. cruciatum anterius
l. cruciatum atlantis
l. cruciatum cruris
l. cruciatum posterius
l. cruciatum tertium genus
l. cruciforme atlantis
ligamenta cuboideonaviculare
l. cuboideonaviculare dorsale
ligamenta cuboideonavicularia
plantaria
l. cuneocuboideum
l. cuneocuboideum dorsale
l. cuneocuboideum interosseum
l. cuneocuboideum plantare
ligamenta cuneometatarsalia
interossea
ligamenta cuneonavicularia dorsalia
l. cuneonavicularia plantaria
l. deltoideum
l. denticulatum

l. ductus venosi
l. duodenorenale
l. epididymidis inferius
ligamenta epididymidis (inferius et superius)
l. epididymidis superius
ligamenta extracapsularia
l. falciforme
l. falciforme hepatis
ligamenta flava
l. fundiforme clitoridis
l. fundiforme penis
l. gastrocolicum
l. gastrolienale
l. gastrophrenicum
l. gastrosplenicum
l. genitoinguinale
ligamenta glenohumeralia
l. glenoidale
l. hepatocolicum
l. hepatoduodenale
l. hepatoesophageum
l. hepatogastricum
l. hepatorenale
l. hyaloideo-capsulare
l. hyoepiglotticum
l. hyothyroideum laterale
l. hyothyroideum medium
l. iliofemorale
l. iliolumbale
l. iliopectineale
l. incudis posterius
l. incudis superius
l. inguinale
ligamenta intercarpalia
l. intercarpalia dorsalia
l. intercarpalia interossea
l. intercarpalia palmaria
l. interclaviculare
ligamenta intercostalia
ligamenta intercuneiformia
ligamenta intercuneiformia dorsalia
ligamenta intercuneiformia interossea
ligamenta intercuneiformia plantaria
l. interfoveolare
l. interspinale
l. intertransversarium
ligamenta intracapsularia
l. ischiocapsulare
l. ischiofemorale
l. jugale
l. laciniatum
l. lacunare
l. laterale articulationis temporomandibularis
l. laterale vesicae
l. latum pulmonis
l. latum uteri
l. lienorenale
l. longitudinale anterius
l. longitudinale posterius
ligamenta longitudinalia
l. lumbocostale
l. mallei anterius
l. mallei laterale

l. mallei superius
l. malleoli lateralis
l. mediale
l. mediale articulationis talocruralis
l. mediale articulationis temporomandibularis
l. mediale puboprostaticum
l. menisci lateralis
l. meniscofemorale anterius
l. meniscofemorale posterius
ligamenta meniscofemoralia
l. metacarpale transversum profundum
l. metacarpale transversum superficiale
ligamenta metacarpalia dorsalia
ligamenta metacarpalia interossea
ligamenta metacarpalia palmaria
l. metatarsale transversum profundum
l. metatarsale transversum superficiale
ligamenta metatarsalia dorsalia
ligamenta metatarsalia interossea
ligamenta metatarsalia plantaria
l. natatorium
ligamenta navicularicuneiformia
l. nuchae
l. orbiculare radii
ligamenta ossiculorum auditorium
ligamenta ossiculorum auditus
l. ovarii proprium
ligamenta palmaria
ligamenta palmaria articulationis interphalangeae manus
ligamenta palmaria articulationis metacarpophalangeae
l. palpebrale externum
l. palpebrale laterale
l. palpebrale mediale
l. patellae
l. pectinatum
l. pectinatum anguli iridocornealis
l. pectinatum iridis
l. pectineale
l. phrenicocolicum
l. phrenicolienale
l. phrenicosplenicum
l. pisohamatum
l. pisometacarpeum
l. plantare longum
ligamenta plantaria
ligamenta plantaria articulationis interphalangeae pedis
ligamenta plantaria articulationis metatarsophalangeae
l. popliteum arcuatum
l. popliteum obliquum
l. pterygospinale
l. pubicum inferius
l. pubicum superius
l. pubocapsulare
l. pubofemorale
l. puboprostaticum
l. puboprostaticum laterale

L

ligamentum *(continued)*
l. puboprostaticum mediale
l. pubovesicale
l. pulmonale
l. quadratum
l. radiatum
l. radiocarpale dorsale
l. radiocarpale palmare
l. reflexum
l. sacrococcygeum anterius
l. sacrococcygeum dorsale superficiale
l. sacrococcygeum laterale
l. sacrococcygeum posterius profundum
l. sacrococcygeum posterius superficiale
l. sacrodurale
ligamenta sacroiliaca anteriora
ligamenta sacroiliaca interossea
ligamenta sacroiliaca posteriora
l. sacroiliacum posterius
l. sacrospinale
l. sacrospinosum
l. sacrotuberale
l. sacrotuberosum
l. serosum
l. sphenomandibulare
l. spirale cochleae
l. spirale ductus cochlearis
l. splenorenale
l. sternoclaviculare anterius
l. sternoclaviculare posterius
ligamenta sternoclavicularia
l. sternocostale intraarticulare
ligamenta sternocostalia radiata
ligamenta sternopericardiaca
l. stylohyoideum
l. stylomandibulare
l. supraspinale
ligamenta suspensoria mammaria
l. suspensorium axillae
l. suspensorium bulbi
l. suspensorium clitoridis
l. suspensorium duodeni
l. suspensorium glandulae thyroideae
l. suspensorium ovarii
l. suspensorium penis
l. talocalcaneare interosseum
l. talocalcaneum
l. talocalcaneum laterale
l. talocalcaneum mediale
l. talocalcaneum posterius
l. talofibulare anterius
l. talofibulare posterius
l. talonaviculare
l. talotibiale anterius
l. talotibiale posterius
l. tarsale externum
l. tarsale internum
ligamenta tarsi
ligamenta tarsi dorsalia
ligamenta tarsi interossea
ligamenta tarsi plantaria

ligamenta tarsometatarsalia
ligamenta tarsometatarsalia dorsalia
ligamenta tarsometatarsalia plantaria
l. temporomandibulare
l. teres femoris
l. teres hepatis
l. teres uteri
l. testis
l. thyroepiglotticum
l. thyrohyoideum laterale
l. thyrohyoideum medianum
l. tibiofibulare anterius
l. tibiofibulare medium
l. tibiofibulare posterius
l. tibionaviculare
ligamenta trachealia
l. transversale cervicis
l. transversum acetabuli
l. transversum atlantis
l. transversum cruris
l. transversum genus
l. transversum humeri
l. transversum pelvis
l. transversum perinei
l. transversum scapulae inferius
l. transversum scapulae superius
l. trapezoideum
l. triangulare
l. triangulare dextrum hepatis
l. triangulare sinistrum hepatis
l. tuberculi costae
l. ulnocarpale palmare
l. umbilicale laterale
l. umbilicale mediale
l. umbilicale medianum
l. uteroovaricum
l. venae cavae sinistrae
l. venosum
l. ventriculare
l. vestibulare
l. vocale

ligand
addressin l.
Fas l.
ligand-binding site
ligand-gated channel
ligandin
ligase chain reaction
ligate
ligation
blunt-end l.
enzyme-catalyzed l.
pole l.
surgical l.
tooth l.
tubal l.
ligator
ligature
elastic l.
intravascular l.
nonabsorbable l.
occluding l.
provisional l.
soluble l.
Stannius l.

suboccluding l.
suture l.
l. wire

light
l. adaptation
l. bath
l. cell of thyroid
l. chain
l. chain-related amyloidosis
cold l.
l. difference
l. differential threshold
l. green SF yellowish
infrared l.
invisible l.
l. liquid petrolatum
l. metal
l. micrograph
l. microscope
minimum l.
polarized l.
reflected l.
l. reflex
refracted l.
l. sense
l. sleep
transmitted l.
l. treatment
l. wire appliance
Wood l.
light-activated resin
light-adapted eye
light-cured resin
lightening
lighthouse lens
light-near dissociation
lightning strip
light-touch palpation
ligneous
l. conjunctivitis
l. struma
l. thyroiditis
lignin
lignoceric acid
likelihood
Likert scale
Lillie
L. allochrome connective tissue
stain
L. azure-eosin stain
L. ferrous iron stain
L. sulfuric acid Nile blue stain
lilliputian hallucination
limb
ampullary membranous l.'s of
semicircular duct
anacrotic l.
anterior l. of internal capsule
anterior l. of stapes
l.'s of bony semicircular canal
bony l.'s of semicircular canal
l. bud
common membranous l. of
membranous semicircular duct

common membranous l. of
semicircular duct
l. of helix
inferior l.
inferior l. of ansa cervicalis
lateral l.
l. lead
long l. of incus
lower l.
medial l.
l. myokymia
pelvic l.
phantom l.
posterior l. of internal capsule
posterior l. of stapes
retrolenticular l. of internal capsule
retrolentiform l. of internal capsule
short l. of incus
simple membranous l. of
semicircular duct
sublenticular l. of internal capsule
sublentiform l. of internal capsule
superior l.
superior l. of ansa cervicalis
thoracic l.
upper l.
limb-girdle muscular dystrophy
limbi (*pl. of* limbus)
limbic
l. lobe
l. system
limb-kinetic apraxia
limbus, pl. **limbi**
l. acetabuli
l. alveolaris
l. anterior palpebrae
l. of cornea
l. corneae
corneal l.
l. fossae ovalis
l. laminae spiralis osseae
l. membranae tympani
l. of osseous spiral lamina
limbi palpebrales
l. penicillatus
l. posterior palpebrae
l. sphenoidalis
l. of sphenoid bone
l. striatus
l. of tympanic membrane
Vieussens l.
lime
air-slaked l.
chlorinated l.
slaked l.
sulfurated l.
l. water
limen, pl. **limina**
difference l.
l. insulae
l. nasi
limerence
limes (L)
l. flocculation (Lf)

L

limes *(continued)*
l. null dose of diphtheria toxin (Lo)
l. reacting dose of diphtheria toxin (Lr)

limina *(pl. of* limen)
liminal
l. stimulus
l. trait
liminometer
limit
critical l.
l. dextrin
l. dextrinase
l. dextrinosis
elastic l.
Hayflick l.
permissible exposure l. (PEL)
proportional l.
quantum l.
short-term exposure l. (STEL)
tolerance l.'s
limited neck dissection
limiting
l. angle
l. decision
l. layer of cornea
l. membrane of retina
l. sulcus
l. sulcus of fourth ventricle
l. sulcus of Reil
Limnatis nilotica
limnemia
limnemic
limnology
limon
limophthisis
limp
limulus lysate test
LINAC
linear accelerator
lincomycin
lincture, linctus
lindane
Lindau
L. disease
L. tumor
Lindner body
line
absorption l.
accretion l.
alveolonasal l.
Amberg lateral sinus l.
l. angle
anocutaneous l.
anterior axillary l.
anterior junction l.
anterior median l.
arcuate l.
arcuate l. of ilium
arcuate l. of rectus sheath
arterial l.
axillary l.
Baillarger l.

base l.
basinasal l.
Beau l.
l. of Bechterew
bismuth l.
black l.
l. of Blaschko
blue l.
Brödel bloodless l.
Burton l.
calcification l. of Retzius
Camper l.
cell l.
cement l.
cervical l.
Chamberlain l.
Chaussier l.
choroid l.
Clapton l.
cleavage l.
Conradi l.
contour l. of Owen
Correra l.
costal l. of pleural reflection
costoclavicular l.
costophrenic septal l.
Crampton l.
Daubenton l.
l. of demarcation
demarcation l. of retina
Dennie l.
dentate l.
developmental l.
Douglas l.
Eberth l.
Egger l.
Ehrlich-Türk l.
epiphysial l.
established cell l.
Farre l.
Feiss l.
Ferry l.
l. of fixation
Fleischner l.
Fraunhofer l.
fulcrum l.
l. of Gennari
germ l.
gluteal l.
Granger l.
growth arrest l.
Gubler l.
gum l.
Haller l.
Hampton l.
Harris l.
Head l.
Hensen l.
highest nuchal l.
high lip l.
Hilton white l.
His l.
Holden l.
Hudson-Stähli l.
Hunter l.

Hunter-Schreger l.
iliopectineal l.
imbrication l. of von Ebner
incremental l.
incremental l. of von Ebner
inferior nuchal l.
inferior temporal l. of parietal bone
infracostal l.
intercondylar l. of femur
intermediate l. of iliac crest
interspinal l.
intertrochanteric l.
intertubercular l.
iron l.
isoelectric l.
l. of Kaes
Kerley A, B, C l.'s
Kilian l.
Langer l.
Lanz l.
lead l.
Looser l.
low lip l.
M l.
Mach l.
mammary l.
mammillary l.
McKee l.
median l.
Mees l.
mercurial l.
Meyer l.
midaxillary l.
midclavicular l.
middle axillary l.
milk l.
Monro l.
Monro-Richter l.
Muehrcke l.
mylohyoid l.
nasobasilar l.
Nélaton l.
neonatal l.
nipple l.
Obersteiner-Redlich l.
oblique l.
oblique l. of mandible
oblique l. of thyroid cartilage
occipital l.
l. of occlusion
Ogston l.
Ohngren l.
orbitomeatal l.
Owen l.
l. pairs
paraspinal l.
parasternal l.
paravertebral l.
Paris l.
Paton l.
pectinate l.
pectineal l. of femur
pectineal l. of pubis
PICC l.

pleural l.
l. of pleural reflection
pleuroesophageal l.
Poirier l.
popliteal l.
postaxillary l.
posterior axillary l.
posterior junction l.
posterior median l.
Poupart l.
preaxillary l.
retentive fulcrum l.
l. of Retzius
Richter-Monro l.
Roser-Nélaton l.
rough l.
sagittal l.
Salter incremental l.
S-BP l.
scapular l.
Schreger l.
semicircular l.
semicircular l. of Douglas
semilunar l.
septal l.
Sergent white l.
Shenton l.
S-N l.
soleal l.
l. for soleus muscle
Spigelius l.
spiral l.
l. spread function (LSF)
stabilizing fulcrum l.
sternal l.
sternal l. of pleural reflection
Stocker l.
subcostal l.
superior nuchal l.
superior temporal l. of parietal bone
supracrestal l.
survey l.
Sydney l.
sylvian l.
temporal l.
temporal l. of frontal bone
tender l.
tension l.
terminal l.
l. test
Topinard l.
tram l.
trapezoid l.
Ullmann l.
vertebral l. of pleural reflection
Vesling l.
vibrating l.
l. of vision
Wegner l.
white l.
white l. of anal canal
white l. of Toldt
Z l.

L

line *(continued)*
l. of Zahn
Zöllner l.
linea, gen. and pl. **lineae**
l. alba
l. anorectalis
l. arcuata
l. arcuata ossis ilii
l. arcuata vaginae musculi recti abdominis
l. aspera
lineae atrophicae
l. axillaris anterior
l. axillaris media
l. axillaris posterior
l. corneae senilis
lineae distractionis
l. epiphysialis
l. glutea anterior
lineae gluteae
l. glutea inferior
l. glutea posterior
l. intercondylaris femoris
l. intermedia cristae iliacae
l. interspinalis
l. intertrochanterica
l. intertubercularis
l. mammillaris
l. mediana anterior
l. mediana posterior
l. medio-axillaris
l. medioclavicularis
l. musculi solei
l. mylohyoidea
l. nigra
l. nuchae inferior
l. nuchae mediana
l. nuchae superior
l. nuchae suprema
l. obliqua
l. obliqua cartilaginis thyroideae
l. obliqua mandibulae
l. parasternalis
l. paravertebralis
l. pectinata canalis analis
l. pectinea femoris
l. poplitea
l. postaxillaris
l. preaxillaris
l. scapularis
l. semicircularis
l. semilunaris
l. spiralis
l. splendens
l. sternalis
l. subcostalis
l. supracristalis
l. temporalis inferior ossis parietalis
l. temporalis ossis frontalis
l. temporalis superior ossis parietalis
l. terminalis pelvis
l. terminalis of pelvis
lineae transversae ossis sacri
l. trapezoidea

lineage
linear
l. absorption coefficient
l. acceleration
l. accelerator (LINAC)
l. amplification
l. amputation
l. atrophy
l. craniectomy
l. energy transfer (LET)
l. epidermal nevus
l. fracture
l. IgA bullous disease in children
l. phonocardiograph
l. scleroderma
l. skull fracture
linearity
linebreeding
lined flap
liner
asbestos l.
cavity l.
LINES
long interspersed element
Lineweaver-Burk
L.-B. equation
L.-B. plot
Lingelsheimia
L. anitrata
Ling method
lingua, pl. **linguae**
l. cerebelli
l. fissurata
l. frenata
l. geographica
l. nigra
l. plicata
lingual
l. aponeurosis
l. arch
l. artery
l. bar
l. bone
l. branch
l. branch of facial nerve
l. crypt
l. embrasure
l. flange
l. follicle
l. frenulum
l. gingiva
l. gingival papilla
l. goiter
l. gyrus
l. hemiatrophy
l. interdental papilla
l. lobe
l. lymph node
l. mucosa
l. muscle
l. nerve
l. occlusion
l. papillae
l. plate
l. plexus

l. quinsy
l. rest
l. salivary gland depression
l. septum
l. splint
l. surface of tooth
l. tonsil
l. vein

lingual-facial-buccal dyskinesia
Linguatula
    L. rhinaria
    L. serrata
linguatuliasis
Linguatulidae
linguiform
lingula, pl. **lingulae**
l. cerebelli
l. of cerebellum
l. of left lung
l. of mandible
l. mandibulae
l. pulmonis sinistri
sphenoidal l.
l. sphenoidalis
lingular
l. artery
l. vein
lingulectomy
linguocervical ridge
linguoclination
linguoclusion
linguodistal
linguofacial (arterial) trunk
linguogingival
l. fissure
l. groove
l. ridge
linguoocclusal
linguopapillitis
linguoplate
linguoversion
liniment
lining cell
linin network
linitis plastica
link
tip l.'s
linkage
l. analysis
l. disequilibrium
genetic l.
l. group
l. map
l. marker
medical record l.
record l.
sex l.
linked
linker
l. DNA
l. scanning
linking number (L)
linnaean system of nomenclature
Linognathus
linoleate

linoleic acid
linolenic acid
linolic acid
linseed oil
lint
lion-jaw bone-holding forceps
lip
lymphocytic interstitial pneumonia
acetabular l.
anterior l. of external os of uterus
anterior l. of uterine os
articular l.
cleft l.
double l.
external l. of iliac crest
glenoidal l.
Hapsburg l.
inner l. of iliac crest
internal l. of iliac crest
large pudendal l.
lateral l. of linea aspera
lower l.
medial l. of linea aspera
l.'s of mouth
outer l. of iliac crest
l. pit
posterior l. of external os of uterus
l. reading
l. reflex
rhombic l.
small pudendal l.
l. sulcus
tympanic l. of limbus of spiral lamina
tympanic l. of spiral limbus
upper l.
vestibular l. of limbus of spiral lamina
vestibular l. of spiral limbus
lipancreatin
liparocele
lipase test
lipectomy
lipedema
lipedematous alopecia
lipemia
alimentary l.
diabetic l.
postprandial l.
l. retinalis
lipemic retinopathy
lipid
l. A
anisotropic l.
anular l.
brain l.
compound l.
l. granulomatosis
l. histiocytosis
isotropic l.
l. keratopathy
l. pneumonia
simple l.
lipidemia
lipid-mobilizing hormone

L

lipidolytic
lipidosis, pl. **lipidoses**
    ceramide lactoside l.
    cerebral l.
    cerebroside l.
    ganglioside l.
    glycolipid l.
    sphingomyelin l.
    sulfatide l.
lipoamide
    l. dehydrogenase
    l. disulfide
    l. reductase (NADH)
lipoarthritis
lipoate acetyltransferase
lipoatrophia
    l. annularis
    l. circumscripta
lipoatrophic diabetes
lipoatrophy
    insulin l.
    partial l.
lipoblast
lipoblastoma
lipoblastomatosis
lipocardiac
lipocatabolic
lipoceratous
lipocere
lipochondria
lipochondrodystrophy
lipochrome
lipoclasis
lipoclastic
lipocrit
lipocyte
lipodermoid
lipodieresis
lipodystrophia progessiva superior
lipodystrophy
    congenital total l.
    familial partial l.
    insulin l.
    membranous l.
    progressive l.
lipoedema
lipofectin
lipofection
lipoferous
lipofibroma
lipofuscin
lipofuscinosis
    ceroid l.
    neuronal ceroid l.
lipogenesis
lipogenic
lipogenous diabetes
lipogranuloma
lipogranulomatosis
    disseminated l.
lipohemia
lipoic acid
lipoid
    l. dermatoarthritis
    l. granuloma

    l. nephrosis
    l. pneumonia
    l. proteinosis
    l. theory of narcosis
lipoidemia
lipoidosis
    cerebroside l.
    l. corneae
    l. cutis et mucosae
    galactosylceramide l.
lipoinjection
lipolipoidosis
lipolysis
lipolytic
lipoma
    l. annulare colli
    l. arborescens
    atypical l.
    l. capsulare
    l. cavernosum
    l. fibrosum
    l. myxomatodes
    l. ossificans
    l. petrificans
    pleomorphic l.
    spindle cell l.
    telangiectatic l.
lipomatoid
lipomatosis
    encephalocraniocutaneous l.
    mediastinal l.
    multiple symmetric l.
    l. neurotica
lipomatous
    l. hypertrophy
    l. infiltration
    l. polyp
lipomeningocele
lipomucopolysaccharidosis
liponucleoproteins
Liponyssus
lipopenia
lipopenic
lipopeptid, lipopeptide
lipophage
lipophagic granuloma
lipophagy
lipophanerosis
lipophil
lipophilic
lipophosphodiesterase
    l. I
    l. II
lipopolysaccharide (LPS)
lipoprotein
    l. (a)
    $alpha_1$-l.
    $beta_1$-l.
    l. electrophoresis
    high density l. (HDL)
    intermediate density l. (IDL)
    l. lipase
    low density l. (LDL)
    l. Lp(a)

malondialdehyde-modified low-density l.
l. polymorphism
very low density l. (VLDL)
l.-X
lipoprotein(a) hyperlipoproteinemia
lipoprotein-associated coagulation inhibitor (LACI)
liposarcoma
liposis
lipositol
liposoluble
liposome
liposuction
tumescent l.
wet-technique l.
liposuctioning
lipothiamide pyrophosphate
lipotrophic
lipotrophy
lipotropic
l. factor
l. hormone (LPH)
l. pituitary l.
lipotropin
lipotropy
lipovaccine
lipovitellin
lipoxenous
lipoxeny
lipoxidase
lipoxygenase
lipoyl dehydrogenase
lipping
lippitude
Lipschütz cell
lipuria
lipuric
liquefacient
liquefaction degeneration
liquefactive necrosis
liquefied phenol
liqueur
liquid (l)
l. air
Cotunnius l.
l. crystal thermography
l. extract
l. glucose
l. human serum
l. paraffin
l. petroleum
l. pitch
l. scintillator
l. ventilation
liquid-liquid chromatography
liquor, pl. **liquores**
l. amnii
l. cerebrospinalis
l. cotunnii
l. entericus
l. folliculi
malt l.
Morgagni l.
mother l.

Scarpa l.
spirituous l.
vinous l.
liquorice
liquorrhea
Lisch nodule
Lisfranc
L. amputation
L. joint
L. ligament
L. operation
L. tubercle
lisinopril
Lison-Dunn stain
lisping
lispro insulin
lissamine rhodamine B 200
Lissauer
L. bundle
L. column
L. fasciculus
L. marginal zone
L. tract
lissencephalia
lissencephalic
lissencephaly
lissive
lissosphincter
lissotrichic, lissotrichous
Lister
L. dressing
L. method
L. tubercle
Listerella
Listeria
L. *denitrificans*
L. *grayi*
L. meningitis
L. *monocytogenes*
listeriosis
listerism
Listing
L. law
L. reduced eye
Liston
L. knife
L. shears
lisuride
liter (l)
literal agraphia
literature
gray l.
lithagogue
litharge
lithectomy
lithiasis
l. conjunctivae
2,8-dihydroxyadenine l.
pancreatic l.
lithic acid
lithium (Li)
l. bromide
l. carbonate
l. carmine
l. citrate

lithium *(continued)*
    effervescent l. citrate
    l. tungstate
Lithobius
lithocholic acid
litholclast
lithogenesis
lithogenic
lithogenous
lithoid
lithokelyphopedion, lithokelyphopedium
lithokelyphos
litholabe
litholapaxy
litholysis
litholyte
litholytic
lithomyl
lithonephritis
lithopedion, lithopedium
lithotome
lithotomist
lithotomy
    high l.
    lateral l.
    marian l.
    median l.
    perineal l.
    l. position
    prerectal l.
    suprapubic l.
    vaginal l.
    vesical l.
lithotresis
lithotripsy
    electrohydraulic shock wave l.
    extracorporeal shock wave l.
    (ESWL)
    shock wave l.
    ultrasonic l.
lithotriptic
lithotriptor
lithotriptoscopy
lithotrite
lithotrity
lithotroph
lithuresis
lithuria
litigious paranoia
litmus
litter
little
    l. ACTH
    L. area
    L. disease
    l. finger
    l. fossa of the cochlear window
    l. fossa of the oval (vestibular) window
    l. head of humerus
    l. league elbow
    L. Leaguer's elbow
    l. toe [V]
littoral cell

Littré
    L. gland
    L. hernia
Litzmann obliquity
live
    l. birth
    l. oral poliovirus vaccine
    l. vaccine
livebirth
liveborn infant
livedo
    postmortem l.
    l. reticularis
    l. reticularis idiopathica
    l. reticularis symptomatica
    l. telangiectatica
    l. vasculitis
livedoid
liver
    l. acinus
    l. breath
    l. bud
    cardiac l.
    l. cell carcinoma
    desiccated l.
    fatty l.
    l. filtrate factor
    l. flap
    hobnail l.
    l. kidney syndrome
    l. *Lactobacillus casei* factor
    lardaceous l.
    left l.
    nutmeg l.
    l. palm
    pigmented l.
    polycystic l.
    posterior l.
    right l.
    l. spot
    l. starch
    l. of sulfur
    wandering l.
    waxy l.
liver-shod clamp
livetin
    alpha-l.
    beta-l.
    gamma-l.
livid
lividity
    postmortem l.
living anatomy
livor
lixivium
LLAT
    lysolecithin-lecithin acyltransferase
LLETZ
    large loop excision of transformation zone of the cervix of the uterus
L-L factor
LLL
    left lower lobe (of lung)
Lloyd reagent

LLQ
    left lower quadrant of abdomen
LM
    licentiate in midwifery
lm
    lumen
LMA
    left mentoanterior position
LMP
    latent membrane protein
    left mentoposterior position
LMT
    left mentotransverse position
LNPF
    lymph node permeability factor
Lo
    limes null dose of diphtheria toxin
LOA
    left occipitoanterior position
load
        electronic pacemaker l.
        genetic l.
        viral l.
load-and-shift maneuver
loading
        carbohydrate l.
        l. dose
        salt l.
        soda l.
Loa loa
lobar
        l. bronchus
        l. nephronia
        l. pneumonia
        l. sclerosis
lobate
lobe
        anterior l. of hypophysis
        azygos l. of right lung
        caudate l.
        cerebral l.
        cuneiform l.
        ear l.
        falciform l.
        flocculonodular l.
        frontal l.
        frontal l. of cerebrum
        glandular l. of hypophysis
        Home l.
        inferior l. of (left / right) lung
        insular l.
        kidney l.
        left l.
        left l. of liver
        left lower l. (of lung) (LLL)
        left upper l. (of lung) (LUL)
        limbic l.
        lingual l.
        lower l. of lung
        l. of mammary gland
        middle l. of prostate
        middle l. of right lung
        nervous l.
        neural l. of hypophysis
        occipital l.

        occipital l. of cerebrum
        parietal l.
        parietal l. of cerebrum
        placental l.
        polyalveolar l.
        posterior l. of hypophysis
        l. of prostate
        pyramidal l. of thyroid gland
        quadrate l.
        renal l.
        Riedel l.
        right l.
        right l. of liver
        right lower l. (RLL)
        right middle l. (RML)
        right upper l. (RUL)
        Spigelius l.
        superior l. of (right/left) lung
        supplemental l.
        temporal l.
        l. of thyroid gland
        upper l. of lung
lobectomy
lobelia
lobeline, lobelin
        l. sulfate
lobi (*pl. of* lobus)
lobitis
Loboa loboi
Lobo disease
lobomycosis
lobopodium, pl. **lobopodia**
lobose, lobous
lobotomy
        prefrontal l.
        transorbital l.
**Lobry de Bruyn-van Ekenstein
    transformation**
Lobstein ganglion
lobster-claw deformity
lobular
        l. capillary hemangioma
        l. carcinoma
        l. carcinoma in situ
        l. glomerulonephritis
        l. neoplasia
lobulate, lobulated
lobule
        ala central l.
        ansiform l.
        anterior lunate l.
        l. of auricle
        biventer l.
        biventral l.
        central l.
        central l. of cerebellum
        conic l. of epididymis
        cortical l. of kidney
        crescentic l. of the cerebellum
        l. of epididymis
        gracile l.
        hepatic l.
        inferior parietal l.
        inferior semilunar l.
        l. of liver

L

lobule *(continued)*
 l. of mammary gland
 paracentral l.
 paramedian l.
 portal l. of liver
 posterior lunate l.
 primary pulmonary l.
 quadrangular l.
 quadrate l.
 renal cortical l.
 respiratory l.
 secondary pulmonary l.
 simple l.
 slender l.
 superior parietal l.
 superior semilunar l.
 l. of testis
 l. of thymus
 l. of thyroid gland
lobulet, lobulette
lobulus, pl. **lobuli**
 l. auriculae
 l. biventer
 l. biventralis
 l. centralis corporis cerebelli
 l. clivi
 l. corticalis renalis
 l. culminis
 l. cuneiformis
 lobuli epididymidis
 l. folii
 l. fusiformis
 lobuli glandulae mammariae
 lobuli glandulae thyroideae
 l. gracilis
 l. hepatis
 l. paracentralis
 l. paramedianus
 l. parietalis inferior
 l. parietalis superior
 l. quadrangularis
 l. quadratus
 l. semilunaris inferior
 l. semilunaris superior
 l. simplex
 lobuli testis
 lobuli thymi
lobus, pl. **lobi**
 l. anterior hypophyseos
 l. appendicularis
 l. azygos pulmonis dextri
 l. caudatus
 lobi cerebri
 l. clivi
 l. dexter
 l. falciformis
 l. flocculonodularis
 l. frontalis
 lobi glandulae mammariae
 lobi glandulae thyroideae
 l. glandularis hypophyseos
 l. hepatis dexter
 l. hepatis sinister
 l. inferior pulmonis dextri et sinistri

 l. insula
 l. insularis
 l. limbicus
 l. linguiformis
 l. medius prostatae
 l. medius pulmonis dextri
 l. nervosus
 l. occipitalis
 l. parietalis
 l. posterior hypophyseos
 l. prostatae
 l. pyramidalis glandulae thyroideae
 l. quadratus
 l. renalis
 l. sinister
 l. superior pulmonis (dextri et
  sinistri)
 l. temporalis
LOCA
 low osmolar contrast agent
local
 l. anaphylaxis
 l. anemia
 l. anesthesia
 l. anesthetic reaction
 l. anesthetics
 l. asphyxia
 l. bloodletting
 l. death
 l. epilepsy
 l. excitatory state
 l. flap
 l. glomerulonephritis
 l. hormone
 l. immunity
 l. sign
 l. stimulant
 l. symptom
 l. syncope
 l. tetanus
 l. tic
localization
 l. agnosia
 auditory l.
 cerebral l.
 germinal l.
 radiotherapy l.
 spatial l.
 stereotactic l.
localization-related epilepsy
localized
 l. amnesia
 l. mucinosis
 l. nodular tenosynovitis
 l. osteitis fibrosa
 l. pemphigoid of Brunsting-Perry
 l. peritonitis
 l. scleroderma
localizing
 l. electrode
 l. symptom
locant
locator
lochia
 l. alba

l. rubra
l. sanguinolenta
l. serosa
lochial
lochiometra
lochiorrhagia
lochiorrhea
loci (*pl. of* locus)
lock
English l.
l. finger
sliding l.
l. stitch
lock-and-key model
locked
l. bite
l. facet
l. knee
l. twins
locked-in syndrome
Locke-Ringer solution
Locke solution
locking suture
lockjaw
Lockwood ligament
LOCM
low osmolar contrast medium
locomotive
locomotor ataxia
locomotorial
locomotorium
locomotory
locular
loculate
loculated
l. empyema
l. pleural effusion
loculation syndrome
loculus, pl. **loculi**
locum
l. tenant
l. tenens
locus, pl. **loci**
l. caeruleus
l. cinereus
cis-acting l.
complex l.
l. of control
l. ferrugineus
genetic l.
marker l.
l. niger
l. perforatus anticus
l. perforatus posticus
sex-linked l.
X-linked l.
Y-linked l.
locust gum
lod
l. method
l. score
Loeb deciduoma
Loeffler
L. bacillus
L. blood culture medium

L. caustic stain
L. methylene blue
L. syndrome I, II
Loevit cell
Loewenthal
L. bundle
L. reaction
L. tract
lofentanil
Löffler
L. disease
L. parietal fibroplastic endocarditis
L. syndrome
Logan bow
logarithm
logarithmic
l. phase
l. phonocardiograph
logetronography
logistic
l. curve
l. model
L. Organ Dysfunction Score
logit transformation
lognormal distribution
logopedia
logopedics
logorrhea
logospasm
logotherapy
Lohlein-Baehr lesion
Lohmann reaction
loiasis
loin
loliism
Lombard voice-reflex test
lomustine (CCNU)
long
l. abductor muscle of thumb
l. adductor muscle
l. association fiber
l. axis
l. axis of body
l. axis view
l. bone
l. buccal nerve
l. central artery
l. chain
l. ciliary nerve
L. coefficient
l. cone technique
l. crus of incus
l. extensor muscle of great toe
l. extensor muscle of thumb
l. extensor muscle of toes
l. fibular muscle
l. flexor muscle of great toe
l. flexor muscle of thumb
l. flexor muscle of toes
L. formula
l. gyrus of insula
l. head
l. incubation hepatitis
l. interspersed element (LINES)
l. levatores costarum muscle

L

long *(continued)*
l. limb of incus
l. muscle of head
l. muscle of neck
l. palmar muscle
l. peroneal muscle
l. pitch helicoidal layer
l. plantar ligament
l. posterior ciliary artery
l. process of malleus
l. pulse
l. QT syndrome
l. radial extensor muscle of wrist
l. root of ciliary ganglion
l. saphenous nerve
l. saphenous vein
l. sight
l. subscapular nerve
l. terminal repeat sequence (LTR)
l. thoracic artery
l. thoracic nerve
l. thoracic vein
l. vinculum
long-acting thyroid stimulator (LATS)
long-chain
l-c acyl-CoA dehydrogenase
l-c fatty acid-CoA ligase
l-c 3-hydroxyacyl-CoA
dehydrogenase deficiency
**long-chain/very long-chain acyl-CoA
dehydrogenase deficiency**
longevity
longissimus
l. capitis muscle
l. cervicis muscle
l. muscle
l. thoracis muscle
longitudinal
l. aberration
l. arch of foot
l. arc of skull
l. bands of cruciform ligament of
atlas
l. canal of modiolus
l. cerebral fissure
l. dissociation
l. duct of epoöphoron
l. fold of duodenum
l. fracture
l. layer of muscle coat of small
intestine
l. layer of muscular coat
l. layer of muscular tunics
l. lie
l. ligament
l. method
l. oval pelvis
l. pontine bundle
l. pontine fasciculi
l. pontine fiber
l. relaxation
l. section
l. sinus
l. study

l. sulcus of heart
l. vertebral venous sinus
longitudinalis
longitype
long-leg arthropathy
Longmire operation
long-term memory (LTM)
longus
l. capitis muscle
l. colli muscle
Lon protease
loop
Biebl l.
bulboventricular l.
capillary l.
cervical l.
cruciform l.
D l.
displacement l.
l. diuretic
l. electrocautery excision procedure
(LEEP)
l. electrosurgical excision procedure
l. excision
gamma l.
Gerdy interatrial l.
Granit l.
hairpin l.
Henle l.
l. of hypoglossal nerve
Hyrtl l.
lenticular l.
memory l.
Meyer-Archambault l.
nephronic l.
peduncular l.
l. resection
l. of spinal nerve
l. stoma
subclavian l.
vector l.
ventricular l.
Vieussens l.
loose
l. association
l. body
l. cartilage
l. skin
loosening of association
Looser
L. line
L. zone
LOP
left occipitoposterior position
lop-ear
loperamide hydrochloride
lophodont
Lophophora williamsii
lophotrichate
lophotrichous
lopremone
Lorain disease
Lorain-Lévi
L.-L. dwarfism

L.-L. infantilism
L.-L. syndrome
lorazepam
lorcainide
lordoscoliosis
lordosis
cervical l.
l. cervicis
l. colli
l. lumbalis
lumbar l.
lordotic
l. albuminuria
l. pelvis
Lorenzo oil
Lorenz sign
Loschmidt number (n_0)
LOT
left occipitotransverse position
lotion
loudness discomfort level
Lou Gehrig disease
Louis
L. angle
L. law
Louis-Bar syndrome
loupe
binocular l.
louping-ill virus
louse, pl. **lice**
biting l.
chewing l.
feather l.
l. fly
sea l.
sucking l.
louse-borne typhus
lousy
lovastatin
Lovén reflex
Lovibond
L. angle
L. profile sign
low
l. convex
l. forceps delivery
l. grade astrocytoma
l. lip line
l. malignant potential tumor
l. molecular weight kininogen
l. molecular weight protein
l. osmolar contrast agent (LOCA)
l. osmolar contrast medium
(LOCM)
l. output failure
l. purine diet
l. residue diet
l. salt diet
l. salt syndrome
l. sodium l.
l. spinal anesthesia
l. wine
low-calorie diet
low-density lipoprotein receptor

low-egg-passage vaccine
Löwenberg
L. canal
L. forceps
L. scala
Lowenstein-Jensen
L.-J. culture medium
L.-J. medium
lower
l. abdominal periosteal reflex
l. airway
l. alveolar point
l. dental arcade
l. esophageal sphincter (LES)
l. extremity
l. eyelid
l. jaw
left l. quadrant of abdomen (LLQ)
l. lid
l. limb
l. lip
l. lobe of lung
l. motor neuron
l. motor neuron dysarthria
l. motor neuron lesion
l. pole
l. pole of testis
l. respiratory tract smear
l. ridge slope
L. ring
L. tubercle
l. uterine segment
l. uterine segment cesarean section
lowest
l. lumbar artery
l. splanchnic nerve
l. thyroid artery
Lowe syndrome
Lowe-Terrey-MacLachlan syndrome
low-fat diet
low-frequency transduction
low-grade squamous intraepithelial lesion
(LGSIL, LSIL)
Lown-Ganong-Levine syndrome
low-pass filter
Lowry-Folin assay
Lowry protein assay
Lowsley tractor
low-tension glaucoma
low-tone hearing loss
loxapine
Loxosceles
loxoscelism
Loxotrema ovatum
lozenge
LPH
lipotropic hormone
L-phase variants
LPN
licensed practical nurse
LPO
left posterior oblique
LPS
lipopolysaccharide

L

Lr
    lawrencium
    limes reacting dose of diphtheria toxin
LRCP
    Licentiate of the Royal College of
        Physicians (of England)
LRCP(E)
    Licentiate of the Royal College of
        Physicians (Edinburgh)
LRCP(I)
    Licentiate of the Royal College of
        Physicians (Ireland)
LRCS
    Licentiate of the Royal College of
        Surgeons (of England)
LRCS(E)
    Licentiate of the Royal College of
        Surgeons (Edinburgh)
LRCS(I)
    Licentiate of the Royal College of
        Surgeons (Ireland)
LRF
    luteinizing hormone-releasing factor
LRFPS
    Licentiate of the Royal Faculty of
        Physicians and Surgeons
LRH
    luteinizing hormone-releasing hormone
LSA
    left sacroanterior position
LSD
    lysergic acid diethylamide
L-serine dehydratase
LSF
    line spread function
LSIL
    low-grade squamous intraepithelial lesion
LSP
    left sacroposterior position
L/S ratio
LST
    left sacrotransverse position
LT
    leukotrienes
LTM
    long-term memory
LTP
    laser trabeculoplasty
LTR
    long terminal repeat sequence
Lu
      Lu antigen
Lubarsch crystal
lubricating cream
lucanthone hydrochloride
Lucas groove
lucensomycin
lucent
lucidification
lucid interval
lucidity
luciferase
luciferin
lucifugal

Lucilia
    L. caesar
    L. illustris
    L. sericata
lucimycin
Lucio
    L. leprosy
    L. leprosy phenomenon
lucipetal
lückenschädel
Lücke test
Lucké virus
Luc operation
Ludwig
    L. angina
    L. angle
    L. ganglion
    L. labyrinth
    L. nerve
    L. stromuhr
Luer-Lok syringe
Luer syringe
lues
    l. venerea
luetic
Luft
    L. disease
    L. potassium permanganate fixative
Lugol iodine solution
Lukes-Collins classification
LUL
    left upper lobe (of lung)
luliberin
lumbago
    ischemic l.
lumbar
    l. appendicitis
    l. artery
    l. branch of iliolumbar artery
    l. cistern
    l. flexure
    l. ganglia
    l. hernia
    l. iliocostal muscle
    l. interspinal muscle
    l. lordosis
    l. lymphatic plexus
    l. (lymphatic) trunk
    l. lymph node
    l. myelogram
    l. nephrectomy
    l. nerve [L1–L5]
    l. part of diaphragm
    l. part of spinal cord
    l. puncture
    l. puncture needle
    l. quadrate muscle
    l. region
    l. rib
    l. rotator muscle
    l. segments L1–L5 of spinal cord
    l. segments of spinal cord L1–5
    l. splanchnic nerve
    l. triangle

l. vein
l. vertebrae [L1–L5]
lumbarization
lumbi (*pl. of* lumbus)
lumboabdominal
lumbocostal
l. ligament
l. triangle of diaphragm
lumbocostoabdominal triangle
lumbodorsal fascia
lumboiliac
lumboinguinal nerve
lumboovarian
lumbosacral
l. angle
l. enlargement
l. enlargement of spinal cord
l. joint
l. (nerve) trunk
l. plexus
lumbotomy incision
lumbrical
l. of foot
l. of hand
lumbricalis
lumbricidal
lumbricide
lumbricoid
lumbricosis
lumbricus
lumbus, pl. **lumbi**
lumen, pl. **lumina, lumens (lm)**
false l.
residual l.
true l.
lumichrome
lumiflavin
lumina (*pl. of* lumen)
luminal
luminalis
luminance
luminescence
luminiferous
luminophore
luminous
l. flux
l. intensity
l. retinoscope
lumirhodopsin
lumisterol
lumpectomy
lumpy jaw
lunacy
Luna-Ishak stain
lunar
l. caustic
l. periodicity
lunare
lunate
l. bone
l. fissure
l. sulcus
l. surface of acetabulum
lunatic
lunatomalacia

Lundh meal
lung
air-conditioner l.
bird-breeder's l.
bird-fancier's l.
black l.
brown l.
l. bud
butterfly l.
cardiac l.
cheese worker's l.
Collier l.
cystic l.
endstage l.
farmer's l.
fibroid l.
l. fluke disease
honeycomb l.
hyperlucent l.
iron l.
malt-worker's l.
mason's l.
miner's l.
mushroom-worker's l.
postperfusion l.
pump l.
quiet l.
shock l.
silo-filler's l.
thresher's l.
unilateral hyperlucent l.
l. unit
uremic l.
vanishing l.
l. volume reduction surgery
welder's l.
wet l.
white l.
l. window
lungworms
lunula, pl. **lunulae**
azure l. of nail
l. of semilunar cusp of
  aortic/pulmonary valve
l. of semilunar valve
l. unguis
lunulae valvularum semilunarium
  valvae aortae/trunci pulmonalis
lunule of nail
Lunyo virus
lupinidine
lupinosis
lupoid
l. hepatitis
l. leishmaniasis
lupulin
lupus
l. anticoagulant
l. band test
chilblain l.
chilblain l. erythematosus
chronic discoid l. erythematosus
cutaneous l. erythematosus
discoid l. erythematosus
disseminated l. erythematosus

L

lupus *(continued)*
    drug-induced l.
    l. erythematosus (LE, L.E.)
    l. erythematosus cell
    l. erythematosus cell test
    l. erythematosus, neonatal
    l. erythematosus panniculitis
    l. erythematosus profundus
    l. livedo
    l. miliaris disseminatus faciei
    neonatal l.
    l. nephritis
    l. pernio
    l. profundus
    l. serpiginosus
    systemic l. erythematosus (SLE)
    l. vulgaris
lupus-like syndrome
LUQ
    left upper quadrant of lung
lura
lural
Luschka
    L. bursa
    L. cartilage
    L. cystic gland
    L. duct
    L. gland
    L. joint
    L. ligament
    L. sinus
    L. tonsil
Luse body
lusitropic
lusitropy
lute
luteal
    l. cell
    l. phase
    l. phase defect
    l. phase deficiency
lutecium
lutein cell
luteinization
luteinize
luteinized unruptured follicle
luteinizing
    l. hormone (LH)
    l. hormone/follicle-stimulating
      hormone-releasing factor
    l. hormone-releasing factor (LH-RF,
      LRF)
    l. hormone-releasing hormone (LH-
      RH, LRH)
    l. principle
luteinoma
Lutembacher syndrome
luteogenic
luteohormone
luteol
luteolin
luteolysin
luteolysis
luteolytic

luteoma
    pregnancy l.
luteoplacental shift
luteotropic, luteotrophic
lutetium
luteus
Lutheran Blood Group, Lu Blood Group
luting agent
lutropin
lututrin
Lutzomyia
    L. flaviscutellata
    L. intermedius
    L. longipalpis
    L. peruensis
Lutz-Splendore-Almeida disease
lux (lx)
luxatio
    l. erecta
    l. perinealis
luxation
    Malgaigne l.
Luxol fast blue
luxus
Luys body
LVET
    left ventricular ejection time
LVN
    licensed vocational nurse
Lw
    lawrencium
lx
    lux
lyase
lycanthropy
lycoctonine
lycopene
lycopenemia
Lycoperdon
lycoperdonosis
lycophora
lycopodium
lye
Lyell
    L. disease
    L. syndrome
Lyme
    L. arthritis
    L. borreliosis
    L. disease
Lymnaea
lymph
    aplastic l.
    blood l.
    l. capillary
    l. cell
    l. circulation
    l. cord
    l. corpuscle
    corpuscular l.
    croupous l.
    dental l.
    l. embolism
    euplastic l.
    fibrinous l.

l. gland
inflammatory l.
intercellular l.
intravascular l.
l. nodule
plastic l.
l. sac
l. scrotum
l. sinus
l. space
tissue l.
vaccine l.
vaccinia l.
l. varix
l. vessels
lympha
lymphaden
lymphadenectomy
lymphadenitis
dermatopathic l.
mesenteric l.
paratuberculous l.
regional l.
regional granulomatous l.
tuberculosis l.
tuberculous l.
lymphadenography
lymphadenoid
lymphadenoma
lymphadenopathy
angioimmunoblastic l. with
dysproteinemia (AILD)
bulky l.
dermatopathic l.
immunoblastic l.
persistent generalized l.
lymphadenopathy-associated virus (LAV)
lymphadenosis
benign l.
lymphadenovarix
lymphagogue
lymphangeitis
lymphangial
lymphangiectasis, lymphangiectasia
cavernous l.
cystic l.
intestinal l.
simple l.
lymphangiectatic
lymphangiectomy
lymphangiitis
lymphangioendothelioma
lymphangiography
lymphangioleiomyomatosis
lymphangiology
lymphangioma
l. cavernosum
l. circumscriptum
l. cysticum
l. simplex
l. tuberosum multiplex
l. xanthelasmoideum
lymphangiomatous
lymphangiomyomatosis
lymphangion

lymphangiophlebitis
lymphangioplasty
lymphangiosarcoma
lymphangiotomy
lymphangitic carcinomatosis
lymphangitis carcinomatosa
lymphapheresis
lymphatic
afferent l.
l. angina
l. corpuscle
l. duct
l. edema
efferent l.
l. filariasis granuloma
l. fistula
l. follicle of larynx
l. follicle of rectum
l. leukemia
l. nodule
l. plexus
l. ring of cardiac part of stomach
l. sarcoma
l. sinus
l. stroma
l. system
l. tissue
l. valvule
l. vessels
lymphaticostomy
lymphatics
lymphatitis
lymphatology
lymphatolysis
lymphatolytic
lymphectasia
lymphedema
congenital l.
hereditary l.
l. praecox
primary l.
lymphedematous keratoderma
lymphemia
lymphization
lymph node, lymphatic node
abdominal l. n.
l. n. of abdominal organ
accessory l. n.
accessory nerve l. n.
anorectal l. n.
anterior axillary l. n.
l. n. of anterior border of omental
foramen
anterior cervical l. n.
anterior deep cervical l. n.
anterior jugular l. n.
anterior mediastinal l. n.
anterior superficial cervical l. n.
anterior tibial l. n.
apical axillary l. n.
appendicular l. n.
l. n. of arch of azygos vein
l. n. around cardia of stomach
axillary l. n.
l. n. of azygos arch

L

lymph node (*continued*)
bifurcation l. n.
brachial l. n.
brachiocephalic l. n.
bronchopulmonary l. n.
buccal l. n.
carinal l. n.
celiac l. n.
central axillary l. n.
central mesenteric l. n.
central superior mesenteric l. n.
colic l. n.
common iliac l. n.
companion l. n. of accessory nerve
cubital l. n.
cystic l. n.
deep anterior cervical l. n.
deep inguinal l. n.
deep lateral cervical l. n.
deep parotid l. n.
l. n. of elbow
external iliac l. n.
facial l. n.
fibular l. n.
foraminal l. n.
gastroduodenal l. n.'s
gluteal l. n.
l. n. of head and neck
hepatic l. n.
hilar l. n.
humeral axillary l. n.
ileocolic l. n.'s
inferior epigastric l. n.'s
inferior mesenteric l. n.'s
inferior phrenic l. n.
inferior tracheobronchial l. n.'s
infraauricular deep parotid l. n.
infraauricular subfascial parotid l. n.
intercostal l. n.'s
interiliac l. n.'s
intermediate lacunar l. n.
intermediate lumbar l. n.'s
internal iliac l. n.'s
interpectoral l. n.'s
intraglandular deep parotid l. n.
intraglandular parotid l. n.'s
intrapulmonary l. n.'s
jugulodigastric l. n.
juguloomohyoid l. n.
juxtaesophageal l. n.'s
juxta-intestinal mesenteric l. n.
lateral axillary l. n.
lateral jugular l. n.
lateral lacunar l. n.
lateral pericardial l. n.
left colic l. n.'s
left gastric l. n.
left gastroepiploic l. n.
left gastroomental l. n.'s
left lumbar l. n.'s
l. n. of ligamentum arteriosum
lingual l. n.
l. n. of lower limb
lumbar l. n.

malar l. n.
mandibular l. n.
mastoid l. n.
medial lacunar l. n.
mesenteric l. n.
mesocolic l. n.
middle colic l. n.
middle group of mesenteric l. n.
middle rectal l. n.
nasolabial l. n.
obturator l. n.
occipital l. n.
pancreatic l. n.
pancreaticoduodenal l. n.
pancreaticosplenic l. n.
paramammary l. n.
pararectal l. n.
parasternal l. n.
paratracheal l. n.
parauterine l. n.
paravaginal l. n.
paravesical l. n.
parietal l. n.
pectoral axillary l. n.
pelvic l. n.
l. n. permeability factor (LNPF)
peroneal l. n.
popliteal l. n.
posterior axillary l. n.
posterior mediastinal l. n.
posterior tibial l. n.
preauricular deep parotid l. n.
prececal l. n.
prelaryngeal l. n.
prepericardial l. n.
pretracheal l. n.
prevertebral l. n.
proximal deep inguinal l. n.
pulmonary l. n.
pyloric l. n.
retroauricular l. n.
retrocecal l. n.
retropharyngeal l. n.
retropyloric l. n.
right colic l. n.
right gastric l. n.
right gastroepiploic l. n.
right gastroomental l. n.
right lumbar l. n.
sacral l. n.
sentinel l. n.
sigmoid l. n.
signal l. n.
splenic l. n.
subaortic l. n.
submandibular l. n.
submental l. n.
subpyloric l. n.
subscapular axillary l. n.
superficial inguinal l. n.
superficial lateral cervical l. n.
superficial parotid l. n.
superior gastric l. n.
superior mesenteric l. n.
superior phrenic l. n.

superior rectal l. n.
superior tracheobronchial l. n.
supraclavicular l. n.
suprapyloric l. n.
thoracic l. n.
thyroid l. n.
tracheal l. n.
l. n. of upper limb
visceral l. n.
visceral l. n. of abdomen

lymphoblast
lymphoblastic
    l. leukemia
    l. lymphoma
lymphoblastoma
    giant follicular l.
lymphoblastosis
lymphocele
lymphocerastism
lymphocinesis, lymphocinesia
lymphocyst
lymphocytapheresis
lymphocyte
    B l.
    cytotoxic T l.
    l. function associated antigen (LFA)
    pre-B l.
    Rieder l.
    T l.
    l. transformation
    transformed l.
    tumor-infiltrating l., tumor-
      infiltrating l.'s
lymphocyte-mediated cytotoxicity
lymphocythemia
lymphocytic
    l. adenohypophysitis
    l. choriomeningitis
    l. choriomeningitis virus
    l. hypophysitis
    l. interstitial pneumonia (lip)
    l. interstitial pneumonitis
    l. leukemia
    l. leukemoid reaction
    l. leukocytosis
    l. leukopenia
    l. series
    l. thyroiditis
lymphocytoblast
lymphocytoma
    benign l. cutis
lymphocytopenia
lymphocytopoiesis
lymphocytosis
lymphocytotoxic antibody
lymphoderma
lymphoduct
lymphoepithelial cyst
lymphogenesis
lymphogenic
lymphogenous
    l. embolism
    l. metastasis
lymphoglandula

lymphogranuloma
    l. benignum
    l. inguinale
    l. malignum
    Schaumann l.
    venereal l.
    l. venereum
    l. venereum antigen
    l. venereum virus
lymphogranulomatosis
lymphography
lymphohistiocytosis
    familial erythrophagocytic l. (FEL)
    familial hemophagocytic l. (FMLH)
lymphoid
    l. cell
    l. hemoblast of Pappenheim
    l. hypophysitis
    l. interstitial pneumonia
    l. leukemia
    l. nodule
    l. polyp
    l. series
    l. system
lymphoidectomy
lymphoidocyte
lymphokine
lymphokinesis
lympholeukocyte
lymphology
lymphoma
    adult T-cell l.
    anaplastic large cell l.
    benign l. of the rectum
    Burkitt l.
    chronic lymphocytic l.
    diffuse small cleaved cell l.
    extranodal marginal zone l.
    follicular l.
    follicular predominantly large cell l.
    follicular predominantly small
      cleaved cell l.
    histiocytic l.
    Hodgkin l.
    immunoblastic l.
    Ki-1+ l.
    large cell l.
    Lennert l.
    lymphoblastic l.
    malignant l.
    mantle cell l.
    marginal zone l.
    Mediterranean l.
    nodular l.
    nodular histiocytic l.
    non-Hodgkin l. (NHL)
    peripheral T-cell l., unspecified
    poorly differentiated lymphocytic l.
    small lymphocytic l.
    T-cell–rich, B-cell l.
    well-differentiated lymphocytic l.
lymphomatoid
    l. granulomatosis
    l. papulosis
    l. polyposis

L

lymphomatosis
lymphomatous
lymphonodus
lymphopathia
lymphopathy
lymphopenia
lymphoplasmacellular disorder
lymphoplasmapheresis
lymphopoiesis
lymphopoietic
lymphoproliferative syndrome
lymphoreticulosis
     benign inoculation l.
lymphorrhagia
lymphorrhea
lymphorrhoid
lymphoscintigraphy
lymphosis
lymphostasis
lymphostatic verrucosis
lymphotaxis
lymphotoxicity
lymphotoxin
lymphotrophy
lymphuria
Lynch syndrome
lynestrenol
lyoenzyme
lyolysis
Lyon hypothesis
lyonization
lyophil
lyophilic colloid
lyophilization
lyophobe
lyophobic colloid
lyosorption
lyotropic series
lypressin
lyra
     l. davidis
     l. uterina
Lys
     lysine
     lysyl
lysate
lyse
lysemia
lysergamide
lysergic acid
     l. a. amide
     l. a. diethylamide (LSD)
     l. a. monoethylamide
lysergide
lysergol
lysin
lysine (K, Lys)
     l. decarboxylase

lysinemia
8-lysine vasopressin
lysinium
lysinogen
lysinogenic
lysinuria
lysinuric protein intolerance
lysis
     bystander l.
lysocephalin
lysogen
lysogenesis
lysogenic
     l. bacterium
     l. induction
     l. strain
lysogenicity
lysogenization
lysogeny
lysokinase
lysolecithin
     l.-lecithin acyltransferase (LLAT)
lysolecithinase
lysophosphatidic acid
     l. a. acyltransferase, 1-acylglycerol-
       3-phosphate acyltransferase
lysophosphatidylcholine
lysophosphatidylserine
lysophospholipase
lysosomal disease
lysosome
     definitive l.
     primary l.'s
     secondary l.'s
lysostaphin
lysotype
lysozyme
Lyssavirus
     Australian bat l.
     European bat l.
lysyl (K, Lys)
     l. hydroxylase
     l. oxidase
     l. 2-oxoglutarate dioxygenase
lysyl-bradykinin
Lyt antigen
Lythoglyphopsis
lytic
lyxitol
lyxoflavin
lyxose
lyxulose
lyze

μ
µ mu
μ_B
  Bohr magneton
μ_N
  nuclear magneton
µµ
  micromicro-
µΩ
  microohm
µCi
  microcurie
µm
  micrometer
µmol
  micromole
µmol/L
  micromolar
µV
M
  morgan
    M antigen
    M band
    M cell
    M concentration
    M line
    M phase
    M protein
    M shell
M.
  mix
M_r
  molecular weight ratio
  relative molecular mass
mµ
  millimicron
m-
  meta-
M2 segment of middle cerebral artery
MA
  mental age
ma
  milliampere
MAA
  macroaggregated albumin
MAB
  monoclonal antibody
MAC
  minimal anesthetic concentration
    MAC complex
Macaca
macaque
Macchiavello stain
MacConkey agar
macerate
maceration
Macewen
  M. sign
  M. symptom
  M. triangle
Mach
  M. band

  M. effect
  M. line
  M. number
Machado-Guerreiro test
Machado-Joseph disease
machine
  anesthesia m.
  heart-lung m.
  panoramic rotating m.
machinery murmur
Machupo virus
Mackay-Marg tonometer
Mackenrodt ligament
Mackenzie
  M. amputation
  M. polygraph
Maclagan
  M. thymol turbidity test
Macleod
  M. rheumatism
  M. syndrome
maclurin
MacNeal tetrachrome blood stain
Macracanthorhynchus
    Macracanthorhynchus hirudinaceus
macrencephaly, macrencephalia
macroadenoma
macroaggregated albumin (MAA)
macroamylase
macroamylasemia
macrobacterium
macrobiosis
macrobiote
macrobiotic diet
macrobiotics
macroblast
macroblepharon
macrobrachia
macrocardia
macrocephalic
macrocephaly
macrocheilia
macrocheiria
macrochemistry
macrochylomicron
macrocnemia
macrococcus
macrocolon
macroconidium, pl. macroconidia
macrocornea
macrocranium
macrocryoglobulin
macrocryoglobulinemia
macrocyst
macrocyte
macrocythemia
  hyperchromatic m.
macrocytic
  m. achylic anemia
  m. anemia of pregnancy
  m. anemia tropical
  m. hyperchromia

M

573

macrocytosis
macrodactylia, macrodactylism, macrodactyly
macrodont
macrodontia, macrodontism
macrodystrophia lipomatosa
macroelements
macroencephalon
macroerythroblast
macroerythrocyte
macroesthesia
macrofollicular adenoma
macrogamete
macrogametocyte
macrogamont
macrogamy
macrogastria
macrogenitosomia
    m. praecox
    m. praecox suprarenalis
macroglia cell
macroglobulin
macroglobulinemia
    Waldenström m.
macroglossia
macrognathia
macrography
macrogyria
macro-Kjeldahl method
macrolabia
macroleukoblast
macrolide
macromastia, macromazia
macromelanosome
macromelia
macromere
macromerozoite
macromineral
macromolecular chemistry
macromolecule
macromonocyte
macromyeloblast
macronormoblast
macronormochromoblast
macronucleus
macronutrient
macronychia
macroorchidism
macroparasite
macropathology
macropenis
macrophage
    activated m.
    alveolar m.
    armed m.
    m. colony-stimulating factor (M-CSF)
    fixed m.
    free m.
    Hansemann m.
    inflammatory m.
    m. inflammatory protein (MIP)
    m. migration inhibition test
    tangible body m.
macrophage-activating factor (MAF)

macrophagocyte
macrophallus
macrophthalmia
macropodia
macropolycyte
macropromyelocyte
macroprosopia
macroprosopous
macropsia
macrorhinia
macroscelia
macroscopic
    m. anatomy
    m. sphincter
macroscopy
macrosigmoid
macrosis
macrosmatic
macrosomia
macrosplanchnic
macrospore
macrostereognosis
macrostomia
macrotia
macrotome
macula, pl. maculae
    maculae acusticae
    m. adherens
    m. albida, pl. maculae albidae
    m. atrophica
    m. cerulea
    m. communicans
    m. communis
    m. corneae
    m. cribrosa, pl. maculae cribrosae
    m. cribrosa inferior
    m. cribrosa media
    m. cribrosa quarta
    m. cribrosa superior
    m. densa
    false m.
    m. flava
    m. gonorrhoica
    honeycomb m.
    m. lactea
    m. lutea
    m. pellucida
    m. of retina
    m. retinae
    m. of saccule
    m. sacculi
    m. tendinea
    m. of utricle
    m. utriculi
    maculae utriculosaccularis
macular, maculate
    m. amyloidosis
    m. area
    m. artery
    m. atrophy
    m. coloboma
    m. corneal dystrophy
    m. degeneration
    m. drusen
    m. erythema

m. evasion
m. fasciculus
m. leprosy
m. retinal dystrophy
m. retinopathy
macule
ash-leaf m.
maculocerebral
maculoerythematous
maculopapule
maculopathy
bull's-eye m.
cystoid m.
familial pseudoinflammatory m.
nicotinic acid m.
solar m.
mad
m. cow disease
M. Hatter syndrome
madarosis
madder
Maddox rod
Madelung
M. deformity
M. disease
M. neck
Madlener operation
madness
Madura
M. boil
M. foot
Madurella
maduromycosis
MAF
macrophage-activating factor
mafenide
Maffucci syndrome
magaldrate
Magendie
M. law
M. space
Magendie-Hertwig
M.-H. sign
M.-H. syndrome
magenstrasse
magenta tongue
maggot
cheese m.
surgical m.
magical thinking
magic forceps
Magill forceps
Magister
M. Chirurgiae (MC, MCh)
magistral
magma reticulare
Magnan
M. sign
M. trombone movement
magnesia
m. and alumina oral suspension
calcined m.
magnesia magma
magnesium (Mg)
m. aluminum silicate

m. bacteriopheophytinate
m. benzoate
m. carbonate
m. chloride
m. citrate
effervescent m. citrate
effervescent m. sulfate
m. hydroxide
m. lactate
m. oxide
m. peroxide
m. phytinates
m. salicylate
m. stearate
m. sulfate
tribasic m. phosphate
m. trisilicate
magnet
m. reaction
m. reflex
superconducting m.
magnetic
m. attraction
m. field
m. field gradient
m. implant
m. inertia
m. resonance angiography (MRA)
m. resonance imaging (MRI)
m. resonance spectroscopy
magnetism
animal m.
magnetocardiography
magnetoencephalogram (MEG)
magnetoencephalography
magnetogyric ratio
magnetometer
magneton
Bohr m. (μ_B)
electron m.
nuclear m. (μ_N)
magnetotherapy
magnification
m. angiography
m. radiography
magnitude
average pulse m.
m. image
peak m.
magnocellular
magnum
Magnus sign
Mahaim fiber
Ma-huang
MAI
Mycobacterium avium-intracellulare
maidenhair tree
maidenhead
maidism
Maier sinus
maim
mainframe
mainstreaming
main succulente

M

maintainer
    space m.
maintenance
    m. dose
    m. drug therapy
    m. medication
maise oil
Maissiat band
maize factor
Majocchi granuloma
major
    m. agglutinin
    m. alar cartilage
    m. amblyoscope
    m. amputation
    m. arterial circle of iris
    m. calices
    m. circulus arteriosus of iris
    m. connector
    m. depression
    m. depressive disorder
    m. duodenal papilla
    m. epilepsy
    m. fissure
    m. forceps
    m. groove
    m. hippocampus
    m. histocompatibility complex
      (MHC)
    m. hypnosis
    m. mood disorder
    m. motor seizure
    m. operation
    m. salivary gland
    m. sublingual duct
    m. surgery
    m. tranquilizer
Makeham hypothesis
mal
    m. de la rosa, m. rosso
    m. del pinto
    m. de Meleda
    m. de mer
    grand m.
    m. morado
    petit m.
    m. rosso (*var. of* m. de la rosa)
mala
malabsorption
    congenital selective glucose and
      galactose m.
    enterocyte cobalamin m.
    fructose m.
    hereditary folate m.
    m. syndrome
Malacarne
    M. pyramid
    M. space
malachite green
malacia
malacic
malacoplakia, malakoplakia
malacosis
malacotic
malactic

maladie
    m. de Roger
    m. des jambes
maladjustment
    social m.
malady
malagma
malaise
malakoplakia (*var. of* malacoplakia)
malalignment
malar
    m. arch
    m. bone
    m. flush
    m. fold
    m. foramen
    m. lymph node
    m. node
    m. point
    m. process
malaria
    acute m.
    airport m.
    algid m.
    autochthonous m.
    benign tertian m.
    bilious remittent m.
    cerebral m.
    chronic m.
    m. comatosa
    double tertian m.
    dysenteric algid m.
    falciparum m.
    gastric algid m.
    induced m.
    intermittent m.
    malariae m.
    malignant tertian m.
    monkey m.
    nonan m.
    ovale m.
    ovale tertian m.
    pernicious m.
    quartan m.
    quotidian m.
    relapsing m.
    remittent m.
    simian m.
    tertian m.
    therapeutic m.
    vivax m.
malarial
    m. cachexia
    m. crescent
    m. fever
    m. hemoglobinuria
    m. knob
    m. periodicity
    m. pigment
    m. pigment stain
malariology
malariotherapy
malarious
Malassez epithelial rest

Malassezia
> *M. furfur*
> *M. ovalis*
> *M. pachydermatis*

malassimilation
malate
> m. dehydrogenase
> m. synthase

malate-aspartate shuttle
malate-condensing enzyme
malathion
malaxation
maldigestion
Maldonado-San Jose stain
male
> m. breast
> m. external genitalia
> genetic human m.
> m. gonad
> m. hermaphroditism
> m. homosexuality
> m. hypogonadism
> m. internal genitalia
> m. pattern alopecia
> m. pattern baldness
> m. pseudohermaphroditism
> m. sterility
> m. urethra
> XX m.
> XXY m.
> XYY m.

Malecot catheter
maleic acid
malemission
maleruption
maleylacetoacetate *cis,trans*-**isomerase**
malformation
> Arnold-Chiari m.
> cystic adenomatoid m.
> mermaid m.
> Michel m.
> venous m.

malfunction
Malgaigne
> M. amputation
> M. fossa
> M. hernia
> M. luxation
> M. triangle

Malherbe calcifying epithelioma
malic
> m. acid
> m. acid dehydrogenase
> m. dehydrogenase
> m. enzyme

malignancy
malignant
> m. anemia
> m. atrophic papulosis
> m. bubo
> m. carcinoid syndrome
> m. catarrhal fever virus
> m. ciliary epithelioma
> m. dysentery
> m. endocarditis

> m. exophthalmos
> m. external otitis
> m. fibrous histiocytoma
> m. glaucoma
> m. granuloma
> m. hepatoma
> m. histiocytosis
> m. hyperphenylalaninemia
> m. hyperpyrexia
> m. hypertension
> m. hyperthermia
> m. jaundice
> m. lentigo melanoma
> m. lymphoma
> m. malnutrition
> m. melanoma in situ
> m. meningioma
> m. midline reticulosis
> m. mixed müllerian tumor
> m. mole syndrome
> m. myopia
> m. nephrosclerosis
> m. pustule
> m. scleritis
> m. smallpox
> m. stupor
> m. tertian fever
> m. tertian malaria
> m. tertian malarial parasite
> m. tumor

malinger
malingerer
malingering
malinterdigitation
Mall
> M. formula
> M. ridge

malleable
mallear
> m. fold
> m. prominence
> m. stripe

mallebrin
mallei (*pl. of* malleus)
malleoincudal
malleolar
> m. articular surface of fibula
> m. articular surface of tibia
> m. groove
> m. stria
> m. sulcus

malleolus, pl. **malleoli**
> external m.
> inner m.
> internal m.
> lateral m.
> m. lateralis
> medial m.
> m. medialis
> outer m.

malleotomy
mallet finger
malleus, pl. **mallei**
Mallory
> M. aniline blue stain

M

Mallory *(continued)*
    M. body
    M. collagen stain
    M. iodine stain
    M. phloxine stain
    M. phosphotungstic acid hematoxylin stain
    M. stain for actinomyces
    M. stain for hemofuchsin
    M. trichrome stain
    M. triple stain
Mallory-Weiss
    M.-W. lesion
    M.-W. syndrome
    M.-W. tear
malnutrition
    malignant m.
    protein m.
malocclusion
malonate semialdehyde
malondialdehyde-modified low-density lipoprotein
Maloney bougie
malonic acid
malonyl-CoA
malonylcoenzyme A
malonyl transacylase
malonylurea
malpighian
    m. body
    m. capsule
    m. cell
    m. corpuscle
    m. gland
    m. glomerulus
    m. layer
    m. nodule
    m. pyramid
    m. rete
    m. stigma
    m. stratum
    m. tubule
    m. tuft
    m. vesicle
malposition
malpractice
malpresentation
malrotation
MALT
    mucosa-associated lymphoid tissue
malt
    m. liquor
    m. sugar
Malta fever
maltase
    acid m.
maltese cross
maltobiose
MALToma
maltose
maltotetrose
malt-worker's lung
malum
    malum articulorum senilis
    malum perforans pedis
    malum venereum
malunion
mamanpian
mamelon
mamelonated
mamelonation
mamillary duct
mamillothalamic tract
mamma, pl. **mammae**
    m. accessoria
    m. erratica
    m. masculina
    supernumerary m.
    m. virilis
mammal
mammalgia
Mammalia
mammaplasty
    augmentation m.
    reconstructive m.
    reduction m.
mammary
    m. branch
    m. calculus
    m. cancer virus of mice
    m. duct
    m. duct ectasia
    m. fistula
    m. fold
    m. gland
    m. line
    m. neuralgia
    m. plexus
    m. region
    m. ridge
    m. souffle
    m. tumor virus of mice
mammectomy
mammiform
mammilla, pl. **mammillae**
mammillaplasty
mammillare
mammillaria
mammillary
    m. artery
    m. body
    m. line
    m. process of lumbar vertebra
    m. tubercle
    m. tubercle of hypothalamus
mammillate
mammillated
mammillation
mammilliform
mammillitis
mammillotegmental fasciculus
mammillothalamic fasciculus
mammogram
mammography
Mammomonogamus
    M. laryngeus
mammoplasty
mammose
mammosomatotroph cell adenoma

mammotomy
mammotroph
mammotropic, mammotrophic
    m. factor
    m. hormone
mammotropin, mammotrophin
Man
    mannose
    mannosyl
managed care
management
    case m.
    component m.
Manchester
    M. operation
    M. ovoid
manchette
Manchurian
    M. hemorrhagic fever
    M. typhus
mandatory minute ventilation
mandelate
mandelic acid
Mandelin reagent
mandelytropine
mandible
mandibula, pl. **mandibulae**
mandibular
    m. arch
    m. axis
    m. canal
    m. cartilage
    m. condyle
    m. dental arcade
    m. dentition
    m. disk
    m. foramen
    m. fossa
    m. glide
    m. guide prosthesis
    m. hinge position
    m. joint
    m. lymph node
    m. movement
    m. nerve [CN V3]
    m. node
    m. notch
    m. process
    m. protraction
    m. reflex
    m. retraction
    m. symphysis
    m. tongue
    m. torus
mandibulectomy
mandibuloacral dysostosis
mandibulofacial
    m. dysostosis
    m. dysotosis syndrome
    m. dysplasia
mandibulomaxillary fixation
mandibulooculofacial syndrome
mandibulopharyngeal
mandibulum
mandragora

mandrake
    wild m.
mandrel, mandril
mandrill
mandrin
mane primo (man. pr.)
maneuver
    Adson m.
    Barlow m.
    Bill m.
    Bracht m.
    Buzzard m.
    Credé m.
    Dix-Hallpike m.
    Ejrup m.
    Hampton m.
    Heimlich m.
    Hillis-Müller m.
    Hueter m.
    Jendrassik m.
    LeCompte m.
    Leopold m.'s
    load-and-shift m.
    Mauriceau m.
    Mauriceau-Levret m.
    McDonald m.
    McRoberts m.
    Müller m.
    Ortolani m.
    Phalen m.
    Pinard m.
    Ritgen m.
    Scanzoni m.
    Sellick m.
    Valsalva m.
    Wigand m.
    Zavanelli m.
manganese (Mn)
manganic
manganous
manganum
mange
    demodectic m.
    sarcoptic m.
mango dermatitis
mangrove fly
mania
    acute m.
maniac
maniacal
manic
    m. episode
    m. excitement
    m. psychosis
manic-depressive
    m.-d. disorder
    m.-d. illness
    m.-d. psychosis
manicky
manifest
    m. content
    m. hyperopia
    m. strabismus
    m. tetany
    m. vector

M

manifestation
    behavioral m.
    neurotic m.
    psychophysiologic m.
    psychotic m.
manifesting
    m. carrier
    m. heterozygote
manikin
maniphalanx
manna
    m. cannellata
    m. communis
    m. in lacrimis
    m. in sortis
    m. sugar
mannand
Mann-Bollman fistula
mannerism
mannite
mannitol hexanitrate
Mannkopf sign
Mann methyl blue-eosin stain
mannoheptulose
mannomustine
mannoprotein
mannosamine
mannosan
mannose (Man)
mannose-binding protein
mannose-1-phosphate guanylyltransferase (GDP)
mannosephosphate isomerase
mannose-6-phosphate receptor (MPR)
mannosidase
mannoside
mannosidosis
mannosyl (Man)
mannuronic acid
Mann-Williamson
    M.-W. operation
    M.-W. ulcer
man-of-war
    Portuguese m.-o.-w.
manometer
    aneroid m.
    dial m.
    differential m.
    mercurial m.
manometric
manometry
    esophageal m.
manoscopy
man. pr.
    mane primo
Manson
    M. disease
    M. eye worm
    M. schistosomiasis
Mansonella
    m. demarquayi
    m. ozzardi
    m. perstans
    m. streptocerca
    m. tucumana

mansonelliasis
mansonellosis
Mansonia
Mansonoides
Mantel-Haenszel test
M^c antigen (*var. of* M$_1$ antigen)
M^g antigen (*var. of* M$_1$ antigen)
M$_1$ antigen
M$_2$ antigen (*var. of* M$_1$ antigen)
mantle
    brain m.
    m. cell lymphoma
    m. layer
    myoepicardial m.
    m. radiotherapy
    m. sclerosis
    m. zone
Mantoux
    M. pit
    M. test
manual
    m. English
    m. pelvimetry
    m. ventilation
    m. visual method
manubriosternal
    m. joint
    m. junction
    m. symphysis
manubrium, pl. **manubria**
    m. mallei
    m. of malleus
    m. sterni
    m. of sternum
manudynamometer
MAO
    monoamine oxidase
MAOI
    monoamine oxidase inhibitor
map
    choroplethic m.
    chromosome m.
    conformational m.
    contig m.
    cytogenetic m.
    m. distance
    fate m.
    genetic m.
    isodemographic m.
    linkage m.
    physical m.
    restriction m.
    sequence-tagged site (STS) m.
    spot m.
map-dot-fingerprint dystrophy
maple
    m. bark disease
    m. sugar
    m. syrup urine
    m. syrup urine disease
maplike skull
mappine
mapping
    cardiac m.
    chromosome m.

m. function
gene m.
S1 nuclease m.
maprotiline
MAPs
microtubule-associated protein
Marañón sign
marantic
m. atrophy
m. edema
m. endocarditis
m. thrombosis
m. thrombus
marasmic
m. kwashiorkor
m. thrombosis
marasmoid
marasmus
nutritional m.
marathon group psychotherapy
marble
m. bone
m. bone disease
Marburg
M. virus
M. virus disease
marc
residue remaining after percolation of a
drug
Marcacci muscle
march
m. fracture
m. hemoglobinuria
Marchand
M. adrenal
M. rest
M. wandering cell
Marchant
Marchant zone
Marchi
M. fixative
M. reaction
M. stain
M. tract
Marchiafava-Bignami disease
Marchiafava-Micheli
M.-M. anemia
M.-M. syndrome
marcid
Marcille triangle
marcor
Marcus
M. Gunn phenomenon
M. Gunn pupil
M. Gunn sign
M. Gunn syndrome
Marek disease virus
marenostrin
Marey law
Marfan
M. disease
M. law
M. syndrome
marfanoid
margarine disease

Margaropus
M. winthemi
margin
acetabular m.
m. of acetabulum
anterior m.
anterior palpebral m.
articular m.
cavity m.
cervical m.
cervical m. of tooth
ciliary m. of iris
corneal m.
costal m.
m.'s of eyelid
falciform m. of saphenous opening
fibular m. of foot
m. of fossa ovalis
free m.
free m. of eyelid
frontal m.
frontal m. of sphenoid
gingival m.
incisal m.
inferior m.
inferolateral m.
inferolateral m. of cerebral
hemisphere
inferomedial m. of cerebral
hemisphere
infraorbital m.
interosseous m.
lacrimal m. of maxilla
lambdoid m. of occipital bone
lateral m.
mastoid m. of occipital bone
medial m.
mesovarian m. of ovary
nasal m. of frontal bone
occipital m.
occipital m. of temporal bone
m. of orbit
orbital m.
orbital m. of eyelid
palpebral m.
parietal m.
parietal m. of frontal bone
parietal m. of greater wing of
sphenoid
posterior palpebral m.
psoas m.
pupillary m. of iris
right m. of heart
m. of safety
sphenoidal m. of temporal bone
squamosal m.
squamosal m. of greater wing of
sphenoid
squamous m.
superior m. of cerebral hemisphere
superomedial m.
supraorbital m.
m. of tongue
ulnar m. of forearm

M

margin (*continued*)
    zygomatic m. of greater wing of sphenoid bone

marginal
    m. arcade
    m. artery of colon
    m. atrial branch of right coronary artery
    m. blepharitis
    m. branch of cingulate sulcus
    m. branch of parietooccipital sulcus
    m. branch [TA] of cingulate sulcus
    m. crest of tooth
    m. fasciculus
    m. gingivitis
    m. gyrus
    m. integrity of amalgam
    m. keratitis
    m. layer
    M. Line Calculus Index (MLC)
    m. mandibular branch of facial nerve
    m. part of orbicularis oris muscle
    m. ray
    m. ridge
    m. ring ulcer of cornea
    m. sinus of placenta
    m. sphincter
    m. sulcus
    m. tentorial branch of internal carotid artery
    m. tubercle
    m. zone
    m. zone lymphoma

margination of placenta

margo, pl. **margines**
    m. acetabularis
    m. anterior
    m. anterior corporis pancreatis
    m. anterior fibulae
    m. anterior pancreatis
    m. anterior pulmonis
    m. anterior radii
    m. anterior testis
    m. anterior tibiae
    m. anterior ulnae
    m. arcuatus hiatus sapheni
    m. ciliaris iridis
    m. dexter cordis
    m. falciformis hiatus sapheni
    m. fibularis pedis
    m. frontalis
    m. frontalis ossis parietalis
    m. frontalis ossis sphenoidalis
    m. incisalis
    m. inferior
    m. inferior cerebri
    m. inferior corporis pancreatis
    m. inferior corporis splenis
    m. inferior hepatis
    m. inferior pancreatis
    m. inferior pulmonis
    m. inferior splenis
    m. inferolateralis

m. inferomedialis hemispherii cerebri
m. infraorbitalis
m. interosseus
m. interosseus fibulae
m. interosseus radii
m. interosseus tibiae
m. interosseus ulnae
m. lacrimalis maxillae
m. lambdoideus ossis occipitalis
m. lambdoideus squamae occipitalis
m. lateralis
m. lateralis antebrachii
m. lateralis humeri
m. lateralis pedis
m. lateralis renis
m. lateralis scapulae
m. lateralis unguis
m. liber
m. liber ovarii
m. liber unguis
m. linguae
m. mastoideus ossis occipitalis
m. mastoideus squamae occipitalis
m. medialis
m. medialis antebrachii
m. medialis cerebri
m. medialis glandulae suprarenalis
m. medialis humeri
m. medialis pedis
m. medialis renis
m. medialis scapulae
m. medialis tibiae
m. mesovaricus ovarii
m. nasalis ossis frontalis
m. occipitalis
m. occipitalis ossis parietalis
m. occipitalis ossis temporalis
m. occultus unguis
m. orbitalis
m. palpebrae
m. parietalis
m. parietalis alaris majoris ossis sphenoidalis
m. parietalis ossis frontalis
m. parietalis ossis sphenoidalis
m. parietalis ossis temporalis
m. parietalis partis squamosae ossis temporalis
m. posterior fibulae
m. posterior partis petrosae ossis temporalis
m. posterior radii
m. posterior testis
m. posterior ulnae
m. pupillaris iridis
m. radialis antebrachii
m. sagittalis ossis parietalis
m. sphenoidalis ossis temporalis
m. squamosus
m. squamosus alaris majoris ossis sphenoidalis
m. squamosus ossis parietalis
m. squamosus ossis sphenoidalis
m. superior corporis pancreatis
m. superior glandulae suprarenalis

m. superior hemispherii cerebri
m. superior pancreatis
m. superior partis petrosae ossis temporalis
m. superior scapulae
m. superior splenis
m. superomedialis
m. supraorbitalis
m. tibialis pedis
m. ulnaris antebrachii
m. uteri
m. zygomaticus alae majoris
m. zygomaticus alaris majoris ossis sphenoidalis
marian lithotomy
Marie ataxia
Marie-Robinson syndrome
Marie-Strümpell disease
marihuana
marine

m. pharmacology
m. soap
Marine-Lenhart syndrome
Marinesco-Garland syndrome
Marinesco-Sjögren syndrome
Marinesco succulent hand
marinobufotoxin
Marion disease
Mariotte

M. blind spot
M. bottle
M. experiment
M. law
mariposia
marital

m. counseling
m. therapy
Marjolin ulcer
marjoram
mark

alignment m.
stretch m.
marked fetal bradycardia
marker

allotypic m.
cell m.
cell surface m.
m. chromosome
DNA m.
m. enzyme
genetic m.
linkage m.
m. locus
oncofetal m.
polymorphic genetic m.
time m.
m. trait
tumor m.
m. X syndrome
Markov process
Marme reagent
marmorated
marmoset virus
marmot
Maroteaux-Lamy syndrome

Marquis reagent
marriage therapy
marrow

bone m.
m. canal
m. cell
gelatinous bone m.
red bone m.
spinal m.
yellow bone m.
marrow-lymph gland
marrow-mesenchyme connection
Marseilles fever
marsh

m. fever
m. gas
Marshall

M. method
M. oblique vein
M. syndrome
M. test
M. vestigial fold
Marshallagia marshalli
Marshall-Marchetti-Krantz operation
Marshall-Marchetti test
marshmallow root
marsupialization
marsupial notch
marsupium
Martegiani

M. area
M. funnel
Martin

M. bandage
M. disease
M. tube
Martin-Bell syndrome
Martin-Gruber anastomosis
Martinotti cell
martius yellow
Martorell syndrome
Maryland coma scale
maschale
maschalyperidrosis
masculine

m. pelvis
m. protest
m. uterus
masculinity
masculinity-femininity scale
masculinization
masculinize
masculinus
mask

ecchymotic m.
Hutchinson m.
laryngeal m.
nonrebreathing m.
tropical m.
masked

m. epilepsy
m. gout
m. hyperthyroidism
m. virus

M

masking
    m. dilemma
    m. level difference
    unsharp m.
masklike face
Maslow hierarchy
masochism
masochist
masochistic personality
Mason-Pfizer virus
mason's lung
MASS
    mitral valve prolapse, aortic anomalies,
      skeletal and skin changes
    MASS syndrome
mass
    m. action principle
    m. action theory
    apperceptive m.
    filar m.
    m. hysteria
    m. infection
    injection m.
    inner cell m.
    intermediate m.
    lateral m. of atlas
    lateral m. of ethmoid bone
    m. law
    molar m.
    molecular m.
    m. movement
    m. number
    m. peristalsis
    pilular m.
    m. reflex
    relative molecular m. (M_r)
    sclerotic cemental m.
    m. screening
    m. sociogenic illness
    m. spectrograph
    tubular excretory m.
massa, pl. massae
    m. intermedia
    m. lateralis atlantis
mass-action ratio
massage
    cardiac m.
    closed chest m.
    external cardiac m.
    gingival m.
    heart m.
    open chest m.
    prostatic m.
    vibratory m.
Masselon spectacles
masseter
    m. muscle
    m. reflex
masseteric
    m. artery
    m. fascia
    m. nerve
    m. tuberosity
    m. vein
masseur

masseuse
massicot
massive
    m. bowel resection syndrome
    m. collapse
Masson
    M. argentaffin stain
    M. trichrome stain
Masson-Fontana ammoniac silver stain
massotherapy
MAST
    military antishock trousers
mast
    m. cell
    m. cell leukemia
    m. leukocyte
mastadenitis
mastadenoma
Mastadenovirus
mastalgia
mastatrophy
mastauxe
mastectomy
    extended radical m.
    modified radical m.
    radical m.
    simple m.
    subcutaneous m.
    total m.
master
    m. cast
    M. of Dental Surgery (M.D.S.)
    m. eye
    m. gland
    M. of Science in Dentistry
      (M.S.D.)
    M. two-step exercise test
mastery motive
mastic
masticate
masticating
    m. cycle
    m. surface
mastication
masticator
    m. nerve
    m. space
masticatory
    m. apparatus
    m. diplegia
    m. force
    m. muscle
    m. nucleus
    m. silent period
    m. spasm
    m. surface
    m. system
mastich, mastiche
Mastigophora
mastigote
mastitis
    chronic cystic m.
    gargantuan m.
    glandular m.
    granulomatous m.

interstitial m.
lactational m.
m. neonatorum
parenchymatous m.
plasma cell m.
puerperal m.
retromammary m.
stagnation m.
submammary m.
suppurative m.
mastoccipital
mastocyte
mastocytogenesis
mastocytoma
mastocytosis
diffuse m.
diffuse cutaneous m.
systemic m.
mastodynia
mastoid
m. abscess
m. air cell
m. angle of parietal bone
m. antrum
m. artery
m. bone
m. border of occipital bone
m. branch of occipital artery
m. branch of posterior auricular artery
m. branch of posterior tympanic artery
m. canaliculus
m. cell
m. cortex
m. emissary vein
m. empyema
m. fontanelle
m. foramen
m. fossa
m. groove
m. lymph node
m. margin of occipital bone
m. notch
m. part of the temporal bone
m. process
m. process of petrous part of temporal bone
m. sinus
m. wall of middle ear
m. wall of tympanic cavity
mastoidal
mastoidale
mastoidectomy
complete m.
modified radical m.
radical m.
simple m.
mastoiditis
sclerosing m.
mastoncus
mastooccipital
mastoparietal
mastopathy
mastopexy

mastoplasia
mastoplasty
mastoptosis
mastorrhagia
mastosquamous
mastosyrinx
mastotomy
masturbate
masturbation
MAT
multifocal atrial tachycardia
mat
m. burn
m. gold
matched groups
matching
impedance m.
maté
mater
arachnoidea m. cranialis
arachnoidea m. encephali
cranial pia m.
pia m. encephali
pia m. spinalis
spinal arachnoid m.
spinal pia m.
materia
m. alba
m. medica
material
base m.
byproduct m.
certified reference m. (CRM)
contrast m.
cross-reacting m. (CRM)
dental m.
genetic m.
impression m.
plastic restoration m.
restorative dental m.
materies morbi
maternal
m. cotyledon
m. death
m. death rate
m. deprivation syndrome
m. dystocia
m. immunity
m. inheritance
m. morbidity
m. mortality ratio
m. placenta
maternal-fetal medicine
maternity hospital
mathematical
m. chaos
m. determinant
m. genetics
m. model
mating
assortative m.
cross m.
m. isolate
nonrandom m.
random m.

M

matrass
matrical
matricaria
matrices (*pl. of* matrix)
matricial
matricide
matrilineal
matrix, pl. **matrices**
    amalgam m.
    m. band
    bone m.
    m. calculus
    cartilage m.
    cell m.
    cytoplasmic m.
    external m.
    m. Gla protein
    identity m.
    m. metalloproteinase
    mitochondrial m.
    m. mitochondrialis
    nail m.
    nuclear m.
    m. retainer
    square m.
    territorial m.
    m. unguis
    m. vesicle
matter
    gray m.
    pontine gray m.
    white m.
mattress suture
maturate
maturation
    m. arrest
    m. factor
    m. index
    m. value
mature
    m. bacteriophage
    m. cataract
    m. cell leukemia
    m. neutrophil
    m. ovarian follicle
maturity-onset diabetes
maturity onset diabetes of youth
matutinal epilepsy
Mauchart ligament
Maurer
    M. cleft
    M. dot
Mauriac syndrome
Mauriceau-Levret maneuver
Mauriceau maneuver
Mauthner sheath
maxilla, pl. **maxillae**
maxillary
    m. angle
    m. antrum
    m. artery
    m. dental arcade
    m. dentition
    m. eminence
    m. gland

    m. hiatus
    m. nerve [CN V2]
    m. plexus
    m. process of embryo
    m. process of inferior nasal concha
    m. protraction
    m. sinus
    m. sinus radiograph
    m. surface of greater wing of sphenoid bone
    m. surface of palatine bone
    m. tuberosity
    m. vein
maxillectomy
maxillitis
maxillodental
maxillofacial prosthetics
maxillojugal
maxillomandibular
    m. fixation
    m. record
    m. registration
    m. relation
    m. traction
maxillopalatine
maxillotomy
maxilloturbinal
maximal
    m. Histalog test
    m. stimulus
    m. thymectomy
Maxim-Gilbert sequencing
Maximow stain for bone marrow
maximum
    m. breathing capacity (MBC)
    glucose transport m.
    m. intensity projection (MIP)
    m. likelihood estimator
    m. occipital point
    m. permissible dose (MPD)
    m. power output
    m. temperature
    m. tolerated dose
    transport m.
    tubular m.
    m. urea clearance
    m. velocity (V_{max})
    m. voluntary ventilation (MVV)
May
    M. apple
    M. apple root
Mayaro virus
Mayer
    M. hemalum stain
    M. mucicarmine stain
    M. mucihematein stain
    M. pessary
    M. reflex
Mayer-Rokitansky-Küster-Hauser syndrome
May-Grünwald stain
May-Hegglin anomaly
mayidism
Mayo
    M. bunionectomy

M. operation
M. vein
Mayo-Robson
M.-R. point
M.-R. position
May-White syndrome
mazamorra
maze
mazindol
mazo-
Mazzoni corpuscle
Mazzotti
M. reaction
M. test
Mb, MbCO, MbO₂
myoglobin and its combinations with CO and oxygen
MBC
maximum breathing capacity
MC
Magister Chirurgiae
mc
millicurie
MCAD
medium-chain acyl-CoA dehydrogenase
McArdle
M. disease
M. syndrome
McArdle-Schmid-Pearson disease
McBurney
M. incision
M. point
M. sign
McCall culdoplasty procedure
McCarey-Kaufmann media
McCarthy reflex
McCrea sound
McCune-Albright syndrome
McDonald maneuver
McGoon technique
MCH
mean corpuscular hemoglobin
MCh
Magister Chirurgiae
MCHC
mean corpuscular hemoglobin concentration
mCi
millicurie
McIndoe operation
McKee line
McKusick metaphyseal dysplasia
MCMI
millon clinical multiaxial inventory
McMurray test
McNemar test
m-cone
MCP-1
monocyte chemoattractant protein-1
McPhail test
MCR
steroid metabolic clearance rate
McRoberts maneuver
M-CSF
macrophage colony-stimulating factor

MCV
mean corpuscular volume
McVay operation
MD
methyldichloroarsine
Md
mendelevium
MDF
myocardial depressant factor
m. dict.
more dicto
MDMA
centrally active phenethylamine derivative related to amphetamine and methamphetamine
MDNCF
monocyte-derived neutrophil chemotactic factor
M.D.S.
Master of Dental Surgery
Me
methyl
Meadows syndrome
meal
Boyden m.
Lundh m.
test m.
m. worm
mean
arithmetic m.
m. calorie
m. corpuscular hemoglobin (MCH)
m. corpuscular hemoglobin concentration (MCHC)
m. corpuscular volume (MCV)
m. electrical axis
m. foundation plane
geometric m.
harmonic m.
m. manifest vector
regression of the m.
standard error of the m. (SEM)
m. temperature
measle
measles
atypical m.
black m.
m. convalescent serum
German m.
hemorrhagic m.
m. immune globulin (human)
m. immunoglobulin
m. mumps, and rubella vaccine (MMR)
three-day m.
tropical m.
m. virus
m. virus vaccine
measly
measure
m.'s of central tendency
Geneva lens m.
measured intelligence
measurement
end-point m.

M

measurement *(continued)*
    kinetic m.
    nasion-pogonion m.
meatal
    m. cartilage
    m. spine
meatometer
meatoplasty
meatorrhaphy
meatoscope
meatoscopy
meatotome
meatotomy
meatus, pl. **meatus**
    acoustic m.
    m. acusticus externus
    m. acusticus externus cartilagineus
    m. acusticus internus
    external acoustic m.
    external auditory m.
    external urinary m.
    fish-mouth m.
    internal acoustic m.
    internal auditory m.
    nasal m.
    m. nasi
    m. nasi inferior
    m. nasi medius
    m. nasi superior
    nasopharyngeal m.
    m. nasopharyngeus
    ureteral m.
    m. urinarius
mebanazine
mebendazole
mebeverine hydrochloride
mebrophenhydramine
mebutamate
mecamylamine hydrochloride
Mecca balsam
mechanical
    m. alternation of the heart
    m. antidote
    m. corepraxy
    m. dysmenorrhea
    m. heart
    m. ileus
    m. intelligence
    m. jaundice
    m. mixture
    m. strabismus
    m. vector
    m. ventilation
    m. vertigo
mechanically balanced occlusion
mechanicoreceptor
mechanics
    body m.
mechanism
    association m.
    countercurrent m.
    defense m.
    double displacement m.
    Douglas m.

    Duncan m.
    gating m.
    immunologic m.
    ordered on-random off m.
    ping-pong m.
    pressoreceptive m.
    proprioceptive m.
    random m.
    re-entrant m.
    Schultze m.
mechanism-based inhibitor
mechanistic school
mechanobullous disease
mechanocardiography
mechanocyte
mechanoelectric transduction
mechanophobia
mechanoreceptor
mechanoreflex
mechanotherapy
mèche
mechlorethamine
    m. hydrochloride
    m., oncovin, procarbazine, and prednisone (MOPP)
mecism
Mecistocirrus
Meckel
    M. band
    M. cartilage
    M. cavity
    M. diverticulum
    M. ganglion
    M. ligament
    M. plane
    M. scan
    M. space
    M. syndrome
Meckel-Gruber syndrome
Mecke reagent
meclastine
meclizine hydrochloride
meclofenamate sodium
meclofenamic acid
meclofenoxate
meclozine hydrochloride
mecometer
meconate
meconial colic
meconic acid
meconin
meconiorrhea
meconium
    m. aspiration
    m. aspiration syndrome
    m. blockage syndrome
    m. ileus
    m. peritonitis
    m. plug
medazepam hydrochloride
medfalan
media (*pl. of* medium)
mediad
medial
    m. accessory olivary nucleus

m. amygdaloid nucleus
m. angle of eye
m. antebrachial cutaneous nerve
m. anterior thoracic nerve
m. arcuate ligament
m. arteriole of retina
m. arteriosclerosis
m. atrial vein
m. basal branch of pulmonary artery
m. basal bronchopulmonary segment [S VII]
m. basal segmental artery
m. bicipital groove
m. border
m. border of foot
m. border of forearm
m. border of humerus
m. border of kidney
m. border of scapula
m. border of suprarenal gland
m. border of tibia
m. brachial cutaneous nerve
m. branch
m. branch of artery of tuber cinereum
m. branch of pontine artery
m. branch of posterior branch of spinal nerve
m. branch of posterior rami of spinal nerve
m. bronchopulmonary segment [S V]
m. calcaneal branch of tibial nerve
m. canthal ligament
m. canthic fold
m. canthus
m. cartilaginous plate
m. central nucleus of thalamus
m. cerebral surface
m. circumflex artery of thigh
m. circumflex femoral artery
m. circumflex femoral vein
m. clunial nerve
m. collateral artery
m. collateral ligament of elbow
m. commisural artery
m. compartment of thigh
m. condyle
m. condyle of femur
m. condyle of tibia
m. cord of brachial plexus
m. crest of fibula
m. crural cutaneous branch of saphenous nerve
m. crural cutaneous nerve
m. crus
m. crus of facial canal
m. crus of the horizontal part of the facial canal
m. crus of major alar cartilage of nose
m. crus of the superficial inguinal ring
m. cuneiform bone

m. cutaneous branch of dorsal branch of posterior intercostal artery
m. cutaneous nerve of arm
m. cutaneous nerve of forearm
m. cutaneous nerve of leg
m. dorsal cutaneous nerve
m. dorsal nucleus of thalamus
m. eminence
m. epicondylar crest
m. epicondylar ridge
m. epicondyle of femur
m. epicondyle of humerus
m. femoral circumflex artery
m. femoral tuberosity
m. fillet
m. forebrain bundle
m. frontal gyrus
m. frontobasal artery
m. geniculate body
m. geniculate nuclei
m. great muscle
m. habenular nucleus
m. hamstring
m. head
m. inferior genicular artery
m. inguinal fossa
m. lacunar lymph node
m. lacunar node
m. lamina of cartilage of pharyngotympanic auditory tube
m. lemniscus
m. ligament of ankle joint
m. ligament of knee
m. ligament of talocrural joint
m. ligament of temporomandibular joint
m. ligament of wrist
m. limb
m. lip of linea aspera
m. longitudinal arch of foot
m. longitudinal bundle
m. longitudinal fasciculus
m. longitudinal stria
m. lumbar intertransversarii muscle
m. lumbar intertransverse muscle
m. lumbocostal arch
m. magnocellular nucleus
m. malleolar artery
m. malleolar branch of posterior tibial artery
m. malleolar facet of talus
m. malleolar network
m. malleolar subcutaneous bursa
m. malleolus
m. mammary branch
m. margin
m. medullary branch of vertebral artery
m. medullary lamina of lentiform nucleus
m. meniscus
m. midpalmar space
m. nasal branch of anterior ethmoidal nerve

M

589

medial *(continued)*

m. nasal fold
m. nasal process
m. nasal prominence
m. nucleus
m. nucleus of thalamus
m. nucleus of trapezoid body
m. occipital artery
m. occipitotemporal gyrus
m. olfactory gyrus
m. orbitofrontal artery
m. palpebral commissure
m. palpebral ligament
m. parabrachial nucleus
m. part of longitudinal arch of foot
m. part of middle lobe vein
m. patellar retinaculum
m. pectoral nerve
m. pericuneate nucleus
m. plantar artery
m. plantar nerve
m. plate of cartilaginous auditory tube
m. plate of pterygoid process
m. pole of ovary
m. popliteal nerve
m. posterior cervical intertransversarii muscle
m. preoptic nucleus
m. process of calcaneal tuberosity
m. pterygoid muscle
m. pterygoid plate
m. puboprostatic ligament
m. rectus muscle
m. reticulospinal tract
m. root of median nerve
m. root of optic tract
m. rotator
m. segment
m. segmental artery
m. septal nucleus
m. striate artery
m. sulcus of crus cerebri
m. superior genicular artery
m. superior olivary nucleus
m. supraclavicular nerve
m. supracondylar crest
m. supracondylar ridge
m. supraepicondylar ridge
m. sural cutaneous nerve
m. surface
m. surface of arytenoid cartilage
m. surface of cerebral hemisphere
m. surface of fibula
m. surface of lung
m. surface of ovary
m. surface of testis
m. surface of tibia
m. surface of toes
m. surface of ulna
m. talocalcaneal ligament
m. tarsal artery
m. tubercle
m. umbilical fold

m. umbilical ligament
m. vastus muscle
m. vein of lateral ventricle
m. ventral nucleus
m. venule of retina
m. vestibular nucleus
m. vestibulospinal tract
m. wall of middle ear
m. wall of orbit
m. wall of tympanic cavity
m. zone

medialecithal
medialis
medialization
median

m. antebrachial vein
m. anterior maxillary cyst
m. aperture of fourth ventricle
m. arcuate ligament
m. atlantoaxial joint
m. bar of Mercier
m. basilic vein
m. callosal artery
m. cephalic vein
m. commissural artery
m. conjugate
m. cricothyroid ligament
m. cubital vein
m. effective dose (ED_{50})
m. eminence
m. glossoepiglottic fold
m. groove of tongue
m. laryngotomy
m. line
m. lithotomy
m. longitudinal raphe of tongue
m. mandibular point
m. maxillary anterior alveolar cleft
m. nerve
m. palatal cyst
m. palatine suture
m. plane
m. preoptic nucleus
m. raphe cyst of the penis
m. relation
m. retruded relation
m. rhinoscopy
m. rhomboid glossitis
m. sacral artery
m. sacral crest
m. sacral vein
m. section
m. sternotomy
m. sulcus of fourth ventricle
m. sulcus of tongue
m. thyrohyoid ligament
m. tongue bud
m. umbilical fold
m. umbilical ligament
m. vein of forearm
m. vein of neck

medianus
mediastinal

m. artery
m. branch

m. branch of internal thoracic
   artery
m. branch of thoracic aorta
m. emphysema
m. fibrosis
m. lipomatosis
m. part of lung
m. part of parietal pleura
m. pleura
m. pleurisy
m. space
m. surface of lung
m. vein
m. window

mediastinitis
fibrosing m.
fibrous m.
idiopathic fibrous m.

mediastinography
gaseous m.

mediastinopericarditis

mediastinoscope

mediastinoscopy
anterior m.
extended m.

mediastinotomy
anterior m.

mediastinum
anterior m.
m. anterius
inferior m.
m. inferius
m. medium
middle m.
posterior m.
m. posterius
superior m.
m. superius
m. of testis
m. testis

mediate
m. auscultation
m. percussion
m. transfusion

mediation

mediator
m. complex
pharmacologic m.'s of anaphylaxis

medicable

medical
m. anatomy
m. biophysics
m. care
m. corps
m. diathermy
m. ethics
m. examiner
m. genetics
m. jurisprudence
m. model
m. mycology
m. pathology
m. psychology
m. record
m. record linkage

m. selection
m. transcriptionist
m. treatment

**Medical Literature Analysis and
Retrieval System (MEDLARS,
MEDLARS-online)**

Medical Officer (M.O.)

medicament

medicamentosus

medicate

medicated

medication
ionic m.
maintenance medication
preanesthetic m.
sublingual m.

medicator

medicephalic

medicinal
m. charcoal
m. chemistry
m. eruption
m. scarlet red
m. soft soap
m. zinc peroxide

medicine
adolescent m.
aerospace m.
alternative m.
American College of Nuclear M.
   (ACNM)
aviation m.
behavioral m.
clinical m.
community m.
comparative m.
complementary m.
defensive m.
desmoteric m.
Digital Imaging and
   Communications in M. (DICOM)
Doctor of Dental M. (DMD)
Doctor of Podiatric M. (DPM)
electrodiagnostic m.
evidence-based m.
experimental m.
family m.
folk m.
forensic m.
geriatric m.
holistic m.
hyperbaric m.
internal m. (IM)
legal m.
maternal-fetal m.
military m.
neonatal m.
nuclear m.
osteopathic m.
patent m.
perinatal m.
physical m.
podiatric m.
preventive m.
proprietary m.

M

591

medicine *(continued)*
    psychosomatic m.
    quack m.
    social m.
    socialized m.
    space m.
    sports m.
    tropical m.
    veterinary m.
medicobiologic, medicobiological
medicochirurgical
medicolegal
medicomechanical
medicophysical
medicopsychology
mediocarpal
medioccipital
mediocolic sphincter
mediodens
mediodorsal nucleus
mediolateral
medionecrosis
    m. of the aorta
    m. aortae idiopathica cystica
mediopubic reflex
mediotarsal
mediotrusion
mediotype
medisect
Mediterranean
    M. erythematous fever
    M. exanthematous fever
    M. lymphoma
    M. spotted fever
medium, pl. **media**
    Acanthamoeba m.
    m. artery
    Balamuth aqueous egg yolk
      infusion m.
    Boeck and Drbohlav Locke-egg-
      serum m.
    clearing m.
    complete m.
    contrast m.
    culture m.
    Czapek-Dox m.
    Diamond TYM m.
    dispersion m.
    Dorset culture egg m.
    Eagle basal m.
    Eagle minimum essential m. (MEM)
    Endo m.
    external m.
    growth m.
    high osmolar contrast m. (HOCM)
    Lash casein hydrolysate-serum m.
    Loeffler blood culture m.
    Lowenstein-Jensen m.
    Lowenstein-Jensen culture m.
    low osmolar contrast m. (LOCM)
    McCarey-Kaufmann media
    motility test m.
    mounting m.
    Mueller-Hinton m.

    NNN m.
    nutrient m.
    passive m.
    selective m.
    separating m.
    Simmons citrate m.
    support m.
    Thayer-Martin m.
    transport m.
    TY1-S-33 m.
    TYSGM-9 m.
    m. vein
medium-chain acyl-CoA dehydrogenase
  (MCAD)
    m.-c. a.-c. d. deficiency
medius
MEDLARS
    Medical Literature Analysis and Retrieval
    System
MEDLARS-online (MEDLINE)
    Medical Literature Analysis and Retrieval
    System
MEDLINE
    MEDLARS-online
medphalan
medrogestone
medroxyprogesterone acetate
medrylamine
medrysone
medulla, pl. **medullae**
    m. of adrenal gland
    m. glandulae suprarenalis
    m. of hair shaft
    m. of kidney
    m. of lymph node
    m. nodi lymphoidei
    m. oblongata
    m. ossium
    m. ossium flava
    m. ossium rubra
    renal m.
    m. renalis
    m. spinalis
    suprarenal m.
    m. of suprarenal gland
medullar
medullary
    m. artery of brain
    m. callus
    m. carcinoma
    m. carcinoma of breast
    m. carcinoma of thyroid
    m. cavity
    m. center
    m. chemoreceptor
    m. cone
    m. cord
    m. fold
    m. groove
    m. laminae of thalamus
    m. layer of thalamus
    m. membrane
    m. plate
    m. pyramid
    m. pyramidotomy

m. ray
m. reticulospinal tract
m. sarcoma
m. sheath
m. space
m. spinal artery
m. sponge kidney
m. stria of fourth ventricle
m. stria of thalamus
m. substance
m. teniae
m. tube
medullated nerve fiber
medullation
medullectomy
medullization
medulloarthritis
medulloblastoma
desmoplastic m.
melanotic m.
medullocell
medulloepithelioma
adult m.
embryonal m.
medullomyoblastoma
medullopontine sulcus
Medusa head
Meeh-Dubois formula
Meeh formula
Mees
M. line
M. stripe
Meesman dystrophy
mefenamic acid
mefenorex hydrochloride
mefexamide
mefloquine
MEG
magnetoencephalogram
megabacterium
megacalycosis
megacardia
megacaryoblast
megacaryocyte
megacephalia
megacephalic
megacephalous
megacephaly
megacins
megacoccus, pl. **megacocci**
megacolon
acquired m.
congenital m.
m. congenitum
idiopathic m.
toxic m.
megacycle
megacystic syndrome
megacystis
megacystitis-megaureter syndrome
megacystitis-microcolon-intestinal hypoperistalsis syndrome
megadactyly, megadactylia, megadactylism
megadolichocolon
megadont

megadontism
megadyne
megaesophagus
megagamete
megagnathia
megahertz (MHz)
megakaryoblast
megakaryocyte
m. growth and development factor
megakaryocytic leukemia
megalecithal
megalgia
megaloblast
megaloblastic anemia
megalocardia
megalocephaly, megalocephalia
megalocheiria, megalochiria
megalocornea
megalocystis
megalocyte
megalocythemia
megalocytic anemia
megalocytosis
megalodactylia, megalodactylism, megalodactyly
megalodont
megalodontia
megaloencephalic
megaloencephalon
megaloencephaly
megaloenteron
megalogastria
megaloglossia
megalographia
megalokaryocyte
megalomania
megalomaniac
megalomelia
megalophthalmos
anterior m.
megalopodia
megalosplanchnic
megalosplenia
megalospore
megalosyndactyly, megalosyndactylia
megaloureter
megalourethra
megamerozoite
meganucleus
megapoietin
megaprosopia
megaprosopous
megarectum
megaseme
megasigmoid
megasomia
megaspore
megathrombocyte
megaureter
primary m.
secondary m.
megavolt
megavoltage
megestrol acetate
meglitinides

M

meglumine
  m. acetrizoate
  m. diatrizoate
  m. iothalamate
megohm
megophthalmus
megoxycyte
megoxyphil, megoxyphile
megrim
meibomian
  m. blepharitis
  m. cyst
  m. gland
  m. sty
meibomitis, meibomianitis
Meige disease
Meigs syndrome
Meinicke test
meiosis
meiotic
  m. division
  m. drive
  m. phase
Meischer syndrome
Meissner
  M. corpuscle
  M. plexus
mel
  honey
  unit of pitch
melagra
melalgia
melamine
  m. formaldehyde
  m. resin
melancholia
  hypochondriacal m.
  involutional m.
melancholic
melancholy
melanemia
melaniferous
melanin
  artificial m., factitious m.
melanism
melanoacanthoma
melanoameloblastoma
melanoblast
melanocyte
melanocyte-stimulating hormone (MSH)
melanocytoma
melanodendrocyte
melanoderma
  m. cachecticorum
  parasitic m.
  racial m.
  senile m.
melanodermatitis
melanogen
melanogenemia
melanogenesis
melanoglossia
melanoid
melanokeratosis
melanoleukoderma colli

melanoliberin
melanoma
  acral lentiginous m.
  amelanotic m.
  benign juvenile m.
  Cloudman m.
  desmoplastic malignant m.
  Harding-Passey m.
  malignant lentigo m.
  malignant m. in situ
  minimal deviation m.
  nodular m.
  subungual m.
  superficial spreading m.
melanomatosis
melanonychia
melanopathy
melanophage
melanophore
melanophore-expanding principle
melanoplakia
melanoprotein
melanorrhagia
melanorrhea
melanosis
  m. coli
  neurocutaneous m.
  oculodermal m.
  pustular m.
  Riehl m.
melanosome
  giant m.
melanostatin
melanotic
  m. freckle
  m. medulloblastoma
  m. neuroectodermal tumor of infancy
  m. pigment
  m. progonoma
melanotonin
melanotrichous
melanotroph
melanotrophin
melanotropin release-inhibiting hormone (MIH)
melanotropin-releasing
  m.-r. factor (MRF)
  m.-r. hormone (MRH)
melanuria
melanuric
melarsoprol
MELAS
  mitochondrial myopathy, encephalopathy, lactacidosis, and stroke
melasma
  m. gravidarum
  m. universale
melatonin
melena
  m. neonatorum
  m. spuria
  m. vera
melenemesis

Meleney
 M. gangrene
 M. ulcer
melengestrol acetate
meletin
melibiase
melibiose
melicera, meliceris
melioidosis
melissa
melissic acid
melissophobia
melitis
melitose
melitracen hydrochloride
melitriose
melittin
Melkersson-Rosenthal syndrome
mellitum, gen. **melliti,** pl. **mellita**
Melnick-Needles
 M.-N. osteodysplasty
 M.-N. syndrome
melodidymus
melomania
melomelia
melon-seed body
meloplasty
melorheostosis
meloschisis
melotia
melphalan
melt
melting
 m. point (m.p.)
 m. temperature
 m. temperature of DNA
Meltzer law
Meltzer-Lyon test
MEM
 Eagle minimum essential medium
member
 inferior m.
 M. of the Royal College of
  Physicians (Edinburgh) (MRCP(E))
 M. of the Royal College of
  Physicians (Ireland) (MRCP(I))
 M. of the Royal College of
  Physicians (of England) (MRCP)
 M. of the Royal College of
  Surgeons (Edinburgh) (MRCS(E))
 M. of the Royal College of
  Surgeons (Ireland) (MRCS(I))
 M. of the Royal College of
  Surgeons (of England) (MRCS)
 superior m.
 virile m.
membra (*pl. of* membrum)
membrana, pl. **membranae**
 m. abdominis
 m. adamantina
 m. adventitia
 m. atlantooccipitalis anterior
 m. atlantooccipitalis posterior
 m. basalis ductus semicircularis
 m. basilaris

 m. capsularis
 m. capsulopupillaris
 m. carnosa
 m. cerebri
 m. choriocapillaris
 m. cordis
 m. cricothyroidea
 m. decidua
 m. eboris
 m. fibroelastica laryngis
 m. fibrosa capsulae articularis
 m. flaccida
 m. fusca
 m. germinativa
 m. granulosa
 m. hyaloidea
 m. hyothyroidea
 membranae intercostales
 m. intercostalis externa
 m. intercostalis interna
 m. interossea antebrachii
 m. interossea cruris
 m. limitans
 m. limitans gliae
 m. mucosa
 m. nictitans
 m. obturatoria
 m. perinei
 m. pituitosa
 m. preformativa
 m. propria ductus semicircularis
 m. propria of semicircular duct
 m. pupillaris
 m. quadrangularis
 m. reticularis organi spiralis
 m. serosa
 m. serotina
 m. spiralis
 m. stapedis
 m. statoconiorum
 m. sterni
 m. striata
 m. succingens
 m. suprapleuralis
 m. synovialis
 m. tectoria (articulationis
  atlantoaxialis medianae)
 m. tectoria ductus cochlearis
 m. tensa
 m. thyrohyoidea
 m. tympani
 m. tympani secundaria
 m. versicolor
 m. vestibularis ductus cochlearis
 m. vibrans
 m. vitellina
 m. vitrea
membranaceous
membranate
membrane
 adamantine m.
 allantoid m.
 alveolocapillary m.
 alveolodental m.
 anal m.

M

membrane *(continued)*
 anterior atlantooccipital m.
 arachnoid m.
 atlantooccipital m.
 m. attack complex
 Barkan m.
 basal m. of semicircular duct
 basement m.
 basilar m. of cochlear duct
 Bichat m.
 Bogros serous m.
 m. bone
 Bowman m.
 Bruch m.
 Brunn m.
 bucconasal m.
 buccopharyngeal m.
 cell m.
 chorioallantoic m.
 choroid m.
 cloacal m.
 closing m.
 Corti m.
 cricothyroid m.
 cricotracheal m.
 cricovocal m.
 croupous m.
 deciduous m.
 Descemet m.
 diphtherial m.
 double m.
 drum m.
 Duddell m.
 dysmenorrheal m.
 egg m.
 elastic m.
 embryonic m.
 enamel m.
 m. enzyme
 epipapillary m.
 epiretinal m.
 exocelomic m.
 m. expansion theory
 external intercostal m.
 extraembryonic m.
 false m.
 fenestrated m.
 fertilization m.
 fetal m.
 fibroelastic m. of larynx
 fibrous m. of joint capsule
 Fielding m.
 flaccid m.
 germ m.
 glassy m.
 glial limiting m.
 Henle fenestrated elastic m.
 Heuser m.
 Hunter m.
 Huxley m.
 hyaline m.
 hyaloid m.
 hyoglossal m.
 inner m.

intercostal m.
internal intercostal m.
internal limiting m.
interosseous m. of forearm
interosseous m. of leg
ivory m.
Jackson m.
keratogenous m.
limiting m. of retina
medullary m.
mitochondrial m.
mucous m.
mucous m. of bronchus
mucous m. of ductus deferens
mucous m. of esophagus
mucous m. of female urethra
mucous m. of gallbladder
mucous m. of large intestine
mucous m. of larynx
mucous m. of male urethra
mucous m. of nose
mucous m. of pharyngotympanic
 auditory tube
mucous m. of pharynx
mucous m. of small intestine
mucous m. of stomach
mucous m. of tongue
mucous m. of trachea
mucous m. of tympanic cavity
mucous m. of ureter
mucous m. of urinary bladder
mucous m. of uterine tube
mucous m. of vagina
Nasmyth m.
nictitating m.
Nitabuch m.
nuclear m.
obturator m.
olfactory m.
oral m.
oronasal m.
oropharyngeal m.
otolithic m.
outer limiting m.
ovular m.
Payr m.
pericardiopleural m.
peridental m.
perineal m.
periodontal m.
periorbital m.
pharyngeal m.
pial-glial m.
pituitary m.
placental m.
plasma m.
pleuropericardial m.
pleuroperitoneal m.
posterior atlantooccipital m.
postsynaptic m.
m. potential
presynaptic m.
primary egg m.
proligerous m.
proper m. of semicircular duct

prophylactic m.
pupillary m.
pyogenic m.
quadrangular m.
Reissner m.
reticular m. of spinal organ
Rivinus m.
round window m.
m. rupture
Ruysch m.
Scarpa m.
schneiderian m.
Schultze m.
secondary egg m.
secondary tympanic m.
semipermeable m.
serous m.
Shrapnell m.
spiral m.
stapedial m.
statoconial m.
sternal m.
striated m.
m. stripping
suprapleural m.
synovial m.
tectorial m.
tertiary egg m.
thyrohyoid m.
Toldt m.
Tourtual m.
tympanic m.
m. of tympanum
undulating m.
undulatory m.
unit m.
urogenital m.
urorectal m.
uteroepichorial m.
vaginal synovial m.
vestibular m.
virginal m.
vitelline m.
vitreous m.
Wachendorf m.
yolk m.
Zinn m.
membrane-coating granule
membranectomy
membranelle
membraniform
membranocartilaginous
membranoid
membranoproliferative glomerulonephritis
membranous
m. ampulla
m. ampullae of the semicircular duct
m. cataract
m. cochlea
m. conjunctivitis
m. dysmenorrhea
m. glomerulonephritis
m. labyrinth

m. lamina of cartilage of pharyngotympanic auditory plate
m. laryngitis
m. layer
m. layer of subcutaneous tissue of abdomen
m. layer of superficial fascia
m. layer of superficial fascia of perineum
m. lipodystrophy
m. neurocranium
m. ossification
m. part of interventricular septum
m. part of male urethra
m. part of nasal septum
m. pharyngitis
m. septum
m. urethra
m. viscerocranium
m. wall of middle ear
m. wall of trachea
m. wall of tympanic cavity
membrum, pl. **membra**
m. inferius
m. muliebre
m. superius
m. virile
memory
affect m.
anterograde m.
m. B cell
long-term m. (LTM)
m. loop
remote m.
retrograde m.
screen m.
selective m.
senile m.
short-term m. (STM)
m. span
subconscious m.
m. T cell
temporary m.
MEN
multiple endocrine neoplasia
MEN1
multiple endocrine neoplasia, type 1
MEN2A
multiple endocrine neoplasia, type 2A
menacme
menadiol
m. diacetate
m. sodium diphosphate
menadione
m. reductase
m. sodium bisulfite
Menangle virus
menaphthone
menaquinone (MK, MQ)
menaquinone-6 (MK-6)
menaquinone-7 (MK-7)
menarche
menarcheal, menarchial
Mendel
M. first law

Mendel *(continued)*
    M. instep reflex
    M. second law
Mendel-Bechterew reflex
Mendeléeff law
mendelevium (Md)
mendelian
    m. character
    m. genetics
    m. inheritance
    M. Inheritance in Man (MIM)
    m. ratio
    m. trait
mendelism
mendelizing
Ménétrier
    M. disease
    M. syndrome
Menge pessary
Mengo
    M. encephalitis
    M. virus
Ménière
    M. disease
    M. syndrome
meningeal
    m. branch
    m. branch of cavernous part of internal carotid artery
    m. branch of cerebral part of internal carotid artery
    m. branch of internal carotid artery
    m. branch of (intracranial part of) vertebral artery
    m. branch of mandibular nerve
    m. branch of maxillary nerve
    m. branch of occipital artery
    m. branch of ophthalmic nerve
    m. branch of spinal nerve
    m. branch of vagus nerve
    m. carcinoma
    m. carcinomatosis
    m. hernia
    m. layer of dura mater
    m. leukemia
    m. neurosyphilis
    m. plexus
    m. vein
meningeocortical
meningeorrhaphy
meninges *(pl. of* meninx)
meningioangiomatosis
meningioma
    cutaneous m.
    malignant m.
    psammomatous m.
meningiomatosis
meningism
meningitic streak
meningitis, pl. **meningitides**
    basilar m.
    cerebrospinal m.
    eosinophilic m.
    epidemic cerebrospinal m.

    epidural m.
    external m.
    internal m.
    listeria m.
    meningococcal m.
    Mollaret m.
    neoplastic m.
    occlusive m.
    otitic m.
    serous m.
    tuberculous m.
meningocele
    spurious m.
    traumatic m.
meningocerebral cicatrix
meningococcal meningitis
meningococcemia
    acute fulminating m.
meningococcus, pl. **meningococci**
meningocortical
meningocyte
meningoencephalitis
    acute primary hemorrhagic m.
    biundulant m.
    chronic progressive syphilitic m.
    eosinophilic m.
    herpetic m.
    mumps m.
    primary amebic m.
    syphilitic m.
meningoencephalocele
meningoencephalomyelitis
meningoencephalopathy
meningomyelitis
meningomyelocele
meningoosteophlebitis
meningoradicular
meningoradiculitis
meningorrhachidian
meningorrhagia
meningosis
meningotyphoid fever
meningovascular
    m. neurosyphilis
    m. syphilis
meninguria
meninx, pl. **meninges**
    m. fibrosa
    m. primitiva
    primitive m.
    m. tenuis
    vascular m.
    m. vasculosa
meniscectomy
menisci *(pl. of* meniscus)
meniscitis
meniscocyte
meniscofemoral ligament
meniscopexy
meniscorrhaphy
meniscotome
meniscus, pl. **menisci**
    articular m.
    m. articularis
    converging m.

diverging m.
lateral m.
m. lateralis
m. lens
medial m.
m. medialis
negative m.
periscopic m.
positive m.
m. sign
tactile m.
m. tactus
Menkes syndrome
menocelis
menometrorrhagia
menopausal syndrome
menopause
premature m.
menophania
Menopon
menorrhagia
menorrhalgia
menotropins
menouria
menoxenia
menses
menstrua (*pl. of* menstruum)
menstrual
m. age
m. colic
m. cycle
m. edema
m. extraction abortion
m. leukorrhea
m. molimina
m. period
m. sclerosis
menstruant
menstruate
menstruation
anovular m.
anovulational m.
nonovulational m.
retained m.
retrograde m.
supplementary m.
suppressed m.
vicarious m.
menstruum, pl. **menstrua**
mensual
mensuration
mental
m. aberration
m. age (MA)
m. apparatus
m. artery
m. branch of inferior alveolar
artery
m. branch of mental nerve
m. canal
m. chronometry
m. deficiency
m. disease
m. disorder
m. disturbance

m. foramen
m. health
m. hospital
m. hygiene
m. illness
m. image
m. impairment
m. impression
m. nerve
m. point
m. process
m. protuberance
m. region
m. retardation
m. scotoma
m. spine
m. symphysis
m. tubercle
mentalis muscle
mentality
mentation
Mentha
menthane
menthol
camphorated m.
menthyl salicylate
mentoanterior position
mentolabial
m. furrow
m. sulcus
mentolabialis
menton
mentoplasty
mentoposterior position (MP)
mentotransverse position
mentum
menyanthes
mepacrine hydrochloride
mepazine acetate
mepenzolate bromide
meperidine hydrochloride
mephenesin
mephentermine sulfate
mephenytoin
mephitic
mephobarbital
mepivacaine hydrochloride
meprobamate
meptazinol
mepyramine maleate
mepyrapone
mEq
milliequivalent
meralgia paresthetica
meralluride
M:E ratio
merbromin
mercaptal
mercaptan
methyl m.
mercaptoacetic acid
mercaptoethanol
2-mercaptoethanol
mercaptol
3-mercaptolactate

M

mercaptolactate-cysteine disulfiduria
mercaptomerin sodium
6-mercaptopurine (Shy)
   -m. ribonucleoside (sI)
6-mercaptopurine, Oncovin (vincristine sulfate), methotrexate, and prednisone (POMP)
3-mercaptopyruvate sulfurtransferase
mercapturic
   m. acid
   m. acid pathway
Mercier
   M. bar
   M. sound
   M. valve
mercocresols
mercumatilin
mercuramide
mercurial
   m. diuretic
   m. line
   m. manometer
   m. stomatitis
mercurialentis
mercurialism
***p*-mercuribenzoate**
mercuric
   m. iodide, red
   m. oleate
   m. oxide, red
   m. oxide, yellow
   m. salicylate
mercuric chloride
   ammoniated m. c.
mercurochrome
mercurophen
mercurophylline sodium
mercurous
   m. chloride
   m. iodide
mercury (Hg)
   ammoniated m.
   m. arc
   m. bichloride
   m. biniodide
   corrosive m. chloride
   m. deutoiodide
   m. perchloride
   m. poisoning
   m. protoiodide
   m. subsalicylate
   m. vapor lamp
   yellow m. iodide
Merendino technique
mereprine
Meretoja syndrome
meridian
   m. of cornea
   m.'s of eyeball
meridianus, pl. **meridiani**
   meridiani bulbi oculi
meridional
   m. aberration
   m. amblyopia

   m. cleavage
   m. fiber of ciliary muscle
merispore
meristematic
meristic
Merkel
   M. cell tumor
   M. corpuscle
   M. filtrum ventriculi
   M. fossa
   M. muscle
   M. tactile cell
   M. tactile disk
mermaid malformation
Mermis
   Mermis nigrescens
meroacrania
meroanencephaly
meroblastic cleavage
merocrine gland
merodiastolic
merogastrula
merogenesis
merogenetic, merogenic
merogony
meromelia
meromicrosomia
meromyosin
   H-m.
   heavy-m.
   L-m.
   light-m.
meront
merorachischisis, merorrhachischisis
merosmia
merosporangium
merosystolic
merotomy
merozoite
merozygote
merphalan
MERRF
   myoclonic epilepsy with ragged red fiber myopathy
Merrifield
   M. knife
   M. synthesis
mersalyl
   m. acid
   m. theophylline
Méry gland
Merzbacher-Pelizaeus disease
mesad
mesal
mesameboid
mesangial
   m. cell
   m. nephritis
   m. proliferative glomerulonephritis
mesangiocapillary glomerulonephritis
mesangium
   extraglomerular m.
mesaortitis
mesareic, mesaraic
mesarteritis

mesaticephalic
mesatipellic, mesatipelvic
    m. pelvis
mesaxon
mescal buttons
mescaline
mesectoderm
mesencephalic
    m. corticonuclear fiber
    m. flexure
    m. nucleus of trigeminal nerve
    m. tegmentum
    m. tract of trigeminal nerve
    m. vein
mesencephalitis
mesencephalon
mesencephalotomy
mesenchyma
mesenchymal
    m. cell
    m. epithelium
    m. tissue
mesenchyme
    interzonal m.
    synovial m.
mesenchymoma, malignant mesenchymoma
    benign m.
    malignant m.
mesenteric
    m. adenitis
    m. artery occlusion
    m. gland
    m. hernia
    m. lymphadenitis
    m. lymph node
    m. vein
mesentericoparietal
    m. fossa
    m. recess
mesenteriolum processus vermiformis
mesenteriopexy
mesenteriorrhaphy
mesenteriplication
mesenteritis
mesenterium dorsale commune
mesenteroaxial volvulus
mesenteron
mesentery
    m. of appendix
    m. of cecum
    m. of lung
    m. of sigmoid colon
    m. of transverse colon
    urogenital m.
mesethmoid bone
mesh graft
meshwork
    trabecular m.
mesiad
mesial
    m. angle
    m. caries
    m. displacement
    m. occlusion
    m. surface of tooth

mesiobuccal
mesiobuccoocclusal
mesiobuccopulpal
mesiocervical
mesioclusion
mesiodens
mesiodistal
mesiodistocclusal (MOD)
mesiogingival
mesiognathic
mesioincisal
mesiolabial
mesiolingual
mesiolinguoocclusal
mesiolinguopulpal
mesioocclusal
mesioocclusion
mesioplacement
mesiopulpal
mesioversion
mesmerism
mesmerize
mesoappendix
mesoarium
mesobilane
mesobilene, mesobilene-
mesobilirubin
mesobilirubinogen
mesobiliviolin
mesoblast
mesoblastema
mesoblastemic
mesoblastic
    m. nephroma
    m. segment
mesocardium, pl. **mesocardia**
    dorsal m.
    ventral m.
mesocarpal
mesocaval shunt
mesocecal
mesocecum
mesocephalic
mesocephalous
Mesocestoides
mesocolic
    m. lymph node
    m. tenia
mesocolon
mesocolopexy
mesocoloplication
meso **compound**
mesocord
mesocuneiform
mesoderm
    branchial m.
    extraembryonic m.
    gastral m.
    intermediate m.
    intraembryonic m.
    lateral m.
    lateral plate m.
    paraxial m.
    primary m.
    prostomial m.

M

mesoderm *(continued)*
    secondary m.
    somatic m.
    somitic m.
    splanchnic m.
    visceral m.
mesodermal factor
mesodermic
mesodiastolic
mesodont
mesoduodenal
mesoduodenum
mesoenteriolum
mesoepididymis
mesogaster
mesogastric
mesogastrium
    dorsal m.
    ventral m.
mesogenic
mesoglia
mesoglial cell
mesogluteal
mesogluteus
mesognathic
mesognathion
mesognathous
mesoileum
mesojejunum
mesolobus
mesolymphocyte
mesomelia
mesomelic dwarfism
mesomere
mesomeric
mesomerism
mesometrium
mesomorph
mesomorphic
meson
mesonephric
    m. adenocarcinoma
    m. duct
    m. fold
    m. rest
    m. ridge
    m. tissue
    m. tubule
mesonephroi *(pl. of* mesonephros)
mesonephroid tumor
mesonephroma
mesonephros, pl. **mesonephroi**
mesoneuritis
    nodular m.
mesoontomorph
mesopexy
mesophil, mesophile
mesophilic
mesophlebitis
mesophragma
mesophryon
mesopic perimetry
mesopneumonium
mesoporphyrins

mesoprocton
mesoprosopic
mesopulmonum
mesorchial
mesorchium
mesorectum
mesoridazine besylate
mesorrhaphy
mesorrhine
mesosalpinx
mesoscope
mesoseme
mesosigmoid
mesosigmoiditis
mesosigmoidopexy
mesosomatous
mesosome
mesosomia
mesostenium
mesosternum
mesosystolic
mesotarsal
mesotendineum
mesotendon
mesothelia (*pl. of* mesothelium)
mesothelial cell
mesothelioma
    benign m.
    benign m. of genital tract
mesothelium, pl. **mesothelia**
mesothorium
mesotropic
mesotympanum
mesouranic
mesovarian
    m. border of ovary
    m. margin of ovary
mesovarium, pl. **mesovaria**
Mesozoa
messenger
    first m.
    messenger RNA (mRNA)
    m. RNA (mRNA)
    second m.
messengerlike RNA
mestanolone
mestenediol
mestranol
mesulphen
mesuranic
MET
    metabolic equivalent
Met
meta- (*m-*)
metaanalysis
metabasis
metabiosis
metabisulfite test
metabolic
    m. acidosis
    m. alkalosis
    m. calculus
    m. coma
    m. craniopathy
    m. disease

m. encephalopathy
m. equivalent (MET)
m. indican
m. pool

metabolimeter
metabolin
metabolism
basal m.
carbohydrate m.
electrolyte m.
energy m.
fat m.
first-pass m.
inborn error of m.
intermediary m.
oxidative m.
primary m.
protein m.
respiratory m.
secondary m.

metabolite
primary m.
secondary m.

metabolize
metabolized vitamin D milk
metabotropic receptor
metacarpal
m. bone [I–V]
m. index
m. vein

metacarpectomy
metacarpi (*pl. of* metacarpus)
metacarpohypothenar reflex
metacarpophalangeal
m. articulation
m. joint

metacarpothenar reflex
metacarpus, pl. **metacarpi**
metacentric chromosome
metacercaria, pl. **metacercariae**
metacestode
metachloral
metachromasia
metachromatic
m. body
m. granule
m. leukodystrophy
m. stain

metachromatism
metachroming
metachromophil, metachromophile
metachronous
metachrosis
metacone
metaconid
metacontrast
metaconule
metacresol
metacryptozoite
metadysentery
metafacial angle
Metagonimus
metaherpetic keratitis
metahypophysial diabetes
metaicteric

metainfective
metakinesis, metakinesia
metal
alkali m.
alkali earth m.
Babbitt m.
base m.
m. base
basic m.
colloidal m.
d'Arcet m.
m. fume fever
fusible m.
heavy m.
m. insert tooth
m. interface
light m.
noble m.
rare earth m.
respiratory m.

metaldehyde
metallic rale
metallocyanide
metalloenzyme
metalloflavodehydrogenase
metalloflavoenzyme
metalloflavoprotein
metalloid
metallophilia
metallophobia
metalloporphyrin
metalloprotein
metalloproteinase
matrix m.

metallothionein
metaluetic
metamer
metamere
metameric nervous system
metamerism
metamorphopsia
metamorphosis
complete m.
fatty m.
heterometabolous m.
holometabolous m.
incomplete m.
retrograde m.

metamorphotic
metamyelocyte
metanephric
m. blastema
m. bud
m. cap
m. diverticulum
m. duct
m. tubule

metanephrine
metanephrogenic, metanephrogenous
m. tissue

metanephros, pl. **metanephroi**
metaneutrophil, metaneutrophile
metanil yellow
metaperiodic acid
metaphase

M

metaphosphoric acid
metaphyseal fibrous cortical defect
metaphysial
    m. dysostosis
    m. dysplasia
metaphysis, pl. **metaphyses**
metaphysitis
metaplasia
    agnogenic myeloid m.
    apocrine m.
    autoparenchymatous m.
    Barrett m.
    coelomic m.
    intestinal m.
    myeloid m.
    primary myeloid m.
    secondary myeloid m.
    squamous m.
    squamous m. of amnion
    symptomatic myeloid m.
metaplasis
metaplastic
    m. anemia
    m. carcinoma
    m. ossification
    m. polyp
metaplexus
metapophysis
metapore
metaprotein
metaproterenol sulfate
metapsychology
metapyretic
metapyrocatechase
metaraminol bitartrate
metarhodopsin
metarteriole
metarubricyte
    pernicious anemia type m.
metastable
metastasis, pl. **metastases**
    biochemical m.
    calcareous m.
    hematogenous m.
    in-transit m.
    lymphogenous m.
    pulsating metastases
    satellite m.
metastasize
metastasizing septicemia
metastatic
    m. abscess
    m. calcification
    m. carcinoid syndrome
    m. carcinoma
    m. choroiditis
    m. mumps
    m. ophthalmia
    m. pneumonia
    m. retinitis
metasternum
metastrongyle
Metastrongylus
metasyphilis
metasyphilitic

metatarsal
    m. artery
    m. bone [I–V]
    m. interosseous ligament
    m. reflex
metatarsalgia
    Morton m.
metatarsectomy
metatarsophalangeal
    m. articulations
    m. joint
metatarsus, pl. **metatarsi**
    m. adductovarus
    m. adductus
    m. atavicus
    m. latus
    m. varus
metathalamus
metathesis
metatroph
metatrophic
metatropic dwarfism
metatypical
metaxalone
Metazoa
metazoonosis
Metchnikoff theory
metencephalic
metencephalon
Metenier sign
metenkephalin
meteorism
meteoropathy
meteorotropic
meter
    m. angle
    potential acuity m. (PAM)
    rate m.
    ventilation m.
    Venturi m.
meter-candle
metered-dose inhaler
metergasia
metergoline
meter-kilogram-second
    m.-k.-s. system
    m.-k.-s. unit
metestrus, metestrum
metformin
methacholine
    m. challenge test
    m. chloride
methacrylate resin
methacrylic acid
methacycline hydrochloride
methadone hydrochloride
methallenestril
methamphetamine
    m. base
    centrally active phenethylamine
      derivative related to amphetamine
      and m. (MDMA)
    m. hydrochloride
methampyrone
methandienone

methandriol
methandrostenolone
methane
Methanobacteriaceae
methanogen
methanol fixative
methantheline bromide
methapyrilene
methaqualone
metharbital
methargen
methazolamide
metHb
    methemoglobin
methdilazine hydrochloride
methemalbumin
methemalbuminemia
methemoglobin (metHb)
    m. reductase
methemoglobinemia
    acquired m.
    congenital m.
    enterogenous m.
    hereditary m.
    primary m.
    secondary m.
methemoglobinuria
methenamine
    m. hippurate
    m. mandelate
    m. salicylate
    m. silver stain
methenamine-silver
methene
N^5,N^{10}-methenyltetrahydrofolate
N^5,N^{10}-methenyltetrahydrofolic acid
methergoline
methicillin sodium
methimazole
methiodal sodium
methionine
    active m.
    m. adenosyltransferase
    m. malabsorption syndrome
    m. sulfoxime
    m. synthase
methionine-activating enzyme
methionyl dipeptidase
methisazone
methitural
methixene hydrochloride
methocarbamol
method
    Abell-Kendall m.
    activated sludge m.
    Altmann-Gersh m.
    Anel m.
    Antyllus m.
    aristotelian m.
    Ashby m.
    auxanographic m.
    Barraquer m.
    Beck m.
    Bier m.
    Billings m.

Born m. of wax plate
   reconstruction
Brasdor m.
Callahan m.
capture-recapture m.
Charters m.
Chayes m.
chloropercha m.
closed circuit m.
Cobb m.
combined m.'s
confrontation m.
cooled-knife m.
copper sulfate m.
correlational m.
Credé m.
cross-sectional m.
Deaver m.
definitive m.
Dick m.
diffusion m.
direct m. for making inlays
disk sensitivity m.
double antibody m.
Edman m.
Eggleston m.
Eicken m.
encu m.
ensu m.
experimental m.
Fick m.
flash m.
flotation m.
Gärtner m.
Gerota m.
glucose oxidase m.
Gruber m.
Hamilton-Stewart m.
Hammerschlag m.
hexokinase m.
Hilton m.
Hirschberg m.
Hung method
immunofluorescence m.
impedance m.
indicator dilution m.
indirect m. for making inlays
indophenol m.
introspective m.
ITO m.
Johnson m.
Keating-Hart m.
Kety-Schmidt m.
Kjeldahl m.
Lamaze m.
Langendorff m.
Lee-White m.
Liborius m.
Ling m.
Lister m.
lod m.
longitudinal m.
macro-Kjeldahl m.
manual visual m.
Marshall m.

M

method *(continued)*
    micro-Astrup m.
    micro-Kjeldahl m.
    microsphere m.
    Moore m.
    Needles split cast m.
    Nikiforoff m.
    Ochsner m.
    open circuit m.
    oral auditory m.
    Orsi-Grocco m.
    Ouchterlony method
    Pachon m.
    paracelsian m.
    parallax m.
    Pavlov m.
    Politzer m.
    Porges m.
    Purmann m.
    Quick m.
    reference m.
    Rehfuss m.
    rhythm m.
    Rideal-Walker m.
    Roux m.
    Sanger m.
    Scarpa m.
    Schäfer m.
    Schede m.
    Schick m.
    Schmidt-Thannhauser m.
    Schweninger m.
    Shaffer-Hartmann m.
    Somogyi m.
    split cast m.
    Stas-Otto m.
    Stewart-Hamilton m.
    Thane m.
    Theden m.
    Thezac-Porsmeur m.
    thiochrome m.
    twin m.
    ultropaque m.
    u-score m.
    Wardrop m.
    Westergren m.
    Wheeler m.
    Wilson m.
    zinc sulfate flotation
      centrifugation m.
methodism
methodology
methohexital sodium
methonium compound
methophenazine
methopholine
methopterin
methorphinan
methoserpidine
methotrexate
methotrimeprazine
methoxamine hydrochloride
methoxsalen
methoxy-

4-methoxybenzoic acid
methoxychlor
methoxyflurane
3-methoxy-4-hydroxymandelic acid
3-methoxy-4-hydroxymandelic acid test
5-methoxyindole-3-acetate
methoxyl
methoxyphenamine hydrochloride
5-methoxytryptamine
methscopolamine bromide
methsuximide
methyclothiazide
methyl (Me)
    active m.
    m. alcohol
    m. aldehyde
    angular m.
    m. blue
    m. bromide
    m. chloride
    m. cysteine hydrochloride
    m. green
    m. green-pyronin stain
    m. hydroxybenzoate
    m. isobutyl ketone
    m. mercaptan
    m. methacrylate
    m. nicotinate
    m. red
    m. salicylate
    m. violet
    m. yellow
2-methylacetoacetyl-CoA thiolase
methylacrylic acid
methylamphetamine hydrochloride
N-**methyl** D-**aspartate (NMDA)**
N-**methyl** D-**aspartic acid**
methylate
methylated spirit *(var. of* industrial
    methylated spirit)
methylation
    restriction m.
methylatropine bromide
methylbenzene
methylbenzethonium chloride
N-**methylcarnosine**
methyl-CCNU
methylcellulose
methylchloroform
3-methylcholanthrene, 20-
    methylcholanthrene
methylcitrate
methylcobalamin
3-methylcrotonyl-CoA
    3-methylcrotonyl-CoA carboxylase
3-methylcrotonyl-CoA
5-methylcytosine
methyldichloroarsine (MD)
methyldopa
methylene
    m. azure
    m. chloride
    m. white
methylene blue
    Kühne m. b.

Loeffler m. b.
new m. b.
polychrome m. b.
3,4-methylenedioxymethamphetamine
methylenesuccinic acid
N^5,N^{10}-**methylenetetrahydrofolate reductase**
methylenophil, methylenophile
methylenophilic, methylenophilous
methylergometrine maleate
methylergonovine maleate
methylglucamine
m. diatrizoate
m. iodipamide
N-**methylglucamine**
3-methylglutaconic aciduria
3-methylglutaconyl-CoA hydratase
methylglyoxalase
methylglyoxal bis(guanylhydrazone)
methylhexaneamine
N-**methylhistidine**
methylkinase
methylmalonate semialdehyde
methylmalonic
m. acid
m. acidemia
m. aciduria
methylmalonyl-CoA
methylmalonyl-CoA epimerase
methylmalonyl-CoA mutase
methylmercury
methylmorphine
methylol riboflavin
methyl orange
methylose
methylparaben
methylpentose
methylphenidate hydrochloride
methylprednisolone
m. acetate
sodium m. succinate
5-methylresorcinol
methylrosaniline chloride
methyl-*tert*-butyl ether (MTBE)
methyltestosterone
17α-methyltestosterone
N^5-**methyltetrahydrofolate**
N^5-methyltetrahydrofolate:homocysteine
methyltransferase
methylthioadenosine
methylthiouracil
methyltocol
methyltransferase
methylxanthines
methyprylon
methysergide maleate
methysticum
metMb
metmyoglobin
metmyoglobin (metMb)
metoclopramide hydrochloride
metocurine iodide
metolazone
metopagus

metopic
m. point
m. suture
metopion
metopism
metopoplasty
metoposcopy
metoprolol tartrate
Metorchis
metoxenous
metoxeny
metra
metratonia
metria
metric system
metrifonate
metriocephalic
metritis
metrizamide
metrizoate sodium
metrocyte
metrodynamometer
metrodynia
metrolymphangitis
metronidazole
metronoscope
metropathia hemorrhagica
metropathic
metropathy
metroperitoneal fistula
metroperitonitis
metrophlebitis
metroplasty
metrorrhagia
metrorrhea
metrosalpingitis
metrostaxis
metrostenosis
metrotomy
metrotrophic test
metyrapone
metyrosine
Meulengracht diet
Mev
one million electron-volts
mevalonate kinase
mevalonic
m. acid
m. aciduria
mevastatin
mevinolin
mexenone
Mexican
M. hat cell
M. hat corpuscle
M. spotted fever
M. tea
M. typhus
mexiletine hydrochloride
Meyenburg
M. complex
M. disease
Meyenburg-Altherr-Uehlinger syndrome
Meyer
M. cartilage

M

Meyer *(continued)*
    M. line
    M. reagent
    M. sinus
Meyer-Archambault loop
Meyer-Betz
    M.-B. disease
    M.-B. syndrome
Meyerhof oxidation quotient
Meyer-Overton
    M.-O. rule
    M.-O. theory of narcosis
Meynert
    M. cell
    M. commissure
    M. decussation
    M. layer
mezlocillin sodium
Mg
    magnesium
mg
    milligram
MGP
    matrix gla protein
MGUS
    monoclonal gammopathy of unknown
    significance
MHA-TP test
MHC
    major histocompatibility complex
        MHC restriction
mho
MHz
    megahertz
MI
    myocardial infarction
mianserin hydrochloride
miasma theory
mibefradil
Mibelli
    M. angiokeratomas
    M. disease
MIC
    minimal inhibitory concentration
micatosis
micellar
micelle
Michaelis
    M. complex
    M. constant (K_m)
Michaelis-Gutmann body
Michaelis-Menten
    M.-M. constant
    M.-M. equation
    M.-M. hypothesis
Michel
    M. malformation
    M. spur
miconazole nitrate
micrencephalia
micrencephalous
micrencephaly

microabscess
    Munro m.
    Pautrier m.
microadenoma
microaerobion
microaerophil, microaerophile
microaerophilic
microaerophilous
microaerosol
microalbuminuria
microanalysis
microanastomosis
microanatomist
microanatomy
microaneurysm
microangiography
microangiopathic hemolytic anemia
microangiopathy
    thrombotic m.
microangioscopy
microarteriography
micro-Astrup method
microatelectasis
microbalance
microbe
microbial
    m. associates
    m. collagenase
    m. genetics
    m. persistence
    m. RNase II
    m. vitamin
microbic
microbicidal
microbicide
microbiologic
microbiologist
microbiology
microbiotic
microbism
    latent m.
microblast
microblepharia
microblepharism
microblepharon
microbody
microbrachia
microbrenner
microcalcifications
microcardia
microcentrum
microcephalia
microcephalic
microcephalism
microcephalous
microcephaly
    encephaloclastic m.
    schizencephalic m.
microcheilia, microchilia
microcheiria, microchiria
microchemistry
microchilia (*var. of* microcheilia)
microchimerism
microchiria (*var. of* microcheiria)
microcide

microcinematography
microcirculation
Micrococcaceae
micrococcal
    m. endonuclease
    m. nuclease
Micrococcus
    M. conglomeratus
    M. luteus
    M. varians
micrococcus, pl. **micrococci**
microcolitis
microcolon
microcolony
microconidium, pl. **microconidia**
microcoria
microcornea
microcoulomb
microcrystalline cellulose
microcurie (μCi)
microcyst
microcystic
    m. disease of renal medulla
    m. epithelial dystrophy
microcyte
microcythemia
microcytic anemia
microcytosis
microdactylia
microdactylous
microdactyly
microdialysis
microdissection
microdont
microdontia, microdontism
microdose
microdrepanocytic anemia
microdrepanocytosis
microdysgenesia
microelectric waves
microelectrode
microelements
microencephaly
microerythrocyte
microetching technique
microevolution
microfibril
microfilament
microfilaremia
microfilaria, pl. **microfilariae**
microfilarial sheath
microfilm
microflora
microfold cell
microfollicular
    m. adenoma
    m. goiter
microgamete
microgametocyte
microgamont
microgamy
microgastria
microgenia
microgenitalism
microglandular adenosis

microglia cell
microgliacyte
microglial cell
microglioma
microgliomatosis
microgliosis
microglobulin
    beta-m.
    beta$_2$-m.
microglossia
micrognathia with peromelia
microgram
micrograph
    electron m.
    light m.
micrography
microgyria
microhemagglutination-Treponema pallidum test
microhematocrit concentration
microhepatia
microheterogeneity
microhm
microincineration
microincision
microinjector
microinvasion
microinvasive carcinoma
microkatal
micro-Kjeldahl method
microkymatotherapy
microlecithal egg
microleukoblast
microliter (μl)
    m.'s of STPD of CO_2 given off per milligram of tissue per hour (Q_{CO2})
microlith
microlithiasis
    pulmonary alveolar m.
micrology
micromanipulation
micromanipulator
micromazia
micromelia
micromelic dwarfism
micromere
micromerozoite
micrometastasis
micrometastatic
    m. disease
micrometer (μm)
    caliper m.
    filar m.
    ocular m.
    slide m.
micrometry
micromicro- (μμ)
micromicrogram
micromicron
microminerals
micromolar (μmol/L)
micromole (μmol)
micromotoscope
micromyelia

M

micromyeloblast
micromyeloblastic leukemia
micron
microneedle
microneme
micronic
micronodular
micronucleus
micronutrients
micronychia
micronystagmus
microohm (μΩ)
microophthalmia transcription factor
   gene
microorganism
microparasite
micropathology
micropenis
microphage
microphagocyte
microphallus
microphobia
microphone
microphonia, microphony
microphonoscope
microphotograph
microphthalmia
      colobomatous m.
microphthalmos
micropipette, micropipet
microplania
microplasia
microplethysmography
micropodia
micropore
microprecipitation test
micropromyelocyte
microprosopia
micropsia
micropuncture
micropyle
microradiography
microrefractometer
microrespirometer
microsaccades
microscintigraphy
microscope
      binocular m.
      color-contrast m.
      comparator m.
      compound m.
      confocal m.
      dark-field m.
      electron m.
      fluorescence m.
      flying spot m.
      infrared m.
      interference m.
      laser m.
      light m.
      opaque m.
      operating m.
      phase m.
      phase-contrast m.
      polarizing m.

      Rheinberg m.
      scanning electron m.
      simple m.
      single m.
      stereoscopic m.
      stroboscopic m.
      surgical m.
      television m.
      ultra-m.
      ultrasonic m.
      ultraviolet m.
      x-ray m.
microscopic, microscopical
      m. anatomy
      m. field
      m. hematuria
      m. polyangiitis
      m. section
      m. sphincter
microscopically controlled surgery
microscopy
      electron m.
      epiluminescence m.
      fluorescence m.
      immersion m.
      immune electron m.
      immunofluorescence m.
      Nomarski interference m.
      surface m.
      time-lapse m.
microseme
microsides
microsmatic
microsome
microsomia
microspectrophotometry
microspectroscope
microsphere method
microspherocytosis
microsphygmy
microsphyxia
microsplanchnic
microsplenia
Microspora
Microsporasida
Microsporida
microsporidia
microsporidian keratoconjunctivitis
microsporidiosis, microsporidiasis
Microsporum
      M. audouinii
      M. canis
      M. canis, var. distortum
      M. ferrugineum
      M. fulvum
      M. gallinae
      M. gypseum
      M. nanum
      M. persicolor
      M. vanbreuseghemi
microstethophone
microstethoscope
microstomia
microsurgery
microsuture

microsyringe
microthelia
microtia
Microtinae
microtine
microtome
microtomy
microtonometer
Microtrombidium
microtropia
microtubule
    subpellicular m.
microtubule-associated protein (MAPs)
microtubule-organizing center
microvascular anastomosis
microvesicle
microvillus, pl. microvilli
    m. inclusion disease
Microviridae
microvolt
microwave therapy
microwelding
microxyphil
microzoon
micrurgical
miction
micturate
micturating cystourethrogram
micturition
    m. reflex
    m. syncope
MID
    minimal infecting dose
mid-
midaxillary line
midazolam hydrochloride
midbody
midbrain
    m. tegmentum
    m. vesicle
midcarpal joint
midclavicular line
middiastolic murmur
middle
    m. atlantoepistrophic joint
    m. axillary line
    m. cardiac vein
    m. carpal joint
    m. cerebellar peduncle
    m. cerebral artery
    m. cervical cardiac nerve
    m. cervical fascia
    m. cervical ganglion
    m. clinoid process
    m. cluneal nerve
    m. colic artery
    m. colic lymph node
    m. colic vein
    m. collateral artery
    m. constrictor muscle of pharynx
    m. costotransverse ligament
    m. cranial fossa
    m. cuneiform bone
    m. ear
    m. esophageal constriction

m. ethmoidal air cell
m. ethmoidal cell
m. ethmoidal sinus
m. finger
m. fossa approach
m. frontal convolution
m. frontal gyrus
m. frontal sulcus
m. genicular artery
m. glossoepiglottic fold
m. gray layer of superior colliculus
m. group of mesenteric lymph node
m. hemorrhoidal artery
m. hemorrhoidal plexus
m. hemorrhoidal vein
m. hepatic vein
m. kidney
m. latency response
m. lobar artery
m. lobar artery of right lung
m. lobe branch of right superior
  pulmonary vein
m. lobe of prostate
m. lobe of right lung
m. lobe syndrome
m. lobe vein
m. macular arteriole
m. mediastinum
m. meningeal artery
m. meningeal artery groove
m. meningeal branch of maxillary
  nerve
m. meningeal nerve
m. meningeal vein
m. nasal concha
m. pain
m. palmar space
m. phalanges of foot and hand
m. piece
m. radioulnar joint
m. rectal artery
m. rectal lymph node
m. rectal node
m. rectal plexus
m. rectal vein
m. sacral artery
m. sacral lymphatic plexus
m. scalene muscle
m. superior alveolar branch of
  infraorbital nerve
m. supraclavicular nerve
m. suprarenal artery
m. talar articular surface of
  calcaneus
m. temporal artery
m. temporal branch of insular part
  of middle cerebral artery
m. temporal branch of lateral
  occipital artery
m. temporal convolution
m. temporal gyrus
m. temporal sulcus
m. temporal vein
m. thyroid vein
m. transverse rectal fold

M

middle *(continued)*
    m. trunk of brachial plexus
    m. turbinated bone
    m. umbilical fold
    m. umbilical ligament
middle-ear effusion
midforceps delivery
midgastric transverse sphincter
midge
midget bipolar cell
midgracile
midgut
midlife crisis
midline
    m. incision
    m. malignant reticulosis granuloma
    m. myelotomy
midmenstrual
midoccipital
midpain
midpalmar space
midplane
midriff
midsagittal
    m. plane
    m. section
midsection
midsigmoid sphincter
midsternum
midtarsal joint
midwife
midwifery
    licentiate in m. (LM)
Miescher
    M. elastoma
    M. granuloma
    M. tubes
MIF
    migration-inhibitory factor
mifepristone
mignon lamp
migraine
    abdominal m.
    acephalgic m.
    basilar m.
    classic m.
    common m.
    complicated m.
    fulgurating m.
    Harris m.
    m. headache
    hemiplegic m.
    ocular m.
    ophthalmoplegic m.
    retinal m.
    m. without headache
migraine-related vestibulopathy
migrating
    m. abscess
    m. tooth
migration
    branch m.
    epithelial m.
    m. inhibition test

    m. inhibitory factor test
    m. of ovum
migration-inhibitory factor (MIF)
migratory
    m. cell
    m. pneumonia
MIH
    melanotropin release-inhibiting hormone
mika operation
Mikulicz
    M. aphthae
    M. cell
    M. clamp
    M. disease
    M. drain
    M. operation
    M. syndrome
Mikulicz-Vladimiroff amputation
mild
    m. fetal bradycardia
    m. mercurial ointment
    m. silver protein
Miles operation
milia (*pl. of* milium)
miliaria
    m. alba
    apocrine m.
    m. crystallina
    m. profunda
    m. rubra
miliary
    m. abscess
    m. aneurysm
    m. embolism
    m. fever
    m. pattern
    m. tuberculosis
milieu
    m. intérieur
    m. interne
    m. therapy
military
    m. antishock trousers (MAST)
    m. medicine
milium, pl. **milia**
milk
    acidophilus m.
    m. anemia
    m. of bismuth
    buddeized m.
    m. of calcium
    certified m.
    certified pasteurized m.
    condensed m.
    m. corpuscle
    m. crust
    m. cyst
    m. duct
    m. factor
    m. fever
    fortified m.
    fortified vitamin D m.
    m. gland
    irradiated vitamin D m.
    lactobacillary m.

m. let-down reflex
m. line
m. of magnesia
metabolized vitamin D m.
modified m.
perhydrase m.
m. ridge
m. sickness
skim m.
skimmed m.
m. spot
m. sugar
m. of sulfur
m. tooth
vitamin D m.
witch's m.
milk-alkali syndrome
milk-ejection reflex
milker's
m. node
m. nodule
milker's nodule virus
Milkman syndrome
milkpox
milk-ring test
milky
m. ascites
m. urine
mill
m. fever
m. wheel murmur
Millard-Gubler syndrome
milled-in
m.-i. curve
m.-i. path
Miller
M. asthma
M. chemicoparasitic theory
Miller-Abbott tube
millet seed
milli-
milliampere (ma)
millibar
millicurie (mc, mCi)
milliequivalent (mEq)
milligram (mg)
millilambert
milliliter (ml)
millimeter (mm)
millimicron (mμ)
millimolar (mM)
millimole (mmol)
milling-in
milliosmole
millipede
millisecond (ms, msec)
millivolt (mV)
Millner needle
Millon
M. Clinical Multiaxial Inventory test
M. reaction
M. reagent
Millon-Nasse test
milphosis

milrinone
Milroy disease
MIM
Mendelian Inheritance in Man
MIM number
mimesis
mimetic
m. muscle
m. paralysis
mimic
m. gene
mimmation
Minamata disease
mind
m. blindness
prelogical m.
subconscious m.
mind-reading
mineral
m. water
m. wax
mineralization
mineralocoid
mineralocorticoid
mineral oil
mineralotropic
miner's
m. asthma
m. cramps
m. disease
m. elbow
m. lung
m. nystagmus
Minerva jacket
mini
miniature
m. scarlet fever
m. stomach
minicore-multicore myopathy
minilaparotomy
minim
minimal
m. air
m. alveolar concentration
m. amplitude nystagmus
m. anesthetic concentration (MAC)
m. brain dysfunction
m. deviation melanoma
m. infecting dose (MID)
m. inhibitory concentration (MIC)
m. lethal dose (MLD)
m. reacting dose (MRD)
minimal-change
m.-c. disease
m.-c. nephrotic syndrome
minimally invasive surgery
minimum
m. light
m. light threshold
m. protein requirement
m. temperature
minimyosin
minithoracotomy
mink enteritis virus

M

Minnesota
  M. Multiphasic Personality Inventory (MMPI)
minocycline
minor
  m. agglutinin
  m. alar cartilage
  m. amputation
  m. arterial circle
  m. calices
  m. circulus arteriosus
  m. connector
  m. duodenal papilla
  m. fissure
  m. forceps
  m. groove
  m. hippocampus
  m. histocompatibility complex
  m. hypnosis
  m. motor seizure
  m. operation
  m. salivary gland
  m. sublingual duct
  m. surgery
  m. tranquilizer
Minot-Murphy diet
minoxidil
mint
minus
  m. lens
  m. strand
minute
  m. output
  m. volume
miodidymus, miodymus
miolecithal
miopragia
miopus
miosis
  paralytic m.
  spastic m.
miostagmin reaction
miotic
MIP
  macrophage inflammatory protein
  maximum intensity projection
miracidium, pl. **miracidia**
Mirchamp sign
mire
mirex
Mirizzi syndrome
mirror
  concave m.
  convex m.
  m. haploscope
  head m.
  m. image
  m.-image dextrocardia
  mouth m.
  m. speech
  van Helmont m.
mirror-image cell
mirror-writing
miryachit

MIS
  mullerian inhibiting substance
misandry
misanthropy
miscarriage
miscarry
miscegenation
miscible
misdiagnosis
misdirection phenomenon
mismatch repair
misogamy
misogyny
misopedia, misopedy
misoprostol
missed
  m. abortion
  m. labor
  m. period
missense
  m. mutation
  m. suppression
mistletoe
MIT
  monoiodotyrosine
Mitchell
  M. procedure
  M. treatment
mite-born typhus
mite typhus
mithramycin
mithridatism
miticidal
miticide
mitigate
mitis
mitochondria (*pl. of* mitochondrion)
mitochondrial
  m. biogenesis
  m. chromosome
  m. disorder
  m. gene
  m. matrix
  m. membrane
  m. myopathy
  m. myopathy, encephalopathy, lactacidosis, and stroke (MELAS)
  m. sheath
mitochondriales
  cristae m.
mitochondrion, pl. **mitochondria**
  m. of hemoflagellates
mitogen
  pokeweed m. (PWM)
mitogenesis
mitogenetic
mitogenic
  m. lectin
mitomycin
mitoplast
mitosis, pl. **mitoses**
  heterotype m.
  multipolar m.
  somatic m.
mitotane

mitotic
 m. cycle
 m. division
 m. figure
 m. index
 m. period
 m. rate
 m. spindle
mitoxantrone hydrochloride
mitral
 m. area
 m. cell
 m. click
 m. commissurotomy
 m. facies
 m. gradient
 m. incompetence
 m. insufficiency
 m. murmur
 m. orifice
 m. regurgitation
 m. stenosis
 m. tap
 m. valve
 m. valve prolapse
 m. valve prolapse, aortic anomalies, skeletal and skin changes (MASS)
 m. valve prolapse syndrome
 m. valvotomy
mitralization
mitramycin
Mitrofanoff principle
Mitsuda
 M. antigen
 M. reaction
Mitsuo phenomenon
mittelschmerz
Mittendorf dot
mivacurium
mix (M.)
mixed
 m. agglutination reaction
 m. agglutination test
 m. aphasia
 m. astigmatism
 m. beat
 m. cell leukemia
 m. chancre
 m. connective-tissue disease
 m. discrete-continuous random variable
 m. disulfide
 m. esotropia
 m. expired gas
 m. function oxygenase
 m. gland
 m. glioma
 m. glycerides
 m. hearing loss
 m. hyperlipemia
 m. hyperlipidemia
 m. hyperlipoproteinemia familial
 m. hypoglycemia
 m. infection

 m. leukemia
 m. lymphocyte culture
 m. lymphocyte culture reaction
 m. lymphocyte culture test
 m. mesodermal tumor
 m. nerve
 m. paralysis
 m. thrombus
 m. tocopherols concentrate
 m. tumor of salivary gland
 m. tumor of skin
 m. venous blood ($\bar{v}$)
mixing
 phenotypic m.
mixotrophy
Mixter clamp
mixture
 Bordeaux m.
 extemporaneous m.
 mechanical m.
 physical m.
 Seidlitz m.
Miyagawa body
Miyagawanella
MK
 menaquinone
MK-6
 menaquinone-6
MK-7
 menaquinone-7
MKS unit (*var. of* meter-kilogram-second unit)
ml
 milliliter
MLC
 Marginal Line Calculus Index
MLC test
MLD
 minimal lethal dose
mlRNA
 messengerlike rna
mM
 millimolar
mm
 millimeter
MMMT
 malignant mixed mullerian tumor
M-mode echocardiography
mmol
 millimole
MMPI
 Minnesota Multiphasic Personality Inventory
 Minnesota Multiphasic Personality Inventory test
MMR
 measles, mumps, and rubella vaccine
MM virus
Mn
 manganese
M'Naghten rule
MND
 motor neuron disease
mneme

M

mnemic, mnemenic
    m. hypothesis
    m. theory
mnemism
mnemonic
mnemonics
MNSs antigen
MNSs blood group
M.O.
    Medical Officer
Mo
    molybdenum
^{99}Mo
    molybdenum-99
MoAb
    monoclonal antibody
mobile
    m. end
    m. part of nasal septum
    m. spasm
mobilization
    stapes m.
mobilize
Mobitz
    M. atrioventricular block
Möbius
    M. sign
    M. syndrome
MOD
    mesiodistocclusal
modal alteration
modality
mode
model
    Adair-Koshland-Némethy-Filmer m.
     (AKNF)
    additive m.
    animal m.
    Armitage-Doll m.
    Bingham m.
    biomedical m.
    biopsychosocial m.
    cloverleaf m.
    computer m.
    concerted m.
    cooperativity m.
    fluid mosaic m.
    m. game
    genetic m.
    induced fit m.
    Koshland-Némethy-Filmer m. (KNF
     model)
    lock-and-key m.
    logistic m.
    mathematical m.
    medical m.
    Monod-Wyman-Changeux m. (MWC
     model)
    multiplicative m.
    multistage m.
    MWC m.
    pathologic m.
    Reed-Frost m.
    Sartwell incubation m.
    statistical m.

modeling
    m. composition
    m. compound
    m. plastic
moderate hypothermia
moderator
    m. band
    m. variable
modern genetics
modification
    behavior m.
    chemical m.
    covalent m.
modified
    m. acid-fast stain
    m. milk
    m. radical hysterectomy
    m. radical mastectomy
    m. radical mastoidectomy
    m. smallpox
    m. trichrome stain
    m. zinc oxide-eugenol cement
modifier
    biologic response m.
    m. gene
modiolus, pl. modioli
    m. of angle of mouth
    m. anguli oris
    m. labii
modulation
    biochemical m.
    m. transfer function (MTF)
modulator
    selective estrogen receptor m.
    (SERM)
modulus
    bulk m.
    m. of elasticity
    m. of volume elasticity
    Young m.
Moeller
    M. glossitis
    M. grass bacillus
mofebutazone
Mogen clamp
mogiarthria
mogilalia
mogiphonia
Mohr
    M. pipette
    M. syndrome
Mohrenheim
    M. fossa
    M. space
Mohs
    M. chemosurgery
    M. fresh tissue chemosurgery
    technique
    M. micrographic surgery
    M. scale
moiety
moist
    m. gangrene
    m. papule
    m. rale

Mokola virus
mol
   mole
molal
molality
molar
   m. absorbancy index
   m. absorption coefficient
   m. absorptivity
   m. behavior
   m. concentration
   m. extinction coefficient
   first m.
   first permanent m.
   m. gas constant (R)
   m. gland
   m. mass
   Moon m.
   mulberry m.
   m. pregnancy
   second m.
   sixth-year m.
   third m.
   m. tooth
   m. tubercle
   twelfth-year m.
molariform
molarity
mold
   m. guide
   pink bread m.
molding
   border m.
   compression m.
   injection m.
   tissue m.
mole (mol)
   carneous m.
   cystic m.
   fleshy m.
   m. fraction
   hairy m.
   hydatid m.
   hydatidiform m.
   invasive m.
molecular
   m. behavior
   m. biology
   m. biophysics
   m. disease
   m. dispersed solution
   m. dispersion
   m. dissociation theory
   m. distillation
   m. epidemiology
   m. formula
   m. genetics
   m. heat
   m. layer
   m. layer of cerebellar cortex
   m. layer of cerebellum
   m. layer of cerebral cortex
   m. layer of olfactory bulb
   m. layer of retina
   m. mass

   m. movement
   m. pathology
   m. rotation
   m. sieve
   m. weight (mol wt, MW)
   m. weight ratio (M_r)
molecularity
molecule
   accessory m.
   adhesion m.
   cell adhesion m. (CAM)
   chimeric m.
   class I, II m.
   costimulatory m.
   endothelial-leukocyte adhesion m.
    (E-LAM)
   gram-molecule
   intercellular adhesion m.-1 (CD 54,
    ICAM-1)
   lectin pathway m.
molilalia
molimina
   menstrual m.
molindone hydrochloride
Molisch test
Mollaret meningitis
Moll gland
mollities
mollusc (*var. of* mollusk)
Mollusca
Molluscipoxvirus
molluscum
   m. body
   m. conjunctivitis
   m. contagiosum
   m. contagiosum virus
   m. corpuscle
mollusk, mollusc
Moloney
   M. test
   M. virus
molt
mol wt
   molecular weight
molybdate
molybdenic, molybdenous
molybdenum (Mo)
   m. cofactor
   m. target tube
molybdenum-99 (^{99}Mo)
molybdic acid
molybdoenzymes
molybdoflavoproteins
molybdopterin
molybdous
molysmophobia
moment
   dipole m.
momism
monad
Monakow
   M. bundle
   M. nucleus
   M. syndrome
   M. tract

M

monamide
monamine
monaminuria
monangle
monarda
monarthric
monarthritis
monarticular
monaster
monatomic
monaural
monaxonic
Mönckeberg
    M. arteriosclerosis
    M. degeneration
    M. medial calcification
    M. sclerosis
Mondini
    M. dysplasia
    M. hearing impairment
Mondonesi reflex
Mondor disease
moneran
monestrous
Monge
    M. disease
    M. Medrano
mongolian
    m. fold
    m. spot
monilethrix
Monilia
Moniliaceae
monilial
moniliasis
moniliform
    m. hair
Moniliformis
monism
monistic
monitor
    cardiac m.
    electronic fetal m.
    Holter m.
    home m.
monitoring
monkey
    m. B virus
    m. hand
    m. malaria
monkey-paw
monkeypox
    m. virus
monkshood
monoacylglycerol
    m. acyltransferase
    m. lipase
monoamelia
monoamide
monoamine
    m. hypothesis
    m. oxidase inhibitor (MAOI)
monoamine oxidase (MAO)
monoaminergic
monoaminuria

monoamniotic
    m. twins
monoassociated
monoauxotroph
monobactam
monobasic
    m. acid
    m. ammonium phosphate
    m. potassium phosphate
monobenzone
monoblast
monobrachius
monobromated, monobrominated
    m. camphor
monocardian
monocephalus
monochlorphenamide
monochorial
    m. twins
monochorionic
    m. diamnionic placenta
    m. monoamnionic placenta
monochroic
monochromasia
monochromasy
monochromatic
    m. aberration
    m. radiation
monochromatism
    blue cone m.
    pi cone m.
    rod m.
monochromatophil, monochromatophile
monochromator
monochromic
monochromophil, monochromophile
monocistronic
monocle
monoclinic
monoclonal
    m. antibody (MAB, MoAb)
    m. gammopathy
    m. gammopathy of undetermined significance
    m. gammopathy of unknown significance (MGUS)
    m. immunoglobulin
    m. peak
    m. protein
monocranius
monocrotic
    m. pulse
monocrotism
monocular
    m. diplopia
    m. heterochromia
monoculus
monocyte
    m. chemoattractant protein
    m. chemoattractant protein-1 (MCP-1)
monocyte-derived neutrophil chemotactic factor (MDNCF)
monocytic
    m. leukemia

m. leukemoid reaction
m. leukocytosis
m. leukopenia
monocytoid cell
monocytopenia
monocytosis
monodactyly, monodactylism
monodisperse
Monod-Wyman-Changeux model (MWC model)
monoethanolamine
monofixation syndrome
monogametic
monogamy
monogenesis
monogenetic
monogenic
monogenous
monogerminal
monoglyceride
monograph
monohydrated
monohydric
m. alcohol
monohydroxysuccinic acid
monoideism
monoinfection
monoiodotyrosine (MIT)
monoisonitrosoacetone
monokine
monolayers
monoleptic fever
monolocular
monomania
monomaniac
monomastigote
monomelic
monomer
monomeric
monometallic
monomicrobic
monomolecular reaction
monomorphic adenoma
monomphalus
monomyoplegia
monomyositis
mononeme
mononeural, mononeuric
mononeuritis multiplex
mononeuropathy multiplex
mononuclear phagocyte system (MPS)
mononucleosis
infectious m.
mononucleotide
monooctanoin
monooxygenases
monoparesis
monoparesthesia
monopathic
monopathy
monopenia
monophagism
monophasia
monophasic complex
monophenol monooxygenase

monophenol oxidase
monophobia
monophthalmos
monophthalmus
monophyletic theory
monophyletism
monophyodont
monoplasmatic
monoplast
monoplastic
monoplegia masticatoria
monoploid
monopodia
monopolar cautery
monopotassium phosphate
monops
monoptychial
monorchia
monorchid
monorchidic
monorchidism
monorchism
monorecidive
m. chancre
monorhinic
monosaccharide
monoscelous
monoscenism
monose
monosodium glutamate (MSG)
monosodium phosphate
monosome
monosomia
monosomic
monosomous
monosomy
monospermy
Monosporium apiospermum
Monostoma
monostome
monostotic fibrous dysplasia
monostratal
monosubstituted
monosymptomatic
monosynaptic
monosyphilide
monoterpenes
monothermia
monothioglycerol
monotocous
monotonic sequence
Monotremata
monotreme
monotrichate
monotrichous
monovalence, monovalency
monovalent antiserum
monovular twins
monoxenic culture
monoxenous
monoxide
monozoic
monozygotic, monozygous
monozygotic twins

M

Monro
   M. doctrine
   M. foramen
   M. line
   M. sulcus
Monro-Kellie doctrine
Monro-Richter line
mons, pl. **montes**
   m. pubis
   m. ureteris
   m. veneris
Monsel solution
Monson curve
monster
montanic acid
montan wax
Monteggia fracture
montelukast sodium
Montenegro test
montes (*pl. of* mons)
Montevideo units
Montgomery
   M. follicle
   M. gland
   M. tubercles
monticulus, pl. **monticuli**
   palmar monticuli
mood
   m. disorder
   m. stabilizing agent
   m. swing
mood-congruent hallucination
mood-incongruent hallucination
moon
   m. face
   m. facies
   M. molar
   m.-shaped face
Moore
   M. lightning streak
   M. method
Mooren ulcer
Mooser body
MOPP
   mechlorethamine, oncovin, procarbazine,
      and prednisone
moral treatment
Morand
   M. foot
   M. spur
Moraxella
   M. anatipestifer
   M. catarrhalis
   M. conjunctivitis
   M. kingae
   M. lacunata
   M. nonliquefaciens
   M. osloensis
   M. phenylpyruvica
morbid
   m. impulse
   m. obesity
   m. thirst
morbidity
   maternal m.

   puerperal m.
   m. rate
morbific
morbigenous
morbility
morbilli
morbilliform
Morbillivirus
   equine m.
morbilous
morbus
   m. Addisonii
morcel
morcellated nephrectomy
morcellation
   m. operation
morcellement
mordant
mor. dict.
   more dicto
Morel ear
Morerastrongylus costaricensis
Morgagni
   M. appendix
   M. cartilage
   M. caruncle
   M. cataract
   M. column
   M. concha
   M. crypt
   M. disease
   M. foramen
   M. foramen hernia
   M. fossa
   M. fovea
   M. frenum
   M. globules
   M. humor
   M. hydatid
   M. lacuna
   M. liquor
   M. nodule
   M. prolapse
   M. retinaculum
   M. sinus
   M. sphere
   M. syndrome
   M. tubercle
   M. valves
   M. ventricle
Morgagni-Adams-Stokes
   M.-A.-S. syncope
   M.-A.-S. syndrome
morgagnian cyst
morgan (M)
Morgan bacillus
Morganella
   M. morganii
morgue
moria
moribund
morin
Morison pouch
Mörner test

morning
    m. after pill
    m. diarrhea
    m. glory
    m. glory anomaly
    m. glory seeds
    m. glory syndrome
    m. sickness
    m. vomiting
moron
Moro reflex
moroxydine
morphea
    m. guttata
    m. linearis
morpheme
morphine
    m. hydrochloride
    m. injector's septicemia
    m. sulfate
morphogenesis
morphogenetic
    m. movement
morphologic
    m. element
morphology
morphometric
morphometry
morphon
morphophysiology
morphosis
morphosynthesis
morphotype
Morquio
    M. disease
    M. syndrome
Morquio-Ullrich disease
morrhuate sodium
mors
    m. thymica
morsicatio buccarum
mor. sol.
morsulus
mortal
mortality
    perinatal m.
    m. rate
mortar kidney
Mortierella
mortification
mortise joint
Morton
    M. metatarsalgia
    M. neuralgia
    M. neuroma
    M. plane
    M. syndrome
    M. toe
mortuary
morula
morulation
moruloid
Morvan
    M. chorea
    M. disease

mosaic
    m. fundus
    m. inheritance
    m. pattern
    m. wart
mosaicism
    cellular m.
    chromosome m.
    gene m.
    germinal m., gonadal m.
Moschcowitz test
moschus
Mosenthal test
Mosler
    M. diabetes
    M. sign
mosquito, pl. mosquitoes
    m. clamp
    m. forceps
moss
    Ceylon m.
    club m.
    Iceland m.
    Irish m.
    muskeag m.
    pearl m.
    peat m.
    sphagnum m.
    m. starch
    M. tube
Mossman fever
Mosso
    M. ergograph
    M. sphygmomanometer
mossy
    m. cell
    m. fiber
    m. foot
most comfortable level
Motais operation
mote
    blood m.'s
moth-eaten alopecia
mother
    m. cell
    m. colony
    m. cyst
    m. liquor
    m. star
    m. surrogate
    surrogate m.
    m. of vinegar
    m. yaw
motile leukocyte
motilin
motility
    m. test
    m. test medium
motion
    brownian m.
    continuous passive m. (CPM, cpm)
    m. sickness
motivation
    extrinsic m.

M

motivation *(continued)*
    intrinsic m.
    personal m.
motive
    achievement m.
    mastery m.
motofacient
motoneuron
motor
    m. abreaction
    m. agraphia
    m. alexia
    m. amusia
    m. aphasia
    m. apraxia
    m. area
    m. ataxia
    m. cell
    m. cortex
    m. dapsone neuropathy
    m. decussation
    m. endplate
    m. fiber
    m. image
    m. impersistence
    m. nerve
    m. nerve of face
    m. neuron
    m. neuron disease (MND)
    m. nucleus
    m. nucleus of facial nerve
    m. nucleus of trigeminal nerve
    m. nucleus of trigeminus
    m. oculi
    m. paralysis
    plastic m.
    m. plate
    m. point
    m. root of ciliary ganglion
    m. root of spinal nerve
    m. root of trigeminal nerve
    m. speech center
    m. system disease
    m. unit
    m. urgency
    m. zone
motorial
motormeter
MOTT
mottle
    quantum m.
mottled
    m. enamel
    m. tooth
mottling
Motulsky dye reduction test
moulage
mould
moult
mounding
Mounier-Kuhn syndrome
mount
mountain
    m. anemia

    m. balm
    m. disease
    m. sickness
mounting
    m. medium
    split cast m.
mourn
mouse
    m. antialopecia factor
    m. cancer
    m. encephalomyelitis
    m. encephalomyelitis virus
    m. hepatitis virus
    joint m.'s
    knockout m.
    m. leukemia viruses
    m. mammary tumor virus
    multimammate m.
    New Zealand mice
    nude m.
    m. parotid tumor virus
    m. poliomyelitis virus
    m. thymic virus
    transgenic m.'s
    m. unit (m.u.)
mousepox virus
mousetail pulse
mouse-tooth forceps
mouth
    m. breathing
    carp m.
    denture sore m.
    m. guard
    m. mirror
    m. rehabilitation
    scabby m.
    sore m.
    m. stick
    tapir m.
    trench m.
    m. of the womb
mouth-to-mouth
    m.-t.-m. respiration
    m.-t.-m. resuscitation
mouthwash
movable
    m. heart
    m. joint
    m. kidney
    m. pulse
    m. spleen
    m. testis
movement
    active m.
    adversive m.
    after-m.
    ameboid m.
    assistive m.
    associated m.
    Bennett m.
    border tissue m.
    bowel m.
    brownian m.
    brownian-Zsigmondy m.
    cardinal ocular m.

choreic m.
ciliary m.
circus m.
cogwheel ocular m.
conjugate m. of eye
decomposition of m.
disconjugate m. of eye
drift m.
fetal m.
fixational ocular m.
flick m.
free mandibular m.
functional mandibular m.'s
fusional m.
hinge m.
intermediary m.
lateral m.
Magnan trombone m.
mandibular m.
mass m.
molecular m.
morphogenetic m.
muscular m.
neurobiotactic m.
non-rapid eye m. (NREM)
opening m.
paradoxical m. of eyelids
paradoxical vocal cord m.
passive m.
pendular m.
protoplasmic m.
rapid eye m. (REM)
reflex m.
resistive m.
saccadic m.
streaming m.
Swedish m.
translatory m.
vermicular m.

Mowry colloidal iron stain
moxa
moxalactam
moxibustion
moxisylyte
moyamoya disease
Mozart ear
MP
    mentoposterior position
m.p.
    melting point
MPD
    maximum permissible dose
MP joint
MPR
    mannose-6-phosphate receptor
MPS
    mononuclear phagocyte system
MPTP
    piperidine derivative
MQ
    menaquinone
MRA
    magnetic resonance angiography
MR angiography

MRCP
    Member of the Royal College of
      Physicians (of England)
MRCP(E)
    Member of the Royal College of
      Physicians (Edinburgh)
MRCP(I)
    Member of the Royal College of
      Physicians (Ireland)
MRCS
    Member of the Royal College of Surgeons
      (of England)
MRCS(E)
    Member of the Royal College of Surgeons
      (Edinburgh)
MRCS(I)
    Member of the Royal College of Surgeons
      (Ireland)
MRD
    minimal reacting dose
MRF
    melanotropin-releasing factor
MRH
    melanotropin-releasing hormone
MRI
    magnetic resonance imaging
mRNA
    messenger RNA
MS
    multiple sclerosis
ms
    millisecond
MS-1 hepatitis
MSB trichrome stain
M.S.D.
    Master of Science in Dentistry
msec
    millisecond
MSG
    monosodium glutamate
MSH
    melanocyte-stimulating hormone
MTBE
    methyl-tert-butyl ether
MTF
    modulation transfer function
m.u.
    mouse unit
mu (μ)
      M. antigen
muC
mucase
Mucha
Mucha-Habermann disease
Much bacillus
muci-
mucicarmine
mucid
muciferous
mucification
muciform
mucigenous
mucihematein
mucilage
mucilaginous gland

M

mucin
    m. clot test
    gastric m.
mucinase
mucinemia
mucinogen granule
mucinoid
    m. degeneration
mucinolytic
mucinosis, metabolic mucinosis
    cutaneous focal m.
    follicular m.
    localized m.
    metabolic m.
    oral focal m.
    papular m.
    reticular erythematous m.
    secondary m.
mucinous
    m. carcinoma
    m. plaque
mucinuria
muciparous gland
mucitis
Muckle-Wells syndrome
muco-
mucoalbuminous cell
mucobuccal fold
mucocele
mucociliary
    m. clearance
    m. clearance rate
mucoclasis
mucocolitis
mucocolpos
mucocutaneous
    m. junction
    m. leishmaniasis
    m. lymph node syndrome
mucoenteritis
mucoepidermoid
    m. carcinoma
    m. tumor
mucoepithelial dysplasia
mucoglobulin
mucoid
    m. adenocarcinoma
    m. colony
    m. impaction of bronchus
    m. medial degeneration
mucolipidosis, pl. mucolipidoses
    m. I, II, III, IV
mucolysis
mucolytic
mucomembranous enteritis
mucopeptide
    m. glycohydrolase
mucoperichondrial flap
mucoperiosteal flap
mucoperiosteum
mucopolysaccharidase
mucopolysaccharide
    m. keratin dystrophy
mucopolysaccharidosis,
  pl. mucopolysaccharidoses

type IH m.
type I H/S m.
type II, III, V, VI, VII m.
type IS m.
type IVA, B m.
mucopolysacchariduria
mucoprotein
    Tamm-Horsfall m.
mucopurulent
mucopus
Mucor
Mucoraceae
Mucorales
mucormycosis
mucosa
    alveolar m.
    m. of bronchi
    bronchial m.
    m. of colon
    m. of ductus deferens
    esophageal m.
    m. of esophagus
    m. of female urethra
    m. of gallbladder
    gastric m.
    gingival m.
    m. of large intestine
    laryngeal m.
    m. of larynx
    lingual m.
    m. of male urethra
    m. of mouth
    nasal m.
    m. of nose
    olfactory m.
    oral m.
    pharyngeal m.
    m. of pharyngotympanic auditory tube
    m. of pharynx
    m. of renal pelvis
    respiratory m.
    m. of seminal gland
    m. of seminal vesicle
    m. of small intestine
    m. of stomach
    m. of tongue
    m. of trachea
    tracheal m.
    m. of tympanic cavity
    m. of ureter
    m. of urethra
    m. of urinary bladder
    m. of uterine tube
    m. of vagina
    vaginal m.
mucosa-associated lymphoid tissue (MALT)
mucosal
    m. disease virus
    m. fold of gallbladder
    m. graft
    m. relief radiography
    m. tunics
    m. wave

mucosanguineous, mucosanguinolent
mucosectomy
mucoserous
>m. cell

mucostatic
mucous
>m. cast
m. cell
m. colitis
m. connective tissue
m. cyst
m. diarrhea
m. gland
m. gland of auditory tube
m. membrane
m. membrane of bronchus
m. membrane of ductus deferens
m. membrane of esophagus
m. membrane of female urethra
m. membrane of gallbladder
m. membrane of large intestine
m. membrane of larynx
m. membrane of male urethra
m. membrane of nose
m. membrane of pharyngotympanic
>auditory tube

>m. membrane of pharynx
m. membrane of small intestine
m. membrane of stomach
m. membrane of tongue
m. membrane of trachea
m. membrane of tympanic cavity
m. membrane of ureter
m. membrane of urinary bladder
m. membrane of uterine tube
m. membrane of vagina
m. neck cell
m. papule
m. patch
m. plaque
m. plug
m. polyp
m. rale
m. sheath of tendon

mucoviscidosis
mucro, pl. **mucrones**
>m. cordis
m. sterni

mucron
mucronate
mucrones (*pl. of* mucro)
mucus
>m. blanket
glairy m.
m. impaction

mud
>m. bed
m. fever

Muehrcke
>M. bands
M. line
M. sign

Mueller electronic tonometer

Mueller-Hinton
>M.-H. agar
M.-H. medium

Muellerius capillaris
muffle furnace
MUGA
>multiple-gated acquisition scan

mu-heavy-chain disease
Muir-Torre syndrome
mulberry
>m. calculus
m. molar
m. ovary
m. spot

Mulder test
Mules operation
mule-spinner's cancer
mulibrey nanism
muliebria
Müller
>M. M.
M. capsule
M. duct
M. fixative
M. law
M. maneuver
M. muscle
M. radial cell
M. sign
M. trigone
M. tubercle

müllerian
>m. adenosarcoma
m. agenesis
m. duct
m. duct inhibitory factor
m. inhibiting factor
m. inhibiting substance
m. regression factor

mulling
multangular
>m. bone

multiarticular
multiaxial
>m. classification
m. joint

multibacillary
multicapsular
multicellular
multicentric reticulohistiocytosis
Multiceps
>*M. multiceps*
M. serialis

multicollinearity
multicolony-stimulating factor (multi-CSF)
multicore disease
multi-CSF
>multicolony-stimulating factor

multicuspidate
multicuspid tooth
multidrug resistance
multienzyme complex
multifactorial inheritance
multifetation
multifid

M

multifidus muscle
multifocal
    m. atrial tachycardia (MAT)
    m. choroiditis
    m. lens
    m. osteitis fibrosa
multiform
    m. layer
    m. layer of cerebral cortex
multiformat camera
multiglandular
multigravida
multiinfarct dementia
multi-infection
multilamellar body
multilaminar primary follicle
multilobar, multilobate, multilobed
multilobular
multilocal
    m. genetics
multilocular
    m. adipose tissue
    m. fat
    m. hydatid cyst
multimammae
multimammate mouse
multinodal
multinodular, multinodulate
    m. goiter
multinomial distribution
multinuclear, multinucleate
    m. leukocyte
multinucleosis
multipara
    grand m.
multiparity
multiparous
multipartial
multipennate muscle
multiphasic screening
multiple
    m. alcohol
    m. amputation
    m. anchorage
    m. chemical sensitivity
    m. ego state
    m. embolism
    m. endocrine adenomatosis
    m. endocrine deficiency syndrome
    m. endocrine neoplasia (MEN)
    m. endocrine neoplasia syndrome, type 1, 2A, 2B
    m. endocrine neoplasia, type 1 (MEN1)
    m. endocrine neoplasia, type 2
    m. endocrine neoplasia, type 2A (MEN2A)
    m. endocrine neoplasia, type 2B
    m. endocrine neoplasia, type 3
    m. epiphyseal dysplasia (EDM)
    m. exostosis
    m. fission
    m. fracture
    m. glandular deficiency syndrome
    m. hamartoma syndrome
    m. idiopathic hemorrhagic sarcoma
    m. intestinal polyposis
    m. lentigines syndrome
    m. marker screen
    m. mucosal neuroma syndrome
    m. myeloma
    m. myelomatosis
    m. neuritis
    m. parasitism
    m. personality
    m. personality disorder
    m. pregnancy
    m. puncture tuberculin test
    m. sclerosis (MS)
    m. self-healing squamous epithelioma
    m. serositis
    m. sleep latency test
    m. stain
    m. sulfatase deficiency
    m. symmetric lipomatosis
    m. system atrophy
    m. vision
multiple-gated acquisition scan (MUGA)
multiplicative
    m. division
    m. growth
    m. model
multiplier
    countercurrent m.
multipolar
    m. cell
    m. mitosis
    m. neuron
multirooted
multirotation
multistage model
multisubstrate
multisynaptic
multivalence, multivalency
multivalent
    m. vaccine
multivariate study
multivesicular body
mummification
mummified pulp
mumps
    m. meningoencephalitis
    metastatic m.
    m. sensitivity test
    m. skin test antigen
    m. virus
    m. virus vaccine
mumpvirus
mumu fever
mumug
Münchausen
    M. syndrome
    M. syndrome by proxy
mung bean nuclease
municipal hospital
Munro
    M. abscess
    M. microabscess
    M. point

m. dilator iridis
m. dilator naris
m. dilator pupillae
m. dilator pylori gastroduodenalis
m. dilator pylori ilealis
m. dilator tubae
musculi dorsi
musculi dorsi proprii
m. ejaculator seminis
m. epicranius
m. epitrochleoanconeus
m. erector clitoridis
m. erector penis
m. erector spinae
m. extensor
m. extensor brevis digitorum
m. extensor brevis pollicis
m. extensor carpi radialis brevis
m. extensor carpi radialis longus
m. extensor carpi ulnaris
m. extensor coccygis
m. extensor digiti minimi
m. extensor digiti quinti proprius
m. extensor digitorum
m. extensor digitorum brevis
m. extensor digitorum brevis manus
m. extensor digitorum communis
m. extensor digitorum longus
m. extensor hallucis brevis
m. extensor hallucis longus
m. extensor indicis
m. extensor indicis proprius
m. extensor longus digitorum
m. extensor longus pollicis
m. extensor minimi digiti
m. extensor ossis metacarpi pollicis
m. extensor pollicis brevis
m. extensor pollicis longus
musculi externi bulbi oculi
musculi faciei
m. fibularis brevis
m. fibularis longus
m. fibularis tertius
m. flexor
m. flexor accessorius
m. flexor brevis digitorum
m. flexor brevis hallucis
m. flexor carpi radialis
m. flexor carpi ulnaris
m. flexor digiti minimi brevis manus
m. flexor digiti minimi brevis pedis
m. flexor digitorum brevis
m. flexor digitorum longus
m. flexor digitorum profundus
m. flexor digitorum sublimis
m. flexor digitorum superficialis
m. flexor hallucis brevis
m. flexor hallucis longus
m. flexor longus digitorum
m. flexor longus hallucis
m. flexor longus pollicis
m. flexor pollicis brevis
m. flexor pollicis longus
m. flexor profundus

m. flexor sublimis
m. frontalis
m. fusiformis
m. gastrocnemius
m. gemellus inferior
m. gemellus superior
m. genioglossus
m. geniohyoglossus
m. geniohyoideus
m. glossopalatinus
m. glossopharyngeus
m. gluteus maximus
m. gluteus medius
m. gluteus minimus
m. gracilis
m. helicis major
m. helicis minor
m. hyoglossus
m. hypopharyngeus
m. iliacus
m. iliacus minor
m. iliocapsularis
m. iliococcygeus
m. iliocostalis
m. iliocostalis cervicis
m. iliocostalis dorsi
m. iliocostalis lumborum
m. iliocostalis thoracis
m. iliopsoas
m. incisivus labii inferioris
m. incisivus labii superioris
m. incisurae helicis
m. infracostalis, pl. musculi infracostales
musculi infrahyoidei
m. infraspinatus
m. intercostales externi, pl. musculi intercostales externi
m. intercostalis internus, pl. musculi intercostales interni
m. intercostalis intimus, pl. musculi intercostales intimi
musculi interossei
musculi interossei dorsalis manus, pl. musculi interossei dorsales manus
musculi interossei dorsalis pedis, pl. musculi interossei dorsales pedis
m. interosseus palmaris, pl. musculi interossei palmares
musculi interosseus plantaris
m. interosseus volaris
musculi interspinales
m. interspinalis cervicis
m. interspinalis lumborum
m. interspinalis thoracis
m. intertragicus
musculi intertransversarii
musculi intertransversarii anteriores cervicis
musculi intertransversarii laterales lumborum
musculi intertransversarii mediales lumborum
musculi intertransversarii posteriores cervicis

M

musculus (*continued*)

musculi intertransversarii thoracis
m. ischiocavernosus
m. ischiococcygeus
m. keratopharyngeus
musculi laryngis
m. laryngopharyngeus
m. latissimus dorsi
m. levator alae nasi
m. levator anguli oris
m. levator anguli scapulae
m. levator ani
m. levator costae, pl. musculi
 levatores costarum
musculi levatores costarum breves
m. levatores costarum breves
musculi levatores costarum longi
m. levatores costarum longi
m. levator glandulae thyroideae
m. levator labii inferioris
m. levator labii superioris
m. levator labii superioris alaeque
 nasi
m. levator palati
m. levator palpebrae superioris
m. levator prostatae
m. levator scapulae
m. levator veli palatini
musculi linguae
m. longissimus
m. longissimus capitis
m. longissimus cervicis
m. longissimus dorsi
m. longissimus thoracis
m. longitudinalis inferior linguae
m. longitudinalis superior linguae
m. longus capitis
m. longus colli
m. lumbricalis manus, pl. musculi
 lumbricales manus
m. lumbricalis pedis, pl. musculi
 lumbricales pedis
m. masseter
m. mentalis
m. multifidus
m. multifidus spinae
m. multipennatus
m. mylohyoideus
m. mylopharyngeus
m. nasalis
m. obliquus auriculae
m. obliquus capitis inferior
m. obliquus capitis superior
m. obliquus externus abdominis
m. obliquus inferior
m. obliquus internus abdominis
m. obliquus superior
m. obturator externus
m. obturator internus
m. occipitalis
m. occipitofrontalis
m. omohyoideus
m. opponens
m. opponens digiti minimi

m. opponens digiti quinti
m. opponens minimi digiti
m. opponens pollicis
m. orbicularis
m. orbicularis oculi
m. orbicularis oris
m. orbicularis palpebrarum
m. orbitalis
m. orbitopalpebralis
musculi ossiculorum auditoriorum
musculi ossiculorum auditus
m. palatoglossus
m. palatopharyngeus
m. palatosalpingeus
m. palatostaphylinus
m. palmaris brevis
m. palmaris longus
m. papillaris
musculi pectinati
m. pectineus
m. pectoralis major
m. pectoralis minor
m. pennatus
musculi perinei
m. peroneocalcaneus
m. peroneus brevis
m. peroneus longus
m. peroneus tertius
m. petropharyngeus
m. petrostaphylinus
m. pharyngopalatinus
m. piriformis
m. plana
m. plantaris
m. platysma
m. platysma myoides
m. pleuroesophageus
m. popliteus
m. procerus
m. pronator
m. pronator pedis
m. pronator quadratus
m. pronator radii teres
m. pronator teres
m. prostaticus
m. psoas major
m. psoas minor
m. pterygoideus externus
m. pterygoideus internus
m. pterygoideus lateralis
m. pterygoideus medialis
m. pterygopharyngeus
m. pterygospinosus
m. puboanalis
m. pubococcygeus
m. puboperinealis
m. puboprostaticus
m. puborectalis
m. pubovaginalis
m. pubovesicalis
m. pyramidalis
m. pyramidalis auriculae
m. pyramidalis nasi
m. pyriformis
m. quadratus

m. quadratus femoris
m. quadratus labii inferioris
m. quadratus labii superioris
m. quadratus lumborum
m. quadratus menti
m. quadratus plantae
m. quadriceps
m. quadriceps extensor femoris
m. quadriceps femoris
m. rectococcygeus
musculi rectourethrales
m. rectouterinus
m. rectovesicalis
m. rectus
m. rectus abdominis
m. rectus capitis anterior
m. rectus capitis anticus major
m. rectus capitis anticus minor
m. rectus capitis lateralis
m. rectus capitis posterior major
m. rectus capitis posterior minor
m. rectus capitis posticus major
m. rectus capitis posticus minor
m. rectus externus
m. rectus femoris
m. rectus inferior
m. rectus internus
m. rectus lateralis
m. rectus medialis
m. rectus superior
m. rectus thoracis
musculi regionis analis
musculi regionis urogenitalis
m. retrahens aurem
m. retrahens auriculam
m. rhomboatloideus
m. rhomboideus major
m. rhomboideus minor
m. risorius
m. rotator
musculi rotatores
musculi rotatores cervicis
musculi rotatores lumborum
musculi rotatores thoracis
m. sacrococcygeus anterior
m. sacrococcygeus dorsalis
m. sacrococcygeus posterior
m. sacrococcygeus ventralis
m. sacrolumbalis
m. sacrospinalis
m. salpingopharyngeus
m. sartorius
m. scalenus anterior
m. scalenus anticus
m. scalenus medius
m. scalenus minimus
m. scalenus posterior
m. scalenus posticus
musculi scapulohumerales
m. semimembranosus
m. semipennatus
m. semispinalis
m. semispinalis capitis
m. semispinalis cervicis
m. semispinalis colli

m. semispinalis dorsi
m. semispinalis thoracis
m. semitendinosus
m. serratus anterior
m. serratus magnus
m. serratus posterior inferior
m. serratus posterior superior
m. skeleti
m. soleus
m. sphincter
m. sphincter ampullae
m. sphincter ampullae
  biliaropancreaticae
m. sphincter ampullae
  hepatopancreaticae
m. sphincter ani externus
m. sphincter ani internus
m. sphincter ductus biliaris
m. sphincter ductus choledochi
m. sphincter ductus pancreatici
m. sphincter oris
m. sphincter palatopharyngeus
m. sphincter pupillae
m. sphincter pylori
m. sphincter urethrae externus
m. sphincter urethrae externus
  femininae
m. sphincter urethrae externus
  masculinae
m. sphincter urethrae internus
m. sphincter urethrovaginalis
m. sphincter vaginae
m. sphincter vesicae
m. spinalis
m. spinalis capitis
m. spinalis cervicis
m. spinalis colli
m. spinalis dorsi
m. spinalis thoracis
musculi splenii
m. splenius capitis
m. splenius cervicis
m. splenius colli
m. stapedius
m. sternalis
m. sternochondroscapularis
m. sternoclavicularis
m. sternocleidomastoideus
m. sternofascialis
m. sternohyoideus
m. sternothyroideus
m. styloauricularis
m. styloglossus
m. stylohyoideus
m. stylolaryngeus
m. stylopharyngeus
m. subclavius
m. subcostalis, pl. musculi subcostales
m. subcutaneus colli
musculi suboccipitales
m. subscapularis
m. supinator
m. supinator longus
m. supinator radii brevis
m. supraclavicularis

M

musculus (*continued*)
musculi suprahyoidei
m. supraspinalis
m. supraspinatus
m. suspensorius duodeni
m. tarsalis inferior
m. tarsalis superior
m. temporalis
m. temporoparietalis
m. tensor fasciae femoris
m. tensor fasciae latae
m. tensor tarsi
m. tensor tympani
m. tensor veli palatini
m. teres major
m. teres minor
m. tetragonus
musculi thoracis
musculi thoracoappendiculares
m. thyroarytenoideus
m. thyroarytenoideus externus
m. thyroarytenoideus internus
m. thyroepiglotticus
m. thyrohyoideus
m. thyropharyngeus
m. tibialis anterior
m. tibialis anticus
m. tibialis gracilis
m. tibialis posterior
m. tibialis posticus
m. tibialis secundus
m. tibiofascialis anterior
m. tibiofascialis anticus
m. trachealis
m. tracheloclavicularis
m. trachelomastoideus
m. tragicus
m. transversalis abdominis
m. transversalis capitis
m. transversalis cervicis
m. transversalis colli
m. transversalis nasi
musculi transversospinales
m. transversus abdominis
m. transversus auriculae
m. transversus linguae
m. transversus menti
m. transversus nuchae
m. transversus perinei profundus
m. transversus perinei superficialis
m. transversus thoracis
m. trapezius
m. triangularis
m. triangularis labii inferioris
m. triangularis labii superioris
m. triangularis sterni
m. triceps
m. triceps brachii
m. triceps coxae
m. triceps surae
m. triticeoglossus
m. unipennatus
m. uvulae
m. vastus externus

m. vastus intermedius
m. vastus internus
m. vastus lateralis
m. vastus medialis
m. ventricularis
m. verticalis linguae
m. vocalis
m. zygomaticus
m. zygomaticus major
m. zygomaticus minor
mushbite
mushroom poisoning
mushroom-worker's lung
musical
m. agraphia
m. alexia
m. murmur
music blindness
musician's cramp
musicotherapy
muskeag moss
Musset sign
mussitation
must
mustard
black m.
m. chlorohydrin
expressed m. oil
m. gas (HD)
hemisulfur m.
nitrogen m. (HN2)
m. oil
M. operation
M. procedure
semisulfur m.
sulfur m.
uracil m.
volatile m. oil
white m.
mustine hydrochloride
mutacism
mutagen
frameshift m.
mutagenesis
cassette m.
insertional m.
site-directed m.
mutagenic
mutant
active m.
amber m.
auxotrophic m.
cold-sensitive m.
conditional-lethal m.
conditionally lethal m.
deficiency m.
m. gene
inactive m.
petite m.
quick-stop m.
silent m.
suppressor-sensitive m.
temperature-sensitive m.
uninducible m.
virulent phage m.

mutarotase
mutarotation
mutase
mutation
>addition m.
>addition-deletion m.
>amber m.
>back m.
>deletion m.
>frameshift m.
>induced m.
>lethal m.
>missense m.
>natural m.
>neutral m.
>new m.
>nonsense m.
>ochre m.
>opal m.
>point m.
>m. rate
>reading-frame-shift m.
>reverse m.
>silent m.
>site specific m.
>somatic m.
>spontaneous m.
>suppressor m.
>transition m.
>transversion m.
>umber m.
>up promoter m.

mutational frequency
mute
mutein
mutilating
>m. keratoderma
>m. leprosy

mutilation
mutism
>akinetic m.
>elective m.
>voluntary m.

muton
mutton-fat keratic precipitate
mutualism
mutualist
mutualistic symbiosis
mutual resistance
mV
>millivolt

MVE virus
>Murray Valley encephalitis virus

MVV
>maximum voluntary ventilation

MW
>molecular weight

MWC model
>Monod-Wyman-Changeux model

myalgia
>epidemic m.
>m. thermica

myasthenia
>m. angiosclerotica
>m. gravis

myasthenic
>m. crisis
>m. facies
>m. reaction
>m. syndrome

myatonia, myatony
>m. congenita

myatrophy
mycelia (*pl. of* mycelium)
mycelian
mycelioid
mycelium, pl. **mycelia**
>aerial m.
>nonseptate m.
>septate m.

mycete
mycetism, mycetismus
>m. cerebralis
>m. choliformis
>m. gastrointestinalis
>m. nervosa
>m. sanguinareus

mycetogenetic, mycetogenic
mycetogenous
mycetoma
mycobacteria
>atypical m.
>Runyon group I, II, III, IV m.

Mycobacteriaceae
mycobacteriosis
Mycobacterium
>M. *abscessus*
>M. *avium*
>M. *avium-intracellulare* (MAI)
>M. *avium-intracellulare complex*
>M. *bovis*
>M. *chelonae*
>M. *chelonae* subsp. *abscessus*
>M. *fortuitum*
>M. *intracellulare*
>M. *kansasii*
>M. *leprae*
>M. *marianum*
>M. *marinum*
>M. *microti*
>M. *paratuberculosis*
>M. *phlei*
>M. *scrofulaceum*
>M. *smegmatis*
>M. *tuberculosis*
>M. *ulcerans*
>M. *vaccae*
>M. *xenopi*

mycobactin
mycocide
mycodermatitis
mycogastritis
mycolic acids
mycologist
mycology
>medical m.

mycophage
Mycoplasma
>M. *buccale*
>M. *faucium*

M

Mycoplasma (*continued*)
  M. fermentans
  M. genitalium
  M. hominis
  M. laidlawii
  M. orale
  M. pharyngis
  M. pneumoniae
  M. salivarium
mycoplasma, pl. **mycoplasmata**
Mycoplasmatales
mycopus
mycose
mycosis, pl. **mycoses**
  m. framboesioides
  m. fungoides
  m. intestinalis
mycostatic
mycosterols
mycotic
  m. aneurysm
  m. endocarditis
  m. keratitis
mycotoxicosis
mycotoxin
mycovirus
mydaleine
mydatoxin
mydriasis
  alternating m.
  amaurotic m.
  paralytic m.
  spastic m.
mydriatic
myectomy
myectopy, myectopia
myelapoplexy
myelatelia
myelauxe
myelemia
myelencephalon
myelic
myelin
  m. body
  m. figure
  m. protein A1
  m. sheath
myelinated
  m. nerve
  m. nerve fiber
myelination
myelinic
  m. degeneration
myelinization
myelinoclasis
myelinogenesis
myelinolysis
  central pontine m.
myelinopathy
myelitic
myelitis
  acute necrotizing m.
  acute transverse m.
  ascending m.

bulbar m.
concussion m.
demyelinated m.
Foix-Alajouanine m.
funicular m.
postinfectious m.
postvaccinal m.
radiation m.
subacute necrotizing m.
systemic m.
transverse m.
myeloarchitectonics
myeloblast
myeloblastemia
myeloblastic leukemia
myeloblastoma
myeloblastosis
myelocele
myelocyst
myelocystic
myelocystocele
myelocystomeningocele
myelocyte
  m. A, B, C
myelocythemia
myelocytic
  m. crisis
  m. leukemia
  m. leukemoid reaction
myelocytoma
myelocytomatosis
myelocytosis
myelodiastasis
myelodysplasia
myelodysplastic syndrome
myelofibrosis
myelogenesis
myelogenic, myelogenetic
  m. leukemia
  m. sarcoma
myelogenous
myelogone, myelogonium
myelogram
  cervical m.
  lumbar m.
myelography
myeloic
myeloid
  m. cell
  m. leukemia
  m. metaplasia
  m. sarcoma
  m. series
  m. tissue
myeloidosis
myelokathexis
myeloleukemia
myelolipoma
myelolymphocyte
myelolysis
myeloma
  Bence Jones m.
  endothelial m.
  giant cell m.
  L-chain m.

multiple m.
m. multiplex
nonsecretory m.
plasma cell m.
myelomalacia
angiodysgenetic m.
myelomatosis
multiple m.
m. multiplex
myelomeningocele
myelomere
myelomonocyte
myelomonocytic leukemia
myeloneuritis
myelonic
myeloparalysis
myelopathic
m. anemia
myelopathy
carcinomatous m.
compressive m.
diabetic m.
paracarcinomatous m.
radiation m.
myeloperoxidase
myelopetal
myelophthisic
m. anemia
myelophthisis
myeloplast
myeloplegia
myelopoiesis
myelopoietic
myeloproliferative syndrome
myeloradiculitis
myeloradiculodysplasia
myeloradiculopathy
myeloradiculopolyneuronitis
myelorrhagia
myelorrhaphy
myeloschisis
myelosclerosis
myelosis
aleukemic m.
chronic nonleukemic m.
erythremic m.
funicular m.
leukemic m.
leukopenic m.
subleukemic m.
myelospongium
myelosyphilis
myelotome
myelotomography
myelotomy
Bischof m.
commissural m.
midline m.
T m.
myelotoxic
myenteric
m. plexus
m. reflex
myenteron
myesthesia

myiasis
accidental m.
African furuncular m.
aural m.
human botfly m.
intestinal m.
nasal m.
ocular m.
tumbu dermal m.
wound m.
mykol
mylabris
mylohyoid
m. artery
m. branch
m. fossa
m. groove
m. line
m. muscle
m. nerve
m. ridge
mylohyoideus
mylopharyngeal
m. part of superior constrictor muscle of pharynx
m. part of superior pharyngeal constrictor muscle of pharynx
myoadenylate deaminase
myoalbumin
myoarchitectonic
myoatrophy
myoblast
myoblastic
myoblastoma
granular cell m.
myobradia
myocardia (*pl. of* myocardium)
myocardial
m. bridge
m. depressant factor (MDF)
m. infarction (MI)
m. insufficiency
m. ischemia
m. rigor mortis
myocardiograph
myocardiopathy
alcoholic m.
chagasic m.
myocardiorrhaphy
myocarditic
myocarditis
acute isolated m.
Fiedler m.
giant cell m.
idiopathic m.
indurative m.
toxic m.
myocardium, pl. **myocardia**
hibernating m.
stunned m.
myocele
myocelialgia
myocelitis
myocellulitis
myocerosis

M

myochrome
myochronoscope
myocinesimeter
myoclonia
    fibrillary m.
myoclonic
    m. astatic epilepsy
    m. epilepsy with ragged red fiber
     myopathy (MERRF)
    m. seizure
myoclonus
    benign m. of infancy
    benign infantile m.
    m. epilepsy
    m. multiplex
    nocturnal m.
    palatal m.
    stimulus sensitive m.
myocolpitis
myocomma, pl. **myocommata**
myocrismus
myocutaneous **flap**
myocyte
    Anitschkow m.
myocytolysis of heart
myocytoma
myodegeneration
myodemia
myodermal flap
myodiastasis
myodynamia
myodynamics
myodynamometer
myodynia
myodystony
myodystrophy, myodystrophia
myoedema
myoelastic theory
myoelectric
myoendocarditis
myoepicardial mantle
myoepithelial cell
myoepithelioma
myoepithelium
myoesthesis, myoesthesia
myofascial
    m. pain-dysfunction syndrome
    m. syndrome
myofascitis
myofibril
myofibrilla, pl. **myofibrillae**
myofibrillar
myofibroblast
myofibroma
myofibromatosis
    infantile m.
myofibrosis cordis
myofibrositis
myofilaments
myofunctional therapy
myogen
myogenesis
myogenic, myogenetic
    m. potential
    m. tonus

myogenous
myoglobin
    carbonmonoxy m.
    m. and its combinations with CO
     and oxygen (Mb, MbCO, MbO$_2$)
myoglobinuria
myoglobulinuria
myognathus
myogram
myograph
    palate m.
myographic
myography
myohemoglobin
myoid cell
myoidema
myoinositol
myoischemia
myokerosis
myokinase
myokinesimeter
myokymia
    facial m.
    generalized m.
    hereditary m.
    limb m.
myolemma
myolipoma
myologia
myologist
myology
    descriptive m.
myolysis
    cardiotoxic m.
myoma
myomalacia
myomatous polyp
myomectomy
    abdominal m.
    left ventricular m.
    vaginal m.
myomelanosis
myomere
myometer
myometrial
    m. arcuate artery
    m. radial artery
myometritis
myometrium
myomitochondrion, pl. **myomitochondria**
myomotomy
myon
myonecrosis
    clostridial m.
myoneme
myoneural
    m. blockade
    m. junction
myoneuroma
myonymy
myopachynsis
myopalmus
myopathic
    m. atrophy

m. facies
m. scoliosis
myopathy
carcinomatous m.
centronuclear m.
distal m.
dysthyroid m.
minicore-multicore m.
mitochondrial m.
myoclonic epilepsy with ragged red fiber m. (MERRF)
myotubular m.
nemaline m.
ocular m.
proximal myotonic m. (PROMM)
rod m.
thyrotoxic m.
myopericarditis
myoperitonitis
myophone
myophosphorylase deficiency glycogenosis
myopia
axial m.
curvature m.
degenerative m.
index m.
malignant m.
night m.
pathologic m.
prematurity m.
senile lenticular m.
simple m.
space m.
transient m.
myopic
m. astigmatism
m. choroidopathy
m. conus
m. crescent
m. degeneration
myoplasm
myoplastic
myoplasty
myopolar
myoprotein
myorrhaphy
myorrhexis
myosalpingitis
myosalpinx
myosarcoma
myosclerosis
myoseptum
myosin
m. filament
m. light chain kinase
myosinogen
myosinose
myositic
myositis
cervical m.
epidemic m.
m. epidemica acuta
m. fibrosa
infectious m.
interstitial m.

m. ossificans
m. ossificans circumscripta
m. ossificans progressiva
proliferative m.
m. purulenta tropica
tropical m.
myospasm, myospasmus
cervical m.
myospherulosis
myosthenometer
myostroma
myostromin
myotactic
myotasis
myotatic
m. contraction
m. irritability
m. reflex
myotenositis
myotenotomy
myothermic
myotome
myotomy
cricopharyngeal m.
Heller m.
myotone
myotonia
m. acquisita
m. atrophica
m. congenita
m. dystrophica
m. neonatorum
myotonic
m. cataract
m. chondrodystrophy
m. dystrophy
m. response
myotonoid
myotonus
myotony
myotrophy
myotube
myotubular myopathy
myotubule
myovascular sphincter
myovenous sphincter
Myoviridae
myrica
myricin
myringa
myringectomy
myringitis
m. bulbosa
bullous m.
myringodermatitis
myringoplasty
myringosclerosis
myringostapediopexy
myringotome
myringotomy
myrinx
myristic acid
myristica oil
myristicin
myristoleic acid

M

myrmecia
myrosinase
myrrh
mysophilia
mysophobia
mytacism
myurous
myxadenitis labialis
myxasthenia
myxedema
      congenital m.
      m. heart
      infantile m.
      operative m.
      pituitary m.
      m. voice
myxedematoid
myxedematous infantilism
myxemia
myxochondrofibrosarcoma
myxochondroma
Myxococcidium stegomyiae
myxocyte
myxofibroma
myxofibrosarcoma
myxoid
      m. cyst
      m. degeneration

myxolipoma
myxoma
      atrial m.
      m. enchondromatosum
      m. fibrosum
      m. lipomatosum
      odontogenic m.
      m. sarcomatosum
myxomatosis
      m. virus
myxomatous degeneration
myxomembranous colitis
myxomycete
Myxomycetes
myxoneuroma
myxopapillary ependymoma
myxopapilloma
myxopoiesis
myxorrhea gastrica
myxosarcoma
Myxospora
Myxosporea
myxovirus
Myxozoa

ν (*var. of* nu)

N
    newton
    nitrogen
N/2
    seminormal
^{13}**N**
    nitrogen-13
^{14}**N**
    nitrogen-14
^{15}**N**
    nitrogen-15
N_A
    Avogadro number
n
    nano-
n
    refractive index
N
    normal concentration
n_0
    loschmidt number
NA
    nomina anatomica
Na
    sodium
^{24}**Na**
    sodium-24
nabilone
nabothian
    n. cyst
    n. follicle
nacreous
    n. ichthyosis
NAD
    nicotinamide adenine dinucleotide
N.A.D.
    no appreciable disease
NAD$^+$
    NAD$^+$ nucleosidase (NADase)
    NAD$^+$ pyrophosphorylase
    NAD$^+$ synthetase
NADase
    NAD$^+$ nucleosidase
NADH
    nicotinamide adenine dinucleotide
    NADH dehydrogenase
    NADH dehydrogenase (quinone)
    NADH-hydroxylamine reductase
nadide
nadir
Nadi reaction
nadolol
NADP
    nicotinamide adenine dinucleotide
        phosphate
NADP$^+$
    nicotinamide adenine dinucleotide
        phosphate
NADPH
    nicotinamide adenine dinucleotide
        phosphate

NADPH-cytochrome c_2 reductase
NADPH dehydrogenase
NADPH dehydrogenase (quinone)
NADPH diaphorase
NADPH-ferrihemoprotein reductase
NAD(P)$^+$ nucleosidase
Naegeli
    N. syndrome
    N. type of monocytic leukemia
Naegleria
nafcillin
    n. sodium
Naffziger
    N. operation
    N. syndrome
naftifine hydrochloride
NAG
    n-acetylglutamate
nagana
Nägele
    N. obliquity
    N. pelvis
    N. rule
Nagel test
Nageotte cell
nail
    n. bed
    egg shell n.
    n. fold
    half and half n.
    Hippocratic n.'s
    ingrown n.
    Küntscher n.
    n. matrix
    parrot-beak n.
    pincer n.
    n. pit
    n. plate
    n. pulse
    racket n.
    reedy n.
    shell n.
    Smith-Petersen n.
    spoon n.
    n. wall
    yellow n.
nailing
nail-patella syndrome
Nair buffered methylene blue stain
Nakanishi stain
naked virus
nalbuphine hydrochloride
nalidixic acid
nalorphine
naloxone hydrochloride
naltrexone
NAME
    NAME syndrome
NANB
    non-A, non-B
    NANB hepatitis

N

NANBNC
    non-A, non-B, non-C
        NANBNC hepatitis
Nance-Insley syndrome
Nance-Sweeney chondrodysplasia
NANC neuron
NANDA
    North American Nursing Diagnosis
        Association
nandrolone
    n. decanoate
    n. phenpropionate
    n. phenylpropionate
nanism
    mulibrey n.
    renal n.
    symptomatic n.
Nannizzia
nano- (n)
nanocephalia
nanocephalous, nanocephalic
nanocephaly
nanocormia
nanogram (ng)
nanoid enamel
nanokatal (nkat)
nanomelia
nanometer (nm)
nanomolar (nM)
nanophthalmia, nanophthalmos
Nanophyetus salmincola
nanukayami fever
nape nevus
napex
naphazoline hydrochloride
naphtha
        coal tar n.
        wood n.
naphthalene
naphthalenol
naphthalin
naphthazoline hydrochloride
naphthol
naphtholate
naphthol yellow S
naphthoquinone
naphthyl
napier
naproxen
napsylate
narceine
narcissism
        primary n.
        secondary n.
narcissistic personality disorder
narcoanalysis
narcohypnia
narcohypnosis
narcolepsy
narcoleptic
    n. tetrad
narcosis
        CO_2 n.
        intravenous n.
        nitrogen n.

narcosynthesis
narcotherapy
narcotic
    n. blockade
    n. hunger
    n. reversal
narcotism
naris, pl. **nares**
    anterior n.
    external n.
    internal n.
    posterior nares
NARP
    neuropathy, ataxia, retinitis pigmentosa
narrow-angle glaucoma
narrowband
nasal
    n. arch
    n. atrium
    n. bone
    n. border of frontal bone
    n. calculus
    n. capsule
    n. catarrh
    n. cavity
    n. crest
    n. crest of horizontal plate of
        palatine bone
    n. crest of palatine process of
        maxilla
    n. duct
    n. feeding
    n. foramen
    n. ganglion
    n. gland
    n. glioma
    n. height
    n. hemorrhage
    n. index
    n. margin of frontal bone
    n. meatus
    n. mucosa
    n. muscle
    n. myiasis
    n. nerve
    n. notch
    n. part of frontal bone
    n. part of pharynx
    n. pharynx
    n. pit
    n. placode
    n. point
    n. polyp
    n. process
    n. reflex
    n. region
    n. ridge
    n. sac
    n. septal branch of superior labial
        branch of facial artery
    n. septal cartilage
    n. septum
    n. spine of frontal bone
    n. surface of maxilla
    n. surface of palatine bone

n. valve
n. venous arch
n. venules of retina
n. vestibule
nasalis muscle
nascent
Nasik vibrio
nasioiniac
nasion-pogonion measurement
nasion-postcondylar plane
nasion soft tissue
Nasmyth
N. cuticle
N. membrane
nasoalveolar cyst
nasoantral
nasobasilar line
nasobregmatic arc
nasociliary
n. nerve
n. root of ciliary ganglion
nasofrontal vein
nasogastric tube
nasojugal fold
nasolabial
n. cyst
n. groove
n. lymph node
n. node
n. sulcus
nasolacrimal
n. canal
n. duct
nasomandibular fixation
nasomaxillary suture
nasomental reflex
naso-occipital arc
naso-oral
nasopalatine
n. duct cyst
n. groove
n. nerve
nasopharyngeal
n. carcinoma
n. groove
n. leishmaniasis
n. meatus
n. passage
nasopharyngolaryngoscope
nasopharyngoscope
nasopharyngoscopy
nasopharynx
nasorostral
nasosinusitis
nasotracheal
n. intubation
n. tube
Nasse law
nasus externus
natal
n. cleft
N. sore
n. tooth
natality
natamycin

nates (*pl. of* natis)
natiform skull
national
N. Formulary (NF)
N. Health Service (N.H.S.)
N. Institutes of Health (NIH)
N. League for Nursing (NLN)
N. Science Foundation (NSF)
natis, pl. **nates**
native
n. albumin
n. protein
natremia, natriemia
natrexone hydrochloride
natriferic
natrium
natriuresis
natriuretic
Nattrassia mangiferae
natural
n. antibody
n. dentition
n. dye
n. focus of infection
n. hemolysin
n. immunity, nonspecific n.
n. killer (NK)
n. killer cell
n. killer cell leukemia
n. killer cell stimulating factor
n. mutation
n. pigment
n. product
n. selection
nature-nurture issue
naturopath
naturopathic
naturopathy
Nauheim
N. bath
N. treatment
naupathia
nausea
epidemic n.
n. gravidarum
nauseant
nauseate
nauseated
nauseous
Nauta stain
navel
navicula
navicular
n. abdomen
n. articular surface of talus
n. (bone)
n. bone of hand
n. fossa of urethra
navigator echo
Nb
niobium
NBT
nitroblue tetrazolium
NBT test

N

Nd
neodymium
NDP
nucleoside diphosphate
ND virus
Nd:YAG laser
Ne
neon
near
n. drowning
n. point
n. point of convergence
n. reaction
n. reflex
n. sight
nearest neighbor frequency
nearsightedness
nearthrosis
near-total thyroidectomy
nebramycin
nebul.
nebula
nebula, pl. **nebulae (nebul.)**
nebularine
nebulin
nebulization
nebulize
nebulizer
jet n.
spinning disk n.
ultrasonic n.
nebulous urine
Necator
necatoriasis
necessary cause
neck
anatomical n. of humerus
buffalo n.
bull n.
dental n.
n. of femur
n. of fibula
n. of gallbladder
n. of glans
n. of hair follicle
n. of humerus
Madelung n.
n. of malleus
n. of mandible
n. of pancreas
n. of radius
n. reflex
n. of rib
n. of scapula
n. sign
stiff n.
surgical n. of humerus
n. of talus
n. of thigh bone
n. of tooth
turkey gobbler n.
n. of (urinary) bladder
n. of uterus
webbed n.

n. of womb
wry n.
necklace
Casal n.
neck-shaft angle
necrectomy
necrobacillosis
necrobiosis
n. lipoidica
n. lipoidica diabeticorum
necrobiotic
necrobiotic xanthogranuloma
necrocytosis
necrogenic
necrogenous
necrogranulomatous
necrologist
necrology
necrolysis
toxic epidermal n. (TEN)
necrolytic migratory erythema
necromania
necrometer
necroparasite
necropathy
necrophagous
necrophilia, necrophilism
necrophilous
necrophobia
necropsy
necrosadism
necroscopy
necrose
necrosectomy
necrosis
acute massive liver n.
acute retinal n. (ARN)
aseptic n.
avascular n.
n. bacillus
bridging hepatic n.
caseation n.
caseous n.
central n.
coagulation n.
colliquative n.
contraction band n.
cystic medial n.
epiphysial aseptic n.
fat n.
fibrinoid n.
focal n.
ischemic n.
laminar cortical n.
liquefactive n.
progressive emphysematous n.
progressive outer retinal n. (PORN)
renal papillary n.
simple n.
subcutaneous fat n. of newborn
suppurative n.
total n.
zonal n.
necrospermia
necrosteon, necrosteosis

necrotic
  n. arachnidism
  n. cirrhosis
  n. cyst
  n. infectious conjunctivitis
  n. inflammation
  n. pulp
necrotizing
  n. angiitis
  n. arteriolitis
  n. cellulitis
  n. encephalitis
  n. encephalomyelopathy
  n. encephalopathy
  n. enterocolitis
  n. fasciitis
  n. hemorrhagic leukomyelitis
  n. inflammation
  n. keratitis
  n. papillitis
  n. scleritis
  n. sialometaplasia
  n. ulcerative gingivitis (NUG)
necrotomy
  osteoplastic n.
needle
  aneurysm n.
  artery n.
  aspirating n.
  atraumatic n.
  n. bath
  n. biopsy
  biopsy n.
  cataract n.
  n. culture
  cutting n.
  Deschamps n.
  Emmet n.
  exploring n.
  n. forceps
  Francke n.
  Frazier n.
  Gillmore n.
  Hagedorn n.
  hypodermic n.
  knife n.
  lumbar puncture n.
  Millner n.
  n. point tracing
  Salah sternal puncture n.
  spatula n.
  stop-n.
  Tuohy n.
  Veress n.
needle-carrier
needle-driver
needle-holder
Needles split cast method
needling
neencephalon
NEEP
  negative end-expiratory pressure
Neer impingement sign
nefopam hydrochloride

negation
negative
  n. accommodation
  n. afterimage
  n. anergy
  n. base excess
  n. catalyst
  n. chemotaxis
  n. chronotropism
  n. control
  n. convergence
  n. cooperativity
  n. cytotaxis
  n. electrode
  n. electrotaxis
  n. end-expiratory pressure (NEEP)
  n. feedback
  n. G
  n. h
  n. image
  n. leukocytotaxia
  n. meniscus
  n. myoclonic seizure
  n. neutrotaxis
  n. phase
  n. photodromy
  n. phototaxis
  n. phototropism
  n. politzerization
  n. pressure
  n. pressure ventilation
  n. reinforcer
  n. S
  n. scotoma
  n. stain
  n. stereotropism
  n. strand virus
  n. supporting reaction
  n. symptom
  n. taxis
  n. thermotaxis
  n. transference
  n. tropism
  n. valence
negatively inotropic
negativism
negatron
Negishi virus
Negri
  N. body
  N. corpuscle
Negro phenomenon
Neisser
  N. coccus
  N. stain
  N. syringe
Neisseria
  N. catarrhalis
  N. caviae
  N. flava
  N. flavescens
  N. gonorrhoeae
  N. haemolysans
  N. meningitidis

N

Neisseria (continued)
    N. sicca
    N. subflava
neisseria, pl. **neisseriae**
Nélaton
    N. catheter
    N. fiber
    N. fold
    N. line
    N. sphincter
Nelson
    N. syndrome
    N. tumor
nem
nemaline myopathy
nemathelminth
Nemathelminthes
nematicidal, nematocidal
nematicide, nematocide
nematization
nematoblast
nematocidal (*var. of* nematicidal)
nematocide (*var. of* nematicide)
nematocyst
Nematoda
nematode
nematodiasis
    cerebrospinal n.
Nematodirella longispiculata
nematoid
nematologist
nematology
nematospermia
neoadjuvant
neoantigens
neoarsphenamine
neoarthrosis
Neoascaris vitulorum
neobiogenesis
neobladder
neoblastic
neocerebellum
neochymotrypsinogen
neocinchophen
neocortex
neocystostomy
neodymium (Nd)
neoencephalon
neofetal
neofetus
neoformation
neogenesis
neogenetic
neokinetic
neolallism
neologism
neomorph, neomorphism
neomycin sulfate
neon (Ne)
neonatal
    n. anemia
    n. apoplexy
    n. calf diarrhea virus
    n. conjunctivitis

    n. death
    n. diagnosis
    n. hepatitis
    n. herpes
    n. hyperbilirubinemia
    n. hypoglycemia
    n. isoerythrolysis
    n. jaundice
    n. line
    n. lupus
    n. medicine
    n. mortality rate
    n. ring
    n. screening
    n. tetanus
    n. tetany
    n. tooth
neonate
neonatologist
neonatology
neoneurotization
neopallium
neophobia
neoplasia
    cervical intraepithelial n.
    lobular n.
    multiple endocrine n. (MEN)
    multiple endocrine n., type 1
      (MEN1)
    multiple endocrine n., type 2
    multiple endocrine n., type 2A
      (MEN2A)
    multiple endocrine n., type 2B
    multiple endocrine n., type 3
    prostatic intraepithelial n. (PIN)
    vaginal intraepithelial n.
    vulvar intraepithelial n.
neoplasm
    histoid n.
    Revised European-American
      Classification of Lymphoid N.'s
      (REAL)
neoplastic
    n. arachnoiditis
    n. meningitis
neopterin
neopyrithiamin
neoretinal b
neoretinene B
Neospora canium
neostigmine
neostomy
neostriatum
neoteny
Neotestudina rosati
neothalamus
neotype
    n. culture
    n. strain
neotyrosine
neovascular glaucoma
neovascularization
    choroidal n.
    classic choroidal n.

net
    Chiari n.
    chromidial n.
    n. flux
    n. knot
Netherton syndrome
netilmicin sulfate
nettle
Nettleshop-Falls albinism
nettling hair
network
    acromial arterial n.
    arteriolar n.
    articular vascular n.
    articular vascular n. of elbow
    articular vascular n. of knee
    calcaneal arterial n.
    chromatin n.
    cytokine n.
    dorsal carpal n.
    dorsal venous n.
    lateral malleolar n.
    linin n.
    medial malleolar n.
    neurofibrillar n.
    patellar n.
    peritarsal n.
    plantar venous n.
    Purkinje n.
    subpapillary n.
    trabecular n.
NeuAc
    n-acetylneuraminic acid
Neubauer artery
Neuberg ester
Neufeld
    N. capsular swelling
    N. reaction
Neumann
    N. disease
    N. law
    N. sheath
neural
    n. arch of vertebra
    n. axis
    n. canal
    n. crest
    n. crest syndrome
    n. cyst
    n. deafness
    n. factor
    n. fold
    n. ganglion
    n. groove
    n. hearing loss
    n. layer of optic part of retina
    n. lobe of hypophysis
    n. part of hypophysis
    n. plate
    n. segment
    n. spine
    n. tube
neuralgia
    atypical facial n.
    atypical trigeminal n.

    epileptiform n.
    facial n.
    n. facialis vera
    Fothergill n.
    geniculate n.
    glossopharyngeal n.
    hallucinatory n.
    Hunt n.
    idiopathic n.
    intercostal n.
    mammary n.
    Morton n.
    occipital n.
    periodic migrainous n.
    sciatic n.
    Sluder n.
    sphenopalatine n.
    stump n.
    suboccipital n.
    supraorbital n.
    symptomatic n.
    trifacial n.
    trigeminal n.
neuralgic amyotrophy
neuralgiform
neuramebimeter
neuraminic acid
neuraminidase
neuranagenesis
neurapophysis
neurapraxia
neurarchy
neurasthenia
    angioparalytic n.
    angiopathic n.
    gastric n.
    n. gravis
    n. praecox
    primary n.
    pulsating n.
    sexual n.
    traumatic n.
neurasthenic
    n. personality
neuraxis
neuraxon, neuraxone
neurectasis, neurectasia, neurectasy
neurectomy
    occipital n.
    presacral n.
    retrogasserian n.
    vestibular n.
neurectopia, neurectopy
neurenteric
    n. canal
    n. cyst
neurepithelium
neuri-
neuridine
neurilemma cell
neurilemoma
    acoustic n.
    Antoni type A, B n.
neurility
neurimotility

N

neurimotor
neurine
neurinoma
    acoustic n.
neuritic plaque
neuritis, pl. **neuritides**
    adventitial n.
    ascending n.
    axial n.
    brachial n.
    central n.
    descending n.
    Eichhorst n.
    endemic n.
    fallopian n.
    interstitial n.
    intraocular n.
    Leyden n.
    multiple n.
    occipital n.
    optic n.
    parenchymatous n.
    retrobulbar n.
    sciatic n.
    segmental n.
    suboccipital n.
    toxic n.
    traumatic n.
neuroallergy
neuroanastomosis
neuroanatomy
neuroarthropathy
neuroaugmentation
neuroaugmentive
neuroaxonal dystrophy
neurobiology
neurobiotactic movement
neurobiotaxis
neuroblast
neuroblastoma
    olfactory n.
neuroborreliosis
neurocardiac
neurocele
neurocentral
    n. joint
    n. suture
    n. synchondrosis
neurochemistry
neurochitin
neurochorioretinitis
neurochoroiditis
neurochronaxic theory
neurocirculatory asthenia
neurocladism
neurocranial granulomatous arteritis
neurocranium
    cartilaginous n.
    membranous n.
neurocristopathy
neurocutaneous
    n. melanosis
    n. syndrome
neurocyte
neurocytolysis

neurocytoma
neurodendrite
neurodendron
neurodermatitis
neurodynamic
neurodynia
neuroectoderm
neuroectodermal junction
neuroectomy
neuroencephalomyelopathy
neuroendocrine
    n. transducer cell
neuroendocrinology
neuroepithelial
    n. body
    n. cell
    n. layer of retina
neuroepithelium
    n. of ampullary crest
    n. of macula
neurofibra, pl. **neurofibrae**
    neurofibrae autonomicae
    neurofibrae postganglionicae
    neurofibrae preganglionicae
    neurofibrae somaticae
neurofibril
neurofibrillar network
neurofibrillary
    n. degeneration
    n. tangle
neurofibroma
    plexiform n.
    storiform n.
neurofibromatosis
    abortive n.
    central type n.
    incomplete n.
neurofilament
neuroganglion
neurogastric
neurogenesis
neurogenic, neurogenetic
    n. airway
    n. atrophy
    n. bladder
    n. claudication
    n. fracture
    n. tonus
neurogenous
neuroglia cell
neurogliacyte
neuroglial, neurogliar
neurogliomatosis
neurogram
neurography
neurohemal organ
neurohistology
neurohormone
neurohumoral
    n. secretion
    n. transmission
neurohypophysial hormone
neurohypophysis
neuroid
neurokeratin

neurolemma cell
neuroleptanalgesia
neuroleptanesthesia
neuroleptic
    n. agent
    n. malignant syndrome
neurolinguistic programming
neurolinguistics
neurologist
neurology
neurolymph
neurolymphomatosis
neurolysin
neurolysis
neurolytic
neuroma
    acoustic n.
    amputation n.
    n. cutis
    false n.
    fibrillary n.
    Morton n.
    plexiform n.
    n. telangiectodes
    traumatic n.
neuromalacia
neuromatosis
neuromelanin
neuromeningeal
neuromere
neuromimetic
neuromuscular
    n. blocking agent
    n. junction
    n. relaxant
    n. spindle
    n. system
neuromyasthenia
    epidemic n.
neuromyelitis optica
neuromyopathy
    carcinomatous n.
neuromyositis
neuron
    autonomic motor n.
    bipolar n.
    gamma motor n.
    ganglionic motor n.
    Golgi type I, II n.
    intercalary n.
    internuncial n.
    lower motor n.
    motor n.
    multipolar n.
    NANC n.
        nonadrenergic, noncholinergic
        neuron
    nonadrenergic, noncholinergic n.
    (NANC neuron)
    polymorphic n.
    postganglionic motor n.
    preganglionic motor n.
    pseudounipolar n.
    sensory n.
    somatic motor n.

    unipolar n.
    upper motor n.
    visceral motor n.
neuronal
    n. ceroid lipofuscinosis
    n. hyperplasia
    n. intestinal dysplasia
    n. migration abnormality
neurone
neuronephric
neuronevus
neuronitis
    vestibular n.
neuronopathy
    sensory n.
    X-linked recessive bulbospinal n.
neuronophage
neuronophagia, neuronophagy
neuron-specific enolase
neuronyxis
neuro-oncology
neuro-ophthalmology
neurootology
neuroparalysis
neuroparalytic
    n. keratitis
    n. keratopathy
neuropath
neuropathia epidemica
neuropathic
    n. albuminuria
    n. arthritis
    n. arthropathy
    n. bladder
    n. joint
neuropathogenesis
neuropathology
neuropathy
    acute motor axonal n.
    acute sensory motor axonal n.
    asymmetric motor n.
    n., ataxia, retinitis pigmentosa
    (NARP)
    auditory n.
    brachial plexus n.
    compression n.
    dapsone n.
    diabetic n.
    diphtherial n.
    entrapment n.
    familial amyloid n.
    giant axonal n.
    Graves optic n.
    heavy metal n.
    hereditary hypertrophic n.
    hereditary sensory radicular n.
    hypertrophic interstitial n.
    ischemic optic n.
    isoniazid n.
    lead n.
    leprous n.
    motor dapsone n.
    onion bulb n.
    symmetric distal n.
    vitamin B_{12} n.

N

neuropeptide
    n. Y
neuropharmacology
neurophilic
neurophonia
neurophysins
neurophysiology
neuropil
neuroplasm
neuroplasty
neuroplegic
neuroplexus
neuropodia
neuropore
    anterior n.
    caudal n.
    cranial n.
    posterior n.
    rostral n.
neuropraxia
neuropsychiatry
neuropsychologic, neuropsychological
    n. disorder
neuropsychology
neuropsychopathic
neuropsychopathy
neuropsychopharmacology
neuroradiology
neuroregulator
neurorelapse
neuroretinitis
    diffuse unilateral subacute n. (DUSN)
    Leber idiopathic stellate n.
    stellate n.
neurorrhaphy
neurosarcocleisis
neurosarcoidosis
neurosarcoma
neuroschwannoma
neurosciences
neurosecretion
neurosecretory
    n. cell
    n. substance
neurosis, pl. **neuroses**
    accident n.
    anxiety n.
    cardiac n.
    character n.
    combat n.
    compensation n.
    compulsive n.
    conversion hysteria n.
    depressive n.
    experimental n.
    hypochondriacal n.
    hysterical n.
    noogenic n.
    obsessional n.
    obsessive-compulsive n.
    oedipal n.
    pension n.
    posttraumatic n.
    torsion n.

    transference n.
    traumatic n.
neurosomatic junction
neurosplanchnic
neurospongium
Neurospora
neurosteroid
neurostimulator
neurosurgeon
neurosurgery
    functional n.
neurosuture
neurosyphilis
    asymptomatic n.
    meningeal n.
    meningovascular n.
    paretic n.
    tabetic n.
neurotaxis
neurotendinous
    n. organ
    n. spindle
neurotensin
neurotension
neurothekeoma
neurothele
neurotherapeutics, neurotherapy
neurotic
    n. disorder
    n. excoriation
    n. manifestation
neuroticism
neurotization
neurotize
neurotmesis
neurotome
neurotomy
    retrogasserian n.
neurotonic reaction
neurotoxic
neurotoxin
neurotransmission
neurotransmitter
    adrenergic n.
    cholinergic n.
neurotrauma
neurotripsy
neurotrophic
    n. atrophy
    n. keratitis
neurotrophy
neurotropic
    n. attraction
    n. virus
neurotropy, neurotropism
neurotrosis
neurotubule
neurovaccine
neurovaricosis, neurovaricosity
neurovascular
    n. bundle of Walsh
    n. flap
    n. sheath
neurovegetative
neurovirus

neurovisceral
neurula, pl. **neurulae**
neurulation
Neusser granule
neutral
    n. axis of straight beam
    n. buffered formalin fixative
    n. element
    n. fat
    n. lipid storage disease
    n. mutation
    n. occlusion
    n. oxide
    n. point
    n. reaction
    n. spirit
    n. stain
    n. zone
neutralization
    n. plate
    n. test
    viral n.
neutralize
neutralizing antibody
neutral red
neutro-
neutroclusion
neutron
    epithermal n.
    n. radiation
neutropenia
    cyclic n.
    periodic n.
neutropenic angina
neutrophil, neutrophile
    band n.
    n. chemotactant factor
    n. granule
    hypersegmented n.
    immature n.
    juvenile n.
    mature n.
    segmented n.
    stab n.
neutrophil-activating
    n.-a. factor
    n.-a. protein
neutrophilia
neutrophilic
    n. eccrine hidradenitis
    n. leukemia
    n. leukocyte
    n. leukocytosis
    n. leukopenia
neutrophilopenia
neutrophilous
neutrotaxis
    indifferent n.
    negative n.
    positive n.
nevi (*pl. of* nevus)
nevocyte
nevoid
    n. amentia
    n. hypertrichosis

nevoxanthoendothelioma
nevus, pl. **nevi**
    acquired n.
    n. anemicus
    n. araneus
    nevi, atrial myxoma, myxoid
      neurofibromas, and n.
    A-type n. cell
    balloon cell n.
    basal cell n.
    bathing trunk n.
    Becker n.
    blue n.
    blue rubber-bleb nevi
    B-type n. cell
    capillary n.
    n. cavernosus
    n. cell
    cellular blue n.
    n. comedonicus
    compound n.
    congenital n.
    C-type n. cell
    dysplastic n.
    epithelioid cell n.
    faun tail n.
    flame n.
    n. flammeus
    giant pigmented n.
    halo n.
    inflammatory linear verrucous
      epidermal n.
    intradermal n.
    Ito n.
    Jadassohn n.
    junction n.
    lentigines, atrial myxoma,
      mucocutaneous myxomas, and blue
      nevi (LAMB)
    linear epidermal n.
    n. lipomatosus
    n. lymphaticus
    nape n.
    oral epithelial n.
    Ota n.
    n. papillomatosus
    pigmented hair epidermal n.
    n. pigmentosus
    n. pilosus
    n. sebaceus
    spider n.
    n. spilus
    spindle cell n.
    Spitz n.
    strawberry n.
    Sutton n.
    n. unius lateris
    Unna n.
    n. vascularis, n. vasculosus
    n. venosus
    verrucous n.
    white sponge n.
    woolly hair n.
nevus vasculosus (*var. of* nevus
    vascularis)

N

new
- n. combination
- n. growth
- N. Hampshire rule
- n. methylene blue
- n. mutation
- N. World leishmaniasis
- n. yellow enzyme
- N. York Heart Association classification
- N. York virus
- N. Zealand mice

newberyite

newborn

Newcastle
- N. disease
- N. disease virus

Newcomer fixative

Newton
- N. disk
- N. law

newton (N)

newtonian
- n. aberration
- n. constant of gravitation
- n. flow
- n. fluid
- n. viscosity

newton-meter

nexins

Neyman-Pearson statistical hypothesis

Nezelof
- N. syndrome
- N. type of thymic alymphoplasia

NF
- National Formulary

ng
- nanogram

NGF
- nerve growth factor
- NGF antiserum

NHL
- non-Hodgkin lymphoma

N.H.S.
- National Health Service

NH₂-terminal

Ni
- nickel

niacin
- n. test

niacinamide

nialamide

nib

nicardipine

niche
- enamel n.
- Haudek n.

nick
- N. procedure
- n. translation

nickel (Ni)
- n. dermatitis

nickeloplasmin

Nickerson-Kveim test

nicking
- arteriovenous n.

niclosamide

nicofuranose

Nicolas-Favre disease

Nicolle stain for capsule

Nicol prism

nicotinamide

nicotinamide adenine dinucleotide (NAD, NADH)

nicotinamide adenine dinucleotide phosphate (NADP, NADP⁺, NADPH)

nicotinamide mononucleotide (NMN)

nicotinate

nicotinehydroxamic acid methiodide

nicotine stomatitis

nicotinic
- n. acid amide
- n. acid maculopathy
- n. cholinergic receptor
- n. receptor

nicotinic acid

nicotinic alcohol

nicotinomimetic

nicotinyl alcohol

nicotinyl tartrate

nicoumalone

nictation

nictitate

nictitating
- n. membrane
- n. spasm

nictitation

nidal

nidation

NIDDM
- non-insulin-dependent diabetes mellitus

nidogen

nidus, pl. **nidi**
- n. avis
- n. hirundinis

Niemann
- N. disease
- N. splenomegaly

Niemann-Pick
- N.-P. C1 disease (NPC)
- N.-P. cell
- N.-P. disease

Niewenglowski ray

nifedipine

nifenazone

nifuraldezone

nifuratel

nifuroxime

nigerose

night
- n. blindness
- n. hospital
- n. myopia
- n. pain
- n. sight
- n. soil
- n. sweat
- n. vision

nightguard

Nightingale
nightmare
nightshade
     deadly n.
night terrors
nigra
nigrities
     nigrities linguae
nigrosin, nigrosine
Nigrospora
nigrostriatal
NIH
     National Institutes of Health
nihilism
     therapeutic n.
nihilistic delusion
nikethamide
Nikiforoff method
Nikolsky sign
nil disease
Nile blue A
nimodipine
nimustine
nine mile fever
ninhydrin reaction
ninhydrin-Schiff stain
ninth cranial nerve [CN IX]
niobium (Nb)
Nipah virus
nipple
     accessory n.
     aortic n.
     n. line
     n. shield
niridazole
nirvana principle
nisin
nisoldipine
Nissen
     N. fundoplication
     N. operation
Nissl
     N. body
     N. degeneration
     N. granule
     N. stain
     N. substance
nit
Nitabuch
     N. layer
     N. membrane
     N. stria
niter
     cubic n.
     n. paper
nitinol filter
niton
nitrate
     n. respiration
nitrazepam
nitrendipine
nitric acid
     fuming n. a.
nitric oxide (NO·)

n. o. reductase
n. o. synthase (NO synthase)
nitridation
nitride
nitrification
nitrile
nitrimuriatic acid
nitrite
nitritoid reaction
nitrituria
nitroblue
     n. tetrazolium (NBT)
     n. tetrazolium test (NBT test)
nitrocellulose
nitrochloroform
nitro dye
nitrofurans
nitrofurantoin polyneuropathy
nitrofurazone
nitrogen (N)
     n. autotrophy
     n. balance
     blood urea n. (BUN)
     n. cycle
     n. distribution
     n. equivalent
     filtrate n.
     n. fixation
     heavy n.
     n. monoxide
     n. mustard (HN2)
     n. narcosis
     nonprotein n. (NPN)
     rest n.
     undetermined n.
     urea n.
     urinary n.
nitrogen-13 (^{13}N)
nitrogen-14 (^{14}N)
nitrogen-15 (^{15}N)
nitrogenase
nitrogen group
nitrogen lag
nitrogenous equilibrium
nitrogen partition
nitroglycerin
nitrohydrochloric acid
nitroid shock
nitromannitol
nitromersol
nitrometer
nitron
nitrophenylsulfenyl (Nps)
nitroprusside test
nitrosamine
nitroso-
S-nitrosohemoglobin
nitrosourea
nitrosyl
nitrous
     n. acid
     n. oxide
nitroxanthic acid
nitroxoline
nitroxy

N

nitroxyl
nitryl
nizatidine
njovera
NK
    natural killer
      NK cell
N.K.
    nomenklatur kommission
nkat
    nanokatal
Nle
    norleucine
NLN
    National League for Nursing
nM
    nanomolar
nm
    nanometer
NMDA
    N-methyl D-aspartate
      NMDA receptor
NMN
    nicotinamide mononucleotide
NMP
    nucleoside 5′-monophosphate
NMR
    nuclear magnetic resonance
      NMR imaging
NNN medium
NO·
    nitric oxide
No
    nobelium
no
    n. appreciable disease (N.A.D.)
    n. reflow phenomenon
Noack syndrome
nobelium (No)
Noble
    n. element
    n. gas
    n. metal
    N. position
    N. stain
Noble-Collip procedure
Nocardia
    N. asteroides
    N. brasiliensis
    N. caviae
    N. dacryolith
    N. farcinica
    N. gibsonii
    N. lurida
    N. madurae
    N. mediterranei
    N. nova
    N. orientalis
    N. otitidiscaviarum
    N. transvalensis
nocardia, pl. **nocardiae**
Nocardiaceae
nocardiasis
nocardioform
Nocardiopsis dassonvillei

nocardiosis
    granulomatous n.
nocebo
nociceptive
    n. reflex
nociceptor
nocifensor reflex
noctalbuminuria
nocte maneque (noct. maneq.)
noctiphobia
noct. maneq.
    nocte maneque
noctograph
nocturia
nocturnal
    n. amblyopia
    n. diarrhea
    n. dyspnea
    n. emission
    n. enuresis
    n. epilepsy
    n. myoclonus
    n. periodicity
    n. vertigo
nodal
    n. bigeminy
    n. bradycardia
    n. fever
    n. plane
    n. point
    n. rhythm
    n. tachycardia
    n. tissue
nodding spasm
node
    anterior tibial n.
    n. of Aschoff and Tawara
    atrioventricular n.
    AV n.
    Babès n.
    buccal n.
    buccinator n.
    n. of Cloquet
    coronary n.
    cystic n.
    delphian n.
    Dürck n.
    fibular n.
    Flack n.
    foraminal n.
    Haygarth n.
    Heberden n.
    hemal n.
    hemolymph n.
    Hensen n.
    intermediate lacunar n.
    jugulodigastric n.
    juguloomohyoid n.
    Keith n.
    Keith and Flack n.
    Koch n.
    lateral lacunar n.
    n. of ligamentum arteriosum
    lymph n. (*See* lymph node, lymph
      node)

malar n.
mandibular n.
medial lacunar n.
middle rectal n.
milker's n.
nasolabial n.
Osler n.
parietal n.
posterior tibial n.
primitive n.
promontorial common iliac n.
n. of Ranvier
Rosenmüller n.
n. of Rouviere
S-A n.
    sinoatrial node
sentinel n.
signal n.
singer's n.
sinoatrial n. (S-A node)
sinuatrial n.
sinus n.
subdigastric n.
subpyloric n.
suprapyloric n.
Tawara n.
teacher's n.
Troisier n.
Virchow n.
visceral n.
vital n.

nodi (*pl. of* nodus)
nodi lymphatici (*pl. of* nodus
  lymphaticus)
nodi lymphoidei (*pl. of* nodus
  lymphoideus)
nodose
n. ganglion
n. rheumatism
nodoventricular fiber
nodular
n. amyloidosis
n. arteriosclerosis
n. body
n. disease
n. episcleritis
n. fasciitis
n. headache
n. hidradenoma
n. histiocytic lymphoma
n. hyperplasia of prostate
n. iritis
n. leprosy
n. lymphoma
n. melanoma
n. mesoneuritis
n. non-X histiocytosis
n. opacity
n. panencephalitis
n. regenerative hyperplasia
n. scleritis
n. sclerosis
n. subepidermal fibrosis
n. transformation of the liver

n. tuberculid
n. vasculitis
nodulation
nodule
aggregated lymphatic n.
aggregated lymphoid n.
aggregated lymphoid n. of small
  intestine
Albini n.
apple jelly n.
Arantius n.
Aschoff n.
benign rheumatoid n.
Bianchi n.
Bohn n.
Busacca n.
Caplan n.
cold n.
Dalen-Fuchs n.
enamel n.
Gamna-Gandy n.
gastric lymphoid n.
Hoboken n.
hot n.
Jeanselme n.
juxtaarticular n.
laryngeal lymphoid n.
Lisch n.
lymph n.
lymphatic n.
lymphoid n.
malpighian n.
milker's n.
Morgagni n.
picker's n.
primary n.
pseudorheumatoid n.
pulp n.
rheumatoid n.
Sakurai-Lisch n.
Schmorl n.
secondary n.
n. of semilunar cusp
n. of semilunar valve
siderotic n.
singer's n.
solitary n. of intestine
solitary lymphatic n.
splenic lymph n.
vocal cord n.
nodulus, pl. **noduli**
n. caroticus
n. lymphaticus
noduli lymphoidei aggregati
  appendicis vermiformis
noduli lymphoidei solitarii
noduli valvularum semilunarium
nodus, pl. **nodi**
n. atrioventricularis
n. buccinatorius
n. sinuatrialis
n. sinuatrialis echo
n. tibialis anterior
nodus lymphaticus, pl. **nodi lymphatici**
nodi lymphatici cavales laterales

N

nodus lymphaticus *(continued)*
nodi lymphatici colici
nodi lymphatici comitantes nervi
  accessorii
nodi lymphatici iliaci communes
  mediales
nodi lymphatici iliaci externi
  laterales
nodi lymphatici iliaci externi
  mediales
nodi lymphatici pancreatici
  superiores
nodi lymphatici paravesiculares
nodi lymphatici postcavales
nodi lymphatici postvesiculares
nodi lymphatici preaortici
nodi lymphatici precavales
nodi lymphatici prevesiculares
nodi lymphatici vesicales laterales
nodus lymphoideus, pl. **nodi lymphoidei**
nodi lymphoidei abdominis
nodi lymphoidei accessorii
nodi lymphoidei anorectales
nodi lymphoidei appendiculares
n. l. arcus venae azygos
nodi lymphoidei axillares
nodi lymphoidei axillares anteriores
nodi lymphoidei axillares apicales
nodi lymphoidei axillares centrales
nodi lymphoidei axillares humerales
nodi lymphoidei axillares laterales
nodi lymphoidei axillares pectorales
nodi lymphoidei axillares posteriores
nodi lymphoidei axillares
  subscapulares
nodi lymphoidei brachiales
nodi lymphoidei brachiocephalici
nodi lymphoidei bronchopulmonales
n. l. buccinatorius
nodi lymphoidei capitis et colli
nodi lymphoidei centrales
nodi lymphoidei cervicales anteriores
nodi lymphoidei cervicales anteriores
  profundi
nodi lymphoidei cervicales anteriores
  superficiales
nodi lymphoidei cervicales laterales
  profundi
nodi lymphoidei cervicales laterales
  superficiales
nodi lymphoidei coeliaci
nodi lymphoidei colici dextri
nodi lymphoidei colici medii
nodi lymphoidei colici sinistri
nodi lymphoidei cubitales
n. l. cysticus
nodi lymphoidei epigastrici inferiores
nodi lymphoidei faciales
n. l. fibularis
n. l. foraminalis
nodi lymphoidei gastrici dextri
nodi lymphoidei gastrici sinistri
nodi lymphoidei gastroomentales
  dextri

nodi lymphoidei gastroomentales
  sinistri
nodi lymphoidei gluteales
nodi lymphoidei hepatici
nodi lymphoidei ileocolici
nodi lymphoidei iliaci communes
nodi lymphoidei iliaci communes
  promontorii
nodi lymphoidei iliaci externi
nodi lymphoidei iliaci interni
nodi lymphoidei inguinales profundi
nodi lymphoidei inguinales
  superficiales
nodi lymphoidei intercostales
nodi lymphoidei interiliaci
nodi lymphoidei interpectorales
nodi lymphoidei intrapulmonales
nodi lymphoidei jugulares anteriores
nodi lymphoidei jugulares laterales
n. l. jugulodigastricus
n. l. juguloomohyoideus
nodi lymphoidei juxtaesophageales
nodi lymphoidei juxtaesophageales
  pulmonales
n. l. lacunaris intermedius
n. l. lacunaris lateralis
n. l. lacunaris medialis
nodi lymphoidei lienales
n. l. ligamenti arteriosi
nodi lymphoidei linguales
nodi lymphoidei lumbales dextri
nodi lymphoidei lumbales intermedii
nodi lymphoidei lumbales sinistri
nodi lymphoidei abdominis
  viscerales
nodi lymphoidei juxtaintestinales
n. l. malaris
n. l. mandibularis
nodi lymphoidei mastoidei
nodi lymphoidei mediastinales
  anteriores
nodi lymphoidei mediastinales
  posteriores
nodi lymphoidei membri inferioris
nodi lymphoidei membri superioris
nodi lymphoidei mesenterici
nodi lymphoidei mesenterici
  inferiores
nodi lymphoidei mesenterici
  superiores
nodi lymphoidei mesocolici
n. l. nasolabialis
nodi lymphoidei obturatorii
nodi lymphoidei occipitales
nodi lymphoidei pancreatici
nodi lymphoidei
  pancreaticoduodenales
nodi lymphoidei pancreaticolienales
nodi lymphoidei pancreaticosplenales
nodi lymphoidei paracolici
nodi lymphoidei paramammarii
nodi lymphoidei pararectales
nodi lymphoidei parasternales
nodi lymphoidei paratracheales
nodi lymphoidei parauterini

nodi lymphoidei paravaginales
nodi lymphoidei parietales
nodi lymphoidei parotidei intraglandulares
nodi lymphoidei parotidei profundi
nodi lymphoidei parotidei profundi infra-auriculares
nodi lymphoidei parotidei profundi preauriculares
nodi lymphoidei parotidei superficiales
nodi lymphoidei pelvis
nodi lymphoidei pericardiales laterales
nodi lymphoidei phrenici inferiores
nodi lymphoidei phrenici superiores
nodi lymphoidei popliteales
nodi lymphoidei precaecales
nodi lymphoidei prelaryngeales
nodi lymphoidei prepericardiaci
nodi lymphoidei pretracheales
nodi lymphoidei prevertebrales
nodi lymphoidei promontorii
n. l. proximalis profundus
nodi lymphoidei pulmonales
nodi lymphoidei pylorici
nodi lymphoidei rectales superiores
n. l. rectalis medius
nodi lymphoidei retrocecales
nodi lymphoidei retropharyngeales
nodi lymphoidei retropylorici
nodi lymphoidei sacrales
nodi lymphoidei sigmoidei
nodi lymphoidei splenici
nodi lymphoidei subaortici
nodi lymphoidei submandibulares
nodi lymphoidei submentales
nodi lymphoidei subpylorici
nodi lymphoidei superiores centrales
nodi lymphoidei supraclaviculares
n. l. suprapyloricus
nodi lymphoidei thoracis
nodi lymphoidei thyroidei
n. l. tibialis posterior
nodi lymphoidei tracheobronchiales inferiores
nodi lymphoidei tracheobronchiales superiores
nodi lymphoidei viscerales

NOE
nuclear Overhauser effect
noematic
noesis
noetic anxiety
noeud vital
Noguchia
n. granulosis
noise
n. pollution
structured n.
white n.
noise-induced hearing loss
noma

Nomarski
N. interference microscopy
N. optics
nomenclatural type
nomenclature
binary n., binomial n.
Cleland n.
Nomenklatur Kommission (N.K.)
nomifensine maleate
Nomina Anatomica (NA)
nominal aphasia
nomogram
blood volume n.
cartesian n.
d'Ocagne n.
Radford n.
Siggaard-Andersen n.
nomograph
nomothetic
n. approach
nomotopic
nonabsorbable
n. ligature
n. surgical suture
nonaccommodative esotropia
nonadrenergic, noncholinergic neuron (NANC neuron)
non–A-E hepatitis
nonallele
nonanatomic tooth
nonan malaria
n-**nonanoic acid**
non-A, non-B (NANB)
non-A, non-B hepatitis
non-A, non-B hepatitis virus
non-A, non-B, non-C (NANBNC)
n.-A, n.-B, n.-C hepatitis (NANBNC hepatitis)
nonapeptide
non-arcon articulator
nonbacterial
n. thrombotic endocarditis
n. verrucous endocarditis
nonbullous congenital ichthyosiform erythroderma
nonbursate
noncariogenic
noncellular
nonchromaffin paraganglioma
nonchromogens
nonclassical phenylketonuria
nonclonogenic cell
noncohesive gold
noncomedogenic
noncommunicating
n. hydrocele
n. hydrocephalus
noncompetitive inhibition
noncomplementary role
non compos mentis
nonconjugative plasmid
noncontained disk herniation
nonconvulsive seizure
noncovalent bond
non–cycle-specific agent

N

nondeciduous placenta
nondepolarizing
    n. block
    n. neuromuscular blocking agent
    n. relaxant
nondiabetic glycosuria
nondirective psychotherapy
nondisease
nondisjunction
    primary n.
    secondary n.
nonelectrolyte
nonepileptic seizure
nonessential amino acids
nonestrogenic
nonfenestrated forceps
nonfilament polymorphonuclear leukocyte
nonfluent aphasia
nongonococcal urethritis
nongranular leukocyte
non-heme iron protein
non-Hodgkin lymphoma (NHL)
nonhomologous chromosome
nonhyperglycemic glycosuria
nonimmune
    n. agglutination
    n. fetal hydrops
    n. serum
nonimmunity
noninfectious
noninfiltrating lobular carcinoma
noninflammatory edema
non-insulin-dependent diabetes mellitus
    (NIDDM)
noninvasive
    n. positive pressure ventilation
nonionic
    n. contrast agent
    n. surfactant
nonisolated proteinuria
nonketotic
    n. hyperglycemia
    n. hyperglycinemia
nonlamellar bone
nonlipid histiocytosis
nonmaleficence
nonmedullated
    n. fiber
nonmotile leukocyte
nonmyelinated
nonneoplastic
nonneurogenic neurogenic bladder
non-newtonian fluid
non-nucleated
nonobstructive
    n. atelectasis
    n. jaundice
nonoccluded virus
nonocclusion
nonoestrogenic
nonorganic aphonia
nonose
nonossifying fibroma
nonosteogenic fibroma
nonovulational menstruation

nonoxynol 9
nonparametric
nonparous
nonparticipant observer
nonpedunculated hydatid
nonpenetrance
nonpenetrant trait
nonpenetrating
    n. keratoplasty
    n. wound
non per os (NPO, n.p.o.)
nonphasic sinus arrhythmia
nonpitting edema
non-PKU hyperphenylalaninemia
nonplasmatic compartment
nonpolar
    n. amino acid
    n. compound
    n. solvent
nonprecipitable antibody
nonprecipitating antibody
nonproprietary name
nonprotein nitrogen (NPN)
nonproteogenic
nonrandom mating
non-rapid eye movement (NREM)
nonreactive depression
nonreassuring fetal status
nonrebreathing
    n. anesthesia
    n. mask
    n. valve
nonrefractive accommodative esotropia
nonrenal azotemia
nonreset nodus sinuatrialis
nonresponder tolerance
nonrigid connector
nonrotation
    n. of intestine
    n. of kidney
nonsaponifiable
nonsecretor
nonsecretory myeloma
nonsense
    n. codon
    n. mutation
    n. suppression
    n. syndrome
    n. triplet
nonseptate mycelium
nonsexual generation
nonshivering thermogenesis
nonspecific
    n. anergy
    n. building-related illness
    n. cholinesterase
    n. immunity
    n. protein
    n. system
    n. therapy
    n. urethritis
    n. vaginitis
nonsteroidal antiinflammatory drug
    (NSAID)

nonstress test
nonsuppressible insulinlike activity (NSILA)
nonthrombocytopenic purpura
nontoxic
    n. goiter
    n. nodular goiter (NTNG)
nontransmural myocardial infarction (NTMI)
nontropical sprue
nontypeable *Haemophilus influenzae*
nonunion
nonuterotropic
nonvalent
nonvascular
nonvenereal syphilis
nonverbal
nonviable
nonvital
    n. pulp
    n. tooth
noogenic neurosis
Noonan syndrome
noradrenaline
    n. acid tartrate
    n. bitartrate
nordazepam
nordefrin hydrochloride
Nordhausen sulfuric acid
norepinephrine bitartrate
norethandrolone
norethindrone acetate
norethisterone
norethynodrel
norfloxacin
norgestrel
norleucine (Nle)
norm
norma, pl. **normae**
    n. anterior
    n. basilaris
    n. facialis
    n. frontalis
    n. inferior
    n. lateralis
    n. occipitalis
    n. posterior
    n. sagittalis
    n. superior
    n. temporalis
    n. ventralis
    n. verticalis
normal
    n. animal
    n. antibody
    n. antithrombin
    n. antitoxin
    n. bite
    n. cholesteremic xanthomatosis
    n. concentration (N)
    n. distribution
    n. electrical axis
    n. hearing
    n. horse serum

    n. human plasma
    n. human serum
    n. human serum albumin
    n. occlusion
    n. opsonin
    n. phosphate
    n. pressure hydrocephalus
    n. solution
    n. tartrate
    n. toxin
    n. value
normalization
normalize
normally posed tooth
normal-tension glaucoma
normative
normeperidine
normetanephrine
normethadone
normobaric
normoblast
normoblastosis
normocapnia
normocephalic
normochromia
normochromic
    n. anemia
normocyte
normocytic anemia
normocytosis
normoerythrocyte
normoglycemia
normoglycemic
    n. glycosuria
normokalemia, normokaliemia
normokalemic periodic paralysis
normospermatogenic sterility
normosthenuria
normotensive
normothermia
normotonic
normotopia
normotopic
normotriglyceridemic abetalipoproteinemia
normovolemia
normoxia
norophthalmic acid
norpipanone
Norrie disease
Norris corpuscle
norsteroids
norsympatol
norsynephrine
North
    N. American blastomycosis
    N. American Nursing Diagnosis Association (NANDA)
    N. Queensland tick fever
    N. Queensland tick typhus
Northern blot analysis
Norton operation
Norton-Simon hypothesis
nortriptyline hydrochloride
norvaline (Nva)

N

Norwalk
    N. agent
    N. virus
Norway itch
Norwegian scabies
Norwood
    N. operation
    N. procedure
noscapine
nose
    brandy n.
    cleft n.
    copper n.
    dog n.
    n. drops
    external n.
    hammer n.
    potato n.
    rum n.
    saddle n.
    toper's n.
nosebleed
nose-bridge-lid reflex
nose-eye reflex
Nosema corneum
Nosematidae
nosematosis
nosepiece
nosetiology
nosoacusis
nosochthonography
nosocomial pneumonia
nosogenesis, nosogeny
nosogenic
nosogeography
nosographic
nosography
nosologic
nosology
    psychiatric n.
nosomania
nosometry
nosomycosis
nosonomy
nosophilia
nosophobia
nosophyte
nosopoietic
Nosopsyllus
nosotaxy
nosotoxic
nosotoxicosis
nosotoxin
nosotrophy
nosotropic
nostalgia
nostomania
nostophobia
nostril
    internal n.
nostrum
NO synthase
    nitric oxide synthase
notal
notancephalia

notanencephalia
notatin
notch
    acetabular n.
    angular n.
    antegonial n.
    anterior n. of auricle
    anterior cerebellar n.
    anterior n. of cerebellum
    anterior n. of ear
    aortic n.
    n. of apex of heart
    auricular n.
    cardiac n.
    n. of cardiac apex
    cardiac n. of left lung
    cardial n.
    n. in cartilage of acoustic meatus
    clavicular n. of sternum
    costal n.
    cotyloid n.
    dicrotic n.
    digastric n.
    ethmoidal n.
    fibular n.
    frontal n.
    greater sciatic n.
    hamular n.
    Hutchinson crescentic n.
    iliosciatic n.
    inferior thyroid n.
    interarytenoid n.
    interclavicular n.
    intercondylar n.
    intertragic n.
    intervertebral n.
    ischiatic n.
    jugular n. of occipital bone
    jugular n. of petrous part of
     temporal bone
    jugular n. of sternum
    Kernohan n.
    lacrimal n.
    lesser sciatic n.
    n. for ligamentum teres
    mandibular n.
    marsupial n.
    mastoid n.
    nasal n.
    pancreatic n.
    parietal n.
    parotid n.
    popliteal n.
    posterior cerebellar n.
    posterior n. of cerebellum
    preoccipital n.
    presternal n.
    pterygoid n.
    pterygomaxillary n.
    radial n.
    Rivinus n.
    n. for round ligament of liver
    sacrosciatic n.
    scapular n.
    semilunar n.

sigmoid n.
sphenopalatine n.
sternal n.
superior thyroid n.
supraorbital n.
suprascapular n.
suprasternal n.
tentorial n.
n. of tentorium
terminal n. of auricle
trochlear n.
tympanic n.
ulnar n.
umbilical n.
vertebral n.

notched
n. tooth
note blindness
notencephalocele
Nothnagel syndrome
no-threshold concept
notifiable disease
notochord
notochordal
n. canal
n. plate
n. process
n. sheath
Notoedres cati
noumenal
nourishment
nous
novobiocin
Novy and MacNeal blood agar
noxa
noxious
noxythiolin
Np
neper
NPC
Niemann-Pick C1 disease
NPH insulin
NPN
nonprotein nitrogen
NPO, n.p.o.
non per os
Nps
nitrophenylsulfenyl
NREM
non-rapid eye movement
nRNA
nuclear RNA
NSAID
nonsteroidal antiinflammatory drug
NS echo
NSF
National Science Foundation
NSILA
nonsuppressible insulinlike activity
N terminus
NTMI
nontransmural myocardial infarction
NTNG
nontoxic nodular goiter

NTP
nucleoside 5′-triphosphate
nu, ν
n. body
nubecula
Nuc
nucleoside
nucha
nuchal
n. arm
n. cord
n. fascia
n. ligament
n. plane
n. region
n. rigidity
n. tubercle
Nuck
N. diverticulum
N. hydrocele
nuclear
n. atom
n. bag
n. bag fiber
n. cataract
n. chain fiber
n. chemistry
n. energy
n. envelope
n. factor-kappa B
n. family
n. fusion
n. hyaloplasm
n. inclusion body
n. jaundice
n. lamina
n. layer of retina
n. magnetic resonance (NMR)
n. magnetic resonance imaging
n. magnetic resonance tomography
n. magneton (μ_N)
n. matrix
n. medicine
n. membrane
n. ophthalmoplegia
n. Overhauser effect (NOE)
n. pacemaker
n. pore
n. reaction
N. Regulatory Commission
n. RNA (nRNA)
n. sap
n. sclerosis
n. spindle
n. stain
nuclear-cytoplasmic ratio
nuclease
azotobacter n.
micrococcal n.
mung bean n.
nucleated
nucleate endonuclease
nucleation
heterogeneous n.
homogeneous n.

N

nuclei (*pl. of* nucleus)
nucleic
  n. acid
  n. acid base
  n. acid hybridization
  n. acid probe
  infectious n. acid
nucleiform
nucleocapsid
nucleochylema
nucleochyme
nucleocortical fiber
nucleofilament
nucleohistone
nucleoid
  Lavdovsky n.
nucleolar
  n. chromosome
  n. organizer
  n. zone
nucleolar-nuclear ratio
nucleoli (*pl. of* nucleolus)
nucleoliform
nucleoloid
nucleolonema
nucleolus, pl. nucleoli
  chromatin n.
  false n.
  n. organizer
  n. organizer region
nucleomicrosome
nucleon
Nucleophaga
nucleophil, nucleophile
nucleophilic
nucleophosphatases
nucleoplasm
nucleoplasmic index
nucleoplasmin
nucleoprotein
nucleoreticulum
nucleorrhexis
nucleosidases
nucleoside (Nuc)
  n. bisphosphate
  n. diphosphate (NDP)
  n. diphosphate kinase
  n. diphosphate sugar
  n. monophosphate
  n. 5′-monophosphate (NMP)
  n. pair
  n. phosphorylase
  n. triphosphate
  n. 5′-triphosphate (NTP)
nucleoskeleton
nucleosome
nucleospindle
nucleotidase
nucleotide
  cyclic n.
  n. deletion
  flavin n.
  n. pair
  n. sequence
nucleotidyltransferase

nucleotoxin
nucleus, pl. nuclei
  abducens n.
  n. of abducens nerve
  n. abducentis
  nuclei accessorii tractus optici
  accessory cuneate n.
  n. of accessory nerve
  accessory olivary nuclei
  accessory nuclei of optic tract
  n. accumbens
  n. acusticus
  n. alae cinereae
  n. ambiguus
  ambiguus n.
  n. amygdalae
  n. amygdalae basalis lateralis
  n. amygdalae basalis medialis
  n. amygdalae centralis
  n. amygdalae corticalis
  n. amygdalae interstitialis
  n. amygdalae lateralis
  n. amygdalae medialis
  amygdaloid n.
  n. ansae lenticularis
  n. of the ansa lenticularis
  n. anterior
  anterior n.
  n. anterior corporis trapezoidei
  nuclei anteriores thalami
  n. anterior hypothalami
  anterior hypothalamic n.
  anterior interpositus n.
  anterior olfactory n.
  anterior periventricular n.
  anterior nuclei of thalamus
  anterior n. of trapezoid body
  n. anterodorsalis
  anterodorsal n. of thalamus
  n. anterolateralis
  anteromedial n.
  n. anteromedialis
  anteromedial n. of thalamus
  n. anteroventralis
  anteroventral n. of thalamus
  arcuate n.
  arcuate n. of thalamus
  n. arcuatus
  n. arcuatus of intermediate
    hypothalamic area
  n. arcuatus of medulla oblongata
  n. arcuatus thalami
  auditory n.
  autonomic nuclei
  basal nuclei
  nuclei basales
  basal n. of Ganser
  n. basalis of Ganser
  basket n.
  basolateral amygdaloid n.
  basomedial amygdaloid n.
  Bechterew n.
  benzene n.
  Blumenau n.
  branchiomotor n.

Burdach n.
caeruleun n.
n. caeruleus
n. campi dorsalis
n. campi medialis
n. campi ventralis
nuclei camporum perizonalium
caudal pontine reticular n.
caudate n.
n. caudatus
central n.
central amygdaloid n.
n. centralis
n. centralis lateralis
n. centralis tegmenti superior
central lateral n. of thalamus
centromedian n.
n. centromedianus
cerebellar n.
nuclei cerebelli
Clarke n.
cochlear nuclei
nuclei cochleares
n. cochlearis anterior
n. cochlearis posterior
nuclei colliculi inferioris
n. commissurae posterioris
convergence n. of Perlia
nuclei corporis geniculati medialis
nuclei corporis mamillaris
n. corporis mammillaris lateralis
n. corporis mammillaris medialis
nuclei corporis trapezoidei
cortical amygdaloid n.
nuclei of cranial nerve
cuneate n.
n. of cuneate fasciculus
n. cuneatus
n. cuneatus accessorius
n. cuneatus, pars centralis
n. cuneatus pars, rostralis
cuneiform n.
n. cuneiformis
n. of Darkschewitsch
Deiters n.
dentate n. of cerebellum
n. dentatus
descending n. of the trigeminus
diploid n.
dorsal n.
dorsal accessory olivary n.
n. dorsales thalami
n. of dorsal field
n. dorsalis
n. dorsalis corporis geniculati
  lateralis
n. dorsalis corporis trapezoidei
n. dorsalis hypothalami
n. dorsalis lateralis
n. dorsalis nervi vagi
dorsal lateral geniculate n.
dorsal motor n. of vagus
dorsal premammillary n.
dorsal septal n.
dorsal n. of thalamus

dorsal thoracic n.
dorsal n. of trapezoid body
dorsal vagal n.
dorsal n. of vagus
dorsolateral n.
dorsomedial n.
dorsomedial hypothalamic n.
dorsomedial n. of hypothalamus
n. dorsomedialis
n. dorsomedialis hypothalami
droplet n.
Edinger-Westphal n.
emboliform n.
n. emboliformis
endolemniscal n.
n. endolemniscalis
endopeduncular n.
n. endopeduncularis
external cuneate n.
facial n.
n. facialis
facial motor n.
n. fasciculi gracilis
fastigial n.
n. fastigii
filiform n.
n. filiformis
n. funiculi cuneati
n. funiculi gracilis
gametic n.
n. gelatinosus
gelatinous n.
geniculatus lateralis n.
germ n.
n. gigantocellularis medullae
  oblongatae
gigantocellular n. of medulla
  oblongata
globosus n.
n. globosus
n. of Goll
gonad n.
gracile n.
n. gracilis
Gudden tegmental n.
gustatory n.
habenular n.
n. habenularis lateralis
n. habenularis medialis
hypoglossal n.
n. of hypoglossal nerve
n. of inferior colliculus
inferior olivary n.
inferior salivary n.
inferior salivatory n.
inferior vestibular n.
intercalated n.
n. intercalatus
intermediolateral n.
n. intermediolateralis
intermediomedial n.
n. intermediomedialis
interpeduncular n.
n. interpeduncularis
n. interpositus

N

nucleus *(continued)*
interpositus n.
n. interpositus anterior
n. interpositus posterior
interstitial n.
interstitial amygdaloid n.
interstitial n. of anterior
  hypothalamus
interstitial n. of Cajal
n. interstitiales fasciculi
  longitudinalis medialis
nuclei interstitiales hypothalami
  anterioris
n. interstitialis
interstitial n. of medial longitudinal
  fasciculus
nuclei intralaminares thalami
intralaminar nuclei of thalamus
Klein-Gumprecht shadow nuclei
lateral n.
lateral amygdaloid n.
lateral cervical n.
lateral cuneate n.
lateral dorsal n.
lateral geniculate n.
n. of lateral geniculate body
lateral habenular n.
n. lateralis
n. lateralis cerebelli
n. lateralis corporis trapezoidei
n. lateralis medullae oblongatae
n. lateralis posterior
nuclei of lateral lemniscus
lateral n. of mammillary body
lateral n. of medulla oblongata
n. of the lateral olfactory tract
lateral parabrachial n.
lateral pericuneate n.
lateral posterior n.
lateral preoptic n.
lateral reticular n.
lateral septal n.
lateral superior olivary n.
lateral n. of thalamus
lateral n. of trapezoid body
lateral tuberal nuclei
lateral vestibular n.
nuclei lemnisci lateralis
n. of lens
lenticular n.
n. lentiformis
n. lentis
n. of Luys
n. of mammillary body
n. masticatorius
masticatory n.
medial n.
medial accessory olivary n.
medial amygdaloid n.
medial central n. of thalamus
medial dorsal n. of thalamus
nucleus mediales thalami
n. of medial field
medial geniculate nucleus

n. of medial geniculate body
medial habenular n.
n. medialis
n. medialis centralis thalami
n. medialis cerebelli
n. medialis corporis trapezoidei
n. medialis magnocellularis
n. medialis thalami
medial magnocellular n.
medial parabrachial n.
medial pericuneate n.
medial preoptic n.
medial septal n.
medial superior olivary n.
medial n. of thalamus
medial n. of trapezoid body
medial ventral n.
medial vestibular n.
median preoptic n.
mediodorsal n.
n. mediodorsalis
n. medioventralis
mesencephalic n. of trigeminal
  nerve
n. mesencephalicus nervi trigemini
Monakow n.
motor n.
motor n. of facial nerve
n. motorius nervi trigemini
motor n. of trigeminal nerve
motor n. of trigeminus
n. nervi abducentis
n. nervi accessorii
n. nervi cochlearis
n. nervi cranialis
n. nervi facialis
n. nervi hypoglossi
n. nervi oculomotorii
n. nervi phrenici
n. nervi trochlearis
n. nervi vestibulocochlearis
n. niger
oculomotor n.
n. of oculomotor nerve
n. olfactorius anterior
n. olivaris accessorius medialis
n. olivaris accessorius posterior
n. olivaris inferior
n. olivaris principalis
n. olivaris superior
n. olivaris superior lateralis
n. olivaris superior medialis
Onuf n.
oral pontine reticular n.
n. of origin
n. originis
parabigeminal n.
n. parabigeminalis
parabrachial n.
n. parabrachiales
n. parabrachialis lateralis
n. parabrachialis medialis
n. paracentralis thalami
paracentral n. of thalamus
paralemniscal n.

n. paralemniscalis
paramedial reticular n.
paranigral n.
n. paranigralis
parapeduncular n.
n. parapeduncularis
paraventricular n.
paraventricular n. of hypothalamus
n. paraventricularis hypothalami
pedunculopontine tegmental n.
n. pericuneatus lateralis
n. pericuneatus medialis
perifornical n.
n. perifornicalis
perihypoglossal nucleus
n. periolivares
periolivary n.
peripeduncular n.
n. peripeduncularis
peritrigeminal n.
n. peritrigeminalis
n. periventricularis posterior
n. periventricularis ventralis
periventricular preoptic n.
n. of perizonal field
Perlia n.
phenanthrene n.
phrenic n.
n. of phrenic nerve
pontine n.
n. pontis
pontobulbar n.
n. pontobulbaris
posterior n.
n. posterior
posterior accessory olivary n.
n. of posterior commissure
n. posterior hypothalami
n. posterior hypothalamic
posterior hypothalamic n.
posterior n. of hypothalamus
posterior interpositus n.
posterior medial n. of thalamus
n. posterior nervi vagi
posterior periventricular n.
posterior thoracic n.
posterior n. of vagus nerve
posterolateral n.
n. posterolateralis
posteromedial n.
n. posteromedialis
precommissural septal n.
pregeniculate n.
n. premammillaris dorsalis
n. premammillaris ventralis
n. preopticus lateralis
n. preopticus medialis
n. preopticus medianus
n. preopticus periventricularis
prerubral n.
pretectal n.
n. pretectales
n. principalis nervi trigemini
principal olivary n.

principal sensory n. of trigeminal nerve
principal sensory n. of the trigeminus
n. of pudendal nerve
n. pulposus
pulvinar n.
n. pulvinares
n. pyramidalis
pyrrole n.
raphe nucleus
nucleus raphes
red n.
reduction n.
reproductive n.
reticular n. of the brainstem
n. reticulares medullae oblongatae
n. reticulares mesencephali
n. reticularis pontis
n. reticularis pontis caudalis
n. reticularis pontis oralis
n. reticularis tegmenti pontis
n. reticularis thalami
reticular n. of medulla oblongata
reticular n. of mesencephalon
reticular n. of pons
reticular n. of thalamus
retroposterior lateral n.
n. reuniens
rhombencephalic gustatory n.
Roller n.
roof n.
n. ruber
n. saguli
sagulum n.
n. salivatorius inferior
n. salivatorius superior
Schwalbe n.
secondary sensory n.
segmentation n.
semilunar n. of Flechsig
n. sensorius superior nervi trigemini
sensory n.
n. septalis precommissuralis
septofimbrial n.
shadow n.
sole n.
n. of solitary tract
somatic n.
somatic motor n.
special visceral efferent n.
special visceral motor n.
sperm n.
spherical n.
n. spinalis nervi trigemini
spinal trigeminal n.
spinal n. of trigeminal nerve
spinal n. of the trigeminus
Spitzka n.
Staderini n.
steroid n.
Stilling n.
subcaeruleus n.
subcuneiform n.
n. subcuneiformis

N

nucleus (*continued*)
  subhypoglossal n.
  n. subhypoglossalis
  subparabrachial n.
  n. subparabrachialis
  subthalamic n.
  n. subthalamicus
  superior central tegmental n.
  superior olivary n.
  superior salivary n.
  superior salivatory n.
  superior vestibular n.
  suprachiasmatic n.
  n. suprachiasmaticus
  supralemniscal n.
  n. supralemniscalis
  n. supramammillaris
  supramammillary n.
  supraoptic n.
  supraoptic n. of hypothalamus
  n. supraopticus
  n. tecti
  tegmental n.
  n. tegmentalis pedunculopontinus
  n. tegmenti
  n. tegmenti pontis caudalis
  n. tegmenti pontis oralis
  terminal n.
  n. terminalis
  n. terminationis
  tetracyclic steroid n.
  thalamic gustatory n.
  n. thoracicus posterior
  n. tractus olfactorii lateralis
  n. tractus solitarii
  n. of trapezoid body
  triangular n.
  triangular n. of septum
  trochlear n.
  n. of trochlear nerve
  trophic n.
  tuberal n.
  n. tuberales laterales
  n. tuberomammillaris
  tuberomammillary n.
  ventral anterior n. of thalamus
  n. ventrales thalami
  n. of ventral field
  ventral intermediate n. of thalamus
  n. ventralis
  n. ventralis anterior
  n. ventralis corporis geniculi
    lateralis
  n. ventralis intermedius
  n. ventralis lateralis
  n. ventralis posterior intermedius
    thalami
  n. ventralis posterior thalami
  n. ventralis posterolateralis
  n. ventralis posteromedialis
  ventral lateral geniculate n.
  ventral lateral n. of thalamus
  ventral posterior intermediate n. of
    thalamus

  ventral posterior lateral n. of
    thalamus
  ventral posterior n. of thalamus
  ventral posterolateral n. of thalamus
  ventral posteromedial n. of thalamus
  ventral premammillary n.
  ventral principal n.
  ventral n. of thalamus
  ventral tier thalamic n.
  ventral n. of trapezoid body
  ventrobasal nucleus
  n. ventrobasales
  ventrolateral n.
  ventromedial n.
  ventromedial n. of hypothalamus
  n. ventromedialis hypothalami
  vestibular nucleus
  n. vestibulares
  n. vestibularis inferior
  n. vestibularis lateralis
  n. vestibularis medialis
  n. vestibularis superior
  vestibulocochlear n.
  n. viscerales nervi oculomotorii
  visceral nuclei of oculomotor nerve

nuclide
nude mouse
Nuel space
NUG
  necrotizing ulcerative gingivitis
Nuhn gland
null
  n. cell
  n. hypothesis
null-cell adenoma
nulligravida
nullipara
nulliparity
nulliparous
numb chin syndrome
number
  atomic n. (*Z*)
  Avogadro n. (N_A)
  Brinell hardness n. (BHN)
  CT n.
  electronic n.
  gold n.
  Hehner n.
  Hogben n.
  Hounsfield n.
  hydrogen n.
  iodine n.
  Kestenbaum n.
  Knoop hardness n.
  Koettstorfer n.
  linking n. (*L*)
  Loschmidt n. (n_0)
  Mach n.
  mass n.
  MIM n.
  Polenské n.
  Reichert-Meissl n.
  Reynolds n.
  saponification n.
  stoichiometric n.

thiocyanogen n.
transport n.
turnover n.
volatile fatty acid n.
wave n.
writhing n.
numbness
numerical
n. aperture
n. hypertrophy
n. taxonomy
nummiform
nummular
n. dermatitis
n. eczema
n. sputum
nummulation
nunnation
nun's murmur
nurse
n. cell
charge n.
clinical n. specialist
community n.
community health n.
dry n.
n. epidemiologist
flight n.
general duty n.
graduate n.
head n.
home health n.
hospital n.
infection control n.
licensed practical n. (LPN)
licensed vocational n. (LVN)
practical n.
n. practitioner
private n.
private duty n.
public health n.
registered n. (RN)
school n.
scrub n.
special n.
student n.
visiting n.
wet n.
nursemaid's elbow
nurse-midwife
certified n.-m. (CNM)
nursing
n. assignment
n. audit
n. bottle caries
n. home
n. model
n. plan of care
n. process
nutation
nutgall
nutmeg
n. liver
nutmeg oil

nutrient
n. agar
n. artery
n. artery of femur
n. artery of fibula
n. artery of humerus
n. artery of radius
n. artery of the tibia
n. artery of ulna
n. canal
n. enema
essential n.
n. foramen
n. medium
trace n.
n. vessel
nutrilites
nutrition
total parenteral n. (TPN)
nutritional
n. amblyopia
n. cirrhosis
n. dropsy
n. edema
n. energy
n. hemosiderosis
n. macrocytic anemia
n. marasmus
n. polyneuropathy
n. type cerebellar atrophy
nutritive
n. equilibrium
nutriture
Nuttallia
nux vomica
Nva
norvaline
nyctalgia
nyctalopia with congenital myopia
nyctanopia
nycterine
nycterohemeral
nycto-
nyctohemeral
nyctophilia
nyctophobia
Nyctotherus
nycturia
Nyhan
nylidrin hydrochloride
nymph
nympha, pl. **nymphae**
nymphal
nymphectomy
nymphitis
nymphocaruncular sulcus
nymphohymenal sulcus
nympholabial
nympholepsy
nymphomania
nymphomaniac
nymphomaniacal
nymphoncus
nymphotomy
nystagmic

N

nystagmiform
nystagmogram
nystagmograph
nystagmography
nystagmoid
nystagmus
    after-n.
    amaurotic n.
    n. blockage syndrome
    Bruns n.
    caloric n.
    cervical n.
    compressive n.
    congenital n.
    conjugate n.
    convergence-retraction n.
    deviational n.
    dissociated n.
    downbeat n.
    dysjunctive n.
    end-point n.
    fast component of n.
    fixation n.
    galvanic n.
    gaze paretic n.
    incongruent n.

    irregular n.
    jerky n.
    labyrinthine n.
    latent n.
    miner's n.
    minimal amplitude n.
    ocular n.
    opticokinetic n.
    optokinetic n.
    palatal n.
    pendular n.
    positional n.
    railroad n.
    rotational n.
    rotatory n.
    seesaw n.
    slow component of n.
    n. test
    upbeat n.
    vertical n.
    vestibular n.
    voluntary n.
nystatin
Nysten law
nyxis

Ω

ohm

O

orotidine
oxygen
    O agglutinin
    O antigen
    O colony
    O shell

^{15}O

oxygen-15

^{16}O

oxygen-16

^{17}O

oxygen-17

^{18}O

oxygen-18

OA

occipitoanterior position

oak apple
oasthouse urine disease
oat
    o. cell
    o. cell carcinoma
oath
oatmeal-tomato paste agar
OAV
    OAV dysplasia
    OAV syndrome
OB
    obstetrics
O'Beirne
    O. sphincter
    O. valve
obeliac
obeliad
obelion
Obermayer test
Obermeier spirillum
Obersteiner-Redlich
    O.-R. line
    O.-R. zone
Ober test
obese
obesity
    android o.
    gynecoid o.
    hypothalamic o.
    hypothalamic o. with hypogonadism
    o. index
    morbid o.
    simple o.
obex
obfuscation
OB/GYN
obidoxime chloride
object
    o. blindness
    o. choice
    o. constancy
    o. glass
    good o.

    o. libido
    o. relationship
    sex o.
    test o.
    transitional o.
objective
    achromatic o.
    apochromatic o.
    immersion o.
    o. optometer
    o. perimetry
    o. probability
    o. psychology
    o. sign
    o. symptom
    o. synonym
objective assessment data
objective vertigo (*var. of* vertigo)
obligate
    o. aerobe
    o. anaerobe
    o. parasite
oblique
    o. amputation
    o. arytenoid muscle
    o. auricular muscle
    o. bandage
    o. bundle of pons
    o. cord of interosseous membrane of forearm
    o. diameter
    o. facial cleft
    o. fiber of muscular layer of stomach
    o. fissure
    o. fissure of lung
    o. fracture
    o. head
    o. illumination
    left posterior o. (LPO)
    o. lie
    o. ligament of elbow joint
    o. line
    o. line of mandible
    o. line of thyroid cartilage
    o. muscle of auricle
    o. part of cricothyroid muscle
    o. pericardial sinus
    o. pontine fasciculus
    o. popliteal ligament
    o. projection
    o. ridge
    o. ridge of trapezium
    right anterior o. (RAO)
    right posterior o. (RPO)
    o. section
    o. sinus of pericardium
    o. vein of left atrium
obliquity
    Litzmann o.
    Nägele o.

O

obliquus
    o. capitis inferior muscle
    o. capitis superior muscle
obliterating
    o. arteritis
    o. endarteritis
obliteration
    osteoplastic o. of the frontal sinus
obliterative
    o. arachnoiditis
    o. bronchitis
    o. pericarditis
oblong
    o. fovea of arytenoid cartilage
    o. pit of arytenoid cartilage
oblongata
obnubilation
OBS
    organic brain syndrome
observer
    nonparticipant o.
    participant o.
obsession
    impulsive o.
    inhibitory o.
obsessional neurosis
obsessive
    o. behavior
    o. personality
obsessive-compulsive
    o.-c. neurosis
    o.-c. personality
    o.-c. personality disorder
obsolescence
obstacle sense
obstetric, obstetrical
    o. binder
    o. conjugate
    o. conjugate diameter
    o. conjugate of pelvic outlet
    o. forceps
    o. hand
    o. palsy
    o. paralysis
    o. position
    o. ultrasound
obstetrician
obstetrics (OB)
    o. and gynecology
obstinate
obstipation
obstruction
    closed loop o.
    ureteropelvic junction o.
    ureterovesical o.
obstructive
    o. appendicitis
    o. dysmenorrhea
    o. hydrocephalus
    o. jaundice
    o. murmur
    o. pneumonia
    o. sleep apnea
    o. thrombus
    o. uropathy

obstruent
obtund
obturating embolism
obturation
    intermittent self-o.
obturator
    o. appliance
    o. artery
    o. branch of pubic branch of inferior epigastric vein
    o. canal
    o. crest
    o. externus muscle
    o. fascia
    o. foramen
    o. groove
    o. hernia
    o. internus muscle
    o. lymph node
    o. membrane
    o. nerve
    o. tubercle
    o. vein
obtuse
obtusion
Occam's razor
occipital
    o. anchorage
    o. angle of parietal bone
    o. artery
    o. aspect
    o. belly of occipitofrontalis muscle
    o. bone
    o. border
    o. border of parietal bone
    o. border of temporal bone
    o. branch
    o. cerebral vein
    o. condyle
    o. emissary vein
    o. fontanelle
    o. forceps
    o. groove
    o. gyrus
    o. horn
    o. horn syndrome
    o. line
    o. lobe
    o. lobe of cerebrum
    o. lobe epilepsy
    o. lymph node
    o. margin
    o. margin of temporal bone
    o. neuralgia
    o. neurectomy
    o. neuritis
    o. operculum
    o. part of corpus callosum
    o. plane
    o. plexus
    o. point
    o. pole
    o. pole of cerebrum
    o. region of head
    o. sinus

o. somite
o. squama
o. stripe
o. triangle
o. vein

occipitalis
o. muscle
occipitalization
occipitoanterior position (OA)
occipitoatloid
occipitoaxial, occipitoaxoid
o. ligament
occipitobregmatic
occipitocollicular tract
occipitofacial
occipitofrontal
o. diameter
o. fasciculus
o. muscle
occipitofrontalis muscle
occipitomastoid suture
occipitomental
o. diameter
o. projection
occipitoparietal
occipitopontine
o. fiber
o. tract
occipitoposterior (OP)
o. position (OP)
occipitotectal
o. fiber
o. tract
occipitotemporal sulcus
occipitothalamic radiation
occipitotransverse position
occiput
occlude
occluded virus
occluder
occluding
o. centric relation record
o. frame
o. ligature
o. paper
o. relation
occlusal
o. adjustment
o. analysis
o. balance
o. caries
o. clearance
o. correction
o. curvature
o. disharmony
o. embrasure
o. force
o. form
o. harmony
o. imbalance
o. path
o. pattern
o. pivot
o. plane
o. position

o. pressure
o. radiograph
o. rest
o. rest bar
o. rim
o. scheme
o. surface of tooth
o. system
o. table
o. trauma
o. vertical dimension
o. wear

occlusion
abnormal o.
afunctional o.
anterior o.
balanced o.
bimaxillary protrusive o.
buccal o.
centric o.
coronary o.
distal o.
eccentric o.
edge-to-edge o.
end-to-end o.
functional o.
gliding o.
hyperfunctional o.
labial o.
lateral o.
lingual o.
mechanically balanced o.
mesenteric artery o.
mesial o.
neutral o.
normal o.
pathogenic o.
physiologic o.
physiologically balanced o.
posterior o.
postnormal o.
protrusive o.
o. of pupil
retrusive o.
o. rim
spherical form of o.
torsive o.
traumatic o.
traumatogenic o.
working o.

occlusive
o. dressing
o. ileus
o. meningitis
occlusometer
occult
o. bleeding
o. blood
o. border of nail
o. carcinoma
o. choroidal neovascularization
o. fracture
o. hydrocephalus
o. posterior laryngeal cleft

O

occupational
> o. disease
> o. hearing loss
> O. Safety and Health Administration (OSHA)
> o. therapy (OT)

Oceanospirillum
ocellus, pl. **ocelli**
ochlophobia
Ochoa law
ochratoxin
> o. A

ochre
> o. codon
> o. mutation

Ochrobactrum
ochrodermia
ochrometer
ochronosis
> exogenous o.

ochronotic arthritis
Ochsner
> O. clamp
> O. method

ocrylate
octacosanoic acid
octad
octafluoropropane
octamethyl pyrophosphoramide (OMPA)
octamylamine
octan
octandioic acid
octanoate
octanoic acid
octanoyl-CoA synthetase
octapeptide
octaploidy
octapressin
octavalent
octavus
Octomitidae
Octomitus hominis
octopamine
octose
octoxynol
octulose
octulosonic acid
octyl gallate
octylphenoxy polyethoxyethanol
ocular
> o. albinism
> o. albinism 1, 2, 3
> o. albinism with late-onset sensorineural deafness
> o. albinism with sensorineural deafness
> o. bobbing
> o. cicatricial pemphigoid
> compensating o.
> o. cone
> o. crisis
> o. cup
> o. dysmetria
> o. flutter

> o. humor
> Huygens o.
> o. hypertelorism
> o. larva migrans
> o. larva migrans granuloma
> o. lens
> o. micrometer
> o. migraine
> o. motor
> o. motor apraxia
> o. muscle
> o. myiasis
> o. myopathy
> o. nystagmus
> o. onchocerciasis
> o. paralysis
> o. pemphigoid
> o. prosthesis
> Ramsden o.
> o. rigidity
> o. scoliosis
> o. sparganosis
> o. tension (Tn)
> o. torticollis
> o. vertigo
> o. vesicle
> wide field o.

ocularist
ocular-mucous membrane syndrome
oculentum, pl. **oculenta**
oculi (*pl. of* oculus)
oculist
oculoauriculovertebral dysplasia
oculobuccogenital syndrome
oculocardiac reflex
oculocephalic reflex
oculocephalogyric reflex
oculocerebrorenal syndrome
oculocutaneous
> o. albinism
> o. syndrome

oculodentodigital dysplasia
oculodermal melanosis
oculodynia
oculoencephalic angiomatosis
oculofacial
oculography
> photosensor o.

oculogravic illusion
oculogyral illusion
oculogyria
oculogyric crisis
oculomandibulodyscephaly
oculomandibulofacial syndrome
oculomotor
> o. nerve [CN III]
> o. nucleus
> o. response
> o. root of ciliary ganglion
> o. sulcus of mesencephalon
> o. system

oculomotorius
oculonasal
oculopathy

oculopharyngeal
    o. dystrophy
    o. syndrome
oculoplethysmography
oculopneumoplethysmography
oculopupillary
oculosympathetic
oculovagal reflex
oculovertebral
    o. dysplasia
    o. syndrome
oculovestibulo-auditory syndrome
oculozygomatic
oculus, pl. **oculi**
    o. dexter (O.D.)
ocytocin
OD
    optic density
O.D.
    oculus dexter
o.d.
odaxesmus
odaxetic
odd chromosome
Oddi sphincter
odds
Odland body
odogenesis
odontagra
odontalgia dentalis
odontalgic
odontectomy
odonterism
odontiasis
odontinoid
odontitis
odontoameloblastoma
odontoblast
odontoblastic
    o. layer
    o. process
odontoblastoma
odontoclast
odontodynia
odontodysplasia
odontogenesis imperfecta
odontogenic
    o. cyst
    o. dysplasia
    o. fibroma
    o. keratocyst
    o. myxoma
odontogeny
odontoid
    o. process
    o. process of epistropheus
    o. vertebra
odontology
    forensic o.
odontoloxia, odontoloxy
odontolysis
odontoma
    ameloblastic o.
    complex o.
    compound o.

odontoneuralgia
odontonomy
odontonosology
odontoparallaxis
odontopathy
odontophobia
odontoplasty
odontoprisis
odontoptosis
odontorrhagia
odontoschism
odontoscope
odontoscopy
odontosis
odontotherapy
odontotomy
    prophylactic o.
odor
odorant binding protein
odoratism
odoriferous gland
odorimeter
odorimetry
odorivection
odorography
odorous
O'Dwyer tube
odynacusis
odynophagia
odynophonia
Oe
    oersted
oedipal
    o. neurosis
    o. period
    o. phase
oedipism
Oedipus complex
Oehl muscle
oenanthal
oersted (Oe)
oesophagostomiasis
Oesophagostomum
    O. apiostomum
    O. brevicaudum
    O. brumpti
    O. columbianum
    O. dentatum
    O. georgianum
    O. quadrispinulatum
    O. radiatum
    O. stephanostomum
    O. venulosum
oestradiol
oestrid
oestriol
oestrogen
oestrone
oestrosis
Oestrus
OFD
    orofaciodigital
    OFD syndrome
official formula
officinal

O

off-label indication
off-vertical rotation
Ofuji disease
Ogilvie syndrome
Ogino-Knaus rule
Ogston line
Ogston-Luc operation
Oguchi disease
Ogura operation
O'Hara forceps
OHI
    oral hygiene index
OHI-S
    simplified oral hygiene index
ohm (Ω)
ohmammeter
Ohm law
ohmmeter
ohne Hauch
Ohngren line
OI
    osteogenesis imperfecta
oi-
oidium, pl. **oidia**
oil
    absolute o.
    o. of American wormseed
    o. of anise
    o. bath
    o. of bay
    o. of bergamot
    betula o.
    o. of bitter almond
    o. of bitter orange
    bitter orange peel o.
    o. of cardamom
    o. of chenopodium
    o. of cherry laurel
    o. of cinnamon
    cinnamon o.
    o. of citronella
    o. of clove
    coal o.
    concrete o.
    o. of coriander
    corn o.
    o. of cubeb
    o. cyst
    o. of dwarf pine needles
    o. embolism
    essential o.
    ethereal o.
    o. of eucalyptus
    fatty o.
    o. of fennel
    fixed o.
    fusel o.
    o. gland
    o. immersion
    joint o.
    jojoba o.
    o. of juniper
    o. of lavender
    o. of lemon
    o. of lemon grass

    Lorenzo o.
    oil of o.
    oil of crispmint
    oil of curled mint
    oil of jojoba
    olive o.
    palm o.
    o. of pennyroyal
    o. of peppermint
    o. pneumonia
    red o.
    o. retention enema
    rock o.
    o. of rose
    o. of spearmint
    o. sugar
    sweet birch o.
    o. tumor
    o. of turpentine
    o. vaccine
    o. of vitriol
    volatile o.
    o. of wormwood
oily granuloma
ointment
    o. base
    blue o.
    eye o.
    hydrophilic o.
    mild mercurial ointment
    ophthalmic o.
Okazaki fragment
OKT cell
olamine
old
    O. World leishmaniasis
    o. yellow enzyme
Oldfield syndrome
oleaginous
oleander
oleandomycin phosphate
oleate
olecranon
    o. bursitis
    o. fossa
    o. process
    o. reflex
olefin
oleic acid
olein
oleo-
oleogomenol
oleogranuloma
oleoma
oleometer
oleopalmitate
oleoresin
oleosaccharum, pl. **oleosacchara**
oleostearate
oleosus
oleotherapy
oleovitamin A and D
oleum terebinthinae
oleyl alcohol
oleyl-CoA, oleyl-coenzyme A

olfactie, olfacty
olfaction
olfactology
olfactometer
olfactometry
olfactophobia
olfactory
    o. agnosia
    o. angle
    o. area
    o. aura
    o. bulb
    o. bundle
    o. cortex
    o. epithelium
    o. esthesioneuroblastoma
    o. fila
    o. foramen
    o. gland
    o. glomerulus
    o. groove
    o. groove of nasal cavity
    o. hallucination
    o. hyperesthesia
    o. hypesthesia
    o. membrane
    o. mucosa
    o. nerve [CN I]
    o. neuroblastoma
    o. organ
    o. peduncle
    o. pit
    o. placode
    o. pyramid
    o. receptor cell
    o. region of mucosa of nose
    o. region of nasal mucosa
    o. region of nose
    o. region of tunica mucosa of nose
    o. root
    o. stria
    o. sulcus
    o. sulcus of nasal cavity
    o. tract
    o. trigone
    o. tubercle
olfacty (*var. of* olfactie)
olibanum
oligamnios
oligemia
oligemic shock
olighidria, oligidria
oligo
oligoamnios
oligocholia
oligochylia
oligochymia
oligoclonal band
oligocystic
oligodactyly, oligodactylia
oligodendria
oligodendroblast
oligodendroblastoma
oligodendrocyte
oligodendroglia cell

oligodendroglioma
    anaplastic o.
    pleomorphic o.
oligodipsia
oligodontia
oligodynamic
oligogalactia
oligoglucan-branching glycosyltransferase
oligo-α-1,6-glucosidase
oligohydramnios
oligohydruria
oligolecithal
oligomenorrhea
oligomer
oligomorphic
oligonephronic
oligonucleotide
oligopepsia
oligopeptide
oligophrenia
    phenylpyruvate o.
oligoplastic
oligopnea
oligoptyalism
oligoria
oligosaccharide
oligosialia
oligospermia, oligospermatism
oligosymptomatic
oligosynaptic
oligothymia
oligotrichia
oligotrichosis
oligotrophia, oligotrophy
oligozoospermatism
oligozoospermia
oliguria
oliva, pl. **olivae**
    o. inferior
    o. superior
olivary
    o. body
    o. eminence
olive
    inferior o.
    o. oil
    superior o.
olive-tipped catheter
olivifugal
olivipetal
olivocerebellar tract
olivocochlear
    o. bundle
    o. fiber
    o. tract
olivopontocerebellar
    o. atrophy
    o. degeneration
olivospinal
    o. fiber
    o. tract
Ollier
    O. disease
    O. graft
    O. theory

O

Ollier-Thiersch graft
Olmsted syndrome
ololiuqui
olophonia
olympian forehead
Ombrédanne operation
ombrophobia
omega-oxidation theory
Omenn syndrome
omenta (*pl. of* omentum)
omental
    o. appendix
    o. branch
    o. bursa
    o. eminence of pancreas
    o. enterocleisis
    o. flap
    o. foramen
    o. sac
    o. tenia
    o. tuber
    o. tuberosity of liver
omentectomy
omentitis
omento-
omentofixation
omentopexy
omentoplasty
omentorrhaphy
omentovolvulus
omentulum
omentum, pl. omenta
    gastrocolic o.
    gastrohepatic o.
    gastrosplenic o.
    greater o.
    lesser o.
    o. majus
    o. minus
omentumectomy
omeprazole
Ommaya reservoir
omn. hor.
    omni hora
omnifocal lens
omni hora (omn. hor.)
omnipotence of thought
omnivorous
omoclavicular triangle
omohyoid muscle
omophagia
omothyroid
omotracheal triangle
OMP
    orotidylic acid
        OMP decarboxylase
        OMP pyrophosphorylase
OMPA
    octamethyl pyrophosphoramide
omphal-, omphalo-
omphalectomy
omphalelcosis
omphalic
omphalitis
omphalo- (*var. of* omphal-)

omphaloangiopagus
omphalocele
omphaloenteric
omphalomesenteric
    o. artery
    o. cord
    o. cyst
    o. duct
    o. duct cyst
omphalopagus
omphalophlebitis
omphalorrhagia
omphalorrhea
omphalorrhexis
omphalos
omphalosite
omphalospinous
omphalotomy
omphalotripsy
omphalovesical
omphalus
Omsk
    O. hemorrhagic fever
    O. hemorrhagic fever virus
Onchocerca volvulus
onchocerciasis
    ocular o.
onchocercid
Onchocercidae
onchocercoma
onchocercosis
Oncocerca
oncocyte
oncocytic
    o. adenoma
    o. carcinoma
    o. hepatocellular tumor
oncocytoma
oncofetal
    o. antigen
    o. marker
oncogene
    ras o.
oncogenesis
oncogenic virus
oncogenous
oncograph
oncography
oncologist
    radiation o.
oncology
    radiation o.
oncolysis
oncolytic
Oncomelania
oncometer
oncometric
oncometry
oncosis
oncosphere embryo
oncostatin M
oncotherapy
oncotic
    o. pressure
oncotomy

oncotropic
Oncovirinae
oncovirus
ondansetron
Ondine curse
one-carbon fragment
one-horned uterus
oneiric
oneirism
oneirocritical
oneirodynia
      o. activa
oneirology
oneirophrenia
one million electron-volts (Mev)
oniomania
onion bulb neuropathy
oniric
onko-
onlay
      o. graft
Onodi cell
on-off phenomenon
onomatomania
onomatophobia
onomatopoiesis
ontogenesis
ontogenetic
ontogenic homeostasis
ontogeny
ontology
Onuf nucleus
onyalai
onychalgia
onychatrophia, onychatrophy
onychauxis
onychectomy
onychia
      o. maligna
      o. sicca
onychoclasis
onychocryptosis
onychodystrophy
onychograph
onychogryposis
onychoheterotopia
onychoid
onychology
onycholysis
onychomadesis
onychomalacia
onychomycosis
onychopathology
onychopathy
onychophagy, onychophagia
onychophosis
onychoptosis
onychorrhexis
onychoschizia
onychosis
onychostroma
onychotillomania
onychotomy
onychotrophy

o'nyong-nyong
      o.-n. fever
      o.-n. virus
onyx
oocyesis
oocyst
oocyte
      primary o.
      secondary o.
oogenesis
oogenetic
oogenic, oogenous
oogonium, pl. oogonia
ookinesis, ookinesia
ookinete
oolemma
oomycosis
oophagia, oophagy
oophoralgia
oophorectomy
oophoritic cyst
oophoritis
oophorocystectomy
oophorocystosis
oophoron
oophoropathy
oophoropexy
oophoroplasty
oophororrhaphy
oophorosalpingectomy
oophorosalpingitis
oophorotomy
oophorrhagia
ooplasm
oosome
oosporangium
oospore
ootheca
ootid
ootype
OP
      occipitoposterior
      occipitoposterior position
opacification
opacifying gallstone
opacity
      nodular o.
      snowball o.
opal
      o. codon
      o. mutation
opalescent
      o. dentin
Opalski cell
opaque
      o. microscope
open
      o. angiography
      o. biopsy
      o. bite
      o. chain compound
      o. chest massage
      o. circuit method
      o. comedo
      o. cordotomy

O

open (*continued*)
    o. dislocation
    o. drainage
    o. drop anesthesia
    o. head injury
    o. heart surgery
    o. hospital
    o. laparoscopy
    o. pneumothorax
    o. reading frame
    o. reduction of fracture
    o. skull fracture
    o. system
    o. tuberculosis
    o. wound
open-angle glaucoma
opening
    access o.
    aortic o.
    o. of aqueduct of midbrain
    o. axis
    cardiac o.
    o. of carotid canal
    caval o. of diaphragm
    o. of cerebral aqueduct
    o. contraction
    o. of coronary sinus
    esophageal o.
    external o.
    o. of external acoustic meatus
    external o. of cochlear canaliculus
    external o. of urethra
    femoral o.
    o. of frontal sinus
    ileocecal o.
    o. of inferior vena cava
    internal acoustic o.
    o. of internal acoustic meatus
    internal urethral o.
    lacrimal o.
    o. movement
    oral o.
    orbital o.
    o. of papillary duct
    pharyngeal o. of eustachian tube
    pharyngeal o. of pharyngotympanic tube
    piriform o.
    o. of pulmonary trunk
    o. of pulmonary veins
    saphenous o.
    o. of smallest cardiac veins
    o. snap
    o. of the sphenoidal sinus
    o. of superior vena cava
    tendinous o.
    tympanic o. of canaliculus for chorda tympani
    tympanic o. of eustachian tube
    tympanic o. of pharyngotympanic auditory tube
    ureteral o.
    urethral o.
    uterine o. of uterine tubes

    o. of uterus
    vaginal o.
    vertical o.
    o. of vestibular canaliculus
operable
opera-glass hand
operant
    o. behavior
    o. conditioning
operate
operating
    o. microscope
    o. table
operation
    Altemeier o.
    Arlt o.
    arterial switch o.
    Ball o.
    Barkan o.
    Bassini o.
    Battista o.
    Belsey Mark o.
    Billroth I, II o.
    Blalock-Hanlon o.
    Blalock-Taussig o.
    bloodless o.
    Bozeman o.
    Bricker o.
    Brock o.
    Brunschwig o.
    Caldwell-Luc o.
    Carmody-Batson o.
    cesarean o.
    commando o.
    concrete o.
    Cotte o.
    cricoid split o.
    Dana o.
    Dandy o.
    Daviel o.
    debulking o.
    decompression o.
    Doyle o.
    Elliot o.
    Emmet o.
    endolymphatic shunt o.
    Estes o.
    fenestration o.
    filtering o.
    Finney o.
    flap o.
    Fontan o.
    formal o.
    Fothergill o.
    Frazier-Spiller o.
    Fredet-Ramstedt o.
    Freund o.
    Gilliam o.
    Gillies o.
    Gil-Vernet o.
    Glenn o.
    Graefe o.
    Gritti o.
    Halsted o.
    Hartmann o.

Heaney o.
Heller o.
Hill o.
Hoffa o.
Hofmeister o.
Hummelsheim o.
Hunter o.
interval o.
Jacobaeus o.
Jansen o.
Kasai o.
Kazanjian o.
Keen o.
Keller-Madlener o.
Kelly o.
Killian o.
Koerte-Ballance o.
Kondoleon o.
Kraske o.
Krönlein o.
Ladd o.
Lambrinudi o.
Laroyenne o.
Lash o.
LeCompte o.
Leriche o.
Lisfranc o.
Longmire o.
Luc o.
Madlener o.
major o.
Manchester o.
Mann-Williamson o.
Marshall-Marchetti-Krantz o.
Mayo o.
McIndoe o.
McVay o.
mika o.
Mikulicz o.
Miles o.
minor o.
morcellation o.
Motais o.
Mules o.
Mustard o.
Naffziger o.
Nissen o.
Norton o.
Norwood o.
Ogston-Luc o.
Ogura o.
Ombrédanne o.
Payne o.
Pólya o.
Pomeroy o.
Potts o.
pubovaginal o.
Putti-Platt o.
radical o. for hernia
Ramstedt o.
Rastelli o.
Récamier o.
Ridell o.
Ripstein o.
Roux-en-Y o.

Saenger o.
Schauta vaginal o.
Schroeder o.
Schuchardt o.
scleral buckling o.
Scott o.
second-look o.
Senning o.
seton o.
Shirodkar o.
Sistrunk o.
Smith o.
Smith-Boyce o.
Smith-Indian o.
Soave o.
Spinelli o.
stapes mobilization o.
Stoffel o.
Stookey-Scarff o.
Sturmdorf o.
subcutaneous o.
Syme o.
talc o.
TeLinde o.
Torek o.
Trendelenburg o.
Urban o.
Waters o.
Waterston o.
Wertheim o.
Whipple o.
Whitehead o.
operative
o. dentistry
o. myxedema
operator gene
opercula (*pl. of* operculum)
opercular
o. fold
o. part
operculated
operculitis
operculum, pl. **opercula**
o. ilei
occipital o.
trophoblastic o.
operon
Lac o.
ophiasis
Ophidia
ophidiasis
ophidiophobia
ophidism
ophritis
ophryitis
ophryogenes
ophryon
Ophryoscolecidae
ophryosis
ophryospinal angle
ophthalmalgia
ophthalmia
catarrhal o.
caterpillar-hair o.
Egyptian o.

O

ophthalmia *(continued)*
    gonorrheal o.
    granular o.
    metastatic o.
    o. neonatorum
    o. nivalis
    o. nodosa
    phlyctenular o.
    purulent o.
    spring o.
    sympathetic o.
    transferred o.
ophthalmic
    o. acid
    o. artery
    o. hyperthyroidism
    o. nerve [CN V1]
    o. ointment
    o. scoliosis
    o. solution
    o. vein
    o. vesicle
ophthalmodynamometer
    Bailliart o.
    suction o.
ophthalmodynamometry
ophthalmolith
ophthalmologist
ophthalmology
ophthalmomalacia
ophthalmomandibulomelic dysplasia
ophthalmomelanosis
ophthalmometer
ophthalmomycosis
ophthalmomyiasis
ophthalmopathy
    endocrine o.
    external o.
    Graves o.
    internal o.
ophthalmoplegia
    chronic progressive external o. (CPEO)
    exophthalmic o.
    o. externa
    external o.
    fascicular o.
    fibrotic o.
    o. interna
    internal o.
    internuclear o. (INO)
    nuclear o.
    orbital o.
    Parinaud o.
    o. partialis
    o. progressiva
    o. totalis
    wall-eyed bilateral internuclear o. (WEBINO)
ophthalmoplegic
    o. migraine
ophthalmoscope
    binocular o.
    demonstration o.

    direct o.
    indirect o.
ophthalmoscopic
ophthalmoscopy
    direct o.
    indirect o.
    o. with reflected light
ophthalmotrope
ophthalmovascular
opianine
opianyl
opiate
    o. intoxication syndrome
    o. receptor
opine
opiocortin
opioid antagonists
opiomelanocortin
opipramol hydrochloride
opisthenar
opisthiobasial
opisthion
opisthionasial
opisthocheilia, opisthochilia
opisthomastigote
opisthorchiasis
opisthorchid
Opisthorchiidae
Opisthorchis
    o. felineus
    o. sinensis
    o. viverrini
opisthotic
opisthotonic
opisthotonoid
opisthotonos, opisthotonus
Opitz
    O. BBB syndrome
    O. G syndrome
opium
    Boston o.
    deodorized o., denarcotized o.
    granulated o.
    powdered o.
    pudding o.
opobalsamum
opodidymus
Oppenheim
    O. disease
    O. reflex
    O. syndrome
oppilative
opponens
    o. digiti minimi muscle
    o. muscle
    o. pollicis muscle
opponent color
opportunistic pathogen
opposer
    o. muscle of little finger
    o. muscle of thumb
oppositional
    o. defiant disorder
opposure
opsin

opsinogen
opsiuria
opsoclonus
opsogen
opsomania
opsonic index
opsonin
    common o.
    immune o.
    normal o.
    specific o.
    thermolabile o.
    thermostable o.
opsonization
opsonocytophagic
opsonometry
opsonophilia
opsonophilic
optic, optical
    o. aberration
    o. activity
    o. agnosia
    o. alexia
    o. antipode
    o. ataxia
    o. axis
    o. canal
    o. capsule
    o. chiasm
    o. cup
    o. decussation
    o. density (OD)
    o. disk
    o. fissure
    o. foramen
    o. groove
    o. illusion
    o. image
    o. iridectomy
    o. isomerism
    o. keratoplasty
    o. layer
    o. nerve [CN II]
    o. nerve glioma
    o. nerve head
    o. nerve hypoplasia
    o. nerve sheath decompression
    o. nerve sheath fenestration
    o. neuritis
    Nomarski o.'s
    o. pachymeter
    o. papilla
    o. part of retina
    o. pit
    o. placode
    o. radiation
    o. recess
    o. righting reflex
    o. rotation
    o. rotatory dispersion (ORD)
    schlieren o.'s
    o. stalk
    o. tract
    o. vesicle
optician

opticianry
opticociliary
opticokinetic nystagmus
opticopupillary
optimism
    therapeutic o.
optimum
    o. dose
    o. pH
    o. temperature
optokinetic nystagmus
optomeninx
optometer
    objective o.
optometrist
optometry
optomyometer
optotypes
OPV
    oral poliovirus vaccine
ora (pl. of os)
ora, pl. orae
    o. serrata retinae
orad
oral
    o. auditory method
    o. biology
    o. cavity
    o. cavity proper
    o. contraceptive
    o. epithelial nevus
    o. erosive lichen planus
    o. fissure
    o. focal mucinosis
    o. hygiene
    o. lactose tolerance test
    o. membrane
    o. mucosa
    o. opening
    o. part of pharynx
    o. pathology
    o. pharynx
    o. phase
    o. physiotherapy
    o. plate
    o. poliovirus vaccine (OPV)
    o. pontine reticular nucleus
    o. primacy
    o. region
    o. shield
    o. smear
    o. stereotypy
    o. submucous fibrosis
    o. surgeon
    o. surgery
    o. tooth
    o. vestibule
orale
Oral Hygiene Index (OHI)
orality
orange
    o. G
    o. wood
Orbeli effect

O

orbicular
o. bone
o. ligament
o. ligament of radius
o. muscle
o. muscle of eye
o. muscle of mouth
o. process
o. zone of hip joint
orbiculare
orbicularis
o. muscle
o. oculi muscle
o. oculi reflex
o. oris muscle
o. phenomenon
o. pupillary reflex
orbiculus ciliaris
orbit
orbita
orbital
o. abscess
o. artery
o. axis
o. branch of maxillary nerve
o. branch of middle meningeal artery
o. branch of pterygopalatine ganglion
o. cavity
o. cellulitis
o. decompression
o. eminence of zygomatic bone
o. exenteration
o. fasciae
o. fat body
o. fat pad
o. gyri
o. height
o. hernia
o. implant
o. index
o. lamina of ethmoid bone
o. layer of ethmoid bone
o. margin
o. margin of eyelid
o. muscle
o. nerve
o. opening
o. ophthalmoplegia
o. part of frontal bone
o. part of inferior frontal gyrus
o. part of lacrimal gland
o. part of optic nerve
o. part of orbicularis oculi muscle
o. plane
o. plate
o. plate of ethmoid bone
o. process of palatine bone
o. region
o. rim
o. septum
o. sulcus
o. surface
o. tubercle
o. width
orbitale
orbitalis muscle
orbitofrontal
o. artery
o. cortex
orbitography
positive contrast o.
orbitomeatal
o. line
o. plane
orbitonasal index
orbitonometer
orbitonometry
orbitopagus
orbitopathy
dysthyroid o.
Graves o.
orbitosphenoid
orbitotomy
Orbivirus
orcein
orchalgia
orchectomy
orchella
orchialgia
orchichorea
orchidectomy
orchidic
orchiditis
orchidometer
orchidopexy
orchidoptosis
orchidorraphy
orchiectomy
orchiepididymitis
orchil
orchiocele
orchiodynia
orchioncus
orchioneuralgia
orchiopathy
orchiopexy
transseptal o.
orchioplasty
orchiorrhaphy
orchiotherapy
orchiotomy
orchis, pl. orchises
orchitic
orchitis
o. parotidea
traumatic o.
o. variolosa
orchotomy
orcin
orcinol test
orciprenaline sulfate
ORD
optic rotatory dispersion
ordeal bean
order
pecking o.

ordered
    o. on-random off mechanism
orderly
ordinal scale
ordinate
orectic
orexia
orexigenic
orf virus
organ
    accessory o.
    accessory o. of the eye
    annulospiral o.
    auditory o.
    Chievitz o.
    circumventricular o.
    Corti o.
    critical o.
    o. culture
    enamel o.
    end o.
    external female genital o.
    external male genital o.
    floating o.
    flower-spray o. of Ruffini
    genital o.
    Golgi tendon o.
    gustatory o.
    o. of hearing
    internal female genital o.
    internal male genital o.
    intromittent o.
    Jacobson o.
    neurohemal o.
    neurotendinous o.
    olfactory o.
    otolithic o.
    ptotic o.
    o. of Rosenmüller
    sense o.
    o. of smell
    spiral o.
    subcommissural o.
    subfornical o. (SFO)
    supernumerary o.
    tactile o.
    target o.
    o. of taste
    o. of touch
    urinary o.
    vascular o. of lamina terminalis
    vestibular o.
    vestibulocochlear o.
    vestigial o.
    o. of vision
    visual o.
    vomeronasal o.
    wandering o.
    Weber o.
    o. of Zuckerkandl
organa (*pl. of* organon) (*pl. of* organum)
organelle
    cell o.
    paired o.'s

organic
    o. acid
    o. brain syndrome (OBS)
    o. catalyst
    o. chemistry
    o. compound
    o. contracture
    o. delusion
    o. dental cement
    o. disease
    o. evolution
    o. hallucinosis
    o. headache
    o. hearing impairment
    o. mental disorder
    o. mood syndrome
    o. murmur
    o. pain
    o. phosphate
    o. principle
    o. stricture
    o. vertigo
organicism
organicist
organidin
organification defect
organism
    calculated mean o. (CMO)
    defective o.
    fastidious o.
    hypothetical mean o. (HMO)
    pleuropneumonia-like o.'s (PPLO)
organization
    health maintenance o.
    preferred provider o.
    pregenital o.
organize
organizer
    nucleolar o.
    nucleolus o.
    primary o.
    procentriole o.
organoaxial
organoferric
organogel
organogenesis
organogenetic, organogenic
organogeny
organography
organoid
    o. tumor
organoleptic
organology
organomegaly
organomercurial
organometallic
organon, pl. **organa**
organonomy
organonymy
organopathy
organopexy, organopexia
organophilic
organophilicity
organophosphate
organosol

O

organotaxis
organotherapy
organotrophic
organotropic
organotropism
organotropy
organ-specific
    o.-s. antigen
organum, pl. **organa**
    o. auditus
    organa genitalia
    organa genitalia feminina externa
    organa genitalia feminina interna
    organa genitalia masculina externa
    organa genitalia masculina interna
    o. gustatorium
    o. gustus
    organa oculi accessoria
    o. olfactus
    organa sensuum
    o. spirale
    o. subcommissurale
    o. subformicale
    o. tactus
    organa urinaria
    o. vasculosum laminae terminalis
    o. vestibulocochleare
    o. visus
    o. vomeronasale
orgasm
orgasmic, orgastic
Oriboca virus
oriens layer
Oriental
    O. boil
    O. button
    O. ringworm
    O. schistosomiasis
    O. sore
    O. ulcer
orientation
    sexual o.
Orientia
    o. tsutsugamushi
orienting
    o. reflex
    o. response
orientomycin
orifice
    anal o.
    aortic o.
    cardiac o.
    cardial o.
    esophagogastric o.
    o. of external acoustic meatus
    external urethral o.
    filling internal urethral o.
    gastroduodenal o.
    golf-hole ureteral o.
    ileal o.
    o. of ileal papilla
    ileocecal o.
    o. of inferior vena cava
    o. of internal acoustic meatus
    internal urethral o.

    left atrioventricular o.
    mitral o.
    pulmonary o.
    pyloric o.
    right atrioventricular o.
    root canal o.
    o. of superior vena cava
    tricuspid o.
    ureteric o.
    o. of uterus
    vaginal o.
    o. of vermiform appendix
    voiding internal urethral o.
orificial
orificium, pl. **orificia**
    o. externum uteri
    o. internum uteri
    o. ureteris
    o. urethrae externum
    o. vaginae
origanum oil
origin
    deep o.
    ectal o.
    ental o.
    pyrexia of unknown o. (PUO)
    real o.
    o. of replication
    superficial o.
oris
orizaba jalap root
Ormond disease
ornate
Ornish
    O. prevention diet
    O. reversal diet
ornithine
    o. acetyltransferase
    o. δ-aminotransferase
    o. carbamoyltransferase
    o. cycle
    o. decarboxylase
    o. transaminase
    o. transcarbamoylase
ornithinemia
ornithinuria
Ornithodoros
    O. coriaceus
    O. erraticus
    O. hermsi
    O. lahorensis
    O. moubata complex
    O. pappilipes
    O. parkeri
    O. rudis
    O. savigni
    O. talajé
    O. tholozani
    O. turicata
    O. venezuelensis
    O. verrucosus
Ornithonyssus
ornithosis
    o. virus
oroantral fistula

orodigitofacial dysostosis
orofacial fistula
orofaciodigital (OFD)
    o. syndrome
orolingual
oronasal
    o. fistula
    o. membrane
oropharyngeal
    o. isthmus
    o. membrane
    o. passage
oropharynx
Oropouche fever
orosomucoid
orotate phosphoribosyltransferase
orotic acid
orotic aciduria
orotidine (O)
    o. 5′-monophosphate
orotidinuria
orotidylate
orotidylic acid (OMP)
    o. a. decarboxylase
    o. a. phosphorylase
    o. a. pyrophosphorylase
orotracheal
    o. intubation
    o. tube
Oroya fever
orphan
    o. disease
    o. drug
    o. product
    o. receptor
    o. virus
orphenadrine citrate
orphenadrine hydrochloride
orris
Orsi-Grocco method
O-R system
Orth
    O. fixative
    O. stain
orthesis
orthetics
orthoacid
orthocaine
orthocephalic
orthocephalous
orthochromatic
orthochromophil, orthochromophile
orthocrasia
orthocytosis
orthodentin
orthodeoxia
orthodigita
orthodontia
orthodontic
    o. appliance
    o. band
    o. therapy
orthodontics
    surgical o.
orthodontist

orthodromic
orthogenesis
orthogenic
orthogenics
orthoglycemic glycosuria
orthognathia
orthognathic, orthognathous
    o. surgery
orthograde conduction
orthokeratology
orthokeratosis
orthokinetics
orthomechanical
orthomechanotherapy
orthomelic
orthometer
orthomolecular
    o. psychiatry
    o. therapy
Orthomyxoviridae
orthopedics
    dental o.
    functional jaw o.
orthopedic surgery
orthopedist
orthopercussion
orthophoria
orthophoric
orthophosphate
    inorganic o.
orthophosphoric acid
orthophrenia
orthopnea position
orthopneic position
Orthopoxvirus
orthoprosthesis
orthopsychiatry
Orthoptera
orthoptic
orthoptics
orthoptist
Orthoreovirus
orthoscope
orthoscopic
    o. lens
    o. spectacles
orthosis, pl. orthoses
    ankle-foot o.
    cervical o.
    cervicothoracic o.
    knee-ankle-foot o.
    thoracolumbosacral o.
    wrist-hand o.
orthostatic
    o. albuminuria
    o. hypopiesis
    o. hypotension
    o. proteinuria
    o. tachycardia
orthostereoscope
orthothanasia
orthotics
orthotist
orthotolidine
orthotonos, orthotonus

O

orthotopic
    o. graft
    o. ureterocele
orthotropic
orthovoltage
Ortolani
    O. maneuver
    O. test
orycenin
O.S.
os, pl. **ossa**
    o. acromiale
    anatomical internal o. of uterus
    o. basilare
    o. breve
    o. calcis
    o. capitatum
    ossa carpi
    o. centrale
    o. centrale tarsi
    o. clitoridis
    o. coccygis
    o. costale
    o. coxae
    ossa cranii
    o. cuboideum
    o. cuneiforme intermedium
    o. cuneiforme laterale
    o. cuneiforme mediale
    ossa digitorum
    o. ethmoidale
    external o. of uterus
    ossa faciei
    o. femoris
    o. frontale
    o. hamatum
    histological internal o. of uterus
    o. hyoideum
    o. iliacum
    o. ilium
    o. incae
    o. incisivum
    incompetent cervical o.
    o. innominatum
    o. intermaxillare
    o. intermedium
    o. intermetatarseum
    o. interparietale
    o. irregulare
    o. ischii
    o. japonicum
    o. lacrimale
    o. longum
    o. lunatum
    o. magnum
    o. malare
    ossa membri inferioris
    ossa membri superioris
    ossa metacarpalia I–V
    ossa metacarpi, pl. ossa metacarpalia
    ossa metatarsalia I–V
    ossa metatarsi, pl. ossa metatarsalia
    o. multangulum majus
    o. multangulum minus
    o. nasale

    o. naviculare
    o. naviculare manus
    o. occipitale
    o. odontoideum
    o. orbiculare
    o. palatinum
    o. parietale
    ossa pedis
    o. pisiforme
    o. planum
    o. pneumaticum
    o. premaxillare
    o. pterygoideum
    o. pubis
    o. pyramidale
    o. sacrum
    o. scaphoideum
    o. sesamoideum, pl. ossa sesamoidea
    o. sphenoidale
    o. subtibiale
    ossa suprasternalia
    o. suturarum
    o. sylvii
    ossa tarsalia
    ossa tarsi
    o. temporale
    o. tibiale posterius
    o. trapezium
    o. trapezoideum
    o. triangulare
    o. tribasilare
    o. trigonum
    o. triquetrum
    o. unguis
    o. uteri externum
    o. uteri internum
    o. vesalianum
    o. zygomaticum
os, pl. **ora**
osazone
oscheal
oscheoplasty
oscillating vision
oscillation
oscillator
oscillatory potential
oscillograph
oscillography
oscillometer
oscillometric
oscillometry
oscillopsia
oscilloscope
    cathode ray o. (CRO)
    storage o.
oscitate
oscitation
osculum, pl. **oscula**
Osgood-Schlatter disease
OSHA
    Occupational Safety and Health
    Administration
Osler
    O. disease

O. node
O. sign
Osler-Vaquez disease
osmate
osmatic
OSMED
    chondrodystrophy with sensorineural
      deafness
osmesis
osmic acid
osmic acid fixative
osmicate
osmication, osmification
osmics
osmiophilic
osmiophobic
osmium tetroxide
osmoceptor
osmodysphoria
osmogram
osmolal clearance
osmolality
    calculated serum o.
osmolar
osmolarity
osmole
osmology
osmometer
osmometry
osmophil, osmophilic
osmophobia
osmophore
osmoreceptor
osmoregulatory
osmose
osmosis
    reverse o.
osmosity
osmotherapy
osmotic
    o. diuresis
    o. diuretic
    o. fragility
    o. nephrosis
    o. pressure
    o. shock
osphresiologic
osphresiology
osphresiophilia
osphresiophobia
osphresis
osphretic
ossa (*pl. of* os)
ossein, osseine
osseocartilaginous
osseomucin
osseomucoid
osseous
    o. ampulla
    o. cell
    o. hydatid cyst
    o. labyrinth
    o. lacuna
    o. part of skeletal system
    o. polyp

o. spiral lamina
o. tissue
ossicle
    Andernach o.
    auditory o.
    Bertin o.
    epactal o.
    Kerckring o.
    ligament of auditory o.
ossicula (*pl. of* ossiculum)
ossicular
    o. chain
    o. reconstruction
ossiculectomy
ossiculotomy
ossiculum, pl. **ossicula**
    ossicula auditus
    ossicula mentalia
ossiferous
ossific
    o. center
ossification
    o. center
    endochondral o.
    intramembranous o.
    membranous o.
    metaplastic o.
ossiform
ossify
ossifying cartilage
osteal
ostealgia
osteanagenesis
osteanaphysis
ostectomy
ostein, osteine
osteitic
osteitis
    alveolar o.
    caseous o.
    central o.
    o. condensans ilii
    condensing o.
    cortical o.
    o. deformans
    o. fibrosa circumscripta
    o. fibrosa cystica
    o. fibrosa disseminata
    focal condensing o.
    hematogenous o.
    localized o. fibrosa
    multifocal o. fibrosa
    o. pubis
    renal o. fibrosa
    sclerosing o.
    o. tuberculosa multiplex cystica
ostemia
ostempyesis
osteoanagenesis
osteoarthritis
    hyperplastic o.
osteoarthropathy
    hypertrophic pulmonary o.
    idiopathic hypertrophic o.

O

osteoarthropathy *(continued)*
    pneumogenic o.
    pulmonary o.
osteoarthrosis
osteoblast
osteoblastic
osteoblastoma
osteocalcin
osteocartilaginous
osteochondritis
    o. deformans juvenilis
    o. deformans juvenilis dorsi
    o. dissecans
    syphilitic o.
osteochondrodysplasia
osteochondrodystrophia deformans
osteochondrodystrophy
osteochondrogenic cell
osteochondroma
osteochondromatosis
    synovial o.
osteochondrosarcoma
osteochondrosis
osteochondrous
osteoclasis, osteoclasia
osteoclast
    o. activating factor
osteoclastic
osteoclastoma
osteocollagenous fiber
osteocranium
osteocystoma
osteocyte
osteodentin
osteodermatopoikilosis
osteodesmosis
osteodiastasis
osteodynia
osteodysplasty
    Melnick-Needles o.
osteodystrophia
osteodystrophy
    Albright hereditary o.
    renal o.
osteoectomy
osteoepiphysis
osteofibroma
osteofibrosis
    periapical o.
osteogen
osteogenesis
    distraction o.
    o. imperfecta (OI)
    o. imperfecta congenita
    o. imperfecta congenita
    o. imperfecta tarda
    o. imperfecta tarda
    Type I, II, III, IV o. imperfecta
osteogenic, osteogenetic
    o. cell
    o. fiber
    o. layer
    o. sarcoma
    o. tissue

osteogenous
osteogeny
osteography
osteohalisteresis
osteohypertrophy
osteoid
    o. osteoma
    o. tissue
osteolipochondroma
osteologia
osteologist
osteology
osteolysis
osteolytic
osteoma
    o. cutis
    dental o.
    giant osteoid o.
    o. medullare
    osteoid o.
    o. spongiosum
osteomalacia
    infantile o.
    juvenile o.
    senile o.
osteomalacic
    o. pelvis
osteomatoid
osteomere
osteometry
osteomyelitis
    chronic diffuse sclerosing o.
    chronic focal sclerosing o.
    Garré o.
    Pseudomonas o.
osteomyelodysplasia
osteomyelofibrotic syndrome
osteon, osteone
osteoncus
osteonecrosis
osteonectin
osteopath
osteopathia
    o. condensans
    o. hemorrhagica infantum
    o. striata
osteopathic
    o. medicine
    o. physician
    o. scoliosis
osteopathology
osteopathy
    alimentary o.
    Doctor of O. (DO)
osteopedion
osteopenia
osteoperiosteal graft
osteoperiostitis
osteopetrosis
    o. acro-osteolytica
    o. with renal tubular acidosis
osteopetrotic
osteophage
osteophlebitis
osteophony

osteophyte
osteoplaque
osteoplast
osteoplastic
    o. amputation
    o. bone flap
    o. craniotomy
    o. necrotomy
    o. obliteration of the frontal sinus
osteoplasty
osteopoikilosis
osteoponin
osteopontin
osteoporosis
    o. circumscripta cranii
    juvenile o.
    posttraumatic o.
osteoporotic
    o. marrow defect
osteoprogenitor cell
osteoprotegerin
osteoradiologist
osteoradiology
osteoradionecrosis
osteorrhaphy
osteosarcoma
    parosteal o.
    periosteal o.
osteosclerosis
osteosclerotic
    o. anemia
osteosis
    parathyroid o.
    renal fibrocystic o.
osteospongioma
osteosteatoma
osteosuture
osteosynthesis
osteothrombosis
osteotome
osteotomy
    "C" sliding o.
    Dwyer o.
    horizontal o.
    Le Fort o.
    sagittal split mandibular o.
    segmental alveolar o.
    sliding oblique o.
    vertical o.
osteotribe
osteotrite
osteotrophy
osteotympanic
ostia (*pl. of* ostium)
ostial
    o. sphincter
ostiomeatal
    o. complex
    o. unit
ostitic
ostitis
ostium, pl. **ostia**
    o. abdominale tubae uterinae
    abdominal o. of uterine tube
    o. anatomicum

    o. aortae
aortic o.
    o. appendicis vermiformis
    o. arteriosum
    o. atrioventriculare dextrum
    o. atrioventriculare sinistrum
    o. cardiacum
    o. histologicum
    o. ileale
    o. ileocecale
    o. internum
    o. pharyngeum tubae auditivae
    o. pharyngeum tubae auditoriae
    o. primum
    o. pyloricum
    o. secundum
    o. sinus coronarii
    o. trunci pulmonalis
    o. tympanicum tubae auditivae
    o. ureteris
    o. urethrae externum
    o. urethrae internum
    o. urethrae internum accipiens
    o. urethrae internum evacuans
    o. uteri
    o. uteri externum
    o. uteri internum
    uterine o. of uterine tubes
    o. uterinum tubae uterinae
    o. vaginae
    o. venae cavae inferioris
    o. venae cavae superioris
    ostia venarum pulmonalium
    o. venosum cordis
    o. of vermiform appendix
ostomate
ostomy
ostosis
ostraceous
ostreotoxism
Ostrum-Furst syndrome
Ostwald solubility coefficient
OT
    occupational therapy
otalgia
    geniculate o.
    reflex o.
otalgic
Ota nevus
Ot antigen
OTC
    over-the-counter
Othello syndrome
other-directed
otic
    o. barotrauma
    o. capsule
    o. ganglion
    o. pit
    o. placode
    o. vesicle
otitic
    o. abscess
    o. hydrocephalus
    o. meningitis

O

otitis
> adhesive o.
> o. desquamativa
> o. externa
> o. interna
> malignant external o.
> o. media
> reflux o. media
> secretory o. media
> serous o. media

otoacoustic emission
otobiosis
Otobius
otocephaly
otocerebritis
otoconium, pl. **otoconia**
otocranial
otocranium
otocyst
Otodectes
otodectic
otodynia
otoencephalitis
otoganglion
otogenic, otogenous
otolaryngologist
otolaryngology
otolithic
> o. crisis
> o. membrane
> o. organ

otoliths, otolites
otologic
otologist
otology
otomandibular
> o. dysostosis
> o. syndrome

otomucormycosis
otomycosis
otoneuralgia
otopalatodigital syndrome
otopathy
otopharyngeal tube
otoplasty
otorhinolaryngology
otorrhea
> cerebrospinal fluid o.

otosalpinx
otosclerosis
otoscope
> Siegle o.

otoscopy
> pneumatic o.

otospondylomegaepiphyseal dysplasia
otospongiosis
otosteal
ototoxic
ototoxicity
> familial aminoglycoside o.

O-**(triethylaminoethyl) cellulose**
otto
> O. disease
> O. pelvis
> o. of rose

Ottoson potential
O.U.
ouabagenin
ouabain
Ouchterlony
> O. method
> O. technique
> O. test

ounce (oz.)
outer
> o. border of iris
> o. cone fiber
> o. limiting layer
> o. limiting membrane
> o. lip of iliac crest
> o. malleolus
> o. nuclear layer
> o. plexiform layer
> o. sheath of optic nerve
> o. spiral sulcus
> o. stripe of renal medulla
> o. table of skull
> o. zone of renal medulla

outlet
> o. forceps delivery
> pelvic o.
> thoracic o.

outlier
outline form
outpatient anesthesia
out of phase
output
> cardiac o.
> maximum power o.
> minute o.
> pacemaker o.
> stroke o.

outstanding ear
ova (*pl. of* ovum)
oval
> o. area of Flechsig
> o. corpuscle
> o. fasciculus
> o. foramen
> o. foramen of heart
> o. fossa
> o. window

ovalbumin
ovale malaria
ovalocytosis
ovaria (*pl. of* ovarium)
ovarialgia
ovarian
> o. amenorrhea
> o. artery
> o. branch of uterine artery
> o. bursa
> o. colic
> o. cortex
> o. cycle
> o. cyst
> o. dysmenorrhea
> o. fimbria
> o. follicle
> o. fossa

o. hormone
o. ligament
o. plexus
o. pregnancy
o. varicocele
o. vein
o. vein syndrome
ovariectomy
ovarioabdominal pregnancy
ovariocele
ovariocentesis
ovariocyesis
ovariodysneuria
ovariogenic
ovariolytic
ovariopathy
ovariorrhexis
ovariosalpingectomy
ovariosalpingitis
ovariostomy
ovariotomy
ovaritis
ovarium, pl. **ovaria**
o. bipartitum
o. disjunctum
o. gyratum
o. lobatum
o. masculinum
ovary
mulberry o.
polycystic o.
third o.
overanxious disorder
overbite
overclosure
overcompensation
overcorrection
overdenture
overdetermination
overdominance
overdominant
overdrive
overeruption
overextension
overflow
o. incontinence
o. wave
overgrafting
overhang
overhanging restoration
overhead projector
overhydration
overjet, overjut
overlap
horizontal o.
o. hybridization
vertical o.
overlay
o. denture
emotional o.
overlearning
overproduction theory
overresponse
overriding
o. aorta

overripe cataract
oversensing
overshoot
over-the-counter (OTC)
overt homosexuality
overtone
psychic o.
overvalued idea
overventilation
overwintering
ovicidal
oviducal
oviduct
oviductal
oviferous
oviform
ovigenesis
ovigenetic, ovigenic
ovigenous
ovigerous
ovigerus
ovine
oviparity
oviparous
oviposit
oviposition
ovipositor
ovist
ovocyte
ovoflavin
ovogenesis
ovoglobulin
ovoid
fetal o.
Manchester o.
ovolarviparous
ovomucin
ovomucoid
ovoplasm
ovoprotogen
ovosiston
ovotestis
ovotransferrin
ovovitellin
ovoviviparous
ovula (*pl. of* ovulum)
ovular
o. membrane
o. transmigration
ovulation
anestrous o.
o. inhibitor
paracyclic o.
ovulational sclerosis
ovulatory
ovule
ovulocyclic porphyria
ovulum, pl. **ovula**
ovum, pl. **ova**
alecithal o.
blighted o.
centrolecithal o.
fertilized o.
isolecithal o.
ova and parasite examination

O

ovum *(continued)*
    Peters o.
    telolecithal o.
Owen line
own control
Owren disease
ox
    o. bots
    o. heart
oxacillin sodium
oxalaldehyde
oxalate calculus
oxalemia
oxalic acid
oxalo
oxaloacetate transacetase
oxaloacetic acid
oxalosis
oxalosuccinic acid
oxalosuccinic carboxylase
oxalourea
oxaluria
oxaluric acid
oxalyl
oxalylurea
oxamniquine
oxanamide
oxandrolone
oxaphenamide
oxazepam
oxazin dye
oxazole
oxazolidinediones
oxazolidinones
oxeladin
Oxford unit
oxiconazole
oxidant
oxidase
    direct o.
    indirect o.
    o. reaction
    terminal o.
    o. test
oxidasis
oxidation
    alpha-o., α-oxidation
    beta-o., β-oxidation
    end o.
    omega-o., ω-oxidation
    terminal o.
α-oxidation *(var. of* alpha-oxidation)
β-oxidation *(var. of* beta-oxidation)
ω-oxidation *(var. of* omega-oxidation)
oxidation-reduction
    o.-r. electrode
    o.-r. indicator
    o.-r. potential (E_0^+)
    o.-r. reaction
    o.-r. system (O-R system)
oxidative
    o. deamination
    o. decarboxylation

    o. metabolism
    o. phosphorylation
oxide
    acid o.
    basic o.
    indifferent o.
    neutral o.
oxidize
oxidized
    o. cellulose
    o. glutathione
oxidoreductase
oxime
    amide o.
oximeter
    cuvette o.
oximetry
    pulse o.
oxirane
oxoacetic acid
oxo acid
3-oxoacid-CoA transferase
3-oxoacyl-ACP reductase
3-oxoacyl-ACP synthase
2-oxoglutarate dehydrogenase
2-oxoglutaric acid
2-oxo-5-guanidovaleric acid
oxolamine
oxolinic acid
oxonium ion
oxophenarsine hydrochloride
5-oxoprolinase
5-oxoproline (Glp)
4-oxoproline reductase
5-oxoprolinuria
17-oxosteroids
oxosuccinic acid
oxotremorine
oxprenolol hydrochloride
OXT
    oxytocin
oxtriphylline
oxyacoia, oxyakoia, oxyecoia
oxyaphia
oxybarbiturates
oxybenzone
oxybiotin
oxybutynin chloride
oxycalorimeter
oxycellulose
oxycephalia
oxycephalic, oxycephalous
oxycephaly
oxychloride
oxychromatic
oxychromatin
oxycodone
11-oxycorticoids
oxyecoia *(var. of* oxyacoia)
oxygen (O)
    o. affinity anoxia
    o. affinity hypoxia
    o. capacity
    o. consumption (Q_O, Q_{O2}, $\dot{V}_{O2}$)
    o. debt

o. deficit
o. deprivation theory of narcosis
o. effect
o. electrode
heavy o.
high pressure o.
hyperbaric o.
o. poisoning
singlet o.
o. tent
o. therapy
o. toxicity
triplet o.
o. utilization coefficient
oxygen-15 (^{15}O)
oxygen-16 (^{16}O)
oxygen-17 (^{17}O)
oxygen-18 (^{18}O)
oxygenase
mixed function o.
oxygenate
oxygenated hemoglobin
oxygenation
apneic o.
hyperbaric o.
oxygen-derived free radical
oxygenic
oxygenize
oxyheme
oxyhemochromogen
oxyhemoglobin (HbO$_2$)
oxyiodide
oxykrinin
oxyluciferin
oxymesterone
oxymetazoline hydrochloride
oxymetholone
oxymorphone hydrochloride
oxymyoglobin
oxynervone
oxyntic
o. cell
o. gland
oxypertine
oxyphenbutazone

oxyphencyclimine hydrochloride
oxyphenisatin acetate
oxyphenonium bromide
oxyphil, oxyphile
o. adenoma
o. cell
o. chromatin
o. granule
oxyphilic
o. carcinoma
o. leukocyte
oxyphonia
oxypolygelatin
oxypurine
oxypurinol
oxyrhine
oxyrygmia
Oxyspirura mansoni
oxytalan
oxytetracycline
oxythiamin
oxytocia
oxytocic
oxytocin (OXT)
arginine o.
o. challenge test
oxyuricide
oxyurid
Oxyuridae
Oxyuris
oz.
ounce
ozena
ozenous
ozocerite
ozokerite
purified o.
ozonator
ozone
ozonide
ozonolysis
ozonometer
ozonoscope
ozostomia

O

π (*var. of* pi)
Ψ

    psi
φ, Φ

    phi
P

    pressure
        P antigen
        P cell
        P element
        P enzyme
        P factor
        P selectin
        P substance of Lewis
        P wave
P-170, P-glycoprotein
^{33}**P**

    phosphorus-33
^{32}**P**

    phosphorus-32
P₁

    parental generation
Pᵢ

      pi cone monochromatism
P

    partial pressure
*P*_B

    barometric pressure
p

    pupil
p-
PA

      PA conduction time
      PA interval
      PA projection
P.A.

    physician assistant
Paas disease
PABA

    p-aminobenzoic acid
pablum
pabular
pabulum
pacchionian

    p. body
    p. corpuscle
    p. depression
    p. gland
    p. granulation
pacefollower
pacemaker

    artificial p.
    demand p.
    diaphragmatic p.
    ectopic p.
    electric cardiac p.
    electronic p.
    external p.
    p. failure
    fixed-rate p.
    nuclear p.
    p. output

    pervenous p.
    p. potential
    runaway p.
    p. sensitivity
    shifting p.
    subsidiary atrial p.
    p. syndrome
    transthoracic p.
    wandering p.
Pacheco parrot disease virus
pachometer
Pachon

    P. method
    P. test
pachyblepharon
pachycephalia
pachycephalic, pachycephalous
pachycephaly
pachycheilia, pachychilia
pachycholia
pachychromatic
pachychymia
pachydactylia
pachydactylous
pachydactyly
pachyderma

    p. laryngis
    p. lymphangiectatica
    p. verrucosa
    p. vesicae
pachydermatosis
pachydermodactyly
pachydermoperiostosis syndrome
pachyglossia
pachygnathous
pachygyria
pachyleptomeningitis
pachymeningitis

    p. externa
    hemorrhagic p.
    hypertrophic cervical p.
    p. interna
    pyogenic p.
pachymeningopathy
pachymeninx
pachymeter

    optic p.
pachynema
pachynsis
pachyntic
pachyonychia congenita
pachyotia
pachyperiostitis
pachyperitonitis
pachypleuritis
pachypodous
pachysomia
pachytene
pachyvaginalitis
pachyvaginitis

    pachyvaginitis cystica
pacing catheter

P

pacinian corpuscle
pacinitis
pack
    cold p.
    dry p.
    hot p.
    wet p.
packed
    p. cell volume
    p. human blood cell
packer
packing
    denture p.
    p. process
paclitaxel
PACS
    picture archive and communication system
pad
    abdominal p.
    dinner p.
    fat p.
    fat p. of ischioanal fossa
    heel p.
    knuckle p.'s
    laparotomy p.
    orbital fat p.
    Passavant p.
    periarterial p.
    pharyngoesophageal p.
    retromolar p.
    sucking p.
    suctorial p.
    threshold p.
Padykula-Herman stain
Paecilomyces lilacinus
paeciloycosis
PAF
    platelet-aggregating factor
PAGE
    polyacrylamide gel electrophoresis
Pagenstecher circle
Paget
    P. cell
    P. disease
Paget-Eccleston stain
pagetic
pagetoid
    p. cell
    p. reticulosis
Paget-von Schrötter syndrome
pagophagia
PAH
    p-aminohippuric acid
Pahvant
    P. Valley fever
    P. Valley plague
pain
    after-p.'s
    bearing-down p.
    expulsive p.
    false p.
    girdle p.
    growing p.
    hunger p.
    intermenstrual p.

    intractable p.
    labor p.
    middle p.
    night p.
    organic p.
    periodic bone p.
    phantom limb p.
    postprandial p.
    psychogenic p.
    p. reaction
    referred p.
    respirophasic p.
    rest p.
    somatoform p.
    p. threshold
    p. tolerance
painful
    p. anesthesia
    p. arc sign
    p. arc syndrome
    p. bruising syndrome
    p. heel
    p. hematuria
    p. paraplegia
    p. point
    p. toe
painless
    p. hematuria
    p. jaundice
pain-pleasure principle
paint
    carbol-fuchsin p.
    Castellani p.
painter's colic
pair
    base p.
    buffer p.
    chromosome p.
    conjugate acid-base p.
    line p.'s
    nucleoside p.
    nucleotide p.
    p. production
paired
    p. allosomes
    p. associates
    p. beats
    p. organelles
pairing
    chromosome p.
pajaroello
Palade granule
palatal
    p. abscess
    p. bar
    p. index
    p. myoclonus
    p. nystagmus
    p. papillomatosis
    p. plate
    p. reflex
    p. seal
    p. shelf
    p. triangle

palate
- bony p.
- Byzantine arch p.
- cleft p.
- falling p.
- Gothic p.
- hard p.
- p. hook
- p. myograph
- pendulous p.
- primary p.
- primitive p.
- secondary p.
- soft p.

palati (*pl. of* palatum)
palatiform
palatinase
palatine
- p. aponeurosis
- p. bone
- p. crest of horizontal process of palatine bone
- p. gland
- p. groove
- p. papilla
- p. process of maxilla
- p. raphe
- p. reflex
- p. ridge
- p. spine
- p. surface of horizontal plate of palatine bone
- p. tonsil
- p. torus
- p. uvula

palatinose
palatitis
palatoethmoidal suture
palatoglossal arch
palatoglossus muscle
palatognathous
palatogram
palatograph
palatomaxillary
- p. index
- p. suture

palatomyograph
palatonasal
palatopharyngeal
- p. arch
- p. muscle
- p. sphincter

palatopharyngeus
- p. muscle

palatopharyngoplasty
palatopharyngorrhaphy
palatoplasty
palatoplegia
palatorrhaphy
palatoschisis
palatouvularis muscle
palatovaginal
- p. canal
- p. groove

palatum, pl. **palati**

- p. durum
- p. fissum
- p. molle
- p. osseum

pale
- p. globe
- p. hypertension
- p. infarct
- p. thrombus

paleencephalon
paleocerebellum
paleocortex
paleokinetic
paleopathology
paleostriatal syndrome
paleostriatum
paleothalamus
Palfyn sinus
palikinesia, palicinesia
palinal
palindrome
palindromia
palindromic
- p. DNA
- p. encephalopathy
- p. sequence

palisade
- p. layer

palladium (Pd)
pallanesthesia
pallesthesia
pallesthetic sensibility
pallial
palliate
palliative treatment
pallidal syndrome
pallidectomy
pallidoamygdalotomy
pallidoansotomy
pallidotomy
pallidum
- dorsal p.
- p. dorsale
- ventral p.
- p. ventrale

pallium
pallor
- cachectic pallor

palm
- p. grasp
- liver p.
- p. oil
- p. wax

palma, pl. **palmae**
- p. manus

palmar
- p. aponeurosis
- p. branch of anterior interosseous nerve
- p. branch of median nerve
- p. branch of ulnar nerve
- p. carpal branch of radial artery
- p. carpal branch of ulnar artery
- p. carpal ligament
- p. carpal tendinous sheath

P

palmar *(continued)*
- p. carpometacarpal ligament
- p. crease
- p. digital vein
- p. fascia
- p. fibromatosis
- p. flexion
- p. interossei
- p. interosseous artery
- p. ligament
- p. ligament of interphalangeal joint of hand
- p. ligament of metacarpophalangeal joint
- p. metacarpal artery
- p. metacarpal ligament
- p. metacarpal vein
- p. monticuli
- p. plate
- p. psoriasis
- p. radiocarpal ligament
- p. reflex
- p. surface of finger
- p. ulnocarpal ligament

palmaris
- p. brevis muscle
- p. longus muscle

palmate fold of cervical canal
palm-chin reflex
palmellin
Palmer acid test
palmi (*pl. of* palmus)
palmic
palmin test
palmitaldehyde
palmitate
palmitic acid
palmitin
palmitin test (*var. of* palmin test)
palmitoleic acid
palmityl alcohol
palmodic
palmomental reflex
palmoplantar keratoderma
palmoscopy
palmus, pl. **palmi**
palpable rale
palpate
palpation
- bimanual p.
- light-touch p.

palpatopercussion
palpatory percussion
palpebra, pl. **palpebrae**
- p. III
- p. inferior
- p. superior
- p. tertia

palpebral
- p. branch of infratrochlear nerve
- p. conjunctiva
- p. fissure
- p. gland
- p. margin

- p. part of lacrimal gland
- p. part of orbicularis oculi muscle
- p. raphe
- p. vein

palpebralis
palpebrate
palpebration
palpebronasal fold
palpitatio cordis
palpitation
PALS
- periarterial lymphatic sheath

palsy
- Bell p.
- birth p.
- brachial birth p.
- bulbar p.
- cerebral p.
- crutch p.
- Dejerine-Klumpke p.
- diver's p.
- double elevator p.
- Erb p.
- extrapyramidal cerebral p.
- facial p.
- Klumpke p.
- lead p.
- obstetric p.
- posticus p.
- pressure p.
- progressive bulbar p.
- progressive supranuclear p.
- scrivener's p.
- shaking p.
- trembling p.

paludal fever
PAM
- potential acuity meter

2-PAM
- 2-pralidoxime

pamaquine
p-**aminohippurate clearance**
pamoate
pampiniform
- p. body
- p. venous plexus

pampinocele
panacea
panacinar emphysema
panagglutinable
panagglutinin
panangiitis
panarteritis
panarthritis
panatrophy
panblastic
panbronchiolitis
- diffuse p.

pancake kidney
pancarditis
pancervical smear
Pancoast
- P. syndrome
- P. tumor

pancolectomy
pancreas, pl. **pancreata**
    p. accessorium
    accessory p.
    anular p.
    Aselli p.
    p. divisum
    dorsal p.
    lesser p.
    p. minus
    small p.
    unciform p.
    uncinate p.
    ventral p.
    Willis p.
    Winslow p.
pancreatalgia
pancreatectomy
pancreatemphraxis
pancreatic
    p. abscess
    p. branch
    p. calculus
    p. cholera
    p. colic
    p. cystoduodenostomy
    p. deoxyribonuclease
    p. diabetes
    p. diarrhea
    p. digestion
    p. diverticulum
    p. dornase
    p. duct
    p. encephalopathy
    p. hyperglycemic hormone
    p. infantilism
    p. island
    p. islets
    p. juice
    p. lithiasis
    p. lymph node
    p. notch
    p. plexus
    p. polypeptide
    p. ribonuclease
    p. RNase
    p. sphincter
    p. steatorrhea
    p. vein
pancreaticoduodenal
    p. arterial arcades
    p. lymph node
    p. transplantation
    p. vein
pancreaticoduodenectomy
    pylorus-preserving p.
pancreaticoenteric recess
pancreaticosplenic lymph node
pancreatin
pancreatitis
    acute hemorrhagic p.
    calcareous p.
    calcific p.
    chronic p.
    chronic fibrosing p.
    chronic relapsing p.
pancreatocholecystostomy
pancreatoduodenectomy
pancreatoduodenostomy
pancreatogastrostomy
pancreatogenic
pancreatogenous diarrhea
pancreatography
pancreatojejunostomy
pancreatolith
pancreatolithectomy
pancreatolithiasis
pancreatolithotomy
pancreatolysis
pancreatolytic
pancreatomegaly
pancreatomy
pancreatopathy
pancreatopeptidase E
pancreatorenal syndrome
pancreatotomy
pancreatropic
pancreectomy
pancrelipase
pancreolith
pancreopathy
pancreozymin
pancreozymin-secretin test
pancuronium bromide
pancytopenia
    congenital p.
    Fanconi p.
pandemic
pandemicity
pandiculation
Pandy
    P. reaction
    P. test
panencephalitis
    nodular p.
    subacute sclerosing p. (SSPE)
panendoscope
panesthesia
Paneth granular cell
pang
    breast p.
panhidrosis
panhydrometer
panhyperemia
panhypopituitarism (PHP)
panhypopituitary dwarfism
panic
    p. attack
    p. disorder
    homosexual p.
panidrosis
panimmunity
panlobular emphysema
panmixis
panmyelophthisis
panmyelosis
Panner disease
panni (*pl. of* pannus)
pannicular hernia

P

panniculectomy
panniculitis
    alpha$_1$-antitrypsin deficiency p.
    cytophagic histiocytic p.
    lupus erythematosus p.
    poststeroid p.
    relapsing febrile nodular
      nonsuppurative p.
    subacute migratory p.
panniculus, pl. **panniculi**
    p. adiposus
    p. adiposus telae subcutaneae
      abdominis
    p. carnosus
    p. carnosus muscle
panning
pannus, pl. **panni**
    corneal p.
    p. crassus
    phlyctenular p.
    p. siccus
    p. tenuis
    trachomatous p.
panophthalmitis
panoptic stain
panoramic
    p. radiograph
    p. rotating machine
    p. x-ray film
panosteitis
panotitis
panphobia
Pansch fissure
pansclerosis
pansinuitis
pansinusitis
panspermia, panspermatism
pansporoblast
pansporoblastic
pansystolic murmur
pant
pantalgia
pantaloon hernia
pantamorphia
pantamorphic
pantanencephaly, pantanencephalia
pantaphobia
pantatrophia, pantatrophy
pantetheine
    p. kinase
    p. 4′-phosphate
pantethine
panthenol
pantoate
pantoate-activating enzyme
pantograph
pantoic acid
pantomogram
pantomograph
pantomography
pantomorphia
pantomorphic
pantonine

pantoscopic
    p. spectacles
    p. tilt
pantothenate synthetase
pantothenic acid
pantothenyl alcohol
pantoyl
pantoyltaurine
pantropic virus
Panum area
panzerherz
PAP
    3-phosphoadenosine 5-phosphate
    PAP technique
Pap
    P. smear
    P. test
papain, papainase
Papanicolaou
    P. examination
    P. smear
    P. smear test
    P. stain
papaveretum
papaverine
papaw
papaya
papayotin
paper
    articulating p.
    p. autoradiography
    chromatography p.
    p. chromatography
    Congo red p.
    filter p.
    high-quality filter p.
    p. mill worker's disease
    niter p.
    occluding p.
    p. plate
    potassium nitrate p.
    saltpeter p.
Papez circuit
papilla, pl. **papillae**
    acoustic p.
    basilar p.
    Bergmeister p.
    bile p.
    p. of breast
    circumvallate papillae
    clavate papillae
    conic papillae
    papillae conicae
    papillae corii
    papillae of corium
    dental p.
    dentinal p.
    p. dentis
    dermal papillae
    p. of dermis
    papillae dermis
    p. ductus parotidei
    p. duodeni major
    p. duodeni minor
    filiform p.

papillae filiformes
papillae foliatae
foliate papillae
fungiform papillae
papillae fungiformes
gingival p.
p. gingivalis
hair p.
ileal p.
p. ilealis
p. incisiva
incisive p.
interdental p.
p. interdentalis
interproximal p.
lacrimal p.
p. lacrimalis
lenticular papillae
lingual papillae
lingual gingival p.
lingual interdental p.
p. lingualis, pl. papillae linguales
major duodenal p.
p. mammae
minor duodenal p.
nerve p.
p. nervi optici
optic p.
palatine p.
parotid p.
p. parotidea
p. of parotid gland
p. pili
renal p.
p. renalis, pl. papillae renales
retrocuspid p.
tactile p.
papillae of tongue
urethral p.
p. urethralis
papillae vallatae, pl. papillae vallatae
vallate papillae
vascular papillae
p. of Vater
papillary, papillate
p. adenocarcinoma
p. adenoma of large intestine
p. carcinoma
p. cystadenoma lymphomatosum
p. cystic adenoma
p. duct
p. foramina of kidney
p. hidradenoma
p. layer
p. muscle
p. muscle dysfunction
p. muscle syndrome
p. process of caudate lobe of liver
p. ridge
p. stasis
p. tumor
papillectomy
papilledema
papilliferous

papilliform
papillitis
foliate p.
necrotizing p.
papilloadenocystoma
papillocarcinoma
papilloma
basal cell p.
p. canaliculum
p. diffusum
duct p.
p. durum
hard p.
Hopmann p.
p. inguinale tropicum
intracystic p.
intraductal p.
inverted p.
p. molle
Shope p.
soft p.
transitional cell p.
urothelial p.
villous p.
p. virus
zymotic p.
papillomatosis
confluent and reticulate p.
florid oral p.
juvenile p.
laryngeal p.
palatal p.
recurrent respiratory p.
subareolar duct p.
papillomatous
Papillomavirus
Papillon-Léage and Psaume syndrome
Papillon-Lefèvre syndrome
papilloretinitis
papillotomy
papillula, pl. **papillulae**
Papovaviridae
papovavirus
PAPP
p-aminopropiophenone
pappataci
p. fever
p. fever viruses
Pappenheimer body
Pappenheim stain
pappus
PAPS
adenosine 3'-phosphate 5'-phosphosulfate
papular
p. acrodermatitis of childhood
p. dermatitis of pregnancy
p. mucinosis
p. tuberculid
p. urticaria
papule
follicular p.
moist p.
mucous p.
piezogenic pedal p.

P

papule *(continued)*
      pruritic urticarial p.'s and plaques of pregnancy (PUPPP)
      split p.
papuloerythematous
papulonecrotic tuberculid
papulopustular
papulopustule
papulosis
      bowenoid p.
      lymphomatoid p.
      malignant atrophic p.
papulosquamous
papulovesicle
papulovesicular
PAPVR
      partial anomalous pulmonary venous return
papyraceous
      p. plate
      p. scar
par
para, para I, para II
para-actinomycosis
paraaminobenzoic acid
paraaortic body
para-appendicitis
parabanic acid
parabasal
      p. body
      p. filament
parabigeminal nucleus
parabiosis
parabiotic
paraboloid condenser
parabrachial nucleus
parabulia
paracanthoma
paracanthosis
paracarcinomatous
      p. encephalomyelopathy
      p. myelopathy
paracarmine stain
paracasein
paracellular transport
paracelsian method
paracenesthesia
paracentesis
paracentetic
paracentral
      p. artery
      p. branch of callosomarginal artery
      p. branch of pericallosal artery
      p. fissure
      p. lobule
      p. nucleus of thalamus
      p. scotoma
      p. sulcus
paracentric inversion
paracervical block anesthesia
paracervix
paracetaldehyde
paracetamol
parachlorophenol

paracholera
parachordal
      p. cartilage
      p. plate
parachroma
parachute
      p. deformity
      p. mitral valve
      p. reflex
parachymosin
paracicatricial emphysema
paracinesia, paracinesis
paracmasis
paracmastic
paracme
paracoccidioidal granuloma
Paracoccidioides brasiliensis
paracoccidioidin
paracoccidioidomycosis
paracolic
      p. gutter
      p. recess
paracolitis
paracolon bacillus
paracolpitis
paracolpium
paracone
paraconid
paracortex
paracousis
paracrine
paracusis, paracusia
      false p.
      p. loci
      Willis p.
paracyclic ovulation
paracyesis
paracystic pouch
paracystitis
paracystium
paracytic
paradenitis
paradental
paradentium
paradidymal
paradidymis, pl. **paradidymides**
paradipsia
paradox
      Weber p.
paradoxical
      p. contraction
      p. diaphragm phenomenon
      p. embolism
      p. extensor reflex
      p. flexor reflex
      p. incontinence
      p. movement of eyelids
      p. patellar reflex
      p. pupil
      p. pupillary phenomenon
      p. pupillary reflex
      p. respiration
      p. triceps reflex
      p. vocal cord movement
paradoxic pulse

paraduodenal
    p. fold
    p. fossa
    p. hernia
    p. recess
paradysentery bacillus
paraesophageal hernia
paraesthesia
paraffin
    p. cancer
    chlorinated p.
    hard p.
    liquid p.
    p. tumor
    p. wax
    white soft p.
    yellow soft p.
paraffinoma
Parafilaria multipapillosa
paraflagellate
paraflagellum, pl. paraflagella
paraflocculus ventralis
parafollicular cell
paraformaldehyde
parafrenal abscess
parafuchsin
paragammacism
paraganglioma
    nonchromaffin p.
paraganglion, pl. paraganglia
paraganglionic cell
paragene
paragenital tubule
parageusia
parageusic
paraglenoid
    p. groove
    p. sulcus
paraglottic space
paragnathus
paragnomen
paragonimiasis
Paragonimus
    P. granuloma
    P. kellicotti
    P. ringeri
    P. westermani
paragonorrheal
paragrammatism
paragraphia
Paraguay tea
parahepatic
parahiatal hernia
parahidrosis
parahippocampal gyrus
parahormone
parahypophysis
parainfluenza viruses
para I, para II (*var. of* para)
parajejunal fossa
parakappacism
parakeratosis
    p. pustulosa
    p. scutularis
parakinesia, parakinesis

paralalia literalis
paralambdacism
paraldehyde
paralemniscal nucleus
paraleprosis
paralepsy
paralexia
paralgesia
paralgia
paralipophobia
parallactic
parallax
    binocular p.
    heteronymous p.
    homonymous p.
    p. method
    stereoscopic p.
    p. test
    vertical p.
parallel
    p. attachment
    p. rays
parallelism
parallelometer
parallergic
paralogia, paralogism, paralogy
    thematic p.
paraluteal cell
paralutein cell
paralysis, pl. paralyses
    acute ascending p.
    p. agitans
    ascending p.
    Brown-Séquard p.
    bulbar p.
    central p.
    compression p.
    crossed p.
    crutch p.
    diphtherial p.
    diver's p.
    Duchenne-Erb p.
    Erb p.
    facial p.
    familial periodic p.
    faucial p.
    flaccid p.
    generalized p.
    ginger p.
    global p.
    glossolabiolaryngeal p.
    glossolabiopharyngeal p.
    glossopalatolabial p.
    glossopharyngeolabial p.
    Gubler p.
    hyperkalemic periodic p.
    hypokalemic periodic p.
    hysterical p.
    immune p.
    immunologic p.
    jake p.
    Klumpke p.
    Landry p.
    lead p.
    mimetic p.

P

paralysis *(continued)*
    mixed p.
    motor p.
    musculospiral p.
    normokalemic periodic p.
    obstetric p.
    ocular p.
    periodic p.
    peripheral facial p.
    postdiphtheritic p.
    posticus p.
    Pott p.
    pressure p.
    progressive bulbar p.
    pseudobulbar p.
    sensory p.
    sleep p.
    sodium-responsive periodic p.
    spastic spinal p.
    spinal p.
    supranuclear p.
    tick p.
    Todd p.
    Todd postepileptic p.
    vasomotor p.
    Zenker p.
paralyssa
paralytic
    p. dementia
    p. ectropion
    p. ileus
    p. miosis
    p. mydriasis
    p. rabies
    p. scoliosis
    p. strabismus
paralyze
paralyzing vertigo
paramagnetic
paramagnetism
paramammary lymph node
paramastigote
paramastoid process
Paramecium
paramedial reticular nucleus
paramedian
    p. artery
    p. incision
    p. lobule
    p. pontine branch of pontine artery
paramedic
paramedical
paramenia
paramesial
paramesonephric duct
parameter
    enzyme p.
    infection transmission p.
    practice p.
paramethadione
paramethasone acetate
parametria (*pl. of* parametrium)
parametrial

parametric
    p. abscess
    p. test
parametritis
parametrium, pl. **parametria**
paramimia
paramnesia
Paramoeba
paramolar
paramorphine
Paramphistomatidae
paramphistomiasis
Paramphistomum
paramusia
paramyloidosis
paramyoclonus multiplex
paramyotonia
    ataxic p.
    congenital p.
paramyotonus
Paramyxoviridae
Paramyxovirus
paranalgesia
paranasal
    p. sinus
paraneoplasia
paraneoplastic
    p. acrokeratosis
    p. encephalomyelopathy
    p. pemphigus
    p. syndrome
paranephric
    p. abscess
    p. body
    p. fat
paranephros, pl. **paranephroi**
paranesthesia
paraneural infiltration
paraneurone
parangi
paranigral nucleus
paranoia
    acute hallucinatory p.
    litigious p.
paranoiac
paranoid
    p. personality
    p. personality disorder
    p. schizophrenia
paranomia
paranuclear
    p. body
paranucleate
paranucleolus
paranucleus
paraomphalic
paraoperative
paraoral
paraovarian
paraoxon
parapancreatic
paraparesis
paraparetic
parapedesis
parapeduncular nucleus

paraperitoneal hernia
parapestis
parapharyngeal
    p. abscess
    p. space
paraphasia
    thematic p.
paraphasic
paraphia
paraphilia
paraphimosis palpebrae
paraphonia
paraphrasia
paraphysial, paraphyseal
    p. body
    p. cyst
paraphysis, pl. **paraphyses**
parapineal
paraplasm
paraplastic
paraplegia
    ataxic p.
    congenital spastic p.
    p. dolorosa
    p. in extension
    p. in flexion
    infantile spastic p.
    painful p.
    Pott p.
    spastic p.
    superior p.
paraplegic
parapneumonic effusion
Parapoxvirus
parapraxia
paraproctitis
paraproctium, pl. **paraproctia**
paraprostatitis
paraprotein
paraproteinemia
parapsoriasis
    p. en plaque
    p. guttata
    p. lichenoides
    p. lichenoides et varioliformis acuta
    small plaque p.
    p. varioliformis
parapsychology
paraquat
pararama
pararectal
    p. fossa
    p. lymph node
    p. pouch
pararenal
pararhotacism
pararosanilin
pararrhythmia
parasaccular hernia
parasacral
parasagittal
    p. plane
    p. section
parasalpingitis
Parascaris equorum

parascarlatina
paraseptal
    p. cartilage
    p. emphysema
parasexuality
parasigmatism
parasinoidal
    p. sinus
parasite
    accidental p.
    autistic p.
    autochthonous p.
    commensal p.
    euroxenous p.
    facultative p.
    heterogenetic p.
    heteroxenous p.
    incidental p.
    inquiline p.
    malignant tertian malarial p.
    obligate p.
    quartan p.
    specific p.
    spurious p.
    stenoxous p.
    temporary p.
    tertian p.
parasite-host ecosystem
parasitemia
parasitic
    p. chylocele
    p. cyst
    p. disease
    p. hemoptysis
    p. leiomyoma
    p. melanoderma
    p. thyroiditis
    p. twin
parasiticidal
parasiticide
parasitism
    multiple p.
parasitize
parasitocenose
parasitogenesis
parasitogenic
parasitoid
parasitologist
parasitology
parasitome
parasitophobia
parasitophorous vacuole
parasitosis
parasitotropic
parasitotropism
parasitotropy
parasol insertion
parasomnia
paraspinal line
parastasis
parasternal
    p. hernia
    p. line
    p. lymph node

P

parastriate
    p. area
    p. cortex
Parastrongylus
parasubiculum
parasympathetic
    p. ganglia
    p. nerve
    p. nervous system
    p. part of autonomic division of
      peripheral nervous system
    p. root of ciliary ganglion
    p. root of otic ganglion
    p. root of pelvic ganglion
    p. root of pterygopalatine ganglion
    p. root of submandibular ganglion
parasympatholytic
parasympathomimetic
parasympathotonia
parasynapsis
parasynovitis
parasyphilis
parasyphilitic
parasyphilosis
parasystole
parasystolic beat
parataxia
parataxic distortion
parataxis
paratenesis
paratenic host
paratenon
paraterminal
    p. body
    p. gyrus
parathion
parathormone
parathymia
parathyrin
parathyroid
    p. gland
    p. hormone (PTH)
    p. hormonelike protein (PLP)
    p. hormone-related peptide (PTHrP)
    p. hormone-related protein
    p. insufficiency
    p. osteosis
    p. tetany
parathyroidectomy
parathyroprival tetany
parathyrotropic, parathyrotrophic
paratope
paratracheal lymph node
paratrichosis
paratripsis
paratrophic
paratuberculous lymphadenitis
paratyphlitis
paratyphoid
    p. bacillus
    p. fever
paraumbilical vein
paraurethral
    p. duct
    p. gland

parauterine lymph node
paravaccinia virus
paravaginal lymph node
paravaginitis
paravalvular
paravenous
paraventricular
    p. nucleus
    p. nucleus of hypothalamus
paravertebral
    p. anesthesia
    p. ganglia
    p. gutter
    p. line
    p. triangle
paravesical
    p. fossa
    p. lymph node
    p. pouch
paraxial
    p. mesoderm
    p. ray
paraxon
Parazoa
parazoon
parchment
    p. crackling
    p. heart
    p. right ventricle
    p. skin
paregoric
pareira
parelectronomic
parencephalia
parencephalitis
parencephalocele
parencephalous
parenchyma
    p. glandulae thyroideae
    p. prostatae
    p. of prostate
    p. testis
    p. of testis
    p. of thyroid gland
parenchymal cell
parenchymatitis
parenchymatous
    p. cartilage
    p. cell of corpus pineale
    p. degeneration
    p. goiter
    p. hemorrhage
    p. mastitis
    p. neuritis
parent
    p. artery
    p. cell
    p. cyst
parental
    p. generation (P_1)
    p. rejection
parenteral
    p. absorption
    p. alimentation

p. hyperalimentation
p. therapy
parenteric fever
Parenti-Fraccaro syndrome
parepicele
parepididymis
parepithymia
parerethisis
paresis
divergence p.
general p.
paresthesia
paresthetic
Paré suture
paretic neurosyphilis
pareunia
pargyline hydrochloride
paridrosis
paries, pl. **parietes**
p. anterior gastris
p. anterior vaginae
p. caroticus cavi tympani
p. externus ductus cochlearis
p. inferior orbitae
p. jugularis cavi tympani
p. labyrinthicus cavi tympani
p. lateralis orbitae
p. mastoideus cavi tympani
p. medialis orbitae
p. membranaceus cavi tympani
p. membranaceus tracheae
p. posterior gastris
p. posterior vaginae
p. superior orbitae
p. tegmentalis cavi tympani
p. tympanicus ductus cochlearis
p. vestibularis ductus cochlearis
parietal
p. abdominal fascia
p. angle
p. bone
p. border
p. border of frontal bone
p. border of sphenoid bone
p. border of squamous part of
temporal bone
p. border of temporal bone
p. branch
p. branch of medial occipital artery
p. branch of middle meningeal
artery
p. branch of superficial temporal
artery
p. cell
p. eminence
p. emissary vein
p. eye
p. fistula
p. foramen
p. hernia
p. layer
p. layer of leptomeninges
p. layer of serous pericardium
p. layer of tunica vaginalis of
testis

p. lobe
p. lobe of cerebrum
p. lobe epilepsy
p. lymph node
p. margin
p. margin of frontal bone
p. margin of greater wing of
sphenoid
p. node
p. notch
p. pelvic fascia
p. peritoneum
p. plate
p. pleura
p. region
p. thrombus
p. tuber
p. vein
p. wall
parietofrontal
parietography
parietomastoid suture
parietooccipital
p. artery
p. branch of anterior cerebral artery
p. branch of posterior cerebral
artery
p. fissure
p. sulcus
parietopontine
p. fiber
p. tract
parietosphenoid
parietosplanchnic
parietosquamosal
parietotemporal
parietovisceral
Parinaud
P. conjunctivitis
P. oculoglandular syndrome
P. ophthalmoplegia
P. syndrome
Paris
P. green
P. line
P. yellow
parity
Park aneurysm
Parker-Kerr suture
Parkes Weber syndrome
Parkinson
P. disease
P. facies
parkinsonian
parkinsonism
Park-Williams fixative
paroccipital
p. process
parodontitis
parodontium
parodynia
parole
parolfactory
p. area
p. sulci

P

parolivary
paromomycin sulfate
paromphalocele
Parona space
paronychia
paroophoritic cyst
paroophoritis
paroöphoron
parorchidium
parorchis
parorexia
parosmia
parosphresia
parosteal
    p. fasciitis
    p. osteosarcoma
parosteitis
parosteosis, parostosis
parostitis
parotic
parotid
    p. abscess
    p. bed
    p. branch
    p. bubo
    p. duct
    p. fascia
    p. gland
    p. notch
    p. papilla
    p. plexus of facial nerve
    p. recess
    p. sheath
    p. space
    p. vein
parotidectomy
parotideomasseteric fascia
parotiditis
    epidemic p.
    postoperative p.
    punctate p.
parotidoauricularis
parotin
parotitis
parous
parovarian
parovariotomy
parovaritis
parovarium
paroxypropione
paroxysm
paroxysmal
    p. cerebral dysrhythmia
    p. cold hemoglobinuria
    p. hypertension
    p. nocturnal dyspnea
    p. nocturnal hemoglobinemia
    p. nocturnal hemoglobinuria
    p. sleep
    p. tachycardia
parricide
parrot
    P. disease
    p. fever

    p. jaw
    p. virus
parrot-beak nail
parry
    P. disease
    p. fracture
pars, pl. **partes**
    p. abdominalis aortae
    p. abdominalis ductus thoracici
    p. abdominalis esophagi
    p. abdominalis musculi pectorales majoris
    p. abdominalis plexus visceralis et ganglii visceralis
    p. abdominalis ureteris
    p. acromialis musculi deltoidei
    partes aequales (part. aeq.)
    p. alaris musculi nasalis
    p. alveolaris mandibulae
    p. amorpha
    p. anterior
    p. anterior commissurae anterioris
    p. anterior commissurae rostralis
    p. anterior faciei diaphragmatis hepatis
    p. anterior fornicis vaginae
    p. anterior linguae
    p. anularis vaginae fibrosae digitorum manus et pedis
    p. aryepiglottica musculi arytenoidei obliqui
    p. ascendens aortae
    p. ascendens duodeni
    p. ascendens musculi trapezii
    p. atlantica arteriae vertebralis
    p. autonomica systematis nervosi peripherici
    p. basalis
    p. basalis arteriae pulmonalis
    p. basalis arteriarum lobarium inferiorum pulmonis sinistri et dextri
    p. basilaris
    p. basilaris ossis occipitalis
    p. basilaris pontis
    p. buccopharyngea musculi constrictoris pharyngei superioris
    p. canalis nervi optici
    p. cardiaca gastricae
    p. cardiaca ventriculi
    p. cartilaginea septi nasi
    p. cartilaginea systematis skeletalis
    p. cartilaginea tubae auditivae
    p. cartilaginea tubae auditoriae
    p. cavernosa
    p. cavernosa arteriae carotidis internae
    p. ceca retinae
    p. centralis systematis nervosi
    p. centralis ventriculi lateralis
    p. ceratopharyngea musculi constrictoris pharyngis medii
    p. cerebralis arteriae carotidis internae

p. cervicalis arteriae carotidis internae
p. cervicalis arteriae vertebralis
p. cervicalis ductus thoracici
p. cervicalis esophagi
p. cervicalis medullae spinalis
p. chondropharyngea musculi constrictoris pharyngei medii
p. ciliaris retinae
p. clavicularis musculi deltoidei
p. clavicularis musculi pectoralis majoris
p. coccygea medullae spinalis
p. cochlearis nervi vestibulocochlearis
p. coeliacoduodenalis musculi (ligamenti) suspensorii duodeni
p. convoluta lobuli corticalis renis
p. corneoscleralis reticuli trabecularis sclerae
partes corporis humani
p. corticalis
p. corticalis arteriae cerebralis mediae
p. costalis diaphragmatis
p. costalis pleurae parietalis
p. cranialis partis parasympathetici divisionis autonomici systematis nervosi
p. craniocervicalis plexuum et gangliorum visceralium
p. cricopharyngea musculi constrictoris pharyngis inferioris
p. cruciformis vaginae fibrosae
p. cuneiformis vomeris
p. cupularis recessus epitympanici
p. cystica
p. descendens aortae
p. descendens duodeni
p. descendens ligamenti iliofemoralis
p. descendens musculi trapezii
p. dextra faciei diaphragmaticae hepatis
p. diaphragmatica pleurae parietalis
p. distalis adenohypophyseos
p. distalis prostatae
p. distalis urethrae prostaticae
partes dorsales musculorum intertransversariorum lateralium lumborum
p. dorsalis pontis
p. duralis fili terminalis
p. endocrina pancreatis
p. exocrina pancreatis
p. extraocularis arteriae et venae centralis retinae
p. fetalis placentae
p. flaccida membranae tympanae
p. frontalis corporis callosi
p. funicularis ductus deferentis
partes genitales femininae externae
partes genitales masculinae externae
p. glossopharyngea musculi constrictoris pharyngis superioris

p. granulosa
p. hepatica
p. hepatis dextra
p. hepatis sinistra
p. horizontalis duodeni
p. iliaca fasciae iliopsoaticae
p. inferior
p. inferior alae lobuli centralis
p. inferior duodeni
p. inferior ganglii vestibularis
p. inferior venae lingularis venae pulmonalis superioris sinistrae
p. infraclavicularis plexus brachialis
p. infralobaris venae posterioris venae pulmonalis superioris dextrae
p. infundibularis
p. inguinalis ductus deferentis
p. insularis
p. insularis arteriae cerebri mediae
p. interarticularis
p. intercartilaginea rimae glottidis
p. intermedia
p. intermedia adenohypophyseos
p. intermedia commissurae bulborum
p. intermedia urethrae masculinae
p. intermembranacea rimae glottidis
partes intersegmentales venarum pulmonum
p. intracranialis arteriae vertebralis
p. intracranialis nervi optici
p. intralaminaris nervi optici intralocularis
p. intralobaris (intersegmentalis) venae posterioris lobi superioris pulmonis dextri
p. intramuralis urethrae masculinae
p. intraocularis nervi optici
p. intrasegmentalis venae pulmonum
p. iridica retinae
p. labialis musculi orbicularis oris
p. lacrimalis musculi orbicularis oculi
p. laryngea pharyngis
p. lateralis arcus pedis longitudinalis
p. lateralis compartimenti antebrachii posterioris (extensorum)
p. lateralis fornicis vaginae
p. lateralis musculorum intertransversariorum posteriorum cervicis
p. lateralis nuclei accumbentis
p. lateralis ossis occipitalis
p. lateralis ossis sacri
p. lateralis venae lobi medii venae pulmonalis dextri superioris
p. libera membri inferioris
p. libera membri superioris
p. lumbalis diaphragmatis
p. lumbalis medullae spinalis
p. marginalis musculi orbicularis oris
p. mastoidea ossis temporalis
p. medialis arcus pedis longitudinalis

P

pars (*continued*)

p. medialis musculorum intertransversariorum posteriorum cervicis
p. medialis nuclei accumbentis
p. medialis venae lobi medii venae pulmonis dextri superioris
p. mediastinalis pleurae parietalis
p. mediastinalis pulmonis
p. membranacea septi interventricularis
p. membranacea septi nasi
p. membranacea urethrae masculinae
p. mobilis septi nasi
p. muscularis septi interventricularis cordis
p. mylopharyngeus musculi constrictoris pharyngis superioris
p. nasalis ossis frontalis
p. nasalis pharyngis
p. nervosa hypophyseos
p. nervosa retinae
p. obliqua musculi cricothyroidei
p. occipitalis corporis callosi
p. olfactoria tunicae mucosae
p. opercularis
p. optica retinae
p. oralis pharyngis
p. orbitalis
p. orbitalis glandulae lacrimalis
p. orbitalis musculi orbicularis oculi
p. orbitalis nervi optici
p. orbitalis ossis frontalis
p. ossea septi nasi
p. ossea systematis skeletalis
p. ossea tubae auditivae
p. ossea tubae auditoriae
p. palpebralis glandulae lacrimalis
p. palpebralis musculi orbicularis oculi
p. parasympathica divisionis automaticae systematis nervosi peripherici
p. patens arteriae umbilicalis
p. pelvica
p. pelvica ductus deferentes
p. pelvica ureteris
p. peripherica systematis nervosi
p. perpendicularis
p. petrosa arteriae carotidis internae
p. petrosa ossis temporalis
p. phallica
p. pharyngea hypophyseos
p. phrenicocoeliaca musculi (ligamenti) suspensorii duodeni
p. pialis fili terminalis
p. pigmentosa
p. plana
p. postcommunicalis arteriae cerebri anterioris
p. posterior commissurae anterioris
p. posterior faciei diaphragmatis hepatis
p. posterior fornicis vaginae

p. posterior linguae
p. postlaminaris nervi optici intraocularis
p. postsulcalis linguae
p. precommunicalis arteriae cerebri anterioris
p. precommunicalis arteriae cerebri posterioris
p. prelaminaris nervi optici intraocularis
p. preprostatica urethrae masculinae
p. presulcalis
p. presulcalis linguae
p. prevertebralis arteriae prevertebralis
p. prima duodeni
p. profunda compartimenti antebrachii anterioris
p. profunda compartimenti cruris posterioris
p. profunda glandulae parotideae
p. profunda glandulae parotidis
p. profunda musculi masseteri
p. profunda musculi sphincteri ani externi
p. profunda partis palpebralis musculi orbicularis oculi
p. prostatica urethrae
p. proximalis prostatae
p. proximalis urethrae prostaticae
p. psoatica fasciae iliopsoaticae
p. pterygopharyngea musculi constrictoris pharyngis superioris
p. pylorica gastris
p. pylorica ventriculi
p. quadrata hepatis
p. radiata lobuli corticalis renis
p. recta musculi cricothyroidei
p. respiratoria tunicae mucosae
p. retrolentiformis capsulae internae
p. retrolentiformis cruris posterior
p. sacralis medullae spinalis
p. scrotalis ductus deferentis
p. secundum duodeni
p. sellaris
p. solealis compartimenti cruris posterioris
p. sphenoidalis arteriae cerebralis mediae
p. spinalis fili terminalis
p. spinalis musculi deltoidei
p. spinalis nervi accessorii
p. spongiosa urethrae masculinae
p. squamosa ossis temporalis
p. sternalis diaphragmatis
p. sternocostalis musculi pectoralis majoris
p. subcutanea musculi sphincteri ani externi
p. sublentiformis capsulae internae
p. sublentiformis cruris posterioris
p. superficialis compartimenti antebrachii anterioris
p. superficialis compartimenti cruris posterioris

p. superficialis glandulae parotideae
p. superficialis musculi masseteri
p. superficialis musculi sphincteri ani externi
p. superior ali lobuli centralis
p. superior duodeni
p. superior faciei diaphragmaticae hepatis
p. superior ganglii vestibularis
p. superior venae lingularis venae pulmonis superioris sinistri
p. supraclavicularis plexus brachialis
p. sympathica (divisionis autonomicae systematis nervosei peripherici)
p. tecta, p. tecta pancreatis, p. tecta renalis, p. tecta ureteralis
p. tecta duodeni
p. tensa membranae tympani
p. terminalis
p. terminalis ilei
p. thoracica aortae
p. thoracica ductus thoracici
p. thoracica esophagi
p. thoracica medullae spinalis
p. thoracica muscularis iliocostalis lumborum
p. thoracica plexuum et ganglionorum visceralium
p. thoracica tracheae
p. thyroepiglottica musculi thyroarytenoidei
p. thyropharyngea musculi constrictoris pharyngis inferioris
p. tibiocalcanea ligamenti collateralis medialis articulationis talocruralis
p. tibiocalcanea ligamenti deltoidei
p. tibionavicularis ligamenti collateralis medialis articulationis talocrucalis
p. tibiotalaris anterior ligamenti collateralis medialis articulationis talocruralis
p. tibiotalaris posterior ligamenti collateralis medialis articulationis talocruralis
p. transversa ligamenti iliofemoralis
p. transversa musculi nasalis
p. transversa musculi trapezii
p. transversa rami sinistri venae portae hepatis
p. transversaria arteriae vertebralis
p. triangularis
p. tricipitalis compartimenti cruris posterioris
p. tuberalis
p. tympanica ossis temporalis
p. umbilicalis rami sinistri venae portae hepatis
p. uterina placentae
p. uterina tubae uterinae
p. uvealis reticuli trabecularis sclerae
p. vagalis nervi accessorii

p. ventralis musculi intertransversarii lateralium lumborum
p. ventralis pontis
p. vertebralis faciei costalis pulmonis
p. vestibularis nervi vestibulocochlearis
partes vicibus (part. vic.)
Parsonage-Turner syndrome
pars-planitis
pars tecta pancreatis (*var. of* pars tecta)
pars tecta renalis (*var. of* pars tecta)
pars tecta ureteralis (*var. of* pars tecta)
part
abdominal p. of aorta
abdominal p. of esophagus
abdominal p. of pectoralis major (muscle)
abdominal p. of peripheral autonomic plexuses and ganglia
abdominal p. of thoracic duct
abdominal p. of ureter
acromial p. of deltoid muscle
alar p. of nasalis muscle
alveolar p. of mandible
anterior p.
anterior p. of anterior commissure of brain
anterior p. of diaphragmatic surface of liver
anterior p. of fornix of vagina
anterior p. of pons
anterior tibiotalar p. of deltoid ligament
anterior tibiotalar p. of medial ligament of ankle joint
anterior p. of tongue
anular p. of fibrous digital sheath of digits of hand and foot
aryepiglottic p. of oblique arytenoid muscle
ascending p. of aorta
ascending p. of duodenum
ascending p. of trapezius muscle
atlantic p. of vertebral artery
autonomic p. of peripheral nervous system
basal p.
basal p. of left and right inferior pulmonary artery
basal p. of occipital bone
basilar p.
basilar p. of occipital bone
basilar p. of pons
bony p. of external acoustic meatus
bony p. of nasal septum
bony p. of pharyngotympanic tube
bony p. of skeletal system
buccopharyngeal p. of superior pharyngeal constrictor
cardiac p. of stomach
cardial p. of stomach
cartilaginous p. of external acoustic meatus
cartilaginous p. of nasal septum

P

part (*continued*)

cartilaginous p. of pharyngotympanic tube

cartilaginous p. of skeletal system

cavernous p. of internal carotid artery

celiacoduodenal p. of suspensory ligament of duodenum

central p. of lateral ventricle

ceratopharyngeal p. of middle constrictor muscle of pharynx

ceratopharyngeal p. of middle pharyngeal constrictor (muscle) of pharynx

cerebral p. of arachnoid

cerebral p. of dura mater

cerebral p. of internal carotid artery

cervical p. of esophagus

cervical p. of internal carotid artery

cervical p. of spinal cord

cervical p. of thoracic duct

cervical p. of vertebral artery

chondropharyngeal p. of middle constrictor muscle of pharynx

chondropharyngeal p. of middle pharyngeal constrictor muscle of pharynx

ciliary p. of retina

clavicular p. of deltoid muscle

clavicular p. of pectoralis major muscle

coccygeal p. of spinal cord

cochlear p. of vestibulocochlear nerve

convoluted p. of kidney lobule

corneoscleral p. of trabecular tissue of sclera

cortical p.

cortical p. of middle cerebral artery

costal p. of diaphragm

costal p. of parietal pleura

cranial p. of parasympathetic part of autonomic division of nervous system

craniocervical p. of peripheral autonomic plexuses and ganglia

cricopharyngeal p. of inferior constrictor muscle of pharynx

cruciform p. of fibrous digital sheath

cruciform p. of fibrous sheath

cuneiform p. of vomer

cupular p. of epitympanic recess

deep p. of anterior compartment of forearm

deep p. of external anal sphincter

deep p. of flexor retinaculum

deep p. of masseter

deep p. of palpebral part of orbicularis oculi

deep p. of parotid gland

deep p. of posterior (flexor) compartment of leg

descending p. of aorta

descending p. of duodenum

descending p. of facial canal

descending p. of iliofemoral ligament

descending p. of trapezius muscle

diaphragmatic p. of parietal pleura

distal p. of anterior lobe of hypophysis

distal p. of prostate

distal p. of prostatic urethra

dorsal p. of intertransversarii laterales lumborum

dorsal p. of pons

dural p. of filum terminale

endocrine p. of pancreas

exocrine p. of pancreas

extraocular p. of central retinal artery and vein

first p. of duodenum

flaccid p. of tympanic membrane

free p. of lower limb

free p. of upper limb

frontal p. of corpus callosum

funicular p. of ductus deferens

glossopharyngeal p. of superior pharyngeal constrictor

hidden p.

hidden p. of duodenum

horizontal p. of duodenum

horizontal p. of facial canal

inferior p.

inferior p. of duodenum

inferior p. of lingular vein

inferior p. of trapezius muscle

inferior p. of vestibular ganglion

inferior p. of vestibulocochlear nerve

infraclavicular p. of brachial plexus

infralobar p. of posterior vein

infrasegmental p.

infundibular p.

inguinal p. of ductus deferens

insular p.

insular p. of middle cerebral artery

intercartilaginous p. of glottic opening

intercartilaginous p. of rima glottidis

intermediate p.

intermediate p. of adenohypophysis

intermediate p. of male urethra

intermediate p. of vestibular bulb

intermembranous p. of glottic opening

intermembranous p. of rima glottidis

intersegmental p. of pulmonary vein

intracranial p. of optic nerve

intracranial p. of vertebral artery

intralaminar p. of intralocular part of optic nerve

intralobar p. of the posterior vein

intramural p. of male urethra

intraocular p. of optic nerve

intrasegmental p. of pulmonary vein

iridial p. of retina

labial p. of orbicularis oris muscle

lacrimal p. of orbicularis oculi muscle
laryngeal p. of pharynx
lateral p. of longitudinal arch of foot
lateral p. of middle lobe vein
lateral p. of occipital bone
lateral p. of posterior cervical intertransversarii muscle
lateral p. of posterior compartment of forearm
lateral p. of sacrum
lateral p. of vaginal fornix
left p. of liver
lumbar p. of diaphragm
lumbar p. of spinal cord
marginal p. of orbicularis oris muscle
mastoid p. of the temporal bone
medial p. of longitudinal arch of foot
medial p. of middle lobe vein
mediastinal p. of lung
mediastinal p. of parietal pleura
membranous p. of interventricular septum
membranous p. of male urethra
membranous p. of nasal septum
mobile p. of nasal septum
muscular p. of interventricular septum
mylopharyngeal p. of superior constrictor muscle of pharynx
mylopharyngeal p. of superior pharyngeal constrictor muscle of pharynx
nasal p. of frontal bone
nasal p. of pharynx
nervous p. of retina
neural p. of hypophysis
oblique p. of cricothyroid (muscle)
occipital p. of corpus callosum
opercular p.
p. of optic nerve in canal
optic p. of retina
oral p. of pharynx
orbital p. of frontal bone
orbital p. of inferior frontal gyrus
orbital p. of lacrimal gland
orbital p. of optic nerve
orbital p. of orbicularis oculi muscle
osseous p. of skeletal system
palpebral p. of lacrimal gland
palpebral p. of orbicularis oculi muscle
parasympathetic p. of autonomic division of peripheral nervous system
patent p. of umbilical artery
pelvic p.
pelvic p. of ductus deferens
pelvic p. of peripheral autonomic plexuses and ganglia
pelvic p. of ureter

pelvic p. of the urogenital sinus
p.'s per billion (ppb)
peripheral p. of nervous system
petrous p. of internal carotid artery
petrous p. of temporal bone
phrenicoceliac p. of suspensory ligament of duodenum
pial p. of filum terminale
pigmented p. of retina
postcommunicating p. of anterior cerebral artery
postcommunicating p. of posterior cerebral artery
posterior p.
posterior p. of anterior commissure of brain
posterior p. of the diaphragmatic surface of the liver
posterior p. of liver
posterior tibiotalar p. of deltoid ligament
posterior tibiotalar p. of medial ligament of ankle joint
posterior p. of tongue
posterior p. of vaginal fornix
postlaminar p. of intraocular part of optic nerve
postsulcal p. of tongue
precommunicating p. of anterior cerebral artery
precommunicating p. of posterior cerebral artery
prelaminar p. of intraocular part of optic nerve
preprostatic p. of male urethra
presulcal p. of tongue
prevertebral p. of vertebral artery
proximal p. of prostate
proximal p. of prostatic urethra
psoatic p. of iliopsoas fascia
pterygopharyngeal p. of superior constrictor muscle of pharynx
pyloric p. of stomach
quadrate p. of liver
radial p. of posterior compartment of forearm
retrolenticular p. of internal capsule
right p. of diaphragmatic surface of liver
right p. of liver
sacral p. of spinal cord
scrotal p. of ductus deferens
second p. of duodenum
soft p.
soleal p. of posterior compartment of leg
sphenoid p. of middle cerebral artery
spinal p. of accessory nerve
spinal p. of arachnoid
spinal p. of deltoid muscle
spinal p. of filum terminale
spongy p. of the male urethra
squamous p. of frontal bone
squamous p. of occipital bone

P

part (*continued*)

squamous p. of temporal bone
sternal p. of diaphragm
sternocostal p. of pectoralis major muscle
straight p. of cricothyroid muscle
subcutaneous p. of external anal sphincter
sublenticular p. of internal capsule
suboccipital p. of vertebral artery
superficial p. of anterior compartment of forearm
superficial p. of external anal sphincter
superficial p. of masseter muscle
superficial p. of parotid gland
superficial p. of posterior compartment of leg
superior p. of diaphragmatic surface of liver
superior p. of duodenum
superior p. of lingular vein
superior p. of vestibular ganglion
superior p. of vestibulocochlear nerve
supraclavicular p. of brachial plexus
supravaginal p. of cervix
sympathetic p. of autonomic division of peripheral nervous system
tense p. of the tympanic membrane
terminal p.
third p. of duodenum
thoracic p. of aorta
thoracic p. of esophagus
thoracic p. of iliocostalis lumborum muscle
thoracic p. of peripheral autonomic plexuses and ganglia
thoracic p. of spinal cord
thoracic p. of thoracic duct
thoracic p. of trachea
thyroepiglottic p. of thyroarytenoid muscle
thyropharyngeal p. of inferior constrictor muscle of pharynx
thyropharyngeal p. of inferior pharyngeal constrictor muscle of pharynx
tibiocalcaneal p. of deltoid ligament
tibiocalcaneal p. of medial ligament of ankle joint
tibionavicular p. of deltoid ligament
tibionavicular p. of medial ligament of ankle joint
tibiotalar p. of medial ligament of ankle joint
transversarial p. of vertebral artery
transverse p. of iliofemoral ligament
transverse p. of left branch of portal vein
transverse p. of nasalis muscle
transverse p. of trapezius muscle
triangular p.

tympanic p. of temporal bone
umbilical p. of left branch of portal vein
uterine p. of uterine tube
uveal p. of trabecular reticulum
uveal p. of trabecular tissue of sclera
vagal p. of accessory nerve
vaginal p. of cervix
ventral p. of intertransversarii laterales lumborum muscle
ventral p. of pons
vertebral p. of the costal surface of the lungs
vertebral p. of diaphragm
vestibular p. of vestibulocochlear nerve

part. aeq.

partes aequales

partes (*pl. of* pars)
parthenogenesis
parthenophobia
partial

p. adrenocortical insufficiency
p. agglutinin
p. anencephaly
p. aneuploidy
p. anodontia
p. anomalous pulmonary venous connection
p. anomalous pulmonary venous return (PAPVR)
p. antigen
p. breech extraction
p. cricoid cleft
p. cystectomy
p. denture
p. denture impression
p. denture retention
p. enterocele
p. epilepsy
p. heart block
p. ileal bypass
p. laryngectomy
p. left ventriculectomy
p. lipoatrophy
p. posterior laryngeal cleft
p. pressure (*P*)
p. sclerectasia
p. seizure
p. thromboplastin time (PTT)
p. volume

partial-thickness

p.-t. burn
p.-t. graft

participant observer
particle

alpha p. (α)
beta p.
chromatin p.
core p.
Dane p.
defective interfering p.
D.I. p.
electron transport p. (ETP)

elementary p.
kappa p.'s
signal recognition p. (SRP)
submitochondrial p.
Zimmermann elementary p.
particulate
p. wear debris
partition
p. chromatography
p. coefficient
partogram
parturient
p. canal
parturifacient
parturition
part. vic.
partes vicibus
parulis, pl. **parulides**
parumbilical
paruresis
parvalbumin
parvilocular cyst
Parvobacteriaceae
parvocellular
parvoline
Parvoviridae
Parvovirus B19
parvule
parvus
PAS
p-aminosalicylic acid
PASA
p-aminosalicylic acid
pascal
Pascal law
Pascheff conjunctivitis
Paschen body
paspalism
passage
blind p.
nasopharyngeal p.
oropharyngeal p.
serial p.
Passalurus ambiguus
Passavant
P. bar
P. cushion
P. pad
P. ridge
passiflora
passion
passional attitudes
passive
p. agglutination
p. anaphylaxis
p. atelectasis
p. clot
p. congestion
p. cutaneous anaphylactic reaction
p. cutaneous anaphylaxis
p. cutaneous anaphylaxis test
p. diffusion
p. duction
p. eruption
p. hemagglutination

p. hyperemia
p. immunity
p. immunization
p. incontinence
p. learning
p. length-tension curve
p. medium
p. movement
p. prophylaxis
p. transference
p. transport
p. tremor
p. vasoconstriction
p. vasodilation
passive-aggressive
p.-a. behavior
p.-a. personality
passivism
passivity
PAS stain
pasta, pl. **pastae**
paste
dermatologic p.
desensitizing p.
paster
Pasteur
P. effect
P. pipette
P. vaccine
Pasteurella
P. *aerogenes*
P. *multocida*
P. *pestis*
P. *pseudotuberculosis*
P. *"SP"*
P. *tularensis*
pasteurella, pl. **pasteurellae**
pasteurellosis
pasteurization
pasteurize
pasteurizer
Pastia sign
pastil, pastille
Sabouraud p.
pastoral counseling
past-pointing
patagium, pl. **patagia**
Patau syndrome
patch
butterfly p.
p. clamp
p. clamping
cotton-wool p.
herald p.
Hutchinson p.
mucous p.
Peyer p.
salmon p.
shagreen p.
smoker's p.
soldier's p.
p. test
patchy atelectasis
Patein albumin
patella, pl. **patellae**

P

patella *(continued)*
 p. alta
 p. baja
 floating p.
 slipping p.
patellar
 p. anastomosis
 p. apprehension sign
 p. fossa of vitreous
 p. ligament
 p. network
 p. retinaculum
 p. surface of femur
 p. tendon reflex
patellectomy
patelliform
patelloadductor reflex
patellofemoral
 p. stress syndrome
 p. syndrome
patency
 probe p.
patent
 p. blue V
 p. ductus arteriosus
 p. medicine
 p. part of umbilical artery
Paterson-Brown-Kelly syndrome
Paterson-Kelly syndrome
path
 p. analysis
 clinical p.
 condyle p.
 generated occlusal p.
 incisal p.
 p. of insertion
 milled-in p.
 occlusal p.
pathema
pathematic aphasia
pathergy
pathetic nerve
pathfinder
pathic
pathoamine
pathobiology
pathocidin
pathoclisis
pathocrinia
pathodontia
pathoformic
pathogen
 behavioral p.
 opportunistic p.
pathogenesis
 drug p.
pathogenic, pathogenetic
 p. occlusion
pathogenicity
pathogeny
pathognomonic symptom
pathognomy
pathognostic

pathologic, pathological
 p. absorption
 p. amenorrhea
 p. amputation
 p. anatomy
 p. calcification
 p. diagnosis
 p. fracture
 p. glycosuria
 p. histology
 p. model
 p. myopia
 p. physiology
 p. protein
 p. retraction ring
 p. sphincter
 p. startle syndrome
pathologist
 speech-language p.
pathology
 anatomic p.
 cellular p.
 clinical p.
 comparative p.
 dental p.
 functional p.
 humoral p.
 medical p.
 molecular p.
 oral p.
 speech p.
 speech-language p.
 surgical p.
pathometric
pathometry
pathomimesis
pathomimicry
pathomiosis
pathomorphism
pathonomia, pathonomy
pathophobia
pathophysiology
pathopoiesis
pathosis
pathotropism
pathway
 4-aminobutyrate p.
 auditory p.
 biochemical p.
 critical p.
 Embden-Meyerhof p.
 Embden-Meyerhof-Parnas p.
 Entner-Douderoff p.
 GABA p.
 hexose monophosphate p.
 lacrimal p.
 mercapturic acid p.
 pentose phosphate p.
 phosphogluconate p.
 polyol p.
 salvage p.
 sorbitol p.
 ubiquitin-protease p.
 visual p.

patient
> p. care information system (PCIS)
> target p.

patient-controlled
> p.-c. analgesia (PCA)
> p.-c. anesthesia

Patois virus
Paton line
patricide
Patrick test
patrilineal
pattern
> airspace-filling p.
> airway p.
> alveolar p.
> ballerina-foot p.
> butterfly p.
> p. distortion amblyopia
> ground-glass p.
> honeycomb p.
> hourglass p.
> interstitial p.
> juvenile p.
> miliary p.
> mosaic p.
> occlusal p.
> reticulonodular p.
> p. retinal dystrophy
> wax p.

patterned alopecia
pattern-sensitive epilepsy
patulin
patulous
pauciarticular
paucibacillary
paucisynaptic
Paul
> P. reaction
> P. test

Paul-Bunnell test
Pauli exclusion principle
Pauling-Corey helix
Pauling theory
pause
> apneic p.
> compensatory p.
> postextrasystolic p.
> preautomatic p.
> respiratory p.
> p. signal
> sinus p.

Pautrier
> P. abscess
> P. microabscess

pavement epithelium
Pavlov
> P. method
> P. pouch
> P. reflex
> P. stomach

pavlovian conditioning
pavor nocturnus
Pavy disease
pawpaw
Payne operation

Payr
> P. clamp
> P. membrane
> P. sign

Pb
> lead

PBG
> porphobilinogen

PBI
> protein-bound iodine
> PBI test

p.c.
> post cibum

PCA
> patient-controlled analgesia
> PCA pump

PCB
> polychlorinated biphenyl

PCIS
> patient care information system

PCMB, *p*CMB
> p-chloromercuribenzoate

P congenitale
PCP
> phencyclidine

PCR
> polymerase chain reaction

PCT
> porphyria cutanea tarda

PCWP
> pulmonary capillary wedge pressure

PD
> phenyldichloroarsine

Pd
> palladium

p.d.
> prism diopter

P-dextrocardiale
PDGF
> platelet-derived growth factor

PDI
> Periodontal Disease Index

PDL
> pulsed dye laser

PEA
> pulseless electrical activity

peach kernel oil
peak
> biclonal p.
> p. expiratory flow
> juxtaphrenic p.
> kilovolt p. (kVp)
> p. kilovoltage (pkV)
> p. magnitude
> monoclonal p.

peak flow rate
peanut oil
pearl
> p. cyst
> Elschnig p.
> enamel p.
> epithelial p.
> Epstein p.
> gouty p.
> P. index

P

pearl (*continued*)
    keratin p.
    Laënnec p.
    p. moss
    squamous p.
    p. worker's disease
pearl-ash
pear-shaped area
peat moss
peau d'orange
peccant humor
peccatiphobia
pecilocin
pecking order
Pecquet
    P. cistern
    P. duct
    P. reservoir
pectase
pecten
    anal p.
    p. analis
    p. band
    p. ossis pubis
    p. pubis
pectenitis
pectenosis
pectic
pectic acid
pectin
    p. lyase
    p. sugar
pectinase
pectinate
    p. fiber
    p. ligament of iridocorneal angle
    p. ligament of iris
    p. line
    p. muscle
    p. zone
pectineal
    p. ligament
    p. line of femur
    p. line of pubis
    p. muscle
pectinesterase
pectineus muscle
pectinic acids
pectiniform septum
pectization
pectora (*pl. of* pectus)
pectoral
    p. and abdominal anterior cutaneous branch of intercostal nerve
    p. axillary lymph node
    p. branch of thoracoacromial artery
    p. fascia
    p. girdle
    p. gland
    p. reflex
    p. region
    p. ridge
    p. vein
pectoralgia

pectoralis
    p. major muscle
    p. minor muscle
pectoriloquy
    aphonic p.
    whispered p.
    whispering p.
pectorodorsalis muscle
pectorodorsal muscle
pectorophony
pectose
pectous
pectus, pl. **pectora**
    p. carinatum
    p. excavatum
    p. recurvatum
pedal system
pedatrophia, pedatrophy
pederast
pederasty
Pederson speculum
pedes (*pl. of* pes)
pedesis
pediatric
    p. dentistry
    p. radiology
pediatrician
pediatrics
pediatrist
pediatry
pedicel
pedicellate
pedicellation
pedicle
    p. of arch of vertebra
    p. flap
    p. graft
    vascular p.
pedicular
pediculate
pediculi (*pl. of* pediculus)
pediculicide
Pediculoides ventricosus
pediculophobia
pediculosis
    p. capitis
    p. corporis
    p. palpebrarum
    p. pubis
pediculous blepharitis
Pediculus
    p. arcus vertebrae
pediculus, pl. **pediculi**
pedicure
pedigree analysis
pediophobia
pediphalanx
pedis
pedodontia
pedodontics
pedodontist
pedodynamometer
pedogenesis
pedogram
pedograph

pedography
pedometer
pedomorphism
pedophilia
pedophilic
peduncle
    cerebral p.
    p. of corpus callosum
    p. of flocculus
    inferior cerebellar p.
    inferior thalamic p.
    lateral thalamic p.
    p. of mammillary body
    middle cerebellar p.
    olfactory p.
    superior cerebellar p.
    ventral thalamic p.
peduncular
    p. ansa
    p. loop
    p. vein
pedunculate
pedunculated
    p. hydatid
    p. polyp
pedunculi (*pl. of* pedunculus)
pedunculomammillary fasciculus
pedunculopontine tegmental nucleus
pedunculotomy
pedunculus, pl. pedunculi
    p. cerebellaris inferior
    p. cerebellaris medius
    p. cerebellaris superior
    p. cerebri
    p. corporis callosi
    p. corporis mammillaris
    p. flocculi
    p. of pineal body
    p. thalami inferior
    p. thalami lateralis
    p. thalami ventralis
    p. vitellinus
peel
    bitter orange p.
    bitter orange p., dried
    bitter orange p., fresh
    face p.
peeling
    chemical p.
peenash
PEEP
    positive end-expiratory pressure
peeping testis
peer review
peg
    rete p.
peg-and-socket
    p.-a.-s. articulation
    p.-a.-s. joint
pegged tooth
PEGs
    polyethylene glycol
pejorism
PEL
    permissible exposure limit

pelade
pelargonic acid
Pel-Ebstein
    P.-E. disease
    P.-E. fever
Pelger-Huët nuclear anomaly
peliosis
    bacterial p.
    p. hepatis
    p. hepatitis
Pelizaeus-Merzbacher disease
pellagra
    infantile p.
    secondary p.
    p. sine p.
pellagra-preventing factor (p-p factor)
pellagroid
pellagrous
Pellegrini disease
Pellegrini-Stieda disease
pellet
    p. implantation
pellicle
    acquired p.
    brown p.
pellicular, pelliculous
Pellizzi syndrome
pellote
pellucid
    p. marginal corneal degeneration
    p. zone
pelma
pelmatic
pelmatogram
pelopathy
pelotherapy
pelta
peltation
pelves (*pl. of* pelvis)
pelvic
    p. abscess
    p. axis
    p. bone
    p. brim
    p. canal
    p. cavity
    p. cellulitis
    p. diaphragm
    p. direction
    p. exenteration
    p. fascia
    p. ganglia
    p. girdle
    p. hematocele
    p. inclination
    p. index
    p. inflammatory disease (PID)
    p. inlet
    p. kidney
    p. limb
    p. lymph node
    p. outlet
    p. part
    p. part of ductus deferens

P

pelvic *(continued)*
    p. part of peripheral autonomic plexuses and ganglia
    p. part of ureter
    p. part of the urogenital sinus
    p. peritonitis
    p. plane of greatest dimensions
    p. plane of inlet
    p. plane of least dimensions
    p. plane of outlet
    p. plexus
    p. pole
    p. presentation
    p. promontory
    p. splanchnic nerve
    p. surface of sacrum
    p. version
pelvicephalography
pelvicephalometry
pelvifixation
pelvilithotomy
pelvimetry
    CT p.
    manual p.
    radiographic p.
pelviolithotomy
pelvioperitonitis
pelvioplasty
pelvioscopy
pelviperitonitis
pelvirectal sphincter
pelvis, pl. **pelves**
    android p.
    anthropoid p.
    assimilation p.
    beaked p.
    brachypellic p.
    caoutchouc p.
    contracted p.
    cordate p.
    cordiform p.
    Deventer p.
    dolichopellic p.
    dwarf p.
    false p.
    flat p.
    frozen p.
    funnel-shaped p.
    p. of gallbladder
    greater p.
    gynecoid p.
    hardened p.
    heart-shaped p.
    inverted p.
    p. justo major
    p. justo minor
    juvenile p.
    kyphoscoliotic p.
    kyphotic p.
    large p.
    lesser p.
    longitudinal oval p.
    lordotic p.
    p. major

    masculine p.
    mesatipellic p.
    p. minor
    Nägele p.
    p. nana
    p. obtecta
    osteomalacic p.
    Otto p.
    p. plana
    platypellic p.
    platypelloid p.
    Prague p.
    pseudoosteomalacic p.
    rachitic p.
    renal p.
    p. renalis
    reniform p.
    Robert p.
    Rokitansky p.
    rostrate p.
    round p.
    rubber p.
    scoliotic p.
    small p.
    spider p.
    split p.
    spondylolisthetic p.
    p. spuria
    transverse oval p.
    true p.
    ureteric p.
    p. vera
pelvisacral
pelviscope
pelvitherm
pelviureterography
pelvivertebral angle
pelvocaliectasis
pelvocephalography
pelvofemoral muscular dystrophy
pelvoscopy
pelvospondylitis ossificans
pemoline
pemphigoid
    benign mucosal p.
    bullous p.
    localized p. of Brunsting-Perry
    ocular p.
    ocular cicatricial p.
pemphigus
    benign familial chronic p.
    Brazilian p.
    p. erythematosus
    p. foliaceus
    p. gangrenosus
    paraneoplastic p.
    p. vegetans
    p. vulgaris
pempidine
pencil tenderness
pendelluft
Pendred syndrome
pendular
    p. movement
    p. nystagmus

pendulous
    p. abdomen
    p. heart
    p. palate
pendulum rhythm
penectomy
penes (*pl. of* penis)
penetrance
    genetic p.
penetrant trait
penetrate
penetrating
    p. keratoplasty
    p. ulcer
    p. wound
penetration
penetrometer
pen grasp
penial
peniaphobia
penicillamine
penicillanate
penicillanic acid
penicillary
penicillate
penicilli (*pl. of* penicillus)
penicillic acid
penicillin
    aluminum p.
    p. amidase
    p. B
    benzyl p.
    buffered crystalline p. G
    chloroprocaine p. O
    p. G
    p. G benzathine
    p. G hydrabamine
    p. G potassium
    p. G potassium
    p. G procaine
    p. G sodium
    p. N
    p. O
    p. phenoxymethyl
    p. V
    p. V benzathine
    p. V hydrabamine
penicillinase
penicillinate
penicilliosis
Penicillium lilacinum
penicilloic acid
penicilloyl polylysine
penicillus, pl. **penicilli**
penicin
penile
    p. epispadias
    p. fibromatosis
    p. hypospadias
    p. implant
    p. prosthesis
    p. raphe
    p. urethra
penillic acids

penin
penis, pl. **penes**
    bifid p.
    buried p.
    clubbed p.
    concealed p.
    p. envy
    p. femineus
    gryposis p.
    p. muliebris
    webbed p.
penischisis
pennate muscle
penniform
pennyroyal
penopubic epispadias
penoscrotal
    p. hypospadias
    p. transposition
penotomy
Penrose drain
pension neurosis
pentabasic
pentachlorophenol
pentad
    Reynolds p.
pentadactyl, pentadactyle
pentaerythritol tetranitrate
pentagastrin test
pentalogy
    p. of Cantrell
    p. of Fallot
pentamer
pentamidine isethionate
pentanoic acid
pentapeptide
pentapiperide fumarate
pentapiperium methylsulfate
pentaquine
Pentastoma
pentastomiasis
Pentastomida
pentatomic
Pentatrichomonas
pentavalent gas gangrene antitoxin
pentazocine
pentetate trisodium calcium
pentetic acid
penthienate bromide
pentifylline
pentitol
pentobarbital
pentolinium tartrate
penton antigen
pentosan
pentose
    p. monophosphate shunt
    p. nucleotide
    p. phosphate cycle
    p. phosphate pathway
pentostatin
pentosuria
    alimentary p.
    essential p.
    primary p.

P

pentoxide
pentoxifylline
pentulose
pentyl
pentylenetetrazol
penumbra
peplomer
peplos
peppermint
    p. camphor
    p. oil
Pepper syndrome
pep pills
pepsic
pepsin
pepsinate
pepsiniferous
pepsinogen
pepsinogenous
pepsinuria
pepstatin
peptic
    p. cell
    p. digestion
    p. esophagitis
    p. gland
    p. ulcer
peptidase
    p. D
    p. P
peptide
    adrenocorticotropic p.
    anionic neutrophil-activating p.
     (ANAP)
    p. antibiotic
    antigen p.
    atrial natriuretic p. (ANP)
    bitter p.
    p. bond
    bradykinin-potentiating p.
    calcitonin gene-related p. (CGRP)
    cyclic p.
    gastric inhibitory p. (GIP)
    glucagonlike p. (GLP-1)
    glucagonlike insulinotropic p. (GLIP)
    heterodetic p.
    heteromeric p.
    homodetic p.
    homomeric p.
    p. hydrolase
    parathyroid hormone-related p.
     (PTHrP)
    phenylthiocarbamoyl p.
    S p.
    sigma p.
    p. synthetase
    vasoactive intestinal p.
peptidergic
peptidoglycan
peptidoid
peptidolytic
peptidyl dipeptidase A
peptidyl leukotrienes
peptidyltransferase
peptization

Peptococcaceae
Peptococcus
    P. aerogenes
    P. constellatus
    P. niger
peptocrinine
peptogenic, peptogenous
peptoid
peptolide
peptolysis
peptolytic
peptone
peptonic
peptonization
Peptostreptococcus
    P. anaerobius
    P. asaccharolyticus
    P. evolutus
    P. foetidus
    P. intermedius
    P. magnus
    P. micros
    P. morbillorum
    P. paleopneumoniae
    P. parvulus
    P. plagarumbelli
    P. productus
    P. putridus
peracephalus
peracid
peracute
per anum
perarticulation
peratodynia
peraxillary
perazine
percentile
percept analysis
perception
    depth p.
    extrasensory p. (ESP)
    simultaneous p.
perceptive
    p. hearing impairment
perceptivity
perceptorium
perceptual expansion
percolation
percolator
percomorph oil
per contiguum
per continuum
percuss
percussion
    auscultatory p.
    bimanual p.
    clavicular p.
    deep p.
    direct p.
    finger p.
    immediate p.
    mediate p.
    Murphy p.
    palpatory p.
    piano p.

p. sound
threshold p.
p. wave
percussor
percutaneous
p. absorption
p. cholangiography
p. endoscopic gastrostomy
p. nephrostomy
p. radiofrequency gangliolysis
p. stimulation
p. transhepatic cholangiography (PTHC)
p. transluminal angioplasty
p. transluminal coronary angioplasty (PTCA)
perencephaly
Perez
P. reflex
P. sign
perfect
p. fungus
p. stage
p. state
perfectionism
perfectionistic personality
perflation
perflubron
perfluorooctyl bromide (PFOB)
perforans
perforated
p. layer of sclera
p. space
p. ulcer
perforating
p. abscess
p. appendicitis
p. artery of deep femoral artery
p. artery of foot
p. artery of hand
p. artery of internal thoracic artery
p. artery of penis
p. branch
p. branch of anterior interosseous artery
p. branch of fibular artery
p. branch of internal thoracic artery
p. branch of palmar metacarpal artery
p. branch of peroneal artery
p. branch of plantar metatarsal artery
p. fiber
p. folliculitis
p. keratoplasty
p. radiate artery of kidney
p. ulcer of foot
p. vein
p. wound
perforation
perforator
perforin
performance
p. intensity

p. status
p. test
performic acid
performic acid reaction
perfrigeration
perfusate
perfuse
perfusion
p. cannula
regional p.
pergolide mesylate
perhexiline maleate
perhydrase milk
perhydrocyclopenta[a]phenanthrene
periaccretio pericardii
periacinal, periacinous
periadenitis mucosa necrotica recurrens
perialveolar wiring
perianal
periangiocholitis
periangitis
periaortic
periaortitis
periapex
periapical
p. abscess
p. cemental dysplasia
p. curettage
p. cyst
p. granuloma
p. osteofibrosis
p. radiograph
p. tissue
periappendiceal abscess
periappendicitis decidualis
periappendicular
periaqueductal gray substance
periarterial
p. lymphatic sheath (PALS)
p. pad
p. plexus
p. plexus of anterior cerebral artery
p. plexus of ascending pharyngeal artery
p. plexus of choroid artery
p. plexuses of coronary artery
p. plexus of facial artery
p. plexus of inferior phrenic artery
p. plexus of inferior thyroid artery
p. plexus of internal thoracic artery
p. plexus of lingual artery
p. plexus of maxillary artery
p. plexus of middle cerebral artery
p. plexus of occipital artery
p. plexus of ophthalmic artery
p. plexus of popliteal artery
p. plexus of posterior auricular artery
p. plexus of subclavian artery
p. plexus of superficial temporal artery
p. plexus of superior thyroid artery
p. plexus of testicular artery
p. plexus of thyroid artery

P

periarterial *(continued)*
    p. plexus of vertebral artery
    p. sympathectomy
periarteritis nodosa
periarthric
periarthritis
periarticular abscess
periatrial
periauricular
periaxial
periaxillary
periaxonal
periblast
peribronchial
peribronchiolar
peribronchiolitis
peribronchitis
peribuccal
peribulbar
peribursal
pericallosal
    p. artery
    p. cistern
pericanalicular fibroadenoma
pericapillary cell
pericardectomy
pericardia (*pl. of* pericardium)
pericardiacophrenic
    p. artery
    p. vein
pericardial, pericardiac
    p. branch of phrenic nerve
    p. branch of thoracic aorta
    p. cavity
    p. decompression
    p. effusion
    p. fremitus
    p. friction rub
    p. friction sound
    p. knock
    p. murmur
    p. pleura
    p. reflex
    p. rub
    p. symphysis
    p. tap
    p. vein
    p. villi
pericardicentesis
pericardiectomy
    radical p.
pericardiocentesis
pericardiology
pericardioperitoneal
    p. canal
pericardiophrenic
pericardiopleural
    p. membrane
pericardiorrhaphy
pericardiostomy
pericardiotomy
pericarditic
pericarditis
    acute fibrinous p.

    adhesive p.
    bacterial p.
    p. calculosa
    carcinomatous p.
    chronic constrictive p.
    constrictive p.
    dry p.
    epistenocardiac p.
    p. epistenocardica
    fibrinous p.
    fibrous p.
    hemorrhagic p.
    internal adhesive p.
    p. obliterans
    obliterative p.
    postmyocardial infarction p.
    postpericardiotomy p.
    posttraumatic p.
    purulent p.
    rheumatic p.
    p. sicca
    tuberculous p.
    uremic p.
    p. villosa
    viral p.
    p. with effusion
pericardium, pl. pericardia
    adherent p.
    bread-and-butter p.
    p. fibrosa
    p. fibrosum
    fibrous p.
    p. serosum
    serous p.
    shaggy p.
    visceral p.
pericardotomy
pericecal
pericellular
pericemental
    p. abscess
    p. attachment
pericentral
    p. fibrosis
    p. scotoma
pericentric inversion
pericholangitis
perichondral, perichondrial
    p. bone
perichondritis
    peristernal p.
    relapsing p.
perichondrium
perichord
perichordal
perichoroidal, perichoroid
    p. space
perichrome
periclaustral lamina
pericolic
    p. membrane syndrome
pericolitis
    p. dextra
    p. sinistra
pericolonitis

pericolpitis
periconchal sulcus
pericorneal
pericoronal
    p. abscess
    p. flap
pericoronitis
pericorpuscular synapse
pericranial
pericranitis
pericranium
pericyazine
pericystic
pericystitis
pericystium
pericyte
pericytial
pericytic venule
peridens
peridental
    p. ligament
    p. membrane
peridentitis
peridentium
periderm, periderma
peridermal, peridermic
peridesmic
peridesmitis
peridesmium
perididymis
perididymitis
peridium
peridiverticulitis
periduodenitis
peridural anesthesia
periencephalitis
perienteric
perienteritis
periependymal
periesophageal
periesophagitis
perifocal
perifollicular
perifolliculitis abscedens et suffodiens
perifornical nucleus
perifuse
perifusion
periganglionic
perigastric
perigastritis
perigemmal
periglandulitis
periglottic
periglottis
perihepatic
perihepatitis
perihernial
perihypoglossal nuclei
peri-implantoclasia
periinfarction block
perijejunitis
perikaryon, pl. perikarya
perikeratic
perikyma, pl. perikymata
perilabyrinthitis

perilaryngeal
perilenticular
periligamentous
perilimbal suction cup
perilunar dislocation
perilymph
perilympha
perilymphangial
perilymphangitis
perilymphatic
    p. duct
    p. fistula
    p. gusher
    p. space
perimeningitis
perimenopause
perimeter
    arc p.
    Goldmann p.
    projection p.
    Tübinger p.
perimetria (*pl. of* perimetrium)
perimetric
perimetritic
perimetritis
perimetrium, pl. perimetria
perimetry
    computed p.
    flicker p.
    kinetic p.
    mesopic p.
    objective p.
    quantitative p.
    scotopic p.
    static p.
perimolysis
perimortem delivery
perimuscular fibrosis
perimyelis
perimyelitis
perimyocarditis
perimyositis
perimysia (*pl. of* perimysium)
perimysial
perimysiitis, perimysitis
perimysium, pl. perimysia
    p. externum
    p. internum
perinatal
    p. death
    p. medicine
    p. mortality
    p. mortality rate
    p. torsion
perinate
perinatologist
perinatology
perinea (*pl. of* perineum)
perineal
    p. artery
    p. body
    p. branch of posterior cutaneous
      nerve of thigh
    p. branch of posterior femoral
      cutaneous nerve

P

perineal (*continued*)
p. fascia
p. flexure of anal canal
p. flexure of rectum
p. hernia
p. hypospadias
p. lithotomy
p. membrane
p. muscle
p. nerve
p. raphe
p. region
p. section
p. space
p. urethrostomy
p. urethrotomy
perineocele
perineometer
perineoplasty
perineorrhaphy
perineoscrotal
perineostomy
perineosynthesis
perineotomy
perineovaginal fistula
perinephria (*pl. of* perinephrium)
perinephrial
perinephric abscess
perinephritis
perinephrium, pl. **perinephria**
perineum, pl. **perinea**
watering-can p.
perineural infiltration
perineuria (*pl. of* perineurium)
perineurial
perineuritis
perineurium, pl. **perineuria**
perineuronal satellite
perinuclear
p. cataract
p. space
periocular
period
absolute refractory p.
amblyogenic p.
critical p.
eclipse p.
effective refractory p.
ejection p.
extrinsic incubation p.
fertile p.
functional refractory p.
gap_0 p.
gap_2 p.
gap_1 p.
incubation p.
induction p.
intrapartum p.
isoelectric p.
isometric p. of cardiac cycle
isometric contraction p.
isometric relaxation p.
isovolumic p.
latency p.

latent p.
masticatory silent p.
menstrual p.
missed p.
mitotic p.
oedipal p.
preejection p.
prepatent p.
prodromal p.
puerperal p.
pulse p.
quarantine p.
refractory p.
relative refractory p.
silent p.
synthesis p.
total refractory p.
vulnerable p.
Wenckebach p.
periodate
periodic
p. acid-Schiff stain
p. arthralgia
p. biopolymer
p. bone pain
p. catatonia
p. disease
p. edema
p. fever
p. filariasis
p. law
p. migrainous neuralgia
p. neutropenia
p. paralysis
p. peritonitis
p. polyserositis
p. system
periodic acid
periodicity
diurnal p.
filarial p.
lunar p.
malarial p.
nocturnal p.
subperiodic p.
periodontal
p. abscess
p. anesthesia
p. atrophy
P. Disease Index (PDI)
p. file
p. ligament
p. ligament fiber
p. membrane
p. pocket
p. probe
Periodontal Index (PI)
periodontia (*pl. of* periodontium)
periodontics
periodontist
periodontitis
apical p.
p. complex
juvenile p.

p. simplex
suppurative p.
periodontium, pl. **periodontia**
periodontoclasia
periodontolysis
periodontosis
periolivary nucleus
periomphalic
perionychium, pl. **perionychia**
perionyx
perioophoritis
perioophorosalpingitis
perioperative
periophthalmic
periophthalmitis
perioral
periorbit
periorbita
periorbital
p. cellulitis
p. membrane
periorchitis hemorrhagica
periost
periostea (*pl. of* periosteum)
periosteal
p. bone
p. bud
p. chondroma
p. elevator
p. ganglion
p. graft
p. implantation
p. layer of dura mater
p. osteosarcoma
p. reaction
p. reflex
p. sarcoma
periosteitis
periosteoma
periosteomedullitis
periosteomyelitis
periosteopathy
periosteophyte
periosteosis
periosteotome
periosteotomy
periosteous
periosteum, pl. **periostea**
alveolar p.
p. alveolare
p. cranii
periostitis
periostoma
periostosis, pl. **periostoses**
periostosteitis
periostotome
periostotomy
periotic
p. bone
p. cartilage
periovaritis
periovular
peripachymeningitis
peripancreatitis
peripapillary

peripartum cardiomyopathy
peripatetic
peripeduncular nucleus
peripenial
peripharyngeal space
peripherad
peripheral
p. aneurysm
p. anterior synechia
p. arteriosclerosis
p. cataract
p. chemoreceptor
p. dysostosis
p. facial paralysis
p. glare
p. iridectomy
p. nervous system
p. ossifying fibroma
p. part of nervous system
p. protein
p. resistance
p. scotoma
p. seal
p. T-cell lymphoma, unspecified
p. vision
peripheralis
peripherin
peripherocentral
periphery
periphlebitic
periphlebitis
Periplaneta
periplasm
periplocin
peripolar cell
peripolesis
periporitis
periportal
p. cirrhosis
p. space of Mall
periproctic
periproctitis
periprostatic
periprostatitis
peripylephlebitis
peripylic
peripyloric
perirectal abscess
perirectitis
perirenal
p. fascia
p. fat capsule
p. insufflation
perirhinal
perirhizoclasia
perisalpingitis
perisalpingoovaritis
perisalpinx
periscopic
p. lens
p. meniscus
perisigmoiditis
perisinuous
perisinusoidal space
perispermatitis serosa

P

perisplanchnic
perisplanchnitis
perisplenic
perisplenitis
perispondylic
perispondylitis
peristalsis
    mass p.
    reversed p.
peristaltic
peristasis
peristatic hyperemia
peristernal perichondritis
peristole
peristolic
peristoma
peristomal, peristomatous
peristome
peristriate
    p. area
    p. cortex
peristrumous
perisynovial
perisystolic
peritarsal network
peritectomy
peritendineum, pl. peritendinea
peritendinitis
    p. calcarea
    p. serosa
peritenon
peritenontitis
perithecium, pl. perithecia
perithelial cell
perithelium, pl. perithelia
    Eberth p.
perithoracic
perithyroiditis
peritomist
peritomy
peritonea (pl. of peritoneum)
peritoneal
    p. button
    p. cavity
    p. dialysis
    p. fossae
    p. insufflation
    p. villi
peritonealgia
peritoneocentesis
peritoneoclysis
peritoneopathy
peritoneopericardial
peritoneopexy
peritoneoplasty
peritoneoscope
peritoneoscopy
peritoneotomy
peritoneovenous shunt
peritoneum, pl. peritonea
    parietal p.
    p. parietale
    urogenital p.
    p. urogenitale

    visceral p.
    p. viscerale
peritonitis
    adhesive p.
    benign paroxysmal p.
    bile p.
    chemical p.
    chyle p.
    circumscribed p.
    p. deformans
    diaphragmatic p.
    diffuse p.
    p. encapsulans
    fibrocaseous p.
    gas p.
    general p.
    localized p.
    meconium p.
    pelvic p.
    periodic p.
    productive p.
    tuberculous p.
peritonsillar abscess
peritonsillitis
peritracheal gland
peritrichal, peritrichate, peritrichic
Peritrichida
peritrichous
peritrigeminal nucleus
peritrochanteric
peritubular
    p. contractile cell
    p. dentin
    p. zone
perityphlic
perityphlitis
    perityphlitis p.
periumbilical
periungual fibroma
periureteral, periureteric
    p. abscess
periureteritis plastica
periurethral abscess
periurethritis
periuterine
periuvular
perivaginitis
perivascular
    p. cuff
    p. fibrous capsule
perivasculitis
perivenous
periventricular
    p. fiber
    p. preoptic nucleus
    p. zone
perivertebral
perivesical
perivisceral cavity
perivisceritis
perivitelline space
periwinkle
perkinism
perlèche
Perlia nucleus

perlingual
Perls
    P. Prussian blue stain
    P. test
permanent
    p. callus
    p. cartilage
    p. restoration
    p. stained smear examination
    p. stricture
    p. threshold shift
    p. tooth
permanganate
permanganic acid
permeability
    p. coefficient
    p. constant
    p. theory of narcosis
    p. vitamin
permeable
permeant
permease
permeate
permeation
permissible exposure limit (PEL)
permissive
    p. cell
    p. hypercapnic ventilation
perniciosiform
pernicious
    p. anemia
    p. anemia type metarubricyte
    p. anemia type prorubricyte
    p. anemia type rubriblast
    p. malaria
    p. vomiting
perniosis
perobrachius
perocephalus
perochirus
perodactyly, perodactylia
perogen
peromelia, peromely
perone
peroneal
    p. anastomotic ramus
    p. artery
    p. bone
    p. border of foot
    p. communicating branch
    p. communicating nerve
    p. compartment of leg
    p. lymph node
    p. muscular atrophy
    p. phenomenon
    p. pulley
    p. retinaculum
    p. trochlea of calcaneus
    p. vein
peroneotibial
peroneus
    p. brevis muscle
    p. longus muscle
    p. tertius muscle
peropus

peroral endoscopy
per os (PO)
perosplanchnia
perosseous
peroxidase
    horseradish p.
    p. reaction
    p. stain
peroxidases
peroxide
peroxisome
peroxyacetyl nitrate
peroxy acid
peroxyformic acid
peroxyl
perpendicular
    p. fasciculus
    p. plate
    p. plate of ethmoid bone
    p. plate of palatine bone
perpetually growing tooth
perphenazine
per primam intentionem
Perrault syndrome
per rectum
persalt
per saltum
persecution complex
persecutory
    p. delusion
    p. type of paranoid disorder
perseveration
Persian
    P. Gulf syndrome
    P. relapsing fever
persic oil
persistence
    lactase p.
    microbial p.
persistent
    p. anterior hyperplastic primary
      vitreous
    p. atrioventricular canal
    p. cloaca
    p. ectopic pregnancy
    p. frontal suture
    p. generalized lymphadenopathy
    p. müllerian duct syndrome
    p. posterior hyperplastic primary
      vitreous
    p. tremor
    p. truncus arteriosus
    p. vegetative state (PVS)
persistently growing tooth
persister
persona
personal
    p. equation
    p. growth laboratory
    p. motivation
    p. probability
    p. space
personality
    affective p.
    antisocial p.

P

personality *(continued)*
    asthenic p.
    authoritarian p.
    avoidant p.
    basic p.
    borderline p.
    compulsive p.
    cyclothymiac p.
    dependent p.
    p. disorder
    dual p.
    p. formation
    hysterical p.
    inadequate p.
    p. integration
    p. inventory
    masochistic p.
    multiple p.
    neurasthenic p.
    obsessive p.
    obsessive-compulsive p.
    paranoid p.
    passive-aggressive p.
    perfectionistic p.
    p. profile
    psychopathic p.
    schizoid p.
    schizotypal p.
    shut-in p.
    syntonic p.
    p. test
    type A, B p.
person-years
perspiration
    insensible p.
    sensible p.
perspiratory gland
perstillation
persuasion
persulfate
persulfide
persulfuric acid
pertactin
pertechnetate
Perthes
    P. disease
    P. test
Pertik diverticulum
pertrochanteric fracture
per tubam
pertussis
    p. immune globulin
    p. immunoglobulin
    p. syndrome
    p. vaccine
pertussis-like syndrome
Peruvian
    P. bark
    P. tarantula
    P. wart
pervaporation
pervasive developmental disorder
pervenous pacemaker

perversion
    polymorphous p.
    sexual p.
pervert
perverted
per vias naturales
pervious
pes, pl. **pedes**
    p. abductus
    p. adductus
    p. anserinus
    p. cavus
    p. equinovalgus
    p. equinovarus
    p. gigas
    p. hippocampi
    p. planus
    p. pronatus
    p. valgus
    p. varus
pescovegetarian
pessary
    p. cell
    p. corpuscle
    cube p.
    diaphragm p.
    doughnut p.
    Dumontpallier p.
    Gariel p.
    Hodge p.
    Mayer p.
    Menge p.
    ring p.
pessimism
    therapeutic p.
pest
pesticemia
pesticide
pestiferous
pestilence
pestilential
pestis
    p. ambulans
    p. bubonica
    p. fulminans
    p. major
    p. minor
    p. siderans
Pestivirus
pestle
PET
    positron emission tomography
peta-
petechia, pl. **petechiae**
    calcaneal petechiae
    Tardieu petechiae
petechial
    p. angiomas
    p. hemorrhage
Peters
    P. anomaly
    P. ovum
pethidine
petiolate, petiolated
petiole

petioled
petiolus epiglottidis
petit
>P. aponeurosis
>P. canal
>P. hernia
>P. herniotomy
>P. lumbar triangle
>p. mal
>p. mal epilepsy
>p. mal seizure
>p. sinus

petite mutant
Petri
>P. dish
>P. dish culture

petrifaction
pétrissage
petroccipital
petrolatum
>heavy liquid p.
>hydrophilic p.
>light liquid p.
>white p.

petroleum
>p. benzin
>p. ether
>p. jelly
>liquid p.

petromastoid
petrooccipital
>p. fissure
>p. joint
>p. synchondrosis

petropharyngeus
petrosa, pl. petrosae
petrosal
>p. bone
>p. branch of middle meningeal artery
>p. foramen
>p. fossa
>p. fossula
>p. ganglion
>p. impression of the pallium
>p. sinus
>p. vein

petrosalpingostaphylinus
petrositis
petrosomastoid
petrosphenoid
petrosphenoidal
>p. fissure
>p. syndrome

petrosquamous, petrosquamosal
>p. fissure
>p. suture

petrostaphylinus
petrotympanic fissure
petrous
>p. bone
>p. part of internal carotid artery
>p. part of temporal bone
>p. pyramid

petrousitis

Pette-Döring disease
Petzval surface
Peutz-Jeghers syndrome
Peutz syndrome
pexin
pexinogen
pexis
Peyer
>P. gland
>P. patch

peyote, peyotl
Peyronie disease
Peyrot thorax
Pezzer catheter
Pfannenstiel incision
Pfaundler-Hurler syndrome
Pfeiffer
>P. phenomenon
>P. syndrome

Pfeifferella
PFFD
>proximal femoral focal deficiency

Pflüger law
PFOB
>perfluorooctyl bromide

Pfuhl sign
PG
>prostaglandin

pg
>picogram

PGA
>prostaglandin A

PGB
>prostaglandin B

PGC
>prostaglandin C

PGD
>prostaglandin D

P-glycoprotein (*var. of* P-170)
PGR
>psychogalvanic response

P_2Gri
>diphosphoglycerate

$1,3-P_2Gri$
>1,3-bisphosphoglycerate

$2,3-P_2Gri$
>2,3-bisphosphoglycerate

PH
>PH conduction time

Ph
>phenyl

Ph1
>philadelphia chromosome

pH
>blood pH
>critical pH
>optimum pH
>pH scale
>pH value

PHA
>phytohemagglutinin

phacoanaphylactic uveitis
phacoanaphylaxis
phacocele
phacocyst

P

phacocystectomy
phacodonesis
phacoemulsification
phacoerysis
phacofragmentation
phacogenic
    p. glaucoma
    p. uveitis
phacoid
phacolysis
phacolytic glaucoma
phacoma
phacomalacia
phacomatosis
phacomorphic glaucoma
phacoscope
Phaenicia sericata
phaeo-
phaeohyphomycosis
phaeomycotic cyst
phage
    beta p.
    defective p.
    Lambda p.
phagedena
    p. gangrenosa
    p. nosocomialis
    p. tropica
phagedenic
    p. ulcer
phago-
phagocyte dysfunction
phagocytic
    p. dysfunction disorders
      immunodeficiency
    p. dysfunction immunodeficiency
    p. index
    p. pneumonocyte
phagocytin
phagocytize
phagocytoblast
phagocytolysis
phagocytolytic
phagocytose
phagocytosis
    induced p.
    spontaneous p.
phagodynamometer
phagolysis
phagolysosome
phagolytic
phagophobia
phagosome
phagotype
phakic eye
phako-
phakoma
phakomatosis
phalangeal
    p. cell
    p. joint
phalangectomy
phalanx, pl. **phalanges**
    distal p. of foot
    distal p. of hand

    p. distalis manus
    p. distalis pedis
    p. media pedis et manus
    middle phalanges of foot and hand
    proximal p. of foot
    proximal p. of hand
    p. proximalis manus
    p. proximalis pedis
    tufted p.
    ungual p.
Phalen maneuver
phallalgia
phallectomy
phalli (*pl. of* phallus)
phallic
    p. phase
    p. tubercle
phallicism
phalliform
phallism
phallocampsis
phallocrypsis
phallodynia
phalloid
phalloidin
phallolysin
phalloncus
phalloplasty
phallotomy
phallotoxins
phallus, pl. **phalli**
phanero-
phanerogenic
phaneromania
phaneroscope
phanerosis
    fatty p.
phanerozoite
phanquone
phantasia
phantasm
phantasmagoria
phantasmology
phantasmoscopia, phantasmoscopy
phantom
    p. aneurysm
    p. corpuscle
    p. limb
    p. limb pain
    Schultze p.
    sensory p.
    p. tumor
phantomize
pharmacal
pharmaceutical, pharmaceutic
    p. biology
    p. chemistry
pharmaceutics
pharmaceutist
pharmacist
    Registered P. (RPh)
pharmacochemistry
pharmacodiagnosis
pharmacodynamic
pharmacodynamics

pharmacoendocrinology
pharmacoepidemiology
pharmacogenetics
pharmacogenomics
pharmacognosist
pharmacognosy
pharmacography
pharmacokinetic
pharmacokinetics
pharmacologic, pharmacological
    p. mediators of anaphylaxis
    p. stress imaging
pharmacologist
    clinical p.
pharmacology
    biochemical p.
    clinical p.
    marine p.
pharmacomania
Pharmacopeia
pharmacopeial
    p. gel
pharmacophilia
pharmacophobia
Pharmacopoeia Germanica (PhG)
pharmacopsychosis
pharmacoresistent epilepsy
pharmacotherapy
pharmacy
    clinical p.
    Doctor of P. (Pharm. D.)
Pharm. D.
    Doctor of Pharmacy
pharyngeal
    p. arch
    p. branch
    p. branch of the artery of pterygoid canal
    p. branch of the ascending pharyngeal artery
    p. branch of descending palatine artery
    p. branch of glossopharyngeal nerve
    p. branch of inferior thyroid artery
    p. branch of pterygopalatine ganglion
    p. branch of recurrent laryngeal nerve
    p. branch of vagus nerve
    p. bursa
    p. calculus
    p. canal
    p. cartilage
    p. flap
    p. fornix
    p. gland
    p. groove
    p. hypophysis
    p. isthmus
    p. lacuna
    p. lymphatic ring
    p. membrane
    p. mucosa
    p. nerve
    p. opening of eustachian tube

    p. opening of pharyngotympanic tube
    p. pituitary
    p. plexus
    p. pouch
    p. pouch syndrome
    p. raphe
    p. recess
    p. reflex
    p. ridge
    p. space
    p. tonsil
    p. tubercle
    p. vein
pharyngectomy
pharynges (*pl. of* pharynx)
pharyngeus
pharyngismus
pharyngitic
pharyngitis
    atrophic p.
    gangrenous p.
    membranous p.
    p. sicca
    ulcerative p.
    ulceromembranous p.
pharyngo-
pharyngobasilar fascia
pharyngobranchial duct
pharyngocele
pharyngoconjunctival
    p. fever
    p. fever virus
pharyngoepiglottic, pharyngoepiglottidean
    p. fold
pharyngoesophageal
    p. constriction
    p. cushion
    p. diverticulum
    p. pad
pharyngoesophagoplasty
pharyngoglossal
pharyngoglossus
pharyngolaryngeal
pharyngolaryngitis
pharyngolith
pharyngomaxillary space
pharyngonasal cavity
pharyngo-oral
pharyngopalatine arch
pharyngopalatinus
pharyngoplasty
pharyngoplegia
pharyngorhinoscopy
pharyngoscope
pharyngoscopy
pharyngospasm
pharyngostaphylinus
pharyngostenosis
pharyngotomy
pharyngotonsillitis
pharyngotympanic
    p. groove
    p. tube
pharynx, pl. **pharynges**

P

pharynx *(continued)*
    laryngeal p.
    nasal p.
    oral p.
phase
    anal p.
    aqueous p.
    cis p.
    continuous p.
    coupling p.
    discontinuous p.
    dispersed p.
    dispersion p.
    eclipse p.
    p. encoding
    eruptive p.
    external p.
    gap_0 p.
    gap_1 p.
    gap_2 p.
    genital p.
    horizontal growth p.
    p. I, II block
    p. image
    in p.
    internal p.
    lag p.
    latency p.
    logarithmic p.
    luteal p.
    M p.
    meiotic p.
    p. microscope
    negative p.
    oedipal p.
    oral p.
    phallic p.
    positive p.
    postmeiotic p.
    postmitotic p.
    postreduction p.
    poststationary p.
    pregenital p.
    premeiotic p.
    premitotic p.
    pre-oedipal p.
    prereduction p.
    radial growth p.
    reduction p.
    p. rule
    S p.
    p. shift
    short luteal p.
    stationary p.
    supernormal recovery p.
    synaptic p.
    trans p.
    vertical growth p.
    vulnerable p.
phasic
    p. reflex
    p. sinus arrhythmia
phasmid
Phasmidia

phasmophobia
phatnorrhagia
PhD
    Doctor of Philosophy
phenacaine hydrochloride
phenacemide
phenacetin (APC)
phenacetolin
phenaceturic acid
phenacridane chloride
phenacyclamine
phenaglycodol
phenanthrene nucleus
phenarsenamine
phenarsone sulfoxylate
phenate
phenazocine
phenazoline hydrochloride
phenazopyridine hydrochloride
phencyclidine (PCP)
phendimetrazine tartrate
phenelzine sulfate
phenetamine
phenethicillin potassium
phenethyl alcohol
phenetsal
pheneturide
phenformin hydrochloride
phenglutarimide hydrochloride
phengophobia
phenicarbazide
phenindamine tartrate
phenindione
pheniramine maleate
phenmethylol
phenmetrazine hydrochloride
phenobarbital
    p. elixir
phenobutiodil
phenocopy
phenodin
phenol
    camphorated p.
    p. coefficient
    liquefied p.
    p. oxidase
phenolase
phenolated
phenolemia
phenology
phenolphthalein
phenol red
phenolsulfonphthalein (PSP)
phenoluria
phenomenology
phenomenon, pl. **phenomena**
    adhesion p.
    AFORMED p.
    Anrep p.
    aqueous influx p.
    Arias-Stella p.
    arm p.
    Arthus p.
    Ascher aqueous influx p.
    Aschner p.

Ashman p.
Aubert p.
Austin Flint p.
autoscopic p.
Babinski p.
Bell p.
Bombay p.
Bordet-Gengou p.
breakoff p., breakaway p.
Brücke-Bartley p.
Capgras p.
centralization p.
cervicolumbar p.
cogwheel p.
constancy p.
crowding p.
Cushing p.
Danysz p.
dawn p.
Debré p.
declamping p.
déjà vu p.
Dejerine hand p.
Denys-Leclef p.
d'Herelle p.
dip p.
Donath-Landsteiner p.
Doppler p.
Duckworth p.
Ehret p.
Ehrlich p.
erythrocyte adherence p.
escape p.
facialis p.
finger p.
Flynn p.
Friedreich p.
Galassi pupillary p.
Gallavardin p.
gap p.
Gärtner vein p.
generalized Shwartzman p.
Gengou p.
gestalt p.
Glover p.
Grasset p.
Grasset-Gaussel p.
Gunn p.
Hamburger p.
Hill p.
hip p.
hip-flexion p.
Hoffmann p.
Houssay p.
Hunt paradoxic p.
immune adherence p.
jaw-winking p.
Jod-Basedow p.
Köbner p.
Koch p.
Kohnstamm p.
Kühne p.
LE p.
Leede-Rumpel p.
leg p.

Lucio leprosy p.
Marcus Gunn p.
misdirection p.
Mitsuo p.
Negro p.
no reflow p.
on-off p.
orbicularis p.
paradoxical diaphragm p.
paradoxical pupillary p.
peroneal p.
Pfeiffer p.
phi p.
Pool p.
pseudo-Graefe p.
psi p.
Pulfrich p.
Purkinje p.
quellung p.
radial p.
Raynaud p.
rebound p.
reclotting p.
red cell adherence p.
reentry p.
release p.
Riddoch p.
Ritter-Rollet p.
R-on-T p.
Rumpel-Leede p.
Rust p.
Sanarelli p.
Sanarelli-Shwartzman p.
Schellong-Strisower p.
Schiff-Sherrington p.
Schüller p.
Schultz-Charlton p.
Sherrington p.
shot-silk p.
Shwartzman p.
Somogyi p.
Soret p.
sparing p.
Splendore-Hoeppli p.
staircase p.
Staub-Traugott p.
steal p.
Strümpell p.
symbiotic fermentation p.
Theobald Smith p.
tibial p.
toe p.
tongue p.
Tournay p.
Tullio p.
two-dimension–three-dimension p.
Twort p.
Twort-d'Herelle p.
Tyndall p.
vacuum disk p.
warmup p.
Wenckebach p.
Westphal-Piltz p.
Wever-Bray p.

phenoperidine

P

phenothiazine
phenotype
phenotypic
    p. mixing
    p. threshold
    p. value
phenoxazine
phenoxazone
phenoxybenzamine hydrochloride
2-phenoxyethanol
phenoxymethylpenicillin
phenozygous
phenpentermine tartrate
phenprobamate
phenprocoumon
phenpropionate
phensuximide
phentermine
phentolamine hydrochloride
phentolamine mesylate
phentolamine test
phenyl (Ph)
    p. alcohol
    p. aminosalicylate
    p. salicylate
phenylacetic acid
phenylaceturic acid
phenylacetylurea
phenylacrylic acid
phenylalaninase
phenylalanine
    p. ammonia-lyase
    p. 4-hydroxylase
    p. 4-monooxygenase
phenylamine
phenylbenzene
phenylbutazone
phenylcarbinol
phenyldichloroarsine (PD)
phenylephrine hydrochloride
phenylethanolamine *N*-methyltransferase (PNMT)
phenylethyl alcohol
phenylethylbarbituric acid
phenylethylmalonamide
phenylethylmalonylurea
phenylglycolic acid
phenylhydrazine hemolysis
phenylindanedione
phenylisothiocyanate (PITC)
phenylketonuria (PKU)
    nonclassical p.
phenyllactic acid
phenylmercuric acetate
phenylmercuric nitrate
phenylpropanolamine
phenylpyruvate oligophrenia
phenylpyruvic acid
phenylpyruvic amentia
phenylthiocarbamide
phenylthiocarbamoyl
    p. peptide
    p. protein
phenylthiohydantoin
phenylthiourea

phenyltoloxamine
phenyltrimethylammonium (PTMA)
phenyramidol hydrochloride
phenytoin
pheochrome
pheochromoblast
pheochromocyte
pheochromocytoma
pheomelanin
pheomelanogenesis
pheomelanosome
pheresis
pheromone
PhG
    Pharmacopoeia Germanica
phi (φ, Φ)
phial
phialide
phialoconidium, pl. **phialoconidia**
Phialophora
Phialophore-type conidiophore
Philadelphia
    P. chromosome
    P. cocktail
philanthropic hospital
philiater
Philip gland
Philippe triangle
Philippine hemorrhagic fever
Phillips catheter
Phillipson reflex
philomimesia
Philopia casei
philoprogenitive
philosopher's stone
philtrum, pl. **philtra**
phimosis, pl. **phimoses**
    p. clitoridis
    p. vaginalis
phimotic
phi phenomenon
phlebalgia
phlebectasia
phlebectomy
phlebeurysm
phlebitic
phlebitis
    adhesive p.
    p. nodularis necrotisans
    septic p.
phleboclysis
    drip p.
phlebodynamics
phlebogram
phlebograph
phlebography
phleboid
phlebolite
phlebolith
phlebolithiasis
phlebology
phlebomanometer
phlebometritis
phlebomyomatosis
phlebophlebostomy

phleboplasty
phleborrhaphy
phlebosclerosis
phlebostasis
phlebostenosis
phlebothrombosis
phlebotomine
phlebotomist
phlebotomize
Phlebotomus
    P. argentipes
    P. chinensis
    P. flaviscutellatus
    P. longipalpis
    P. major
    P. noguchi
    P. orientalis
    P. papatasii
    P. perniciosus
    P. sergenti
    P. verrucarum
phlebotomus
    p. fever
    p. fever viruses
phlebotomy
    bloodless p.
Phlebovirus
phlegm
phlegmasia
    phlegmasia cerulea dolens
phlegmatic
phlegmon
phlegmonous
    p. abscess
    p. enteritis
    p. erysipelas
    p. ulcer
phlogiston theory
phlogosin
phlogotherapy
phlorizin
    p. diabetes
    p. glycosuria
phloroglucin, phloroglucinol, phloroglucol
phloxine
phlyctenula, pl. phlyctenulae
phlyctenular
    p. conjunctivitis
    p. keratitis
    p. ophthalmia
    p. pannus
phlyctenule
phlyctenulosis
PhNCS protein
phobia
    school phobia
    simple p.
    social p.
    specific p.
phobic
phobophobia
phocomelia, phocomely
phocomelic dwarfism
pholcodine
pholedrine

Phoma
phon
phonacoscope
phonacoscopy
phonal
phonarteriogram
phonarteriography
phonasthenia
phonation
phonatory
phoneme
phonemic regression
phonendoscope
phonetic balance
phonetics
phoniatrics
phonic
phonoangiography
phonocardiogram
phonocardiograph
    linear p.
    logarithmic p.
    spectral p.
    stethoscopic p.
phonocardiography
phonocatheter
phonogram
phonology
phonomania
phonometer
phonomyoclonus
phonomyography
phonopathy
phonophobia
phonophore
phonophotography
phonopsia
phonoreceptor
phonoscope
phonoscopy
phonosurgery
phorbin
phorbol
phoresis
phoresy
phoria
Phormia regina
Phoroptor
phorozoon
phosgene oxime (CX)
phosphagen
phosphagenic
phosphamic acid
phosphamidase
phosphastat
phosphatase
    acid p.
    alkaline p.
    leukocyte alkaline p. (LAP)
    p. unit
phosphate
    p. acetyltransferase
    bone p.
    codeine p.
    cyclic p.

P

phosphate *(continued)*
  dexamphetamine sodium p.
  p. diabetes
  dihydrogen p.
  disodium p.
  energy-rich p.
  high-energy p.
  inorganic p. (Pi)
  monopotassium p.
  monosodium p.
  normal p.
  organic p.
  p. tetany
  triple p.
  trisodium p.
phosphated
phosphatemia
phosphatic
phosphatidal
phosphatidase
phosphatidate phosphatase
phosphatide
phosphatidic acid
phosphatidolipase
phosphatidyl (Ptd)
phosphatidylcholine (PtdCho)
phosphatidylethanolamine (PtdEth)
  p. cytidylyltransferase
phosphatidylglycerol
phosphatidylinositol (PtdIns)
  p. 4,5-bisphosphate (PIP$_2$,
    PtdIns(4,5)P$_2$)
  p. 4-phosphate
  p. synthase
phosphatidylserine (PtdSer)
phosphaturia
phosphene
  accommodation p.
phosphide
phosphine
phosphite
phosphoacylase
3′-phosphoadenosine 5′-phosphate (PAP)
3′-phosphoadenosine 5′-phosphosulfate
5-phospho-alpha-D-ribosyl-1-pyrophosphate
  (PPRibp, PPRP, PRPP)
phosphoamidase
phosphoamides
phosphoarginine
phosphocholine
  p. cytidylyltransferase
  p. diacylglycerol transferase
phosphocreatine
phosphodiesterases
  spleen p.
phosphodiester hydrolase
phosphodismutase
phospho*enol*pyruvate carboxykinase
phospho*enol*pyruvic acid
  phospho*enol*pyruvic acid
    carboxykinase
phosphoethanolamine cytidylyltransferase
1-phosphofructaldolase
1-phosphofructokinase

6-phosphofructokinase
phosphogalactoisomerase
phosphoglucokinase
phosphoglucomutase
phosphogluconate dehydrogenase
phosphogluconate pathway
6-phosphogluconolactonase
6-phospho-D-glucono-δ-lactone
phosphoglyceracetals
phosphoglycerate kinase
phosphoglyceric acid
phosphoglyceride
phosphoglyceromutase
phosphohexokinase
phosphohexomutase
phosphohexose isomerase
phosphohexose isomerase deficiency
phosphohydrolase
phosphoinositide
phosphokinase
phospholipase
  p. A$_1$, A$_2$, B, C, D
phospholipid syndrome
phosphomutase
phosphonecrosis
phosphonium
O-**phosphono-**
N^{ω}-**phosphonocreatine**
4′-phosphopantetheine
phosphopenia
phosphopentose epimerase
phosphopentose isomerase
phosphophorin
phosphoprotein
phosphopyruvate hydratase
phosphor
  photostimulable p.
  p. plate
phosphorated
phosphorescence
phosphorescent
phosphorhidrosis
phosphoriboisomerase
5-phosphoribose 1-diphosphate
5-phosphoribosylamine
phosphoribosylglycineamide synthetase
phosphoribosyltransferase
phosphoribulokinase
phosphoribulose epimerase
phosphoric acid
  cyclic p. a.
  dilute p. a.
  glacial p. a.
phosphoridrosis
phosphorism
phosphorized
phosphoroclastic
  p. cleavage
  p. reaction
phosphorolysis
phosphorous
phosphorous acid
phosphorpenia
phosphoruria

phosphorus
> amorphous p.
> p. pentoxide
> red p.

phosphorus-32 (^{32}P)
phosphorus-33 (^{33}P)
phosphoryl
phosphorylase
> p. *a*
> p. *b*
> p. kinase
> nucleoside p.
> p. phosphatase

phosphorylase-rupturing enzyme (PR enzyme)
phosphorylases
phosphorylation
> oxidative p.
> substrate-level p.

phosphorylcholine
phosphorylethanolamine glyceridetransferase
***O*-phosphoserine**
phosphosphingosides
phosphosugar
phosphotransacetylase
phosphotransferases
phosphotriose isomerase
phosphotungstic
> p. acid
> p. acid hematoxylin (PTAH)
> p. acid stain

phosphovitin
phosphuresis
phosphureted hydrogen
phosphuria
phosvitin
phot
photalgia
photaugiaphobia
photechic effect
photesthesia
photic
> p. driving
> p. stimulation

photic-sneeze reflex
photism
photoablation
photoactinic
photoaging
photoallergic sensitivity
photoallergy
photoautotroph
photoautotrophic
Photobacterium
> p. *phosphoreum*

photobacterium, pl. **photobacteria**
photobiology
photobiotic
photobleach
photocatalyst
photo cell
photoceptor
photochemical
photochemistry

photochemotherapy
photochromic
> p. lens
> p. spectacles

photochromogens
photocoagulation
photocoagulator
> laser p.
> xenon-arc p.

photodermatitis
photodistribution
photodromy
> negative p.
> positive p.

photodynamic
> p. sensitization
> p. therapy

photodynia
photodysphoria
photoelectric
> p. absorption
> p. effect

photoelectrometer
photoelectron
photoerythema
photoesthetic
photofluorography
photogastroscope
photogen
photogenesis
photogenic, photogenous
> p. epilepsy

photohemotachometer
photoheterotroph
photoheterotrophic
photoinactivation
photokeratoscope
photokinesis
photokinetic
photokinetics
photokymograph
photolithotroph
photoluminescent
photolyase
photolysis
photolyte
photolytic
photomacrography
photomania
photometer
> flame p.
> flicker p.

photometry
photomicrograph
photomicrography
photomultiplier tube
photomyoclonus
> hereditary p.

photon (hν)
> p. density

photo-patch test
photopathy
photopeak
photoperceptive
photoperiodism

P

photophobia
photophobic
photophore
photophoresis
    extracorporeal p.
photophosphorylation
photophthalmia
photopia
photopic
    p. adaptation
    p. eye
    p. vision
photopsia
photopsin
photopsy
photoptarmosis
photoradiation therapy
photoreaction
photoreactivating enzyme
photoreactivation
photoreceptive
photoreceptor cell
photorefractive keratectomy (PRK)
photorespiration
photoretinitis
photoretinopathy
photoscan
photosensitive
photosensitivity
photosensitization
photosensor oculography
photostable
photostethoscope
photostimulable phosphor
photostress test
photosynthesis
    bacterial p.
phototaxis
    negative p.
    positive p.
phototherapeutic keratectomy (PTK)
phototherapy
photothermal
phototimer
phototoxic
    p. sensitivity
phototoxicity
phototroph
phototropism
    negative p.
    positive p.
photuria
PHP
    panhypopituitarism
phragmoplast
phren
phrenalgia
phrenectomy
phrenemphraxis
phrenetic
phrenic
    p. ampulla
    p. ganglion
    p. nerve
    p. nucleus

    p. pleura
    p. plexus
    p. pressure test
    p. vein
phrenicectomy
phreniclasia
phrenicoabdominal branch of phrenic nerve
phrenicoceliac part of suspensory ligament of duodenum
phrenicocolic ligament
phrenicocostal sinus
phrenicoexeresis
phrenicogastric
phrenicoglottic, phrenoglottic
phrenicohepatic
phrenicolienal ligament
phrenicomediastinal recess
phreniconeurectomy
phrenicopleural fascia
phrenicosplenic, phrenosplenic
    p. ligament
phrenicotomy
phrenicotripsy
phrenocardia
phrenocolic
phrenogastric
    p. ligament
phrenoglottic (*var. of* phrenicoglottic)
phrenograph
phrenohepatic
phrenologist
phrenology
phrenopericardial angle
phrenoplegia
phrenoptosia
phrenosin
phrenosinic acid
phrenospasm
phrenosplenic (*var. of* phrenicosplenic)
phrenotropic
phrygian cap
phrynoderma
phrynolysin
PHS
    Public Health Service
pH-stat
o-phthalaldehyde
phthalein
phthalic acid
phthaloyl
phthalyl
phthalylsulfacetamide
phthalylsulfathiazole
phthinoid chest
phthiriophobia
Phthirus
phthisiologist
phyco-
Phycomycetes
phycomycetosis
phycomycosis
    subcutaneous p.
phyla (*pl. of* phylum)
phylacagogic

phylaxis
phyletic
phyllode
phyllodes tumor
phylloquinone
    p. K
    p. reductase
phyloanalysis
phylogenesis
phylogenetic, phylogenic
phylogeny
phylum, pl. phyla
phymatoid
phymatorrhysin
Physa
Physalia
    P. physalis
physaliferous
physaliform
physaliphore
physaliphorous cell
physalis
Physaloptera
physalopteriasis
physeal
physiatrician
physiatrics
physiatrist
physiatry
physic
physical
    p. age
    p. allergy
    p. anthropology
    p. diagnosis
    p. elasticity of muscle
    p. examination
    p. fitness
    p. half-life
    p. map
    p. medicine
    p. mixture
    p. sign
    p. therapy (PT)
physician
    American College of Nuclear P.'s
    (ACNP)
    p. assistant (P.A.)
    attending p.
    family p.
    hospital-based p.
    osteopathic p.
    resident p.
physician-assisted suicide
Physick pouch
physicochemical
physics
    radiation p.
physiogenic
physiognomy
physiognosis
physiologic, physiological
    p. age
    p. albuminuria
    p. amenorrhea

    p. anatomy
    p. anemia
    p. anisocoria
    p. antidote
    p. chemistry
    p. congestion
    p. cup
    p. dead space (V_D)
    p. drive
    p. dwarfism
    p. elasticity of muscle
    p. equilibrium
    p. excavation
    p. homeostasis
    p. hypertrophy
    p. icterus
    p. incompatibility
    p. jaundice
    p. leukocytosis
    p. occlusion
    p. rest position
    p. retraction ring
    p. saline
    p. sclerosis
    p. scotoma
    p. sphincter
    p. tremor
    p. unit
    p. vertigo
physiologically balanced occlusion
physiologicoanatomical
physiologist
physiology
    comparative p.
    general p.
    hominal p.
    pathologic p.
physiopathologic
physiopathology
physiopsychic
physiopyrexia
physiotherapeutic
physiotherapist
physiotherapy
    oral p.
physique
physis
physocele
Physocephalus sexalatus
physocephaly
physometra
Physopsis
physopyosalpinx
physostigma
physostigmine salicylate
phytanate
    p. α-oxidase
phytanic acid
6-phytase
phytate
phytic acid
phytin
phytoagglutinin
phytobezoar
phytochemistry

P

phytodermatitis
Phytoflagellata
phytohemagglutinin (PHA)
phytoid
phytol
phytolectin
Phytomastigina
Phytomastigophorasida
Phytomastigophorea
phytomenadione
phytomitogen
phytonadione
phytophagous
phytophotodermatitis
phytopneumoconiosis
phytoporphyrin
phytosis
phytosphingosine
phytosterol
phytosterolemia
phytotoxic
phytotoxin
phytotrichobezoar
phytyl alcohol
PI
    periodontal index
Pi
    inorganic phosphate
p*I*
    isoelectric point
pi, π
pia
    p. mater
    p. mater cranialis
    p. mater encephali
    p. mater spinalis
pia-arachnitis
pia-arachnoid
pial
    p. filament
    p. funnel
    p. part of filum terminale
pial-glial membrane
pian bois
pianist's cramp
piano percussion
piano-player's cramp
piarachnoid
piblokto, pibloktog
pica
Picchini syndrome
PICC line
Pick
    P. atrophy
    P. body
    P. bundle
    P. cell
    P. disease
    P. syndrome
picker's nodule
Pickles chart
pickling
pickwickian syndrome
picogram (pg)
picokatal (pkat)

picolinic acid
picolinuric acid
picometer (pm)
picomolar (pM)
picomole (pmol)
Picornaviridae
picornavirus
picramic acid
Picrasma
picrate
picric acid
picrocarmine stain
picroformol
    p. fixative
picro-Mallory trichrome stain
picronigrosin stain
picrotoxin
picrotoxinin
picryl
pictograph
picture
    p. archive and communication
      system (PACS)
    p. element
    p. frame vertebra
PID
    pelvic inflammatory disease
Pidgin Sign English (PSE)
piebald
    p. eyelash
    p. skin
piebaldism
piebaldness
piece
    end p.
    Fab p.
    Fc p.
    middle p.
    principal p.
piedra
    black p.
    p. nostras
    white p.
Piedraia
pieds terminaux
Pierini
Pierre Robin syndrome
piesimeter, piesometer
    Hales p.
piesis
piezochemistry
piezoelectric
    p. effect
    p. transducer
piezoelectricity
piezogenic pedal papule
piezometer
pig
    p. skin
pigbel
pigeon
    p. breast
    p. chest
pigment
    bile p.

p. cell
p. cell of iris
p. cell of retina
p. cell of skin
chymotropic p.
p. cirrhosis
p. dispersion syndrome
p. epithelium
p. epithelium of optic retina
formalin p.
hematogenous p.
hepatogenic p.
p. induration of the lung
malarial p.
melanotic p.
natural p.
respiratory p.
visual p.
wear-and-tear p.

pigmentary
p. cirrhosis
p. glaucoma
p. retinopathy

pigmentation
arsenic p.
exogenous p.

pigmented
p. ameloblastoma
p. dermatofibrosarcoma protuberans
p. epulis
p. hair epidermal nevus
p. keratic precipitate
p. layer of ciliary body
p. layer of iris
p. layer of retina
p. liver
p. part of retina
p. purpuric lichenoid dermatosis
p. villonodular synovitis
p. villonodular tenosynovitis

pigmentolysin
pigmentum nigrum
pigmy
Pignet formula
pigtail catheter
pilar, pilary
p. cyst
p. tumor of scalp

pile
sentinel p.
thermoelectric p.

pileous gland
piles
pileus
pili (*pl. of* pilus)
piliferous cyst
pilimiction
pilin
pill
bread p.
morning after p.
pep p.'s

pillar
anterior p. of fauces
anterior p. of fornix

p. cell
p. cell of Corti
Corti p.
p. of fauces
p. of fornix
p. of iris
posterior p. of fauces
posterior p. of fornix

pillet
pill mass
pill-rolling tremor
pilocarpine
pilocarpus
pilocystic
pilocytic astrocytoma
piloerection
piloid
p. astrocytoma
p. gliosis

pilomatrixoma
pilomotor
p. fiber
p. reflex

pilon fracture
pilonidal
p. cyst
p. fistula
p. sinus

pilose
pilosebaceous
pilosis
Piltz sign
pilula, pl. **pilulae**
pilular
p. mass

pilule
pilus, pl. **pili**
pili annulati
F pili
I pili
pili multigemini
R pili
pili torti

pimaricin
pimelic acid
pimelorrhea
pimelorthopnea
pimenta, pimento
p. oil

pimozide
pimple
PIN
prostatic intraepithelial neoplasia

pin
p. amalgam
p. implant
Steinmann p.

pinacyanol
Pinard maneuver
pincement
pincer nail
pinch
p. graft

pincushion distortion
Pindborg

P

Pindborg tumor
pindolol
pine
> p. oil
> p. tar
> white p.

pineal
> p. body
> p. cell
> p. cyst
> p. eye
> p. gland
> p. habenula
> p. recess
> p. stalk

pinealectomy
pinealocyte
pinealoma
> ectopic p.
> extrapineal p.

pinealopathy
pineapple
Pinel system
pine-needle oil
pineoblastoma
pineocytoma
ping-pong
> p.-p. bone
> p.-p. fracture
> p.-p. mechanism

pinguecula, pinguicula
pinhole pupil
piniform
pink
> p. bread mold
> p. disease

pinkeye
Pinkus tumor
pinledge
pinna, pl. **pinnae**
> p. nasi

pinnal
pinniped
pinocyte
pinocytosis
pinocytotic vesicle
pinosome
Pins
> P. sign
> P. syndrome

pint
pinta
> p. fever

pintids
pinus
pinworm vaginitis
Piophila casei
piorthopnea
PIP
> proximal interphalangeal
> > PIP joint

PIP$_2$
> phosphatidylinositol 4,5-bisphosphate

pipamazine
pipamperone

pipazethate
pipe
> p. bone
> p. stem cirrhosis

pipecolic acid
pipecolinic acid
pipecuronium
pipecuronium bromide
pipenzolate methylbromide
piper
piperacillin sodium
piperazine
> p. adipate
> p. calcium edetate
> p. citrate
> p. estrone sulfate
> p. tartrate

piperazine diethanesulfonic acid (PIPES)
Piper forceps
piperidine
> p. derivative (MPTP)

piperidolate hydrochloride
piperocaine hydrochloride
piperoxan hydrochloride
PIPES
> piperazine diethanesulfonic acid

pipe-smoker's cancer
pipestem
> p. artery
> p. fibrosis

pipette, pipet
> blowout p.
> graduated p.
> Mohr p.
> Pasteur p.
> serologic p.

pipobroman
piposulfan
pipradrol hydrochloride
piprinhydrinate
pipsyl (Ips)
piqûre diabetes
pirbuterol
Pirenella
pirenzepine
piretanide
piribedil
Pirie bone
piriform
> p. aperture
> p. area
> p. cortex
> p. fossa
> p. muscle
> p. neuron layer
> p. opening
> p. recess
> p. sinus

piriformis muscle
Pirogoff
> P. amputation
> P. angle
> P. triangle

piromen
Piroplasma

Piroplasmida
piroplasmosis
piroxicam olamine
pirprofen
Pirquet
    P. index
    P. reaction
    P. test
pisciform cataract
pisiform
    p. bone
    p. joint
pisohamate ligament
pisometacarpal ligament
pisotriquetral joint
pisounciform ligament
pisouncinate ligament
pistol-shot
    p.-s. femoral sound
piston pulse
pit
    anal p.
    articular p. of head of radius
    p. of atlas for dens
    auditory p.
    buccal p.
    p. caries
    central p.
    coated p.
    commisural p.
    costal p. of transverse process
    p. and fissure caries
    gastric p.
    granular p.
    p. of head of femur
    inferior articular p. of atlas
    inferior costal p.
    iris p.
    lens p.
    lip p.
    Mantoux p.
    nail p.
    nasal p.
    oblong p. of arytenoid cartilage
    olfactory p.
    optic p.
    otic p.
    preauricular p.
    primitive p.
    pterygoid p.
    p. of stomach
    sublingual p.
    superior articular p. of atlas
    superior costal p.
    suprameatal p.
    triangular p. of arytenoid cartilage
    trochlear p.
pit-1
PITC
    phenylisothiocyanate
pitch
    Burgundy p.
    liquid p.
    unit of p. (mel)

    p. wart
    white p.
pitchblende
pitch-worker's cancer
pith
pithecoid theory
pithode
Pitot tube
Pitres
    P. area
    P. sign
Pitressin
pitted keratolysis
pitting edema
Pittsburgh
    P. pneumonia
    P. pneumonia agent
pituicyte
pituicytoma
pituita
pituitarism
pituitarium
pituitary
    p. adamantinoma
    p. adenoma
    p. ameloblastoma
    anterior p.
    p. apoplexy
    p. cachexia
    desiccated p.
    p. diverticulum
    p. dwarf
    p. dwarfism
    p. dystopia
    p. fossa
    p. gigantism
    p. gland
    p. gonadotropic hormone
    p. growth hormone
    p. infantilism
    p. membrane
    p. myxedema
    pharyngeal p.
    posterior p.
    p. stalk
    p. stalk section
pituitous
pityriasis
    p. alba
    p. alba atrophicans
    p. capitis
    p. circinata
    p. lichenoides
    p. lichenoides chronica
    p. lichenoides et varioliformis acuta
    (PLEVA)
    p. linguae
    p. maculata
    p. nigra
    p. rosea
    p. rubra pilaris
    p. versicolor
pityroid

P

755

Pityrosporum
>*P. orbiculare*
>*P. ovale*

pivalate

pivot
>adjustable occlusal p.
>p. joint
>occlusal p.
>p. shift test

pix

pixel

PJ interval

P-K
>P.-K. antibody
>P.-K. test

PK
>pyruvate kinase

pkat
>picokatal

PKU
>phenylketonuria

pkV
>peak kilovoltage

PL
>placental lactogen

place
>p. coding
>p. theory

placebo
>active p.

placenta
>accessory p.
>p. accreta
>p. accreta vera
>adherent p.
>anular p.
>battledore p.
>bidiscoidal p.
>p. biloba
>p. bipartita
>central p. previa
>chorioallantoic p.
>chorioamnionic p.
>p. circumvallata
>cotyledonary p.
>deciduate p.
>dichorial diamnionic p.
>p. diffusa
>p. dimidiata
>disperse p.
>Duncan p.
>p. duplex
>endotheliochorial p.
>endothelio-endothelial p.
>epitheliochorial p.
>p. extrachorales
>p. fenestrata
>fetal p.
>p. fetalis
>p. gonadotropin
>hemochorial p.
>hemoendothelial p.
>horseshoe p.
>incarcerated p.
>p. increta

labyrinthine p.
>p. marginata
>maternal p.
>p. membranacea
>monochorionic diamnionic p.
>monochorionic monoamnionic p.
>p. multiloba
>p. multipartita
>nondeciduous p.
>p. panduraformis
>p. percreta
>p. previa
>p. previa centralis
>p. previa marginalis
>p. previa partialis
>p. protein
>p. reflexa
>p. reniformis
>retained p.
>ring-shaped p.
>Schultze p.
>p. spuria
>succenturiate p.
>supernumerary p.
>total p. previa
>p. triloba
>p. tripartita
>p. triplex
>twin p.
>p. uterina
>p. velamentosa
>villous p.
>zonary p.

placentagonadotropin

placental
>p. barrier
>p. circulation
>p. dysfunction
>p. dysfunction syndrome
>p. dysmature
>p. dystocia
>p. growth hormone
>p. lactogen (PL)
>p. lobe
>p. membrane
>p. parasitic twin
>p. plasmodium
>p. polyp
>p. presentation
>p. septa
>p. sign
>p. site trophoblastic tumor
>p. souffle
>p. sulfatase deficiency
>p. thrombosis
>p. transfusion
>p. transfusion syndrome

Placentalia

placentation

placentitis

placentoma

placentotherapy

Placido da Costa disk

placode
>auditory p.

epibranchial p.
lens p.
nasal p.
olfactory p.
optic p.
otic p.
plafond
plagiocephalic
plagiocephalism
plagiocephalous
plagiocephaly
plague
ambulatory p.
p. bacillus
black p.
bubonic p.
glandular p.
hemorrhagic p.
larval p.
Pahvant Valley p.
p. pneumonia
pneumonic p.
pulmonic p.
p. septicemia
septicemic p.
sylvatic p.
p. vaccine
plain film
plakalbumin
plakins
plan
subjective, objective, assessment,
and p. (SOAP)
plana (*pl. of* planum)
planchet
Planck
P. constant (*h*)
P. theory
plane
Addison clinical p.
Aeby p.
auriculoinfraorbital p.
axial p.
axiolabiolingual p.
axiomesiodistal p.
bite p.
Broca visual p.
Camper p.
canthomeatal p.
coronal p.
cove p.
datum p.
Daubenton p.
equatorial p.
eye-ear p.
facial p.
first parallel pelvic p.
fourth parallel pelvic p.
Frankfort p.
Frankfort horizontal p.
frontal p.
guide p.
horizontal p.
p. of incidence
infraorbitomeatal p.

p. of inlet
interspinal p.
interspinous p.
intertubercular p.
p. joint
labiolingual p.
p. of least pelvic dimensions
mean foundation p.
Meckel p.
median p.
p. of midpelvis
midsagittal p.
Morton p.
nasion-postcondylar p.
nodal p.
nuchal p.
occipital p.
occlusal p.
p. of occlusion
orbital p.
orbitomeatal p.
p. of outlet
parasagittal p.
p. of pelvic canal
pelvic p. of greatest dimensions
pelvic p. of inlet
pelvic p. of least dimensions
pelvic p. of outlet
popliteal p. of femur
principal p.
p. of reference
p. of regard
sagittal p.
second parallel pelvic p.
spectacle p.
sternal p.
subcostal p.
supracrestal p.
supracristal p.
supraorbitomeatal p.
suprasternal p.
p. suture
temporal p.
third parallel pelvic p.
tooth p.
transaxial p.
transpyloric p.
transverse p.
p. wart
wide p.
planigraphy
planimeter
planimetry
planithorax
plankter
plankton
planktonic
planocellular
planoconcave lens
planoconvex lens
planography
planomania
Planorbis
planovalgus

P

plant
p. agglutinin
p. antitoxin
p. casein
p. indican
p. RNase
p. toxin
p. viruses

planta, pl. **plantae**
p. pedis

plantago
p. ovata coating
p. seed

plantain seed

plantalgia

plantar
p. aponeurosis
p. arterial arch
p. calcaneocuboid ligament
p. calcaneonavicular ligament
p. cuboideonavicular ligament
p. cuneocuboid ligament
p. cuneonavicular ligament
p. digital vein
p. fascia
p. fasciitis
p. fibromatosis
p. flexion
p. interossei interosseous muscle
p. ligament
p. ligament of interphalangeal joint of foot
p. ligament of metatarsophalangeal joint
p. metatarsal artery
p. metatarsal ligament
p. metatarsal vein
p. muscle
p. muscle reflex
p. quadrate muscle
p. region
p. space
p. surface of foot
p. surface of toe
p. tarsal ligament
p. tarsometatarsal ligament
p. tendon sheath of fibularis longus muscle
p. tendon sheath of peroneus longus muscle
p. venous arch
p. venous network
p. wart

plantarflexor compartment of leg

plantaris
p. muscle

plantigrade

planula, pl. **planulae**
invaginate p.

planum, pl. **plana**
plana coronalia
plana frontalia
horizontal plana
plana horizontalia
p. interspinale

p. intertuberculare
p. medianum
p. occipitale
p. orbitale
p. popliteum
plana sagittalia
p. semilunatum
p. sphenoidale
p. sternale
p. subcostale
p. supracristale
p. temporale
p. transpyloricum
plana transversalia

planuria

plaque
atheromatous p.
bacterial p.
bacteriophage p.
dental p.
Hollenhorst p.
P. Index
mucous p.
neuritic p.
pleural p.
Randall p.
senile p.

plasm

plasma
p. accelerator globulin
p. albumin
antihemophilic p.
blood p.
p. cell
p. cell balanitis
p. cell gingivitis
p. cell hepatitis
p. cell leukemia
p. cell mastitis
p. cell myeloma
p. expander
p. factor X
p. fibronectin
fresh frozen p. (FFP)
p. hydrolysate
p. iodoprotein disorder
p. labile factor
p. layer
p. marinum
p. membrane
muscle p.
normal human p.
p. protein
p. renin activity (PRA)
salted p.
p. scalpel
p. stain
p. substitute
p. therapy
p. thromboplastin antecedent (PTA)
p. thromboplastin component (PTC)
p. thromboplastin factor (PTF)
p. thromboplastin factor B

plasmablast

plasma cell dyscrasia

plasmacrit test
plasmacyte
plasmacytoblast
plasmacytoma
plasmacytosis
plasmagene
plasmakinins
plasmalemma
plasmalogen
plasmal reaction
plasmals
plasmapheresis
plasmapheretic
plasmatic
    p. compartment
plasmatic stain (*var. of* plasma stain)
plasmatogamy
plasmenic acid
plasmic stain (*var. of* plasma stain)
plasmid
    bacteriocinogenic p.
    conjugative p.
    F p.
    infectious p.
    nonconjugative p.
    R p.
    resistance p.
    transmissible p.
plasminogen activator
plasminokinase
plasminoplastin
plasmin prothrombins conversion factor (PPCF)
plasmocytic leukemoid reaction
plasmodia (*pl. of* plasmodium)
plasmodial
    p. trophoblast
plasmodiotrophoblast
Plasmodium
    P. aethiopicum
    P. berghei
    P. brazilianum
    P. cynomolgi
    P. falciparum
    P. knowlesi
    P. kochi
    P. malariae
    P. ovale
    P. vivax
plasmodium, pl. plasmodia
    placental p.
Plasmodromata
plasmogamy
plasmogen
plasmokinin
plasmolemma
plasmolysis
plasmolytic
plasmolyze
plasmon
plasmorrhexis
plasmoschisis
plasmosin
plasmotomy
plasmotropic

plasmotropism
plasmotype
plasmozyme
plastein
plaster
    p. bandage
    p. of Paris
    p. splint
plastic
    p. anatomy
    Bingham p.
    p. bronchitis
    p. corpuscle
    p. cyclitis
    p. envelope culture
    p. induration
    p. iritis
    p. lymph
    modeling p.
    p. motor
    p. pleurisy
    p. restoration material
    p. section stain
    p. surgery
    p. tooth
plasticity
plastid
    blood p.
plastochromanol-3, plastochromanol E_3
plastochromenol-8
plastogamy
plastoquinone (PQ)
plastoquinone-9, plastoquinone E_9 (PQ-9)
plastron
plate
    alar p. of neural tube
    amorphous selenium p.
    anal p.
    axial p.
    basal p. of neural tube
    base p.
    blood p.
    bone p.
    buttress p.
    cardiogenic p.
    cell p.
    chorionic p.
    cloacal p.
    compression p.
    cribriform p. of ethmoid bone
    cutis p.
    dorsal p. of neural tube
    dorsolateral p. of neural tube
    end p.
    epiphysial p.
    equatorial p.
    ethmovomerine p.
    flat p.
    floor p.
    foot p.
    frontal p.
    growth p.
    horizontal p. of palatine bone
    Kühne p.
    lateral p.

P

plate *(continued)*
    lateral cartilaginous p.
    lateral p. of cartilaginous auditory tube
    lateral pterygoid p.
    lateral p. of pterygoid process
    lingual p.
    medial cartilaginous p.
    medial p. of cartilaginous auditory tube
    medial pterygoid p.
    medial p. of pterygoid process
    medullary p.
    p. of modiolus
    motor p.
    muscle p.
    nail p.
    neural p.
    neutralization p.
    notochordal p.
    oral p.
    orbital p.
    orbital p. of ethmoid bone
    palatal p.
    palmar p.
    paper p.
    papyraceous p.
    parachordal p.
    parietal p.
    perpendicular p.
    perpendicular p. of ethmoid bone
    perpendicular p. of palatine bone
    phosphor p.
    polar p.
    prechordal p.
    prochordal p.
    pterygoid p.
    quadrigeminal p.
    roof p.
    secondary spiral p.
    segmental p.
    selenium p.
    sieve p.
    spiral p.
    stigmal p.
    suction p.
    tarsal p.
    tectal p.
    terminal p.
    p. thrombosis
    tympanic p. of temporal bone
    urethral p.
    ventral p.
    ventral p. of neural tube
    vertical p.
    visceral p.
    wing p.
plateau
    p. iris
    p. pulse
    ventricular p.
Plateau-Talbot law
platelet
    p. actomyosin

    p. aggregation test
    p. cofactor I, II
    p. factor 3
    p. tissue factor
platelet-activating factor
platelet-aggregating factor (PAF)
platelet-derived growth factor (PDGF)
plateletpheresis
platelike atelectasis
plating
    compression p.
    replica p.
platinic
platinous
platinum (Pt)
    p. black
    p. foil
    p. group
platybasia
platycephaly
platycnemia
platycnemic
platycnemism
platycrania
platycyte
platyglossal
platyhelminth
Platyhelminthes
platyhieric
platymeric
platymorphia
platyopia
platyopic
platypellic pelvis
platypelloid pelvis
platypnea
platyrrhine
platyrrhiny
platysma, pl. **platysmas**
    p. muscle
platysmata
platyspondylia, platyspondylisis
platystencephaly
play therapy
pleasure
    P. curve
    p. principle
plectridium
pledget
pledgetted suture
pleiotropic gene
pleiotropy, pleiotropia
    functional p.
    structural p.
Pleistophora
pleochroic
pleochroism
pleochromatic
pleochromatism
pleocytosis
pleomastia, pleomazia
pleomorphic
    p. adenoma
    p. lipoma

p. oligodendroglioma
p. xanthoastrocytoma
pleomorphism
pleomorphous
pleonasm
pleonosteosis
Leri p.
pleoptics
pleoptophor
plerocercoid
Plesiomonas shigelloides
plesiomorphic
plesiomorphism
plesiomorphous
plessesthesia
plessimeter
plessimetric
plessor
plethora
plethoric
plethysmograph
body p.
digital p.
pressure p.
volume-displacement p.
plethysmographic goggle
plethysmography
impedance p.
venous occlusion p.
plethysmometry
pleura, pl. **pleurae**
cervical p.
costal p.
p. costalis
diaphragmatic p.
p. diaphragmatica
mediastinal p.
p. mediastinalis
parietal p.
p. parietalis
p. pericardiaca
pericardial p.
phrenic p.
p. phrenica
p. pulmonalis
pulmonary p.
visceral p.
p. visceralis
pleuracentesis
pleural
p. calculus
p. canal
p. cavity
p. cupula
p. effusion
p. fluid
p. fremitus
p. friction rub
p. isthmus
p. line
p. plaque
p. poudrage
p. pressure
p. rale
p. reaction

p. recess
p. rub
p. sinus
p. space
p. stripe
p. tap
p. villi
pleural crackles
pleuralgia
pleurapophysis
pleurectomy
pleurisy
adhesive p.
benign dry p.
bilateral p.
chronic p.
costal p.
diaphragmatic p.
double p.
dry p.
encysted p.
epidemic benign dry p.
epidemic diaphragmatic p.
fibrinous p.
hemorrhagic p.
interlobular p.
mediastinal p.
plastic p.
productive p.
proliferating p.
pulmonary p.
purulent p.
sacculated p.
serofibrinous p.
serous p.
suppurative p.
typhoid p.
visceral p.
wet p.
p. with effusion
pleuritic
p. pneumonia
p. rub
pleuritis
pleuritogenous
pleurocele
pleurocentesis
pleurocentrum
pleuroclysis
pleurodesis
pleurodynia
epidemic p.
pleuroesophageal
p. line
p. muscle
pleuroesophageus muscle
pleurogenic
pleurogenous
pleurography
pleurohepatitis
pleurolith
pleurolysis
pleuropericardial
p. canal
p. fold

P

pleuropericardial *(continued)*
    p. hiatus
    p. membrane
    p. murmur
pleuropericarditis
pleuroperitoneal
    p. canal
    p. cavity
    p. fold
    p. hiatus
    p. membrane
    p. shunt
pleuropneumonectomy
pleuropneumonia-like organisms (PPLO)
pleuropulmonary
pleuroscopy
pleurotomy
pleurotyphoid
pleurovenous shunt
pleurovisceral
PLEVA
    pityriasis lichenoides et varioliformis
      acuta
plexal
plexectomy
plexiform
    p. layer
    p. layer of cerebral cortex
    p. layer of retina
    p. neurofibroma
    p. neuroma
pleximeter
plexitis
    brachial p.
plexogenic
    p. pulmonary arteriopathy
plexometer
plexopathy
plexor
plexus, pl. **plexuses**
    abdominal aortic plexuses
    acromial p.
    p. annularis
    anterior coronary periarterial p.
    anular p.
    aortic lymphatic p.
    p. aorticus
    areolar venous p.
    p. arteriae choroideae
    arterial p.
    articular vascular p.
    ascending pharyngeal p.
    Auerbach p.
    autonomic plexus
    p. autonomicus brachialis
    axillary lymphatic p.
    basilar venous p.
    Batson p.
    brachial p.
    brachial autonomic p.
    p. brachialis
    cardiac p.
    p. cardiacus profundus
    p. caroticus internus

cavernous p. of clitoris
cavernous p. of conchae
cavernous nervous p.
cavernous p. of penis
celiac p.
cervical p.
p. cervicalis
choroid p.
p. choroideus
p. choroideus ventriculi lateralis
p. choroideus ventriculi quarti
p. choroideus ventriculi tertii
choroid p. of fourth ventricle
choroid p. of lateral ventricle
choroid p. of third ventricle
ciliary ganglionic p.
coccygeal p.
p. coccygeus
common carotid nervous p.
p. coronarii cordis
coronary p.
Cruveilhier p.
deep cardiac p.
deferential p.
p. of ductus deferens
enteric p.
esophageal p.
Exner p.
external carotid p.
external iliac lymphatic p.
external maxillary p.
facial p.
femoral p.
p. gangliosus ciliaris
gastric plexus of autonomic system
p. gastrici systematis autonomici
gastric nervous plexus
p. gulae
Haller p.
Heller p.
hemorrhoidal p.
hepatic p.
iliac p.
inferior dental p.
inferior hemorrhoidal plexus
inferior hypogastric p.
inferior mesenteric p.
inferior rectal p.
inferior thyroid p.
inferior vesical venous p.
inguinal lymphatic p.
intermesenteric p.
internal carotid venous p.
internal mammary p.
internal maxillary p.
internal thoracic lymphatic p.
intracavernous p.
p. intraparotideus nervi facialis
intraparotid p. of facial nerve
ischiadic p.
Jacobson p.
Jacques p.
jugular lymphatic p.
Leber p.
lingual p.

lumbar lymphatic p.
lumbosacral p.
lymphatic p.
p. lymphaticus
p. lymphaticus axillaris
p. lymphaticus iliacus externus
p. lymphaticus inguinalis
p. lymphaticus jugularis
p. lymphaticus lumbalis
p. lymphaticus sacralis medius
p. mammarius
p. mammarius internus
mammary p.
p. maxillaris externus
p. maxillaris internus
maxillary p.
Meissner p.
meningeal p.
p. meningeus
middle hemorrhoidal plexus
middle rectal p.
middle sacral lymphatic p.
myenteric p.
nerve p.
p. nervorum gastricorum
p. nervorum lumbalium
p. nervorum spinalium
p. nervosus
p. nervosus aorticus abdominalis
p. nervosus aorticus thoracicus
p. nervosus arteriae carotidis
  internae
p. nervosus cardiacus
p. nervosus cardiacus superficialis
p. nervosus caroticus communis
p. nervosus caroticus externus
p. nervosus cavernosus
p. nervosus celiacus
p. nervosus cervicalis posterior
p. nervosus deferentialis
p. nervosus dentalis inferior
p. nervosus dentalis superior
p. nervosus entericus
p. nervosus esophageus
p. nervosus femoralis
p. nervosus hepaticus
p. nervosus hypogastricus inferior
p. nervosus hypogastricus superior
p. nervosus iliacus
p. nervosus intermesentericus
p. nervosus lienalis
p. nervosus lumbosacralis
p. nervosus mesentericus inferior
p. nervosus mesentericus superior
p. nervosus myentericus
p. nervosus ovaricus
p. nervosus pancreaticus
p. nervosus pelvicus
p. nervosus pharyngeus
p. nervosus prostaticus
p. nervosus pulmonalis
p. nervosus rectalis inferiores
p. nervosus rectalis medius
p. nervosus rectalis superior
p. nervosus renalis

p. nervosus splenicus
p. nervosus submucosus
p. nervosus subserosus
p. nervosus suprarenalis
p. nervosus tympanicus
p. nervosus uretericus
p. nervosus uterovaginalis
occipital p.
ovarian p.
pampiniform venous p.
pancreatic p.
parotid p. of facial nerve
pelvic p.
periarterial p.
periarterial p. of anterior cerebral
  artery
periarterial p. of ascending
  pharyngeal artery
periarterial p. of choroid artery
periarterial plexuses of coronary
  artery
periarterial p. of facial artery
periarterial p. of inferior phrenic
  artery
periarterial p. of inferior thyroid
  artery
periarterial p. of internal thoracic
  artery
p. periarterialis
p. periarterialis arteriae auricularis
  posterioris
p. periarterialis arteriae cerebri
  anterioris
p. periarterialis arteriae cerebri
  mediae
p. periarterialis arteriae choroideae
p. periarterialis arteriae facialis
p. periarterialis arteriae lingualis
p. periarterialis arteriae maxillaris
p. periarterialis arteriae occipitalis
p. periarterialis arteriae ophthalmicae
p. periarterialis arteriae pharyngeae
  ascendentis
p. periarterialis arteriae phrenicae
  inferioris
p. periarterialis arteriae popliteae
p. periarterialis arteriae subclaviae
p. periarterialis arteriae temporalis
  superficialis
p. periarterialis arteriae testicularis
p. periarterialis arteriae thoracicae
  internae
p. periarterialis arteriae thyroideae
  superioris
p. periarterialis arteriae vertebralis
periarterial p. of lingual artery
periarterial p. of maxillary artery
periarterial p. of middle cerebral
  artery
periarterial p. of occipital artery
periarterial p. of ophthalmic artery
periarterial p. of popliteal artery
periarterial p. of posterior auricular
  artery
periarterial p. of subclavian artery

P

plexus *(continued)*
periarterial p. of superficial temporal artery
periarterial p. of superior thyroid artery
periarterial p. of testicular artery
periarterial p. of thyroid artery
periarterial p. of vertebral artery
pharyngeal p.
phrenic p., p. phrenicus
popliteal p., p. popliteus
posterior auricular p.
posterior cervical p.
posterior coronary p.
prostaticovesical venous p.
prostatic venous p.
pterygoid venous p.
p. pudendalis
p. pudendus nervosus
pulmonary p.
Quénu hemorrhoidal p.
Ranvier p.
rectal p.
rectal venous p.
Remak p.
renal p.
sacral p.
p. sacralis
sacral venous p.
Santorini p.
Sappey p.
sciatic p.
solar p.
spermatic p.
spinal nerve p.
p. of spinal nerve
splenic p.
Stensen p.
stroma p.
subclavian p.
submucosal p.
suboccipital venous p.
subserous p.
superficial cardiac p.
superficial temporal p.
superior dental p.
superior hemorrhoidal p.
superior hypogastric p.
superior mesenteric p.
superior rectal p.
superior thyroid p.
suprarenal p.
sympathetic plexuses
testicular p.
thoracic aortic p.
p. thyroideus inferior
tympanic p.
unpaired thyroid venous p.
ureteric p.
uterine venous p.
uterovaginal p.
vaginal venous p.
vascular p.
p. vascularis cavernosus conchae

p. vasculosus
p. venosus
p. venosus areolaris
p. venosus basilaris
p. venosus canalis hypoglossi
p. venosus caroticus internus
p. venosus foraminis ovalis
p. venosus pampiniformis
p. venosus prostaticovesicalis
p. venosus prostaticus
p. venosus pterygoideus
p. venosus rectalis
p. venosus sacralis
p. venosus suboccipitalis
p. venosus thyroideus impar
p. venosus uterinus
p. venosus vaginalis
p. venosus vertebralis
p. venosus vertebralis externus anterior
p. venosus vertebralis externus posterior
p. venosus vertebralis internus anterior
p. venosus vertebralis internus posterior
p. venosus vesicalis
p. venosus vesicalis inferior
venous p.
venous p. of bladder
venous p. of canal of hypoglossal nerve
venous p. of foramen ovale
vertebral p.
p. vertebralis
vertebral venous p.
p. vesicalis
vesical nervous p.
vesicular venous p.
plexus viscerales
Walther p.
plexus phrenicus *(var. of* phrenic plexus)
plexus popliteus *(var. of* popliteal plexus)
plica, pl. **plicae**
plicae adiposae pleurae
plicae alares plicae synovialis infrapatellaris
plicae ampullares tubae uterinae
p. anterior faucium
p. aryepiglottica
p. axillaris
plicae cecales
p. cecalis vascularis
p. chordae tympani
p. choroidea
plicae ciliares
plicae circulares intestini tenuis
p. duodenalis inferior
p. duodenalis superior
p. duodenojejunalis
p. duodenomesocolica
p. epigastrica
plicae epiglotticae
p. fimbriata faciei inferioris linguae
plicae gastricae

plicae gastropancreaticae
p. glossoepiglottica lateralis
p. glossoepiglottica mediana
p. gubernatrix
p. hypogastrica
p. ileocecalis
p. incudis
p. inguinalis
p. interdigitalis
p. interureterica
plicae iridis
p. lacrimalis
p. longitudinalis duodeni
p. lunata
plicae malleares anterior et posterior
p. membranae tympani
plicae mucosae vesicae biliaris
p. nervi laryngei superioris
p. palatina transversa
plicae palmatae canalis cervicis uteri
p. palpebronasalis
p. paraduodenalis
p. posterior faucium
plicae recti
p. rectouterina
p. rectovaginalis
p. salpingopalatina
p. salpingopharyngea
plicae semilunares coli
plicae semilunares of colon
p. semilunaris
p. semilunaris of conjunctiva
p. semilunaris conjunctivae
p. semilunaris of eye
p. spiralis ductus cystici
p. stapedialis
p. sublingualis
p. synovialis
p. synovialis infrapatellaris
p. synovialis patellaris
plicae transversales recti
p. triangularis
plicae tubariae tubae uterinae
p. tubopalatina
p. umbilicalis lateralis
p. umbilicalis medialis
p. urachi
p. ureterica
p. uterovesicalis
p. venae cavae sinistrae
p. ventricularis
p. vesicalis transversa
p. vesicouterina
p. vestibularis
p. vestibuli
p. villosa
p. vocalis
plicate
plication
plicotomy
ploidy
plombage
plosive
plot
double-reciprocal p.

Eadie-Hofstee p.
funnel p.
Hanes p.
Hill p.
Lineweaver-Burk p.
Ramachandran p.
Scatchard p.
Woolf-Lineweaver-Burk p.
PLP
parathyroid hormonelike protein
pyridoxal 5-phosphate
plug
Dittrich p.
epithelial p.
laminated epithelial p.
meconium p.
mucous p.
Traube p.'s
plugger
automatic p.
back-action p.
foot p.
root canal p.
plugging instrument
plumbago
plumbic
plumbism
plumbum
Plummer disease
Plummer-Vinson syndrome
plumose
pluricausal
pluriglandular
plurilocular
plurinuclear
pluripotent
p. cell
pluriresistant
plus
p. lens
p. strand
plutomania
plutonism
plutonium (Pu)
Pm
promethium
pM
picomolar
pm
picometer
PMA index
PMIS
postmyocardial infarction syndrome
P mitrale
PML
progressive multifocal leukoencephalopathy
pmol
picomole
PMR
proportional mortality ratio
PMS
premenstrual syndrome
pneo-
pneocardiac reflex

P

pneopneic reflex
pneuma
pneumarthrogram
pneumarthrography
pneumarthrosis
pneumatic
    p. antishock garment
    p. bone
    p. dilator
    p. otoscopy
    p. retinopexy
    p. space
    p. tire injury
    p. tonometer
pneumatics
pneumatism
pneumatists
pneumatization
pneumatized bone
pneumatocardia
pneumatocele
    extracranial p.
    intracranial p.
pneumatoenteric recess
pneumatohemia
pneumatometer
pneumatorrhachis
pneumatoscope
pneumatosis
    p. coli
    p. cystoides intestinalis
pneumaturia
pneumatype
pneumoarthrography
pneumobacillus
pneumobulbar
pneumocardial
pneumocele
    extracranial p.
    intracranial p.
pneumocentesis
pneumocephalus
pneumocholecystitis
pneumococcal
    p. empyema
    p. polysaccharide
    p. vaccine
pneumococcal/suppurative keratitis
pneumococcemia
pneumococci (*pl. of* pneumococcus)
pneumococcidal
pneumococcolysis
pneumococcosis
pneumococcosuria
pneumococcus, pl. **pneumococci**
    Fraenkel p.
pneumocolon
pneumoconiosis, pneumokoniosis,
  pl. **pneumoconioses**
    bauxite p.
    coal worker's p.
    collagenous p.
    p. siderotica
pneumocranium
Pneumocystis carinii **pneumonia**

pneumocystography
pneumocystosis
pneumocyte
pneumoderma
pneumodynamics
pneumoempyema
pneumoencephalogram
pneumoencephalography
pneumoenteric recess
pneumogastric nerve
pneumogastrography
pneumogenic osteoarthropathy
pneumogram
pneumograph
pneumography
pneumohemia
pneumohemopericardium
pneumohemothorax
pneumohydrometra
pneumohydropericardium
pneumohydroperitoneum
pneumohydrothorax
pneumohypoderma
pneumokoniosis (*var. of* pneumoconiosis)
pneumolith
pneumolithiasis
pneumology
pneumolysis
pneumomalacia
pneumomassage
pneumomediastinum
pneumomelanosis
pneumomycosis
pneumomyelography
pneumonectomy
pneumonia
    acute interstitial p.
    alcoholic p.
    anaerobic p.
    apex p.
    apical p.
    aspiration p.
    atypical p.
    bacterial p.
    bilious p.
    bronchial p.
    caseous p.
    central p.
    chemical p.
    chronic eosinophilic p.
    community-acquired p.
    congenital p.
    core p.
    deglutition p.
    desquamative p.
    desquamative interstitial p. (DIP)
    p. dissecans
    double p.
    embolic p.
    eosinophilic p.
    fibrous p.
    Friedländer bacillus p.
    gangrenous p.
    giant cell p.
    Hecht p.

hospital-acquired p.
hypostatic p.
influenza p.
influenzal virus p.
p. interlobularis purulenta
interstitial plasma cell p.
intrauterine p.
lipid p.
lipoid p.
lobar p.
lymphocytic interstitial p. (lip)
lymphoid interstitial p.
p. malleosa
metastatic p.
migratory p.
nosocomial p.
obstructive p.
oil p.
Pittsburgh p.
plague p.
pleuritic p.
Pneumocystis carinii p.
postobstructive p.
primary atypical p.
purulent p.
rheumatic p.
septic p.
staphylococcal p.
streptococcal p.
suppurative p.
terminal p.
tularemic p.
typhoid p.
unresolved p.
uremic p.
usual interstitial p. (UIP)
usual interstitial p. of Liebow
p. virus of mice
wandering p.
woolsorter's p.
pneumonic
p. plague
pneumonitis
acute interstitial p.
hypersensitivity p.
lymphocytic interstitial p.
radiation p.
uremic p.
pneumonocele
pneumonocentesis
pneumonococcal
pneumonococcus
pneumonoconiosis, pneumonokoniosis
pneumonocyte
granular p.'s
phagocytic p.
pneumonomelanosis
pneumonopathy
eosinophilic p.
pneumonopexy
pneumonopleuritis
pneumonorrhaphy
pneumonotomy
pneumo-orbitography

pneumopericardium
tension p.
pneumoperitoneum
pneumoperitonitis
pneumopexy
pneumophagia
pneumopleuritis
pneumopyelography
pneumoradiography
pneumoresection
pneumoretroperitoneum
pneumoroentgenography
pneumorrhachis
pneumoscope
pneumoserothorax
pneumosilicosis
pneumotachogram
pneumotachograph
Fleisch p.
Silverman-Lilly p.
pneumotachometer
pneumothermomassage
pneumothorax
artificial p.
catamenial p.
extrapleural p.
iatrogenic p.
open p.
pressure p.
p. simplex
spontaneous p.
tension p.
therapeutic p.
traumatic p.
pneumotomy
pneumoventricle
Pneumovirus
pneusis
pnigophobia
PNMT
phenylethanolamine n-methyltransferase
PNP
psychogenic nocturnal polydipsia
PNP syndrome
PNPB
positive-negative pressure breathing
PO
per os
P/O
P/O quotient
P/O ratio
Po
polonium
pock
pocket
gingival p.
infrabony p.
intrabony p.
periodontal p.
Rathke p.
retraction p.
rheumatoid p.
Seessel p.
subcrestal p.
Tröltsch p.'s

P

pocketed calculus
pockmark
poculum diogenis
podagra
podagral, podagric, podagrous
podalgia
podalic
    p. extraction
    p. version
podarthritis
podedema
podiatric medicine
podiatrist
podiatry
    Doctor of P. (DP)
podismus
poditis
    tourniquet p.
podobromidrosis
podocyte
pododynamometer
pododynia
podofilox
podogram
podograph
podolite
podologist
podology
podomechanotherapy
podometer
podophyllin
podophyllotoxin
podophyllum
    Indian p.
    p. resin
podospasm, podospasmus
Podoviridae
POEMS
    polyneuropathy, organomegaly,
    endocrinopathy, monoclonal
    gammopathy, and skin changes
      POEMS syndrome
pogoniasis
pogonion
Pogonomyrmex
poietin
poikiloblast
poikilocyte
poikilocythemia
poikilocytosis
poikilodentosis
poikiloderma
    p. atrophicans vasculare
    p. of Civatte
    p. congenitale
poikilotherm
poikilothermic, poikilothermal,
  poikilothermous
poikilothermy, poikilothermism
poikilothrombocyte
poikilothymia
point
    p. A, B
    absorbent p.
    alveolar p.

p. angle
anterior focal p.
apophysary p.
apophysial p.
auricular p.
axial p.
boiling p. (b.p.)
Cannon p.
Capuron p.
cardinal p.
central-bearing p.
Clado p.
clinical end p.
cold-rigor p.
congruent p.
conjugate p.
contact p.
p. of convergence
craniometric p.
critical p.
p. deletion
dew p.
p. of elbow
end p.
p. epidemic
equivalence p.
far p.
p. of fixation
flash p.
focal p.
freezing p.
fusing p.
Guéneau de Mussy p.
gutta-percha p.
Hallé p.
heat-rigor p.
incident p.
incisal p.
isoelectric p. (IEP, p*I*)
isoionic p.
isosbestic p.
J p.
jugal p.
lower alveolar p.
malar p.
p. of maximal impulse
maximum occipital p.
Mayo-Robson p.
McBurney p.
median mandibular p.
melting p. (m.p.)
mental p.
metopic p.
motor p.
Munro p.
p. mutation
nasal p.
near p.
neutral p.
nodal p.
occipital p.
p. of ossification
painful p.
posterior focal p.
power p.

preauricular p.
pressure p.
primary p. of ossification
principal p.
p. of proximal contact
p. of regard
retention p.
secondary p. of ossification
silver p.
p. source
spinal p.
subnasal p.
Sudeck critical p.
supra-auricular p.
supranasal p.
supraorbital p.
sylvian p.
p. system test types
tender p.
trigger p.
triple p.
Trousseau p.
Valleix p.
Weber p.
zygomaxillary p.
pointillage
pointing
Poirier
P. gland
P. line
poise
Poiseuille
P. law
P. space
P. viscosity coefficient
Poiseuille
poison
acrid p.
arrow p.
fish p.
fugu p.
p. ivy
p. oak
respiratory p.
p. sumac
poisoning
ackee p.
acute lead p.
acute mercury p.
bacterial food p.
blood p.
carbon disulfide p.
carbon monoxide p.
chronic lead p.
chronic mercury p.
crotalaria p.
cyanide p.
Datura p.
djenkol p.
ergot p.
food p.
lead p.
mercury p.
mushroom p.
oxygen p.

radiation p.
Salmonella food p.
scombroid p.
silver p.
Staphylococcus food p.
systemic p.
tetraethyl p.
thallium p.
turpentine p.
poisonous
Poisson distribution
Poisson-Pearson formula
Poitou colic
poker
p. back
p. spine
pokeweed mitogen (PWM)
Poland syndrome
polar
p. amino acid
p. anemia
p. body
p. cataract
p. cell
p. compound
p. fiber
p. frontal artery
p. globule
p. hypogenesis
p. plate
p. presentation
p. ring
p. solvent
p. star
p. temporal artery
p. zone
polarimeter
polarimetry
polariscope
polariscopic
polariscopy
polarity
polarization
polarize
polarized light
polarizer
polarizing microscope
polarography
poldine methylsulfate
pole
abapical p.
animal p.
anterior p. of eyeball
anterior p. of lens
cephalic p.
frontal p.
frontal p. of cerebrum
germinal p.
inferior p.
inferior p. of kidney
inferior p. of testis
lateral p.
p. ligation
lower p.
lower p. of testis

P

pole *(continued)*
    medial p. of ovary
    occipital p.
    occipital p. of cerebrum
    pelvic p.
    posterior p. of eyeball
    posterior p. of lens
    superior p.
    superior p. of kidney
    superior p. of testis
    temporal p.
    temporal p. of cerebrum
    upper p.
    upper p. of testis
    vegetal p., vegetative p.
    vitelline p.
Polenské number
poli (*pl. of* polus)
policeman
polio
polioclastic
poliodystrophia cerebri progressiva infantilis
poliodystrophy
    progressive cerebral p.
polioencephalitis
    p. infectiva
    inferior p.
    superior p.
    superior hemorrhagic p.
polioencephalomeningomyelitis
polioencephalomyelitis
polioencephalopathy
poliomyelitis
    acute anterior p.
    acute bulbar p.
    chronic anterior p.
    p. immune globulin (human)
    p. immunoglobulin
    p. vaccines
    p. virus
poliomyeloencephalitis
poliomyelopathy
poliosis
    ciliary p.
poliovirus hominis
poliovirus vaccine
polishing
    p. brush
Politzer
    P. bag
    P. luminous cone
    P. method
politzerization
    negative p.
polka fever
polkissen of Zimmermann
pollakidipsia
pollakiuria
pollen
    p. antigen
    p. extract

pollenosis
pollex, pl. **pollices**
    p. pedis
pollicization
pollinosis
pollutant
pollution
    air p.
    noise p.
polocyte
polonium (Po)
poloxalene
poloxalkol
polster
polus, pl. **poli**
    p. anterior bulbi oculi
    p. anterior lentis
    p. frontalis
    p. inferior
    p. inferior renis
    p. inferior testis
    poli lienalis inferior et superior
    p. occipitalis
    p. posterior bulbi oculi
    p. posterior lentis
    poli renales inferior et superior
    p. superior
    p. superior renis
    p. superior testis
    p. temporalis
poly
Pólya
    P. gastrectomy
    P. operation
poly(A)
    poly(A) polymerase
polyacid
polyacrylamide gel electrophoresis (PAGE)
polyadenitis maligna
polyadenopathy
polyadenosis
polyadenous
polyadenylation
poly(adenylic acid)
polyalcohol
polyallelism
polyalveolar lobe
polyamine-methylene resin
polyamine oxidase
poly(amino acids)
polyangiitis
    microscopic p.
polyanion
polyarteritis nodosa
polyarthric
polyarthritis
    p. chronica
    p. chronica villosa
    epidemic p.
    p. rheumatica acuta
    vertebral p.
polyarticular
polyasplenia
polyauxotroph

polyavitaminosis
polyaxial joint
polybasic acid
polyblennia
polycarbophil
polycarboxylate cement
polycardia
polycentric
polycheiria, polychiria
polychlorinated biphenyl (PCB)
polychondritis
    chronic atrophic p.
    relapsing p.
polychromasia
polychromatic
    p. cell
    p. radiation
polychromatocyte
polychromatophil, polychromatophile
    p. cell
polychromatophilia
polychromatophilic
polychromatosis
polychrome methylene blue
polychromemia
polychromia
polychromophil
polychromophilia
polychylia
polycistronic
polyclinic
polyclonal
    p. activator
    p. antibody
    p. gammopathy
polyclonia
polycoria
polycrotic
polycrotism
polycyesis
polycystic
    p. disease of kidney
    p. kidney
    p. liver
    p. liver disease
    p. ovary
    p. ovary syndrome
polycythemia
    compensatory p.
    p. hypertonica
    relative p.
    p. rubra
    p. rubra vera
    p. vera
polydactylism
polydactylous
polydactyly
polydentia
polydipsia
    hysterical p.
    psychogenic p.
    psychogenic nocturnal p. (PNP)
polydispersoid
polydysplasia
polydystrophic

polydystrophy
    pseudo-Hurler p.
polyembryony
polyendocrine deficiency syndrome
polyendocrinopathy
polyene
polyenic acid
polyenoic acid
polyergic
polyester resin
polyesthesia
polyestradiol phosphate
polyestrous
polyethylene glycol (PEGs)
polyfructose
polygalactia
polygalacturonase
poly(gamma-glutamic acid)
polyganglionic
polygene
polygenic inheritance
polyglactin 910
polyglandular
poly-β-glucosaminidase
polyglutamate
poly(glutamic acid)
poly(glycolic acid)
polygnathus
polygraph
    Mackenzie p.
polygyria
polyhedral body
polyhexoses
polyhidrosis
polyhybrid
polyhydramnios
polyhydric
polyhypermenorrhea
polyhypomenorrhea
polyisoprenes
polyisoprenoids
polykaryocyte
polylactosamines
polyleptic fever
polylinker
polylogia
polymastia
polymastigote
polymegethism
polymelia
polymenorrhea
polymer
    cross-linked p.
    p. fume fever
polymerase
    p. alpha
    p. beta
    p. chain reaction (PCR)
    p. gamma
    Taq p.
polymeria
polymeric
polymerization
polymerize
polymetacarpalia, polymetacarpalism

P

polymetatarsalia, polymetatarsalism
polymicrolipomatosis
polymitus
polymorph
polymorphic
    p. genetic marker
    p. neuron
    p. reticulosis
    p. superficial keratitis
polymorphism
    balanced p.
    corneal endothelial p.
    DNA p.
    genetic p.
    lipoprotein p.
    restriction fragment length p. (RFLP)
    restriction length p., fragment length p.
    restriction-site p.
polymorphocellular
polymorphocytic leukemia
polymorphonuclear leukocyte
polymorphous
    p. layer
    p. light eruption
    p. low-grade carcinoma of salivary gland
    p. perversion
polymyalgia
    p. arteritica
    p. rheumatica
polymyoclonus
polymyositis
polymyxin
    p. B sulfate
polynesic
polyneural
polyneuralgia
polyneuritis
    acute idiopathic p.
    chronic familial p.
    infectious p.
    postinfectious p.
polyneuronitis
polyneuropathy
    acute inflammatory p.
    alcoholic p.
    arsenical p.
    axonal p.
    axon loss p.
    buckthorn p.
    chronic inflammatory demyelinating p. (CIDP)
    critical illness p.
    demyelinating p.
    diabetic p.
    isoniazid p.
    nitrofurantoin p.
    nutritional p.
    progressive hypertrophic p.
    segmental demyelinating p.
    uremic p.
polynoxylin
polynuclear, polynucleate

polynucleosis
polynucleotidases
polynucleotide
    p. methyltransferases
    p. phosphorylase
    p. thioltransferases
polynucleotide methylases
polyodontia
polyol
    p. dehydrogenases
    p. pathway
Polyomavirus
polyoma virus
polyoncosis, polyonchosis
polyonychia
polyopia, polyopsia
polyorchism, polyorchidism
polyostotic fibrous dysplasia
polyotia
polyovular ovarian follicle
polyovulatory
polyoxyethylene alcohol
polyoxyl 40 stearate
polyp
    adenomatous p.
    bleeding p.
    bronchial p.
    cardiac p.
    cellular p.
    choanal p.
    cystic p.
    dental p.
    fibroepithelial p.
    fibrous p.
    fleshy p.
    gelatinous p.
    Hopmann p.
    hydatid p.
    hyperplastic p.
    inflammatory p.
    juvenile p.
    laryngeal p.
    lipomatous p.
    lymphoid p.
    metaplastic p.
    mucous p.
    myomatous p.
    nasal p.
    osseous p.
    pedunculated p.
    placental p.
    pulp p.
    regenerative p.
    retention p.
    sessile p.
    tooth p.
    vascular p.
polypapilloma
polypathia
polypectomy snare
polypeptide
    gastric inhibitory p. (GIP)
    glucose-dependent insulinotropic p.
    pancreatic p.

trefoil p.
vasoactive intestinal p. (VIP)
polyphagia
polyphalangism
polyphallic
polypharmacy
polyphenic gene
polyphenol oxidase
polyphobia
polyphosphorylase
polyphrasia
polyphyletic theory
polyphyletism
polyphyodont
polypi (*pl. of* polypus)
polypiform
polyplasmia
polyplastic
Polyplax
polyploid
polyploidy
polypnea
polypodia
polypoid adenoma
polyporous
Polyporus
polyposia
polyposis
adenomatous p. coli
familial adenomatous p. (FAP)
familial p. coli
lymphomatoid p.
multiple intestinal p.
polypotome
polypotrite
polypous
p. endocarditis
p. gastritis
polypragmasy
polyprenols
polyptychial
polypus, pl. **polypi**
polyradiculitis
polyradiculomyopathy
polyradiculoneuropathy
acute inflammatory demyelinating p.
polyradiculopathy
diabetic p.
polyribonucleotide nucleotidyltransferase
polyribosomes
polyrrhea
polysaccharide
p. conjugated vaccine
pneumococcal p.
specific soluble p.
p. sulfate ester
polyscelia
polyscope
polyserositis
familial paroxysmal p.
familial recurrent p.
periodic p.
recurrent p.
polysinusitis
polysomes

polysomia
polysomic
polysomnogram
polysomnography
polysomy
polysorbate 80
polyspermia, polyspermism
polyspermy
polysplenia syndrome
polysteraxic
polystichia
polysulfide rubber
polysuspensoid
polysymbrachydactyly
polysynaptic
polysyndactyly
polytendinitis
polytene chromosome
polytenization
polyterpene
polythelia
polythiazide
polytocous
polytomography
polytrichia
polytrichosis
polytrophic
poly(U)
polyuridylic acid
polyunguia
polyuria test
poly(uridylic acid) (poly(U))
polyuronides
polyvalent
p. allergy
p. antiserum
p. serum
p. vaccine
polyvidone
polyvinyl
p. alcohol
p. chloride (PVC)
polyvinylpyrrolidone (PVP)
polyvinylpyrrolidone-iodine complex
polyzoic
polyzygotic twin
pomade acne
pomatum
POMC
proopiomelanocortin
pomegranate
Pomeroy operation
POMP
6-mercaptopurine, Oncovin (vincristine
sulfate), methotrexate, and prednisone
Pompe disease
pompholyx
ponceau de xylidine
ponderal index
pond fracture
Ponfick shadow
pono-
ponograph
ponopalmosis
ponophobia

P

ponos
pons, pl. **pontes**
    p. basilaris pontis
    p. cerebelli
    pontes grisei caudolenticulares
    p. hepatis
    p. varolii
pontic
ponticulus
    p. hepatis
    p. nasi
    p. promontorii
pontine, pontile
    p. angle
    p. angle tumor
    p. artery
    p. cistern
    p. corticonuclear fiber
    p. flexure
    p. gray matter
    p. hemorrhage
    p. nucleus
    p. vein
pontobulbar
    p. body
    p. nucleus
pontocerebellar
    p. cistern
    p. fiber
    p. recess
pontocerebellum
ponto-geniculo-occipital spike
pontomedullary groove
pontomesencephalic vein
pontoreticulospinal tract
pool
    abdominal p.
    gene p.
    metabolic p.
    P. phenomenon
    vaginal p.
pooled serum
Pool-Schlesinger sign
poorly
    p. compliant bladder
    p. crystalline hydroxyapatite
    p. differentiated lymphocytic
      lymphoma
popliteal
    p. arch
    p. artery
    p. communicating nerve
    p. entrapment syndrome
    p. fascia
    p. fossa
    p. groove
    p. line
    p. lymph node
    p. muscle
    p. notch
    p. plane of femur
    p. plexus
    p. region
    p. space

    p. surface of femur
    p. vein
popliteus
    p. muscle
POPOP
    1,4-bis(5-phenyloxazol-2-yl)benzene
poppy oil
population
    p. genetics
    p. pyramid
POR
    problem-oriented record
porcelain
    p. gallbladder
    p. inlay
porcine
    p. graft
    p. hemagglutinating encephalomyelitis
      virus
    p. valve
porcupine skin
pore
    alveolar p.
    auditory p.
    dilated p.
    external acoustic p.
    external auditory p.
    gustatory p.
    interalveolar p.
    internal acoustic p.
    Kohn p.
    nuclear p.
    skin p.
    slit p.
    sweat p.
    taste p.
Porges-Meier test
Porges method
pori (*pl. of* porus)
poria (*pl. of* porion)
Porifera
porins
poriomania
porion, pl. **poria**
PORN
    progressive outer retinal necrosis
pornolagnia
porocephaliasis
Porocephalidae
porocephalosis
Porocephalus
    p. armillatus
poroconidium
porokeratosis
    actinic p.
poroma
    eccrine p.
porosis, pl. **poroses**
    cerebral p.
porosity
porospore
porotic
porous
porphin, porphine

P

position *(continued)*
    left occipitotransverse p. (LOT)
    left sacroanterior p. (LSA)
    left sacroposterior p. (LSP)
    left sacrotransverse p. (LST)
    lithotomy p.
    mandibular hinge p.
    Mayo-Robson p.
    mentoanterior p.
    mentoposterior p. (MP)
    mentotransverse p.
    Noble p.
    obstetric p.
    occipitoanterior p. (OA)
    occipitoposterior p. (OP)
    occipitotransverse p., p.
      occipitotransverse position
    occlusal p.
    orthopnea p.
    orthopneic p.
    physiologic rest p.
    postural p., postural resting p.
    prone p.
    protrusive p.
    rest p.
    reverse Trendelenburg p.
    right frontoanterior p. (RFA)
    right frontoposterior p. (RFP)
    right frontotransverse p. (RFT)
    right mentoanterior p. (RMA)
    right mentoposterior p. (RMP)
    right mentotransverse p. (RMT)
    right occipitoanterior p. (ROA)
    right occipitoposterior p. (ROP)
    right occipitotransverse p. (ROT)
    right sacroanterior p. (RSA)
    right sacroposterior p. (RSP)
    right sacrotransverse p. (RST)
    Rose p.
    sacroanterior p. (SA)
    sacroposterior p. (SP)
    sacrotransverse p.
    Scultetus p.
    semi-Fowler p.
    semiprone p.
    p. sense
    Simon p.
    Sims p.
    supine p.
    terminal hinge p.
    Trendelenburg p.
    Valentine p.
    Walcher p.
positional
    p. cloning
    p. nystagmus
    p. vertigo
    p. vertigo of Bárány
positioner
positive
    p. accommodation
    p. afterimage
    p. afterpotential
    p. anergy

    p. chemotaxis
    p. chronotropism
    p. contrast orbitography
    p. control
    p. convergence
    p. cooperativity
    p. cytotaxis
    p. electrode
    p. electron
    p. electrotaxis
    p. end-expiratory pressure (PEEP)
    p. feedback
    p. G
    p. hydrotropism
    p. meniscus
    p. neutrotaxis
    p. phase
    p. photodromy
    p. phototaxis
    p. phototropism
    p. ray
    p. reinforcer
    p. scotoma
    p. stain
    p. stereotropism
    p. supporting reaction
    p. symptom
    p. taxis
    p. thermotaxis
    p. transference
    p. tropism
    p. valence
positively inotropic
positive-negative pressure breathing (PNPB)
positron emission tomography (PET)
posologic
posology
post
    p. cibum (p.c.)
    p. dam
    p. dam area
    p. implant
postacetabular
postadolescence
postadrenalectomy syndrome
postanal
    p. dimple
    p. gut
postanesthetic
postapoplectic
postarsphenamine jaundice
postauricular incision
postaxial
postaxillary line
postbrachial
postcapillary venules
postcardinal
postcardiotomy syndrome
postcava
postcaval ureter
postcentral
    p. area
    p. fissure
    p. gyrus

p. sulcal artery
p. sulcus
postcholecystectomy syndrome
postchroming
postcibal
postclavicular
postcloacal gut
postcoital
    p. contraception
    p. test
postcoitus
postcommissural fiber
postcommissurotomy syndrome
postcommunicating
    p. part of anterior cerebral artery
    p. part of posterior cerebral artery
postconcussion syndrome
postcordial
postcostal anastomosis
postcrown
postcubital
postdam
postdate pregnancy
postdiastolic
postdicrotic
postdiphtheritic paralysis
postdormital
postdormitum
postdrive depression
postductal
postencephalitic
postepileptic
posterior
    p. accessory olivary nucleus
    p. acoustic stria
    p. alveolar artery
    p. ampullar nerve
    p. antebrachial cutaneous nerve
    p. antebrachial nerve
    p. antebrachial region
    p. anterior jugular vein
    p. aphasia
    p. arch of atlas
    p. articular facet of dens
    p. articular surface of dens
    p. asynclitism
    p. atlanto-occipital membrane
    p. auricular artery
    p. auricular groove
    p. auricular muscle
    p. auricular nerve
    p. auricular plexus
    p. auricular vein
    p. axillary fold
    p. axillary line
    p. axillary lymph node
    p. basal branch
    p. basal bronchopulmonary segment S X
    p. basal segmental artery
    p. belly of digastric muscle
    p. blepharitis
    p. border of eyelid
    p. border of fibula

p. border of petrous part of temporal bone
p. border of radius
p. border of testis
p. border of ulna
p. brachial cutaneous nerve
p. brachial region
p. branch
p. branch of great auricular nerve
p. branch of inferior pancreaticoduodenal artery
p. branch of lateral cerebral sulcus
p. branch of medial antebrachial cutaneous nerve
p. branch of medial cutaneous nerve of forearm
p. branch of obturator artery
p. branch of obturator nerve
p. branch of recurrent ulnar artery
p. branch of renal artery
p. branch of right branch of portal vein
p. branch of right hepatic duct
p. branch of right superior pulmonary vein
p. branch of spinal nerve
p. branch of superior thyroid artery
p. branch of ulnar recurrent artery
p. bronchopulmonary segment S II
p. canaliculus of chorda tympani
p. cardinal vein
p. carpal region
p. cecal artery
p. central convolution
p. central gyrus
p. centriole
p. cerebellar notch
p. cerebellomedullary cistern
p. cerebral artery
p. cervical intertransversarii muscle
p. cervical intertransverse muscle
p. cervical plexus
p. cervical region
p. chamber of eyeball
p. choroidal artery
p. choroiditis
p. circumflex humeral artery
p. circumflex humeral vein
p. clinoid process
p. column
p. column cordotomy
p. column of spinal cord
p. commissure of the larynx
p. communicating artery
p. compartment of arm
p. compartment of forearm
p. compartment of leg
p. compartment of thigh
p. condyloid foramen
p. conjunctival artery
p. cord of brachial plexus
p. coronary plexus
p. costotransverse ligament
p. cranial fossa
p. cricoarytenoid ligament

P

posterior *(continued)*
p. cricoarytenoid muscle
p. cruciate ligament
p. crural region
p. crus of stapes
p. cubital region
p. curvature
p. cusp of left atrioventricular valve
p. cusp of mitral valve
p. cusp of right atrioventricular valve
p. cusp of tricuspid valve
p. cutaneous nerve of arm
p. cutaneous nerve of forearm
p. cutaneous nerve of thigh
p. dental artery
p. descending coronary artery
p. division of brachial plexus
p. elastic layer
p. embryotoxon
p. ethmoidal air cell
p. ethmoidal artery
p. ethmoidal cell
p. ethmoidal nerve
p. external arcuate fiber
p. extremity of spleen
p. facial vein
p. fascicle of palatopharyngeus muscle
p. fasciculus proprius
p. femoral cutaneous nerve
p. focal point
p. fontanelle
p. fossa approach
p. funiculus
p. gastric artery
p. gastric branch of posterior vagal trunk
p. glandular branch of superior thyroid artery
p. gray commissure
p. hepatic segment I
p. horn
p. humeral circumflex artery
p. hypothalamic area
p. hypothalamic nucleus
p. hypothalamic region
p. inferior cerebellar artery
p. inferior cerebellar artery syndrome
p. inferior iliac spine
p. inferior nasal branch of greater palatine nerve
p. inferior nasal nerve
p. intercondylar area of tibia
p. intercostal artery 1–11
p. intercostal vein
p. intermediate groove
p. intermediate sulcus
p. interosseous artery
p. interosseous nerve
p. interpositus nucleus
p. interventricular branch of right coronary artery

p. interventricular groove
p. interventricular sulcus
p. intestinal portal
p. intraoccipital joint
p. intraoccipital synchondrosis
p. junction line
p. knee region
p. labial artery
p. labial branch of internal perineal artery
p. labial branch of perineal artery
p. labial commissure
p. labial nerve
p. labial vein
p. lacrimal crest
p. laryngeal cleft
p. lateral nasal artery
p. layer of rectus sheath
p. leukoencephalopathy syndrome
p. ligament of fibular head
p. ligament of head of fibula
p. ligament of incus
p. ligament of knee
p. limb of internal capsule
p. limb of stapes
p. limiting lamina of cornea
p. limiting layer of cornea
p. lip of external os of uterus
p. liver
p. lobe of hypophysis
p. longitudinal bundle
p. longitudinal ligament
p. lunate lobule
p. marginal vein
p. medial nucleus of thalamus
p. median fissure of the medulla oblongata
p. median fissure of spinal cord
p. median line
p. median sulcus of medulla oblongata
p. median sulcus of spinal cord
p. mediastinal artery
p. mediastinal lymph node
p. mediastinum
p. medullary velum
p. meningeal artery
p. meniscofemoral ligament
p. myocardial infarction
p. nares
p. nasal apertures
p. nasal spine of horizontal plate of palatine bone
p. neck region
p. nephrectomy
p. neuropore
p. notch of cerebellum
p. nucleus
p. nucleus of hypothalamus
p. nucleus of vagus nerve
p. occipitoaxial ligament
p. occlusion
p. palatal seal
p. palatal seal area
p. palatine arch

p. palatine foramina
p. palatine spine
p. palpebral margin
p. pancreaticoduodenal artery
p. paracentral gyrus
p. parietal artery
p. parolfactory sulcus
p. parotid vein
p. part
p. part of anterior commissure of brain
p. part of the diaphragmatic surface of the liver
p. part of liver
p. part of tongue
p. part of vaginal fornix
p. pelvic exenteration
p. perforated substance
p. pericallosal vein
p. periventricular nucleus
p. peroneal artery
p. pillar of fauces
p. pillar of fornix
p. pituitary
p. pole of eyeball
p. pole of lens
p. polymorphous corneal dystrophy
p. primary division
p. probability
p. process of septal cartilage
p. process of talus
p. pyramid of the medulla
p. quadrigeminal body
p. ramus of lateral cerebral sulcus
p. ramus of lateral sulcus of cerebrum
p. ramus of spinal nerve
p. recess
p. recess of tympanic membrane
p. region of arm
p. region of elbow
p. region of forearm
p. region of knee
p. region of leg
p. region of neck
p. region of thigh
p. region of wrist
p. renal segment
p. rhinoscopy
p. rhizotomy
p. root of spinal nerve
p. sacroiliac ligament
p. sacrosciatic ligament
p. sagittal diameter
p. scalene muscle
p. scapular nerve
p. scleritis
p. sclerotomy
p. scrotal branch of internal pudendal artery
p. scrotal branch of perineal artery
p. scrotal nerve
p. scrotal vein
p. segment
p. segmental artery

p. semicircular canal
p. septal artery of nose
p. septal branch of nose
p. septal branch of sphenopalatine artery
p. sinus of tympanic cavity
p. spinal artery
p. spinal sclerosis
p. spinocerebellar tract
p. staphyloma
p. sternoclavicular ligament
p. subcapsular cataract
p. superior alveolar artery
p. superior alveolar branch of maxillary nerve
p. superior fissure
p. superior iliac spine
p. superior lateral nasal branch of maxillary nerve
p. superior lateral nasal branch of pterygopalatine ganglion
p. superior medial nasal branch of maxillary nerve
p. superior medial nasal branch of pterygopalatine ganglion
p. supraclavicular nerve
p. surface
p. surface of arm
p. surface of arytenoid cartilage
p. surface of cornea
p. surface of elbow
p. surface of eyelids
p. surface of fibula
p. surface of forearm
p. surface of iris
p. surface of kidney
p. surface of leg
p. surface of lens
p. surface of lower limb
p. surface of pancreas
p. surface of petrous part of temporal bone
p. surface of prostate
p. surface of radius
p. surface of scapula
p. surface of shaft of humerus
p. surface of suprarenal gland
p. surface of thigh
p. surface of tibia
p. surface of ulna
p. symblepharon
p. synechia
p. talar articular surface
p. talocalcaneal ligament
p. talofibular ligament
p. talotibial ligament
p. tegmental decussation
p. temporal artery
p. temporal branch of middle cerebral artery
p. thalamic radiation
p. thoracic nerve
p. thoracic nucleus
p. tibial lymph node
p. tibial muscle

P

779

posterior *(continued)*
- p. tibial node
- p. tibial recurrent artery
- p. tibial vein
- p. tibiofibular ligament
- p. tibiotalar ligament
- p. tibiotalar part of deltoid ligament
- p. tibiotalar part of medial ligament of ankle joint
- p. tooth
- p. tooth form
- p. transverse temporal gyrus
- p. triangle of neck
- p. trigeminothalamic tract
- p. tubercle
- p. tympanic artery
- p. urethra
- p. urethral valves
- p. urethritis
- p. uveitis
- p. vaginal hernia
- p. vaginismus
- p. vein of corpus callosum
- p. vein of left ventricle
- p. vein of septum pellucidum
- p. vestibular branch of vestibulocochlear artery
- p. vitrectomy
- p. wall of middle ear
- p. wall of stomach
- p. wall of tympanic cavity
- p. wall of vagina

posterius
posteroanterior
- p. projection

posteroclusion
posteroexternal
posterointernal
posterolateral
- p. central artery
- p. fissure
- p. fontanelle
- p. groove
- p. nucleus
- p. sulcus
- p. thoracotomy
- p. tract

posteromedial
- p. central artery
- p. frontal branch of callosomarginal artery
- p. nucleus

posteromedian
posteroparietal
posterosuperior
posterotemporal
posteruption cuticle
postesophageal
postestrus, postestrum
postextrasystolic
- p. pause
- p. T wave

postfebrile

postganglionic
- p. fiber
- p. motor neuron
- p. nerve fiber

postgastrectomy syndrome
postglenoid foramen
posthemiplegic
- p. athetosis
- p. chorea

posthemorrhagic anemia
posthepatic
posthepatitic cirrhosis
posthetomy
posthioplasty
posthippocampal fissure
posthitis
postholith
posthyoid
posthypnotic
- p. amnesia
- p. psychosis
- p. suggestion

posthypoglycemic hyperglycemia
postictal
posticus
- p. palsy
- p. paralysis

postinfarction ventricular septal defect
postinfectious
- p. bradycardia
- p. myelitis
- p. polyneuritis
- p. psychosis

postinfluenzal
postischial
post-kala azar dermal leishmanoid
postlaminar part of intraocular part of optic nerve
postlingual
- p. deafness
- p. fissure

post-lumbar puncture syndrome
postlunate fissure
postmalarial
postmalaria neurologic syndrome
post-marketing surveillance
postmastoid
postmature infant
postmaturity syndrome
postmedian
postmediastinal
postmediastinum
postmeiotic phase
postmeningitic hydrocephalus
postmenopausal atrophy
postminimus
postmitotic phase
postmortem
- p. clot
- p. delivery
- p. examination
- p. hypostasis
- p. livedo
- p. lividity
- p. rigidity

p. suggillation
p. thrombus
p. wart
postmyocardial
    p. infarction pericarditis
    p. infarction syndrome (PMIS)
postnarial
postnaris
postnasal drip
postnatal life
postnecrotic cirrhosis
postneuritic
postnormal occlusion
postobstructive pneumonia
postocular
postoperative
    p. bronchopneumonia
    p. parotiditis
    p. pressure alopecia
    p. tetany
postoral arch
postorbital
postpalatal seal
postpalatine
postparalytic
postpartum
    p. alopecia
    p. amenorrhea
    p. atony
    p. blues
    p. cardiomyopathy
    p. estrus
    p. hemorrhage
    p. hypertension
    p. pituitary necrosis syndrome
    p. psychosis
    p. tetanus
postparturient hemoglobinuria
postperfusion lung
postpericardiotomy
    p. pericarditis
    p. syndrome
postpharyngeal space
postphlebitic syndrome
postpneumonic
postprandial
    p. lipemia
    p. pain
postprimary tuberculosis
postpuberal, postpubertal
postpuberty
postpubescent
postpyknotic
postpyloric sphincter
postpyramidal fissure
postreduction phase
postremal chamber of eyeball
postrenal albuminuria
postrhinal fissure
postrolandic
postrubella syndrome
postsacral
postscapular
postscarlatinal
postsphenoid bone

postsphygmic
postsplenic
poststationary phase
post-steady state
post-stenotic dilation
poststeroid panniculitis
postsulcal part of tongue
postsynaptic membrane
posttarsal
posttecta
postterm infant
postthrombotic syndrome
posttibial
posttranscriptional
posttranslational
posttransplant lymphoproliferative disease
posttransverse
posttraumatic
    p. arterial thrombosis
    p. delirium
    p. dementia
    p. epilepsy
    p. headache
    p. hydrocephalus
    p. leptomeningeal cyst
    p. neck syndrome
    p. neurosis
    p. osteoporosis
    p. pericarditis
    p. psychosis
    p. stress disorder
    p. stress syndrome
    p. syndrome
    p. venous thrombosis
posttrematic
posttussis suction sound
posttussive suction
posttyphoid
postulate
    Ampère p.
    Avogadro p.
    Ehrlich p.
    Koch p.'s
postural
    p. albuminuria
    p. contraction
    p. drainage
    p. hypotension
    p. ischemia
    p. position
    p. reflex
    p. set
    p. sway response
    p. syncope
    p. tremor
    p. version
    p. vertigo
posture
    p. sense
    Stern p.
posturography
    dynamic p.
postuterine
postvaccinal
    p. encephalitis

P

postvaccinal (*continued*)
    p. encephalomyelitis
    p. myelitis
postvalvar, postvalvular
potable
    p. water
Potain
Potain sign
potamophobia
potash
    caustic p.
    sulfurated p.
potassic
potassium (K)
    p. acetate
    p. acid tartrate
    p. alum
    p. aminosalicylate
    p. antimonyltartrate
    p. atractylate
    p. bicarbonate
    p. bichromate
    p. bitartrate
    p. bromide
    p. chlorate
    p. chloride
    p. citrate
    p. cyanide
    dibasic p. phosphate
    p. dichromate
    effervescent p. citrate
    p. ferrocyanide
    p. gluconate
    p. guaiacolsulfonate
    p. hydroxide
    p. hypophosphite
    p. inhibition
    p. iodate
    p. iodide
    p. metaphosphate
    monobasic p. phosphate
    p. nitrate
    p. nitrate paper
    penicillin G p.
    p. perchlorate
    p. permanganate
    p. phosphate
    p. rhodanate
    p. sodium tartrate
    p. sorbate
    p. sparing diuretic
    p. succinate
    p. sulfate
    p. sulfocyanate
    p. tartrate
    p. thiocyanate
potassium-39 (^{39}K)
potassium-40 (^{40}K)
potassium-42 (^{42}K)
potassium-43 (^{43}K)
potato
    p. dextrose agar
    p. nose
    p. tumor of neck

pot curare
potency
    sexual p.
potent
potential
    action p.
    p. acuity meter (PAM)
    after-p.
    bioelectric p.
    biotic p.
    brain p.
    brainstem auditory evoked p.
    chemical p.
    cochlear p.
    compound action p.
    demarcation p.
    early receptor p. (ERP)
    endocochlear p.
    p. energy
    evoked p.
    excitatory junction p. (EJP)
    excitatory postsynaptic p. (EPSP)
    generator p.
    inhibitory junction p. (IJP)
    inhibitory postsynaptic p. (IPSP)
    injury p.
    membrane p.
    myogenic p.
    oscillatory p.
    Ottoson p.
    oxidation-reduction p. ($E_0{}^+$)
    pacemaker p.
    redox p.
    S p.
    somatosensory evoked p.
    spike p.
    summating p.
    thermodynamic p.
    transmembrane p.
    ventricular late p.
    visual evoked p.
    zeta p.
    zoonotic p.
potentiation
potentiator
potentiometer
potentiometric titration
potion
Pott
    P. abscess
    P. aneurysm
    P. curvature
    P. disease
    P. fracture
    P. paralysis
    P. paraplegia
Potter
    P. disease
    P. facies
    P. syndrome
    P. version
Potter-Bucky diaphragm
Potts
    P. anastomosis

P. clamp
P. operation
pouch
antral p.
branchial p.
Broca p.
p. culture
deep perineal p.
Denis Browne p.
Douglas p.
p. of Douglas
endodermal p.
Hartmann p.
Heidenhain p.
hepatorenal p.
hypophyseal p.
ileoanal p.
Kock p.
laryngeal p.
Morison p.
paracystic p.
pararectal p.
paravesical p.
Pavlov p.
pharyngeal p.
Physick p.
Prussak p.
Rathke p.
rectouterine p.
rectovaginouterine p.
rectovesical p.
Seessel p.
superficial inguinal p.
superficial perineal p.
ultimobranchial p.
uterovesical p.
vesicouterine p.
Willis p.
pouchitis
poudrage
pleural p.
poultice
poultry handler's disease
poultryman's itch
pound (lb)
poundal
Poupart
P. ligament
P. line
povidone-iodine
Powassan
P. encephalitis
P. virus
powder
bleaching p.
powdered
p. gold
p. ipecac
p. opium
p. stomach
power
back vertex p.
carbon dioxide combining p.
equivalent p.
p. failure

p. injector
p. point
resolving p.
statistical p.
pox
Kaffir p.
Poxviridae
poxvirus officinalis
Pozzi muscle
PP
pyrophosphate
PP$_i$
inorganic pyrophosphatase
P.p.
punctum proximum
p-p
p.-p. factor
ppb
parts per billion
PPCA
proserum prothrombin conversion accelerator
PPCF
plasmin prothrombins conversion factor
PPD
purified protein derivative of tuberculin
P-P interval
PPLO
pleuropneumonia-like organisms
ppm
PPO
2,5-diphenyloxazole
P1, P2, P3, P4 segment of posterior cerebral artery
PPRibp, PPRP
5-phospho-alpha-D-ribosyl-1-pyrophosphate
P pulmonale
PQ
plastoquinone
PQ-9
plastoquinone-9
PQ interval
PR
PR enzyme
PR interval
PR segment
P.r.
punctum remotum
Pr
presbyopia
PRA
plasma renin activity
practical
p. anatomy
p. nurse
p. units
practice
extramural p.
family p.
general p.
group p.
p. guidelines
intramural p.
p. parameter

P

practitioner
Prader-Willi syndrome
pragmatics
pragmatism
Prague pelvis
2-pralidoxime (2-PAM)
pralidoxime chloride
pramoxine hydrochloride
prandial
praseodymium
Pratt
    P. dilator
    P. symptom
Prausnitz-Küstner
    P.-K. antibody
    P.-K. reaction
pravastatin
    p. sodium
praxiology
praxis
prazepam
praziquantel
prazosin hydrochloride
preagonal
prealbumin
    thyroxine-binding p. (TBPA)
preanal
preanesthetic medication
preantiseptic
preaortic
preaseptic
preauricular
    p. deep parotid lymph node
    p. groove
    p. pit
    p. point
    p. sinus
    p. sulcus
preautomatic pause
preaxial
preaxillary line
pre-B lymphocyte
precalciferol
precancer
precancerous lesion
precapillary anastomosis
precardiac
precardinal
precartilage
precautions
precava
prececal lymph node
prececocolic fascia
precentral
    p. area
    p. cerebellar vein
    p. fissure
    p. gyrus
    p. sulcal artery
    p. sulcus
precervical sinus
prechiasmatic sulcus
prechordal plate
prechroming
precipitable

precipitant
precipitate
    keratic p.
    p. labor
    mutton-fat keratic p.
    pigmented keratic p.
    red p.
    sweet p.
    white mercuric p.
    yellow p.
precipitated
    p. calcium carbonate
    p. sulfur
precipitating
    p. antibody
    p. cause
precipitation
    p. curve
    double antibody p.
    immune p.
    p. test
precipitin
    p. reaction
    p. test
precipitinogen
precipitinogenoid
precipitogen
precipitoid
precipitophore
precision
    p. attachment
    p. rest
preclinical
precocious
    p. pseudopuberty
    p. puberty
precocity
precognition
precollagenous fiber
precommissural
    p. bundle
    p. fiber
    p. septal area
    p. septal nucleus
    p. septum
precommunical
    p. segment of anterior cerebral
      artery
    p. segment of posterior cerebral
      artery
precommunicating
    p. part of anterior cerebral artery
    p. part of posterior cerebral artery
preconceptual stage
preconscious
preconvulsive
precordia
precordial
    p. catch syndrome
    p. electrocardiography
    p. lead
precordialgia
precordium
precorneal film

precostal
    p. anastomosis
precritical
preculminate fissure
precuneal
    p. artery
    p. branch of anterior cerebral artery
precuneate
precuneus
precursor
precursory cartilage
predentin
pre-Descemet corneal dystrophy
prediabetes
prediastole
prediastolic
predicrotic
predictive
    p. validity
    p. value
predigestion
predispose
predisposing
    p. cause
    p. factor
predisposition
prednisolone
    p. acetate
    p. butylacetate
    p. sodium phosphate
    p. succinate
    p. tebutate
prednisone
    cyclophosphamide, doxorubicin
    (Adriamycin), vincristine, p.
    (CHOP)
    mechlorethamine, oncovin,
    procarbazine, and p. (MOPP)
prednylidene
predormital
predormitum
predorsal bundle
preductal
preeclampsia
    superimposed p.
preejection period
preepiglottic space
preeruptive
preexcitation
    p. syndrome
    ventricular p.
preextraction record
preferred provider organization
preformation theory
prefrontal
    p. area
    p. cortex
    p. leukotomy
    p. lobotomy
    p. vein
preganglionic
    p. motor neuron
    p. nerve fiber
pregeniculate nucleus

pregenital
    p. organization
    p. phase
pregnancy
    abdominal p.
    aborted ectopic p.
    ampullar p.
    p. cell
    cervical p.
    chemical p.
    combined p.
    compound p.
    cornual p.
    p. diabetes
    ectopic p.
    extraamniotic p.
    extrachorial p.
    extramembranous p.
    extrauterine p.
    fallopian p.
    false p.
    p. gingivitis
    heterotopic p.
    heterotropic p.
    higher order p.
    p. hormone
    hydatid p.
    hysterical p.
    interstitial p.
    intraligamentary p.
    intramural p.
    intraperitoneal p.
    p. luteoma
    molar p.
    multiple p.
    mural p.
    ovarian p.
    ovarioabdominal p.
    persistent ectopic p.
    postdate p.
    prolonged p.
    secondary abdominal p.
    spurious p.
    tubal p.
    tuboabdominal p.
    tuboovarian p.
    tubouterine p.
    p. tumor
    twin p.
    uterine p.
    uteroabdominal p.
pregnancy-induced hypertension
pregnane
pregnanediol
pregnanedione
pregnanetriol
pregnant
pregnene
pregneninolone
pregnenolone succinate
pregranulosa cell
prehallux
prehelicine
prehemataminic acid
prehensile

prehension
prehormone
prehyoid gland
preictal
preinduction
preinfarction
>p. angina
>p. syndrome

preinterparietal bone
prekallikrein
prelacrimal
prelaminar
>p. branch of spinal branch of dorsal branch of posterior intercostal artery
>p. part of intraocular part of optic nerve

prelaryngeal lymph node
preleptotene
preleukemia
prelimbic
preliminary impression
prelingual deafness
preload
>ventricular p.

prelogical
>p. mind
>p. thinking

premalignant
premammary abscess
premaniacal
premature
>p. alopecia
>p. beat
>p. birth
>p. contact
>p. contraction
>p. delivery
>p. ejaculation
>p. labor
>p. membrane rupture
>p. menopause
>p. ovarian failure
>p. senility syndrome
>p. systole

prematurity myopia
premaxilla
premaxillary
>p. bone
>p. suture

premedication
premeiotic phase
premelanosome
premenstrual
>p. dysphoric disorder
>p. edema
>p. salivary syndrome
>p. syndrome (PMS)
>p. tension
>p. tension syndrome

premenstruum
premitochondria
premitotic phase
premolar tooth
premonocyte

premorbid
premotor
>p. area
>p. cortex
>p. syndrome

premunition
premunitive
premyeloblast
premyelocyte
prenaris, pl. **prenares**
prenatal
>p. diagnosis
>p. life
>p. screening

preneoplastic
prenodular fissure
Prentice rule
prenyl
prenylamine
prenylation
preoccipital notch
pre-oedipal phase
preoperative record
preoptic
>p. area
>p. region

preoral gut
preosteoblast
preoxygenation
prep
prepalatal
prepancreatic artery
prepapillary sphincter
preparation
>cavity p.
>corrosion p.
>cytologic filter p.
>heart-lung p.

prepared
>p. chalk
>p. ipecacuanha
>p. mutton tallow
>p. suet

preparturient
prepatellar
>p. bursa
>p. bursitis

prepatent period
prepericardial lymph node
preperitoneal
prephenic acid
prepiriform gyrus
preplacental
preponderance
>directional p.

prepontine cistern
prepotential
preprocollagen
preproinsulin
preproprotein
preprostate urethral sphincter
preprostatic
>p. part of male urethra
>p. sphincter

preprotein

prepsychotic
prepuberal
prepubescent
prepuce
    p. of clitoris
    hooded p.
    p. of penis
    ventral apron p.
preputia (*pl. of* preputium)
preputial
    p. calculus
    p. gland
    p. sac
preputiotomy
preputium, pl. **preputia**
    p. clitoridis
    p. penis
prepyloric
    p. sphincter
    p. vein
prepyramidal
    p. fissure
    p. tract
prerectal lithotomy
prereduced
prereduction phase
prerenal
    p. albuminuria
    p. azotemia
preretinal
pre-rolandic artery
prerubral
    p. field
    p. nucleus
presacral
    p. anesthesia
    p. fascia
    p. nerve
    p. neurectomy
    p. sympathectomy
presbyacousia
presbyacusis, presbyacusia
presbyastasis
presbyatrics
presbycusis
presbyopia (Pr)
presbyopic
prescribe
prescription
    shotgun p.
presenile
    p. dementia
    p. spontaneous gangrene
presenility
presenium
present
presentation
    acromion p.
    breech p.
    brow p.
    cephalic p.
    compound p.
    face p.
    footling p.
    frank breech p.

    full breech p.
    head p.
    incomplete foot p.
    knee p.
    pelvic p.
    placental p.
    polar p.
    shoulder p.
    sincipital p.
    transverse p.
    vertex p.
presenting symptom
preseptal cellulitis
preservative
presomite embryo
presphenoid bone
presphygmic
prespinal
presplenic fold
prespondylolisthesis
pressor
    p. amine
    p. base
    p. fiber
    p. nerve
    p. substance
pressoreceptive mechanism
pressoreceptor
    p. nerve
    p. reflex
    p. system
pressosensitive
pressosensitivity
    reflexogenic p.
pressure (P)
    abdominal p.
    absolute p.
    acoustic p.
    p. alopecia
    p. amaurosis
    p. anesthesia
    atmospheric p.
    p. atrophy
    back p.
    barometric p. (P_B)
    biting p.
    blood p. (BP)
    central venous p. (CVP)
    cerebrospinal p.
    p. collapse
    continuous positive airway p.
      (CPAP)
    coronary perfusion p.
    critical p.
    detrusor p.
    diastolic p.
    differential blood p.
    Donders p.
    p. dressing
    effective osmotic p.
    p. epiphysis
    p. gangrene
    gauge p.
    hydrostatic p.
    intracranial p. (ICP)

P

pressure *(continued)*
    intraocular p.
    leak point p.
    negative p.
    negative end-expiratory p. (NEEP)
    occlusal p.
    oncotic p.
    osmotic p.
    p. palsy
    p. paralysis
    partial p. (*P*)
    p. plethysmograph
    pleural p.
    p. pneumothorax
    p. point
    positive end-expiratory p. (PEEP)
    pulmonary p.
    pulmonary capillary wedge p. (PCWP)
    pulp p.
    pulse p.
    p. pulse differentiation
    p. reversal
    selection p.
    p. sense
    solution p.
    p. sore
    standard p.
    p. stasis
    systolic p.
    transmural p.
    transpulmonary p.
    transthoracic p.
    p. ulcer
    p. urticaria
    vapor p.
    ventricular filling p.
    p. waveform
    wedge p.
    zero end-expiratory p. (ZEEP)
pressure-controlled
    p.-c. respirator
    p.-c. ventilation
pressure-support ventilation
pressure-volume index
pre–steady state
presternal
    p. notch
    p. region
presternum
prestriate area
presulcal part of tongue
presumed ocular histoplasmosis
presumptive region
presuppurative
presynaptic membrane
presystole
presystolic
    p. gallop
    p. murmur
    p. thrill
pretarsal
pretecta

pretectal
    p. area
    p. nucleus
    p. region
pretectoolivary fiber
pretectum
preterm
    p. infant
    p. membrane rupture
prethyroid, prethyroideal, prethyroidean
pretibial
    p. fever
pretracheal
    p. fascia
    p. layer of cervical fascia
    p. lymph node
pretrematic
pretympanic
prevalence
preventive
    p. dentistry
    p. dose
    p. medicine
    p. treatment
prevertebral
    p. fascia
    p. ganglia
    p. layer of cervical fascia
    p. lymph node
    p. part of vertebral artery
prevesical
previllous
    p. chorion
    p. embryo
Prevotella
    P. bivia
    P. denticola
    P. disiens
    P. heparinolytica
    P. intermedia
    P. melaninogenica
    P. oralis
    P. oris
prezone
priapism
priapus
Pribnow box
Price-Jones curve
prickle
    p. cell
    p. cell layer
prickly heat
prilocaine hydrochloride
primacy
    genital p.
    oral p.
primal
    p. repression
    p. scene
primaquine phosphate
    p. p. sensitivity
primaquine sensitivity
primary
    p. adhesion
    p. adrenocortical insufficiency

p. aerodontalgia
p. alcohol
p. aldosteronism
p. amebic meningoencephalitis
p. amenorrhea
p. amide
p. amine
p. amputation
p. amyloidosis
p. anesthetic
p. atelectasis
p. atypical pneumonia
p. biliary cirrhosis
p. brain vesicle
p. bronchus
p. bubo
p. carcinoma
p. cardiomyopathy
p. caries
p. carnitine deficiency
p. cementum
p. center of ossification
p. choana
p. coccidioidomycosis
p. color
p. complex
p. constriction
p. curvature of vertebral column
p. dementia
p. dental lamina
p. dentin
p. dentition
p. deviation
p. digestion
p. digit of foot
p. disease
p. dried yeast
p. drive
p. dye test
p. dysmenorrhea
p. egg membrane
p. embryonic cell
p. erythroblastic anemia
p. extrapulmonary coccidioidomycosis
p. fissure of cerebellum
p. gain
p. generalized epilepsy
p. gout
p. hair
p. hemochromatosis
p. hemorrhage
p. herpetic gingivostomatitis
p. herpetic stomatitis
p. hydrocephalus
p. hyperoxaluria and oxalosis
p. hyperparathyroidism
p. hypertension
p. hyperthyroidism
p. hypogammaglobulinemia
p. hypogonadism
p. idiopathic macular atrophy
p. immune response
p. impression
p. interatrial foramen
p. irritant

p. irritant dermatitis
p. labial groove
p. lateral sclerosis
p. lymphedema
p. lysosome
p. macular atrophy of skin
p. medical care
p. megaureter
p. mesoderm
p. metabolism
p. metabolite
p. methemoglobinemia
p. myeloid metaplasia
p. narcissism
p. neurasthenia
p. neuroendocrine carcinoma of the skin
p. neuronal degeneration
p. nodule
p. nondisjunction
p. oocyte
p. organizer
p. ossification center
p. ovarian follicle
p. palate
p. pentosuria
p. pigmentary degeneration of retina
p. point of ossification
p. process
p. progressive cerebellar degeneration
p. proteose
p. pulmonary lobule
p. radiation
p. ray
p. reaction
p. refractory anemia
p. reinforcement
p. rejection
p. renal calculus
p. renal tubular acidosis
p. sclerosing cholangitis
p. screw-worm
p. senile dementia
p. sensation
p. sequestrum
p. sex character
p. shock
p. skin graft
p. sodium phosphate
p. spermatocyte
p. structure
p. syphilis
p. telangiectasia
p. tooth
p. tuberculosis
p. union
p. villus
p. visual area
p. visual cortex
p. vitreous

primase (dnaG)
primate
primer extension
primerite

primidone
primigravida
    elderly p.
primipara
primiparity
primiparous
primite
primitive
    p. aorta
    p. choana
    p. chorion
    p. costal arch
    p. furrow
    p. groove
    p. gut
    p. knot
    p. meninx
    p. neuroectodermal tumor
    p. node
    p. palate
    p. perivisceral cavity
    p. pit
    p. reticular cell
    p. ridge
    p. streak
primordia
primordial
    p. cartilage
    p. cyst
    p. dwarfism
    p. germ cell
    p. gigantism
    p. kidney
    p. ovarian follicle
primordium
    genital p.
primosome
primula
primulin
primus
princeps, pl. **principes**
    p. cervicis
    p. cervicis artery
    p. pollicis
    p. pollicis artery
Princeteau tubercle
principal
    p. artery of thumb
    p. focus
    p. olivary nucleus
    p. optic axis
    p. piece
    p. plane
    p. point
    p. sensory nucleus of trigeminal nerve
    p. sensory nucleus of the trigeminus
principes (*pl. of* princeps)
principle
    active p.
    antianemic p.
    Bernoulli p.
    bitter p.
    closure p.

    consistency p.
    Fick p.
    follicle-stimulating p.
    founder p.
    hematinic p.
    Huygens p.
    p. of inertia
    Le Chatelier p.
    luteinizing p.
    mass action p.
    melanophore-expanding p.
    Mitrofanoff p.
    nirvana p.
    organic p.
    pain-pleasure p.
    Pauli exclusion p.
    pleasure p.
    proximate p.
    reality p.
    repetition-compulsion p.
    ultimate p.
Pringle disease
Prinzmetal angina
prion
    p. protein (PrP)
prior probability
prism
    p. cover test
    p. diopter (p.d.)
    enamel p.
    Fresnel p.
    Nicol p.
    Risley rotary p.
    p. vergence test
prisma, pl. **prismata**
    prismata adamantina
prismatic
prison fever typhus
privacy
private
    p. antigen
    p. blood group
    p. duty nurse
    p. hospital
    p. nurse
privet cough
privileged site
PRK
    photorefractive keratectomy
PRL
    prolactin
p.r.n.
    pro re nata
proaccelerin
proacrosin
proacrosomal granule
proactinium
proactivator
proactive inhibition
proal
proamnion
probability
    conditional p.
    p. curve
    joint p.

objective p.
personal p.
posterior p.
prior p.
p. sample
subjective p.
probacteriophage
defective p.
proband
probang
probe
Bowman p.
p. gorget
nucleic acid p.
p. patency
periodontal p.
radioactive p.
p. syringe
vertebrated p.
viral p.
probenecid
probilifuscins
probiosis
probiotic
problem
problem-oriented record (POR)
proboscis, pl. **proboscides**
Probstymayria vivipara
probucol
procainamide hydrochloride
procaine hydrochloride
procapsid
procarbazine hydrochloride
procarboxypeptidase
procarcinogens
Procaryotae
procaryote
procaryotic
procatarctic
procatarxis
procedure
back table p.
Batista p.
Belsey p.
Chamberlain p.
Clagett p. for empyema
Collis-Belsey p.
commando p.
Damus-Kaye-Stancel p.
dideoxy p.
Dor p.
Eloesser p.
endorectal pull-through p.
Ewart p.
Fontan p.
Girdlestone p.
Harada-Ito p.
Hummelsheim p.
Jatene p.
Kestenbaum p.
Konno p.
Konno-Rastan p.
lateral tarsal strip p.
loop electrocautery excision p.
(LEEP)

loop electrosurgical excision p.
McCall culdoplasty p.
Mitchell p.
Mustard p.
Nick p.
Noble-Collip p.
Norwood p.
Puestow p.
push-back p.
Putti-Platt p.
Reichel-Pólya stomach p.
Rittenhouse-Manogian p.
Ross p.
sacrocolpopexy p.
sacrospinous vaginal vault
suspension p.
shelf p.
Sugiura p.
Thal p.
Vineberg p.
Walsh p.
procelia
procelous
procentriole
p. organizer
procephalic
procercoid
procerus muscle
process
A.B.C. p.
accessory p. of lumbar vertebra
acromial p.
agene p.
alar p.
alveolar p. of maxilla
anterior clinoid p.
anterior p. of malleus
apical p.
articular p.
ascending p.
auditory p.
basilar p.
basilar p. of occipital bone
binary p.
Budde p.
Burns falciform p.
calcaneal p. of cuboid
caudate p.
ciliary p.
Civinini p.
clinoid p.
cochleariform p.
complex learning p.
condylar p. of mandible
condyloid p.
conoid p.
coracoid p.
coronoid p.
coronoid p. of the mandible
coronoid p. of the ulna
costal p.
dendritic p.
dental p.
ensiform p.

P

process (*continued*)

ethmoidal p. of inferior nasal concha
falciform p. of sacrotuberous ligament
Folli p.
follian p.
foot p.
frontal p. of maxilla
frontal p. of zygomatic bone
frontonasal p.
frontosphenoidal p.
funicular p.
globular p.
hamular p. of lacrimal bone
hamular p. of sphenoid bone
head p.
inferior articular p.
Ingrassia p.
intrajugular p.
jugular p. of occipital bone
lacrimal p. of inferior nasal concha
lateral p. of calcaneal tuberosity
lateral p. of malleus
lateral nasal p.
lateral p. of septal nasal cartilage
lateral p. of talus
Lenhossék p.
lenticular p. of incus
long p. of malleus
malar p.
mammillary p. of lumbar vertebra
mandibular p.
Markov p.
mastoid p.
mastoid p. of petrous part of temporal bone
maxillary p. of embryo
maxillary p. of inferior nasal concha
medial p. of calcaneal tuberosity
medial nasal p.
mental p.
middle clinoid p.
muscular p. of arytenoid cartilage
nasal p.
notochordal p.
odontoblastic p.
odontoid p.
odontoid p. of epistropheus
olecranon p.
orbicular p.
orbital p. of palatine bone
packing p.
palatine p. of maxilla
papillary p. of caudate lobe of liver
paramastoid p.
paroccipital p.
posterior clinoid p.
posterior p. of septal cartilage
posterior p. of talus
primary p.
progressive p.

pterygoid p. of sphenoid bone
pterygospinous p.
pyramidal p. of palatine bone
Rau p.
Ravius p.
retromandibular p. of parotid gland
p. schizophrenia
secondary p.
sheath p. of sphenoid bone
short p. of malleus
slender p. of malleus
sphenoid p.
sphenoidal p. of palatine bone
sphenoid p. of septal nasal cartilage
spinous p. of sphenoid
spinous p. of tibia
spinous p. of vertebra
Stieda p.
stochastic p.
styloid p. of fibula
styloid p. of radius
styloid p. of temporal bone
styloid p. of third metacarpal bone
styloid p. of ulna
superior articular p.
superior articular p. of sacrum
supracondylar p. of humerus
supraepicondylar p.
temporal p. of zygomatic bone
Tomes p.
transverse p. of vertebra
trochlear p.
uncinate p. of cervical vertebra
uncinate p. of ethmoid bone
uncinate p. of first thoracic vertebra
uncinate p. of pancreas
vaginal p.
vaginal p. of peritoneum
vaginal p. of sphenoid bone
vaginal p. of testis
vermiform p.
vocal p.
vocal p. of arytenoid cartilage
xiphoid p.
zygomatic p. of frontal bone
zygomatic p. of maxilla
zygomatic p. of temporal bone

processing
processor

speech p.

processus, pl. **processus**

p. accessorius vertebrae lumbalis
p. alveolaris maxillae
p. anterior mallei
p. articularis
p. articularis superior ossis sacri
p. ascendens
p. brevis
p. calcaneus ossis cuboidei
p. caudatus
p. ciliaris
p. clinoideus
p. clinoideus anterior
p. clinoideus medius
p. clinoideus posterior

p. cochleariformis
p. condylaris mandibulae
p. coracoideus
p. coronoideus
p. coronoideus mandibulae
p. coronoideus ulnae
p. costalis
p. ethmoidalis conchae nasalis
  inferioris
p. falciformis ligamenti
  sacrotuberalis
p. ferreini
p. frontalis maxillae
p. frontalis ossis zygomatici
p. gracilis
p. intrajugularis
p. jugularis ossis occipitalis
p. lacrimalis conchae nasalis
  inferioris
p. lateralis mallei
p. lateralis tali
p. lateralis tuberis calcanei
p. lenticularis incudis
p. mammillaris vertebrae lumbalis
p. mastoideus
p. mastoideus partis petrosae ossis
  temporalis
p. maxillaris conchae nasalis
  inferioris
p. medialis tuberis calcanei
p. muscularis cartilaginis
  arytenoideae
p. orbitalis ossis palatini
p. palatinus ossis maxillae
p. papillaris lobi caudati hepatis
p. paramastoideus
p. posterior cartilaginis septi nasi
p. posterior tali
p. pterygoideus ossis sphenoidalis
p. pterygospinosus
p. pyramidalis ossis palatini
p. ravii
p. retromandibularis
p. retromandibularis glandulae
  parotidis
p. sphenoidalis cartilaginis septi nasi
p. sphenoidalis ossis palatini
p. spinosus
p. spinosus vertebrae
p. styloideus ossis metacarpalis III
p. styloideus ossis temporalis
p. styloideus radii
p. styloideus ulnae
p. supraepicondylaris humeri
p. temporalis ossis zygomatici
p. transversus vertebrae
p. trochleariformis
p. trochlearis
p. uncinatus ossis ethmoidalis
p. uncinatus pancreatis
p. uncinatus vertebrae cervicalis
p. uncinatus vertebrae thoracicae
  primae
p. vaginalis ossis sphenoidalis
p. vaginalis peritonei

p. vaginalis of peritoneum
p. vermiformis
p. vocalis cartilaginis arytenoideae
p. xiphoideus
p. zygomaticus maxillae
p. zygomaticus ossis frontalis
p. zygomaticus ossis temporalis
procheilia, prochilia
procheilon, prochilon
prochiral
prochirality
prochlorperazine
prochondral
prochordal plate
prochymosin
procidentia uteri
procollagen
  p. aminoproteinase
  p. carboxyproteinase
proconvertin
procreate
procreation
procreative
proctalgia fugax
proctatresia
proctectasia
proctectomy
proctitis
  chronic ulcerative p.
  epidemic gangrenous p.
  idiopathic p.
proctocele
proctoclysis
proctococcypexy
proctocolectomy
proctocolitis
proctocolonoscopy
proctocolpoplasty
proctocystocele
proctocystoplasty
proctocystotomy
proctodeal
proctodeum, pl. **proctodea**
proctodynia
proctologic
proctologist
proctology
proctoparalysis
proctoperineoplasty
proctopexy
proctophobia
proctoplasty
proctoplegia
proctopolypus
proctoptosia, proctoptosis
proctorrhagia
proctorrhaphy
proctorrhea
proctoscope
  Tuttle p.
proctoscopy
proctosigmoid
proctosigmoidectomy
proctosigmoiditis
proctosigmoidoscope

P

proctosigmoidoscopy
proctospasm
proctostasis
proctostat
proctostenosis
proctostomy
proctotome
proctotomy
proctotresia
proctovalvotomy
procumbent
procursive
    p. chorea
    p. epilepsy
procurvation
procyclidine hydrochloride
procyclidine methochloride
prodigiosin
α-prodine hydrochloride
prodromal
    p. period
    p. stage
prodrome
prodromic, prodromous
    p. sign
prodromus, pl. **prodromi**
prodrug
product
    cleavage p.
    double p.
    end p.
    fibrin/fibrinogen degradation p.
     (FDP)
    fission p.
    p. inhibition
    natural p.
    orphan p.
    spallation p.
    substitution p.
productive
    p. inflammation
    p. peritonitis
    p. pleurisy
product-moment correlation
proelastase
proemial
proencephalon
proenkephalin
proenzyme
proerythroblast
proerythrocyte
proestrogen
proestrum
proestrus
profenamine hydrochloride
Profeta law
profibrinolysin
proficiency
    p. sample
    p. testing
profilactin
profile
    biochemical p.
    biophysical p.
    facial p.

    personality p.
    p. record
    test p.
    urethral pressure p.
profilin
profilometer
proflavine (hemi)sulfate
proformiphen
profound hypothermia
profunda
    p. brachii artery
    p. femoris artery
    p. femoris vein
profundus
profusion
progabide
progastrin
progenia
progenitalis
progenitor
progeny
progeria
    p. with cataract
    p. with microphthalmia
progestational hormone
progesterone
    p. challenge test
    p. receptor
    p. unit
progestin
progestogen
proglossis
proglottid
proglottis, pl. **proglottides**
prognathic
prognathism
    basilar p.
prognathous
prognose
prognosis
    denture p.
prognostic
prognosticate
prognostician
progonoma
    p. of jaw
    melanotic p.
prograde
program
programmable hearing aid
programmed cell death
programming
    neurolinguistic p.
progranulocyte
progress curve
progressive
    p. bacterial synergistic gangrene
    p. bulbar palsy
    p. bulbar paralysis
    p. cataract
    p. cerebellar tremor
    p. cerebral poliodystrophy
    p. choroidal atrophy
    p. circumscribed cerebral atrophy
    p. cleavage

p. emphysematous necrosis
p. familial scleroderma
p. hypertrophic polyneuropathy
p. infantile spinal muscular atrophy
p. lipodystrophy
p. multifocal leukoencephalopathy (PML)
p. outer retinal necrosis (PORN)
p. pigmentary dermatosis
p. process
p. spinal amyotrophy
p. spinal muscular atrophy
p. staining
p. subcortical encephalopathy
p. supranuclear palsy
p. tapetochoroidal dystrophy
p. vaccinia
proguanil hydrochloride
prohormone
proinsulin
projectile vomiting
projection
p. angiogram
anteroposterior p.
AP p.
apical lordotic p.
axial p.
base p.
Caldwell p.
cross-table lateral p.
enamel p.
erroneous p.
false p.
p. fiber
Fischer p.
frog-leg lateral p.
Granger p.
half-axial p.
Haworth p.
lateral p.
left anterior oblique p. (LAO)
maximum intensity p. (MIP)
oblique p.
occipitomental p.
PA p.
p. perimeter
posteroanterior p.
Rhese p.
Stenvers p.
submental vertex p.
submentovertical p.
p. system
Towne p.
visual p.
Waters p.
projective
p. identification
p. test
Prokaryotae
prokaryote
prokaryotic
prolabial
prolabium
prolactin (PRL)

p. cell
p. unit
prolactin-inhibiting factor
prolactinoma
prolactin-producing adenoma
prolamine
prolapse
p. of the corpus luteum
first-degree p.
mitral valve p.
Morgagni p.
second-degree p.
p. of umbilical cord
p. of the uterus, third-degree p.
valvular p.
prolective
prolepsis
proleptic
proleukocyte
prolidase
proliferate
proliferating
p. cell nuclear antigen
p. pleurisy
p. systematized angioendotheliomatosis
p. tricholemmal cyst
proliferation
p. cyst
diffuse mesangial p.
gingival p.
p. therapy
proliferative, proliferous
p. arthritis
p. bronchiolitis
p. choroiditis
p. cyst
p. dermatitis
p. fasciitis
p. gingivitis
p. glomerulonephritis
p. inflammation
p. intimitis
p. myositis
p. retinopathy
prolific
proligerous
p. disk
p. membrane
prolinase
proline
p. aminopeptidase
p. dehydrogenase
p. dipeptidase
p. iminopeptidase
p. oxidase
p. racemase
D-p. reductase
prolonged
p. action tablet
p. pregnancy
prolyl
p. dipeptidase
p. hydroxylase
prolylglycine dipeptidase

P

promastigote
promegaloblast
prometaphase banding
promethazine hydrochloride
promethazine theoclate
promethestrol dipropionate
promethium (Pm)
prominence
Ammon p.
canine p.
cardiac p.
p. of facial canal
forebrain p.
frontonasal p.
hepatic p.
hypothenar p.
laryngeal p.
lateral nasal p.
p. of lateral semicircular canal
mallear p.
medial nasal p.
spiral p. of cochlear duct
styloid p.
thenar p.
tubal p.
p. of venous valvular sinus
prominens
prominent heel
prominentia, pl. **prominentiae**
p. canalis facialis
p. canalis semicircularis lateralis
p. laryngea
p. mallearis
p. spiralis ductus cochlearis
p. styloidea
promitochondria
PROMM
proximal myotonic myopathy
promonocyte
promontorial common iliac node
promontorium, pl. **promontoria**
p. cavi tympani
p. ossis sacri
promontory
pelvic p.
sacral p.
p. of the sacrum
tympanic p.
p. of tympanic cavity
promoter
promoting agent
promotion
health p.
prompt insulin zinc suspension
promyelocyte
pronasion
pronate
pronation
p. of foot
p. of forearm
pronator
p. muscle
p. quadratus muscle
p. reflex
p. ridge

p. teres muscle
p. teres syndrome
p. tuberosity
pronephric
p. duct
p. tubule
pronephros, pl. **pronephroi**
prone position
pronograde
pronometer
pronormoblast
pronucleus, pl. **pronuclei**
female p.
male p.
proof spirit
proopiomelanocortin (POMC)
prootic
pro-oxidants
propafenone
propagate
propagated thrombus
propagation
propagative
propalinal
propamidine
propane
propanedioic acid
1,2,3-propanetriol
propanidid
propanoic acid
propanol
propanoyl
propantheline bromide
proparacaine hydrochloride
proparathyroid hormone
propatyl nitrate
propene
propentdyopent
propenyl
propepsin
propeptone
proper
p. cochlear artery
p. fasciculi
p. ligament of ovary
p. membrane of semicircular duct
p. palmar digital artery
p. palmar digital nerve
p. plantar digital artery
p. plantar digital nerve
p. substance
properdin
p. factor B, D
p. system
properitoneal inguinal hernia
property emergence
prophage
defective p.
prophase
prophenpyridamine maleate
prophylactic
p. membrane
p. odontotomy
p. treatment
prophylaxis, pl. **prophylaxes**

active p.
chemical p.
dental p.
passive p.
propicillin
propiocortin
propiolactone
propionate
Propionibacterium
    P. acnes
    P. freudenreichii
    P. jensenii
    P. propionicus
propionic acid
propionic acidemia
propionyl
propionyl-CoA
    propionyl-CoA carboxylase
propionylglycine
propitocaine hydrochloride
proplasia
proplasmacyte
proplexus
propofol
proportional
    p. assist ventilation
    p. counter
    p. limit
    p. mortality ratio (PMR)
proportionate
    p. dwarfism
    p. infantilism
propositus, pl. **propositi**
propoxyphene hydrochloride
propoxyphene napsylate
propranolol hydrochloride
proprietary
    p. hospital
    p. medicine
proprietary name
proprioception
proprioceptive
    p. mechanism
    p. reflex
    p. sensibility
proprioceptive-oculocephalic reflex
proprioceptor
propriospinal
proproteins
proptometer
proptosis
proptotic
propulsion
propyl
    p. alcohol
    p. gallate
    p. hydroxybenzoate
propylcarbinol
propylene glycol
propylhexedrine
propyliodone
propylparaben
propylthiouracil (PTU)
propyromazine

pro rat. aet.
    pro ratione aetatis
pro ratione aetatis (pro rat. aet.)
pro re nata (p.r.n.)
prorennin
prorsad
prorubricyte
    pernicious anemia type p.
proscillaridin
proscolex
prosecretin
prosecretion granule
prosect
prosector
prosectorium
prosencephalon
proserum prothrombin conversion accelerator (PPCA)
prosodemic
prosody
prosopagnosia
prosopagus
prosopectasia
prosoplasia
prosopoanoschisis
prosopopagus
prosoposchisis
prosopothoracopagus
prospective fate
prostacyclin
prostaglandin (PG)
    p. A (PGA)
    p. B (PGB)
    p. C (PGC)
    p. D (PGD)
    p. E_1, E_2
    p. endoperoxide synthase
    p. $F_{2\alpha}$
    p. $F_{2\alpha}$ tromethamine
prostanoic acid
prostanoids
prostata
prostatalgia
prostate
    female p.
    p. gland
prostatectomy
prostate-specific antigen (PSA)
prostatic
    p. adenoma
    p. branch of inferior vesical artery
    p. branch of middle rectal artery
    p. calculus
    p. catheter
    p. duct
    p. ductule
    p. fluid
    p. intraepithelial neoplasia (PIN)
    p. massage
    p. sheath
    p. sinus
    p. urethra
    p. utricle
    p. venous plexus
prostaticovesical venous plexus

P

prostatism
prostatitis
prostatocystitis
prostatodynia
prostatolith
prostatolithotomy
prostatomegaly
prostatomy
prostatorrhea
prostatoseminalvesiculectomy
prostatotomy
prostatovesiculectomy
prostatovesiculitis
prosternation
prostheon
prosthesis, pl. prostheses
    auditory p.
    cardiac valve p.
    cochlear p.
    definitive p.
    dental p.
    heart valve p.
    hybrid p.
    mandibular guide p.
    ocular p.
    penile p.
    provisional p.
    surgical p.
    testicular p.
    tilting disk valve p.
prosthetic
    p. dentistry
    p. group
    p. valve
prosthetics
    dental p.
    maxillofacial p.
prosthetist
prosthetophacos
prosthion
prosthodontia
prosthodontics
prosthodontist
Prosthogonimus macrorchis
prosthokeratoplasty
prostomial mesoderm
prostration
    heat p.
protactinium
protalbumose
protaminase
protamine
    p. sulfate
    p. zinc insulin
protanomaly
protanopia
protean
protease
    p. inhibitor
    Lon p.
    tricorn p.
protection
    p. test
protective
    p. block

    p. colloid
    p. laryngeal reflex
    p. protein
    p. spectacles
    p. zone
protector
    hearing p.'s
Proteeae
protein
    p. 4.1
    p. A
    acute phase p.
    acyl carrier p. (ACP)
    amyloid p.
    androgen binding p. (ABP)
    antitermination p.
    antitumor p.
    antiviral p. (AVP)
    autologous p.
    basic p.
    Bence Jones p.
    bone Gla p. (BGP)
    p. C
    cAMP receptor p. (CRP)
    capping p.
    catabolite gene activator p. (CAP)
    cholesterol ester transport p.
    circumsporozoite p.
    cis-acting p.
    compound p.
    conjugated p.
    copper p.
    corticosteroid-binding p.
    C-reactive p. (CRP)
    denatured p.
    derived p.
    docking p.
    encephalithogenic p.
    eosinophil cationic p. (ECP)
    extrinsic p.
    p. factor
    fatty acid–binding p.
    p. fever
    fibrous p.
    foreign p.
    G p.
    G-p.
    glial fibrillary acidic p.
    globular p.
    GTP binding p.
    heat shock p. (hsp)
    heterologous p.
    homologous p.
    immune p.
    integral p.
    intrinsic p.
    iron-sulfur p.
    p. kinase C
    p. kinases
    latent membrane p. (LMP)
    low molecular weight p.
    M p.
    macrophage inflammatory p. (MIP)
    p. malnutrition
    mannose-binding p.

matrix Gla p. (MGP)
p. metabolism
microtubule-associated p. (MAPs)
monoclonal p.
monocyte chemoattractant p.
monocyte chemoattractant p.-1
  (MCP-1)
muscle p.
myelin p. A1
native p.
neutrophil-activating p.
non-heme iron p.
nonspecific p.
odorant binding p.
p. p53
parathyroid hormonelike p. (PLP)
parathyroid hormone-related p.
pathologic p.
peripheral p.
phenylthiocarbamoyl p.
PhNCS p.
p. phosphatase
placenta p.
plasma p.
prion p. (PrP)
protective p.
PTC p.
purified placental p.
p. quotient
receptor p.
retinol-binding p.
p. S
S p.
serum p.
p. shock
p. shock therapy
simple p.
stimulatory p. 1 (SP1)
structure p.
surfactant-specific p.
p. synthesis
Tamm-Horsfall p.
thrombospondin-related adhesive p.
thyroxine-binding p. (TBP)
unwinding p.
vitamin D–binding p. (DBP)
whey p.
Z-p.
proteinaceous
proteinase
  Clostridium histolyticum p. B
protein-bound
  p.-b. iodine (PBI)
  p.-b. iodine test
protein hydrolysate
protein-losing enteropathy
proteinogenic
proteinoid
proteinosis
  lipoid p.
  pulmonary alveolar p.
proteinuria
  Bence Jones p.
  gestational p.
  isolated p.

nonisolated p.
orthostatic p.
postural p.
protensity
proteoclastic
proteogenic
proteoglycan
  p. I
proteohormone
proteolipids
proteolysis
proteolytic
proteometabolic
proteometabolism
Proteomyxidia
proteopectic, proteopexic
proteopepsis
proteopexis
proteose
  primary p.
  secondary p.
proteosome
Proteus
  P. inconstans
  P. mirabilis
  P. morganii
  P. rettgeri
  P. vulgaris
prothipendyl
prothoracic gland
prothrombase
prothrombin
  p. accelerator
  p. and proconvertin test
  p. time
prothrombinase
prothrombinogen
prothrombinopenia
prothrombokinase
protirelin
protist
Protista
protium
protoactinium
protoalbumose
protoalkaloid
protobiology
protocatechuic acid
protochordal knot
protocol
  Bruce p.
protocone
protoconid
protocoproporphyria hereditaria
Protoctista
protoderm
protodiastolic gallop
protoduodenum
protoerythrocyte
protofilament
protogen A
protogonoplasm
protokylol hydrochloride
protoleukocyte
protolysate

P

protomer
protomerite
protometrocyte
proton
    p. pump
    p. pump inhibitor
protoneuron
protonymph
protooncogene
protopathic sensibility
protopectin
protopianoma
protoplasm
    totipotential p.
protoplasmic, protoplasmatic
    p. astrocyte
    p. astrocytoma
    p. movement
protoplasmolysis
protoplast
protoporphyria
    erythropoietic p.
protoporphyrinogen type III
    p. t. i. oxidase
protoporphyrin type III
protoproteose
protosalt
protospore
protostoma
protostome
protosulfate
prototaxic
Prototheca
protothecosis
prototroph
prototrophic
    p. strain
prototrophism
prototype
protoveratrine A and B
protovertebra
protovertebral
protoxide
protozoa (*pl. of* protozoon)
protozoal
protozoan cyst
protozoiasis
protozoicide
protozoologist
protozoology
protozoon, pl. **protozoa**
protozoophage
protraction
    mandibular p.
    maxillary p.
protractor
protriptyline hydrochloride
protrude
protruded disk
protruding
    p. ear
    p. tooth
protrusio acetabuli
protrusion
    bimaxillary p.

    bimaxillary dentoalveolar p.
    double p.
protrusive
    p. excursion
    p. jaw relation
    p. occlusion
    p. position
    p. record
protrusive interocclusal record (*var. of* interocclusal record)
protrypsin
protuberance
    Bichat p.
    external occipital p.
    internal occipital p.
    mental p.
protuberant abdomen
protuberantia
    p. laryngea
    p. mentalis
    p. occipitalis externa
    p. occipitalis interna
proud flesh
prourokinase
Proust
    P. law
    P. space
provertebra
Providencia
    P. alcalifaciens
    P. rettgeri
    P. stuartii
provirus
provisional
    p. callus
    p. cortex
    p. denture
    p. ligature
    p. prosthesis
    p. restoration
provitamin
    p. A, D_2, D_3
provocation typhoid
provocative
    p. test
    p. Wassermann test
Prowazek body
Prowazek-Greeff body
Prowazekia
proxemics
proximad
proximal
    p. border of nail
    p. caries
    p. centriole
    p. contact
    p. deep inguinal lymph node
    p. femoral focal deficiency (PFFD)
    p. interphalangeal (PIP)
    p. interphalangeal joint
    p. medial striate artery
    p. myotonic myopathy (PROMM)
    p. part of prostate
    p. part of prostatic urethra
    p. phalanx of foot

p. phalanx of hand
p. radioulnar articulation
p. radioulnar joint
p. spiral septum
p. splenorenal shunt
p. tibiofibular joint
p. urethral sphincter
proximalis
proximate
p. cause
p. contact
p. principle
proximoataxia
proximobuccal
proximolabial
proximolingual
proxymetacaine hydrochloride
prozone reaction
prozygosis
PrP
prion protein
PRPP
5-phospho-alpha-D-ribosyl-1-pyrophosphate
p. synthetase
prune
p. belly
p. belly syndrome
prune-juice
p.-j. expectoration
p.-j. sputum
Prunus
p. serotina
p. virginiana
prurigo
actinic p.
p. aestivalis
Besnier p.
p. gestationis
Hebra p.
p. mitis
p. nodularis
p. simplex
summer p.
pruritic
p. urticarial papules and plaques of pregnancy (PUPPP)
pruritus
p. aestivalis
p. ani
aquagenic p.
bath p.
essential p.
p. gravidarum
p. hiemalis
senile p.
p. senilis
symptomatic p.
p. vulvae
Prussak
P. fiber
P. pouch
P. space
Prussian blue stain
prussiate

prussic acid
PSA
prostate-specific antigen
psalterial cord
psalterium, pl. **psalteria**
psammocarcinoma
psammoma
p. body
Virchow p.
psammomatous meningioma
psammous
PSA velocity
PSE
Pidgin Sign English
psellism
pseudacromegaly
pseudagraphia
pseudalbuminuria
Pseudallescheria boydii
pseudallescheriasis
Pseudamphistomum
pseudangina
pseudankylosis
pseudarthrosis
pseudelminth
pseudesthesia
pseudoacanthosis nigricans
pseudoacephalus
pseudoachondroplasia
pseudoachondroplastic spondyloepiphysial dysplasia
pseudoactinomycosis
pseudoagglutination
pseudoagrammatism
pseudoagraphia
pseudo-ainhum
pseudoalbuminuria
pseudoalkaloids
pseudoallelic
pseudoallelism
pseudo-alopecia areata
pseudoanaphylactic shock
pseudoanaphylaxis
pseudoanemia
pseudoaneurysm
pseudoangina
pseudoanodontia
pseudoappendicitis
pseudoapraxia
pseudoarthrosis
pseudoauthenticity
pseudobacillus
pseudobacterium
pseudobulbar paralysis
pseudocartilage
pseudocartilaginous
pseudocast
pseudocele
pseudocelom
pseudocephalocele
pseudochancre
pseudocholinesterase
atypical p.
p. deficiency
typical p.

P

801

pseudochorea
pseudochromesthesia
pseudochromidrosis, pseudochromhidrosis
pseudochylous ascites
pseudocirrhosis
pseudoclonus
pseudocoarctation of the aorta
pseudocolloid
pseudocollusion
pseudocoma
pseudocowpox virus
pseudocoxalgia
pseudocrisis
pseudocroup
pseudocryptorchism
pseudocumene
pseudocumol
pseudocyesis
pseudocylindroid
pseudocyst
pseudodeciduosis
pseudodementia
pseudodextrocardia
pseudodiabetes
pseudodiastolic
pseudodigitoxin
pseudodiphtheria
pseudodipsia
pseudodiverticulum
pseudodominance
pseudodysentery
pseudoephedrine hydrochloride
pseudoepitheliomatous hyperplasia
pseudoerysipelas
pseudoesthesia
pseudoexfoliation
  pseudoexfoliation of lens capsule
pseudoexfoliation syndrome
pseudoexfoliative glaucoma
pseudofluctuation
pseudofolliculitis
pseudofracture
pseudofructose
pseudofusion beat
pseudoganglion
pseudo-Gaucher cell
pseudogene
pseudogeusesthesia
pseudogeusia
pseudoglanders
pseudoglioma
pseudoglobulin
pseudoglomerulus
pseudoglucosazone
pseudogout
pseudo-Graefe
  p.-G. phenomenon
  p.-G. sign
pseudogynecomastia
pseudohematuria
pseudohemoptysis
pseudohermaphrodite
pseudohermaphroditism
  female p.
  male p.

pseudohernia
pseudoheterotopia
pseudo-Hurler
  p.-H. disease
  p.-H. polydystrophy
pseudohydrocephaly
pseudohydronephrosis
pseudohyperkalemia
pseudohyperparathyroidism
pseudohypertelorism
pseudohypertrophic muscular dystrophy
pseudohypertrophy
pseudohypha
pseudohyponatremia
pseudohypoparathyroidism
  p. type Ia, I b
pseudoicterus
pseudoileus
pseudoinfarction
pseudoinfluenza
pseudointraligamentous
pseudoisochromatic
pseudoisoenzymes
pseudojaundice
pseudokeratin
pseudolepromatous leishmaniasis
pseudolipoma
pseudolithiasis
pseudologia phantastica
pseudolymphocyte
pseudolymphocytic choriomeningitis virus
pseudolymphoma
  cutaneous p.
pseudolysogenic strain
pseudolysogeny
pseudomalignancy
pseudomamma
pseudomania
pseudomasturbation
pseudomegacolon
pseudomelanosis
pseudomembrane
pseudomembranous
  p. bronchitis
  p. colitis
  p. conjunctivitis
  p. enteritis
  p. enterocolitis
  p. gastritis
  p. inflammation
pseudomeningitis
pseudomenstruation
pseudometaplasia
pseudomnesia
pseudomonad
Pseudomonas
  P. acidovorans
  P. aeruginosa
  P. cepacia
  P. diminuta
  P. fluorescens
  P. mallei
  P. maltophilia
  P. osteomyelitis
  P. piscicida

P. *pseudoalcaligenes*
P. *pseudomallei*
P. *putrefaciens*
P. *stutzeri*
P. *vesicularis*
pseudomonilethrix
pseudomonomolecular
pseudomorph
pseudomucinous cyst
pseudomycelium
pseudomyopia
pseudomyxoma peritonei
pseudonarcotic
pseudoneoplasm
pseudoneurogenic bladder
pseudoneuroma
pseudoneurotic schizophrenia
pseudonit
pseudoosteomalacia
pseudoosteomalacic pelvis
pseudopapilledema
pseudoparalysis
    arthritic general p.
    congenital atonic p.
pseudoparaplegia
    Basedow p.
pseudoparasite
pseudoparenchyma
pseudoparesis
pseudopelade of Brocq
pseudopericarditis
pseudoperoxidase
pseudophacos
pseudophakia
pseudophakodonesis
pseudophotesthesia
pseudophyllid
Pseudophyllidea
pseudoplastic fluid
pseudoplatelet
pseudopocket
pseudopod
pseudopodium, pl. **pseudopodia**
pseudopolydystrophy
pseudopolyp
pseudoporphyria
pseudopregnancy
pseudoprognathism
pseudo psychosis
pseudopterygium
pseudoptosis
pseudopuberty
    precocious p.
pseudorabies virus
pseudoreaction
pseudoreplica
pseudoretinitis pigmentosa
pseudorheumatism
pseudorheumatoid nodule
pseudorickets
pseudorosette
pseudorubella
pseudosarcoma
pseudosarcomatous fasciitis
pseudoscarlatina

pseudosclerosis
pseudoseizure
pseudosmallpox
pseudosmia
***Pseudostertagia* bullosa**
pseudostoma
pseudostrabismus
pseudostratified epithelium
pseudotabes
    pupillotonic p.
pseudotruncus arteriosus
pseudotubercle
pseudotubercular yersiniosis
pseudotuberculosis
pseudotubular degeneration
pseudotumor
    p. cerebri
    inflammatory p.
pseudounimolecular
pseudounipolar
    p. cell
    p. neuron
pseudouridine
pseudovacuole
pseudovariola
pseudoventricle
pseudovitamin B_{12}
pseudovomiting
pseudoxanthoma cell
pseudoxanthoma elasticum
psi (Ψ)
    p. phenomenon
psicose
psilocin
Psilocybe
psilocybin
psilosis
psilothin
psilotic
P-sinistrocardiale
psittacine
psittacosis
    p. inclusion body
    p. virus
psoas
    p. abscess
    p. major muscle
    p. margin
    p. minor muscle
psoatic part of iliopsoas fascia
psomophagia, psomophagy
psoralen
psorenteritis
Psorergates
psoriasiform
psoriasis
    p. annularis
    p. annulata
    p. arthropica
    p. circinata
    p. diffusa
    diffused p.
    exfoliative p.
    flexural p.
    generalized pustular p. of Zambusch

P

psoriasis *(continued)*
    p. geographica
    p. guttata
    p. gyrata
    p. nummularis
    palmar p.
    p. punctata
    pustular p.
psoriatic arthritis
Psoroptes
psoroptic acariasis
PSP
    phenolsulfonphthalein
psychalgalia
psychalgia
psychalia
psychanopsia
psychataxia
psyche
psychedelic
    p. drug
    p. therapy
psychiatric nosology
psychiatrist
psychiatry
    analytic p.
    biologic p.
    child p.
    community p.
    contractual p.
    cross-cultural p.
    descriptive p.
    dynamic p.
    existential p.
    forensic p.
    industrial p.
    orthomolecular p.
    psychoanalytic p.
    social p.
psychic
    p. blindness
    p. contagion
    p. determinism
    p. energy
    p. force
    p. impotence
    p. inertia
    p. overtone
    p. seizure
    p. tic
    p. trauma
psychical
psychism
psychoacoustics
psychoactive
psychoallergy
psychoanalysis
    active p.
    adlerian p.
    freudian p.
    jungian p.
psychoanalyst
psychoanalytic
    p. psychiatry

    p. psychotherapy
    p. situation
    p. therapy
psychoauditory
psychobiology
psychocardiac reflex
psychocatharsis
psychochrome
psychochromesthesia
psychodiagnosis
Psychodidae
psychodometry
psychodrama
psychodynamics
psychodysleptic drug
psychoendocrinology
psychoexploration
psychogalvanic
    p. reaction
    p. reflex
    p. response (PGR)
    p. skin reflex
    p. skin response
psychogalvanometer
psychogender
psychogenesis
psychogenic, psychogenetic
    p. hearing impairment
    p. nocturnal polydipsia (PNP)
    p. nocturnal polydipsia syndrome
    p. pain
    p. pain disorder
    p. polydipsia
    p. purpura
    p. seizure
    p. torticollis
    p. tremor
    p. vomiting
psychogeny
psychogeusic
psychogogic
psychographic
psychography
psychohistory
psychokinesis, psychokinesia
psycholinguistics
psychologic, psychological
    p. tests
psychologist
psychology
    adlerian p.
    analytic p.
    animal p.
    atomistic p.
    behavioral p.
    behavioristic p.
    child p.
    clinical p.
    cognitive p.
    community p.
    comparative p.
    constitutional p.
    counseling p.
    criminal p.
    depth p.

developmental p.
dynamic p.
educational p.
environmental p.
existential p.
experimental p.
forensic p.
genetic p.
gestalt p.
health p.
holistic p.
humanistic p.
individual p.
industrial p.
medical p.
objective p.
subjective p.
psycholytic drug
psychometrics
psychometry
psychomotor
p. epilepsy
p. retardation
p. seizure
p. test
psychoneuroimmunology
psychoneurosis maidica
psychoneurotic
psychonomic
psychonomy
psychonosology
psychonoxious
psycho-oncology
psychopath
psychopathic personality
psychopathologist
psychopathology
psychopathy
psychopharmaceutical
psychopharmacology
psychophysical
psychophysics
psychophysiologic
p. manifestation
psychophysiologic disorder (*var. of*
psychosomatic disorder)
psychophysiology
psychoprophylaxis
psychorelaxation
psychormic
psychosensory, psychosensorial
p. aphasia
psychoses (*pl. of* psychosis)
psychosexual
p. development
p. dysfunction
psychosine
psychosis, pl. **psychoses**
affective p.
alcoholic psychoses
bipolar p.
Cheyne-Stokes p.
depressive p.
drug p.
febrile p.

functional p.
hysterical p.
ICU p.
infection-exhaustion p.
Korsakoff p.
manic p.
manic-depressive p.
posthypnotic p.
postinfectious p.
postpartum p.
posttraumatic p.
pseudo p.
puerperal p.
schizoaffective p.
senile p.
situational p.
toxic p.
traumatic p.
Windigo p., Wittigo p.
psychosocial dwarfism
psychosomatic
p. disorder
p. medicine
psychosomimetic
psychostimulant
psychosurgery
psychosynthesis
psychotechnics
psychotherapeutic
psychotherapeutics
psychotherapist
psychotherapy
anaclitic p.
autonomous p.
brief p.
contractual p.
directive p.
dyadic p.
dynamic p.
existential p.
group p.
heteronomous p.
hypnotic p.
intensive p.
marathon group p.
nondirective p.
psychoanalytic p.
reconstructive p.
suggestive p.
supportive p.
transactional p.
psychotic
p. disorder
p. manifestation
psychotogen
psychotogenic
psychotomimetic drug
psychotropic
p. agent
p. drug
psychroalgia
psychroesthesia
psychrometer
sling p.
psychrometry

P

psychrophile, psychrophil
psychrophilic
psychrophobia
psychrophore
psyllium hydrophilic mucilloid
psyllium seed
PT
> physical therapy

Pt
> platinum

PTA
> plasma thromboplastin antecedent
>> PTA stain

PTAH
> phosphotungstic acid hematoxylin

ptarmic
ptarmus
PTC
> plasma thromboplastin component
>> PTC protein
>> PTC peptide

PTCA
> percutaneous transluminal coronary
> angioplasty

Ptd
> phosphatidyl

PtdCho
> phosphatidylcholine

PtdEth
> phosphatidylethanolamine

PtdIns
> phosphatidylinositol

PtdIns(4,5)P$_2$
> phosphatidylinositol 4,5-bisphosphate

PtdSer
> phosphatidylserine

PTE
> pulmonary thromboembolism

PTEA
> pulmonary thromboendarterectomy

pteridine
pterin deaminase
pterion
pteroic acid
pteropterin
pteroylmonoglutamic acid
pteroyltriglutamic acid
pterygium
> p. colli
> p. syndrome
> p. unguis

pterygo-
pterygoid
> p. branch of maxillary artery
> p. branch of posterior deep
>   temporal artery
> p. canal
> p. chest
> p. depression
> p. fissure
> p. fossa
> p. fovea
> p. hamulus
> p. lamina
> p. nerve

> p. notch
> p. pit
> p. plate
> p. process of sphenoid bone
> p. ridge of sphenoid bone
> p. tubercle
> p. tuberosity of mandible
> p. venous plexus

pterygomandibular
> p. ligament
> p. raphe
> p. space

pterygomaxillare
pterygomaxillary
> p. fissure
> p. fossa
> p. notch

pterygomeningeal artery
pterygopalatine
> p. canal
> p. fossa
> p. ganglion
> p. groove
> p. nerve

pterygopharyngeal part of superior
  constrictor muscle of pharynx
pterygospinal ligament
pterygospinous
> p. ligament
> p. process

PTF
> plasma thromboplastin factor

PTH
> parathyroid hormone

PTHC
> percutaneous transhepatic cholangiography

pthiriasis
> pthiriasis pubis

Pthirus
PTHrP
> parathyroid hormone-related peptide

PTK
> phototherapeutic keratectomy

PTMA
> phenyltrimethylammonium

ptomaine
ptomainemia
ptomatine
ptomatropine
ptosed
ptosis, pl. **ptoses**
> p. adiposa
> aponeurogenic p.
> p. sympathetica

ptotic organ
6-PTS
> 6-pyruvoyltetrahydropterin synthase

PTT
> partial thromboplastin time

PTU
> propylthiouracil

p53 tumor suppressor gene
ptyalagogue
ptyalectasis
ptyalin

ptyalism
ptyalocele
ptyalography
ptyalolith
ptyalolithiasis
ptyalolithotomy
ptychotis oil
ptyocrinous
Pu
    plutonium
pubarche
puberal, pubertal
puberty
    delayed p.
    precocious p.
    true precocious p.
pubes
pubescence
pubescent
pubic
    p. angle
    p. arch
    p. artery
    p. body
    p. bone
    p. branch of inferior epigastric
      artery
    p. branch of inferior epigastric vein
    p. branch of obturator artery
    p. crest
    p. hair
    p. ramus
    p. region
    p. spine
    p. symphysis
    p. tubercle
pubiotomy
pubis
public
    p. antigen
    p. health
    p. health dentistry
    p. health nurse
    p. hospital
Public Health Service (PHS)
puboanalis muscle
pubocapsular ligament
pubococcygeal muscle
pubococcygeus muscle
pubofemoral
    p. ligament
puboperinealis muscle
puboprostatic
    p. ligament
    p. muscle
puboprostaticus muscle
puborectal
    p. muscle
puborectalis muscle
pubourethral triangle
pubovaginal
    p. muscle
    p. operation
pubovaginalis muscle

pubovesical
    p. ligament
    p. muscle
pubovesicalis muscle
Puchtler-Sweat stain
pudding opium
puddle sign
pudendal
    p. anesthesia
    p. canal
    p. cleavage
    p. cleft
    p. hematocele
    p. hernia
    p. nerve
    p. sac
    p. slit
    p. vein
pudendum, pl. pudenda
    p. femininum
    p. muliebre
pudic nerve
puerile respiration
puerpera, pl. puerperae
puerperal
    p. eclampsia
    p. fever
    p. hemoglobinemia
    p. mastitis
    p. morbidity
    p. period
    p. psychosis
    p. sepsis
    p. septicemia
    p. tetanus
puerperant
puerperium, pl. puerperia
Puestow procedure
puff
    veiled p.
puffball
Pulex
    P. cheopis
    P. fasciatus
    P. irritans
    P. penetrans
    P. serraticeps
Pulfrich phenomenon
pulicicide, pulicide
pulley
    anular p.
    cruciform p.
    p. of humerus
    muscular p.
    peroneal p.
    p. of talus
pullulanase
pullulate
pullulation
pulmo, pl. pulmones
    p. dexter
    p. sinister
pulmoaortic
pulmolith

P

pulmonary
  p. acinus
  p. adenomatosis
  p. alveolar microlithiasis
  p. alveolar proteinosis
  p. alveolus
  p. amebiasis
  p. anthrax
  p. arc
  p. area
  p. artery
  p. artery anastomosis
  p. artery aneurysm
  p. artery atresia
  p. artery banding
  p. artery catheter
  p. bleb
  p. branch of autonomic nervous system
  p. branch of pulmonary nerve plexus
  p. bulla
  p. capillary wedge pressure (PCWP)
  p. cavity
  p. circulation
  p. cirrhosis
  p. collapse
  p. cone
  p. conus
  p. distomiasis
  p. dysmaturity syndrome
  p. edema
  p. embolism
  p. emphysema
  p. encephalopathy
  p. fistula
  p. glomangiosis
  p. glomus
  p. groove
  p. hamartoma
  p. heart
  p. hypertension
  p. hypostasis
  p. incompetence
  p. insufficiency
  p. ligament
  p. lymph node
  p. murmur
  p. orifice
  p. osteoarthropathy
  p. pleura
  p. pleurisy
  p. plexus
  p. pressure
  p. ridge
  p. schistosomiasis
  p. siderosis
  p. sinus
  p. stenosis
  p. sulcus
  p. talcosis
  p. thromboendarterectomy (PTEA)
  p. toilet
  p. transpiration
  p. trunk

  p. tuberculosis
  p. tularemia
  p. valve
  p. vein
  p. ventilation
pulmonectomy
pulmones (*pl. of* pulmo)
pulmonic
  p. plague
  p. regurgitation
  p. tularemia
  p. valve
pulmonic murmur (*var. of* pulmonary murmur)
pulmonis
pulmonitis
pulmonocoronary reflex
pulp
  p. abscess
  p. amputation
  p. atrophy
  p. calcification
  p. calculus
  p. canal
  p. cavity
  p. cavity of crown
  p. chamber
  coronal p.
  crown p.
  dead p.
  dental p.
  dentinal p.
  digital p.
  digital p. of hand
  enamel p.
  exposed p.
  p. of finger
  p. horn
  mummified p.
  necrotic p.
  p. nodule
  nonvital p.
  p. polyp
  p. pressure
  putrescent p.
  radicular p.
  red p.
  red p. of spleen
  root p.
  splenic p.
  p. stone
  p. test
  p. of toe
  tooth p.
  vertebral p.
  vital p.
  white p.
  white p. of spleen
pulpa
  p. alba splenica
  p. coronalis
  p. dentis
  p. digiti manus
  p. lienis
  p. radicularis

p. rubra splenica
p. splenica
pulpalgia
pulpal wall
pulpar cell
pulpectomy
pulpifaction
pulpiform
pulpify
pulpitis
 hyperplastic p.
 hypertrophic p.
 irreversible p.
 reversible p.
 suppurative p.
pulpit spectacles
pulpless tooth
pulpodontia
pulposus
pulpotomy
pulpy
pulsate
pulsatile hematoma
pulsatility index
pulsating
 p. empyema
 p. metastases
 p. neurasthenia
pulsation
 balloon counter p.
 suprasternal p.
pulsator
pulse
 abdominal p.
 alternating p.
 anacrotic p.
 anadicrotic p.
 bigeminal p.
 bisferious p.
 bulbar p.
 cannonball p.
 capillary p.
 carotid p.
 catacrotic p.
 catadicrotic p.
 collapsing p.
 cordy p.
 Corrigan p.
 coupled p.
 p. curve
 p. deficit
 dicrotic p.
 entoptic p.
 filiform p.
 gaseous p.
 p. generator
 p. granuloma
 guttural p.
 hard p.
 p. height analyzer
 intermittent p.
 irregular p.
 jugular p.
 labile p.
 long p.

monocrotic p.
mousetail p.
movable p.
nail p.
p. oximetry
paradoxic p.
p. period
piston p.
plateau p.
p. pressure
quadrigeminal p.
Quincke p.
radial p.
radiofrequency p.
p. rate
respiratory p.
reversed paradoxical p.
Riegel p.
sequence p.
p. sequence
soft p.
sustained p.
tense p.
p. therapy
thready p.
trigeminal p.
triphammer p.
undulating p.
unequal p.
vagus p.
venous p.
vermicular p.
water-hammer p.
p. wave
p. wave duration
wiry p.
pulse-chase experiment
pulsed
 p. dye laser (PDL)
 p. laser
pulsed-field gel electrophoresis
pulseless
 p. disease
 p. electrical activity (PEA)
pulsellum
pulsimeter, pulsometer
pulsion diverticulum
pulsus
 p. abdominalis
 p. alternans
 p. anadicrotus
 p. bigeminus
 p. bisferiens
 p. caprisans
 p. catacrotus
 p. catadicrotus
 p. celer
 p. celerrimus
 p. cordis
 p. debilis
 p. differens
 p. duplex
 p. durus
 p. filiformis
 p. fluens

P

pulsus *(continued)*
 p. formicans
 p. fortis
 p. frequens
 p. heterochronicus
 p. inaequalis
 p. incongruens
 p. infrequens
 p. intercidens
 p. intercurrens
 p. irregularis perpetuus
 p. magnus
 p. mollis
 p. monocrotus
 p. myurus
 p. paradoxus
 p. parvus
 p. parvus et tardus
 p. quadrigeminus
 p. respiratione intermittens
 p. tardus
 p. tremulus
 p. trigeminus
 p. vacuus
 p. venosus
pultaceous
pulverization
pulverize
pulverulent
pulvinar nucleus
pulvinate
pumice
pump
 breast p.
 calcium p.
 calf p.
 Carrel-Lindbergh p.
 constant infusion p.
 dental p.
 p. failure
 hydrogen p.
 intraaortic balloon p.
 ion p.
 jet ejector p.
 p. lung
 PCA p.
 proton p.
 saliva p.
 sodium p.
 sodium-potassium p.
 stomach p.
pumped laser
pump-oxygenator
puna
punch
 p. biopsy
 p. card
 p. graft
punchdrunk syndrome
puncta (*pl. of* punctum)
punctate
 p. basophilia
 p. cataract
 p. hemorrhage

 p. hyalosis
 p. keratitis
 p. keratoderma
 p. parotiditis
 p. retinitis
punctiform
punctuation codon
punctum, pl. **puncta**
 p. cecum
 p. coxale
 p. dolorosum
 p. fixa
 kissing puncta
 lacrimal p.
 p. lacrimale
 p. luteum
 p. mobile
 p. ossificationis
 p. ossificationis primarium
 p. ossificationis secundarium
 p. proximum (P.p.)
 p. remotum (P.r.)
 p. vasculosum
puncture
 Bernard p.
 cisternal p.
 p. diabetes
 diabetic p.
 lumbar p.
 Quincke p.
 spinal p.
 sternal p.
 tracheoesophageal p.
 p. wound
pungent
PUO
 pyrexia of unknown origin
pupa, pl. **pupae**
pupil (p)
 Adie p.
 amaurotic p.
 Argyll Robertson p.
 artificial p.
 Bumke p.
 catatonic p.
 cat's eye p.
 fixed p.
 Gunn p.
 Holmes-Adie p.
 Horner p.
 Hutchinson p.
 keyhole p.
 Marcus Gunn p.
 paradoxical p.
 pinhole p.
 Robertson p.
 seclusion of p.
 tadpole-shaped p.
 tonic p.
pupilla, pl. **pupillae**
pupillary
 p. axis
 p. block
 p. block glaucoma
 p. border of iris

p. distance
p. light-near dissociation
p. margin of iris
p. membrane
p. reflex
relative afferent p. defect
p. ruff
p. zone
pupillary-skin reflex
pupillography
pupillometer
pupillometry
pupillomotor
pupillostatometer
pupillotonic pseudotabes
pupiparous
PUPPP
pruritic urticarial papules and plaques of pregnancy
Pur
purine
pure
p. absence
p. aphasias
p. autonomic failure
chemically p. (c.p.)
p. color
p. culture
p. random drift
p. red cell anemia
p. red cell aplasia
p. tone audiogram
pure-tone
p.-t. audiometer
p.-t. average
purgation
purgative
saline p.
purge
purging cassia
purified
p. cotton
p. ozokerite
p. placental protein
p. protein derivative of tuberculin (PPD)
p. water
puriform
purine (Pur)
p. base
p. body
p. ribonucleoside
purine-free diet
purinemia
purine-nucleoside phosphorylase
purine-restricted diet
purity
radiochemical p.
radioisotopic p.
radionuclidic p.
radiopharmaceutical p.
Purkinje
P. cell
P. cell layer
P. conduction

P. corpuscle
P. effect
P. fiber
P. figure
P. images
P. network
P. phenomenon
P. shift
P. system
Purkinje-Sanson image
Purmann method
puromucous
puromycin
purple
visual p.
purpura
allergic p.
anaphylactoid p.
p. angioneurotica
p. annularis telangiectodes
factitious p.
fibrinolytic p.
p. fulminans
Henoch p.
Henoch-Schönlein p.
hyperglobulinemic p.
idiopathic thrombocytopenic p. (ITP)
immune thrombocytopenic p.
nonthrombocytopenic p.
psychogenic p.
p. pulicans, p. pulicosa
p. rheumatica
Schönlein p.
p. senilis
p. simplex
p. symptomatica
thrombocytopenic p.
thrombopenic p.
thrombotic thrombocytopenic p.
p. urticans
Waldenström p.
purpura pulicosa (*var. of* purpura pulicans)
purpurea glycosides A
purpuric
purpurin
purpurinuria
purr
pursed lips breathing
purse-string
p.-s. corepexy
p.-s. instrument
p.-s. suture
Purtscher
P. disease
P. retinopathy
purulence, purulency
purulent
p. conjunctivitis
p. cyclitis
p. encephalitis
p. inflammation
p. ophthalmia
p. pericarditis
p. pleurisy

P

purulent *(continued)*
    p. pneumonia
    p. retinitis
    p. synovitis
puruloid
pus
    p. basin
    blue p.
    p. cell
    cheesy p.
    p. corpuscle
    curdy p.
    green p.
    ichorous p.
    laudable p.
    sanious p.
    p. tube
push-back procedure
pustulant
pustular
    p. blepharitis
    p. melanosis
    p. psoriasis
pustulation
pustule
    malignant p.
    spongiform p. of Kogoj
pustulocrustaceous
pustulosis
    p. palmaris et plantaris
    p. vacciniformis acuta
putamen
Putnam-Dana syndrome
putrefaction
putrefactive
putrefy
putrescence
putrescent pulp
putrescine
putrid bronchitis
Putti-Platt
    P.-P. operation
    P.-P. procedure
putty kidney
Puumala virus
PUVA
PVA fixative
PVC
    polyvinyl chloride
PVM virus
PVP
    polyvinylpyrrolidone
PVS
    persistent vegetative state
PWM
    pokeweed mitogen
pyarthrosis
pyelectasis, pyelectasia
pyelitic
pyelitis
pyelocaliceal
pyelocaliectasis
pyelocalyceal
pyelocystitis

pyelofluoroscopy
pyelogram
pyelography
    antegrade p.
    intravenous p. (IVP)
    retrograde p.
pyelolithotomy
pyelolymphatic
pyelonephritic kidney
pyelonephritis
    acute p.
    ascending p.
    chronic p.
    xanthogranulomatous p.
pyelonephrosis
pyeloplasty
    capsular flap p.
    Culp p.
    disjoined p., dismembered p.
    Foley Y-plasty p.
    Scardino vertical flap p.
pyeloplication
pyeloscopy
pyelostomy
pyelotomy
    extended p.
pyelotubular reflux
pyeloureterectasis
pyeloureterography
pyelovenous backflow
pyemesis
pyemia
    cryptogenic p.
    portal p.
pyemic
    p. abscess
    p. embolism
Pyemotes tritici
pyencephalus
pyesis
pygal
pygalgia
pygmalionism
pygmy
pygoamorphus
pygodidymus
pygomelus
pygopagus
pyknic
pyknodysostosis
pyknoepilepsy
pyknolepsy
pyknomorphous
pyknophrasia
pyknosis
pyknotic
pyla
pylar
pylephlebitis
pylethrombophlebitis
pylethrombosis
pylic
pylon
pyloralgia
pylorectomy

pylori (*pl. of* pylorus)
pyloric
    p. antrum
    p. artery
    p. branch of anterior vagal trunk
    p. canal
    p. cap
    p. constriction
    p. gland
    p. incompetence
    p. insufficiency
    p. lymph node
    p. orifice
    p. part of stomach
    p. sphincter
    p. stenosis
    p. vein
pyloristenosis
pyloritis
pyloroduodenitis
pylorogastrectomy
pyloromyotomy
pyloroplasty
    Finney p.
    Heineke-Mikulicz p.
    Jaboulay p.
pyloroptosis, pyloroptosia
pylorospasm
pylorostenosis
pylorostomy
pylorotomy
pylorus, pl. **pylori**
pylorus-preserving
  pancreaticoduodenectomy
Pym fever
pyocele
pyocelia
pyocephalus
    circumscribed p.
    external p.
    internal p.
pyochezia
pyocin
pyococcus
pyocolpocele
pyocolpos
pyocyanic
pyocyanogenic
pyocyanolysin
pyocyst
pyocystis
pyocyte
pyoderma
    p. gangrenosum
    secondary p.
    p. vegetans
pyogen
pyogenesis
pyogenic, pyogenetic
    p. arthritis
    p. bacterium
    p. fever
    p. granuloma
    p. infection
    p. membrane

    p. pachymeningitis
    p. salpingitis
pyogenous
pyohemia
pyohemothorax
pyoid
pyometra
pyometritis
pyomyositis
    tropical p.
pyonephritis
pyonephrolithiasis
pyonephrosis
pyo-ovarium
pyopericarditis
pyopericardium
pyoperitoneum
pyoperitonitis
pyophysometra
pyopneumocholecystitis
pyopneumohepatitis
pyopneumopericardium
pyopneumoperitoneum
pyopneumoperitonitis
pyopneumothorax
    subdiaphragmatic p.
    subphrenic p.
pyopoiesis
pyopoietic
pyopyelectasis
pyorrhea
pyosalpingitis
pyosalpingo-oophoritis
pyosalpingo-oothecitis
pyosalpinx
pyosemia
pyosepticemia
pyosis
pyospermia
pyostatic
pyostomatitis vegetans
pyothorax
pyourachus
pyoureter
Pyr
    pyrimidine
pyracin
pyramid
    anterior p.
    cerebellar p.
    Ferrein p.
    Lallouette p.
    p. of light
    Malacarne p.
    malpighian p.
    p. of medulla oblongata
    medullary p.
    olfactory p.
    petrous p.
    population p.
    posterior p. of the medulla
    renal p.
    p. sign
    p. of thyroid
    p. of tympanum

P

pyramid *(continued)*
    p. of vermis
    p. of vestibule
pyramidal
    p. auricular muscle
    p. bone
    p. cataract
    p. cell
    p. cell layer
    p. eminence
    p. fiber
    p. fracture
    p. layer
    p. lobe of thyroid gland
    p. muscle
    p. muscle of auricle
    p. process of palatine bone
    p. radiation
    p. tract
    p. tractotomy
pyramidale
pyramidalis muscle
pyramides (*pl. of* pyramis)
pyramidotomy
    medullary p.
    spinal p.
pyramin, pyramine
pyramis, pl. **pyramides**
    p. of cerebellum
    p. medullae oblongatae
    p. renalis, pl. pyramides renales
    p. tympani
    p. vestibuli
pyran
pyranone
pyranose
pyrantel pamoate
pyrathiazine hydrochloride
pyrazinamide
pyrazolone
pyrectic
pyrenemia
Pyrenochaeta romeroi
pyrenoid
pyrethrin
pyrethroid
pyrethrolone
pyrethrum
pyretic
pyretogen
pyretogenesis
pyretogenetic, pyretogenic
pyretogenous
pyretotherapy
pyrexia
    p. of unknown origin (PUO)
pyrexial
pyrexiophobia
pyribenzyl methyl sulfate
pyridine
pyridinium
pyridinoline
pyridofylline
pyridostigmine bromide

pyridoxal
    p. kinase
    p. 5-phosphate (PLP)
pyridoxamine 5-phosphate
pyridoxamine-phosphate oxidase
4-pyridoxic acid
pyridoxine 4-dehydrogenase
pyridoxine dependency with seizure
pyriform
    p. aperture wiring
    p. apparatus
pyrilamine maleate
pyrimethamine
pyrimidine (Pyr)
    p. base
    p. dimer
    p. 5'-nucleotidase
    p. transferase
pyrin
pyrithiamin
pyroboric acid
pyrocalciferol
pyrocatechase
pyrocatechin
pyrocatechol
pyrogallic acid
pyrogallol
pyrogallolphthalein
pyrogen
    endogenous p. (EP)
    exogenous p.'s
    leukocytic p.'s
pyrogenic
pyroglobulin
pyroglutamic acid
pyroligneous
    p. alcohol
    p. spirit
    p. vinegar
pyrolysis
pyromania
pyromaniac
pyromen
pyrometer
    resistance p.
pyrone
pyronin
    p. B, G, Y
pyroninophilia
pyrophobia
pyrophosphatase
    inorganic p. (PP$_i$)
pyrophosphate (PP)
    ^{99m}Tc p.
pyrophosphokinases
pyrophosphoric acid
pyrophosphorylases
pyrophosphotransferases
pyropoikilocytosis
    hereditary p.
pyroscope
pyrosis
pyrotherapy
pyrotic
pyrotoxin

pyroxylic spirit
pyroxylin
pyrrhol cell
pyrrobutamine phosphate
pyrrol
      p. blue
      p. cell
pyrrolase
pyrrole nucleus
pyrrolidine
pyrrolidine-2-carboxylate
pyrrolidone-5-carboxylate
5-pyrrolidone-2-carboxylic acid
pyrroline
1-pyrroline-5-carboxylate dehydrogenase
pyrroline-2-carboxylate reductase
pyrroline-5-carboxylate reductase
pyruvaldoxine
pyruvate
      active p.

      p. carboxylase
      p. decarboxylase
      p. dehydrogenase
      p. dehydrogenase
      p. dehydrogenase complex
      p. kinase (PK)
      p. kinase deficiency
      p. oxidase
      p. oxidation factor
pyruvic
      p. acid
      p. aldehyde
pyruvic-malic carboxylase
6-pyruvoyltetrahydropterin synthase (6-PTS)
pyrvinium pamoate
Pythium insidiosum
pythogenesis
pythogenic, pythogenous
pyuria

P

Q
 coulomb
  Q angle
  Q bands
  Q disk
  Q enzyme
  Q fever
  Q tip test
  Q wave
Q
 blood flow
Q_{CO_2}
 microliters of STPD of CO_2 given off per
  milligram of tissue per hour
Q_O, Q_{O2}
 oxygen consumption
$-Q_6$
 ubiquinone-6
$-Q_{10}$
 ubiquinone-10
q
 quodque
QALY
 quality-adjusted life years
Q-banding
Q-banding stain
QF
 quality factor
QH_2
 ubiquinol
q.i.d.
 quater in die
QNB
 quinuclidinyl benzilate
Q.R.
 quantum rectum
QRB interval
QR interval
QRS
  Q. complex
  Q. interval
q.s.
 quantum satis
QS_2 interval
Q-switched laser
QT interval
Q-TWiST
quackery
quack medicine
quadrangular
  q. cartilage
  q. lobule
  q. membrane
  q. space
  q. therapy
quadrant
  left upper q. of lung (LUQ)
  right lower q. (RLQ)
  right upper q. (RUQ)
quadrantanopia

quadrantic
  q. hemianopia
  q. scotoma
quadrate
  q. ligament
  q. lobe
  q. lobule
  q. muscle
  q. muscle of loins
  q. muscle of sole
  q. muscle of thigh
  q. muscle of upper lip
  q. part of liver
  q. pronator muscle
quadratus
  q. femoris muscle
  q. lumborum fascia
  q. lumborum muscle
  q. muscle
  q. plantae muscle
quadribasic
quadriceps
  q. femoris muscle
  q. muscle of thigh
  q. reflex
quadricepsplasty
quadricuspid
quadridigitate
quadrigeminal
  q. artery
  q. body
  q. cistern
  q. lamina
  q. plate
  q. pulse
  q. rhythm
quadrigeminum
quadrigeminus
quadrigeminy
quadrilateral space
quadriparesis
quadripedal extensor reflex
quadriplegia
quadriplegic
quadripolar
quadrisect
quadrisection
quadritubercular
quadrivalent
quadruped
quadruple
  q. amputation
  q. rhythm
quadruplet
quail bronchitis virus
qualitative
  q. alteration
  q. analysis
  q. trait
quality
  q. control
  q. control chart

quality *(continued)*
    q. factor (QF)
    q. of life
quality-adjusted life years (QALY)
quality assurance
quanta *(pl. of* quantum)
quantal effect
quantile
quantitative
    q. alteration
    q. analysis
    q. genetics
    q. hypertrophy
    q. perimetry
Quant sign
quantum, pl. **quanta**
    q. efficiency
    q. limit
    q. mottle
    q. rectum (Q.R.)
    q. requirement
    q. satis (q.s.)
    q. sink
    q. sufficiat
    q. theory
    q. vis (q.v.)
    q. yield
Quaranfil virus
quarantine period
quark
quart
quartan
    double q.
    q. fever
    q. malaria
    q. parasite
    triple q.
quartisect
quartz glass
quasi-continuous wave laser
quasidominance
quasidominant
quassation
quassia
quater in die (q.i.d.)
quaternary
    q. carbon atom
    q. structure
    q. syphilis
quaternary ammonium ion *(var. of* amine)
Quatrefages angle
quazepam
quebrachine
quebracho
Queckenstedt-Stookey test
Queensland tick typhus
quellung
    q. phenomenon
    q. reaction
    q. test
quenching
    fluorescence q.
Quénu hemorrhoidal plexus

Quénu-Muret sign
quercetin
quercus
querulent
questionnaire
    Holmes-Rahe q.
quick
    q. cure resin
    Q. method
    Q. test
quickening
quicklime
quicksilver
quick-stop mutant
quiescent
quiet
    q. hip disease
    q. iritis
    q. lung
quilted suture
quin-2
quina
quinacrine chromosome banding stain
quinacrine hydrochloride
quinaldic acid
quinaldine red
quinaldinic acid
quinaquina
quinate dehydrogenase
quinazoline
quince
Quincke
    Q. pulse
    Q. puncture
    Q. sign
quinestradiol, quinestradol
quinestrol
quinethazone
quingestanol acetate
quinhydrone electrode
quinic acid
quinidine
    q. polygalacturonate
    q. sulfate
quinine
    q. bisulfate
    q. carbacrylic resin
    q. carbacrylic resin test
    q. ethylcarbonate
    q. sulfate
    q. and urea hydrochloride
    q. urethan
quininism
Quinlan test
quinocide hydrochloride
quinol
quinoline
quinolinic acid
quinolinol
quinolizidine
quinology
quinolone
quinone reductase
quinovose
quinquedigitate

quinquetubercular
quinquevalent
quinquina
quinsy
    lingual q.
quintan fever
quintuplet
quinuclidinyl benzilate (QNB)
quisqualate receptor
quisqualic acid
quodque (q)
quorum sensing
quotidian
    q. fever
    q. malaria
quotient
    achievement q.

Q

    Ayala q.
    cognitive laterality q. (CLQ)
    extremal q.
    intelligence q. (IQ)
    Meyerhof oxidation q.
    P/O q.
    protein q.
    respiratory q. (RQ)
    spinal q.
quoties opus sit (quot. op. sit.)
quot. op. sit.
    quoties opus sit
q.v.
    quantum vis

ρ (*var. of* rho)

R
- roentgen
  - R antigen
  - R enzyme
  - R factor
  - R pili
  - R plasmid
  - R wave

R
- molar gas constant

r
- radius
- roentgen

r
- racemic

Ra
- radium

²²⁶Ra
- radium-226

rabbeting

rabbit
- r. fever
- r. fibroma
- r. fibroma virus
- r. myxoma virus

rabbitpox virus

rabid

rabies
- dumb r.
- furious r.
- r. immune globulin
- r. immunoglobulin
- paralytic r.
- r. vaccine
- r. vaccine, Flury strain egg-passage
- r. virus
- r. virus, Flury strain
- r. virus, Kelev strain

rabiform

rac-

raccoon eyes

racefemine

racemase

racemate

raceme

racemic (*r*)
- r. calcium pantothenate

racemization

racemose
- r. aneurysm
- r. gland
- r. hemangioma

racephedrine hydrochloride

rachial

rachicentesis

rachides (*pl. of* rachis)

rachidial

rachidian

rachilysis

rachiocentesis

rachiochysis

rachiopagus

rachioplegia

rachiotome

rachiotomy

rachipagus

rachis, pl. **rachides**

rachischisis
- r. partialis
- r. totalis

rachitic
- r. diet
- r. pelvis
- r. rosary
- r. scoliosis

rachitis
- r. fetalis
- r. fetalis annularis
- r. fetalis micromelica
- r. intrauterina
- r. tarda

rachitism

rachitis uterina

rachitogenic

rachitome

racial melanoderma

racket
- r. amputation
- r. nail

racquet hypha

rad

radarkymography

radectomy

Radford nomogram

radiability

radiable

radiad

radial
- r. acceleration
- r. aplasia-thrombocytopenia syndrome
- r. border of forearm
- r. bursa
- r. clubhand
- r. collateral artery
- r. collateral ligament
- r. collateral ligament of elbow joint
- r. collateral ligament of wrist joint
- r. eminence of wrist
- r. flexor muscle of wrist
- r. fossa of humerus
- r. groove
- r. growth phase
- r. immunodiffusion (RID)
- r. index artery
- r. keratotomy
- r. nerve
- r. notch
- r. part of posterior compartment of forearm
- r. phenomenon
- r. pulse
- r. recurrent artery
- r. reflex

radial (*continued*)
r. scar
r. sclerosing lesion
r. styloid tendovaginitis
r. tuberosity
r. tunnel syndrome
r. vein
radialis
r. indicis artery
radian
radiant
r. energy
r. heat
r. intensity
r. layer
radiate
r. carpal ligament
r. crown
r. layer of tympanic membrane
r. ligament
r. ligament of head of rib
r. ligament of wrist
r. sternocostal ligament
radiatio, pl. **radiationes**
r. acustica
r. corporis callosi
r. inferior thalami
r. optica
r. pyramidalis
r. thalami anterior
r. thalamica posterior
r. thalami centralis
radiation
acoustic r.
afterloading r.
alpha r.
r. anemia
annihilation r.
anterior thalamic r.
background r.
beta r.
r. biology
r. biophysics
r. burn
r. caries
r. cataract
central thalamic r.
Cerenkov r.
characteristic r.
r. chimera
r. of corpus callosum
corpuscular r.
r. dermatosis
electromagnetic r.
gamma r.
geniculocalcarine r.
Gratiolet r.
hemibody r.
heterogeneous r.
homogeneous r.
hyperfractionated r.
hypofractionated r.
inferior thalamic r.
ionizing r.

K-r.
L-r.
monochromatic r.
r. myelitis
r. myelopathy
neutron r.
occipitothalamic r.
r. oncologist
r. oncology
optic r.
r. physics
r. pneumonitis
r. poisoning
polychromatic r.
posterior thalamic r.
primary r.
pyramidal r.
r. risk
scattered r.
secondary r.
r. sickness
r. therapy
r. weighting factor
Wernicke r.
radical
acid r.
carboxymethyl r. (CM-)
coenzyme A r. (CoAS–)
color r.
r. cystectomy
free r.
r. hysterectomy
r. mastectomy
r. mastoidectomy
r. neck dissection
r. operation for hernia
oxygen-derived free r.
r. pericardiectomy
radices (*pl. of* radix)
radicle
radicotomy
radicula
radiculalgia
radicular
r. abscess
r. cyst
r. filum
r. pulp
r. syndrome
radiculectomy
radiculitis
acute brachial r.
radiculoganglionitis
radiculomeningomyelitis
radiculomyelopathy
radiculoneuropathy
radiculopathy
diabetic thoracic r.
radiectomy
radiferous
radii (*pl. of* radius)
radioactive
r. atom
r. constant
r. cyanocobalamin

r. equilibrium
r. iodide uptake test
r. iodine
r. isotope
r. probe
r. thyroxine
radioactive cow
radioactivity
artificial r.
induced r.
radioallergosorbent test (RAST)
radioautogram
radioautography
radiobicipital reflex
radiobiology
radiocalcium
radiocarbon
radiocardiogram
radiocardiography
radiocarpal
r. articulation
r. joint
radiocephalpelvimetry
radiochemical purity
radiochemistry
radiochlorine
radiocholangiography
radiocholecystography
radiocineangiocardiography
radiocineangiography
radiocinematography
radiocobalt
radiocurable
radiodense
radiodensity
radiodermatitis
radiodiagnosis
radiodigital
radioelectrophysiologram
radioelectrophysiolograph
radioelectrophysiolography
radioelement
radioepithelitis
radiofrequency pulse
radiogallium
radiogenesis
radiogenic
radiogenics
radiogold colloid
radiogram
radiograph
bitewing r.
cephalometric r.
decubitus r.
lateral decubitus r.
lateral oblique r.
lateral ramus r.
lateral skull r.
maxillary sinus r.
occlusal r.
panoramic r.
periapical r.
scout r.
submental vertex r.
submentovertex r.

Towne projection r.
transcranial r.
Trendelenburg r.
Waters view r.
radiographer
radiographic
r. parallel line shadow
r. pelvimetry
radiography
advanced multiple-beam
equalization r. (AMBER)
air-gap r.
bedside r.
computed r.
digital r. (DR)
electron r.
filmless r.
magnification r.
mucosal relief r.
portable r.
scanning equalization r.
sectional r.
serial r.
spot-film r.
radiohumeral
radioimmunity
radioimmunoassay (RIA)
radioimmunodiffusion
radioimmunoelectrophoresis
radioimmunoprecipitation (RIP)
radioimmunosorbent test (RIST)
radioiodinated serum albumin (RISA)
radioiodine
radioiron
radioisotope
radioisotopic purity
radiolabeled thyroxine
radiolead
radiolesion
radioligand
radiologic, radiological
r. anatomy
r. enteroclysis
r. sphincter
radiologist
radiology
American College of R. (ACR)
cardiovascular r.
chest r.
diagnostic r.
interventional r.
pediatric r.
therapeutic r.
radiolucency
radiolucent
radiolus
radiometer
radiomicrometer
radiomimetic
radiomuscular
radionecrosis
radioneuritis
radionitrogen
radionuclide
r. angiocardiography

R

radionuclide *(continued)*
r. angiography
r. cisternography
r. ejection fraction
r. generator
r. ventriculography
radionuclidic purity
radiopacity
radiopalmar
radiopaque
radiopathology
radiopelvimetry
radioperiosteal reflex
radiopharmaceutical
r. chemistry
r. purity
r. synovectomy
radiophobia
radiophosphorus
radiopill
radiopotassium
radioprotectant
radioreceptor
r. assay
radioresistant
radioscopy
radiosensitive
radiosensitivity
radiosensitization
radiosensitizer
radiosodium
radiostereoscopy
radiostrontium
radiosulfur
radiosurgery
radiotelemetering capsule
radiotelemetry
radiotherapeutic
radiotherapeutics
radiotherapist
radiotherapy
r. localization
mantle r.
radiothermy
radiothyroidectomy
radiothyroxin
radiotoxemia
radiotracer
radiotransparent
radiotropic
radioulnar
r. articular disk
r. disk
r. syndesmosis
radisectomy
radium, radium-226 (Ra)
r. beam therapy
r. emanation
radius, pl. **radii (r)**
r. fixus
r. of lens
r. lentis

thrombocytopenia and absent r.
(TAR)
radix, pl. **radices**
r. accessoria
r. anterior nervi spinalis
r. arcus vertebrae
r. brevis ganglii ciliaris
r. buccalis
r. clinica dentis
r. cranialis nervi accessorii
r. dentis
r. dorsalis nervi spinalis
r. facialis
r. inferior ansae cervicalis
r. inferior nervi vestibulocochlearis
r. lateralis nervi mediani
r. lateralis tractus optici
r. linguae
r. longa ganglii ciliaris
r. medialis nervi mediani
r. medialis tractus optici
r. mesenterii
r. motoria nervi spinalis
r. motoria nervi trigemini
r. nasi
r. nasociliaris ganglii ciliaris
r. nervi facialis
r. nervi oculomotorii ad ganglion
ciliare
radices nervi trigemini
r. oculomotoria ganglii ciliaris
radices parasympathicae gangliorum
pelvicorum
r. parasympathica ganglii ciliaris
r. parasympathica ganglii otici
r. parasympathica ganglii
submandibularis
r. penis
r. pili
r. posterior nervi spinalis
r. pulmonis
r. sensoria ganglii ciliaris
r. sensoria ganglii pterygopalatini
r. sensoria ganglii sublingualis
r. sensoria ganglii submandibularis
r. sensoria nervi spinalis
r. sensoria nervi trigemini
r. spinalis nervi accessorii
r. superior ansae cervicalis
r. superior nervi vestibulocochlearis
r. sympathica ganglii ciliaris
r. sympathica ganglii otici
r. sympathica ganglii pterygopalatini
r. sympathica ganglii sublingualis
r. sympathica ganglii
submandibularis
r. unguis
r. ventralis nervi spinalis
r. vestibularis
radon (Rn)
Raeder paratrigeminal syndrome
raffinose
rage
sham r.
ragpicker's disease

ragsorter's disease
Rahe-Holmes social readjustment rating
  scale
Rahn-Otis sample
Raillietina
raillietiniasis
railroad nystagmus
rainbow symptom
Rainey corpuscle
RAI test
Raji
  R. cell
  R. cell radioimmune assay
rale
  amphoric r.
  atelectatic r.
  bubbling r.
  cavernous r.
  clicking r.
  consonating r.
  crackling r.
  crepitant r.
  dry r.
  gurgling r.
  guttural r.
  metallic r.
  moist r.
  mucous r.
  palpable r.
  pleural r.
  sibilant r.
  Skoda r.
  sonorous r.
  subcrepitant r.
  vesicular r.
  whistling r.
raloxifene
Ramachandran plot
ramal
Raman
  R. effect
  R. spectrum
Rambourg
  R. chromic acid-phosphotungstic
    acid stain
  R. periodic acid-chromic
    methenamine-silver stain
rami (*pl. of* ramus)
ramicotomy
ramification
ramify
ramisection
ramitis
ramose, ramous
ramp
Ramsay Hunt syndrome
Ramsden ocular
Ramstedt operation
ramulus, pl. **ramuli**
ramus, pl. **rami**
  ramus mammarii mediales rami
    cutanei anterioris ramorum ventral
  r. glandulares
    anterior/lateralis/posterior arteriae
    thyroideae supe

ramus mammarii mediales ramorum
  perforantium arteriae thoracicae in
r. accessorius arteriae meningeae
  mediae
r. acetabularis
r. acromialis arteriae suprascapularis
r. acromialis arteriae
  thoracoacromialis
rami ad pontem
rami alveolares superiores anteriores
  nervi infraorbitalis
rami alveolares superiores posteriores
  nervi maxillaris
r. alveolaris superior medius nervi
  infraorbitalis
r. anastomoticus
r. anastomoticus arteriae meningeae
  mediae cum arteriae lacrimali
r. anterior
r. anterior arteriae renalis
anterior r. of cervical nerve
r. anterior descendens
rami anteriores nervorum cervicalium
rami anteriores nervorum lumbalium
rami anteriores nervorum sacralium
rami anteriores nervorum thoracis
r. anterior lateralis
anterior r. of lateral sulcus of
  cerebrum
anterior r. of lumbar nerve
r. anterior nervi spinalis
anterior r. of sacral nerve
anterior r. of spinal nerve
r. anterior sulci lateralis cerebri
anterior r. of thoracic nerve
r. apicalis lobi inferioris arteriae
  pulmonalis dextrae
r. apicalis venae pulmonalis dextrae
  superioris
r. apicoposterior venae pulmonalis
  sinistrae superioris
rami articulares
rami articulares arteriae descendentis
  genicularis
r. ascendens
r. ascendens arteriae superficialis
  cervicalis
r. ascendens sulci lateralis cerebri
ascending r. of lateral sulcus of
  cerebrum
rami atriales
r. atrialis anastomoticus ramus
  circumflexus arteriae coronariae
  sinistrae
r. atrialis intermedius arteriae
  coronariae dextrae
r. atrialis intermedius arteriae
  coronariae sinistrae
rami auriculares anteriores arteriae
  temporalis superficialis
r. auricularis arteriae auricularis
  posterioris
r. auricularis arteriae occipitalis
r. auricularis nervi vagi
r. basalis anterior

ramus *(continued)*

r. basalis anterior venae basalis superioris
r. basalis lateralis
r. basalis medialis
r. basalis posterior
r. basalis tentorii arteriae carotidis internae
rami bronchiales
rami bronchiales segmentorum
rami buccales nervi facialis
rami calcanei
rami calcanei laterales nervi suralis
rami calcanei mediales nervi tibialis
r. calcarinus arteriae occipitalis medialis
rami capsulae internae
rami capsulares arteriae renalis
rami capsulares arteriorum intrarenalium
rami cardiaci cervicales inferiores nervi vagi
rami cardiaci cervicales superiores nervi vagi
rami cardiaci thoracici gangliorum thoracicorum
rami cardiaci thoracici nervi vagi
r. cardiacus
rami caroticotympanici
r. carpalis dorsalis arteriae radialis
r. carpalis dorsalis arteriae ulnaris
r. carpalis palmaris arteriae radialis
r. carpalis palmaris arteriae ulnaris
r. carpeus dorsalis arteriae radialis
r. carpeus dorsalis arteriae ulnaris
r. carpeus palmaris arteriae radialis
r. carpeus palmaris arteriae ulnaris
rami caudae nuclei caudati
rami celiaci nervi vagi
rami celiaci trunci vagi posterioris
rami centrales anteromediales
cephalic arterial rami
r. cervicalis nervi facialis
r. chiasmaticus
rami choroidei
rami choroidei posteriores arteriae cerebri posteriores laterales et mediales
r. choroidei posteriores laterales
r. choroidei posteriores mediales
r. choroidei ventriculi lateralis
r. choroidei ventriculi tertii
r. choroideus ventriculi quarti
r. cingularis
r. cingularis arteriae callosomarginalis
r. circumflexus arteriae coronariae sinistrae
r. circumflexus fibularis arteriae tibialis posterioris
r. circumflexus peronealis arteriae tibialis posterioris
r. clavicularis arteriae thoracoacromialis

rami clivales
rami clivales partis cerebralis arteriae carotidis internae
r. cochlearis arteriae labyrinthi
r. cochlearis arteriae vestibulocochlearis
r. colicus arteriae ileocolicae
r. collateralis arteriarum intercostalium posteriorum III–XI
r. collateralis nervorum intercostalium
r. colli nervi facialis
r. communicans, pl. rami communicantes
r. communicans arteriae fibularis
r. communicans arteriae peroneae
r. communicans cum chorda tympani
r. communicans cum nervo glossopharyngeo
r. communicans fibularis nervi fibularis communis
r. communicans ganglii otici cum chorda tympani
r. communicans ganglii otici cum nervo auriculotemporali
r. communicans ganglii otici cum nervo pterygoideo mediali
r. communicans ganglii otici cum ramo meningeo nervi mandibularis
r. communicans nervi facialis cum nervo glossopharyngeo
r. communicans nervi facialis cum plexu tympanico
r. communicans nervi fibularis communis cum nervo cutaneo surae mediali
r. communicans nervi glossopharyngei cum ramo auriculari nervi vagi
r. communicans nervi intermedii cum plexu tympanico
r. communicans nervi interossei antebrachii anterioris cum nervi ulnari
r. communicans nervi lacrimalis cum nervo zygomatico
r. communicans nervi laryngei interni cum nervo laryngeo recurrente
r. communicans nervi laryngei recurrentis cum ramo laryngeo interno
r. communicans nervi laryngei superioris cum nervo laryngeo recurrenti
r. communicans nervi lingualis cum chorda tympani
r. communicans nervi mediani cum nervo ulnari
r. communicans nervi nasociliaris cum ganglio ciliari
r. communicans nervi peronei communis cum nervo cutaneo surae mediali

R

r. communicans nervi radialis cum
nervi ulnari
r. communicans peroneus nervi
peronei communis
r. communicans plexus tympanici
cum ramo auriculari nervi vagi
r. communicans ulnaris nervi
radialis
rami communicantes (*pl. of* r.
communicans)
rami communicantes albi
rami communicantes ganglii
sublingualis cum nervo linguali
rami communicantes grisei
rami communicantes of sympathetic
part of autonomic division of
nervous system
communicating rami of sympathetic
trunk
rami corporis amygdaloidei
r. corporis callosi dorsalis
rami corporis geniculati lateralis
r. costalis lateralis arteriae
thoracicae internae
r. cricothyroideus (arteriae thyroideae
superioris)
rami cruris posterioris capsulae
internae
rami cutanei anteriores nervi
femoralis
rami cutanei anteriores pectoralis et
abdominalis nervorum
intercostalium
rami cutanei cruris mediales nervi
sapheni
r. cutaneus anterior abdominalis
nervi intercostalis
r. cutaneus anterior nervi
iliohypogastrici
r. cutaneus anterior (pectoralis et
abdominalis) nervorum
thoracicorum
r. cutaneus anterior pectoralis nervi
intercostalis
r. cutaneus lateralis
r. cutaneus lateralis
abdominalis/pectoralis nervorum
intercostalium
r. cutaneus lateralis nervi
iliohypogastrici
r. cutaneus lateralis ramorum
posteriorum arteriae intercostalium
r. cutaneus medialis rami dorsalis
arteriarum intercostalium
posteriorum III–XI
r. cutaneus medialis ramorum
dorsalium nervorum thoracicorum
r. cutaneus nervi mixti
r. cutaneus rami anterioris nervi
obturatorii
r. deltoideus
r. deltoideus arteriae profundae
brachii
r. deltoideus arteriae
thoracoacromialis

dental r.
rami dentales
rami dentales arteriae alveolaris
inferioris
rami dentales arteriae alveolaris
superioris posterioris
rami dentales inferiores
rami dentales inferiores plexus
dentalis inferioris
rami dentales superiores
rami dentales superiores plexus
dentalis superioris
r. descendens
r. descendens arteriae circumflexae
femoris lateralis
r. descendens arteriae circumflexae
femoris medialis
r. descendens arteriae occipitalis
r. descendens arteriae segmentalis
anterioris pulmonis dextri et
sinistri
r. descendens arteriae segmentalis
posterioris pulmonis dextri et
sinistri
r. descendens rami superficialis
arteriae transversae cervicis
r. dexter
r. dexter arteriae hepaticae propriae
r. dexter venae portae hepatis
r. digastricus nervi facialis
rami dorsales
rami dorsales arteriae intercostalis
supremae
rami dorsales arteriae subcostalis
r. dorsales arteriae subcostalis
rami dorsales arteriarum
intercostalium posteriorum primae
et secundae
rami dorsales linguae arteriae
lingualis
rami dorsales nervi ulnaris
r. dorsalis
r. dorsalis arteriae lumbalis
r. dorsalis arteriarum intercostalium
posteriorum III–XI
r. dorsalis nervi spinalis
r. dorsalis venarum intercostalium
posteriorum IV–XI
dorsal primary r. of spinal nerve
rami duodenales arteriae
pancreaticoduodenalis superioris
anterioris
rami epiploicae
rami esophageales
rami esophageales aortae thoracicae
rami esophageales arteriae gastricae
sinistrae
rami esophageales arteriae thyroideae
inferioris
rami esophageales gangliorum
thoracicorum
rami esophageales partis thoracicae
aortae
rami esophagei

ramus *(continued)*

rami esophagei nervi laryngei
   recurrentis
rami esophagei nervi vagi
r. externus nervi laryngei superioris
r. externus trunci nervi accessorii
rami fauciales nervi lingualis
r. femoralis nervi genitofemoralis
r. frontalis anteromedialis
r. frontalis anteromedialis arteriae
   callosomarginalis
r. frontalis arteriae meningeae
   mediae
r. frontalis arteriae temporalis
   superficialis
r. frontalis intermediomedialis
r. frontalis intermediomedialis
   arteriae callosomarginalis
r. frontalis posteromedialis
r. frontalis posteromedialis arteriae
   callosomarginalis
rami ganglii submandibularis
rami communicantes ganglii
   submandibularis cum nervo linguali
r. ganglii trigeminalis
rami ganglionares
r. ganglionares trigeminales arteriae
   carotidis internae
rami ganglionici nervi maxillaris
rami gastrici anteriores nervi vagi
rami gastrici anteriores trunci
   vagalis anterioris
rami gastrici posteriores nervi vagi
rami gastrici posteriores trunci
   vagalis posterioris
r. genitalis nervi genitofemoralis
rami genus capsulae internae
rami gingivales inferiores plexus
   dentalis inferioris
rami gingivales superiores plexus
   dentalis superioris
rami glandulares
rami glandulares arteriae facialis
rami glandulares arteriae thyroideae
   inferioris
rami glandulares ganglii
   submandibularis
r. glandularis anterior arteriae
   thyroideae superioris
r. glandularis posterior arteriae
   thyroideae superioris
rami globi pallidi
gray rami communicantes
rami hepatici nervi vagi
rami hepatici trunci vagi anterior
r. hypothalamicus
r. iliacus arteriae iliolumbalis
r. inferior
r. inferior arteriae gluteae superioris
inferior dental rami
rami inferiores nervi transversi
   cervicalis
rami inferiores nervi transversi colli
r. inferior nervi oculomotorii

r. inferior ossis pubis
inferior pubic r.
r. infrahyoideus arteriae thyroideae
   superioris
r. infrapatellaris nervi sapheni
rami inguinales arteriarum
   pudendarum externarum
   profundarum
rami intercostales anteriores
rami intercostales anteriores arteriae
   thoracicae internae
rami interganglionares trunci
   sympathici
r. intermedius arteriae hepaticae
   propriae
internal r. of accessory nerve
r. internus nervi laryngei superioris
r. internus trunci nervi accessorii
rami interventriculares septales
rami interventriculares septales
   arteriae coronariae sinistrae/dextrae
r. interventricularis anterior arteriae
   coronariae sinistrae
r. interventricularis posterior arteriae
   coronariae dextrae
ischial r.
ischiopubic r.
r. of ischium
rami isthmi faucium nervi lingualis
rami labiales anteriores arteriae
   pudendae externae profundae
rami labiales inferiores nervi
   mentalis
rami labiales nervi mentalis
rami labiales posteriores arteriae
   perinealis
rami labiales posteriores arteriae
   pudendae internae
rami labiales superiores nervi
   infraorbitalis
r. labialis inferior arteriae facialis
r. labialis superior arteriae facialis
rami laryngopharyngei ganglii
   cervicalis superioris
rami laterales
rami laterales arteriae pontis
rami laterales arteriarum centralium
   anterolateralium
rami laterales arteriarum tuberis
   cinerei
rami laterales rami sinistri venae
   portae hepatis
rami laterales ramorum dorsalium
   nervorum spinalis
r. lateralis ductus hepatici sinistri
r. lateralis interventricularis anterioris
   arteriae coronariae sinistrae
r. lateralis nasi arteriae facialis
r. lateralis nervi supraorbitalis
r. lateralis rami lobaris medii
   arteriae pulmonalis dextrae
r. lateralis ramorum dorsalium
   nervorum thoracicorum
rami lienales arteriae lienalis
rami linguales

rami linguales nervi glossopharyngei
rami linguales nervi hypoglossi
rami linguales nervi lingualis
r. lingualis nervi facialis
r. lingularis inferior
r. lingularis superior
r. lingularis venae pulmonis sinistrae superioris
rami lobi caudati rami sinistri venae portae hepatis
r. lobi medii arteriae pulmonalis dextrae
r. lobi medii venae pulmonalis dextrae superioris
r. lumbalis arteriae iliolumbalis
rami malleolares laterales arteriae fibularis (peronei)
rami malleolares mediales arteriae tibialis posterioris
rami mammarii
rami mammarii laterales
rami mammarii laterales arteriae thoracicae lateralis
rami mammarii laterales ramorum cutaneorum lateralis nervorum thoracicorum
rami mammarii laterales ramorum cutaneorum lateralium nervorum intercostalium
rami mammarii mediales
rami mammarii mediales ramorum cutaneorum anteriorum nervorum int
r. of mandible
r. mandibulae
r. marginalis
r. marginalis dexter
r. marginalis mandibulae nervi facialis
r. marginalis sinister arteriae coronariae sinistrae
r. marginalis sulci cinguli
r. marginalis sulci parietooccipitalis
r. marginalis tentorii arteriae carotidis internae
r. marginalis tentorii partis cavernosae arteriae carotidis internae
ramus mastoidei arteriae auricularis posterioris
ramus mastoidei arteriae tympanicae posterioris
r. mastoideus arteriae occipitalis
r. meatus acustici interni
ramus mediales
ramus mediales arteriae pontis
ramus mediales arteriarum centralium anterolateralium
ramus mediales arteriarum tuberis cinerei
ramus mediales rami sinistri venae portae hepatis
r. medialis ductus hepatici sinistri
r. medialis nervi supraorbitalis

r. medialis rami lobaris medii arteriae pulmonalis dextrae
r. medialis ramorum dorsalium nervorum spinalis
ramus mediastinales
ramus mediastinales aortae thoracicae
ramus mediastinales arteriae thoracicae internae
ramus medullares laterales
ramus medullares laterales (partis intracranialis) arteriae vertebralis
ramus medullares mediales
ramus medullares mediales arteriae vertebralis
ramus membranae tympani nervi auriculotemporalis
ramus meningei
r. meningeus accessorius
r. meningeus accessorius arteriae meningeae mediae
r. meningeus anterior arteriae ethmoidalis anterioris
r. meningeus anterior arteriae vertebralis
r. meningeus arteriae carotidis internae
r. meningeus arteriae occipitalis
r. meningeus arteriae vertebralis
r. meningeus medius nervi maxillaris
r. meningeus nervi mandibularis
r. meningeus nervi maxillaris
r. meningeus nervi vagi
r. meningeus nervorum spinalium
r. meningeus partis cavernosae arteriae carotidis internae
r. meningeus partis cerebralis arteriae carotidis internae
r. meningeus posterior
r. meningeus recurrens nervi ophthalmici
ramus mentales nervi mentalis
r. mentalis arteriae alveolaris inferioris
ramus musculares
ramus musculares arteriae vertebralis
ramus musculares nervi accessorii
ramus musculares nervi axillaris
ramus musculares nervi fibularis profundi
ramus musculares nervi fibularis superficialis
ramus musculares nervi interossei antebrachii anterior
ramus musculares nervi mediani
ramus musculares nervi musculocutanei
ramus musculares nervi radialis
ramus musculares nervi tibialis
ramus musculares nervi ulnaris
ramus musculares nervorum intercostalium
ramus musculares nervorum perinealium

ramus *(continued)*

ramus musculares nervorum
spinalium
ramus musculares partis
supraclavicularis plexus brachialis
ramus musculares rami anterioris
nervi obturatorii
ramus musculares rami posterioris
nervi obturatorii
r. musculi stylopharyngei nervi
glossopharyngei
r. mylohyoideus arteriae alveolaris
inferioris
ramus nasales anteriores laterales
arteriae ethmoidalis anterioris
ramus nasales externi nervi
ethmoidalis anterioris
ramus nasales externi nervi
infraorbitalis
ramus nasales interni
ramus nasales interni nervi
ethmoidalis anterioris
ramus nasales interni nervi
infraorbitalis
ramus nasales laterales nervi
ethmoidalis anterioris
ramus nasales mediales nervi
ethmoidalis anterioris
ramus nasales posteriores inferiores
nervi palatini majoris
ramus nasales posteriores superiores
laterales ganglii pterygopalatini
ramus nasales posteriores superiores
laterales nervi maxillaris
ramus nasales posteriores superiores
mediales ganglii pterygopalatini
ramus nasales posteriores superiores
mediales nervi maxillaris
rami communicantes nervi
auriculotemporalis cum nervo
faciali
rami communicantes nervi lingualis
cum nervo hypoglosso
r. nervi oculomotorii arteriae
communicantis posterioris
rami communicantes nervorum
spinalium
r. nodi atrioventricularis
r. nodi sinuatrialis arteriae
coronariae dextrae
ramus nucleorum hypothalamicorum
r. obturatorius arteriae epigastricae
inferioris
r. obturatorius rami pubici arteriae
epigastricae inferioris
ramus occipitales arteriae auricularis
posterioris
ramus occipitales arteriae occipitis
ramus occipitales nervi auricularis
posterioris
r. occipitalis
r. occipitotemporalis
ramus omentales
ramus orbitales nervi maxillaris

r. orbitalis arteriae meningeae
mediae
r. orbitalis ganglii pterygopalatini
r. ossis ischii
ramus ovarici arteriae uterinae
r. palmaris nervi interossei
antebrachii anterioris
r. palmaris nervi mediani
r. palmaris nervi ulnaris
r. palmaris profundus arteriae
ulnaris
r. palmaris superficialis arteriae
radialis
ramus palpebrales nervi
infratrochlearis
ramus pancreatici
ramus pancreatici arteriae
pancreaticoduodenalis superioris
ramus pancreatici arteriae splenicae
r. paracentrales
ramus paracentrales arteriae
callosomarginalis
ramus parietales
r. parietalis arteriae meningeae
mediae
r. parietalis arteriae occipitalis
medialis
r. parietalis arteriae temporalis
superficialis
r. parieto-occipitalis
r. parieto-occipitalis arteriae
occipitalis medialis
ramus parotidei
r. parotidei arteriae temporalis
superficialis
ramus parotidei nervi
auriculotemporalis
ramus parotidei venae facialis
ramus partis retrolentiformis capsulae
internae
ramus pectorales arteriae
thoracoacromialis
ramus pedunculares
r. perforans
r. perforans arteriae fibularis
r. perforans arteriae interossei
anterioris
ramus perforantes arcus palmaris
profundi
ramus perforantes arteriae thoracicae
internae
ramus perforantes arteriarum
metacarpalium palmarium
ramus perforantes arteriarum
metatarsearum plantarium
ramus pericardiaci aortae thoracicae
r. pericardiacus nervi phrenici
ramus perineales nervi cutanei
femoris posterioris
peroneal anastomotic r.
r. petrosus arteriae meningeae
mediae
ramus pharyngeales
ramus pharyngeales arteriae
pharyngeae ascendentis

ramus pharyngeales arteriae
 thyroideae inferioris
ramus pharyngei
ramus pharyngei nervi
 glossopharyngei
ramus pharyngei nervi laryngei
 recurrentis
ramus pharyngei nervi vagi
r. pharyngeus arteriae canalis
 pterygoidei
r. pharyngeus arteriae palatinae
 descendentis
r. pharyngeus ganglii pterygopalatini
ramus phrenicoabdominales nervi
 phrenici
r. plantaris profundus arteriae
 dorsalis pedis
r. posterior arteriae obturatoriae
r. posterior arteriae
 pancreaticoduodenalis inferioris
r. posterior arteriae recurrentis
 ulnaris
r. posterior arteriae renalis
r. posterior arteriae thyroideae
 superioris
r. posterior descendens
r. posterior ductus hepatici dextri
ramus posteriores
posterior r. of lateral cerebral
 sulcus
posterior r. of lateral sulcus of
 cerebrum
r. posterior nervi auricularis magni
r. posterior nervi cutanei antebrachii
 medialis
r. posterior nervi obturatorii
r. posterior nervi spinalis
r. posterior rami dextri venae
 portae hepatis
posterior r. of spinal nerve
r. posterior sulci lateralis cerebri
r. posterior sulcus lateralis cerebri
r. posterior venae pulmonalis
 dextrae superioris
ramus precuneales arteriae cerebri
 anterioris
r. prelaminaris rami spinalis rami
 dorsalis arteriae intercostalis
 posterioris
ramus profundi arteriae transversae
 cervicis
r. profundus
r. profundus arteriae circumflexae
 femoris medialis
r. profundus arteriae gluteae
 superioris
r. profundus arteriae plantaris
 medialis
r. profundus arteriae scapularis
 descendentis
r. profundus arteriae transversae
 colli
r. profundus nervi plantaris lateralis
r. profundus nervi radialis
r. profundus nervi ulnaris

ramus prostatici arteriae rectalis
 mediae
ramus prostatici arteriae vesicalis
 inferioris
ramus pterygoidei arteriae maxillaris
r. pterygoideus arteriae temporalis
 profundae posterioris
pubic r.
r. pubicus arteriae epigastricae
 inferioris
r. pubicus arteriae obturatoriae
r. pubicus venae epigastricae
 inferioris
ramus pulmonales plexi nervosi
 pulmonalis
ramus pulmonales systematis
 autonomici
ramus pulmonales thoracici
 gangliorum thoracicorum
r. pyloricus trunci vagalis anterioris
ramus radiculares
ramus renales nervi vagi
r. renalis nervi splanchnici minoris
ramus sacrales laterales arteriae
 sacralis medianae
r. saphenus arteriae descendentis
 genicularis
ramus scrotales anteriores arteriae
 pudendae externae profundae
ramus scrotales posteriores arteriae
 perinealis
ramus scrotales posteriores arteriae
 pudendae internae
ramus septales
ramus septales anteriores arteriae
 ethmoidalis anterioris
r. septi nasi arteriae labialis
 superioris
r. septi posterioris nasalis
r. sinister
r. sinister arteriae hepaticae propriae
r. sinister venae portae hepatis
r. sinus carotici
r. sinus carotici nervi
 glossopharyngei [CN IX]
r. sinus cavernosi
r. sinus cavernosi arteriae carotidis
 arteriae
r. sinus cavernosi arteriae carotidis
 internae
r. sinus cavernosi partis cavernosae
 arteriae carotidis internae
ramus spinales
ramus splenici arteriae splenicae
r. stapedius arteriae stylomastoideae
r. stapedius arteriae tympanicae
 posterioris
ramus sternales arteriae thoracicae
 internae
ramus sternocleidomastoidei arteriae
 occipitalis
r. sternocleidomastoideus arteriae
 thyroideae superioris
r. stylohyoideus nervi facialis

ramus *(continued)*
ramus subendocardiales fasciculi
atrioventricularis
ramus subscapulares arteriae axillaris
ramus substantiae nigrae
r. superficialis
r. superficialis arteriae circumflexae
femoris medialis
r. superficialis arteriae gluteae
superioris
r. superficialis arteriae plantaris
medialis
r. superficialis arteriae transversae
cervicis
r. superficialis arteriae transversae
colli
r. superficialis nervi plantaris
lateralis
r. superficialis nervi radialis
r. superficialis nervi ulnaris
r. superior
r. superior arteriae gluteae superioris
superior dental ramus
rami superiores
r. superior nervi oculomotorii
r. superior nervi transversalis
cervicalis
r. superior ossis pubis
superior pubic r.
r. superior venae pulmonalis
dextrae/sinistrae inferioris
r. suprahyoideus arteriae lingualis
r. sympathicus ad ganglion
submandibulare
ramus temporales anteriores
ramus temporales intermedii
ramus temporales intermedii arteriae
occipitalis lateralis
ramus temporales medii arteriae
occipitalis lateralis
ramus temporales nervi facialis
ramus temporales posteriores
ramus temporales superficiales nervi
auriculotemporalis
r. temporalis anterior
r. temporalis medius partis insularis
arteriae cerebrae mediae
r. temporalis posterior arteriae
cerebri mediae
r. tentorii
ramus terminales arteriae cerebri
medii
ramus thalamici
r. thalamicus
ramus thymici
ramus thymici arteriae thoracicae
internae
r. thyrohyoideus ansae cervicalis
r. tonsillae cerebellae
ramus tonsillares nervi
glossopharyngei
ramus tonsillares nervi palatini
minores
r. tonsillaris arteriae facialis

ramus tracheales
ramus tracheales arteriae thyroideae
inferioris
ramus tracheales nervi laryngei
recurrentis
ramus tractus optici
r. transversus arteriae circumflexae
femoris lateralis
r. transversus arteriae circumflexae
femoris medialis
r. tubarius
r. tubarius arteriae ovaricae
r. tubarius arteriae uterinae
r. tubarius plexus tympanici
ramus tuberis cinerei
r. ulnaris nervi cutanei antebrachii
medialis
ramus ureterici
ramus ureterici arteriae ovaricae
ramus ureterici arteriae renalis
ramus ureterici arteriae suprarenalis
inferioris
ramus ureterici arteriae testicularis
ramus ureterici partis patentis
arteriae umbilicalis
ventral ramus of cervical nerve
ramus ventrales nervorum
cervicalium
ramus ventrales nervorum lumbalium
ramus ventrales nervorum sacralium
ramus ventrales nervorum thoracis
r. ventralis
r. ventralis nervi spinalis
ventral ramus of lumbar nerve
ventral primary ramus of cervical
spinal nerves
ventral primary ramus of lumbar
spinal nerves
ventral primary ramus of sacral
spinal nerves
ventral primary r. of spinal nerve
ventral primary ramus of thoracic
spinal nerve
ventral ramus of sacral nerve
ventral r. of spinal nerve
ventral ramus of thoracic nerve
r. vermis superior
ramus vestibulares arteriae labyrinthi
r. vestibularis posterior arteriae
vestibulocochlearis
white ramus communicantes
ramus zygomatici nervi facialis
r. zygomaticofacialis nervi
zygomatici
r. zygomaticotemporalis nervi
zygomatici
ramycin
rancid
rancidify
rancidity
Randall
R. plaque
R. stone forceps
random
r. coil

r. mating
r. mating equilibrium
r. mechanism
r. pattern flap
r. sample
r. sampling
r. variable
r. wave
randomization
randomized controlled trial (RCT)
Raney
R. alloy
R. catalyst
R. nickel
range
r. of accommodation
r. of convergence
therapeutic r.
Ranikhet disease
ranine
r. anastomosis
r. artery
r. tumor
ranitidine
rank
rank-difference correlation
Ranke
R. angle
R. complex
R. formula
Rankin clamp
Rankine scale
Ransohoff sign
RANTES
ranula
ranular
Ranvier
R. cross
R. disk
R. plexus
R. segment
RAO
right anterior oblique
Raoult law
rape
rapeseed oil
raphania
raphe
amnionic r.
r. anococcygea
anogenital r.
r. corporis callosi
iliococcygeal r.
lateral palpebral r.
r. linguae
median longitudinal r. of tongue
r. medullae oblongatae
r. of medulla oblongata
r. musculi iliococcygeus
r. nuclei
r. palati
palatine r.
palpebral r.
r. palpebralis lateralis
penile r.

r. penis
r. of penis
perineal r.
r. perinei
pharyngeal r.
r. pharyngis
r. of pons
r. pontis
pterygomandibular r.
r. pterygomandibularis
r. retinae
scrotal r.
r. scroti
r. of scrotum
Stilling r.
raphespinal fiber
rapid
r. canities
r. decompression
r. eye movement (REM)
r. eye movement sleep
r. film changer
r. plasma reagin test
rapidly progressive glomerulonephritis
Rapoport-Luebering shunt
Rapoport test
Rappaport
R. acinus
R. classification
rapport
rapture of the deep
rare
r. earth
r. earth element
r. earth metal
rare-earth screen
rarefaction
rarefy
RAS
reticular activating system
r. oncogene
rasceta
rash
antitoxin r.
black currant r.
butterfly r.
caterpillar r.
crystal r.
diaper r.
heat r.
hydatid r.
Murray Valley r.
serum r.
summer r.
wildfire r.
rasion
Rasmussen
r. encephalitis
Rasmussen
Rasmussen
R. aneurysm
R. syndrome
raspatory
raspberry tongue

R

RAST
 radioallergosorbent test
Rastelli operation
rat
 albino r.
 r. mite dermatitis
 Wistar r.
rat-bite
 r.-b. disease
 r.-b. fever
rate
 abortion r.
 age-specific r.
 attack r.
 average flow r.
 basal metabolic r. (BMR)
 birth r.
 case fatality r.
 concordance r.
 r. constant (k)
 critical r.
 death r.
 r. equation
 erythrocyte sedimentation r. (ESR)
 fatality r.
 fetal death r.
 fetal heart r.
 five-year survival r.
 general fertility r.
 glomerular filtration r. (GFR)
 gross reproduction r.
 growth r.
 growth r. of population
 hazard r.
 heart r.
 inception r.
 incidence r.
 infant mortality r.
 initial r.
 lethality r.
 maternal death r.
 r. meter
 mitotic r.
 morbidity r.
 mortality r.
 mucociliary clearance r.
 mutation r.
 neonatal mortality r.
 overall catalytic r. of an enzyme
   (k_{cat})
 peak flow r.
 perinatal mortality r.
 pulse r.
 recurrence r.
 repetition r.
 respiratory r.
 sedimentation r.
 shear r.
 slew r.
 steady-state r.
 steroid metabolic clearance r.
   (MCR)
 steroid production r.
 steroid secretory r.

 stillbirth r.
 voiding flow r.
Rathke
 R. bundle
 R. cleft cyst
 R. diverticulum
 R. pocket
 R. pouch
 R. pouch tumor
rating of perceived exertion
ratio
 absolute terminal innervation r.
 accommodative convergence-
   accommodation r. (AC/A)
 A/G r.
   albumin-globulin ratio
 albumin-globulin r. (A/G ratio)
 ALT:AST r.
 amylase-creatinine clearance r.
 body-weight r.
 cardiothoracic r.
 case fatality r.
 r. of decayed and filled surface
   (RDFS)
 r. of decayed and filled teeth
   (RDFT)
 extraction r. (E)
 fertility r.
 flux r.
 functional terminal innervation r.
 grid r.
 gyromagnetic r.
 hand r.
 international normalized r. (INR)
 IRI/G r.
 K:A r.
   ketogenic-antiketogenic ratio
 ketogenic-antiketogenic r. (K:A ratio)
 lecithin/sphingomyelin r. (L/S ratio)
 L/S r.
   lecithinsphingomyelin ratio
 magnetogyric r.
 mass-action r.
 maternal mortality r.
 M:E r.
 mendelian r.
 molecular weight r. (M_r)
 nuclear-cytoplasmic r.
 nucleolar-nuclear r.
 P/O r.
 proportional mortality r. (PMR)
 respiratory exchange r.
 r. scale
 segregation r.
 sex r.
 signal-to-noise r.
 standardized mortality r.
 systolic/diastolic r.
 therapeutic r.
 variance r.
 ventilation/perfusion r. ($\dot{V}a/\dot{Q}$)
 waist-hip r.
 zeta sedimentation r. (ZSR)

rational
  r. formula
  r. therapy
rationalization
ratsbane
rattle
  death r.
rattlesnake
Rattus
Rauber layer
Rau process
Rauscher
  R. leukemia virus
RAV
  rous-associated virus
Ravius process
raw score
ray
  actinic r.
  alpha r.
  anode r.
  becquerel r.
  beta r.
  cathode r.
  chemical r.
  cosmic r.
  direct r.
  r. fungus
  gamma r.
  glass r.
  grenz r.
  H r.
  hard r.
  incident r.
  indirect r.
  infrared r.
  intermediate r.
  marginal r.
  medullary r.
  Niewenglowski r.
  parallel r.'s
  paraxial r.
  positive r.
  primary r.
  reflected r.
  roentgen r.
  secondary r.
  soft r.
  supersonic r.
  r. therapeutics
  ultrasonic r.
  ultraviolet r.
  W r.
  x-r.
Rayer disease
rayl
Rayleigh
  R. equation
  R. test
Raynaud
  R. disease
  R. phenomenon
  R. sign
  R. syndrome

Rb
  rubidium
R-banding stain
rbc
  red blood cell
RBF
  renal blood flow
R.C.P.
  Royal College of Physicians
R.C.P.(E), R.C.P.(Edin)
  Royal College of Physicians (Edinburgh)
R.C.P.(I)
  Royal College of Physicians (Ireland)
R.C.P.S.C.
  Royal College of Physicians and Surgeons of Canada
R.C.S.
  Royal College of Surgeons (England)
R.C.S.(E), R.C.S.(Edin)
  Royal College of Surgeons (Edinburgh)
R.C.S.(I)
  Royal College of Surgeons (Ireland)
RCT
  randomized controlled trial
RD
  registered dietician
RDA
  recommended daily allowance
RDFS
  ratio of decayed and filled surface
RDFT
  ratio of decayed and filled teeth
RDH
  Registered Dental Hygienist
RDPA
  right descending pulmonary artery
R.E.
  right eye
Re
  rhenium
react
reactance (X)
reactant
  acute phase r.
reaction
  accelerated r.
  acid r.
  acute phase r.
  acute situational r.
  acute stress r.
  adverse r.
  alarm r.
  aldehyde r.
  alkaline r.
  allergic r.
  amphoteric r.
  anamnestic r.
  anaphylactic r.
  anaplerotic r.
  antigen-antibody r. (AAR)
  anxiety r.
  Arias-Stella r.
  arousal r.
  Arthus r.
  Ascoli r.

R

reaction *(continued)*
associative r.
basic r.
Bence Jones r.
Berthelot r.
bi bi r.
Bittorf r.
biuret r.
Bloch r.
Bordet and Gengou r.
Brunn r.
Burchard-Liebermann r.
Cannizzaro r.
capsular precipitation r.
Carr-Price r.
catalatic r.
catastrophic r.
cell-mediated r.
r. center
chain r.
Chantemesse r.
cholera-red r.
chromaffin r.
circular r.
cocarde r., cockade r.
colloidal gold r.
complement-fixation r.
consensual r.
constitutional r.
conversion r.
cross-r.
cutaneous graft versus host r.
cytotoxic r.
Dale r.
dark r.
decidual r.
delayed r.
depot r.
depressive r.
dermotuberculin r.
diazo r.
digitonin r.
Dische r.
dissociative r.
dopa r.
dystonic r.
early r.
echo r.
Ehrlich benzaldehyde r.
Ehrlich diazo r.
eosinopenic r.
error-prone polymerase chain r.
eye-closure pupil r.
false-negative r.
false-positive r.
Fenton r.
Fernandez r.
ferric chloride r. of epinephrine
Feulgen r.
fight or flight r.
first-order r.
fixation r.
flocculation r.
focal r.

Folin r.
r. formation
Forssman antigen-antibody r.
fragment r.
Frei-Hoffmann r.
fright r.
fuchsinophil r.
furfurol r.
galvanic skin r.
gel diffusion r.
Gell and Coombs r.
gemistocytic r.
general adaptation r.
Gerhardt r.
graft versus host r. (GVHR)
group r.
Gruber r.
Gruber-Widal r.
Günning r.
Haber-Weiss r.
harlequin r.
heel-tap r.
hemoclastic r.
Henle r.
Herxheimer r.
Hill r.
homograft r.
hunting r.
hypersensitivity r.
id r.
r. of identity
immediate hypersensitivity r.
immune r.
incompatible blood transfusion r.
indirect pupillary r.
intracutaneous r.
iodate r. of epinephrine
iodine r. of epinephrine
irreversible r.
Jaffe r.
Jarisch-Herxheimer r.
Jolly r.
Kiliani-Fischer r.
late r.
lengthening r.
lepromin r.
leukemoid r.
lid-closure r.
Liebermann-Burchard r.
ligase chain r.
local anesthetic r.
Loewenthal r.
Lohmann r.
magnet r.
Marchi r.
Mazzotti r.
Millon r.
miostagmin r.
Mitsuda r.
mixed agglutination r.
mixed lymphocyte culture r.
monomolecular r.
myasthenic r.
Nadi r.
near r.

negative supporting r.
nested polymerase chain r.
Neufeld r.
neurotonic r.
neutral r.
ninhydrin r.
nitritoid r.
r. of nonidentity
nuclear r.
oxidase r.
oxidation-reduction r.
pain r.
Pandy r.
r. of partial identity
passive cutaneous anaphylactic r.
Paul r.
performic acid r.
periosteal r.
peroxidase r.
phosphoroclastic r.
Pirquet r.
plasmal r.
pleural r.
polymerase chain r. (PCR)
Porter-Silber r.
positive supporting r.
Prausnitz-Küstner r.
precipitin r.
primary r.
prozone r.
psychogalvanic r.
quellung r.
reversed Prausnitz-Küstner r.
reverse transcriptase polymerase
  chain r. (RT-PCR)
reversible r.
Sakaguchi r.
Schardinger r.
Schultz r.
Schultz-Charlton r.
Schultz-Dale r.
serum r.
shortening r.
Shwartzman r.
skin r.
specific r.
startle r.
Straus r.
stress r.
supporting r.
symptomatic r.
thermoprecipitin r.
r. time
transcription-based chain r.
Treponema pallidum
  immobilization r.
triketohydrindene r.
type III hypersensitivity r.
unimolecular r.
vaccinoid r.
Voges-Proskauer r.
Wassermann r. (W.r.)
Weidel r.
Weil-Felix r.
Weinberg r.

Wernicke r.
wheal-and-erythema r.
wheal-and-flare r.
white r.
whitegraft r.
Widal r.
xanthoprotein r.
Yorke autolytic r.
zero-order r.
Zimmermann r.

reactivate
reactivation tuberculosis
reactive
r. airway disease
r. arthritis
r. astrocyte
r. attachment disorder
r. cell
r. change
r. depression
r. hyperemia
r. perforating collagenosis
r. schizophrenia
reactivity
reading
lip r.
speech r.
reading frame
blocked r. f.
closed r. f.
open r. f.
unidentified r. f. (URF)
reading-frame-shift mutation
readthrough
reagent
amino acid r.
Benedict-Hopkins-Cole r.
biuret r.
Cleland r.
diazo r.
Dische r.
Dische-Schwarz r.
Drabkin r.
Dragendorff r.
Edlefsen r.
Edman r.
Ehrlich diazo r.
Erdmann r.
Esbach r.
Exton r.
Fehling r.
Folin r.
Fouchet r.
Froehde r.
Frohn r.
Girard r.
Günzberg r.
Hahn oxine r.
Hammarsten r.
Ilosvay r.
Kasten fluorescent Schiff r.'s
Lloyd r.
Mandelin r.
Marme r.
Marquis r.

reagent *(continued)*
    Mecke r.
    Meyer r.
    Millon r.
    Nessler r.
    Rosenthaler-Turk r.
    Sanger r.
    Schaer r.
    Scheibler r.
    Schiff r.
    Scott-Wilson r.
    sulfhydryl r.
    Sulkowitch r.
    Uffelmann r.
    Wurster r.

reagin
    atopic r.

reaginic
    r. antibody

REAL
    Revised European-American Classification of Lymphoid Neoplasms
    REAL classification

real
    r. focus
    r. image
    r. origin

reality
    r. adaptation
    r. principle
    r. testing

reality awareness
real-time
    r.-t. echocardiography
    r.-t. ultrasonography

reamer
    engine r.
    intramedullary r.

rearrangement
    Amadori r.

reassignment
    sex r.

reattachment
Réaumur scale
rebase
rebound
    r. phenomenon
    r. tenderness

rebreathing
    r. anesthesia
    r. technique

Rebuck skin window technique
recalcification
recall
    r. bias

Récamier operation
recanalization
recapitulation theory
receiver
    r. operating characteristic (ROC)
    r. operating characteristic curve

receptaculum, pl. **receptacula**
    r. chyli

    r. ganglii petrosi
    r. pecqueti

receptive
    r. aphasia
    r. field

receptor
    adrenergic r.
    alpha-adrenergic r.
    AMPA r.
    angiotensin r.
    ANP clearance r.
    asialoglycoprotein r.
    B cell r.
    beta-adrenergic r.
    cholinergic r.
    epidermal growth factor r. (EGFR)
    estrogen r.
    Fas r.
    Fc r.
    kainate r.
    laminin r.
    L-AP$_4$ r.
    low-density lipoprotein r.
    mannose-6-phosphate r. (MPR)
    metabotropic r.
    muscarinic r.
    nicotinic r.
    nicotinic cholinergic r.
    NMDA r.
    opiate r.
    orphan r.
    progesterone r.
    r. protein
    quisqualate r.
    retinoic acid r.
    retinoid X r.
    ryanodine r.
    scavenger r.
    sensory r.
    r. site
    stretch r.
    T cell antigen r.

receptosome
recess
    anterior r.
    anterior r. of tympanic membrane
    azygoesophageal r.
    cecal r.
    cerebellopontine r.
    cochlear r.
    costodiaphragmatic r.
    costomediastinal r.
    duodenojejunal r.
    elliptical r. of bony labyrinth
    epitympanic r.
    hepatoenteric r.
    hepatorenal r. of subhepatic space
    Hyrtl epitympanic r.
    inferior duodenal r.
    inferior ileocecal r.
    inferior omental r.
    inferior r. of omental bursa
    infundibular r.
    intersigmoid r.
    Jacquemet r.

lateral r. of fourth ventricle
mesentericoparietal r.
optic r.
pancreaticoenteric r.
paracolic r.
paraduodenal r.
parotid r.
pharyngeal r.
phrenicomediastinal r.
pineal r.
piriform r.
pleural r.
pneumatoenteric r.
pneumoenteric r.
pontocerebellar r.
posterior r.
posterior r. of tympanic membrane
Reichert cochlear r.
retrocecal r.
retroduodenal r.
Rosenmüller r.
sacciform r. of distal radioulnar
   joint
sacciform r. of elbow joint
saccular r. of bony labyrinth
sphenoethmoidal r.
spherical r. of bony labyrinth
splenic r.
subhepatic r.
subphrenic r.
subpopliteal r.
superior azygoesophageal r.
superior duodenal r.
superior ileocecal r.
superior r. of lesser peritoneal sac
superior omental r.
superior r. of omental bursa
superior r. of tympanic membrane
supraoptic r.
suprapineal r.
supratonsillar r.
triangular r.
Tröltsch r.
tubotympanic r.
r. of tympanic cavity
utricular r. of bony labyrinth
utricular r. of membranous labyrinth
vertebromediastinal r.

recession
angle r.
clitoral r.
gingival r.
tendon r.

recessitivity
recessive
r. character
r. inheritance
r. trait

recessus, pl. **recessus**
r. anterior
r. anterior membranae tympanicae
r. cochlearis
r. costodiaphragmaticus
r. costomediastinalis
r. duodenalis inferior

r. duodenalis superior
r. ellipticus labyrinthi ossei
r. epitympanicus
r. hepatorenalis recessus subhepatici
r. ileocecalis inferior
r. ileocecalis superior
r. inferior omentalis
r. infundibuli
r. infundibuliformis
r. intersigmoideus
r. lateralis ventriculi quarti
r. lienalis
r. membranae tympanicae
r. paraduodenalis
r. parotideus
r. pharyngeus
r. phrenicomediastinalis
r. pinealis
r. piriformis
r. pleurales
r. posterior
r. posterior membranae tympanicae
r. retrocecalis
r. retroduodenalis
r. sacciformis articulationis
r. sacciformis articulationis
   radioulnaris distalis
r. saccularis larbyrinthi ossei
r. sphenoethmoidalis
r. sphericus labyrinthi ossei
r. splenicus
r. subhepaticus
r. subphrenicus
r. subpopliteus
r. superior bursae omentalis
r. superior membranae tympanicae
r. supraopticus
r. suprapinealis
r. triangularis
r. utricularis labyrinthi membranacei
r. utricularis labyrinthi ossei
r. vertebromediastinalis

recidivation
recidivism
recidivist
recipe
recipient
recipiomotor
reciprocal
r. anchorage
r. arm
r. beat
r. bigeminy
r. force
r. inhibition
r. innervation
r. rhythm
r. transfusion
r. translocation
reciprocating rhythm
reciprocation
reciprocity law
recirculation
Recklinghausen disease
reclination

R

reclotting phenomenon
recognition time
recoil
    r. atom
    r. wave
recollection
recombinant
    r. DNA
    r. human interleukin-11 (rhIL-11)
    r. strain
    r. vector
recombination
    r. fraction
    genetic r.
    homologous r.
    site-specific r.
recombinatorial repair
recommended daily allowance (RDA)
recon
reconstitution
reconstruction
    ossicular r.
reconstructive
    r. mammaplasty
    r. psychotherapy
    r. surgery
record
    anesthesia r.
    r. base
    centric interocclusal r.
    eccentric interocclusal r.
    face-bow r.
    functional chew-in r.
    hospital r.
    interocclusal r., protrusive
      interocclusal r.
    r. linkage
    maxillomandibular r.
    medical r.
    occluding centric relation r.
    preextraction r.
    preoperative r.
    problem-oriented r. (POR)
    profile r.
    protrusive r.
    r. rim
    terminal jaw relation r.
    three-dimensional r.
recording
    clinical r.
    depth r.
recovery
    creep r.
    inversion r.
    r. room
    r. score
    short TI inversion r. (STIR)
    spontaneous r.
    r. stroke
    ultrasonic egg r.
recreational drug
recrudescence
recrudescent
    r. typhus
    r. typhus fever

recruiting response
recruitment
recta
rectal
    r. alimentation
    r. ampulla
    r. anesthesia
    r. column
    r. fold
    r. plexus
    r. reflex
    r. shelf
    r. sinus
    r. valve
    r. valvotomy
    r. venous plexus
rectalgia
rectangular amputation
rectectomy
rectified
    r. spirit
    r. tar oil
    r. turpentine oil
rectifier tube
rectify
rectoabdominal
rectocardiac reflex
rectocele
rectoclysis
rectococcygeal muscle
rectococcygeus muscle
rectococcypexy
rectocolitis
rectolabial fistula
rectolaryngeal reflex
rectoperineal
rectoperineorrhaphy
rectopexy
rectophobia
rectoplasty
rectorrhaphy
rectosacral fascia
rectoscope
rectoscopy
rectosigmoid
    r. junction
    r. sphincter
rectostenosis
rectostomy
rectotome
rectotomy
rectourethral
    r. fistula
    r. muscle
rectouterine
    r. fold
    r. muscle
    r. pouch
rectouterinus muscle
rectovaginal
    r. fistula
    r. septum
rectovaginouterine pouch
rectovesical
    r. fascia

r. fistula
r. fold
r. muscle
r. pouch
r. septum
rectovesicalis muscle
rectovestibular fistula
rectovulvar fistula
rectum
rectus
r. abdominis muscle
r. capitis anterior muscle
r. capitis lateralis muscle
r. capitis posterior major muscle
r. capitis posterior minor muscle
r. femoris muscle
r. muscle of abdomen
r. muscle of thigh
r. sheath
recumbent
recuperate
recuperation
recurrence
r. rate
r. risk
recurrent
r. abortion
r. albuminuria
r. aphthous stomatitis
r. aphthous ulcers
r. appendicitis
r. artery of Heubner
r. branch of spinal nerve
r. caries
r. corneal erosion
r. encephalopathy
r. fever
r. herpetic stomatitis
r. hypopyon
r. interosseous artery
r. jaundice of pregnancy
r. laryngeal nerve
r. meningeal branch of spinal nerve
r. meningeal nerve
r. nerve
r. polyserositis
r. pyogenic cholangitis
r. radial artery
r. respiratory papillomatosis
r. scarring aphthae
r. stricture
r. ulcerative stomatitis
r. ulnar artery
recurring digital fibroma of childhood
recurvation
red
r. atrophy
r. blood cell (rbc)
r. blood cell cast
r. bone marrow
r. cell adherence phenomenon
r. cell adherence test
r. cell cast
r. corpuscle
R. Cross

r. degeneration
r. fever
r. fiber
r. gum
r. half-moon
r. hepatization
r. imported fire ant
r. induration
r. infarct
r. lead
r. muscle
r. nucleus
r. oil
r. oxide of lead
r. precipitate
r. pulp
r. pulp cord
r. pulp of spleen
r. reflex
r. strawberry tongue
r. sweat
r. thrombus
r. tide
r. vision
r., white, and blue sign
r. wine
redia, pl. **rediae**
redifferentiation
redintegration
redox
r. electrode
r. indicator
r. potential
r. system
redressement forcé
redressment
reduce
reduced
r. coenzyme A (CoASH)
r. enamel epithelium
r. eye
r. glutathione
r. hematin
r. hemoglobin
r. interarch distance
reducible hernia
reducing
r. diet
r. enzyme
r. sugar
r. valve
reductant
reductase
GMP r.
guanylic acid reductase
5α-reductase inhibitor
reductic acid
reduction
r. of chromosome
closed r. of fractures
r. deformity
r. division
r. en masse
r. left ventriculoplasty
r. mammaplasty

R

reduction (*continued*)
    r. nucleus
    open r. of fracture
    r. phase
    selective r.
    tuberosity r.
redundancy
    terminal r.
reduplicated cataract
reduplication
reduvid, reduviid
Reduviidae
reed
    R. cell
    r. instrument theory
Reed-Frost
    R.-F. model
    R.-F. theory of epidemics
Reed-Sternberg cell
reedy nail
reefing
    stomach r.
reenactment
re-entrant mechanism
reentry
    r. phenomenon
    r. theory
Rees-Ecker fluid
refect
refection
refeeding gynecomastia
reference
    r. electrode
    r. method
    r. value
referred
    r. pain
    r. sensation
Refetoff syndrome
refine
reflect
reflectance
reflected
    r. color
    r. inguinal ligament
    r. light
    r. ray
reflecting retinoscope
reflection coefficient
reflector
reflex
    abdominal r.
    abdominocardiac r.
    Abrams heart r.
    accommodation r.
    Achilles r.
    Achilles tendon r.
    acoustic r.
    acousticopalpebral r.
    acquired r.
    acromial r.
    adductor r.
    allied r.
    anal r.

r. angina
ankle r.
antagonistic r.
aortic r.
aponeurotic r.
r. arc
Aschner r.
Aschner-Dagnini r.
r. asthma
attitudinal r.
auditory oculogyric r.
auricular r.
auriculopalpebral r.
auriculopressor r.
auropalpebral r.
axon r.
Babinski r.
back of foot r.
Bainbridge r.
Barkman r.
basal joint r.
Bechterew-Mendel r.
behavior r.
Benedek r.
Bezold-Jarisch r.
biceps femoris r.
Bing r.
bladder r.
blink r.
body righting r.
brachioradial r.
Brain r.
bregmocardiac r.
Brissaud r.
bulbocavernosus r.
bulbomimic r.
Capps r.
cardiac depressor r.
carotid sinus r.
celiac plexus r.
cephalopalpebral r.
Chaddock r.
chain r.
chin r.
Chodzko r.
ciliospinal r.
clasping r.
cochleo-orbicular r.
cochleopalpebral r.
cochleopupillary r.
cochleostapedial r.
conditioned r. (CR)
conjunctival r.
consensual light r.
contralateral r.
r. control
corneal r.
costal arch r.
costopectoral r.
r. cough
cough r.
craniocardiac r.
cremasteric r.
crossed adductor r.
crossed extension r.

crossed knee r.
crossed r. of pelvis
crossed spino-adductor r.
cuboidodigital r.
cutaneous r.
cutaneous pupil r.
cutaneous-pupillary r.
darwinian r.
deep abdominal r.
deep tendon r. (DTR)
defense r.
deglutition r.
Dejerine r.
delayed r.
depressor r.
r. detrusor contraction
diffused r.
digital r.
diving r.
dorsal r.
dorsum of foot r.
dorsum pedis r.
r. dyspepsia
elbow r.
enterogastric r.
epigastric r.
r. epilepsy
erector-spinal r.
esophagosalivary r.
external oblique r.
eye r.
eyeball compression r.
eyeball-heart r.
eye-closure r.
facial r.
faucial r.
femoral r.
femoroabdominal r.
Ferguson r.
finger-thumb r.
flexor r.
forced grasping r.
front-tap r.
fundus r.
gag r.
Galant r.
galvanic skin r.
gastrocolic r.
gastroileac r.
Geigel r.
Gifford r.
gluteal r.
Gordon r.
grasp r.
grasping r.
great-toe r.
Guillain-Barré r.
gustatory-sudorific r.
H r.
r. headache
hepatojugular r.
Hering-Breuer r.
Hoffmann r.
hypochondrial r.
hypogastric r.

inborn r.
r. incontinence
r. inhibition
innate r.
interscapular r.
intrinsic r.
inverted radial r.
investigatory r.
ipsilateral r.
r. iridoplegia
Jacobson r.
jaw r.
jaw-working r.
Joffroy r.
Kisch r.
knee r.
knee-jerk r.
labyrinthine r.
labyrinthine righting r.
lacrimal r.
lacrimogustatory r.
laryngeal r.
laryngospastic r.
latent r.
laughter r.
let-down r.
lid r.
Liddell-Sherrington r.
r. ligament
light r.
lip r.
Lovén r.
lower abdominal periosteal r.
magnet r.
mandibular r.
mass r.
masseter r.
Mayer r.
McCarthy r.
mediopubic r.
Mendel-Bechterew r.
Mendel instep r.
metacarpohypothenar r.
metacarpothenar r.
metatarsal r.
micturition r.
milk-ejection r.
milk let-down r.
Mondonesi r.
Moro r.
r. movement
muscular r.
myenteric r.
myotatic r.
nasal r.
nasomental r.
near r.
neck r.
r. neurogenic bladder
nociceptive r.
nocifensor r.
nose-bridge-lid r.
nose-eye r.
oculocardiac r.
oculocephalic r.

reflex *(continued)*
 oculocephalogyric r.
 oculovagal r.
 olecranon r.
 Oppenheim r.
 optic righting r.
 orbicularis oculi r.
 orbicularis pupillary r.
 orienting r.
 r. otalgia
 palatal r.
 palatine r.
 palmar r.
 palm-chin r.
 palmomental r.
 parachute r.
 paradoxical extensor r.
 paradoxical flexor r.
 paradoxical patellar r.
 paradoxical pupillary r.
 paradoxical triceps r.
 patellar tendon r.
 patelloadductor r.
 Pavlov r.
 pectoral r.
 Perez r.
 pericardial r.
 periosteal r.
 pharyngeal r.
 phasic r.
 Phillipson r.
 photic-sneeze r.
 pilomotor r.
 plantar muscle r.
 pneocardiac r.
 pneopneic r.
 postural r.
 pressoreceptor r.
 pronator r.
 proprioceptive r.
 proprioceptive-oculocephalic r.
 protective laryngeal r.
 psychocardiac r.
 psychogalvanic r.
 psychogalvanic skin r.
 pulmonocoronary r.
 pupillary r.
 pupillary-skin r.
 quadriceps r.
 quadripedal extensor r.
 radial r.
 radiobicipital r.
 radioperiosteal r.
 rectal r.
 rectocardiac r.
 rectolaryngeal r.
 red r.
 Remak r.
 renal r.
 righting r.
 Roger r.
 rooting r.
 Rossolimo r.
 scapular r.

 scapulohumeral r.
 scapuloperiosteal r.
 Schäffer r.
 semimembranosus r.
 semitendinosus r.
 shot-silk r.
 sinus r.
 skin r.
 skin-muscle r.
 skin-pupillary r.
 snapping r.
 snout r.
 sole tap r.
 spinal r.
 spinoadductor r.
 stapedial r.
 Starling r.
 startle r.
 static r.
 statokinetic r.
 statotonic r.
 sternobrachial r.
 stretch r.
 Strümpell r.
 styloradial r.
 suckling r.
 superficial r.
 supination r.
 supinator longus r.
 supporting r.
 supraorbital r.
 suprapatellar r.
 supraumbilical r.
 swallowing r.
 r. sympathetic dystrophy (RSD)
 r. symptom
 synchronous r.
 r. tachycardia
 tarsophalangeal r.
 tendo Achillis r.
 tendon r.
 tensor tympani r.
 r. therapy
 thumb r.
 tonic r.
 trace conditioned r.
 trained r.
 triceps r.
 triceps surae r.
 trigeminofacial r.
 trochanter r.
 Trömner r.
 ulnar r.
 unconditioned r.
 upper abdominal periosteal r.
 urinary r.
 utricular r.
 vagovagal r.
 vasopressor r.
 venorespiratory r.
 vesical r.
 vestibuloocular r.
 vestibulospinal r.
 visceral traction r.
 viscerogenic r.

visceromotor r.
viscerosensory r.
viscerotrophic r.
visual orbicularis r.
vomiting r.
Weingrow r.
Westphal pupillary r.
white pupillary r.
wink r.
withdrawal r.
wrist clonus r.

reflexogenic
r. pressosensitivity
r. zone

reflexogenous
reflexograph
reflexology
reflexometer
reflexophil, reflexophile
reflexotherapy
reflux
abdominojugular r.
esophageal r., gastroesophageal r., r. reflux
r. esophagitis
hepatojugular r.
intrarenal r.
r. nephropathy
r. otitis media
pyelotubular r.
ureterorenal r.
vesicoureteral r.

reformat
refract
refractable
refracted light
refracting angle of a prism
refraction
double r.
dynamic r.
static r.

refractionist
refractionometer
refractive
r. accommodative esotropia
r. amblyopia
r. ametropia
r. index (n)
r. keratoplasty
r. keratotomy

refractivity
refractometer
refractometry
refractory
r. anemia
r. cast
r. flask
r. investment
r. period
r. rickets
r. state

refracture
refrangible
refresh
refrigerant

refrigeration anesthesia
refringence
refringency
refringent
Refsum
R. disease
R. syndrome

refusion
regainer
Regaud fixative
regenerate
regeneration
aberrant r.
guided tissue r.

regenerative polyp
regimen
regio, pl. **regiones**
r. abdominis
r. abdominis lateralis
r. analis
r. antebrachialis anterior
r. antebrachialis posterior
r. antebrachii anterior
r. antebrachii posterior
r. axillaris
r. brachialis anterior
r. brachialis posterior
r. brachii anterior
r. buccalis
r. calcanea
r. capitis
r. carpalis anterior
r. carpalis posterior
regiones cervicales
r. cervicalis anterior
r. cervicalis lateralis
r. cervicalis posterior
r. colli posterior
r. corporis
r. cruralis posterior
r. cruris anterior
r. cubitalis anterior
r. cubitalis posterior
r. deltoidea
r. dorsalis
r. dorsi
r. epigastrica
r. facialis
r. femoralis posterior
r. femoris
r. femoris anterior
r. femoris posterior
r. frontalis capitis
r. genus anterior
r. genus posterior
r. glutealis
r. hypochondriaca
r. infraclavicularis
r. inframammaria
r. infraorbitalis
r. infrascapularis
r. inguinalis
r. lateralis abdominis
r. lumbalis
r. mammaria

R

regio *(continued)*
    regiones membri inferioris
    regiones membri superioris
    r. mentalis
    r. nasalis
    r. nuchalis
    r. occipitalis capitis
    r. olfactoria tunicae mucosae nasi
    r. oralis
    r. orbitalis
    r. parietalis capitis
    r. pectoralis
    r. perinealis
    r. plantaris
    r. presternalis
    r. pubica
    r. respiratoria tunicae mucosae nasi
    r. sacralis
    r. scapularis
    r. sternocleidomastoidea
    r. suralis
    r. talocruralis
    r. tarsalis
    r. temporalis capitis
    regiones thoracicae anteriores et
      laterales
    r. umbilicalis
    r. urogenitalis
    r. vertebralis
    r. zygomatica

region
    abdominal r.
    anal r.
    ankle r.
    anterior antebrachial r.
    anterior r. of arm
    anterior brachial r.
    anterior carpal r.
    anterior cervical r.
    anterior crural r.
    anterior cubital r.
    anterior r. of elbow
    anterior r. of forearm
    anterior hypothalamic r.
    anterior r. of knee
    anterior knee r.
    anterior r. of leg
    anterior r. of neck
    anterior r. of thigh
    anterior thoracic r.
    anterior r. of wrist
    axillary r.
    r. of back
    r. of body
    buccal r.
    calcaneal r.
    r. of chest
    chromosomal r.
    complementarity determining r.
    constant r.
    deltoid r.
    dorsal hypothalamic r.
    epigastric r.
    face r.

r. of face
femoral r.
framework r.
frontal r. of head
gluteal r.
r. of head
heel r.
hinge r.
hypervariable r.
hypochondriac r.
I r.
iliac r.
r. of inferior limb
inframammary r.
infraorbital r.
infrascapular r.
inguinal r.
r. of interest
intermediate hypothalamic r.
K r.
lateral r. of abdominal r.
lateral cervical r.
lateral hypothalamic r.
lateral r. of neck
lateral thoracic r.
r. of lower limb
lumbar r.
mammary r.
mental r.
nasal r.
r. of neck
nuchal region
nucleolus organizer r.
occipital r. of head
r. of olfactory mucosa
olfactory r. of mucosa of nose
olfactory r. of nasal mucosa
olfactory r. of nose
olfactory r. of tunica mucosa of
  nose
oral r.
orbital r.
parietal r.
pectoral r.
perineal r.
plantar r.
popliteal r.
posterior antebrachial r.
posterior r. of arm
posterior brachial r.
posterior carpal r.
posterior cervical r.
posterior crural r.
posterior cubital r.
posterior r. of elbow
posterior r. of forearm
posterior hypothalamic r.
posterior r. of knee
posterior knee r.
posterior r. of leg
posterior r. of neck
posterior neck r.
posterior r. of thigh
posterior r. of wrist
preoptic r.

presternal r.
presumptive r.
pretectal r.
pubic r.
r. of respiratory mucosa
respiratory r. of mucosa of nasal cavity
respiratory r. of tunica mucosa of nose
sacral r.
scaffold-associated r. (SAR)
scapular r.
sternocleidomastoid r.
suboccipital r.
r. of superior limb
sural r.
temporal r. of head
umbilical r.
r. of upper limb
urogenital r.
variable r.
vertebral r.
Wernicke r.
zygomatic r.

regional
r. anatomy
r. anesthesia
r. enteritis
r. enterocolitis
r. granulomatous lymphadenitis
r. hypothermia
r. lymphadenitis
r. perfusion
regional ileitis (*var. of* distal ileitis)
regiones (*pl. of* regio)
register
Registered Dental Hygienist (RDH)
registered dietician (RD)
registered nurse (RN)
registration
maxillomandibular r.
tissue r.
registry
regnancy
regression
r. analysis
r. of the mean
phonemic r.
regressive-reconstructive approach
regressive staining
regular
r. astigmatism
R. insulin
R. insulin injection
regulation
enzyme r.
gene r.
regulator
r. gene
growth r.
humoral r.
regulatory
r. albuminuria
r. sequence
regulon

regurgitant
r. fraction
r. murmur
regurgitate
regurgitation
aortic r.
ischemic mitral r.
r. jaundice
mitral r.
pulmonic r.
valvular r.
rehabilitation
mouth r.
rehearsal
Rehfuss
R. method
R. stomach tube
rehydration
Reichel-Pólya stomach procedure
Reichert
R. cartilage
R. cochlear recess
Reichert-Meissl number
Reichstein
R. compound
R. substance
Reid baseline
Reifenstein syndrome
Reil
R. ansa
R. band
R. ribbon
R. triangle
reimplantation
extravesical r.
ureteral r.
Reinecke salt
reinfection tuberculosis
reinforced anchorage
reinforcement
primary r.
secondary r.
reinforcer
negative r.
positive r.
Reinke
R. crystalloid
R. space
reinnervation
reinoculation
Reinsch test
reintegration
reinversion
Reis-Bücklers corneal dystrophy
Reisseisen muscle
Reissner
R. fiber
R. membrane
Reiter
R. disease
R. syndrome
R. test
rejection
accelerated r.
acute cellular r.

rejection *(continued)*
    allograft r.
    chronic allograft r.
    first-set r.
    hyperacute r.
    parental r.
    primary r.
    second set r.
rejuvenescence
relapse
relapsing
    r. appendicitis
    r. febrile nodular nonsuppurative
      panniculitis
    r. fever
    r. malaria
    r. perichondritis
    r. polychondritis
relation
    acquired centric r.
    acquired eccentric r.
    buccolingual r.
    centric jaw r.
    dynamic r.
    eccentric r.
    intermaxillary r.
    maxillomandibular r.
    median r.
    median retruded r.
    occluding r.
    protrusive jaw r.
    rest jaw r.
    ridge r.
    static r.
    unstrained jaw r.
relational threshold
relationship
    dose-response r.
    dual r.
    Haldane r.
    hypnotic r.
    object r.
    sadomasochistic r.
relative
    r. accommodation
    r. afferent pupillary defect
    r. biologic effectiveness
    r. dehydration
    r. humidity
    r. immunity
    r. incompetence
    r. leukocytosis
    r. molecular mass (M_r)
    r. polycythemia
    r. refractory period
    r. risk
    r. scotoma
    r. sensitivity
    r. specificity
    r. viscosity
relax
relaxant
    depolarizing r.
    muscle r.

    neuromuscular r.
    nondepolarizing r.
    smooth muscle r.
relaxation
    r. atelectasis
    cardioesophageal r.
    isometric r.
    isovolumetric r.
    isovolumic r.
    longitudinal r.
    r. response
    spin-lattice r.
    spin-spin r.
    r. suture
    r. time
    transverse r.
relaxin
relearning
released substance
release phenomenon
releasin
releasing
    r. factor (RF)
    r. hormone (RH)
reliability
    r. coefficient
    equivalent form r.
    interjudge r.
    interrater r.
    test-retest r.
relief
    r. area
    r. chamber
relieve
reline
relocation test
REM
    rapid eye movement
      REM behavior disorder
      REM sleep
      REM syndrome
rem
    roentgen-equivalent-man
Remak
    R. fiber
    R. ganglia
    R. nuclear division
    R. plexus
    R. reflex
    R. sign
remediable
remedial
remedy
remineralization
reminiscence
reminiscent aura
remission
    spontaneous r.
remit
remittence
remittent
    r. malaria
    r. malarial fever
remnant

remodeling
>heart chamber r.

remote
>r. afterloading brachytherapy
>r. memory

removable
>r. bridge
>r. partial denture

ren, pl. **renes**

renal
>r. adenocarcinoma
>r. agenesis
>r. amyloidosis
>r. artery
>r. ballottement
>r. blood flow (RBF)
>r. branch of lesser splanchnic nerve
>r. branch of vagus nerve
>r. calculus
>r. capsulotomy
>r. cast
>r. cell carcinoma
>r. colic
>r. collar
>r. column
>r. corpuscle
>r. cortex
>r. cortical adenoma
>r. cortical lobule
>r. cortical scan
>r. diabetes
>r. epistaxis
>r. failure
>r. fascia
>r. fibrocystic osteosis
>r. ganglia
>r. glycosuria
>r. hematuria
>r. hemorrhage
>r. hypertension
>r. hypoplasia
>r. impression on liver
>r. impression of spleen
>r. infantilism
>r. insufficiency
>r. labyrinth
>r. lobe
>r. medulla
>r. nanism
>r. osteitis fibrosa
>r. osteodystrophy
>r. papilla
>r. papillary necrosis
>r. pelvis
>r. plasma flow (RPF)
>r. plexus
>r. portal system
>r. pyramid
>r. reflex
>renal carbuncle
>r. retinopathy
>r. rickets
>r. segment
>r. sinus
>r. surface of spleen
>r. surface of suprarenal gland
>r. threshold
>r. transplantation
>r. tubular acidosis
>r. vein

renal-splanchnic steal
renal-splenic venous shunt
renaturation
Renaut body
renculus
Rendu-Osler-Weber syndrome
renes (*pl. of* ren)
renicapsule
renicardiac
reniculus, pl. **reniculi**
reniform pelvis
renin
renin-angiotensin-aldosterone system
renin-angiotensin system
reninism
>primary r.

reniportal
rennase
rennet
rennin
renninogen, rennogen
renocutaneous
renogastric
renogenic
renogram
renography
renointestinal
renomegaly
renopathy
renoprival
renopulmonary
renotrophic
renotrophin
renotropic
renotropin
renovascular hypertension
Renpenning syndrome
ren. sem.
Renshaw cell
renunculus
Reoviridae
REO virus
Reovirus
reovirus-like agent
repair
>chemical r.
>r. enzyme
>error-prone r.
>excision r.
>mismatch r.
>recombinatorial r.
>SOS r.

repand
reparative
>r. dentin
>r. giant cell granuloma
>r. granuloma

repellent
reperfusion injury

R

repetition
  r. rate
  r. time (TR)
repetition-compulsion principle
repetitive
  r. DNA
  r. strain disorder
  r. stress disorder
replacement
  r. bone
  cephalic r.
  r. fibrosis
  r. therapy
replant
replantation
  intentional r.
repletion
replica plating
replicase
replicate
replication
  bidirectional r.
  conservative r.
  semiconservative r.
  r. site
  unidirectional r.
replicative
  r. form
  r. intermediate
replicator
replicon
repolarization
reportable disease
reporting bias
repositio
reposition
repositioning
  gingival r.
  jaw r.
  muscle r.
repositor
representation
  internal r.
repressed
repressible enzyme
repression
  catabolite r.
  end product r.
  enzyme r.
  primal r.
repressor
  active r.
  r. gene
  inactive r.
reproducibility
reproduction
  asexual r.
  cytogenic r.
  sexual r.
  somatic r.
  vegetative r.
reproductive
  r. assimilation
  r. cycle

  r. nucleus
  r. system
reptilase
Reptilia
repullulation
repulsion
required arch length
requirement
  minimum protein r.
  quantum r.
RES
  reticuloendothelial system
resazurin
rescinnamine
research
resect
resectable
resection
  abdominoperineal r. (APR)
  gum r.
  loop r.
  muscle r.
  root r.
  scleral r.
  transurethral r.
  wedge r.
resectoscope
  r. electrode
  r. sheath
reserpine
reserve
  r. air
  alkali r.
  breathing r.
  cardiac r.
  r. force
  r. tooth germ
reservoir
  r. bag
  r. host
  r. of infection
  Ommaya r.
  Pecquet r.
  r. of spermatozoa
  vitelline r.
reset nodus sinuatrialis
resident physician
residua (*pl. of* residuum)
residual
  r. abscess
  r. affinity
  r. air
  r. body
  r. body of Regaud
  r. capacity
  r. cleft
  r. cyst
  r. error
  r. inhibition
  r. inhibitor
  r. lumen
  r. ovary syndrome
  r. ridge
  r. schizophrenia

r. urine
r. volume (RV)
residue
day r.
r. remaining after percolation of a
drug (marc)
residuum, pl. residua
resilience
resin
r. acid
acrylic r.
activated r.
anion-exchange r.
autopolymer r.
autopolymerizing r.
carbacrylamine r.
cation-exchange r.
r. cement
chemically cured r.
cholestyramine r.
cold cure r.
cold-curing r.
composite r.
copolymer r.
cross-linked r.
direct filling r.
dual-cure r.
epoxy r.
gum r.
heat-curing r.
Indian podophyllum r.
ion-exchange r.
ipomea r.
jalap r.
light-activated r.
light-cured r.
melamine r.
methacrylate r.
podophyllum r.
polyamine-methylene r.
polyester r.
quick cure r.
quinine carbacrylic r.
self-curing r.
resinates
resines
resinic acid
resinoid
resinol
resinous
resistance
airway r.
bacteriophage r.
dicumarol r.
drug r.
expiratory r.
r. factor
r. form
impact r.
inductive r.
insulin r.
multidrug r.
mutual r.
peripheral r.
r. plasmid

r. pyrometer
synaptic r.
systemic vascular r.
r. thermometer
thyrotropin r.
total peripheral r. (TPR)
resistance-inducing factor (RIF)
resistance-transfer factor (RTF)
resistance-transferring episome
resistant ovary syndrome
resistive movement
resistivity
resistor
resolution acuity
resolvase
resolve
resolvent
resolving power
resonance
amphoric r.
bandbox r.
bellmetal r.
cavernous r.
cracked-pot r.
electron paramagnetic r. (EPR)
electron spin r.
hydatid r.
nuclear magnetic r. (NMR)
skodaic r.
r. theory of hearing
tympanitic r.
vesicular r.
vesiculotympanitic r.
vocal r. (VR)
wooden r.
resonant frequency
resonator
resorb
resorcin
resorcinol
r. monoacetate
r. phthalic anhydride
r. test
resorcinolphthalein sodium
resorption
r. atelectasis
bone r.
gingival r.
horizontal r.
internal r.
r. lacunae
ridge r.
root r.
respirable
r. aerosol
respiration
abdominal r.
aerobic r.
amphoric r.
anaerobic r.
artificial r.
assisted r.
Biot r.
bronchial r.
bronchovesicular r.

respiration *(continued)*
    cavernous r.
    Cheyne-Stokes r.
    cogwheel r.
    controlled r.
    costal r.
    diffusion r.
    electrophrenic r.
    external r.
    forced r.
    internal r.
    interrupted r.
    jerky r.
    Kussmaul r.
    Kussmaul-Kien r.
    labored r.
    mouth-to-mouth r.
    nitrate r.
    paradoxical r.
    puerile r.
    stertorous r.
    sulfate r.
    thoracic r.
    tissue r.
    tubular r.
    vesicular r.
    vesiculocavernous r.

respirator
    cuirass r.
    Drinker r.
    pressure-controlled r.
    tank r.
    volume-controlled r.

respiratory
    r. acidosis
    r. airway
    r. alkalosis
    r. apparatus
    r. arrhythmia
    r. ataxia
    r. bronchioles
    r. burst
    r. capacity
    r. center
    r. chain
    r. coefficient
    r. dead space
    r. distress syndrome of the newborn
    r. distress syndrome type II
    r. enteric orphan virus
    r. enzyme
    r. epithelium
    r. exchange ratio
    r. failure
    r. frequency
    r. gating
    r. hippus
    r. inhibitor
    r. insufficiency
    r. lobule
    r. metabolism
    r. metal
    r. minute volume (RMV)
    r. mucosa

    r. murmur
    r. pause
    r. pigment
    r. poison
    r. pulse
    r. quotient (RQ)
    r. rate
    r. region of mucosa of nasal cavity
    r. region of tunica mucosa of nose
    r. scleroma
    r. sound
    r. syncytial virus
    r. system
    r. therapy
    r. tract

respire

respirometer
    Dräger r.
    Wright r.

respirophasic pain

respondent
    r. behavior
    r. conditioning

response
    acute phase r.
    anamnestic r.
    auditory brainstem r. (ABR)
    automatic auditory brainstem r.
    r. bias
    biphasic r.
    blink r.
    booster r.
    brainstem auditory evoked r.
     (BAER)
    brainstem evoked r. (BSER)
    conditioned r.
    Cushing r.
    depletion r.
    early-phase r.
    evoked r.
    flight or fight r.
    galvanic skin r. (GSR)
    Henry-Gauer r.
    r. hierarchy
    immune r.
    isomorphic r.
    late auditory-evoked r.
    late-phase r.
    level-dependent frequency r.
    middle latency r.
    myotonic r.
    oculomotor r.
    orienting r.
    postural sway r.
    primary immune r.
    psychogalvanic r. (PGR)
    psychogalvanic skin r.
    recruiting r.
    relaxation r.
    secondary immune r.
    somatosensory evoked r. (SER)
    sonomotor r.
    stringent r.
    target r.
    triple r.

unconditioned r.
visual evoked r. (VER)
response-produced cue
rest
    adrenal r.
    r. area
    bed r.
    r. bite
    r. body
    cingulum r.
    incisal r.
    r. jaw relation
    lingual r.
    Malassez epithelial r.
    Marchand r.
    mesonephric r.
    r. nitrogen
    occlusal r.
    r. pain
    r. position
    precision r.
    r. seat
    r. of Serres
    r. vertical dimension
    Walthard cell r.
    wolffian r.
restenosis
restiform
    r. body
    r. eminence
resting
    r. cell
    r. length
    r. saliva
    r. stage
    r. tidal volume
    r. tremor
    r. wandering cell
restitope
restitution
restless
    r. leg
    r. leg syndrome
Reston virus
restoration
    acid-etched r.
    combination r.
    compound r.
    direct acrylic r.
    direct composite resin r.
    overhanging r.
    permanent r.
    provisional r.
    root canal r.
    silicate r.
    temporary r.
restorative
    r. dental material
    r. dentistry
restored cycle
restrained beam
restraint
restriction
    asymmetric fetal growth r.
    r. endonuclease

R

    r. enzyme
    fetal growth r.
    r. fragment length polymorphism
    (RFLP)
    lactase r.
    r. length polymorphism
    r. map
    r. methylation
    MHC r.
    r. site
    symmetric fetal growth r.
restriction-site polymorphism
restrictive cardiomyopathy
restructured cell
resuscitate
    do not r.
resuscitation
    cardiopulmonary r. (CPR)
    mouth-to-mouth r.
retained
    r. menstruation
    r. placenta
    r. products of conception
retainer
    continuous bar r.
    direct r.
    extracoronal r.
    Hawley r.
    indirect r.
    intracoronal r.
    matrix r.
    space r.
retardate
retardation
    intrauterine growth r.
    mental r.
    psychomotor r.
    viscoelastic r.
retarded dentition
retarder
retch
retching
rete, pl. **retia**
    r. acromiale arteriae
      thoracoacromialis
    r. arteriosum
    r. articulare cubiti
    r. articulare genus
    r. calcaneum
    r. canalis hypoglossi
    r. carpale dorsale
    r. carpi posterius
    r. cord
    r. cutaneum corii
    r. cyst of ovary
    r. foraminis ovalis
    Haller r.
    r. halleri
    r. malleolare laterale
    r. malleolare mediale
    malpighian r.
    r. mirabile
    r. ovarii
    r. patellare
    r. peg

rete (*continued*)
   r. ridge
   r. subpapillare
   r. testis
   r. vasculosum articulare
   r. venosum dorsale manus
   r. venosum dorsale pedis
   r. venosum plantare
retention
   r. area
   r. arm
   r. cyst
   denture r.
   direct r.
   r. form
   r. groove
   indirect r.
   r. jaundice
   partial denture r.
   r. point
   r. polyp
   r. suture
   r. vomiting
retentive
   r. circumferential clasp arm
   r. fulcrum line
retia (*pl. of* rete)
retial
reticula (*pl. of* reticulum)
reticular, reticulated
   r. activating system (RAS)
   r. bone
   r. cartilage
   r. cell
   r. corpuscle
   r. degeneration
   r. erythematous mucinosis
   r. fiber
   r. formation
   r. lamina
   r. layer of corium
   r. membrane of spinal organ
   r. nucleus of the brainstem
   r. nucleus of medulla oblongata
   r. nucleus of mesencephalon
   r. nucleus of pons
   r. nucleus of thalamus
   r. substance
   r. tissue
reticularis cell
reticulation
reticulin
reticulocyte
reticulocytopenia
reticulocytosis
reticuloendothelial
   r. cell
   r. system (RES)
reticuloendothelioma
reticuloendothelium
reticulohistiocytoma
reticulohistiocytosis
   multicentric r.

reticuloid
   actinic r.
reticulonodular pattern
reticulopenia
reticulosis
   benign inoculation r.
   leukemic r.
   malignant midline r.
   midline malignant reticulosis r.
   pagetoid r.
   polymorphic r.
reticulospinal tract
reticulotomy
reticulum, pl. **reticula**
   agranular endoplasmic r.
   r. cell sarcoma
   Ebner r.
   endoplasmic r. (ER)
   Golgi internal r.
   granular endoplasmic r.
   Kölliker r.
   rough-surfaced endoplasmic r.
   sarcoplasmic r.
   smooth-surfaced endoplasmic r.
   stellate r.
   trabecular r.
   r. trabeculare sclerae
   trans-Golgi r.
retiform
   r. cartilage
   r. tissue
retina
   detached r.
   detachment of r.
   flecked r.
   fleck r. of Kandori
   leopard r.
   shot-silk r.
   tigroid r.
retinaculum, pl. **retinacula**
   antebrachial flexor r.
   r. of articular capsule of hip
   r. capsulae articularis coxae
   caudal r.
   r. caudale
   r. cutis
   r. cutis mammae
   extensor r.
   retinacula of extensor muscle
   flexor r.
   flexor r. of forearm
   flexor r. of lower limb
   r. of flexor muscle
   inferior extensor r.
   inferior r. of extensor muscle
   inferior fibular r.
   inferior peroneal r.
   lateral patellar r.
   medial patellar r.
   Morgagni r.
   r. musculorum extensorum
   r. musculorum extensorum inferius
   r. musculorum extensorum superius
   r. musculorum fibularium
   r. musculorum fibularium inferius

r. musculorum fibularium superius
r. musculorum flexorum
r. musculorum flexorum membri inferioris
r. musculorum peroneorum
r. musculorum peroneorum inferius
r. musculorum peroneorum superius
retinacula of nail
r. patellae laterale
r. patellae mediale
patellar r.
peroneal r.
retinacula of peroneal muscle
r. of skin
superior extensor r.
superior r. of extensor muscle
superior fibular r.
superior peroneal r.
suspensory r. of breast
r. tendinum
retinacula unguis

retinal
r. adaptation
r. anlage tumor
r. blood vessel
r. camera
r. cones
r. dehydrogenase
r. detachment
r. disparity
r. dysplasia
r. embolism
r. fold
r. image
r. isomerase
r. migraine
r. reductase

11-*cis*-retinal
***trans*-retinal**
retinaldehyde
r. dehydrogenase
r. isomerase
r. reductase

retinectomy
retinene
r.-1
r.-2

retinitis
albuminuric r.
circinate r.
diabetic r.
r. exudativa
exudative r.
leukemic r.
metastatic r.
neuropathy, ataxia, r. pigmentosa (NARP)
r. pigmentosa
r. proliferans
punctate r.
purulent r.
r. sclopetaria
secondary r.
septic r.
serous r.

simple r.
r. syphilitica, syphilitic r.
retinoblastoma
retinochoroid
retinochoroiditis
bird shot r.
r. juxtapapillaris
retinodialysis
retinoic
retinoic acid
retinoic acid receptor
13-*cis*-retinoic acid
retinoid X receptor
retinol
r. dehydrogenase
11-*cis*-retinol
retinol-binding protein
retinopapillitis
r. of premature infants
retinopathy
arteriosclerotic r.
central angiospastic r.
central serous r.
circinate r.
compression r.
diabetic r.
dysproteinemic r.
electric r.
external exudative r.
hypertensive r.
Leber idiopathic stellate r.
leukemic r.
lipemic r.
macular r.
pigmentary r.
r. of prematurity
proliferative r.
r. punctata albescens
Purtscher r.
renal r.
rubella r.
sickle cell r.
solar r.
toxemic r. of pregnancy
toxic r.
transient r.
traumatic r.
venous-stasis r.
whiplash r.
retinopexy
fluid r.
gas r.
pneumatic r.
retinopiesis
retinoschisis
juvenile r.
senile r.
retinoscope
luminous r.
reflecting r.
retinoscopy
cylinder r.
fogging r.
retinotomy
retinyl phosphate

retoperithelium
retort
Retortamonas
retract
retractile testis
retraction
    gingival r.
    mandibular r.
    r. pocket
    r. syndrome
retractor
    Desmarres r.
retrad
retrahens
    r. aurem
    r. auriculam
retreat from reality
retrenchment
retrieval
retroactive inhibition
retroadductor space
retroauricular
    r. fold
    r. lymph node
retrobuccal
retrobulbar
    r. abscess
    r. anesthesia
    r. fat
    r. neuritis
retrocalcaneal bursa
retrocalcaneobursitis
retrocaval ureter
retrocecal
    r. abscess
    r. lymph node
    r. recess
retrocedent gout
retrocervical
retrocession
retrochiasmatic area
retroclusion
retrocochlear hearing loss
retrocolic
retrocollic
retroconduction
retrocursive
retrocuspid papilla
retrodeviation
retrodisplacement
retroduodenal
    r. artery
    r. fossa
    r. recess
retroesophageal
retrofilling
retroflected
retroflection
retroflex
    r. bundle of Meynert
    r. fasciculus
retroflexed
retroflexion of iris

retrogasserian
    r. neurectomy
    r. neurotomy
retrognathic
retrognathism
retrograde
    r. amnesia
    r. aortography
    r. beat
    r. block
    r. cardioplegia
    r. chromatolysis
    r. cystourethrogram
    r. degeneration
    r. ejaculation
    r. embolism
    r. hernia
    r. intussusception
    r. memory
    r. menstruation
    r. metamorphosis
    r. P wave
    r. pyelography
    r. urography
    r. VA conduction
retrography
retrogression
retrohyoid bursa
retroiliac ureter
retroinguinal space
retroinhibition
retroiridian
retrojection
retrojector
retrolental fibroplasia
retrolenticular
    r. limb of internal capsule
    r. part of internal capsule
retrolentiform limb of internal capsule
retrolingual
retromammary mastitis
retromandibular
    r. fossa
    r. process of parotid gland
    r. vein
retromastoid
retromolar
    r. fossa
    r. pad
    r. triangle
retromorphosis
retromylohyoid space
retronasal
retro-ocular
retroperitoneal
    r. fibrosis
    r. hernia
    r. space
    r. vein
retroperitoneum
retroperitonitis
    idiopathic fibrous r.
retropharyngeal
    r. abscess

r. lymph node
r. space
retropharynx
retroplacental
retroplasia
retroposed
retroposition
retroposon
retroposterior lateral nucleus
retropubic
r. hernia
r. space
retropulsion
retropyloric lymph node
retrorectal
r. lamina of endopelvic fascia
r. lamina of hypogastric sheath
retrosigmoid approach
retrospection
retrospective falsification
retrospondylolisthesis
retrosternal
r. hernia
r. space
retrosteroid
retrotarsal fold
retrouterine
retroversioflexion
retroversion
retroverted
retroviral vector
Retroviridae
retrovirus
retrozonular space
retrusion
retrusive
r. excursion
r. occlusion
Rett syndrome
return
r. extrasystole
partial anomalous pulmonary
venous r. (PAPVR)
total anomalous pulmonary
venous r. (TAPVR)
venous r.
returning cycle
Retzius
R. cavity
R. fiber
R. gyrus
R. ligament
R. space
R. stria
R. veins
reunient
Reuss
R. formula
R. test
revaccination
revascularization
reverberating circuit
reverberation
Reverdin graft

reversal
adrenaline r.
epinephrine r.
narcotic r.
pressure r.
sex r.
reverse
r. banding
r. bevel
r. curve
r. Eck fistula
r. genetics
r. Kingsley splint
r. mutation
r. osmosis
r. passive hemagglutination
r. pupillary block
r. transcriptase
r. transcriptase polymerase chain
reaction (RT-PCR)
r. transcription
r. Trendelenburg position
r. triodothyronine (RT$_3$)
reversed
r. anaphylaxis
r. coarctation
r. paradoxical pulse
r. passive anaphylaxis
r. peristalsis
r. phase chromatography
r. Prausnitz-Küstner reaction
r. reciprocal rhythm
r. shunt
reversed-three sign
reversible
r. calcinosis
r. colloid
r. decortication
r. hydrocolloid
r. pulpitis
r. reaction
r. shock
reversion
revertant
review
drug utilization r.
Revilliod sign
revised
R. European-American Classification
of Lymphoid Neoplasms (REAL)
revivescence
revivification
revolutions per minute (rpm)
revulsion
reward
rewarming
Reye syndrome
Reymond
Reynolds
R. number
R. pentad
RF
releasing factor
RFA
right frontoanterior position

R

RFLP
> restriction fragment length polymorphism

RFP
> right frontoposterior position

RFT
> right frontotransverse position

RH
> releasing hormone

Rh
> R. antigen
> R. antigen incompatibility
> R. blocking test
> R. factor
> R. null syndrome

Rha
> l-rhamnose

rhabarberone
rhabditiform larva
Rhabditis-like
rhabdocyte
rhabdoid
rhabdomyoblast
rhabdomyolysis
> acute recurrent r.
> exertional r.
> familial paroxysmal r.
> idiopathic paroxysmal r.

rhabdomyoma
rhabdomyosarcoma
> embryonal r.

rhabdophobia
rhabdosarcoma
rhabdosphincter
Rhabdoviridae
rhabdovirus
Rhadinovirus
rhagades
rhagadiform
rhagiocrine cell
L-rhamnose (Rha)
rhamnoside
rhamnoxanthin
Rhamnus
rhaphania
rhaphe
RH$_o$(D)
> R. immune globulin

Rh$_o$(D) immunoglobulin
rhe
rhegma
rhegmatogenous
> r. retinal detachment

rheic
Rheinberg microscope
rhenium (Re)
rheobase
rheobasic
rheocardiography
rheochrysidin
rheoencephalogram
rheoencephalography
rheogram
rheologist
rheology
rheometer

rheometry
rheopexy
rheostat
rheostosis
rheotaxis
rheotropism
Rhese projection
rhestocythemia
rhesus disease
Rhesus factor
rheum
rheumatalgia
rheumatic
> r. arteritis
> r. carditis
> r. chorea
> r. endocarditis
> r. fever
> r. heart disease
> r. pericarditis
> r. pneumonia
> r. valvulitis

rheumatid
rheumatism
> articular r.
> cerebral r.
> chronic r.
> gonorrheal r.
> r. of the heart
> inflammatory r.
> Macleod r.
> muscular r.
> nodose r.
> subacute r.
> tuberculous r.

rheumatismal
rheumatoid
> r. arteritis
> r. arthritis
> r. disease
> r. factor
> r. nodule
> r. pocket
> r. spondylitis

rheumatologist
rheumatology
rhigotic
rhIL-11
> recombinant human interleukin-11

rhinal
> r. fissure
> r. sulcus

rhinalgia
rhinedema
rhinencephalic
rhinencephalon
rhinenchysis
rhinion
rhinism
rhinitis
> acute r.
> allergic r.
> atrophic r.
> r. caseosa
> caseous r.

chronic r.
gangrenous r.
hypertrophic r.
r. medicamentosa
scrofulous r.
r. sicca
vasomotor r.
rhinoanemometer
rhinocele
rhinocephaly, rhinocephalia
Rhinocladiella
rhinocleisis
rhinodymia
rhinodynia
rhinoestrosis
Rhinoestrus purpureus
rhinogenous
rhinokyphosis
rhinolalia
r. aperta
r. clausa
rhinolite
rhinolith
rhinolithiasis
rhinologic
rhinologist
rhinology
rhinomanometer
rhinomanometry
rhinomycosis
rhinonecrosis
rhinopathy
rhinopharyngeal
rhinopharyngolith
rhinopharynx
rhinophonia
rhinophyma
rhinoplasty
rhinopneumonitis
rhinorrhea
cerebrospinal fluid r.
gustatory r.
rhinosalpingitis
rhinoscleroma
rhinoscope
rhinoscopic
rhinoscopy
anterior r.
median r.
posterior r.
rhinosinusitis
rhinosporidiosis
Rhinosporidium seeberi
rhinostenosis
rhinotomy
rhinotracheitis
Rhinovirus
bovine r.'s
equine r.'s
rhinovirus
Rhipicephalus sanguineus
rhizoid
rhizome
rhizomelia

rhizomelic
r. chondrodysplasia punctata
r. dwarfism
rhizomeningomyelitis
Rhizomucor
rhizoplast
Rhizopoda
Rhizopodasida
Rhizopodea
rhizopterin
Rhizopus
rhizotomy
anterior r.
facet r.
posterior r.
trigeminal r.
rho, ρ
r. factor
rhodamine B
rhodanate
rhodanese
rhodanic acid
rhodanile blue
rhodeose
Rhodesian trypanosomiasis
rhodin
rhodium
Rhodnius
r. prolixus
Rhodococcus equi
rhodogenesis
rhodophylactic
rhodophylaxis
rhodopsin
meta-r. I. II, III
r. kinase
Rhodotorula
rhombencephalic
r. gustatory nucleus
r. isthmus
r. tegmentum
rhombencephalon
rhombic
r. groove
r. lip
rhomboatloideus
rhombocele
rhomboid, rhomboidal
r. fossa
r. impression
r. ligament
r. major muscle
r. minor muscle
r. sinus
rhomboideus
rhombomere
rhonchal, rhonchial
r. fremitus
rhonchus, pl. **rhonchi**
cavernous r.
sibilant r.
sonorous r.
rhopheocytosis
rhoptry, pl. **rhoptries**
rhotacism

R

rhubarb
Rhus
- *R.* dermatitis
- *R. toxicodendron* antigen
- *R. venenata* antigen

rhypophobia
rhythm
- agonal r.
- alpha r.
- atrioventricular junctional r.
- AV junctional r.
- basic electrical r. (BER)
- Berger r.
- beta r.
- bigeminal r.
- cantering r.
- chaotic r.
- circadian r.
- circus r.
- coronary nodal r.
- coronary sinus r.
- coupled r.
- delta r.
- diurnal r.
- ectopic r.
- escape r.
- gallop r.
- idiojunctional r.
- idionodal r.
- idioventricular r.
- junctional r.
- lower nodal r.
- r. method
- nodal r.
- pendulum r.
- quadrigeminal r.
- quadruple r.
- reciprocal r.
- reciprocating r.
- reversed reciprocal r.
- sinus r.
- systolic gallop r.
- theta r.
- tic-tac r.
- trainwheel r.
- trigeminal r.
- triple r.
- ultradian r.
- upper nodal r.
- ventricular r.

rhythmic chorea
rhytide
rhytidectomy
rhytidoplasty
rhytidosis
- r. retinae

RIA
- radioimmunoassay

rib
- rib notching
- r. spreader

Ribas-Torres disease
ribavirin
ribbon
- r. arch
- r. arch appliance
- Reil r.

Ribes ganglion
ribitol
ribityl
rib [I–XII]
- bicipital r.
- bifid r.
- cervical r.
- false r.
- first r. [I]
- floating r. [XI–XII]
- lumbar r.
- slipping r.
- true r. [I–VII]
- vertebral r.
- vertebrochondral r.
- vertebrosternal r.

riboflavin, riboflavine
- r. deficiency
- r. kinase
- methylol r.
- r. unit

riboflavin 5′-phosphate
ribofuranose
9-β-D-ribofuranosyladenine
1-β-D-ribofuranosylcytosine
9-β-D-ribofuranosylguanine
9-β-ribofuranosylpurine
ribofuranosylthymine
1-β-D-ribofuranosyluracil
ribo-2-hexulose
ribonuclease (RNase)
- RNase α
- RNase A
- alkaline RNase
- *Bacillus subtilis* r.
- r. D (RNase D)
- *Escherichia coli* RNase I
- RNase I, II, III
- microbial RNase II
- RNase N_1, N_2
- RNase P
- pancreatic r.
- pancreatic RNase
- plant RNase
- RNase T_1. T_2
- RNase U_2. U_4
- yeast RNase

ribonucleic acid (RNA)
- acceptor RNA
- antisense RNA
- chromosomal RNA
- heterogeneous nuclear RNA (hnRNA)
- informational RNA
- initiation tRNA
- messenger RNA
- messengerlike RNA (mlRNA)
- nuclear RNA (nRNA)
- RNA polymerase
- ribosomal r. a. (rRNA)
- ribosomal RNA
- small nuclear RNA (snRNA)
- soluble RNA (sRNA)

starter tRNA
suppressor tRNA
template RNA
transfer RNA (tRNA)
ribonucleinase
ribonucleoprotein (RNP)
ribonucleoside
ribonucleotide reductase
ribophorins
ribopyranose
ribose
ribose-5-phosphate
riboside
ribosomal ribonucleic acid (rRNA)
ribosomal RNA
ribosome
ribosome-lamella complex
ribosuria
ribosyl
ribosylation
ADP r.
1-ribosylorotate
ribosylpurine
ribosylthymidine
ribothymidine (Thd)
ribothymidine 5′-diphosphate (TDP)
ribothymidylic acid (rTMP, TMP)
ribotide
Ribot law of memory
ribovirus
ribozyme
ribulose
ribulose-1,5-bisphosphate carboxylase
ribulose-phosphate 3-epimerase
Ricco law
rice
r. body
r. diet
r. disease
r. itch
r. starch
rice-field fever
rice-Tween agar
rice-water stool
Richards-Rundle syndrome
Richter
R. hernia
R. syndrome
Richter-Monro line
ricin
ricin-blocked antibody
ricinism
ricinoleate
ricinoleic acid
rickets
acute r.
adult r.
celiac r.
familial hypophosphatemic r.
hemorrhagic r.
hereditary hypophosphatemic r.
late r.
refractory r.
renal r.

scurvy r.
vitamin D-resistant r.
Rickettsia
R. *africae*
R. *akari*
R. *australis*
R. *burnetii*
R. *canis*
R. *conorii*
R. *honei*
R. *japonica*
R. *mooseri*
R. *prowazekii*
R. *psittaci*
R. *rickettsii*
R. *sennetsu*
R. *sibirica*
R. *slovaca*
R. *tsutsugamushi*
R. *typhi*
R. vaccine, attenuated
rickettsial
rickettsialpox
rickettsiosis
vesicular r.
rickettsiostatic
rickety
Rickles test
RID
radial immunodiffusion
Rida virus
Riddoch phenomenon
Rideal-Walker
R.-W. coefficient
R.-W. method
Ridell operation
rider's
r. bone
r. bursa
r. leg
r. muscle
ridge
alveolar r.
apical ectodermal r.
basal r.
bicipital r.
buccocervical r.
buccogingival r.
bulbar r.
bulboventricular r.
dental r.
dermal r.
epidermal r.
epipericardial r.
r. extension
external oblique r.
ganglion r.
genital r.
gluteal r.
gonadal r.
interpapillary r.
key r.
lateral epicondylar r.
lateral supracondylar r.
lateral supraepicondylar r.

ridge *(continued)*
  linguocervical r.
  linguogingival r.
  Mall r.
  mammary r.
  marginal r.
  medial epicondylar r.
  medial supracondylar r.
  medial supraepicondylar r.
  mesonephric r.
  milk r.
  mylohyoid r.
  nasal r.
  oblique r.
  oblique r. of trapezium
  palatine r.
  papillary r.
  Passavant r.
  pectoral r.
  pharyngeal r.
  primitive r.
  pronator r.
  pterygoid r. of sphenoid bone
  pulmonary r.
  r. relation
  residual r.
  r. resorption
  rete r.
  skin r.
  sphenoidal r.
  superciliary r.
  supplemental r.
  supraorbital r.
  taste r.
  temporal r.
  transverse r.
  transverse palatine r.
  transverse r. of sacrum
  trapezoid r.
  triangular r.
  urogenital r.
  wolffian r.

riding embolism

Ridley
  R. circle
  R. sinus

Riedel
  R. disease
  R. lobe
  R. struma
  R. thyroiditis

Rieder
  R. cell
  R. cell leukemia
  R. lymphocyte

Riegel pulse

Rieger
  R. anomaly
  R. syndrome

Riehl melanosis

RIF
  resistance-inducing factor

rifampicin

rifampin

rifamycin, rifomycin

Rift
  R. Valley fever
  R. Valley fever virus

Riga-Fede disease

right
  r. angle clamp
  r. anterior lateral hepatic segment [VI]
  r. anterior medial hepatic segment [V]
  r. atrial branch of right coronary artery
  r. atrioventricular orifice
  r. atrioventricular valve
  r. atrium of heart
  r. auricle
  r. auricular appendage
  r. axis deviation
  r. border of heart
  r. branch
  r. branch of hepatic artery proper
  r. branch of portal vein
  r. bundle of atrioventricular bundle
  r. colic artery
  r. colic flexure
  r. colic lymph node
  r. colic vein
  r. coronary artery
  r. crus of atrioventricular bundle
  r. crus of diaphragm
  r. descending pulmonary artery (RDPA)
  r. duct of caudate lobe of liver
  r. eye (R.E.)
  r. fibrous trigone
  r. flexural artery
  r. frontoanterior position (RFA)
  r. frontoposterior position (RFP)
  r. frontotransverse position (RFT)
  r. gastric artery
  r. gastric lymph node
  r. gastric vein
  r. gastroepiploic artery
  r. gastroepiploic lymph node
  r. gastroepiploic vein
  r. gastroomental artery
  r. gastroomental lymph node
  r. gastroomental vein
  r. heart
  r. heart bypass
  r. hepatic artery
  r. hepatic duct
  r. hepatic vein
  r. inferior pulmonary vein
  r. lateral division of liver
  r. and left fibrous rings of heart
  r. or left lateral decubitus film
  r. and left pulmonary surface of heart
  r. and left ventricles of heart
  r. liver
  r. lobe
  r. lobe of liver
  r. lower lobe (RLL)

r. lower quadrant (RLQ)
r. lumbar lymph node
r. lymphatic duct
r. main bronchus
r. marginal branch
r. margin of heart
r. medial division of liver
r. mentoanterior position (RMA)
r. mentoposterior position (RMP)
r. mentotransverse position (RMT)
r. middle lobe (RML)
r. occipitoanterior position (ROA)
r. occipitoposterior position (ROP)
r. occipitotransverse position (ROT)
r. ovarian vein
r. parasternal impulse
r. part of diaphragmatic surface of liver
r. part of liver
r. posterior lateral hepatic segment [VII]
r. posterior medial hepatic segment [VIII]
r. posterior oblique (RPO)
r. pulmonary artery
r. sacroanterior position (RSA)
r. sacroposterior position (RSP)
r. sacrotransverse position (RST)
r. sagittal fissure
r. splicing junction
r. superior intercostal vein
r. superior pulmonary vein
r. suprarenal vein
r. testicular vein
r. triangular ligament of liver
r. upper lobe (RUL)
r. upper quadrant (RUQ)
r. ventricle
r. ventricular failure
r. ventricular hypoplasia

right-eyed
right-footed
right-handed
righting reflex
right-to-left shunt
rigid

r. connector
r. dysarthria

rigidity

cadaveric r.
catatonic r.
cerebellar r.
clasp-knife r.
cogwheel r.
decerebrate r.
decorticate r.
lead-pipe r.
nuchal r.
ocular r.
postmortem r.
scleral r.

rigor

acid r.
calcium r.
heat r.

r. mortis
myocardial r. mortis

Riley-Day syndrome
riluzole
rim

bite r.
occlusal r.
occlusion r.
orbital r.
record r.

rima, pl. **rimae**

r. glottidis
r. oris
r. palpebrarum
r. pudendi
r. respiratoria
r. vestibuli
r. vocalis
r. vulvae

rimantadine
Rimini test
rimose
rimula
Rindfleisch fold
ring

abdominal r.
r. abscess
amnion r.
annuloplasty r.
anterior limiting r.
Balbani r.
benzene r.
Bickel r.
Cannon r.
cardiac lymphatic r.
casting r.
choroidal r.
r. chromosome
ciliary r.
common tendinous r. of extraocular muscle
r. compound
conjunctival r.
constriction r.
crural r.
deep inguinal r.
r. enhancement
external inguinal r.
femoral r.
fibrocartilaginous r. of tympanic membrane
fibrous r.
fibrous r. of intervertebral disk
r. finger
Fleischer r.
Fleischer-Strümpell r.
Flieringa r.
gestational r.
glaucomatous r.
Graefenberg r.
greater r. of iris
internal inguinal r.
r. of iris
Kayser-Fleischer r.
lesser r. of iris

ring *(continued)*
    Liesegang r.
    r. ligament
    Lower r.
    lymphatic r. of cardiac part of stomach
    neonatal r.
    pathologic retraction r.
    r. pessary
    pharyngeal lymphatic r.
    physiologic retraction r.
    polar r.
    r. precipitin test
    right and left fibrous r.'s of heart
    Schatzki r.
    Schwalbe r.
    scleral r.
    r. scotoma
    signet r.
    r. of Soemmerring
    subcutaneous r.
    superficial inguinal r.
    r. syringe
    tonsillar r.
    tracheal r.
    tympanic r.
    r. ulcer of cornea
    umbilical r.
    vascular r.
    Vieussens r.
    Vossius lenticular r.
    Waldeyer throat r.
    Zinn r.
ringed hair
Ringer
    R. injection
    R. lactate
    R. solution
ring-knife
ringlike corneal dystrophy
ring-shaped placenta
ring-wall lesion
ringworm
    r. of beard
    black-dot r.
    r. of body
    crusted r.
    r. of foot
    honeycomb r.
    r. of nails
    Oriental r.
    r. of scalp
    scaly r.
    Tokelau r.
Rinne test
Riolan
    R. anastomosis
    R. arc
    R. arcade
    R. bone
    R. bouquet
    R. muscle
RIP
    radioimmunoprecipitation

riparian
Ripault sign
ripe cataract
ripening
Ripstein operation
RISA
    radioiodinated serum albumin
rise time
risk
    attributable r.
    competing r.
    empiric r.
    r. factor
    radiation r.
    recurrence r.
    relative r.
Risley rotary prism
risorius
    r. muscle
RIST
    radioimmunosorbent test
ristocetin
risus
    r. caninus
    r. sardonicus
Ritgen maneuver
ritodrine
Rittenhouse-Manogian procedure
Ritter opening tetanus
Ritter-Rollet phenomenon
ritual
ritualistic behavior
rituximab
rivalry
    binocular r.
    r. of retina
    sibling r.
Riva-Rocci sphygmomanometer
Rivea corymbosa
river blindness
Rivero-Carvallo effect
Rivers cocktail
Rivière salt
Rivinus
    R. canal
    R. duct
    R. gland
    R. incisure
    R. membrane
    R. notch
rivus lacrimalis
riziform
RLL
    right lower lobe
RLQ
    right lower quadrant
RMA
    right mentoanterior position
RML
    right middle lobe
RMP
    right mentoposterior position
RMT
    right mentotransverse position

R

RMV
respiratory minute volume
RN
registered nurse
Rn
radon
RNA
ribonucleic acid
RNA
R. enzyme
R. splicing
R. tumor virus
R. virus
RNase
ribonuclease
RNase D
ribonuclease d
RNP
ribonucleoprotein
ROA
right occipitoanterior position
Roach clasp
Roaf syndrome
Robert pelvis
Robertshaw tube
robertsonian translocation
Robertson pupil
Roberts syndrome
Robinow
R. dwarfism
R. syndrome
Robinson
R. catheter
R. index
Robin syndrome
Robison
R. ester
R. ester dehydrogenase
Robison-Embden ester
robotic
robustness
ROC
receiver operating characteristic
ROC curve
roccellin
Rochalimaea
R. henselae
R. quintana
Rochelle salt
rocket immunoelectrophoresis
rock oil
Rocky
R. Mountain spotted fever
R. Mountain spotted fever vaccine
rod
analyzing r.
Auer r.
basal r.
r. cell of retina
Corti r.
r. disk
enamel r.
r. fiber
germinal r.
r. granule

Maddox r.
r. monochromatism
r. myopathy
r. nuclear cell
surgical r.
r. vision
Rodentia
rodenticide
rodent ulcer
roentgen (R, r)
r.-equivalent-man (rem)
r.-equivalent-physical
r. ray
r. unit
roentgenkymogram
roentgenkymograph
roentgenkymography
roentgenogram
roentgenograph
roentgenography
roentgenologist
roentgenology
roentgenometer
roentgenometry
roentgenoscope
roentgenoscopy
roentgenotherapy
Roesler-Dressler infarct
roetheln (*var. of* röteln)
Roger
R. Anderson pin fixation appliance
R. bruit
R. disease
R. murmur
R. reflex
Rogers sphygmomanometer
Röhrer index
Rohr stria
Rokitansky
R. disease
R. hernia
R. pelvis
Rokitansky-Aschoff sinus
Rokitansky-Küster-Hauser syndrome
rolandic
r. epilepsy
r. sulcal artery
Rolando
R. angle
R. area
R. cell
R. column
R. gelatinous substance
R. substance
R. tubercle
role
complementary r.
r. conflict
gender r.
noncomplementary r.
sex r.
sick r.
role-playing
rolitetracycline

roll
    iliac r.
    scleral r.
    r. sulfur
    r. tube
roller
    r. bandage
    R. nucleus
rollerball electrode
Rolleston rule
Rollet stroma
rolling circle
roll-tube culture
Romaña sign
Roman fever
Romano-Ward syndrome
Romanowsky blood stain
Romberg
    R. disease
    R. sign
    R. syndrome
    R. test
rombergism
Römer test
rongeur
Rønne nasal step
R-on-T phenomenon
roof
    r. of fourth ventricle
    r. of mouth
    r. nucleus
    r. of orbit
    r. plate
    r. of skull
    r. of tympanic cavity
    r. of tympanum
roofplate
rooming-in
room temperature (RT)
root
    r. abscess
    accessory r. of tooth
    r. amputation
    anatomical r.
    anterior r. of spinal nerve
    r. apex
    r. avulsion
    black r.
    buccal r. of tooth
    r. canal file
    r. canal orifice
    r. canal plugger
    r. canal restoration
    r. canal spreader
    r. canal therapy
    r. canal of tooth
    r. canal treatment
    r. caries
    r. caries index
    clinical r. of tooth
    cochlear r. of VIII nerve
    conjoined nerve r.
    cranial r. of accessory nerve
    Culver r.
    r. dehiscence

    dorsal r. of spinal nerve
    r. end cyst
    r. end granuloma
    facial r.
    r. of facial nerve
    r. filament
    r. of foot
    r. foramen
    hair r.
    inferior r. of ansa cervicalis
    lateral r. of median nerve
    lateral r. of optic tract
    long r. of ciliary ganglion
    r. of lung
    May apple r.
    medial r. of median nerve
    medial r. of optic tract
    r. of mesentery
    motor r. of ciliary ganglion
    motor r. of spinal nerve
    motor r. of trigeminal nerve
    r. of nail
    nasociliary r. of ciliary ganglion
    nerve r.
    r. of nose
    oculomotor r. of ciliary ganglion
    olfactory r.
    r. of olfactory tract
    parasympathetic r. of ciliary ganglion
    parasympathetic r. of otic ganglion
    parasympathetic r. of pelvic ganglion
    parasympathetic r. of pterygopalatine ganglion
    parasympathetic r. of submandibular ganglion
    r. of penis
    r. planing
    posterior r. of spinal nerve
    r. pulp
    r. resection
    r. resorption
    sensory r. of ciliary ganglion
    sensory r. of pterygopalatine ganglion
    sensory r. of spinal nerve
    sensory r. of sublingual ganglion
    sensory r. of submandibular ganglion
    sensory r. of trigeminal nerve
    r. sheath
    short r. of ciliary ganglion
    spinal r. of accessory nerve
    superior r. of ansa cervicalis
    sympathetic r. of ciliary ganglion
    sympathetic r. of otic ganglion
    sympathetic r. of pterygopalatine ganglion
    sympathetic r. of sublingual ganglion
    sympathetic r. of submandibular ganglion
    tegmental r. of tympanic cavity
    r. tip

r. of tongue
r. of tooth
r. of trigeminal nerve
tuberous r.
ventral r. of spinal nerve
vestibular r.
vestibular r. of vestibulocochlear
nerve
root-form implant
rooting reflex
rootlet
ROP
right occipitoposterior position
ropalocytosis
rope burn
Ropes test
Rorschach test
rosacea
granulomatous r.
hypertrophic r.
tuberculoid r.
rosacea-like tuberculid
Rosai-Dorfman disease
rosanilin dye
rosaprostol
rosary
rachitic r.
Roscoe-Bunsen law
Rose
r. bengal
r. bengal radioactive (^{131}I) test
r. cold
r. hip
r. oil
R. position
r. spot
Rose-Bradford kidney
rosemary oil
Rosenbach
R. law
R. sign
R. test
Rosenbach-Gmelin test
Rosenmüller
R. fossa
R. gland
R. node
R. recess
R. valve
Rosenthal
R. canal
R. fiber
R. vein
Rosenthaler-Turk reagent
roseola
epidemic r.
idiopathic r.
r. infantilis, r. infantum
syphilitic r.
roseola infantum (*var. of* roseola
infantilis)
Roser-Nélaton line
rosette
E r.
EAC r.

Homer-Wright r.
r. test
Wintersteiner r.
rosette-forming cell
Rose-Waaler test
rosin
p-**rosolic acid**
Ro spatula
Ross
R. cycle
R. procedure
R. River fever
R. River virus
Ross-Jones test
Rossolimo
R. reflex
R. sign
rostellum
armed r.
unarmed r.
rostra (*pl. of* rostrum)
rostrad
rostral
r. lamina
r. layer
r. neuropore
r. transtentorial herniation
rostralis
rostrate pelvis
rostriform
rostrum, pl. **rostra, rostrums**
r. corporis callosi
r. of corpus callosum
sphenoidal r.
r. sphenoidale
r. of the sphenoid bone
ROT
right occipitotransverse position
rot
rotamase
rotamer
rotameter
rotary joint
rotating
r. anode
r. anode tube
rotation
r. flap
intestinal r.
molecular r.
off-vertical r.
optic r.
specific optic r.
r. therapy
rotational
r. axis
r. nystagmus
rotator
r. cuff of shoulder
medial r.
r. muscle
rotatores
r. cervicis muscle
r. lumborum muscle

R

rotatores *(continued)*
  r. muscle
  r. thoracis muscle
rotatory
  r. nystagmus
  r. tic
rotavirus
Rotch sign
rote learning
röteln, roetheln
rotenone
Rothera nitroprusside test
Rothia
  R. dentocariosa
Rothmund syndrome
Rothmund-Thomson syndrome
Roth spot
Rotor syndrome
rotoscoliosis
rototome
rotoxamine
Rouget
  R. bulb
  R. muscle
Rouget-Neumann sheath
rough
  r. colony
  r. line
roughage
rough-surfaced endoplasmic reticulum
Roughton-Scholander
  R.-S. apparatus
  R.-S. syringe
Rougnon-Heberden disease
rouleau, pl. **rouleaux**
  r. formation
round
  r. bur
  r. cell sarcoma
  r. eminence
  r. fasciculus
  r. foramen
  r. heart
  r. ligament of elbow joint
  r. ligament of femur
  r. ligament of liver
  r. ligament of uterus
  r. pelvis
  r. pronator muscle
  r. window
  r. window membrane
rounded atelectasis
roundworm
Rous
  R. sarcoma
  R. sarcoma virus
  R. tumor
Rous-associated virus (RAV)
Roussy-Lévy
  R.-L. disease
  R.-L. syndrome
Roux
  R. method
  R. stain

Roux-en-Y
  R.-en-Y. anastomosis
  R.-en-Y. operation
Rovsing sign
Royal College of Physicians (R.C.P.)
Royal College of Physicians (Edinburgh) (R.C.P.(E), R.C.P.(Edin))
Royal College of Physicians (Ireland) (R.C.P.(I))
Royal College of Physicians and Surgeons of Canada (R.C.P.S.C.)
Royal College of Surgeons (Edinburgh) (R.C.S.(E), R.C.S.(Edin))
Royal College of Surgeons (England) (R.C.S.)
Royal College of Surgeons (Ireland) (R.C.S.(I))
royal touch
RPF
  renal plasma flow
RPh
  Registered Pharmacist
rpm
  revolutions per minute
RPO
  right posterior oblique
RPR test
RQ
  respiratory quotient
R-R interval
rRNA
  ribosomal ribonucleic acid
RSA
  right sacroanterior position
RSD
  reflex sympathetic dystrophy
RSP
  right sacroposterior position
RST
  right sacrotransverse position
RST segment
RSV
  rous sarcoma virus
Rs virus
RT
  room temperature
RT$_3$
  reverse triodothyronine
RTF
  resistance-transfer factor
rTMP
  ribothymidylic acid
RT-PCR
  reverse transcriptase polymerase chain reaction
RU-486
Ru
  ruthenium
rub
  friction r.
  pericardial r.
  pericardial friction r.
  pleural r.
  pleural friction r.
  pleuritic r.

Rubarth disease virus
rubber
    r. dam
    r. dam clamp
    r. dam clamp forceps
    r. pelvis
    r. policeman
    r. tissue
rubber-bulb syringe
rubber-shod clamp
rubbing alcohol
rubeanic acid
rubedo
rubefacient
rubefaction
rubella
    r. cataract
    r. HI test
    r. retinopathy
    r. virus
    r. virus vaccine, live
rubellin
rubeola virus
rubeosis
    rubeosis iridis diabetica
rubescent
rubidium (Rb)
rubidomycin (daunorubicin)
rubin S, rubine
Rubinstein-Taybi syndrome
Rubin test
Rubivirus
Rubner
    R. laws of growth
    R. test
rubor
rubratoxin
rubredoxin
rubriblast
    pernicious anemia type r.
rubric
rubricyte
rubrobulbar tract
rubroolivary fiber
rubropontine tract
rubroreticular
    r. fasciculi
    r. tract
rubrospinal
    r. decussation
    r. tract
Rubulavirus
ructus
rudiment
rudimentary
rudimentum, pl. **rudimenta**
    r. hippocampi
Rud syndrome
ruff
    pupillary r.
Ruffini corpuscle
rufous
    r. albinism
ruga, pl. **rugae**
    rugae of gallbladder

    gastric rugae
    r. gastrica
    r. palatina
    rugae of stomach
    rugae of vagina
    vaginal rugae
    rugae vaginales
    rugae vesicae biliaris
rugal column of vagina
rugger jersey vertebra
rugine
rugitus
rugose
rugosity
rugous
Ruhemann purple
RUL
    right upper lobe
rule
    Abegg r.
    American Law Institute r.
    r. of bigeminy
    Chargaff r.
    Clark weight r.
    Cowling r.
    Durham r.
    Gibb phase r.
    Goriaew r.
    Haase r.
    Hückel r.
    Ingelfinger r.
    isoprene r.
    Jackson r.
    Le Bel-van't Hoff r.
    Liebermeister r.
    Meyer-Overton r.
    M'Naghten r.
    Nägele r.
    New Hampshire r.
    r. of nines
    Ogino-Knaus r.
    r. of outlet
    phase r.
    Prentice r.
    Rolleston r.
    Schütz r.
    stopping r.
    Trusler r. for pulmonary artery banding
    Young r.
ruler
    isometric r.
rum-blossom
ruminant
rumination disorder
ruminative
Ruminococcus
Rummel tourniquet
rum nose
Rumpel-Leede
    R.-L. phenomenon
    R.-L. sign
    R.-L. test
run
runaway pacemaker

R

Runeberg formula
runner's knee
running time
runoff
runt disease
runting syndrome
Runyon
    R. classification
    R. group I, II, III, IV mycobacteria
rupia
rupioid
rupture
    artificial membrane r.
    membrane r.
    premature membrane r.
    preterm membrane r.
    spontaneous membrane r.
ruptured
    r. aneurysm
    r. disk
RUQ
    right upper quadrant
rural cutaneous leishmaniasis
Rushton body
Russell
    R. body
    R. effect
    R. Periodontal Index
    R. sign
    R. syndrome
    R. traction
Russell's
    R. viper
    R. viper venom
    R. viper venom clotting time

Russian
    R. autumn encephalitis
    R. autumn encephalitis virus
    R. fly
    R. influenza
    R. spring-summer encephalitis,
      Eastern subtype
    R. spring-summer encephalitis virus
    R. spring-summer encephalitis,
      Western subtype
    R. tick-borne encephalitis
Rust phenomenon
rusty sputum
ruthenium (Ru)
    r. red
rutherford
rutidosis
rutin
rutinose
rutoside
Ruysch
    R. membrane
    R. muscle
    R. tube
    R. vein
RV
    residual volume
R_f value
ryanodine receptor
Ryan stain
rye
    R. classification
    r. smut
Ryle tube

σ (*var. of* sigma)

S

    S antigen
    S factor
    S peptide
    S phase
    S potential
    S protein
    S sign of Golden
    S unit of streptomycin
    S wave

S
    spherical lens

^{35}**S**
    sulfur-35

S$_1$
    first heart sound

S$_2$
    second heart sound

S$_3$
    third heart sound

S$_4$
    fourth heart sound

S$_7$
    summation gallop

S$_f$
    flotation constant

S
    entropy

s
    steady state

s̄
    without

s
    selection coefficient

S1 nuclease mapping

SA
    sacroanterior position

S-A
    sinuatrial
    S-A block
    S-A node

sabadilla

saber
    s. shin
    s. tibia

saber-sheath trachea

Sabia virus

Sabin-Feldman dye test

Sabin vaccine

sabot heart

Sabouraud
    S. dextrose agar
    S. pastil

Sabouraud-Noiré instrument

sabulous

saburra

saburral

sac
    abdominal s.
    air s.
    allantoic s.
    alveolar s.
    amnionic s.
    aneurysmal s.
    aortic s.
    chorionic s.
    conjunctival s.
    cupular blind s.
    dental s.
    endolymphatic s.
    gestational s.
    heart s.
    hernial s.
    Hilton s.
    lacrimal s.
    lesser peritoneal s.
    lymph s.
    nasal s.
    omental s.
    preputial s.
    pudendal s.
    tear s.
    tooth s.
    vestibular blind s.
    vitelline s.
    yolk s.

saccade

saccadic movement

saccate

saccharase

saccharate

saccharephidrosis

saccharic

saccharic acid

saccharide

sacchariferous

saccharification

saccharify

saccharimeter

saccharin

saccharine

saccharogen amylase

saccharolytic

saccharometabolic

saccharometabolism

saccharometer

Saccharomyces

Saccharomycetaceae

Saccharomycetales

saccharopine dehydrogenase

saccharopinuria

saccharose

saccharum
    s. canadense
    s. lactis

sacci (*pl. of* saccus)

sacciform
    s. recess of distal radioulnar joint
    s. recess of elbow joint

saccular
    s. aneurysm
    s. bronchiectasis
    s. duct

S

saccular *(continued)*
    s. gland
    s. nerve
    s. recess of bony labyrinth
    s. spot
sacculated
    s. aneurysm
    s. pleurisy
sacculation of colon
saccule
    laryngeal s.
    s. of larynx
sacculocochlear
sacculus, pl. **sacculi**
    s. alveolaris
    s. communis
    s. endolymphaticus
    s. lacrimalis
    s. laryngis
    s. proprius
    s. vestibuli
saccus, pl. **sacci**
    s. conjunctivalis
    s. endolymphaticus
    s. lacrimalis
    s. reuniens
    s. vaginalis
Sachs-Georgi test
sacra (*pl. of* sacrum)
sacrad
sacral
    s. anesthesia
    s. canal
    s. cornu
    s. crest
    s. flexure
    s. flexure of rectum
    s. foramina
    s. ganglia
    s. hiatus
    s. horn
    s. index
    s. kyphosis
    s. lymph node
    s. nerve [S1–S5]
    s. part of spinal cord
    s. plexus
    s. promontory
    s. region
    s. splanchnic nerve
    s. triangle
    s. tuberosity
    s. vein
    s. venous plexus
    s. vertebrae [S1–S5]
sacralgia
sacralization
sacrectomy
sacred bone
sacroanterior position (SA)
sacrococcygeal
    s. disk
    s. joint

    s. junction
    s. teratoma
sacrococcygeus
sacrocolpopexy procedure
sacrodural ligament
sacrodynia
sacrogenital fold
sacroiliac
    s. articulation
    s. joint
sacroiliitis
sacrolumbalis
sacrolumbar
sacropelvic surface of ilium
sacroposterior position (SP)
sacrosciatic notch
sacrospinal
sacrospinous
    s. ligament
    s. vaginal vault suspension
       procedure
sacrotomy
sacrotransverse position
sacrotuberous ligament
sacrouterine fold
sacrovaginal fold
sacrovertebral
sacrovesical fold
sacrum, pl. **sacra**
    assimilation s.
SACT
    sinoatrial conduction time
SAD
    seasonal affective disorder
saddle
    s. back
    s. block anesthesia
    s. embolism
    s. head
    s. joint
    s. nose
    Turkish s.
saddleback caterpillar
sadism
sadist
sadistic
sadomasochism
sadomasochistic relationship
Saemisch
    S. section
    S. ulcer
Saenger operation
Saethre-Chotzen syndrome
safe sex
safety
    s. lens
    s. spectacles
SAF fixative
safflower oil
saffron
safranin O
safrole
sage
sagitta

sagittal
  s. axis
  s. border of parietal bone
  s. crest
  s. fontanelle
  s. groove
  s. line
  s. plane
  s. section
  s. split mandibular osteotomy
  s. sulcus
  s. suture
  s. synostosis
sagittalis
sago spleen
sagulum nucleus
Saigon cinnamon
sailor's skin
sail sound
Saint
  S. Anthony dance
  S. Anthony fire
  S. Ignatius itch
  S. John dance
  S. triad
  S. Vitus dance
Sakaguchi reaction
Saksenaea vasiformis
Sakurai-Lisch nodule
sakushu fever
sal, pl. **sales**
  s. alembroth
  s. ammoniac
  s. diureticum
  s. soda
  s. volatile
salaam
  s. attack
  s. convulsion
  s. spasm
Salah sternal puncture needle
salbutamol
sales (*pl. of* sal)
salicin
salicyl
  s. aldehyde
salicylamide
salicylanilide
salicylate
salicylated
salicylazosulfapyridine
salicylic acid collodion
salicylic aldehyde
salicylism
salicylize
salicylsalicylic acid
salicylsulfonic acid
salicyluric acid
salient
salifiable
salify
saligenin
salimeter
saline
  s. agglutinin

physiologic s.
  s. purgative
  s. solution
  s. water
Salinem
  S. fever
  S. infection
salinometer
Salisbury common cold viruses
saliva
  chorda s.
  s. ejector
  ganglionic s.
  s. pump
  resting s.
  sympathetic s.
salivant
salivary
  s. calculus
  s. colic
  s. corpuscle
  s. digestion
  s. duct
  s. fistula
  s. gland
  s. gland hormone
  s. gland virus
  s. gland virus disease
salivate
salivation
salivator
salivolithiasis
Salk vaccine
Salla disease
Salmonella
  S. enterica subsp. *choleraesuis*
  S. enterica subsp. *enteritidis*
  S. enterica subsp. *paratyphi A*
  S. enterica subsp. *paratyphi B*
  S. enterica subsp. *typhi*
  S. enterica subsp. *typhimurium*
  S. food poisoning
  S. typhi
  S. typhosa
salmonellosis
salmon patch
salol
salpingectomy
  abdominal s.
salpinges (*pl. of* salpinx)
salpingian
salpingioma
salpingitic
salpingitis
  chronic interstitial s.
  foreign body s.
  gonorrheal s.
  s. isthmica nodosa
  pyogenic s.
salpingocele
salpingocyesis
salpingography
salpingolysis
salpingoneostomy
salpingo-oophorectomy

S

salpingo-oophoritis
salpingo-oophorocele
salpingo-ovariectomy
salpingopalatine fold
salpingoperitonitis
salpingopexy
salpingopharyngeal
    s. fold
    s. muscle
salpingopharyngeus muscle
salpingoplasty
salpingorrhagia
salpingorrhaphy
salpingoscopy
salpingostomy
salpingotomy
    abdominal s.
salpinx, pl. **salpinges**
    s. uterina
salsalate
salt
    acid s.
    s. action
    artificial Carlsbad s.
    artificial Kissingen s.
    artificial Vichy s.
    basic s.
    bile s.
    bone s.
    s. bridge
    common s.
    s. depletion
    s. depletion syndrome
    diazonium s.
    double s.
    s. dye
    s. edema
    effervescent s.
    Epsom s.
    s. fever
    Glauber s.
    hexazonium s.
    s. loading
    Reinecke s.
    Rivière s.
    Rochelle s.
    Seignette s.
    s. sensitivity
    smelling s.
    s. solution
    s. substitute
    table s.
    tetrazonium s.
    s. wasting
    s. water boil
    s. water soap
    s. of wisdom
salt-and-pepper fundus
saltation
saltatory
    s. chorea
    s. conduction
    s. evolution
    s. spasm
salt-depletion crisis

salted
    s. plasma
    s. serum
Salter-Harris classification of epiphysial plate injuries
Salter incremental line
salting in
salting out
salt-losing
    s.-l. defect
    s.-l. nephritis
    s.-l. syndrome
saltpeter
    Chilean s.
    s. paper
salubrious
saluresis
saluretic
salutarium
salutary
salute
    allergic s.
salvage
    s. chemotherapy
    s. cystectomy
    s. pathway
    s. therapy
salve
salvia
Salzmann nodular corneal degeneration
SAM
    s-adenosyl-l-methionine
samandarine
samarium (Sm)
sambucus
sAMP
    adenylosuccinic acid
sample
    cluster s.
    end-tidal s.
    Haldane-Priestley s.
    probability s.
    proficiency s.
    Rahn-Otis s.
    random s.
    stratified s.
sampling
    s. bias
    biologic s.
    chemical s.
    continuous interleaved s.
    haphazard s.
    random s.
    snowball s.
Samter syndrome
San
    S. Joaquin Valley disease
    S. Joaquin Valley fever
    S. Miguel sea lion virus
Sanarelli phenomenon
Sanarelli-Shwartzman phenomenon
sanative
sanatorium
sanatory
Sanchez Salorio syndrome

sand
s. bath
s. body
brain s.
hydatid s.
intestinal s.
s. tumor
urinary s.

sandal
s. foot
s. strap dermatitis

sandalwood oil

sandfly
s. fever
s. fever viruses

Sandhoff disease

Sandifer syndrome

Sandison-Clark chamber

sandpaper
s. disk
s. gallbladder

Sandström body

sandworm disease

sane

Sanfilippo syndrome

Sanger
S. method
S. reagent

sanguifacient

sanguiferous

sanguification

sanguinarine

sanguine

sanguineous
s. cyst

sanguinolent

sanguinopurulent

Sanguisuga

sanguivorous

sanies

saniopurulent

sanioserous

sanious pus

sanitarian

sanitarium

sanitary

sanitation

sanitization

sanity

Sansom sign

Sanson images

santal oil

Santini booming sound

santonin

Santorini
S. canal
S. cartilage
S. concha
S. duct
S. fissure
S. incisures
S. labyrinth
S. major caruncle
S. minor caruncle
S. muscle

S. plexus
S. tubercle
S. vein

São Paulo fever

Sao Paulo typhus

sap
cell s.
nuclear s.

saphena

saphenectomy

saphenous
s. branch of descending genicular artery
s. hiatus
s. nerve
s. opening
s. vein

sapogenin

saponaceous

saponatus

saponification number

saponify

saponins

Sappey
S. fiber
S. plexus
S. vein

sapphism

sapremia

saprobe

saprobic

saprodontia

saprogen

saprogenic, saprogenous

saprophilous

saprophyte
facultative s.

saprophytic

saprozoic

saprozoonosis

SAR
scaffold-associated region

Sar
sarcosine

saralasin acetate

Sarcina ventriculi

sarcine

sarcoblast

Sarcocystis
S. bovih'ominis
S. fusiformis
S. hominis
S. lindemanni
S. miescheriana
S. suihominis
S. tenella

sarcocystosis

sarcode

Sarcodina

sarcogenic cell

sarcoglia

sarcoid
Boeck s.
Spiegler-Fendt s.

sarcoidal granuloma

S

sarcoidosis
hypercalcemic s.
sarcolemma
sarcolemmal, sarcolemmic, sarcolemmous
sarcology
sarcolysine
sarcoma
alveolar soft part s.
ameloblastic s.
angiolithic s.
avian s.
botryoid s.
endometrial stromal s.
Ewing s.
fascicular s.
giant cell s.
giant cell monstrocellular s. of
  Zülch
granulocytic s.
immunoblastic s.
Jensen s.
juxtacortical osteogenic s.
Kaposi s.
leukocytic s.
lymphatic s.
medullary s.
multiple idiopathic hemorrhagic s.
myelogenic s.
myeloid s.
osteogenic s.
periosteal s.
reticulum cell s.
round cell s.
Rous s.
spindle cell s.
synovial s.
telangiectatic osteogenic s.
Sarcomastigophora
sarcomatoid carcinoma
sarcomatosis
sarcomatous
sarcomere
sarconeme
sarcoplasm
sarcoplasmic reticulum
sarcoplast
sarcopoietic
Sarcopsylla penetrans
Sarcopsyllidae
Sarcoptes scabiei
sarcoptic
s. acariasis
s. mange
sarcoptid
sarcosine (Sar)
s. dehydrogenase
sarcosinemia
sarcosis
sarcosome
sarcostosis
sarcotic
sarcotripsy
sarcotubules
sarcous
sardonic grin

sargramostim
sarin
sarmassation
sarsaparilla
SART
sinoatrial recovery time
sartorius
s. bursae
s. muscle
Sartwell incubation model
sassafras
sat.
saturated
satellite
s. abscess
s. cell
s. cell of skeletal muscle
chromosome s.
s. DNA
s. metastasis
perineuronal s.
satellite-rich heterochromatin
satellitosis
satiation
satiety center
sat. sol.
saturated solution
Sattler
S. elastic layer
S. veil
saturate
saturated (sat.)
s. color
s. fat
s. fatty acid
s. hydrocarbon
s. solution (sat. sol.)
saturation
s. analysis
s. index
secondary s.
s. sound pressure level (SSPL)
saturnine
s. colic
s. encephalopathy
s. gout
saturnism
satyriasis
satyrism
saucerization
saucer-shaped cataract
Saundby test
sauriasis
sausage finger
Savage
S. perineal body
S. syndrome
Savary bougie
saw
Gigli s.
Stryker s.
saxitoxin
Sb
antimony

SBE
  subacute bacterial endocarditis
S-BP line
SBS
  shaken baby syndrome
Sc
  scandium
s.c.
  subcutaneous
scab
scabbard trachea
scabby mouth
scabicidal
scabicide
scabies
  crusted s.
  Norwegian s.
scabrities
  s. unguium
scaffold-associated region (SAR)
scala, pl. **scalae**
  Löwenberg s.
  s. media
  s. tympani
  s. vestibuli
scalar electrocardiogram
scald
scalded
  s. mouth syndrome
  s. skin syndrome
scalding
scale
  absolute s.
  activities of daily living s. (ADL)
  adaptive behavior s.
  Ångström s.
  Baumé s.
  Bayley S. of Infant Development
  Binet s.
  Binet-Simon s.
  Brazelton Neonatal Behavioral
    Assessment s.
  Cattell Infant Intelligence S.
  Celsius s.
  centigrade s.
  Charrière s.
  Columbia Mental Maturity S.
  coma s.
  digital gray s.
  expanded disability status s. (EDSS)
  Fahrenheit s.
  French s. (F)
  Gaffky s.
  gray s.
  Guttman s.
  Hamilton anxiety rating s.
  Hamilton depression rating s.
  hardness s.
  homigrade s.
  interval s.
  Karnofsky s.
  Kelvin s.
  Kurtzke multiple sclerosis
    disability s.
  Leiter International Performance S.

  Likert s.
  masculinity-femininity s.
  Mohs s.
  ordinal s.
  pH s.
  Rahe-Holmes social readjustment
    rating s.
  Rankine s.
  ratio s.
  Réaumur s.
  Shipley-Hartford s.
  Sörensen s.
  Stanford-Binet intelligence s.
  Wechsler-Bellevue s.
  Wechsler intelligence s.
  Zubrod s.
scalene
  s. hiatus
  s. tubercle
  s. tubercle of Lisfranc
scalenectomy
scalenotomy
scalenus
  s. anterior muscle
  s. anterior syndrome
  s. medius muscle
  s. minimus muscle
  s. posterior muscle
scaler
  hoe s.
  ultrasonic s.
scaling
scalloping
scalp
  s. contusion
  s. hair
  s. infection
  s. laceration
  s. muscle
scalpel
  plasma s.
scalpriform
scalprum
scaly ringworm
scammony
scamping speech
scan
  CT s.
  duplex Doppler s.
  EMI s.
  Meckel s.
  multiple-gated acquisition s.
    (MUGA)
  renal cortical s.
  sector s.
  ventilation-perfusion s.
scandium (Sc)
scanner
scanning
  s. electron microscope
  s. equalization radiography
  s. speech
  transvaginal s.
scanogram
Scanzoni maneuver

S

scapha
scaphocephalic
scaphocephalism
scaphocephalous
scaphocephaly
scaphohydrocephalus, scaphohydrocephaly
scaphoid
    s. abdomen
    s. bone
    s. fossa
    s. fossa of sphenoid bone
    s. tuberosity
scapi (*pl. of* scapus)
scapula, pl. scapulae
    s. alata
    s. elevata
    winged s.
scapulalgia
scapular
    s. line
    s. notch
    s. reflex
    s. region
scapulary
scapulectomy
scapuloclavicular
scapulocostal syndrome
scapulodynia
scapulohumeral
    s. atrophy
    s. muscle
    s. muscular dystrophy
    s. reflex
scapuloperiosteal reflex
scapulopexy
scapus, pl. scapi
    s. penis
    s. pili
scar
    s. cancer
    s. cancer of the lung
    s. carcinoma
    cigarette-paper s.
    s. emphysema
    hypertrophic s.
    papyraceous s.
    radial s.
Scardino vertical flap pyeloplasty
scarf
    s. bandage
    s. sign
scarification
    s. test
scarify
scarlatina
    s. anginosa
    anginose s.
    s. hemorrhagica
    s. latens
    s. maligna
    s. rheumatica
    s. simplex
scarlatinal nephritis
scarlatinella
scarlatiniform erythema

scarlatinoid
scarlet
    s. fever
    s. fever antitoxin
    s. fever erythrogenic toxin
    s. ¯red
    s. red sulfonate
Scarpa
    S. fascia
    S. fluid
    S. foramina
    S. ganglion
    S. habenula
    S. hiatus
    S. liquor
    S. membrane
    S. method
    S. sheath
    S. staphyloma
    S. triangle
scarring alopecia
Scatchard plot
scatemia
scatologic
scatology
scatoma
scatophagy
scatoscopy
scatter
    Compton s.
scattered radiation
scattergram
scatula
scavenger
    s. cell
    s. receptor
Scedosporium
    S. *apiospermum*
    S. *inflatum*
    S. *prolificans*
scelalgia
scene
    primal s.
scent
Schacher ganglion
Schaeffer-Fulton stain
Schaer reagent
Schäfer method
Schäffer reflex
Schaffer test
Schamberg fever
Schapiro sign
Schardinger
    S. dextrin
    S. enzyme
    S. reaction
scharlach red
Schatzki ring
Schaudinn fixative
Schaumann
    S. body
    S. lymphogranuloma
    S. syndrome
Schauta vaginal operation
Schede method

schedule
    continuous reinforcement s.
    fixed-interval reinforcement s.
    fixed-ratio reinforcement s.
    intermittent reinforcement s.
    s. of reinforcement
    variable-interval reinforcement s.
scheduled drug
Scheele green
Scheibe hearing impairment
Scheibler reagent
Scheie syndrome
Scheiner experiment
Schellong-Strisower phenomenon
Schellong test
schema, pl. **schemata**
    body s.
schematic eye
schematograph
scheme
    occlusal s.
schemochromes
Schenck disease
Scheuermann disease
Schick
    S. method
    S. test
    S. test toxin
Schiff
    S. base
    S. reagent
Schiff-Sherrington phenomenon
Schilder disease
Schiller test
Schilling
    S. band cell
    S. blood count
    S. index
    S. test
    S. type of monocytic leukemia
Schindler disease
schindylesis
schindyletic joint
Schiötz tonometer
Schirmer test
schistocelia
schistocormia
schistocystis
schistocyte
schistocytosis
schistoglossia
schistomelia
schistorrhachis
Schistosoma
    S. haematobium
    S. intercalatum
    S. japonicum
    S. malayensis
    S. mansoni
    S. mattheei
    S. mekongi
schistosomal dermatitis
schistosome granuloma
schistosomia

schistosomiasis
    Asiatic s.
    bladder s.
    cutaneous s. japonica
    ectopic s.
    s. haematobium
    s. intercalatum
    intestinal s.
    s. japonica
    Manson s.
    s. mansoni
    s. mekongi
    Oriental s.
    pulmonary s.
    urinary s.
schistosomulum, pl. **schistosomula**
schistosternia
schistothorax
schizamnion
schizaxon
schizencephalic microcephaly
schizencephaly
schizoaffective
    s. psychosis
schizocyte
schizocytosis
schizogenesis
schizogony
schizogyria
schizoid
    s. personality
    s. personality disorder
schizoidism
schizomycete
schizomycetic
schizont
schizonticide
schizonychia
schizophasia
schizophrenia
    acute s.
    ambulatory s.
    catatonic s.
    childhood s.
    disorganized s.
    hebephrenic s.
    latent s.
    paranoid s.
    process s.
    pseudoneurotic s.
    reactive s.
    residual s.
    simple s.
schizophrenic
schizophreniform disorder
schizotonia
schizotrichia
Schizotrypanum cruzi
schizotypal
    s. personality
    s. personality disorder
schizozoite
schlammfieber
Schlatter disease
Schlemm canal

Schlesinger sign
schlieren optics
Schmidel anastomosis
Schmid-Fraccaro syndrome
Schmidt
    S. diet
    S. syndrome
Schmidt-Lanterman
    S.-L. cleft
    S.-L. incisure
Schmidt-Strassburger diet
Schmidt-Thannhauser method
Schmorl
    S. ferric-ferricyanide reduction stain
    S. jaundice
    S. nodule
    S. picrothionin stain
Schneider
    S. carmine
    S. first rank symptom
schneiderian
    s. first rank symptom
    s. membrane
Schnitzler syndrome
Schober test
Scholander apparatus
Scholz disease
Schönbein test
Schönlein-Henoch syndrome
Schönlein purpura
school
    biometrical s.
    dogmatic s.
    dynamic s.
    hippocratic s.
    iatromathematical s.
    mechanistic s.
    s. nurse
    s. phobia
Schott treatment
schradan
Schreger line
Schridde cancer hair
Schroeder operation
Schuchardt operation
Schüffner
    S. dot
    S. granule
Schüller
    S. disease
    S. duct
    S. phenomenon
    S. syndrome
Schultz
    S. reaction
    S. stain
Schultz-Charlton
    S.-C. phenomenon
    S.-C. reaction
Schultz-Dale reaction
Schultze
    S. cell
    S. fold
    S. mechanism
    S. membrane

    S. phantom
    S. placenta
    S. sign
Schütz
    S. bundle
    S. law
    S. rule
Schwabach test
Schwalbe
    S. corpuscle
    S. nucleus
    S. ring
    S. space
Schwann
    S. cell
    S. cell unit
    S. white substance
schwannoma
    acoustic s.
    vestibular s.
schwannosis
Schwartz
    S. syndrome
    S. tractotomy
Schwartz-Jampel disease
Schweninger-Buzzi anetoderma
Schweninger method
sciage
sciatic
    s. bursa of gluteus maximus
    s. foramen
    s. hernia
    s. nerve
    s. neuralgia
    s. neuritis
    s. plexus
    s. scoliosis
    s. spine
sciatica
SCID
    severe combined immunodeficiency
SCID mouse
    severe combined immunodeficient mouse
science
    behavioral s.
scientific theory
scientometrics
scillaren
    s. A, B
scillaricide
scilliroside
scimitar sign
scinticisternography
scintigram
scintigraphic angiography
scintigraphy
scintillascope
scintillating scotoma
scintillation
    s. camera
    s. counter
scintillator
    liquid s.
scintillometer
scintimammography

scintiphotograph
scintiphotography
scintiscan
scintiscanner
scintography
scion
scirrhosity
scirrhous carcinoma
scirrhus
scission
scissiparity
scissor gait
scissors
> de Wecker s.
> Smellie s.

scissors-shadow
scissura, pl. scissurae
> s. pilorum

scissure
sclera, pl. scleras, sclerae
> blue s.

scleradenitis
scleral
> s. buckling operation
> s. ectasia
> s. resection
> s. rigidity
> s. ring
> s. roll
> s. spur
> s. staphyloma
> s. sulcus
> s. vein
> s. venous sinus

scleras (*pl. of* sclera)
scleratogenous
sclerectasia
> partial s.
> total s.

sclerectomy
scleredema adultorum
sclerema neonatorum
sclerencephaly, sclerencephalia
scleritis
> anterior s.
> anular s.
> brawny s.
> deep s.
> gelatinous s.
> malignant s.
> necrotizing s.
> nodular s.
> posterior s.

scleroatrophy
scleroblastema
sclerochoroidal
sclerochoroiditis
> s. anterior
> s. posterior

scleroconjunctival
sclerocornea
sclerocorneal junction
sclerocystic disease of the ovary
sclerodactyly, sclerodactylia

scleroderma
> linear s.
> localized s.
> progressive familial s.
> systemic s.

sclerodermatous
sclerogenous, sclerogenic
scleroid
scleroiritis
sclerokeratitis
sclerokeratoiritis
scleroma
> respiratory s.

scleromalacia
scleromere
sclerometer
scleromyxedema
scleronychia
sclero-oophoritis
sclerophthalmia
scleroplasty
scleroprotein
sclerosal
sclerosant
sclerose
sclerosing
> s. adenosis
> s. agent
> s. hemangioma
> s. inflammation
> s. keratitis
> s. leukoencephalitis
> s. mastoiditis
> s. osteitis
> s. therapy

sclerosis, pl. scleroses
> Alzheimer s.
> amyotrophic lateral s. (ALS)
> arterial s.
> arteriocapillary s.
> arteriolar s.
> bone s.
> Canavan s.
> central areolar choroidal s.
> combined s.
> diffuse infantile familial s.
> disseminated s.
> endocardial s.
> glomerular s.
> hippocampal s.
> idiopathic hypercalcemic s. of infant
> insular s.
> laminar cortical s.
> lateral spinal s.
> lobar s.
> mantle s.
> menstrual s.
> Mönckeberg s.
> multiple s. (MS)
> nodular s.
> nuclear s.
> ovulational s.
> physiologic s.
> posterior spinal s.
> primary lateral s.

S

sclerosis *(continued)*
    systemic s.
    tuberous s.
    unicellular s.
    valvular s.
    vascular s.
    s. of white matter
sclerostenosis
Sclerostoma
sclerostomy
sclerotherapy
sclerothrix
sclerotia (*pl. of* sclerotium)
sclerotic
    s. body
    s. cemental mass
    s. coat
    s. dentin
    s. gastritis
    s. kidney
    s. stomach
    s. tooth
sclerotica
sclerotium, pl. **sclerotia**
sclerotome
sclerotomy
    anterior s.
    posterior s.
sclerotrichia
sclerotylosis
sclerous
SCM
    sternocleidomastoid muscle
scoleces (*pl. of* scolex)
scoleciasis
scoleciform
scolecoid
scolecology
scolex, pl. **scoleces**
scoliokyphosis
scoliometer
scoliosis
    coxitic s.
    empyemic s.
    habit s.
    myopathic s.
    ocular s.
    ophthalmic s.
    osteopathic s.
    paralytic s.
    rachitic s.
    sciatic s.
    static s.
scoliotic pelvis
scoliotone
Scolopendra
scombroid poisoning
s-cone
scoop
scopine
scopolamine
    s. hydrobromide
    s. methylbromide

Scopolia
    S. japonica
scopoline
scopometer
scopophilia
scopophobia
Scopulariopsis
scorbutic anemia
scorbutigenic
scorbutus
scordinema
score
    APACHE s.
    Apgar s.
    Bishop s.
    discrimination s.
    Dubowitz s.
    Gleason s.
    Jarman s.
    Logistic Organ Dysfunction S.
    raw s.
    recovery s.
    standard s.
    symptom s.
scorpion
Scorpionida
scotochromogens
scotograph
scotoma, pl. **scotomata**
    absolute s.
    anular s.
    arcuate s.
    Bjerrum s.
    cecocentral s.
    central s.
    color s.
    flittering s.
    glaucomatous nerve-fiber bundle s.
    hemianopic s.
    mental s.
    negative s.
    paracentral s.
    pericentral s.
    peripheral s.
    physiologic s.
    positive s.
    quadrantic s.
    relative s.
    ring s.
    scintillating s.
    Seidel s.
    sickle s.
    zonular s.
scotomatous
scotometer
scotometry
scotophilia
scotophobia
scotopia
scotopic
    s. adaptation
    s. eye
    s. perimetry
    s. vision
scotopsin

scotoscopy
Scott operation
Scott-Wilson reagent
scotty dog
scout
    s. film
    s. radiograph
scrape
scrapie
scraping
scratch test
screen
    Bjerrum s.
    s. defense
    s.-film contact
    fluorescent s.
    Hess s.
    intensifying s.
    s. memory
    multiple marker s.
    rare-earth s.
    tangent s.
    triple s.
    vestibular s.
screening
    s. audiometry
    carrier s.
    cytologic s.
    familial s.
    mass s.
    multiphasic s.
    neonatal s.
    prenatal s.
    s. test
screw
    afterloading s.
    s. artery
    s. elevator
    s. joint
screwdriver tooth
screw-worm
    primary s.-w.
    secondary s.-w.
scribe
Scribner shunt
scrivener's palsy
scrobiculate
scrobiculus cordis
scrofula
scrofuloderma
scrofulous
    s. keratitis
    s. rhinitis
scroll
    s. bone
    s. ear
scrota (*pl. of* scrotum)
scrotal
    s. artery
    s. hernia
    s. hypospadias
    s. part of ductus deferens
    s. raphe
    s. septum
    s. swelling

    s. tongue
    s. vein
scrotectomy
scrotiform
scrotitis
scrotoplasty
scrotum, pl. **scrota**
    lymph s.
    watering-can s.
scrub
    s. nurse
    s. typhus
scruple
SCUBA
    self-contained underwater breathing
    apparatus
Scultetus
    S. bandage
    S. position
scum
scurf
scurvy
    Alpine s.
    hemorrhagic s.
    infantile s.
    land s.
    s. rickets
    sea s.
scuta (*pl. of* scutum)
scutate
scute
    tympanic s.
scutiform
Scutigera
scutulum, pl. **scutula**
scutum, pl. **scuta**
scybalous
scybalum, pl. **scybala**
scyphiform
scyphoid
SD
    streptodornase
SDA
    specific dynamic action
SDS
    sodium dodecyl sulfate
Se
    selenium
sea
    s. gull murmur
    s. louse
    s. nettle
    s. scurvy
    s. sickness
    s. urchin granuloma
    s. wasp
seabather's eruption
sea-blue
    s.-b. histiocyte
    s.-b. histiocyte disease
seal
    border s.
    s. finger
    palatal s.
    peripheral s.

S

seal (*continued*)
    posterior palatal s.
    postpalatal s.
    velopharyngeal s.
sealant
    dental s.
    fissure s.
sealed jar technique
seamstress's cramp
searcher
Seashore test
seasickness
season
seasonal affective disorder (SAD)
seat
    basal s.
    rest s.
seatworm
sebaceous
    s. adenoma
    s. cyst
    s. epithelioma
    s. follicle
    s. gland
    s. horn
sebaceus
sebiagogic
sebiferous
Sebileau
    S. hollow
    S. muscle
sebiparous
seborrhea
    s. capitis
    eczematoid s.
    s. faciei
    s. furfuracea
    s. oleosa
    s. sicca
    s. squamosa neonatorum
seborrheic
    s. blepharitis
    s. dermatitis
    s. eczema
    s. keratosis
    s. verruca
sebum
sec
    second
Secernentasida
Secernentia
Seckel
    S. dwarfism
    S. syndrome
seclusion of pupil
secobarbital
second (sec)
    s. cervical vertebra
    s. cranial nerve [CN II]
    s. cuneiform bone
    cycles per s. (cps)
    s. finger
    s. gas effect
    s. heart sound (S$_2$)

s. incisor
s. law of thermodynamics
s. messenger
s. molar
s. parallel pelvic plane
s. part of duodenum
s. set rejection
s. sight
s. signaling system
s. sound
s. temporal convolution
s. tibial muscle
s. toe [II]
s. tooth
secondarily generalized tonic-clonic seizure
secondary
    s. abdominal pregnancy
    s. adhesion
    s. adrenocortical insufficiency
    s. aerodontalgia
    s. agammaglobulinemia
    s. alcohol
    s. aldosteronism
    s. amenorrhea
    s. amide
    s. amine
    s. amputation
    s. amyloidosis
    s. anesthetic
    s. antibody deficiency
    s. aortic area
    s. atelectasis
    s. axis
    s. calcium phosphate
    s. carcinoma
    s. cardiomyopathy
    s. caries
    s. cartilaginous joint
    s. cataract
    s. cementum
    s. center of ossification
    s. choana
    s. coccidioidomycosis
    s. constriction
    s. curvature of vertebral column
    s. dementia
    s. dentin
    s. dentition
    s. deviation
    s. dextrocardia
    s. digestion
    s. disease
    s. drive
    s. drowning
    s. dye test
    s. dysmenorrhea
    s. egg membrane
    s. elaboration
    s. encephalitis
    s. failure
    s. fissure of cerebellum
    s. gain
    s. generalized epilepsy
    s. glaucoma

s. gout
s. hemochromatosis
s. hemorrhage
s. host
s. hydrocephalus
s. hyperparathyroidism
s. hypertension
s. hyperthyroidism
s. hypogammaglobulinemia
s. hypogonadism
s. hypothyroidism
s. immune response
s. immunodeficiency
s. infection
s. interatrial foramen
s. lysosome
s. medical care
s. megaureter
s. mesoderm
s. metabolism
s. metabolite
s. methemoglobinemia
s. myeloid metaplasia
s. narcissism
s. nodule
s. nondisjunction
s. oocyte
s. ossification center
s. ovarian follicle
s. palate
s. pellagra
s. point of ossification
s. process
s. proteose
s. pulmonary lobule
s. pyoderma
s. radiation
s. ray
s. refractory anemia
s. reinforcement
s. renal calculus
s. renal tubular acidosis
s. retinitis
s. saturation
s. screw-worm
s. sensory cortex
s. sensory nucleus
s. sex character
s. spermatocyte
s. spiral lamina
s. spiral plate
s. structure
s. suture
s. syphilis
s. telangiectasia
s. thrombus
s. tuberculosis
s. tympanic membrane
s. union
s. villus
s. visual area
s. visual cortex
s. vitreous
s. X zone

second-degree
s.-d. AV block
s.-d. burn
s.-d. prolapse
second-look operation
second-order conditioning
secosteroid
secreta
secretagogue
secretase
secrete
secretin
s. family
s. test
secretion
cytocrine s.
external s.
neurohumoral s.
secretogogue
secretomotor, secretomotory
s. nerve
secretor
s. factor
secretory
s. canaliculus
s. carcinoma
s. component
s. cyst
s. duct
s. granule
s. immunoglobulin
s. immunoglobulin A
s. nerve
s. otitis media
sectile
sectio, pl. **sectiones**
section
abdominal s.
attached cranial s.
axial s.
cesarean s.
classical cesarean s.
coronal s.
cross s.
detached cranial s.
diagonal s.
frontal s.
frozen s.
Latzko cesarean s.
longitudinal s.
lower uterine segment cesarean s.
median s.
microscopic s.
midsagittal s.
oblique s.
parasagittal s.
perineal s.
pituitary stalk s.
Saemisch s.
sagittal s.
serial s.
thin s.
transverse s.
ultrathin s.

S

sectional
 s. impression
 s. radiography
sectiones (*pl. of* sectio)
sector
 s. echocardiography
 s. iridectomy
 s. scan
sectoranopia
sectorial
secular equilibrium
secundigravida
secundina, pl. **secundinae**
secundines
secundipara
sedate
sedation
sedative
SEDC
 spondyloepiphyseal dysplasia congenita
sedigitate
sediment
sedimentary cataract
sedimentate
sedimentation
 s. coefficient
 s. constant
 s. rate
 s. velocity
sedimentator
sedimentometer
sedimentum lateritium
sedoheptulose
sedoxantrone trihydrochloride
seed
Seeligmüller sign
seesaw
 s. murmur
 s. nystagmus
Seessel
 S. pocket
 S. pouch
segment
 A1, A2 s. of anterior cerebral artery
 abnormal ST s.
 anterior s.
 anterior basal s. [S VIII]
 anterior (bronchopulmonary) s. [S III]
 anterior inferior renal s.
 anterior ocular s.
 anterior superior renal s.
 apical s. [S I]
 apicoposterior s. [SI + SII]
 arterial s. of kidney
 s. bronchopulmonale basale posterius S X
 bronchopulmonary s.
 cardiac s.
 cervical s. of spinal cord [C1–C8]
 coccygeal s. of spinal cord [Co]
 hepatic s.
 s. I
 inferior s.

inferior lingular s. [S V]
inferior renal s.
interannular s.
intermaxillary s.
internodal s.
Lanterman s.
lateral s.
lateral basal s. [S IX]
lateral bronchopulmonary s. S IV
(left anterior) lateral hepatic s. [III]
left medial hepatic s. [IV]
left posterior lateral hepatic s. III
s. of liver
lower uterine s.
lumbar s.'s L1–L5 of spinal cord
lumbar s.'s of spinal cord L1–5
medial s.
medial basal bronchopulmonary s. [S VII]
medial bronchopulmonary s. [S V]
mesoblastic s.
M2 s. of middle cerebral artery
neural s.
posterior s.
posterior basal bronchopulmonary s. S X
posterior bronchopulmonary s. S II
posterior hepatic s. I
posterior renal s.
P1, P2, P3, P4 s. of posterior cerebral artery
PR s.
precommunical s. of anterior cerebral artery
precommunical s. of posterior cerebral artery
Ranvier s.
renal s.
right anterior lateral hepatic s. [VI]
right anterior medial hepatic s. [V]
right posterior lateral hepatic s. [VII]
right posterior medial hepatic s. [VIII]
RST s.
s.'s of spinal cord [C1–Co]
s. of spleen
ST s.
subapical s.
subsuperior s.
superior s.
superior lingular bronchopulmonary s. S IV
superior renal s.
sympathetic s.
upper uterine s.
venous s. of the kidney
segmenta (*pl. of* segmentum)
segmental
 s. alveolar osteotomy
 s. anesthesia
 s. artery of kidney
 s. artery of liver
 s. atelectasis
 s. bronchus

s. demyelinating polyneuropathy
s. fracture
s. glomerulonephritis
s. medullary artery
s. neuritis
s. plate
s. sphincter
s. tubule
s. zone
segmentation
  s. cavity
  s. nucleus
segmentectomy
segmented
  s. cell
  s. leukocyte
  s. neutrophil
segmenter
Segmentina
segmenting body
segmentum, pl. **segmenta**
  s. A1, A2 arteriae cerebri anterioris
  s. anterius
  s. apicale
  s. bronchopulmonale
  s. bronchopulmonale anterius S III
  s. bronchopulmonale apicale S I
  s. bronchopulmonale apicoposterius [SI + II]
  s. bronchopulmonale basale anterius [S VIII]
  s. bronchopulmonale basale laterale [S IX]
  s. bronchopulmonale basale mediale S VII
  s. bronchopulmonale laterale S IV
  s. bronchopulmonale lingulare superius[S IV]
  s. bronchopulmonale mediale S V
  s. bronchopulmonale posterius S II
  s. cardiacum
  segmenta cervicalia C1–C5
  segmenta cervicalia medullae spinalis
  segmenta coccygea medullae spinalis
  segmenta hepatis
  s. hepatis anterius laterale dextrum [VI]
  s. hepatis anterius laterale sinistrum [III]
  s. hepatis anterius mediale dextrum [V]
  s. hepatis mediale sinistrum [IV]
  s. hepatis posterius I
  s. hepatis posterius laterale dextrum [VII]
  s. hepatis posterius laterale sinistrum [II]
  s. hepatis posterius mediale dextrum [VIII]
  s. I, II, III, IV
  s. inferius
  s. internodale
  s. laterale
  segmenta lienis

  s. lingulare bronchopulmonale inferius S V
  segmenta lumbalia L1–L5
  segmenta lumbalia medullae spinalis
  s. mediale
  segmenta medullae spinalis C1–Co
  segmenta medullae spinalis cervicalia C1–C8
  s. medullae spinalis coccygeum [Co]
  segmenta medullae spinalis lumbaria L1–L5
  s. oculare anterius
  s. posterius
  s. P1, P3, P4 arteriae cerebri posterioris
  s. renale anterius inferius
  s. renale anterius superius
  s. renale inferius
  s. renale posterius
  s. renale superius
  segmenta renalia
  segmenta sacralia medullae spinalis
  s. subapicale
  s. subsuperius
  segmenta thoracica medullae spinalis
segregation
  s. analysis
  s. ratio
segregator
Seidel
  S. scotoma
  S. sign
Seidlitz mixture
Seignette salt
Seiler cartilage
Seip syndrome
seismocardiogram
seismotherapy
seizure
  absence s.
  akinetic s.
  anosognosic s.
  astatic s.
  atonic s.
  atypical absence s.
  audiogenic s.
  automotor s.
  autonomic s.
  clonic s.
  complex motor s.
  complex partial s.
  convulsive s.
  dileptic s.
  early s.
  electrographic s.
  epileptic s.
  febrile s.
  focal motor s.
  gelastic s.
  generalized tonic-clonic s.
  grand mal s.
  hypermotor s.
  hypomotor s.
  jacksonian s.

S

seizure *(continued)*
    late s.
    major motor s.
    minor motor s.
    myoclonic s.
    negative myoclonic s.
    nonconvulsive s.
    nonepileptic s.
    partial s.
    petit mal s.
    psychic s.
    psychogenic s.
    psychomotor s.
    secondarily generalized tonic-clonic s.
    simple partial s.
    subclinical s.
    tonic s.
    tonic-clonic s.
    versive s.
selaphobia
Seldinger technique
selectin
    E s.
    L s.
    P s.
selection
    artificial s.
    s. coefficient *(s)*
    medical s.
    natural s.
    s. pressure
    sexual s.
selective
    s. angiography
    s. estrogen receptor modulator (SERM)
    s. grinding
    s. hypoaldosteronism
    s. immunoglobulin A deficiency
    s. inattention
    s. inhibition
    s. injection
    s. medium
    s. memory
    s. norepinephrine reuptake inhibitor
    s. reduction
    s. serotonin reuptake inhibitor
    s. stain
    s. termination
selegiline
selene unguium
selenium (Se)
    s. plate
    s. sulfide
selenocysteine
selenodont
selenomethionine
Selenomonas
self
    subliminal s.
self-accusation
self-analysis
self-awareness

self-centeredness
self-commitment
self-contained underwater breathing apparatus (SCUBA)
self-control
self-curing resin
self-differentiation
self-discovery
self-efficacy
self-fertilization
self-infection
selfish DNA
self-knowledge
self-limited disease
self-love
self-poisoning
self-registering thermometer
self-regulation
self-retaining catheter
self-stimulation
self-tolerance
Selivanoff test
sella
    empty s.
    s. turcica
sellar diaphragm
Sellick maneuver
Selters water
SEM
    standard error of the mean
semantic aphasia
semantics
semeiopathic *(var. of* semiopathic*)*
semeiosis *(var. of* semiosis*)*
semeiotic *(var. of* semiotic*)*
semeiotics *(var. of* semiotics*)*
semelincident
semen, pl. **semina**
semens
semenuria
semialdehyde
semicanal
    s. of auditory tube
    s. for tensor tympani muscle
semicanalis, pl. **semicanales**
    s. musculi tensoris tympani
    s. tubae auditivae
    s. tubae auditoriae
semicartilaginous
Semichon acid carmine stain
semicircular
    s. canal
    s. canal of bony labyrinth
    s. duct
    s. line
    s. line of Douglas
semi-closed circle
semicoma
semicomatose
semiconductor
semiconscious
semiconservative replication
semicrista incisiva
semidecussation
semidirect lead

semiflexion
semi-Fowler position
semihorizontal heart
semilente insulin
semilunar
- s. bone
- s. cartilage
- s. conjunctival fold
- s. cusp
- s. fascia
- s. fasciculus
- s. fibrocartilage
- s. fold
- s. fold of colon
- s. ganglion
- s. hiatus
- s. line
- s. notch
- s. nucleus of Flechsig
- s. valve

semilunare
semiluxation
semimembranosus
- s. muscle
- s. reflex

semimembranous bursa
semina (*pl. of* semen)
seminal
- s. capsule
- s. colliculus
- s. duct
- s. fluid
- s. gland
- s. granule
- s. hillock
- s. lake
- s. vesical cyst
- s. vesicle

semination
seminiferous
- s. epithelium
- s. tubule
- s. tubule dysgenesis

seminoma
- spermacytic s.

seminomatous
seminormal (N/2)
seminuria
semiopathic, semeiopathic
semiorbicular
semiosis, semeiosis
semiotic, semeiotic
semiotics, semeiotics
semioval center
semipennate muscle
semipenniform
semipermeable membrane
semipolar bond
semipronation
semiprone position
semiquinone
semispinal
- s. muscle
- s. muscle of head
- s. muscle of neck
- s. muscle of thorax

semispinalis
- s. capitis muscle
- s. cervicis muscle
- s. muscle
- s. thoracis muscle

Semisulcospina
semisulcus
semisulfur mustard
semisupination
semisupine
semisynthetic
semisystematic name
semitendinosus
- s. muscle
- s. reflex

semitendinous
semitertian
semitrivial name
semivalent
semivertical heart
Semliki Forest virus
Semon-Hering theory
Semple vaccine
semustine
Sendai virus
Senear-Usher
- S.-U. disease
- S.-U. syndrome

Seneca snakeroot
Senecio
senecioic acid
seneciosis
senega
senegal gum
senescence
- dental s.

senescent
Sengstaken-Blakemore tube
senile
- s. amyloidosis
- s. arteriosclerosis
- s. atrophoderma
- s. atrophy
- s. cataract
- s. chorea
- s. degeneration
- s. delirium
- s. dementia
- s. dental caries
- s. deterioration
- s. dwarfism
- s. emphysema
- s. gangrene
- s. halo
- s. hemangioma
- s. involution
- s. keratoderma
- s. keratoma
- s. keratosis
- s. lenticular myopia
- s. lentigo
- s. melanoderma
- s. memory

S

senile *(continued)*
- s. nephrosclerosis
- s. osteomalacia
- s. plaque
- s. psychosis
- s. retinoschisis
- s. sebaceous hyperplasia
- s. tremor
- s. vaginitis
- s. wart

senility
senior synonym
senium
senna
Sennetsu fever
Senning operation
sennoside
- s. A, B

sensate
sensation
- delayed s.
- general s.
- girdle s.
- s. level
- primary s.
- referred s.
- s. time

sense
- chemical s.
- color s.
- s. of equilibrium
- geometric s.
- s. of identity
- joint s.
- kinesthetic s.
- light s.
- muscular s.
- obstacle s.
- s. organ
- position s.
- posture s.
- pressure s.
- seventh s.
- space s.
- special s.
- static s.
- s. strand
- tactile s.
- temperature s.
- thermal s.
- thermic s.
- time s.
- visceral s.
- weight s.

sensibility
- articular s.
- bone s.
- cortical s.
- deep s.
- dissociation s.
- electromuscular s.
- epicritic s.
- pallesthetic s.
- proprioceptive s.

- protopathic s.
- splanchnesthetic s.
- vibratory s.

sensible
- s. heat
- s. perspiration
- s. temperature

sensiferous
sensigenous
sensimeter
sensing
- quorum s.

sensitive
sensitivity
- acquired s.
- analytic s.
- antibiotic s.
- clinical s.
- contrast s.
- diagnostic s.
- idiosyncratic s.
- induced s.
- multiple chemical s.
- pacemaker s.
- photoallergic s.
- phototoxic s.
- primaquine s.
- relative s.
- salt s.
- spectral s.
- s. training group

sensitization
- autoerythrocyte s.
- covert s.
- photodynamic s.

sensitize
sensitized
- s. antigen
- s. cell
- s. culture

sensitizer
sensitizing
- s. dose
- s. injection

sensitometry
sensomobile
sensomobility
sensomotor
sensor
sensoria (*pl. of* sensorium)
sensorial area
sensoriglandular
sensorimotor
- s. area
- s. theory

sensorimuscular
sensorineural hearing loss
sensorium, pl. **sensoria**
sensorivascular
sensorivasomotor
sensory
- s. acuity level
- s. alexia
- s. amblyopia
- s. amusia

s. aphasia
s. ataxia
s. cell
s. cortex
s. crossway
s. decussation of medulla oblongata
s. deprivation
s. ganglion
s. hearing impairment
s. image
s. inattention
s. nerve
s. neuron
s. neuronopathy
s. nucleus
s. paralysis
s. phantom
s. precipitated epilepsy
s. receptor
s. root of ciliary ganglion
s. root of pterygopalatine ganglion
s. root of spinal nerve
s. root of sublingual ganglion
s. root of submandibular ganglion
s. root of trigeminal nerve
s. speech center
s. tract
s. urgency

sensu

s. lato
s. stricto

sensual
sensualism
sensuality
sentient
sentiment
sentinal node biopsy
sentinel

s. animal
s. event
s. gland
s. loop sign
s. lymph node
s. node
s. pile
s. tag

sentisection
Seoul virus
separating

s. medium
s. wire

separation

s. anxiety
s. anxiety disorder
jaw s.
s. of retina
sternochondral s.
s. of teeth

separator
Sephadex
sepsis, pl. **sepses**

intestinal s.
s. lenta
puerperal s.
s. syndrome

sept-
septa (*pl. of* septum)
septal

s. area
s. artery
s. bone
s. branch
s. cell
s. cusp of right atrioventricular valve
s. cusp of tricuspid valve
s. gingiva
s. line
s. nasal cartilage

septan
Septata
septate

s. hymen
s. mycelium
s. uterus
s. vagina

septectomy
septemia
septic

s. abortion
s. arthritis
s. endocarditis
s. fever
s. infarct
s. intoxication
s. phlebitis
s. pneumonia
s. retinitis
s. shock
s. wound

septicemia

acute fulminating meningococcal s.
anthrax s.
cryptogenic s.
metastasizing s.
morphine injector's s.
plague s.
puerperal s.
typhoid s.

septicemic

s. abscess
s. plague

septicopyemia
septicopyemic
septivalent
septodermoplasty
septofimbrial nucleus
septomarginal

s. fasciculus
s. trabecula
s. tract

septonasal
septooptic dysplasia
septoplasty
septorhinoplasty
septostomy

atrial s.
balloon s.

septulum, pl. **septula**

S

septulum *(continued)*
    septula of testis
    s. testis
septum, pl. **septa**
    s. accessorium
    alveolar s.
    anteromedial intermuscular s.
    aortopulmonary s.
    atrioventricular s.
    s. atrioventriculare
    Bigelow s.
    bony nasal s.
    bulbar s.
    s. bulbi urethrae
    s. canalis musculotubarii
    cartilaginous s.
    s. cervicale intermedium
    s. clitoridis
    Cloquet s.
    comblike s.
    s. of corpora cavernosa of clitoris
    s. corporum cavernosorum clitoridis
    crural s.
    distal spiral s.
    s. endovenosum
    endovenous s.
    femoral s.
    s. femorale
    s. of frontal sinus
    gingival s.
    s. glandis
    s. of glans penis
    hanging s.
    interalveolar s.
    s. interalveolare
    interatrial s.
    s. interatriale
    interdental s.
    interlobular s.
    intermediate cervical s.
    s. intermedium
    intermuscular s.
    s. intermusculare
    s. intermusculare vastoadductorium
    interpulmonary s.
    septa interradicularia mandibulae et maxillae
    interradicular septa of maxilla and mandible
    interventricular s.
    s. interventriculare
    intraalveolar septa
    s. linguae
    lingual s.
    s. lucidum
    s. mediastinale
    s. membranaceum ventriculorum
    membranous s.
    s. mobile nasi
    s. musculare ventriculorum
    s. of musculotubal canal
    nasal s.
    s. nasi
    s. nasi osseum

    orbital s.
    s. orbitale
    pectiniform s.
    s. pectiniforme
    s. pellucidum
    s. penis
    s. of pharyngotympanic tube
    placental septa
    precommissural s.
    s. primum
    proximal spiral s.
    rectovaginal s.
    s. rectovaginale
    rectovesical s.
    s. rectovesicale
    scrotal s.
    s. scroti
    s. secundum
    sinus s.
    s. sinuum frontalium
    s. sinuum sphenoidalium
    s. of sphenoidal sinus
    spiral s.
    spiral bulbar s.
    s. spurium
    s. of testis
    s. of tongue
    transparent s.
    transverse s.
    s. tubae
    urogenital s.
    urorectal s.
    ventricular s.
sequela, pl. **sequelae**
sequence
    Alu s.
    chi s.
    coding s.
    s. hypothesis
    insertion s.
    intervening s.
    s. ladder
    leader s.
    long terminal repeat s. (LTR)
    monotonic s.
    nucleotide s.
    palindromic s.
    pulse s.
    s. pulse
    regulatory s.
    Shine-Dalgarno s.
    termination s.
    twin reversed arterial perfusion s. (TRAP)
sequence-tagged
    s.-t. site (STSs)
    s.-t. site (STS) map
sequencing
    dideoxy s.
    Maxim-Gilbert s.
sequential
    s. analysis
    s. anastomosis
    s. multichannel autoanalyzer (SMA)
sequestra (*pl. of* sequestrum)

sequestral
sequestration
  bronchopulmonary s.
  s. cyst
sequestrectomy
sequestrotomy
sequestrum, pl. **sequestra**
  primary s.
sequoiosis
SER
  somatosensory evoked response
Ser
  serine
sera (*pl. of* serum)
seralbumin
serendipity
Sergent white line
serial
  s. extraction
  s. film changer
  s. interval
  s. passage
  s. radiography
  s. section
series, pl. **series**
  aromatic s.
  erythrocytic s.
  fatty s.
  granulocytic s.
  Hofmeister s.
  homologous s.
  lymphocytic s.
  lymphoid s.
  lyotropic s.
  myeloid s.
  small bowel s.
  thrombocytic s.
  upper gastrointestinal s. (UGI)
  upper GI s.
serine (Ser)
  s. carboxypeptidase
  s. deaminase
  s. dehydrase
  L-s. dehydratase
  s. hydrolases
  s. protease inhibitor
  s. sulfhydrase
seriograph
seriography
serioscopy
seriscission
SERM
  selective estrogen receptor modulator
serocolitis
seroconversion
serocystic
serodiagnosis
seroenteritis
seroepidemiology
serofast
serofibrinous
  s. inflammation
  s. pleurisy
serofibrous
serogroup

serologic pipette
serology
seroma
seromembranous
seromucoid
  acid s.
seromucous
  s. cell
  s. gland
seromyotomy
seronegative
seropositive
seropurulent
seropus
seroreversion
serosa
  s. of colon
  s. of esophagus
  s. of gallbladder
  s. of large intestine
  s. of liver
  s. of parietal pleura
  s. of peritoneum
  s. of serous pericardium
  s. of small intestine
  s. of the spleen
  s. of stomach
  s. of urinary bladder
  s. of uterine tube
  s. of uterus
  s. of visceral pleura
serosamucin
serosanguineous
seroserous
serositis
  multiple s.
serosity
serosynovial
serosynovitis
serotaxis
serotherapy
serotina
serotonergic
serotonin norepinephrine reuptake inhibitor
serotype
  heterologous s.
  homologous s.
serous
  s. cell
  s. coat
  s. coat of peritoneum
  s. cyst
  s. demilune
  s. diarrhea
  s. gland
  s. hemorrhage
  s. inflammation
  s. iritis
  s. layer of peritoneum
  s. ligament
  s. membrane
  s. meningitis
  s. otitis media
  s. pericardium

S

serous *(continued)*
    s. pleurisy
    s. retinitis
    s. synovitis
    s. tunic
serovaccination
serovar
serozyme
serpentaria
serpentine aneurysm
serpent ulcer of cornea
serpiginous
    s. choroidopathy
    s. corneal ulcer
    s. keratitis
    s. ulcer
serpigo
serpins
serrate, serrated
    s. suture
Serratia
    s. *marcescens*
serration
serratus
    s. anterior muscle
    s. posterior inferior muscle
    s. posterior superior muscle
serrefine
serrenoeud
Serres
    S. angle
    S. gland
serrulate, serrulated
Sertoli
    S. cell
    S. column
Sertoli-cell-only syndrome
Sertoli-Leydig cell tumor
Sertoli-stromal cell tumor
sertraline
serum, pl. **serums, sera**
    s. accelerator
    s. accelerator globulin
    s. accident
    s. agar
    s. albumin
    anticomplementary s.
    antiepithelial s.
    antilymphocyte s.
    antirabies s.
    antireticular cytotoxic s.
    antitoxic s.
    bacteriolytic s.
    blood s.
    convalescent s.
    Coombs s.
    s. disease
    dried human s.
    s. eruption
    foreign s.
    s. hepatitis (SH)
    s. hepatitis virus
    human measles immune s.
    human pertussis immune s.

    human scarlet fever immune s.
    hyperimmune s.
    immune s.
    inactivated s.
    s. lactis
    liquid human s.
    measles convalescent s.
    muscle s.
    s. nephritis
    nonimmune s.
    normal horse s.
    normal human s.
    polyvalent s.
    pooled s.
    pooled blood s.
    s. protein
    s. prothrombin conversion
      accelerator (SPCA)
    s. rash
    s. reaction
    salted s.
    s. shock
    s. sickness
    specific s.
    s. therapy
    thyrotoxic s.
    truth s.
serumal calculus
serum-fast
serum glutamic-oxaloacetic transaminase (SGOT)
serum glutamic-pyruvic transaminase (SGPT)
serums (*pl. of* serum)
servation
Servetus circulation
service
    denture s.
    National Health S. (N.H.S.)
    Public Health S. (PHS)
    United States Public Health S.
      (USPHS)
servomechanism
seryl
sesame oil
sesamoid
    s. bone
    s. cartilage of cricopharyngeal
      ligament
    s. cartilage of larynx
    s. cartilage of nose
sesquihydrate
sesquiterpene
sessile
    s. hydatid
    s. polyp
sesterterpene
set
    haploid s.
    s. of idiotopes
    learning s.
    postural s.
seta, pl. **setae**
setaceous

Setaria
  s. cervi
  s. equina
setback
setiferous
setigerous
seton
  s. operation
  s. wound
setting
  s. expansion
  s. sun sign
set-up
seven-day fever
seventh
  s. cranial nerve [CN VII]
  s. sense
Sever disease
severe
  s. combined immunodeficiency (SCID)
  s. combined immunodeficient mouse (SCID mouse)
  s. postanoxic encephalopathy
Severinghaus electrode
severity of illness
sevoflurane
sevum
sewer gas
sex
  s. assignment
  s. cell
  s. chromatin
  s. chromosome
  s. chromosome imbalance
  s. cord
  s. determination
  s. factor
  s. hormone
  s. hormone-binding globulin (SHBG)
  s. linkage
  s. object
  s. ratio
  s. reassignment
  s. reversal
  s. role
  safe s.
  s. steroid-binding globulin
sexdigitate
sex-influenced inheritance
sexivalent
sex-limited inheritance
sex-linked
  s.-l. character
  s.-l. inheritance
  s.-l. locus
sexology
sextan
sexual
  s. abuse
  s. deviation
  s. dimorphism
  s. disorder
  s. dwarfism
  s. dysfunction

  s. generation
  s. gland
  s. infantilism
  s. instinct
  s. intercourse
  s. life
  s. neurasthenia
  s. orientation
  s. perversion
  s. potency
  s. preference
  s. reproduction
  s. selection
sexuality
  infantile s.
sexualization
sexually transmitted disease (STD)
Sézary
  S. cell
  S. erythroderma
  S. syndrome
SFO
  subfornical organ
S$_7$ gallop
SGO
  Surgeon General's Office
SGOT
  serum glutamic-oxaloacetic transaminase
SGPT
  serum glutamic-pyruvic transaminase
SH
  serum hepatitis
shadow
  acoustic s.
  s. cell
  s. corpuscle
  Gumprecht s.
  hilar s.
  s. nucleus
  Ponfick s.
  radiographic parallel line s.
  s. test
shadow-casting
Shaffer-Hartmann method
shaft
  s. of clavicle
  s. of femur
  s. of fibula
  hair s.
  s. of humerus
  s. of metacarpal
  s. of metatarsal
  s. of phalanx
  s. of radius
  s. of tibia
  s. of ulna
shaggy
  s. aorta
  s. chorion
  s. pericardium
shagreen
  s. patch
  s. skin
shake
  s. culture

S

shake *(continued)*
    smelter's s.'s
    s. test
shaken baby syndrome (SBS)
shaking palsy
shallow breathing
sham
    s. feeding
    s. rage
sham-movement vertigo
shank
shaping
shared
    s. epitope
    s. psychotic disorder
shark liver oil
sharp
    s. spoon
Sharpey fiber
Sharpey-Schäfer
shave biopsy
Shaver disease
shaving cramp
shawl muscle
SHBG
    sex hormone-binding globulin
shear
    s. flow
    s. rate
    s. stress
    s. thinning
shearing edge
shears
    Liston s.
sheath
    anterior tarsal tendinous s.
    axillary s.
    carotid s.
    carpal tendinous s.
    caudal s.
    common flexor s. of hand
    common peroneal tendon s.
    crural s.
    dentinal s.
    dorsal carpal tendinous s.
    dural s.
    dural s. of optic nerve
    enamel rod s.
    external s. of optic nerve
    external root s.
    s. of eyeball
    fascial s. of extraocular muscle
    fascial s. of eyeball
    femoral s.
    fenestrated s.
    fibrous s.
    fibrous digital s. of foot
    fibrous digital s. of hand
    fibrous digital s. of toes
    fibrous s. of digits of hand
    fibrous tendon s.
    fibular tarsal tendinous s.
    Henle s.
    Hertwig s.

Huxley s.
infundibuliform s.
inner s. of optic nerve
internal s. of optic nerve
internal root s.
intertubercular tendon s.
s. of Key and Retzius
s. ligament
Mauthner s.
medullary s.
microfilarial s.
mitochondrial s.
mucous s. of tendon
myelin s.
Neumann s.
neurovascular s.
notochordal s.
outer s. of optic nerve
palmar carpal tendinous s.
parotid s.
periarterial lymphatic s. (PALS)
plantar tendon s. of fibularis longus
    muscle
plantar tendon s. of peroneus
    longus muscle
s. process of sphenoid bone
prostatic s.
rectus s.
resectoscope s.
root s.
Rouget-Neumann s.
Scarpa s.
s. of Schwann
s. of Schweigger-Seidel
s. of styloid process
synovial s.
synovial s. of digits of foot
synovial s. of digits of hand
synovial tendon s.
synovial s. of toes
tail s.
tendinous s. of abductor pollicis
    longus and extensor pollicis brevis
    muscle
tendinous s. of extensor carpi
    radialis muscle
tendinous s. of extensor carpi
    ulnaris muscle
tendinous s. of extensor digiti
    minimi muscle
tendinous s. of extensor digitorum
    and extensor indicis muscle
tendinous s. of extensor digitorum
    longus muscle of foot
tendinous s. of extensor hallucis
    longus muscle
tendinous s. of extensor pollicis
    longus muscle
tendinous s. of flexor carpi radialis
    muscle
tendinous s. of flexor digitorum
    longus muscle (of foot)
tendinous s. of flexor hallucis
    longus muscle

tendinous s. of flexor pollicis longus muscle
tendinous s. of superior oblique muscle
tendinous s. of tibialis anterior muscle
tendinous s. of tibialis posterior muscle
s. of thyroid gland
tibial tarsal tendinous s.
vascular s.
s. of vessels
Waldeyer s.

sheathed artery
Sheehan syndrome
sheep bot
sheep-pox virus
shelf

Blumer s.
dental s.
palatal s.
s. procedure
rectal s.
vocal s.

shell

cytotrophoblastic s.
diffusion s.
K s.
L s.
M s.
s. nail
O s.
s. shock

shellac

s. base

Shemin cycle
Shenton line
Shepherd fracture
Sherman-Bourquin unit of vitamin B$_2$
Sherman-Munsell unit
Sherman unit
Sherrington

S. law
S. phenomenon

sherry wine
Shibley sign
shield

embryonic s.
nipple s.
oral s.

shift

antigenic s.
axis s.
chemical s.
chloride s.
Doppler s.
s. to the left
luteoplacental s.
permanent threshold s.
phase s.
Purkinje s.
s. to the right
temporary threshold s.
threshold s.

shifting

s. dullness
s. pacemaker

Shiga

S. bacillus
S. toxin

Shiga-Kruse bacillus
Shigalike toxin
Shigella

S. boydii
S. dysenteriae
S. flexneri
S. sonnei

shigellosis
shikimate dehydrogenase
shim
shimamushi disease
shin

s. bone
s. bone fever
saber s.
toasted s.'s

Shine-Dalgarno sequence
shingles
shin-splints
ship

s. beriberi
Fabricius s.
s. fever

Shipley-Hartford scale
shipping fever virus
shipyard eye
Shirodkar operation
shiver
shivering thermogenesis
shock

anaphylactic s.
anaphylactoid s.
anesthetic s.
s. antigen
break s.
cardiac s.
cardiogenic s.
chronic s.
counter-s.
cultural s.
declamping s.
deferred s.
delayed s.
diastolic s.
electric s.
endotoxin s.
hemorrhagic s.
histamine s.
hypovolemic s.
s. index
insulin s.
irreversible s.
s. lung
nitroid s.
oligemic s.
osmotic s.
primary s.
protein s.
pseudoanaphylactic s.

S

897

shock (*continued*)
 reversible s.
 septic s.
 serum s.
 shell s.
 spinal s.
 systolic s.
 s. therapy
 toxic s.
 s. treatment
 vasogenic s.
 s. wave lithotripsy
 wet s.
shocking dose
shoddy fever
Shone
 S. anomaly
 S. complex
 S. syndrome
shook jong
Shope
 S. fibroma
 S. fibroma virus
 S. papilloma
 S. papilloma virus
shop typhus
short
 s. abductor muscle of thumb
 s. adductor muscle
 s. association fiber
 s. bone
 s. central artery
 s. chain
 s. ciliary nerve
 s. circumferential artery
 s. crus of incus
 s. extensor muscle of great toe
 s. extensor muscle of thumb
 s. extensor muscle of toes
 s. fibular muscle
 s. flexor muscle of great toe
 s. flexor muscle of little finger
 s. flexor muscle of little toe
 s. flexor muscle of thumb
 s. flexor muscle of toe
 s. gastric artery
 s. gastric vein
 s. gyri of insula
 s. head
 s. head of biceps brachii
 s. head of biceps femoris
 s. increment sensitivity index
 s. incubation hepatitis
 s. interspersed element (SINES)
 s. levatores costarum muscle
 s. limb of incus
 s. palmar muscle
 s. peroneal muscle
 s. pitch helicoidal layer
 s. posterior ciliary artery
 s. process of malleus
 s. radial extensor muscle of wrist
 s. root of ciliary ganglion
 s. saphenous nerve

 s. saphenous vein
 s. sight
 s. TI inversion recovery
 s. vinculum
 s. wave diathermy
short-bowel syndrome
short-chain acyl-CoA dehydrogenase
 short-chain acyl-CoA dehydrogenase
 deficiency
shortening reaction
shortsightedness
short-term
 s.-t. exposure limit (STEL)
 s.-t. memory (STM)
shot-feel
shotgun prescription
shot-silk
 s.-s. phenomenon
 s.-s. reflex
 s.-s. retina
shotted suture
shoulder
 s. apprehension sign
 s. blade
 s. dystocia
 frozen s.
 s. girdle
 s. joint
 s. presentation
shoulder-girdle syndrome
shoulder-hand syndrome
show
Shprintzen syndrome
Shrapnell membrane
shudder
 carotid s.
Shulman syndrome
shunt
 arteriovenous s.
 AV s.
 Blalock s.
 Blalock-Taussig s.
 cavopulmonary s.
 s. cyanosis
 Denver s.
 dialysis s.
 Dickens s.
 distal splenorenal s.
 Glenn s.
 H s.
 hexose monophosphate s.
 jejunoileal s.
 left-to-right s.
 LeVeen s.
 mesocaval s.
 s. muscle
 pentose monophosphate s.
 peritoneovenous s.
 pleuroperitoneal s.
 pleurovenous s.
 portacaval s.
 portal-systemic s.
 proximal splenorenal s.
 Rapoport-Luebering s.
 renal-splenic venous s.

reversed s.
right-to-left s.
Scribner s.
Torkildsen s.
tracheoesophageal s.
transjugular intrahepatic
  portosystemic s. (TIPS)
Warburg-Dickens-Horecker s.
Warburg-Lipmann-Dickens-
  Horecker s.
Warren s.
Waterston s.

shut-in personality
shuttle
glycerophosphate s.
malate-aspartate s.
s. vector

Shwachman-Diamond syndrome
Shwachman syndrome
Shwartzman
S. phenomenon
S. reaction

Shy
6-mercaptopurine

Shy-Drager syndrome
SI
international system of units

Si
silicon

sI
6-mercaptopurine ribonucleoside

Sia
sialic acid

SIADH
syndrome of inappropriate secretion of
  antidiuretic hormone

sialaden
sialadenitis
sialadenotropic
sialagogue
sialectasis
sialemesis, sialemesia
sialic acid (Sia)
sialidase
sialidosis
sialine
sialism, sialismus
sialoadenectomy
sialoadenitis
sialoadenotomy
sialoaerophagy
sialoangiectasis
sialoangiitis
sialocele
sialodochitis
sialodochoplasty
sialogenous
sialoglycosphingolipid
sialogogue
sialogram
sialography
sialolith
sialolithiasis
sialolithotomy

sialometaplasia
necrotizing s.

sialometry
sialorrhea
sialoschesis
sialosemiology, sialosemeiology
sialosis
sialostenosis
Siamese twin
sib
sibling

Siberian tick typhus
sibilant rale
sibilus
sibling (sib)
s. rivalry

sibship
Sibson
S. aortic vestibule
S. aponeurosis
S. fascia
S. groove
S. muscle

sicca
s. complex
s. syndrome

siccant
siccative
sicchasia
siccolabile
siccostabile, siccostable
sick
s. building syndrome
s. euthyroid syndrome
s. headache
s. role
s. sinus syndrome

sickle
s. cell
s. cell anemia
s. cell C disease
s. cell crisis
s. cell dactylitis
s. cell hemoglobin (Hb S)
s. cell retinopathy
s. cell test
s. cell-thalassemia disease
s. cell trait
s. form
s. scotoma

sicklemia
sickling
sickness
acute African sleeping s.
aerial s.
African sleeping s.
air s.
altitude s.
balloon s.
black s.
caisson s.
car s.
cave s.
chronic African sleeping s.
chronic mountain s.

S

sickness *(continued)*
    decompression s.
    East African sleeping s.
    falling s.
    green tobacco s.
    Indian s.
    Jamaican vomiting s.
    milk s.
    morning s.
    motion s.
    mountain s.
    radiation s.
    sea s.
    serum s.
    sleeping s.
    space s.
    West African sleeping s.
side
    balancing s.
    s. chain
    s. effect
    working s.
side-chain theory
sideration
sideroachrestic anemia
sideroblast
sideroblastic anemia
siderocyte
siderofibrosis
siderogenous
sideropenia
sideropenic dysphagia
siderophage
siderophil, siderophile
siderophilin
siderophilous
siderophore
siderosilicosis
siderosis
    pulmonary s.
siderotic
    s. cataract
    s. nodule
SIDS
    sudden infant death syndrome
Siegert sign
Siegle otoscope
siemens
sieve
    s. bone
    molecular s.
    s. plate
sievert (Sv)
SIF
    somatotropin release-inhibiting factor
Sig.
    label
Siggaard-Andersen nomogram
sigh
sight
    s. blindness
    day s.
    far s.
    long s.

    near s.
    night s.
    second s.
    short s.
sigma, σ
    s. effect
    s. factor
    s. peptide
sigmatism
sigmoid
    s. artery
    s. colon
    s. flexure
    s. fossa
    s. groove
    s. kidney
    s. lymph node
    s. notch
    s. sinus
    s. sulcus
    s. vein
    s. volvulus
sigmoidectomy
sigmoidicity
sigmoiditis
sigmoidopexy
sigmoidoproctostomy
sigmoidorectostomy
sigmoidoscope
sigmoidoscopy
sigmoidostomy
sigmoidotomy
sigmoidovesical fistula
sigmoscope
sign
    Aaron s.
    Abadie s. of tabes dorsalis
    Abrahams s.
    accessory s.
    antecedent s.
    assident s.
    Auenbrugger s.
    Aufrecht s.
    Auspitz s.
    Babinski s.
    Baccelli s.
    Ballance s.
    Bamberger s.
    Bamberger-Pins-Ewart s.
    banana s.
    Bárány s.
    Barré s.
    Bassler s.
    Bastedo s.
    Battle s.
    B6 bronchus s.
    beak s.
    Bechterew s.
    Beevor s.
    Bergman s.
    Biederman s.
    Bielschowsky s.
    Biot breathing s.
    Bird s.
    Bjerrum s.

s. blindness
blue dot s.
Blumberg s.
Bonhoeffer s.
Bozzolo s.
Branham s.
Braxton Hicks s.
Broadbent s.
Brockenbrough s.
Brudzinski s.
burning drops s.
calcium s.
Calkins s.
Cantelli s.
Carman s.
Carnett s.
Carvallo s.
catheter coiling s.
Chaddock s.
Chadwick s.
chandelier s.
Chaussier s.
Chvostek s.
Claybrook s.
clenched fist s.
Collier tucked lid s.
colon cutoff s.
Comby s.
comet tail s.
commemorative s.
contralateral s.
conventional s.
Corrigan s.
Courvoisier s.
crescent s.
Cruveilhier-Baumgarten s.
Cullen s.
Dalrymple s.
Dance s.
Danforth s.
Darier s.
Dejerine s.
Delbet s.
de Musset s.
D'Éspine s.
dimple s.
doll's eye s.
Dorendorf s.
double bubble s.
double ring s.
double track s.
drawer s.
drooping lily s.
Drummond s.
Duchenne s.
Dupuytren s.
Duroziez s.
Ebstein s.
s. of edema of lower eyelid
Epstein s.
Ewart s.
Ewing s.
Faget s.
fan s.
Fischer s.

fissure s.
flag s.
Forchheimer s.
Fothergill s.
Friedreich s.
Froment s.
Gaenslen s.
Gauss s.
Glasgow s.
gloved-finger s.
Goggia s.
Goldstein toe s.
Goodell s.
Gordon s.
Gorlin s.
Gower s.
Graefe s.
Grasset s.
Grey Turner s.
Griesinger s.
Grocco s.
groove s.
Gunn crossing s.
Guyon s.
halo s.
halo s. of hydrops
Hamman s.
Hawkins impingement s.
Hegar s.
Heim-Kreysig s.
Hennebert s.
Higoumenakia s.
Hill s.
Hoagland s.
Hoffmann s.
Homans s.
Hoover s.
iconic s.
impingement s.
indexical s.
inferior triangle s.
Jackson s.
Joffroy s.
Kehr s.
Kerandel s.
Kernig s.
Kestenbaum s.
knuckle s.
Kocher s.
Kreysig s.
Kussmaul s.
Lancisi s.
Landolfi s.
Lasègue s.
Legendre s.
lemon s.
Leri s.
Leser-Trélat s.
Lhermitte s.
local s.
Lorenz s.
Lovibond profile s.
Macewen s.
Magendie-Hertwig s.
Magnan s.

sign *(continued)*
    Magnus s.
    Mannkopf s.
    Marañón s.
    Marcus Gunn s.
    McBurney s.
    meniscus s.
    Metenier s.
    Mirchamp s.
    Möbius s.
    Mosler s.
    Muehrcke s.
    Müller s.
    Munson s.
    Murphy s.
    Musset s.
    neck s.
    Neer impingement s.
    Néri s.
    Nikolsky s.
    objective s.
    s. of the orbicularis
    Osler s.
    painful arc s.
    Pastia s.
    patellar apprehension s.
    Payr s.
    Perez s.
    Pfuhl s.
    physical s.
    Piltz s.
    Pins s.
    Pitres s.
    placental s.
    Pool-Schlesinger s.
    Potain s.
    prodromic s.
    pseudo-Graefe s.
    puddle s.
    pyramid s.
    Quant s.
    Quénu-Muret s.
    Quincke s.
    Ransohoff s.
    Raynaud s.
    red, white, and blue s.
    Remak s.
    reversed-three s.
    Revilliod s.
    Ripault s.
    Romaña s.
    Romberg s.
    Rosenbach s.
    Rossolimo s.
    Rotch s.
    Rovsing s.
    Rumpel-Leede s.
    Russell s.
    Sansom s.
      rf s.
      hapiro s.
      hlesinger s.
      hultze s.
      imitar s.

    Seeligmüller s.
    Seidel s.
    sentinel loop s.
    setting sun s.
    S s. of Golden
    Shibley s.
    shoulder apprehension s.
    Siegert s.
    silhouette s. of Felson
    Skoda s.
    Snellen s.
    spinal s.
    spine s.
    Steinberg thumb s.
    Stellwag s.
    Sternberg s.
    Stewart-Holmes s.
    Stierlin s.
    Straus s.
    string s.
    subjective s.
    Sumner s.
    superior triangle s.
    ten Horn s.
    Thomson s.
    Tinel s.
    Toma s.
    Topolanski s.
    Tournay s.
    Traube s.
    Trendelenburg s.
    Tresilian s.
    trough s.
    Trousseau s.
    Trunecek s.
    Uhthoff s.
    Vierra s.
    Vipond s.
    vital s.
    von Graefe s.
    Weber s.
    Weiss s.
    Wernicke s.
    Westermark s.
    Wilder s.
    Winterbottom s.
    wrist s.

signal
    arrest s.
    contralateral routing of s.
    s. lymph node
    s. node
    pause s.
    s. recognition particle (SRP)
    termination s.
    s. void
signal-processing circuit
signal-to-noise ratio
signature
signed English
signet
    s. ring
    s. ring cell
signet-ring cell carcinoma
significant

siguatera
SIH
    somatotropin release-inhibiting hormone
silastic band
sildenafil
silent
    s. allele
    s. area
    s. electrode
    s. gallstone
    s. gap
    s. ischemia
    s. mutant
    s. mutation
    s. myocardial infarction
    s. period
silhouette sign of Felson
silica
    s. gel
    s. granuloma
silicate
    s. cement
    s. restoration
silicatosis
siliceous
silicic
silicic acid
silicic anhydride
silicious
silicoanthracosis
silicofluoride
silicon (Si)
    amorphous s.
silicon dioxide
    colloidal s. d.
silicone
    s. implant
    s.-related disease problems
silicoproteinosis
silicosiderosis
silicosis
silicotic granuloma
silicotuberculosis
siliqua olivae
silk
    floss s.
    surgical s.
    virgin s.
silo-filler's
    s.-f. disease
    s.-f. lung
silver
    s. cell
    s. chloride
    colloidal s. iodide
    s. cone
    s. fluoride
    fused s. nitrate
    s. impregnation
    s. iodate
    s. lactate
    mild s. protein
    s. nitrate
    s. oxide
    s. picrate

    s. point
    s. poisoning
    s. protein stain
    strong s. protein
    s. sulfadiazine
    toughened s. nitrate
silver-ammoniac silver stain
silver-fork
    s.-f. deformity
    s.-f. fracture
silverized catgut
Silverman-Lilly pneumotachograph
Silver-Russell
    S.-R. dwarfism
    S.-R. syndrome
Silverskiöld syndrome
silver-tin alloy
silvol
Simbu virus
simethicone
simian
    s. crease
    s. fissure
    s. hand
    s. hemorrhagic fever
    s. malaria
    s. vacuolating virus No. 40 (SV40)
    s. virus (SV)
similia similibus curantur
similimum, simillimum
Simmonds disease
Simmons citrate medium
Simonart
    S. band
    S. ligament
Simon position
Simons disease
Simonsiella
simple
    s. absence
    s. acne
    s. anchorage
    s. anisocoria
    s. beam
    s. bone cyst
    s. color
    s. conjunctivitis
    s. crus of semicircular duct
    s. diplopia
    s. dislocation
    s. endometrial hyperplasia
    s. fission
    s. glaucoma
    s. goiter
    s. heterochromia
    s. hyperopic astigmatism
    s. hypertrophy
    s. joint
    s. lipid
    s. lobule
    s. lymphangiectasis
    s. mastectomy
    s. mastoidectomy
    s. membranous limb of semicircular duct

S

simple (*continued*)
  s. microscope
  s. myopia
  s. myopic astigmatism
  s. necrosis
  s. obesity
  s. partial seizure
  s. phobia
  s. protein
  s. pulmonary eosinophilia
  s. retinitis
  s. schizophrenia
  s. skull fracture
  s. squamous epithelium
  s. ulcer
  s. urethritis
simple-central anisocoria
simplex
  syphilis, toxoplasmosis, other
    infections, rubella, cytomegalovirus
    infection, and herpes s.
    (STORCH)
Simplexvirus
Simplified Oral Hygiene Index (OHI-S)
Simpson
  S. forceps
  S. uterine sound
Sims
  S. position
  S. uterine sound
simulated hypertrophy
simulation
  computer s.
simulator
Simulium
  S. damnosum
  S. neavei
  S. ochraceum
  S. rugglesi
simultagnosia
simultanagnosia
simultaneous
  s. communication
  s. contrast
  s. perception
SIMV
  synchronized intermittent mandatory
    ventilation
simvastatin
sincalide
sincipital
  s. presentation
sinciput, pl. **sincipita**
Sindbis
  S. fever
  S. virus
Sinding-Larsen-Johansson syndrome

  terspersed element

903

  node
  nodule

single
  s. ascertainment
  s. bond
  s. gel diffusion precipitin test in
    one dimension
  s. gel diffusion precipitin test in
    two dimensions
  s. immunodiffusion
  s. microscope
  s. photon emission computed
    tomography (SPECT)
  s. ventricle
  s. vial fixative
single-strand break
single-stranded nucleate endonuclease
singlet
  s. oxygen
  s. state
singleton
singular foramen
singultation
singultous
singultus
sinigrase, sinigrinase
sinister
sinistrad
sinistral
sinistrality
sinistrocardia
sinistrocerebral
sinistrocular
sinistrogyration
sinistromanual
sinistropedal
sinistrorotation
sinistrorse
sinistrotorsion
sinistrous
Sin Nombre virus
sinoatrial
  s. block
  s. conduction time (SACT)
  s. node (S-A node)
  s. recovery time (SART)
sinoauricular block
sinography
sinopulmonary
sinovaginal
sinoventricular conduction
sinter
sinuatrial (S-A)
  s. chamber
  s. nodal artery
  s. nodal branch of right coronary
    artery
  s. node
  s. node artery
  s. (S-A) nodal branch of right
    coronary artery
sinus, pl. **sinuses**
  s. alae parvae
  anal s.
  s. anales
  anterior s.
  s. aortae

aortic s.
Arlt s.
s. arrest
s. arrhythmia
barber's pilonidal s.
s. barotrauma
basilar s.
s. block
s. bradycardia
Breschet s.
s. caroticus
carotid s.
s. cavernosus
cavernous s.
cerebral s.
cervical s.
circular s.
s. circularis
coccygeal s.
s. coronarius
coronary s.
costomediastinal s.
cranial s.
dermal s.
s. durae matris
dural venous s.
s. of dura mater
Englisch s.
s. epididymidis
s. of epididymis
ethmoidal s.
s. ethmoidales
s. ethmoidales anteriores
s. ethmoidales mediae
s. ethmoidales posteriores
frontal s.
s. frontalis
Guérin s.
s. histiocytosis with massive
  lymphadenopathy
Huguier s.
inferior longitudinal s.
inferior petrosal s.
inferior sagittal s.
s. intercavernosi anterior et posterior
intercavernous sinus
jugular s.
s. jugularis
s. lactiferi
lactiferous s.
laryngeal s.
s. laryngeus
lateral s.
s. lienis
longitudinal s.
longitudinal vertebral venous s.
Luschka s.
lymph s.
lymphatic s.
Maier s.
marginal s. of placenta
mastoid s.
s. maxillaris
maxillary s.
Meyer s.

middle ethmoidal s.
Morgagni s.
s. of nail
s. nerve of Hering
s. node
s. node artery
oblique pericardial s.
oblique s. of pericardium
s. obliquus pericardii
occipital s.
s. occipitalis
Palfyn s.
paranasal s.
s. paranasales
parasinoidal s.
s. pause
Petit s.
petrosal s.
s. petrosus inferior
s. petrosus superior
phrenicocostal s.
pilonidal s.
piriform s.
pleural s.
s. pocularis
s. posterior cavi tympani
posterior s. of tympanic cavity
preauricular s.
precervical s.
prostatic s.
s. prostaticus
pulmonary s.
s. of pulmonary trunk
rectal s.
s. rectus
s. reflex
renal s.
s. renalis
s. reuniens
rhomboid s.
s. rhythm
Ridley s.
Rokitansky-Aschoff s.
s. sagittalis inferior
s. sagittalis superior
scleral venous s.
s. septum
sigmoid s.
s. sigmoideus
sphenoidal s.
s. sphenoidalis
sphenoparietal s.
s. sphenoparietalis
splenic s.
s. standstill
straight s.
superior longitudinal s.
superior petrosal s.
superior sagittal s.
s. tachycardia
tarsal s.
s. tarsi
tentorial s.
terminal s.
s. terminalis

S

sinus *(continued)*
   s. tonsillaris
   Tourtual s.
   transverse s.
   transverse pericardial s.
   transverse s. of pericardium
   s. transversus
   s. transversus pericardii
   s. trunci pulmonalis
   s. tubercle
   s. tympani
   tympanic s.
   s. unguis
   urogenital s.
   s. urogenitalis
   uterine s.
   uteroplacental s.
   Valsalva s.
   s. of the vena cava
   s. venarum cavarum
   s. venosus
   s. venosus sclerae
   s. venosus syndrome
   venous s.
   venous s. of sclera
   s. vertebrales longitudinales
sinusitis
sinusoid
   uterine s.
sinusoidal
   s. capillary
sinusotomy
sinuvertebral nerve
si op. sit
si opus sit (s.o.s.)
siphon
siphonage
Siphona irritans
Siphonaptera
Siphoviridae
Sipple syndrome
Sippy diet
sireniform
sirenomelia
siriasis
sirup *(var. of* syrup)
SISI test
sismotherapy
sisomicin sulfate
sister chromatid exchange
Sistrunk operation
sit
   si opus s. (s.o.s.)
site
   acceptor s.
   acceptor splicing s.
   active s.
   allosteric s.
   ...dy-combining s.
   n-binding s.
   age s.
   le s.
   unologically privileged s.
   nd-binding s.

   privileged s.
   receptor s.
   replication s.
   restriction s.
   sequence-tagged s. (STSs)
   s. specific mutation
   switching s.
site-directed mutagenesis
site-specific recombination
sitostane
β-sitosterol
sitosterolemia
sitotaxis
sitotoxin
sitotoxism
sitotropism
in situ
situation
   s. anxiety
   psychoanalytic s.
situational
   s. psychosis
   s. test
situs
   s. inversus
   s. inversus viscerum
   s. perversus
   s. solitus
   s. transversus
sitz bath
SI units
sixth
   s. cranial nerve [CN VI]
   s. disease
   s. ventricle
sixth-year molar
sizer
Sjögren
   S. disease
   S. syndrome
Sjögren-Larsson syndrome
Sjöqvist tractotomy
SK
   streptokinase
skatole
skatoxyl
skein
   s. cell
   choroid s.
skeletal
   s. dysplasia
   s. extension
   s. muscle
   s. muscle fiber
   s. muscle tissue
   s. survey
   s. system
   s. traction
skeletology
skeleton
   appendicular s.
   s. appendiculare
   articulated s.
   axial s.
   s. axiale

cardiac s.
cardiac fibrous s.
s. of eyelid
facial s.
fibrous s. of heart
s. of free inferior limb
s. of free superior limb
gill arch s.
s. hand
s. of heart
jaw s.
thoracic s.
s. thoracicus
s. thoracis
visceral s.
Skene
    S. gland
    S. tubule
skeneitis, skenitis
skeneoscope
skew
    s. deviation
    s. distribution
    s. form
skiascopy
Skillern fracture
skim milk
skin
    alligator s.
    s. botfly
    bronzed s.
    deciduous s.
    s. dose
    elastic s.
    farmer's s.
    fish s.
    s. flap
    s. furrow
    glabrous s.
    glossy s.
    golfer's s.
    s. graft
    s. groove
    hidden nail s.
    s. ligament
    loose s.
    parchment s.
    piebald s.
    pig s.
    porcupine s.
    s. pore
    s. reaction
    s. reflex
    s. ridge
    sailor's s.
    shagreen s.
    s. sulci
    s. tag
    s. of teeth
    s. test
    thick s.
    thin s.
    toad s.
    s. traction

    s. writing
    yellow s.
skinbound disease
skin-muscle reflex
Skinner box
skinnerian conditioning
skin-puncture test
skin-pupillary reflex
skip area
skipped generation
Sklowsky symptom
Skoda
    S. rale
    S. sign
    S. tympany
skodaic resonance
skull
    s. base surgery
    cloverleaf s.
    s. fracture
    maplike s.
    natiform s.
    steeple s.
    tower s.
skullcap
sky blue
SL
    spinal length
sl, pl. **slyke**
slab-off
    s.-o. lens
slaked lime
slant culture
slaty anemia
SLE
    systemic lupus erythematosus
sleep
    s. apnea
    s. apnea syndrome
    s. deficit
    s. dissociation
    s. drunkenness
    electric s.
    electrotherapeutic s.
    s. epilepsy
    hypnotic s.
    light s.
    s. paralysis
    paroxysmal s.
    s. phase delay syndrome
    rapid eye movement s.
    REM s.
    s. spindle
    s. terror
    s. terror disorder
    winter s.
sleep-induced apnea
sleepiness
sleeping sickness
sleeplessness
sleeptalking
sleepwalker
sleepwalking

S

sleeve
s. graft
nerve root s.
SLE-like syndrome
slender
s. fasciculus
s. lobule
s. process of malleus
slew rate
slide
s. micrometer
s. tracheoplasty
sliding
s. esophageal hiatal hernia
s. filament hypothesis
s. hook
s. lock
s. oblique osteotomy
slime fever
sling
s. psychrometer
slipped hernia
slipping
s. patella
s. rib
s. rib cartilage
slit
Cheatle s.
filtration s.
s. lamp
s. pore
pudendal s.
s. ventricle syndrome
vulvar s.
slitlamp
Gullstrand s.
slope
s. culture
lower ridge s.
slotted attachment
slough
sloughing ulcer
slow
s. channel-blocking agent
s. combustion
s. component of nystagmus
s. fever
s. virus
s. virus disease
slow-reacting
s.-r. factor of anaphylaxis (SRF-A)
s.-r. substance (SRS)
s.-r. substance of anaphylaxis
SLR factor
Sluder neuralgia
sludge
activated s.
sludged blood
ish layer

ch
of sl)
me

Sm
samarium
SMA
sequential multichannel autoanalyzer
small
s. artery
s. bowel
s. bowel enema
s. bowel series
s. calorie (cal)
s. canal of chorda tympani
s. cardiac vein
s. cell carcinoma
s. cleaved cell
s. deep petrosal nerve
s. increment sensitivity index
s. increment sensitivity index test (SISI test)
s. interarch distance
s. intestine
s. lymphocytic lymphoma
s. nuclear RNA
s. pancreas
s. pelvis
s. plaque parapsoriasis
s. pudendal lip
s. saphenous vein
s. sciatic nerve
s. trochanter
smaller
s. muscle of helix
s. pectoral muscle
s. posterior rectus muscle of head
s. psoas muscle
smallest
s. cardiac vein
s. scalene muscle
s. splanchnic nerve
smallpox
confluent s.
discrete s.
fulminating s.
hemorrhagic s.
malignant s.
modified s.
s. vaccine
varicelloid s.
s. virus
West Indian s.
Sm antigen
smear
alimentary tract s.
bronchoscopic s.
buccal s.
cervical s.
colonic s.
cul-de-sac s.
s. culture
cytologic s.
duodenal s.
ectocervical s.
endocervical s.
endometrial s.
esophageal s.
fast s.

gastric s.
lateral vaginal wall s.
lower respiratory tract s.
oral s.
pancervical s.
Pap s.
Papanicolaou s.
sputum s.
urinary s.
vaginal s.
VCE s.
smegma
s. clitoridis
s. preputii
smegmalith
smell
smell-brain
Smellie scissors
smelling salt
smelter's
s. chills
s. fever
s. shakes
Smith
S. fracture
S. operation
Smith-Boyce operation
Smith-Indian operation
Smith-Lemli-Opitz syndrome
Smith-Petersen
Smith-Petersen nail
Smith-Riley syndrome
smog
smoker's
s. patch
s. tongue
smooth
s. broach
s. chorion
s. colony
s. diet
s. leprosy
s. muscle
s. muscle relaxant
s. muscle tissue
s. muscular sphincter
s. surface caries
smooth-surfaced endoplasmic reticulum
smudge cell
smut
Sn
tin
¹¹³Sn
tin-113
S-N-A angle
snail
s. fever
s. track degeneration
snake
snakeroot
Canada s.
European s.
Seneca s.
Texas s.
Virginia s.

snap
closing s.
s. finger
opening s.
snapping
s. hip
s. reflex
snare
cold s.
galvanocaustic s.
S-N-B angle
SNE
subacute necrotizing encephalomyelopathy
Sneddon syndrome
Sneddon-Wilkinson disease
sneeze
sneezing gas
Snellen
S. sign
S. test types
Snell law
sniff test
S-N line
snore
snout reflex
snow
s. blindness
s. conjunctivitis
snowball
s. opacity
s. sampling
snowman abnormality
snowshoe hare virus
snRNA
small nuclear rna
snub-nose dwarfism
snuff
snuffbox
anatomic s.
snuffle
Snyder test
SOAP
subjective, objective, assessment, and plan
soap
animal s.
Castile s.
curd s.
domestic s.
green s.
hard s.
insoluble s.
marine s.
medicinal soft s.
salt water s.
soft s.
soluble s.
superfatted s.
tallow s.
soapstone
soapsuds enema
Soave operation
socaloin
social
s. adaptation
s. control

social *(continued)*
s. instinct
s. intelligence
s. maladjustment
s. medicine
s. network therapy
s. phobia
s. psychiatry
s. therapy
socialization
socialized medicine
socia parotidis
socioacusis
sociocentric
sociocentrism
sociocosm
sociogenesis
sociogram
sociomedical
sociometric distance
sociometry
sociopath
sociopathy
socket
dry s.
eye s.
s. joint
tooth s.
SOD
superoxide dismutase
soda
baking s.
caustic s.
s. lime
s. loading
washing s.
sodic
sodium (Na)
s. acetate
s. acid carbonate
s. acid citrate
s. acid phosphate
s. alginate
s. *p*-aminohippurate
s. *p*-aminophenylarsonate
s. aminosalicylate
s. antimonylgluconate
s. antimonyl tartrate
s. arsanilate
s. ascorbate
s. aurothiomalate
s. aurothiosulfate
s. benzoate
s. bicarbonate
s. biphosphate
s. bisulfite
s. borate
s. bromide
s. cacodylate
s. carbonate
s. carboxymethyl cellulose
s. chloride
s. chromate Cr 51
s. citrate

s. citrate, acid
s. cromoglycate
s. dehydrocholate
s. diatrizoate
dibasic s. phosphate
s. dihydrogen phosphate
s. dimethylarsenate
s. dodecyl sulfate (SDS)
effervescent s. phosphate
exsiccated s. sulfite
s. fluoride
s. fluosilicate
s. folate
s. fusidate
s. glycerophosphate
s. group
s. hexafluorosilicate
s. hydrogen carbonate
s. hydrogen sulfite
s. hydroxide
s. hypochlorite
s. hypophosphite
s. hyposulfite
s. ichthyolsulfonate
s. indigotin disulfonate
s. iodide
s. iodide iodine-131
s. lactate
s. lauryl sulfate
s. levothyroxine
s. liothyronine
s. metabisulfite
s. methicillin
s. methylarsonate
s. methylprednisolone succinate
s. nitrate
s. nitrite
s. nitroferricyanide
s. nitroprusside
s. orthophosphate
s. perborate
s. peroxide
s. pertechnetate
s. phosphate
s. phosphate ^{32}P
s. polyanhydromannuronic acid sulfate
s. polystyrene sulfonate
s. potassium tartrate
pravastatin s.
primary s. phosphate
s. propionate
s. psylliate
s. pteroylglutamate
s. pump
s. pyroborate
s. pyrosulfite
s. rhodanate
s. ricinate
s. ricinoleate
s. salicylate
s. silicofluoride
s. stearate
s. sulfate
s. sulfite

s. sulfocyanate
s. sulforicinate
s. sulforicinoleate
s. tartrate
s. taurocholate
s. tetraborate
s. tetradecyl sulfate
s. thiocyanate
s. thiosulfate
s. tungstoborate

sodium-24 (^{24}Na)
sodium-potassium pump
sodium-responsive periodic paralysis
sodoku
sodomist, sodomite
sodomy
Soemmerring

S. ganglion
S. ligament
S. muscle
S. spot

soft

s. cataract
s. chancre
s. corn
s. diet
s. drusen
s. palate
s. papilloma
s. part
s. pulse
s. ray
s. soap
s. sore
s. sulfur
s. tissue window
s. tubercle
s. ulcer
s. water

software
Sohval-Soffer syndrome
soil

night s.

soja
sokosho
sol.

solution

Solanaceae
solanaceous
solanochromene
solapsone
solar

s. blindness
s. cheilitis
s. comedo
s. dermatitis
s. elastosis
s. energy
s. fever
s. ganglia
s. keratosis
s. lentigo
s. maculopathy
s. plexus
s. retinopathy

s. therapy
s. treatment
s. urticaria

solasulfone
solation
solder
soldering
soldier's patch
sole

s. of foot
s. nucleus
s. tap reflex

soleal

s. line
s. part of posterior compartment of leg

Solenoglypha
solenoid
Solenopotes capillatus
solenopsin A
Solenopsis

s. invicta
s. richteri

sole-plate ending
soleus muscle
solid

s. edema
s. phase immunoassay

solidism
solidist
solidistic
solid-state detector
solidus
soliped
solipsism
solitariospinal tract
solitary

s. bone cyst
s. bundle
s. fasciculus
s. fibrous tumor
s. follicle
s. gland
s. lymphatic follicle
s. lymphatic nodule
s. nodule of intestine
s. osteocartilaginous exostosis
s. tract

soln.

solution

solubility

s. test

soluble

s. antigen
s. ferric phosphate
s. glass
s. gun cotton
s. ligature
s. RNA
s. soap
s. specific substance (SSS)
s. starch
s. tartar

solum
solute

solutio
solution (sol., soln.)
    acetic s.
    amaranth s.
    aqueous s.
    Benedict s.
    Burow s.
    chemical s.
    colloidal s.
    s. of contiguity
    s. of continuity
    Dakin s.
    disclosing s.
    Earle s.
    ethereal s.
    Fehling s.
    ferric and ammonium acetate s.
    Fonio s.
    Gallego differentiating s.
    Gey s.
    Hanks s.
    Hartman s.
    Hartmann s.
    Hayem s.
    Krebs-Ringer s.
    lactated Ringer s.
    Lange s.
    Locke s.
    Locke-Ringer s.
    Lugol iodine s.
    molecular dispersed s.
    Monsel s.
    normal s.
    ophthalmic s.
    s. pressure
    Ringer s.
    saline s.
    salt s.
    saturated s. (sat. sol.)
    standard s., standardized s.
    supersaturated s.
    test s.
    Tyrode s.
    volumetric s. (VS)
    Weigert iodine s.
solvate
solvation
solvent
    amphiprotic s.
    s. drag
    s. ether
    fat s.
    s. inhalation
    nonpolar s.
    polar s.
    universal s.
solvolysis
soma
soman
somasthenia
somatagnosia
somatalgia
somatasthenia
somatesthesia
somatesthetic

somatic
    s. agglutinin
    s. antigen
    s. artery
    s. cell
    s. cell genetics
    s. cell hybridization
    s. crossing-over
    s. death
    s. delusion
    s. layer
    s. mesoderm
    s. mitosis
    s. motor neuron
    s. motor nucleus
    s. mutation
    s. mutation theory of cancer
    s. nerve
    s. nerve fiber
    s. nucleus
    s. reproduction
    s. sensory cortex
    s. swallow
    s. teniasis
somaticosplanchnic
somaticovisceral
somatist
somatization disorder
somatochrome
somatocrinin
somatoform
    s. disorder
    s. pain
somatogenic
somatoliberin
somatology
somatomammotropin
    human chorionic s.
somatomedin
somatomedins
somatometry
somatopagus
somatopathic
somatopathy
somatopause
somatophrenia
somatoplasm
somatopleure
somatoprosthetics
somatopsychic
somatopsychosis
somatoscopy
somatosensory
    s. aura
    s. evoked potential
    s. evoked response (SER)
somatosensory cortex (*var. of* somatic sensory cortex)
somatosexual
somatostatin
somatostatinoma
somatotherapy
somatotopagnosis
somatotopic
somatotopy

somatotropes
somatotroph
somatotrophic
somatotropic hormone (STH)
somatotropin
    s. release-inhibiting factor (SIF, SRIF)
    s. release-inhibiting hormone (SIH)
somatotropin-releasing
    s.-r. factor (SRF)
    s.-r. hormone (SRH)
somatotype
somatotypology
somatrem
somatropin
somesthesia
somesthetic
    s. area
    s. system
somite
    s. cavity
    occipital s.
somitic mesoderm
somnambulance
somnambulic epilepsy
somnambulism
somnambulist
somnambulistic trance
somnifacient
somniferous
somnific
somniloquence, somniloquism
somniloquist
somniloquy
somnolence, somnolency
somnolent
somnolentia
somnolescent
somnolism
Somogyi
    S. effect
    S. method
    S. phenomenon
    S. unit
Sondermann canal
sone
Songo fever
sonicate
sonication
sonic wave
sonification
sonifier
sonify
sonochemistry
sonogram
sonograph
sonographer
sonography
sonolucent
sonomicrometer
sonomotor response
sonorous rale
soot wart
sophisticate
sophoretin

sopor
soporiferous
soporific
soporose, soporous
sorbefacient
sorbic acid
sorbin
sorbinose
sorbitan
sorbite
sorbitol pathway
D-sorbitol-6-phosphate dehydrogenase
sorbitose
L-sorbose
sordes
sore
    bed s.
    canker s.
    cold s.
    Delhi s.
    desert s.
    hard s.
    Lahore s.
    s. mouth
    Natal s.
    Oriental s.
    pressure s.
    soft s.
    s. throat
    tropical s.
    veldt s.
    venereal s.
soremouth virus
Sörensen scale
Soret
    S. band
    S. phenomenon
soroche
    chronic s.
sorption
Sorsby
    S. macular degeneration
    S. syndrome
SOS
    S. gene
    S. repair
s.o.s.
    si opus sit
sotalol hydrochloride
Sotos syndrome
souffle
    cardiac s.
    fetal s.
    funic s.
    funicular s.
    mammary s.
    placental s.
    umbilical s.
    uterine s.
sound
    s. abatement
    adventitious breath s.
    after-s.
    amphoric voice s.
    anvil s.

S

sound (*continued*)
    atrial s.
    auscultatory s.
    bell s.
    bowel s.
    breath s.
    bronchial breath s.
    bronchovesicular breath s.
    Campbell s.
    cannon s.
    cardiac s.
    cavernous voice s.
    coconut s.
    complex s.
    cracked-pot s.
    Davis interlocking s.
    double-shock s.
    eddy s.
    ejection s.
    s. field
    first heart s. (S_1)
    fourth heart s. (S_4)
    friction s.
    gallop s.
    heart s.
    hippocratic succussion s.
    Jewett s.
    Korotkoff s.
    Le Fort s.
    McCrea s.
    Mercier s.
    muscle s.
    percussion s.
    pericardial friction s.
    pistol-shot femoral s.
    posttussis suction s.
    s. pressure level (SPL)
    respiratory s.
    sail s.
    Santini booming s.
    second s.
    second heart s. (S_2)
    Simpson uterine s.
    Sims uterine s.
    splitting of heart s.
    succussion s.
    tambour s.
    third s.
    third heart s. (S_3)
    tic-tac s.
    to-and-fro s.
    tracheal breath s.
    van Buren s.
    vesicular breath s.
    waterwheel s.
    water-whistle s.
    Winternitz s.
    xiphisternal crunching s.
soundex code
South
    S. African tick-bite fever
    S. African type porphyria
    S. American blastomycosis
    S. American trypanosomiasis

Southern blot analysis
Southey tube
soya
soybean oil
SP
    sacroposterior position
SP1
    stimulatory protein 1
sp.
    species
spa
space
    s. adaptation syndrome
    alveolar dead s.
    anatomic dead s.
    antecubital s.
    anterior clear s.
    apical s.
    axillary s.
    Berger s.
    Bogros s.
    Böttcher s.
    Bowman s.
    Burns s.
    capsular s.
    cartilage s.
    cavernous s.
    cavernous s. of corpora cavernosa
    cavernous s. of corporus
      spongiosum
    central palmar s.
    Chassaignac s.
    Cloquet s.
    Colles s.
    corneal s.
    Cotunnius s.
    dead s.
    deep perineal s.
    denture s.
    disk s.
    Disse s.
    s. of Donders
    endolymphatic s.
    epidural s.
    episcleral s.
    epitympanic s.
    extradural s.
    extradural s.
    extraperitoneal s.
    filtration s.
    Fontana s.
    freeway s.
    gingival s.
    haversian s.
    Henke s.
    His perivascular s.
    infraglottic s.
    interalveolar s.
    intercostal s.
    interfascial s.
    interglobular s.
    interglobular s. of Owen
    intermembrane s.
    interocclusal rest s.
    interosseous metacarpal s.

interosseous metatarsal s.
interpleural s.
interproximal s.
interradicular s.
interseptovalvular s.
intersheath s. of optic nerve
intervaginal subarachnoid s. of optic
  nerve
intervillous s.
intraretinal s.
s. of iridocorneal angle
Kiernan s.
Kretschmann s.
Kuhnt s.
lateral central palmar s.
lateral midpalmar s.
lateral pharyngeal s.
leeway s.
leptomeningeal s.
lymph s.
Magendie s.
s. maintainer
Malacarne s.
masticator s.
Meckel s.
medial midpalmar s.
mediastinal s.
s. medicine
medullary s.
middle palmar s.
midpalmar s.
Mohrenheim s.
muscular s. of retroinguinal
  compartment
s. myopia
Nuel s.
paraglottic s.
parapharyngeal s.
Parona s.
parotid s.
perforated s.
perichoroidal s.
perilymphatic s.
perineal s.
perinuclear s.
peripharyngeal s.
periportal s. of Mall
perisinusoidal s.
perivitelline s.
personal s.
pharyngeal s.
pharyngomaxillary s.
physiologic dead s. (V$_D$)
plantar s.
pleural s.
pneumatic s.
Poiseuille s.
popliteal s.
postpharyngeal s.
preepiglottic s.
Proust s.
Prussak s.
pterygomandibular s.
quadrangular s.
quadrilateral s.

Reinke s.
respiratory dead s.
s. retainer
retroadductor s.
retroinguinal s.
retromylohyoid s.
retroperitoneal s.
retropharyngeal s.
retropubic s.
retrosternal s.
retrozonular s.
Retzius s.
Schwalbe s.
s. sense
s. sickness
spinal epidural space
subarachnoid s.
subchorial s.
subdural s.
subgingival s.
subhepatic s.
subphrenic s.
superficial perineal s.
suprahepatic s.
suprasternal s.
Tarin s.
Tenon s.
thenar s.
Traube semilunar s.
Trautmann triangular s.
vascular s. of retroinguinal
  compartment
vertebral epidural s.
Virchow-Robin s.
Waldeyer s.
Westberg s.
zonular s.
spaced tooth
spacing
  third s.
spade
  s. finger
  s. hand
spagyric
spagyrist
spall
Spallanzani law
spallation product
span
  attention s.
  memory s.
Spanish
  S. fly
  S. influenza
sparganoma
sparganosis
  ocular s.
sparganum
sparing
  s. action
  s. phenomenon
sparteine
spasm
  s. of accommodation
  affect s.

spasm *(continued)*
    anorectal s.
    Bell s.
    cadaveric s.
    canine s.
    carpopedal s.
    diffuse esophageal s.
    epidemic transient diaphragmatic s.
    epileptic s.
    esophageal s.
    facial s.
    habit s.
    hemifacial s.
    infantile s.
    intention s.
    masticatory s.
    mobile s.
    muscle s.
    nictitating s.
    nodding s.
    salaam s.
    saltatory s.
    winking s.

spasmodic
    s. asthma
    s. dysmenorrhea
    s. dysphonia
    s. laryngitis
    s. stricture
    s. tic
    s. torticollis

spasmogen
spasmogenic
spasmolysis
spasmolytic
spasmophilic diathesis
spasmus
    s. coordinatus
    s. glottidis
    s. nictitans
    s. nutans

spastic
    s. anemia
    s. aphonia
    s. colon
    s. diplegia
    s. dysarthria
    s. dysphonia
    s. ectropion
    s. entropion
    s. flat foot
    s. gait
    s. hemiplegia
    s. ileus
    s. miosis
    s. mydriasis
    s. paraplegia
    s. speech
    s. spinal paralysis

spasticity
    clasp-knife s.

spatia interglobularia (*pl. of* spatium interglobulare)

spatial
    s. acuity
    s. contiguity
    s. formula
    s. localization
    s. vector
    s. vectorcardiography

spatium, pl. **spatia**
    spatia anguli iridocornealis
    s. endolympha'ticum
    s. episclerale
    s. extradura'le
    s. extraperitonea'le
    s. intercostale
    s. interfasciale
    s. interglobulare, pl. spatia interglobularia
    spatia interossea metacarpi
    spatia interossea metatarsi
    s. intervaginale bulbi oculi
    s. intervaginale subarachnoidale nervi optici
    s. lateropharyngeum
    s. leptomeningeum
    s. parapharyngeum
    s. perichoroideum
    s. peridurale
    s. perilymphaticum
    s. perinei profundum
    s. perinei superficiale
    s. peripharyngeum
    s. pharyngeum laterale
    s. retroinguinale
    s. retroperitoneale
    s. retropharyngeum
    s. retropubicum
    s. retrozonulare
    s. subarachnoideum
    s. subdurale
    s. supraspinale
    spatia zonularia

spatula
    iris s.
    s. needle
    Ro s.

spatulate
spatulated
spatulation
spay
SPCA
    serum prothrombin conversion accelerator
speaking tube
spearmint oil
special
    s. anatomy
    s. hospital
    s. nurse
    s. sense
    s. somatic afferent column
    s. visceral efferent column
    s. visceral efferent nucleus
    s. visceral motor nucleus

specialist
specialization
specialize

specialized transduction
specialty
speciation
species, pl. **species (sp., spp.)**
    s. tolerance
    type s.
species-specific
    s.-s. antigen
specific
    s. absorbance
    s. absorption coefficient
    s. action
    s. active immunity
    s. activity
    s. anergy
    s. antigen
    s. antiserum
    s. bactericide
    s. building-related illness
    s. capsular substance
    s. cause
    s. cholinesterase
    s. compliance
    s. disease
    s. dynamic action (SDA)
    s. epithet
    s. extinction
    s. granule
    s. gravity (sp. gr.)
    s. heat
    s. hemolysin
    s. immune globulin (human)
    s. immunity
    s. indication
    s. opsonin
    s. optic rotation
    s. parasite
    s. passive immunity
    s. phobia
    s. reaction
    s. serum
    s. soluble polysaccharide
    s. soluble sugar
    s. therapy
    s. transduction
specificity
    analytic s.
    s. constant
    diagnostic s.
    relative s.
    substrate s.
specillum, pl. **specilla**
specimen
    cytologic s.
SPECT
    single photon emission computed
    tomography
spectacle plane
spectacles
    bifocal s.
    clerical s.
    divers' s.
    divided s.
    Franklin s.
    half-glass s.

    hemianopic s.
    lid crutch s.
    Masselon s.
    orthoscopic s.
    pantoscopic s.
    photochromic s.
    protective s.
    pulpit s.
    safety s.
    stenopeic s.
    stenopeic s.
    telescopic s.
spectinomycin hydrochloride
spectra (*pl. of* spectrum)
spectral
    s. phonocardiograph
    s. sensitivity
spectrin
spectrochemistry
spectrocolorimeter
spectrofluorometer
spectrogram
spectrograph
    mass s.
spectrography
spectrometer
spectrometry
    clinical s.
spectrophobia
spectrophotofluorimetry
spectrophotometer
spectrophotometry
    atomic absorption s.
    flame emission s.
spectropolarimeter
spectroscope
    direct vision s.
spectroscopic
spectroscopy
    clinical s.
    infrared s.
    magnetic resonance s.
spectrum, pl. **spectra**
    absorption s.
    antimicrobial s.
    broad s.
    chromatic s.
    color s.
    continuous s.
    excitation s.
    fluorescence s.
    fortification s.
    frequency s.
    infrared s.
    invisible s.
    Raman s.
    thermal s.
    ultraviolet s.
    visible s.
    vocal s.
    wide s.
specular
    s. glare
    s. image
speculum, pl. **specula**

S

speculum *(continued)*
    bivalve s.
    Cooke s.
    duckbill s.
    eye s.
    s. forceps
    Kelly rectal s.
    Pederson s.
    stop-s.
speech
    alaryngeal s.
    s. audiogram
    s. audiometer
    s. awareness threshold
    s. bulb
    s. center
    cerebellar s.
    clipped s.
    cued s.
    s. detection threshold
    echo s.
    esophageal s.
    explosive s.
    helium s.
    mirror s.
    s. pathology
    s. processor
    s. reading
    s. reception threshold
    scamping s.
    scanning s.
    slurring s.
    spastic s.
    staccato s.
    subvocal s.
    syllabic s.
    tracheoesophageal s.
speech-language
    s.-l. pathologist
    s.-l. pathology
speed
spelencephaly
Spens syndrome
sperm
    s. aster
    s. cell
    s. crystal
    s. nucleus
spermaceti
spermacytic seminoma
spermagglutination
sperm-aster
spermatic
    s. cord
    s. duct
    s. filament
    s. fistula
    s. plexus
    s. vein
spermatid
spermatin
spermatoblast
spermatocele
spermatocidal

spermatocide
spermatocyst
spermatocytal
spermatocyte
    primary s.
    secondary s.
spermatocytogenesis
spermatogenesis
spermatogenetic
spermatogenic
spermatogenous
spermatogeny
spermatogone
spermatogonium
spermatoid
spermatology
spermatolysin
spermatolysis
spermatolytic
spermatophobia
spermatophore
spermatopoietic
spermatorrhea
spermatoxin
spermatozoal, spermatozoan
spermatozoon, pl. **spermatozoa**
spermaturia
spermia (*pl. of* spermium)
spermicidal
spermicide
spermidine
spermiduct
spermin crystal
spermine
spermiogenesis
spermism
spermist
spermium, pl. **spermia**
spermolith
spermolysis
Spermophilus
spermotoxin
SPF
    sun protection factor
sp. gr.
    specific gravity
sph.
    spherical
sphacelate
sphacelation
sphacelism
sphacelous
sphacelus
Sphaeroltilus
sphagnum moss
sphenethmoid
sphenion
sphenobasilar
sphenoccipital
sphenocephaly
sphenoethmoid
sphenoethmoidal
    s. recess
    s. suture
    s. synchondrosis

sphenoethmoidectomy
sphenofrontal suture
sphenoid
    s. angle
    s. bone
    s. part of middle cerebral artery
    s. process
    s. process of septal nasal cartilage
sphenoidal
    s. angle of parietal bone
    s. border of temporal bone
    s. concha
    s. crest
    s. emissary foramen
    s. fissure
    s. fontanelle
    s. herniation
    s. lingula
    s. margin of temporal bone
    s. process of palatine bone
    s. ridge
    s. rostrum
    s. sinus
    s. sinus aperture
    s. spine
    s. turbinated bone
    s. yoke
sphenoidale
sphenoiditis
sphenoidostomy
sphenoidotomy
sphenomalar
sphenomandibular ligament
sphenomaxillary
    s. fissure
    s. fossa
    s. suture
sphenooccipital
    s. joint
    s. suture
    s. synchondrosis
spheno-orbital suture
sphenopalatine
    s. artery
    s. foramen
    s. ganglion
    s. neuralgia
    s. notch
sphenoparietal
    s. sinus
    s. suture
sphenopetrosal
    s. fissure
    s. synchondrosis
sphenorbital
sphenosalpingostaphylinus
sphenosquamosal
sphenosquamous suture
sphenotemporal
sphenotic
    s. center
    s. foramen
sphenoturbinal
sphenovomerine
    s. suture

sphenozygomatic
    s. suture
sphere
    attraction s.
    Morgagni s.
spherical (sph.)
    s. aberration
    s. amalgam
    s. form of occlusion
    s. lens (S)
    s. nucleus
    s. recess of bony labyrinth
spherocylinder
spherocylindrical lens
spherocyte
spherocytic
    s. anemia
    s. jaundice
spherocytosis
    hereditary s.
spheroid, spheroidal
    s. articulation
    s. colony
    s. degeneration
    s. joint
spherometer
spherophakia
spheroplast
spheroprism
spherospermia
spherule
sphincter
    s. of ampulla
    anal s.
    anatomic s.
    angular s.
    s. angularis
    s. ani
    s. ani tertius
    antral s.
    s. antri
    s. of antrum
    anular s.
    artificial s.
    basal s.
    bicanalicular s.
    s. of biliaropancreatic ampulla
    Boyden s.
    canalicular s.
    choledochal s.
    colic s.
    s. of common bile duct
    s. constrictor cardiae
    duodenal s.
    duodenojejunal s.
    external anal s.
    external urethral s.
    external urethral s. of female
    external urethral s. of male
    extrinsic s.
    first duodenal s.
    functional s.
    s. of gastric antrum
    Glisson s.
    s. of hepatic flexure of colon

S

sphincter *(continued)*
 hepatopancreatic s.
 s. of hepatopancreatic ampulla
 hypertensive upper esophageal s.
 Hyrtl s.
 ileal s.
 ileocecocolic s.
 iliopelvic s.
 inferior esophageal s.
 s. intermedius
 internal anal s.
 internal urethral s.
 intrinsic s.
 lower esophageal s. (LES)
 macroscopic s.
 marginal s.
 mediocolic s.
 microscopic s.
 midgastric transverse s.
 midsigmoid s.
 s. muscle
 s. muscle of pancreatic duct
 s. muscle of pupil
 s. muscle of pylorus
 s. muscle of urethra
 s. muscle of urinary bladder
 muscular s. supracollicularis
 myovascular s.
 myovenous s.
 Nélaton s.
 O'Beirne s.
 s. oculi
 Oddi s.
 s. of Oddi dysfunction
 s. oris
 ostial s.
 palatopharyngeal s.
 pancreatic s.
 s. of pancreatic duct
 pathologic s.
 pelvirectal s.
 s. of the pharyngeal isthmus
 physiologic s.
 postpyloric s.
 prepapillary s.
 preprostate urethral s.
 preprostatic s.
 prepyloric s.
 proximal urethral s.
 s. pupillae
 pyloric s.
 radiologic s.
 rectosigmoid s.
 segmental s.
 smooth muscular s.
 striated muscular s.
 superior esophageal s.
 supracollicular s.
 s. of third portion of duodenum
 unicanalicular s.
 s. urethrae externus
 urethrovaginal s.
 s. vaginae
 Varolius s.

 velopharyngeal s.
 s. vesicae
 s. vesicae biliaris
sphincteral
sphincteralgia
sphincterectomy
sphincterial, sphincteric
sphincterismus
sphincteritis
sphincteroid tract of ileum
sphincterolysis
sphincteroplasty
sphincteroscope
sphincteroscopy
sphincterotome
sphincterotomy
 external s.
 transduodenal s.
sphinganine
(4*E*)-sphingenine
sphingol
sphingolipid
sphingolipidosis
 cerebral s.
sphingolipodystrophy
sphingomyelinase
sphingomyelin lipidosis
sphingomyelin phosphodiesterase
sphingomyelins
sphingosine
sphygmic interval
sphygmocardiograph
sphygmocardioscope
sphygmochronograph
sphygmogram
sphygmograph
sphygmographic
sphygmography
sphygmoid
sphygmomanometer
 Mosso s.
 Riva-Rocci s.
 Rogers s.
sphygmomanometry
sphygmometer
sphygmometroscope
sphygmo-oscillometer
sphygmopalpation
sphygmophone
sphygmoscope
 Bishop s.
sphygmoscopy
sphygmosystole
sphygmotonograph
sphygmotonometer
sphygmoviscosimetry
spica, pl. **spicae**
 s. bandage
 s. cast
spicula (*pl. of* spiculum)
spicular
spicule
spiculum, pl. **spicula**
spider
 s. angioma

arterial s.
s. cell
s. finger
s. hemangioma
s. nevus
s. pelvis
s. telangiectasia
vascular s.
spider-burst
Spiegelberg criteria
Spiegler-Fendt sarcoid
Spielmeyer acute swelling
Spielmeyer-Sjögren disease
Spielmeyer-Stock disease
Spielmeyer-Vogt disease
spigelian hernia
Spigelius
S. line
S. lobe
spike
ponto-geniculo-occipital s.
s. potential
s. and wave complex
spill
cellular s.
spillway
spilus
spin
s. density
s. echo
spina, pl. **spinae**
s. angularis
s. bifida
s. bifida aperta
s. bifida cystica
s. bifida manifesta
s. bifida occulta
s. dorsalis
erector spinae
s. frontalis
spinae geniorum inferior et superior
s. helicis
s. iliaca anterior inferior
s. iliaca anterior superior
s. iliaca posterior inferior
s. iliaca posterior superior
s. ischiadica
s. meatus
s. mentalis inferior et superior
s. nasalis anterior corporis maxillae
s. nasalis ossis frontalis
s. nasalis posterior laminae
    horizontalis ossis palatini
s. ossis sphenoidalis
spinae palatinae
s. peronealis
s. pubis
s. scapulae
s. suprameatalis
s. suprameatica
s. trochlearis
s. tympanica major
s. tympanica minor
spinach stool

spinal
s. accessory nerve
s. analgesia
s. anesthesia
s. anesthetic
s. apoplexy
s. arachnoid mater
s. artery
s. ataxia
s. block
s. branch
s. canal
s. column
s. concussion
s. cord
s. cord concussion
s. curvature
s. decompression
s. dura mater
s. dysraphism
s. epidural space
s. fusion
s. ganglion
s. headache
s. induction
s. instability
s. lamina
s. lemniscus
s. length (SL)
s. marrow
s. muscle
s. muscle of head
s. muscle of neck
s. muscle of thorax
s. muscular atrophy
s. muscular atrophy, type I, II, III
s. nerve
s. nerve plexus
s. nucleus of trigeminal nerve
s. nucleus of the trigeminus
s. paralysis
s. part of accessory nerve
s. part of arachnoid
s. part of deltoid muscle
s. part of filum terminale
s. pia mater
s. point
s. puncture
s. pyramidotomy
s. quotient
s. reflex
s. root of accessory nerve
s. shock
s. sign
s. stroke
s. tap
s. tract
s. tractotomy
s. tract of trigeminal nerve
s. trigeminal nucleus
s. vein
spinalis
s. capitis muscle
s. cervicis muscle

S

spinalis (*continued*)
    s. muscle
    s. thoracis muscle
spinate
spindle
    aortic s.
    s. cataract
    s. cell
    s. cell carcinoma
    s. cell lipoma
    s. cell nevus
    s. cell sarcoma
    central s.
    cleavage s.
    s. fiber
    His s.
    Krukenberg s.
    Kühne s.
    mitotic s.
    muscle s.
    neuromuscular s.
    neurotendinous s.
    nuclear s.
    sleep s.
spindle-celled layer
spindle-shaped muscle
spine
    alar s.
    angular s.
    anterior inferior iliac s.
    anterior nasal s. (ANS)
    anterior nasal s. of maxilla
    anterior superior iliac s.
    bamboo s.
    s. cell
    cleft s.
    dendritic s.
    dorsal s.
    s. fusion
    greater tympanic s.
    s. of helix
    hemal s.
    Henle s.
    iliac s.
    ischiadic s.
    ischial s.
    lesser tympanic s.
    meatal s.
    mental s.
    nasal s. of frontal bone
    neural s.
    palatine s.
    poker s.
    posterior inferior iliac s.
    posterior nasal s. of horizontal plate
      of palatine bone
    posterior palatine s.
    posterior superior iliac s.
    pubic s.
    s. of scapula
    sciatic s.
    s. sign
    sphenoidal s.
    s. of sphenoid bone

    Spix s.
    suprameatal s.
    thoracic s.
    trochlear s.
Spinelli operation
spin-lattice relaxation
spinnbarkeit
spinning disk nebulizer
spinoadductor reflex
spinobulbar
spinocerebellar
    s. ataxia
    s. tract
spinocerebellum
spinocervical tract
spinocervicothalamic tract
spinocollicular
spinocostalis
spinocuneate fiber
spinoglenoid ligament
spinogracile fiber
spinohypothalamic fiber
spinomesencephalic fiber
spinomuscular
spinoneural
spinoolivary
    s. fiber
    s. tract
spinoperiaqueductal fiber
spinoreticular
    s. fiber
    s. tract
spinose
spinotectal
    s. fiber
    s. tract
spinothalamic
    s. cordotomy
    s. tract
    s. tractotomy
spinotransversarius
spinous
    s. layer
    s. process of sphenoid
    s. process of tibia
    s. process of vertebra
spinovestibular tract
spin-spin relaxation
spintharicon
spinthariscope
spiperone
spiracle
spiradenoma
    eccrine s.
spiral
    s. bandage
    s. bulbar septum
    s. canal of cochlea
    s. canal of modiolus
    s. cochlear ganglion
    s. computed tomography
    s. crest
    s. crest of cochlear duct
    s. CT
    Curschmann s.

s. fold of cystic duct
s. foraminous tract
s. fracture
s. ganglion of cochlea
s. groove
s. hyphae
s. joint
s. ligament of cochlea
s. ligament of cochlear duct
s. line
s. membrane
s. modiolar artery
s. organ
s. plate
s. prominence of cochlear duct
s. septum
s. suture
s. of Tillaux
s. tip catheter
s. tubule
s. valve of cystic duct
s. vein of modiolus
spiramycin
spirem, spireme
spirilla (*pl. of* spirillum)
Spirillaceae
spirillar
spirillicidal
spirillosis
Spirillum
S. fever
S. *minus*
Obermeier S.
Vincent S.
S. *volutans*
spirillum, pl. **spirilla**
spirit
ardent s.
aromatic ammonia s.
industrial methylated s.,
methylated s.
s. lamp
neutral s.
proof s.
pyroligneous s.
pyroxylic s.
rectified s.
s. thermometer
vital s.
wine s.
wood s.
spirituous
s. liquor
Spirocerca lupi
Spirochaeta
S. *obermeieri*
S. *plicatilis*
Spirochaetaceae
Spirochaetales
spirochetal jaundice
spirochete
spirochetemia
spirocheticide
spirochetolysis

spirochetosis
bronchopulmonary s.
spirochetotic
spirogram
spirograph
spiro-index
spirometer
chain-compensated s.
Krogh s.
Tissot s.
wedge s.
Spirometra
S. *mansoni*
S. *mansonoides*
spirometry
forced s.
spironolactone test
spiroscope
spirostan
Spiruroidea
spiruroid larva migrans
spissitude
spitting
spittle
Spitzer theory
Spitzka
S. marginal tract
S. marginal zone
S. nucleus
Spitz nevus
Spix spine
SPL
sound pressure level
splanchnapophysial, splanchnapophyseal
splanchnapophysis
splanchnectopia
splanchnesthesia
splanchnesthetic sensibility
splanchnic
s. afferent column
s. anesthesia
s. cavity
s. efferent column
s. layer
s. mesoderm
s. nerve
s. wall
splanchnicectomy
splanchnicotomy
splanchnocele
splanchnocranium
splanchnography
splanchnolith
splanchnologia
splanchnology
splanchnomegaly
splanchnomicria
splanchnopathy
splanchnopleural
splanchnopleure
splanchnopleuric
splanchnoptosis, splanchnoptosia
splanchnosclerosis
splanchnoskeletal
splanchnoskeleton

splanchnosomatic
splanchnotomy
splanchnotribe
splay
spleen
>   accessory s.
>   s. deoxyribonuclease
>   diffuse waxy s.
>   s. endonuclease
>   floating s.
>   lardaceous s.
>   movable s.
>   s. phosphodiesterases
>   sago s.
>   sugar-coated s.
>   waxy s.

splen accessorius
splenalgia
Splendore-Hoeppli phenomenon
splenectopia, splenectopy
splenelcosis
spleneolus
splenetic
splenia (*pl. of* splenium)
splenial gyrus
splenic
>   s. anemia
>   s. artery
>   s. branch of splenic artery
>   s. cell
>   s. cord
>   s. corpuscle
>   s. flexure
>   s. flexure syndrome
>   s. hilum
>   s. index
>   s. leukemia
>   s. lymph follicle
>   s. lymph node
>   s. lymph nodule
>   s. plexus
>   s. portal venography
>   s. pulp
>   s. recess
>   s. sinus
>   s. trabecula
>   s. vein

spleniculus
spleniform
spleniserrate
splenitis
splenium, pl. **splenia**
>   s. corporis callosi
>   s. of corpus callosum

splenius
>   s. capitis muscle
>   s. cervicis muscle
>   s. muscle
>   s. muscle of head
>   s. muscle of neck

splenocele
splenocleisis
splenocolic
splenodynia
splenogonadal fusion

splenohepatomegaly, splenohepatomegalia
splenoid
splenolymphatic
splenoma
splenomalacia
splenomedullary
splenomegaly, splenomegalia
>   congestive s.
>   Egyptian s.
>   hemolytic s.
>   hyperreactive malarious s.
>   Niemann s.
>   tropical s.

splenomyelogenous
splenomyelomalacia
splenonephric
splenopancreatic
splenopathy
splenopexy, splenopexia
splenophrenic
splenoportogram
splenoportography
splenoptosis, splenoptosia
splenorenal ligament
splenorrhagia
splenorrhaphy
splenosis
>   thoracic s.

splenotomy
splenotoxin
splenule
splenulus, pl. **splenuli**
splenunculus, pl. **splenunculi**
spliceosome
splicing
>   alternative s.

splint
>   acid etch cemented s.
>   active s.
>   air s.
>   airplane s.
>   anchor s.
>   Anderson s.
>   backboard s.
>   Balkan s.
>   cap s.
>   coaptation s.
>   Cramer wire s.
>   Denis Browne s.
>   dynamic s.
>   Essig s.
>   Frejka pillow s.
>   functional s.
>   Gunning s.
>   inflatable s.
>   interdental s.
>   Kingsley s.
>   labial s.
>   ladder s.
>   lingual s.
>   plaster s.
>   reverse Kingsley s.
>   Stader s.
>   surgical s.
>   Taylor s.

Thomas s.
Tobruk s.
wire s.
splinted abutment
splintered fracture
splinter hemorrhage
splinting
split
s. brain
s. cast method
s. cast mounting
s. fat
s. gene
s. hand
s. papule
s. pelvis
s. renal function test
s. tolerance
split-skin graft
split-thickness graft
splitting
s. enzyme
s. of heart sound
split-virus vaccine
spodogenous
spodogram
spodography
spodophorous
spoke-shave
spondaic
spondee
Spondweni virus
spondylalgia
spondylarthritis
spondylitic
spondylitis
ankylosing s.
s. deformans
rheumatoid s.
tuberculous s.
spondyloepiphyseal
s. dysplasia
s. dysplasia congenita (SEDC)
s. dysplasia tarda
spondylolisthesis
spondylolisthetic pelvis
spondylolysis
spondylomalacia
spondylopathy
spondyloptosis
spondylopyosis
spondyloschisis
spondylosis
cervical s.
hyperostotic s.
spondylosyndesis
spondylothoracic
spondylous
sponge
absorbable gelatin s.
Bernays s.
s. biopsy
compressed s.
contraceptive s.
s. tent

spongia
spongiform
s. encephalopathy
s. pustule of Kogoj
spongioblast
spongioblastoma
spongiocyte
spongioid
spongiose
spongiosis
spongiositis
spongy
s. body of penis
s. bone
s. degeneration of infancy
s. layer of female urethra
s. layer of vagina
s. part of the male urethra
s. spot
s. substance
s. urethra
spontaneous
s. abortion
s. agglutination
s. amputation
s. breech extraction
s. cephalic delivery
s. combustion
s. correction of placenta previa
s. evolution
s. fracture
s. gangrene of newborn
s. generation
s. membrane rupture
s. mutation
s. phagocytosis
s. pneumothorax
s. recovery
s. remission
s. version
spoon
cataract s.
Daviel s.
s. nail
sharp s.
Volkmann s.
sporadic
sporadin
sporangiophore
sporangium
spore
black s.
sporicidal
sporicide
sporidium, pl. **sporidia**
sporoagglutination
sporoblast
sporocyst
Sporocystinea
sporodochium
sporogenesis
sporogenous
sporogeny
sporogony
sporont

S

sporophore
sporoplasm
sporotheca
Sporothrix
sporotrichosis
sporotrichositic chancre
Sporotrichum
sporozoan
Sporozoasida
Sporozoea
sporozoite
sporozoon
sports medicine
sporular
sporulation
sporule
spot
  acoustic s.
  Bitot s.
  blind s.
  blood s.
  blue s.
  Brushfield s.
  café au lait s.
  cherry-red s.
  corneal s.
  cotton-wool s.
  De Morgan s.
  Elschnig s.
  s. film
  flame s.
  focal s.
  Fordyce s.
  Fuchs black s.
  hot s.
  hypnogenic s.
  Koplik s.
  liver s.
  s. map
  Mariotte blind s.
  milk s.
  mongolian s.
  mulberry s.
  rose s.
  Roth s.
  saccular s.
  Soemmerring s.
  spongy s.
  Tardieu s.
  Tay cherry-red s.
  temperature s.
  tendinous s.
  s. test for infectious mononucleosis
  Trousseau s.
  utricular s.
  white s.
  yellow s.
spot-film radiography
spotted fever
spousal abuse
spp.
  species
sprain
  s. fracture
spray

spreader
  gutta-percha s.
  rib s.
  root canal s.
spreading
  s. depression
  s. factor
Sprengel deformity
spring
  s. conjunctivitis
  s. finger
  s. lancet
  s. ligament
  s. ophthalmia
sprout
  syncytial s.
sprue
  celiac s.
  nontropical s.
  tropical s.
sprue-former
spud
Spumavirinae
Spumavirus
spun glass hair
spur
  calcarine s.
  s. cell
  s. cell anemia
  Fuchs s.
  Grunert s.
  heel s.
  Michel s.
  Morand s.
  scleral s.
  vascular s.
spurious
  s. ankylosis
  s. cast
  s. meningocele
  s. parasite
  s. pregnancy
Spurling test
sputum, pl. sputa
  s. aerogenosum
  globular s.
  green s.
  nummular s.
  prune-juice s.
  rusty s.
  s. smear
SQ
  subcutaneous
squalamine lactate
squalene
  s. epoxidase
  s. synthase
squama, pl. squamae
  frontal s.
  s. frontalis
  occipital s.
  s. occipitalis
  temporal s.
  s. temporalis
squamatization

S

squame
squamocellular
squamocolumnar junction
squamofrontal
squamomastoid suture
squamo-occipital
squamoparietal suture
squamopetrosal
squamosa, pl. squamosae
squamosal
    s. border
    s. border of parietal bone
    s. margin
    s. margin of greater wing of
      sphenoid
squamosphenoid
squamotemporal
squamotympanic fissure
squamous
    s. alveolar cell
    s. border
    s. border of parietal bone
    s. border of sphenoid bone
    s. cell
    s. cell carcinoma
    s. cell hyperplasia
    s. margin
    s. metaplasia
    s. metaplasia of amnion
    s. odontogenic tumor
    s. part of frontal bone
    s. part of occipital bone
    s. part of temporal bone
    s. pearl
    s. suture
squamozygomatic
square
    s. knot
    s. matrix
    s. wave stimuli
squill
squint
    convergent s.
    divergent s.
    external s.
    s. hook
    internal s.
squinting eye
squirrel plague conjunctivitis
Sr
    strontium
sr
    steradian
^{85}Sr
    strontium-85
^{87m}Sr
    strontium-87m
^{89}Sr
    strontium-89
^{90}Sr
    strontium-90
SRF
    somatotropin-releasing factor
SRF-A
    slow-reacting factor of anaphylaxis

SRH
    somatotropin-releasing hormone
SRIF
    somatotropin release-inhibiting factor
sRNA
    soluble rna
S romanum
SRP
    signal recognition particle
SRS
    slow-reacting substance
SRS-A
    slow-reacting substance of anaphylaxis
ss
    steady state
SSPE
    subacute sclerosing panencephalitis
SSPL
    saturation sound pressure level
SSS
    soluble specific substance
ST
    ST junction
    ST segment
St.
    St. John's wort
    St. Louis encephalitis virus
stab
    s. cell
    s. culture
    s. drain
    s. neutrophil
    s. wound
stabilate
stabile
stabilimeter
stability
    denture s.
    detrusor s.
    dimensional s.
    endemic s.
    enzootic s.
    suspension s.
stabilization
stabilized baseplate
stabilizer
    endodontic s.
stabilizing
    s. circumferential clasp arm
    s. fulcrum line
stable
    s. colloid
    s. disease
    s. equilibrium
    s. factor
    s. fracture
    s. isotope
staccato speech
stachybotryotoxicosis
stachydrine
stachyose
stactometer
Staderini nucleus
Stader splint

stadiometer
stadium, pl. **stadia**
staff
    attending s.
    s. cell
    consulting s.
    house s.
staff of Aesculapius
Stafne bone cyst
stage
    algid s.
    Arneth s.
    bell s.
    bud s.
    cap s.
    cold s.
    defervescent s.
    end s.
    eruptive s.
    exoerythrocytic s.
    genital s.
    imperfect s.
    incubative s.
    intuitive s.
    s. of invasion
    s.'s of labor
    latent s.
    perfect s.
    preconceptual s.
    prodromal s.
    resting s.
    Tanner s.
    trypanosome s.
    tumor s.
    vegetative s.
stagger
staggered spondaic word test
staggers
staghorn calculus
staging
    Jewett and Strong s.
    TNM s.
stagnant
    s. anoxia
    s. hypoxia
stagnation
    s. mastitis
Stahl ear
stain
    Abbott s. for spores
    acetoorcein s.
    acid s.
    Ag-AS s.
    Albert s.
    Altmann anilin-acid fuchsin s.
    auramine O fluorescent s.
    basic fuchsin-methylene blue s.
    Bauer chromic acid leucofuchsin s.
    Becker s. for spirochetes
    Bennhold Congo red s.
    Berg s.
    Best carmine s.
    Bielschowsky s.
    Biondi-Heidenhain s.
    Birch-Hirschfeld s.

Bodian copper-PROTARGOL s.
Borrel blue s.
Bowie s.
Brown-Brenn s.
Cajal astrocyte s.
carbol-thionin s.
C-banding s.
centromere banding s.
chromate s. for lead
chrome alum hematoxylin-
  phloxine s.
Ciaccio s.
contrast s.
Cresylecht violet s.
Da Fano s.
Dane s.
DAPI s.
diazo s. for argentaffin granule
Dieterle s.
differential s.
double s.
Ehrlich acid hematoxylin s.
Ehrlich aniline crystal violet s.
Ehrlich triacid s.
Ehrlich triple s.
Einarson gallocyanin-chrome alum s.
Eranko fluorescence s.
Feulgen s.
Field rapid s.
Fink-Heimer s.
Flemming triple s.
fluorescence plus Giemsa s.
fluorescent s.
Fontana s.
Fontana-Masson silver s.
Foot reticulin impregnation s.
Fouchet s.
Fraser-Lendrum s. for fibrin
Friedländer s. for capsule
G-banding s.
Giemsa chromosome banding s.
Glenner-Lillie s. for pituitary
Golgi s.
Gomori aldehyde fuchsin s.
Gomori chrome alum hematoxylin-
  phloxine s.
Gomori-Jones periodic acid-
  methenamine-silver s.
Gomori methenamine-silver s.'s
  (GMS)
Gomori nonspecific acid
  phosphatase s.
Gomori nonspecific alkaline
  phosphatase s.
Gomori one-step trichrome s.
Gomori silver impregnation s.
Goodpasture s.
Gordon and Sweet s.
Gram s.
Gram-chromotrope s.
green s.
Gridley s.
Gridley s. for fungi
Grocott-Gomori methenamine-
  silver s.

Hale colloidal iron s.
Heidenhain azan s.
Heidenhain iron hematoxylin s.
hematoxylin and eosin s.
hematoxylin-malachite green-basic
  fuchsin s.
hematoxylin-phloxine B s.
Hirsch-Peiffer s.
Hiss s.
Holmes s.
Hortega neuroglia s.
Hucker-Conn s.
immunofluorescent s.
India ink capsule s.
intravital s.
iodine s.
Jenner s.
Kasten fluorescent Feulgen s.
Kasten fluorescent PAS s.
Kinyoun s.
Kleihauer s.
Klinger-Ludwig acid-thionin s. for
  sex chromatin
Klüver-Barrera Luxol fast blue s.
Kokoskin s.
Kossa s.
Kronecker s.
lactophenol cotton blue s.
Laquer s. for alcoholic hyalin
lead hydroxide s.
Leishman s.
Lendrum phloxine-tartrazine s.
Lepehne-Pickworth s.
Levaditi s.
Lillie allochrome connective
  tissue s.
Lillie azure-eosin s.
Lillie ferrous iron s.
Lillie sulfuric acid Nile blue s.
Lison-Dunn s.
Loeffler caustic s.
Luna-Ishak s.
Macchiavello s.
MacNeal tetrachrome blood s.
malarial pigment s.
Maldonado-San Jose s.
Mallory s. for actinomyces
Mallory aniline blue s.
Mallory collagen s.
Mallory s. for hemofuchsin
Mallory iodine s.
Mallory phloxine s.
Mallory phosphotungstic acid
  hematoxylin s.
Mallory trichrome s.
Mallory triple s.
Mann methyl blue-eosin s.
Marchi s.
Masson argentaffin s.
Masson-Fontana ammoniac silver s.
Masson trichrome s.
Maximow s. for bone marrow
Mayer hemalum s.
Mayer mucicarmine s.
Mayer mucihematein s.

May-Grünwald s.
metachromatic s.
methenamine silver s.
methyl green-pyronin s.
modified acid-fast s.
modified trichrome s.
Mowry colloidal iron s.
MSB trichrome s.
multiple s.
Nair buffered methylene blue s.
Nakanishi s.
Nauta s.
negative s.
Neisser s.
neutral s.
Nicolle s. for capsule
ninhydrin-Schiff s.
Nissl s.
Noble s.
nuclear s.
Orth s.
Padykula-Herman s.
Paget-Eccleston s.
panoptic s.
Papanicolaou s.
Pappenheim s.
paracarmine s.
PAS s.
periodic acid-Schiff s.
Perls Prussian blue s.
peroxidase s.
phosphotungstic acid s.
picrocarmine s.
picro-Mallory trichrome s.
picronigrosin s.
plasma s., plasmatic s., plasmic s.
plastic section s.
port-wine s.
positive s.
Prussian blue s.
PTA s.
Puchtler-Sweat s.
Q-banding s.
quinacrine chromosome banding s.
Rambourg chromic acid-
  phosphotungstic acid s.
Rambourg periodic acid-chromic
  methenamine-silver s.
R-banding s.
Romanowsky blood s.
Roux s.
Ryan s.
Schaeffer-Fulton s.
Schmorl ferric-ferricyanide
  reduction s.
Schmorl picrothionin s.
Schultz s.
selective s.
Semichon acid carmine s.
silver-ammoniac silver s.
silver protein s.
Stirling modification of Gram s.
supravital s.
Taenzer s.
Takayama s.

stain (*continued*)
 telomeric R-banding s.
 thioflavin T s.
 Tizzoni s.
 Toison s.
 toluidine blue s.
 trichrome s.
 trypsin G-banding s.
 ultrafast Pap s.
 Unna s.
 Unna-Pappenheim s.
 Unna-Taenzer s.
 uranyl acetate s.
 urate crystals s.
 van Ermengen s.
 van Gieson s.
 Verhoeff elastic tissue s.
 vital s.
 von Kossa s.
 Wachstein-Meissel s. for calcium-
  magnesium-ATPase
 Warthin-Starry silver s.
 Weber s.
 Weigert s. for actinomyces
 Weigert s. for elastin
 Weigert s. for fibrin
 Weigert-Gram s.
 Weigert iron hematoxylin s.
 Weigert s. for myelin
 Weigert s. for neuroglia
 Wilder s. for reticulum
 Williams s.
 Wright s.
 Ziehl s.
 Ziehl-Neelsen s.
staining
 progressive s.
 regressive s.
stains-all
staircase phenomenon
stalagmometer
stalk
 allantoic s.
 body s.
 connecting s.
 s. of epiglottis
 infundibular s.
 optic s.
 pineal s.
 pituitary s.
 yolk s.
stalked hydatid
stammer
stammering of the bladder
Stamnosoma
standard
 s. atmosphere
 s. bicarbonate
 s. cell
 s. deviation
 s. error of difference
 s. error of the mean (SEM)
 s. limb lead
 s. pressure

uDiquitin

 s. score
 s. serologic tests for syphilis
 s. solution
 s. substance
 s. temperature
 s. urea clearance
 s. volume
standardization of a test
standardized mortality ratio
standardized solution (*var. of* standard
 solution)
standby pulse generator
standing
 s. plasma test
standstill
 atrial s.
 auricular s.
 cardiac s.
 sinus s.
 ventricular s.
Stanford-Binet intelligence scale
Stanley cervical ligament
stannic
stannic chloride
stannic oxide
Stannius ligature
stannous
 s. fluoride
stannum
stanolone
stanozolol
stapedectomy
stapedes
stapedial
 s. artery
 s. branch of posterior tympanic
  artery
 s. branch of stylomastoid artery
 s. fold
 s. membrane
 s. reflex
stapedii (*pl. of* stapedius)
stapediotenotomy
stapediovestibular
stapedius, pl. **stapedii**
 s. muscle
stapedotomy
stapes, pl. **stapes**
 s. mobilization
 s. mobilization operation
staphylectomy
staphyledema
staphyline
staphylion
staphylococcal
 s. blepharitis
 s. enterotoxin
 s. pneumonia
 s. scalded skin syndrome
staphylococcemia
staphylococci (*pl. of* staphylococcus)
staphylococcic
staphylococcolysin
staphylococcolysis
staphylococcosis, pl. **staphylococcoses**

Staphylococcus
 S. antitoxin
 S. *aureus*
 S. *epidermidis*
 S. food poisoning
 S. *haemolyticus*
 S. *hominis*
 S. *pyogenes albus*
 S. *pyogenes aureus*
 S. *saprophyticus*
 S. *simulans*
 S. species, coagulase-negative
 S. vaccine
staphylococcus, pl. **staphylococci**
staphylodialysis
staphylohemia
staphylohemolysin
staphylokinase
staphylolysin
staphyloma
 anterior s.
 anular s.
 ciliary s.
 corneal s.
 equatorial s.
 intercalary s.
 posterior s.
 Scarpa s.
 scleral s.
 uveal s.
staphylomatous
staphyloopsonic index
staphylopharyngorrhaphy
staphyloplasty
staphyloptosis
staphylorrhaphy
staphylotoxin
stapling
 gastric s.
star
 daughter s.
 lens s.
 mother s.
 polar s.
 venous s.
 Verheyen s.
 Winslow s.
starch
 animal s.
 s. equivalent
 s. glycerite
 s. gum
 liver s.
 moss s.
 rice s.
 soluble s.
 s. sugar
starch-eating
starch-iodine test
stare
Stargardt disease
Starling
 S. curve
 S. hypothesis

 S. law
 S. reflex
Starr-Edwards valve
start codon
starter tRNA
starting friction
startle
 s. disease
 s. epilepsy
 s. reaction
 s. reflex
starvation
 s. acidosis
 s. diabetes
starve
stasimorphia
stasis, pl. **stases**
 s. cirrhosis
 s. dermatitis
 s. eczema
 intestinal s.
 papillary s.
 pressure s.
 s. ulcer
 venous s.
Stas-Otto method
stat
stat.
 statin
statampere
statcoulomb
state
 absent s.
 activated s.
 anxiety tension s.
 apallic s.
 carrier s.
 central excitatory s.
 convulsive s.
 decerebrate s.
 decorticate s.
 dreamy s.
 eunuchoid s.
 excited s.
 ground s.
 s. hospital
 hypnoid s.
 hypnotic s.
 hypometabolic s.
 imperfect s.
 lacunar s.
 local excitatory s.
 multiple ego s.
 perfect s.
 persistent vegetative s. (PVS)
 post-steady s.
 pre–steady s.
 refractory s.
 singlet s.
 steady s. (s, ss)
 triplet s.
 twilight s.
 vegetative s.
state-dependent learning
statfarad

S

stathenry
stathmokinesis
static
    s. arthropathy
    s. ataxia
    s. bone cyst
    s. compliance
    s. friction
    s. gangrene
    s. hysteresis
    s. infantilism
    s. perimetry
    s. reflex
    s. refraction
    s. relation
    s. scoliosis
    s. sense
    s. system
    s. tremor
statim
statin (stat.)
statins
station
    s. test
stationary
    s. anchorage
    s. cataract
    s. phase
statistic
    descriptive s.
    inferential s.
    vital s.
statistical
    s. genetics
    s. model
    s. power
statistical significance
statoacoustic
    s. nerve
statoconial membrane
statoconium, pl. **statoconia**
statokinetic reflex
statokinetics
statolith
statometer
statosphere
statotonic reflex
stature
    brittle hair, impaired intellect,
    decreased fertility, short s. (BIDS)
status
    s. anginosus
    s. arthriticus
    s. asthmaticus
    s. choleraicus
    s. choreicus
    s. cribrosus
    s. criticus
    s. dysmyelinisatus
    s. dysraphicus
    s. epilepticus
    s. hemicranicus
    s. hypnoticus
    s. lacunaris
    s. lymphaticus

    s. marmoratus
    nonreassuring fetal s.
    performance s.
    s. praesens
    s. spongiosus
    s. sternuens
    s. thymicolymphaticus
    s. thymicus
    s. vertiginosus
statvolt
Staub-Traugott
    S.-T. effect
    S.-T. phenomenon
Stauffer syndrome
staurion
STD
    sexually transmitted disease
steady
    s. state (s, ss)
    s. state approximation
steady-state
    s.-s. rate
    s.-s. velocity
steal
    coronary s.
    iliac s.
    s. phenomenon
    renal-splanchnic s.
    subclavian s.
steam-fitter's asthma
steapsin
stearal
stearaldehyde
stearate
stearic acid
stearin
stearrhea
stearyl alcohol
stearyl-CoA
    stearyl-CoA desaturase
stearyl-coenzyme A
steatite
steatitis
steatocystoma multiplex
steatogenesis
steatolysis
steatolytic
steatonecrosis
steatopyga, steatopygia
steatopygous
steatorrhea
    biliary s.
    intestinal s.
    pancreatic s.
steatosis
    s. cardiaca
    s. cordis
    hepatic s.
steatozoon
Steele-Richardson-Olszewski
    S.-R.-O. disease
    S.-R.-O. syndrome
Steell murmur
Steenbock unit
steeple skull

steering wheel injury
stege
stegnosis
stegnotic
Steinberg thumb sign
Steinert disease
Stein-Leventhal syndrome
Steinmann pin
steinstrasse
Stein test
STEL
    short-term exposure limit
stella, pl. **stellae**
    s. lentis hyaloidea
    s. lentis iridica
stellate
    s. abscess
    s. block
    s. cataract
    s. cell of cerebral cortex
    s. cell of liver
    s. ganglion
    s. hair
    s. ligament
    s. neuroretinitis
    s. reticulum
    s. skull fracture
    s. vein
    s. venule
stellectomy
stellula, pl. **stellulae**
    stellulae vasculosae
    stellulae verheyenii
    stellulae winslowii
Stellwag sign
stem
    brain s.
    s. bronchus
    s. cell
    s. cell factor
    s. cell leukemia
    infundibular s.
sten.
Stender dish
Stenger test
stenion
stenobregmatic
stenocardia
stenocephalia
stenocephalous, stenocephalic
stenocephaly
stenochoria
stenocompressor
stenocrotaphy, stenocrotaphia
Steno duct
stenopeic, stenopaic
    s. disk
    s. iridectomy
    s. spectacles
    s. spectacles
stenosal
    s. murmur
stenosed
stenosing tenosynovitis
stenosis, pl. **stenoses**

    aortic s.
    bronchial s.
    buttonhole s.
    calcific nodular aortic s.
    congenital pyloric s.
    coronary ostial s.
    Dittrich s.
    double aortic s.
    fish-mouth mitral s.
    hypertrophic pyloric s.
    idiopathic hypertrophic subaortic s.
    idiopathic subglottic s.
    infundibular s.
    laryngeal s.
    mitral s.
    muscular subaortic s.
    pulmonary s.
    pyloric s.
    subaortic s.
    subvalvar aortic s.
    supravalvar s.
    supravalvular s.
    tricuspid s.
stenostenosis
stenostomia
stenothermal
stenothorax
stenotic
Stenotrophomonas
    s. maltophilia
stenoxenous
stenoxous parasite
Stensen
    S. duct
    S. foramen
    S. plexus
    S. vein
stent
    expandable s.
    s. graft
Stenvers
    S. projection
    S. view
step
    Krönig s.
    Rønne nasal s.
stephanial
stephanion
Stephanofilaria stilesi
Stephanurus dentatus
steppage
    s. gait
steradian (sr)
sterane
stercobilin
l-**stercobilinogen**
stercolith
stercoraceous
    s. vomiting
stercoral
    s. abscess
    s. appendicitis
    s. ulcer
stercorin
stercoroma

stercorous
sterculia gum
stercus
stere
stereoagnosis
stereoanesthesia
stereoarthrolysis
stereocampimeter
stereochemical
    s. formula
    s. isomerism
stereochemistry
stereocilium, pl. **stereocilia**
stereocinefluorography
stereocolpogram
stereocolposcope
stereoelectroencephalography
stereoencephalometry
stereognosis
stereognostic
stereogram
stereograph
stereography
stereoisomer
stereoisomeric
stereoisomerism
stereology
stereometer
stereometry
stereo-orthopter
stereopathy
stereophorometer
stereophotomicrograph
stereopsis
stereoradiography
stereoroentgenography
stereoscope
stereoscopic
    s. acuity
    s. microscope
    s. parallax
    s. vision
stereoscopy
stereoselective
stereospecific
stereotactic, stereotaxic
    s. brachytherapy
    s. cordotomy
    s. instrument
    s. localization
    s. surgery
stereotaxis
stereotaxy
stereotropic
stereotropism
    negative s.
    positive s.
stereotypy
    oral s.
steric
    s. hindrance
sterid
sterigma, pl. **sterigmata**
sterile
    s. abscess

    s. cyst
    s. insect technique
sterility
    aspermatogenic s.
    dysspermatogenic s.
    female s.
    male s.
    normospermatogenic s.
sterilization
    discontinuous s.
    fractional s.
    intermittent s.
sterilize
sterilizer
    glass bead s.
    hot salt s.
sterna (*pl. of* sternum)
sternad
sternal
    s. angle
    s. artery
    s. articular surface of clavicle
    s. bar
    s. branch of internal thoracic artery
    s. cartilage
    s. end of clavicle
    s. extremity of clavicle
    s. facet of clavicle
    s. joint
    s. line
    s. line of pleural reflection
    s. membrane
    s. muscle
    s. notch
    s. part of diaphragm
    s. plane
    s. puncture
    s. synchondrosis
sternalgia
sternalis
    s. muscle
Sternberg
    S. cell
    S. sign
Sternberg-Reed cell
sternebra, pl. **sternebrae**
sternen
sternobrachial reflex
sternochondral separation
sternochondroscapularis
sternochondroscapular muscle
sternoclavicular
    s. angle
    s. articular disk
    s. disk
    s. joint
    s. ligament
    s. muscle
sternoclavicularis
sternocleidal
sternocleidomastoid
    s. branch of occipital artery
    s. branch of superior thyroid artery
    s. muscle (SCM)

s. region
s. vein
sternocleidomastoideus
sternocostal
    s. articulations
    s. head of pectoralis major muscle
    s. joint
    s. part of pectoralis major muscle
    s. surface of heart
    s. triangle
sternocostalis muscle
sternodynia
sternofascialis
sternoglossal
sternohyoideus
sternohyoid muscle
sternoid
sternomanubrial junction
sternomastoid
    s. artery
    s. muscle
sternopagia
sternopericardial ligament
sternoschisis
sternothyroideus
sternothyroid muscle
sternotomy
    median s.
sternotracheal
sternotrypesis
sternovertebral
Stern posture
sternum, pl. **sterna**
sternutation
sternutator
sternutatory
steroid
    s. acne
    anabolic s.
    s. cell tumor
    s. diabetes
    s. fever
    s. hormone
    s. hydroxylases
    s. metabolic clearance rate (MCR)
    s. 21-monooxygenase
    s. monooxygenases
    s. nucleus
    s. production rate
    s. 5α-reductase
    s. secretory rate
    s. sulfatase deficiency
    s. withdrawal syndrome
steroidal
steroidogenesis
steroidogenic diabetes
sterol
stertor
    hen-cluck s.
stertorous
    s. breathing
    s. respiration
stethalgia
stetharteritis
stethograph

stethomyitis
stethomyositis
stethoparalysis
stethoscope
    binaural s.
    Bowles-type s.
    differential s.
stethoscopic
    s. phonocardiograph
stethoscopy
Stevens-Johnson syndrome
Stewart-Hamilton method
Stewart-Holmes sign
Stewart-Morel syndrome
Stewart test
Stewart-Treves syndrome
STH
    somatotropic hormone
sthenia
sthenic
sthenometer
sthenometry
stibamine glucoside
stibenyl
stibialism
stibiated
stibiation
stibium
stibocaptate
stibogluconate sodium
stibonium
stibophen
stichochrome cell
Stickler syndrome
sticky-ended DNA
Stieda process
Stierlin sign
sties (*pl. of* sty)
stiff
    s. heart syndrome
    s. man syndrome
    s. neck
    s. toe
stigma, pl. **stigmas, stigmata**
    follicular s.
    malpighian stigma
    s. ventriculi
stigmal plate
stigmastane
stigmata (*pl. of* stigma)
stigmatic
stigmatism
stigmatization
stilbamidine
stilbazium iodide
stilbene
stilbestrol
Stiles-Crawford effect
stilet
still
    S. disease
    s. layer
    S. murmur
stillbirth rate
stillborn infant

Still-Chauffard syndrome
Stilling
    S. canal
    S. column
    S. gelatinous substance
    S. nucleus
    S. raphe
stilus (*var. of* stylus)
stimulant
    diffusible s.
    general s.
    local s.
stimulation
    dorsal column s.
    fetal scalp s.
    Ganzfeld s.
    percutaneous s.
    photic s.
    vagal nerve s.
stimulator
    long-acting thyroid s. (LATS)
stimulatory protein 1 (SP1)
stimulus, pl. **stimuli**
    adequate s.
    aversive s.
    conditioned s.
    s. control
    discriminant s.
    s. generalization
    heterologous s.
    heterotopic s.
    homologous s.
    inadequate s.
    liminal s.
    maximal s.
    s. sensitive myoclonus
    square wave stimuli
    subliminal s.
    s. substitution
    subthreshold s.
    supramaximal s.
    s. threshold
    threshold s.
    train-of-four s.
    unconditioned s.
    s. word
sting
stinger
stinging caterpillar
stink weed
stippled
    s. epiphysis
    s. tongue
stippling
    geographic s. of nail
    Ziemann s.
STIR
    short ti inversion recovery
Stirling modification of Gram stain
stirrup
stitch
    s. abscess
    lock s.
STM
    short-term memory

Stobo antigen
stochastic
    s. independence
    s. process
stock
    s. culture
    s. strain
    s. vaccine
Stocker line
Stockholm syndrome
stocking anesthesia
Stoffel operation
stoichiology
stoichiometric
    s. number
stoichiometry
stoke
stoker's cramps
Stokes
    S. amputation
    S. basket
    S. law
Stokes-Adams
    S.-A. disease
    S.-A. syndrome
stolon
stoma, pl. **stomas, stomata**
    Fuchs s.
    loop s.
stomach
    s. ache
    bilocular s.
    s. bubble
    cascade s.
    drain-trap s.
    s. drops
    hourglass s.
    leather-bottle s.
    miniature s.
    Pavlov s.
    powdered s.
    s. pump
    s. reefing
    sclerotic s.
    thoracic s.
    s. tooth
    trifid s.
    s. tube
    wallet s.
    water-trap s.
stomachal
stomachalgia
stomachic
stomachodynia
stomal
    s. ulcer
stomas (*pl. of* stoma)
stomata (*pl. of* stoma)
stomatal
stomatalgia
stomatic
stomatitis
    angular s.
    aphthous s.
    epidemic s.

fusospirochetal s.
gangrenous s.
gonococcal s.
lead s.
s. medicamentosa
mercurial s.
nicotine s.
primary herpetic s.
recurrent aphthous s.
recurrent herpetic s.
recurrent ulcerative s.
ulcerative s.
vesicular s.
stomatocyte
stomatocytosis
stomatodeum
stomatodynia
stomatodysodia
stomatognathic system
stomatologic
stomatologist
stomatology
stomatomalacia
stomatomycosis
stomatonecrosis
stomatopathy
stomatoplasty
stomatorrhagia
stomatoscope
stomatosis
stomion
stomocephalus
stomodeal
stomodeum
Stomoxys calcitrans
stone
artificial s.
s. basket
bladder s.'s
s. heart
philosopher's s.
pulp s.
tear s.
vein s.
stone-mason's disease
Stookey-Scarff operation
stool
butter s.
currant jelly s.
fatty s.
rice-water s.
spinach s.
Trélat s.'s
stop codon
stopping rule
storage
s. disease
s. oscilloscope
storax
STORCH
syphilis, toxoplasmosis, other infections, rubella, cytomegalovirus infection, and herpes simplex
storiform neurofibroma

storm
thyroid s.
Stout wiring
stove-pipe colon
STPD
strabismal
strabismic amblyopia
strabismologist
strabismus
A-s.
accommodative s.
alternate day s.
alternating s.
A-pattern s.
comitant s.
concomitant s.
convergent s.
cyclic s.
divergent s.
incomitant s.
kinetic s.
manifest s.
mechanical s.
paralytic s.
vertical s.
X-s.
straddling embolism
straight
s. artery
s. back syndrome
s. conjugate
s. gyrus
s. muscle
s. part of cricothyroid muscle
s. seminiferous tubule
s. sinus
s. tubule of testis
s. venules of kidney
strain
auxotrophic s.
carrier s.
cell s.
congenic s.
s. fracture
s. gauge
HFR s.
hypothetical mean s. (HMS)
isogenic s.
lysogenic s.
neotype s.
prototrophic s.
pseudolysogenic s.
recombinant s.
stock s.
type s.
wild-type s.
strait
inferior s.
superior s.
straitjacket
stramonium
strand
anticoding s.
antiparallel s.
antisense s.

strand (*continued*)
    coding s.
    complementary s.
    minus s.
    plus s.
    sense s.
    viral s.
strangalesthesia
strangle
strangulated hernia
strangulation
strangury
strap
    s. cell
    s. muscle
Strassburg test
strata (*pl. of* stratum)
stratification
stratified
    s. ciliated columnar epithelium
    s. epithelium
    s. sample
    s. squamous epithelium
    s. thrombus
stratiform fibrocartilage
stratigraphy
stratum, pl. strata
    s. aculeatum
    s. basale
    s. basale epidermidis
    s. cerebrale retinae
    s. cinereum colliculi superioris
    s. circulare membranae tympani
    s. circulare musculi detrusoris
        vesicae
    s. circulare tunicae muscularis
    s. circulare tunicae muscularis coli
    s. circulare tunicae muscularis
        intestini tenuis
    s. circulare tunicae muscularis recti
    s. circulare tunicae muscularis
        ventriculi
    s. compactum
    s. corneum epidermidis
    s. corneum unguis
    s. cutaneum membranae tympani
    s. cylindricum
    s. disjunctum
    s. fibrosum
    s. fibrosum capsulae articularis
    s. fibrosum panniculi adiposi telae
        subcutaneae
    s. fibrosum vaginae tendinis
    s. functionale
    s. ganglionare nervi optici
    s. ganglionicum
    s. germinativum
    s. germinativum unguis
    s. granulare
    s. granulosum corticis cerebelli
    s. granulosum epidermidis
    s. granulosum folliculi ovarici
        vesiculosi
    s. granulosum ovarii

s. griseum colliculi superioris
s. griseum intermedium
s. griseum profundum
s. griseum profundum colliculis
    superioris
s. griseum superficiale
strata gyri dentati
s. helicoidale brevis gradus
s. helicoidale longi gradus
strata hippocampi
s. interolivare lemnisci
s. lemnisci
s. limitans externum
s. limitans internum
s. longitudinale tunicae muscularis
s. longitudinale tunicae muscularis
    coli
s. longitudinale tunicae muscularis
    intestini tenuis
s. longitudinale tunicae muscularis
    recti
s. longitudinale tunicae muscularis
    ventriculi
s. lucidum
strata magnocellularia
malpighian s.
s. medullare intermedium
s. medullare profundum
s. moleculare
s. moleculare corticis cerebelli
s. moleculare et substratum
    lacunosum
s. moleculare retinae
s. multiforme
s. musculosum panniculi adiposi
    telae subcutaneae
s. neuroepitheliale retinae
s. neurofibrarum
s. neuronorum piriformium
s. nucleare externum
s. nucleare internum
strata nuclearia externa et interna
    retinae
s. opticum
s. oriens
s. papillare corii
strata parvocellularia
s. pigmenti bulbi
s. pigmenti corporis ciliaris
s. pigmenti iridis
s. pigmenti retinae
s. plexiforme externum
s. plexiforme internum
s. purkinjense corticis cerebelli
s. pyramidale
s. radiatum
s. radiatum membranae tympani
s. reticulare corii
s. reticulare cutis
s. segmentorum externorum et
    internorum
s. spinosum epidermidis
s. spongiosum
s. subcutaneum

s. synoviale
s. zonale
Straus
S. reaction
S. sign
strawberry
s. birthmark
s. cervix
s. gallbladder
s. hemangioma
s. nevus
s. tongue
straw itch
streak
angioid s.
s. culture
germinal s.
s. gonad
gonadal s.
s. hyperostosis
Knapp s.
meningitic s.
Moore lightning s.
primitive s.
stream
hair s.
streaming movement
streblodactyly
street
s. drug
s. virus
Streeter developmental horizon
strength
associative s.
biting s.
compressive s.
fatigue s.
ionic s.
tensile s.
ultimate s.
yield s.
strength-duration curve
strephosymbolia
strepitus
streptavidin
strepticemia
streptidine
Streptobacillus moniliformis
streptobiosamine
streptobiose
streptocerciasis
streptococcal
s. empyema
s. fibrinolysin
s. pneumonia
s. toxic shock syndrome
streptococcemia
streptococci (*pl. of* streptococcus)
streptococcic
streptococcosis
Streptococcus
S. agalactiae
alpha-hemolytic S.'s
S. anginosus
beta-hemolytic S.'s

S. bovis
S. constellatus
S. durans
S. erythrogenic toxin
S. faecalis
group A S.'s (GAS)
group B S.'s
hemolytic S.'s
S. intermedius
S. lactis
S. lactis R factor
S. M antigen
S. milleri
S. mitis
S. morbillorum
S. mutans
S. pneumoniae
S. pyogenes
S. salivarius
S. sanguis
viridans S.'s
S. viridans
streptococcus, pl. **streptococci**
streptodornase (SD)
streptofuranose
streptokinase (SK)
streptokinase-streptodornase
streptolysin O
Streptomyces
S. albus
S. gibsonii
S. somaliensis
Streptomycetaceae
streptomycete
streptomycin
s. units
streptomycin A
streptomycosis
streptonivicin
streptose
streptosepticemia
streptothrichosis
streptotrichiasis
streptotrichosis
streptozocin
streptozotocin
stress
s. breaker
s. echocardiography
s. fiber
s. fracture
s. immunity
s. inoculation
life s.
s. reaction
s. riser
shear s.
s. shielding
tensile s.
s. test
s. ulcer
s. urinary incontinence (SUI)
yield s.
stress-bearing area

S

stress-broken
    s.-b. connector
    s.-b. joint
stress-strain curve
stretch
    s. mark
    s. receptor
    s. reflex
stretcher
stria, pl. **striae**
    acoustic s.
    anterior acoustic s.
    striae atrophicae
    auditory s.
    brown s.
    striae ciliares
    s. cochlearis anterior
    s. cochlearis intermedia
    s. cochlearis posterior
    striae cutis distensae
    diagonalis s.
    s. diagonalis
    s. externa medullae renalis
    s. fornicis
    Gennari s.
    striae gravidarum
    intermediate acoustic s.
    s. of internal granular layer
    s. of internal pyramidal layer
    s. interna medullae renalis
    Knapp s.
    s. laminae granularis internae
    s. laminae molecularis
    s. laminae pyramidalis internae
    striae lancisi
    Langhans s.
    lateral longitudinal s.
    s. longitudinalis lateralis
    s. longitudinalis medialis
    s. mallearis
    malleolar s.
    medial longitudinal s.
    striae medullares ventriculi quarti
    s. medullaris thalami
    medullary s. of fourth ventricle
    medullary s. of thalamus
    s. of molecular layer
    s. nasi transversa
    Nitabuch s.
    s. occipitalis
    striae olfactoriae
    olfactory s.
    striae parallelae
    posterior acoustic s.
    striae retinae
    Retzius s.
    Rohr s.
    s. spinosa
    s. tecta
    tectal s.
    terminal s.
    s. terminalis
    s. vascularis of cochlear duct
    s. vascularis ductus cochlearis
    ventral acoustic s.
    s. ventriculi tertii
    Wickham s.
    striae of Zahn
striatal
striate
    s. area
    s. atrophy of skin
    s. body
    s. cortex
    s. keratopathy
    s. vein
striated
    s. border
    s. duct
    s. membrane
    s. muscle
    s. muscular sphincter
striation
    basal s.
    tabby cat s.
    tigroid s.
striatonigral fiber
striatum
    dorsal s.
    s. dorsale
    ventral s.
    s. ventrale
stricture
    anastomotic s.
    anular s.
    bridle s.
    contractile s.
    functional s.
    organic s.
    permanent s.
    recurrent s.
    spasmodic s.
    temporary s.
    urethral s.
stricturoplasty
stricturotome
stricturotomy
strident
stridor
    congenital s.
    s. dentium
    expiratory s.
    inspiratory s.
    laryngeal s.
    s. serraticus
stridulous
string
    auditory s.
    s. sign
    s. test
stringed instrument theory
stringent
    s. factor
    s. response
striola
strionigral fiber
strip
    abrasive s.
    amalgam s.

celluloid s.
lightning s.
stripe
s. of Gennari
Hensen s.
inner s. of renal medulla
mallear s.
Mees s.
occipital s.
outer s. of renal medulla
pleural s.
tracheal wall s.
vascular s.
stripped atom
stripper
vein s.
stripper's asthma
stripping
membrane s.
strobila, pl. **strobilae**
strobilocercus
strobiloid
stroboscope
stroboscopic
s. disk
s. microscope
stroboscopy
stroke
effective s.
heart s.
heat s.
mitochondrial myopathy,
encephalopathy, lactacidosis, and s.
(MELAS)
s. output
recovery s.
spinal s.
sun s.
s. volume
s. work index
stroking
stroma, pl. **stromata**
s. glandulae thyroideae
s. iridis
s. of iris
lymphatic s.
nerve s.
s. ovarii
s. of ovary
s. plexus
Rollet s.
s. of thyroid gland
s. of vitreous
s. vitreum
stromal
s. corneal dystrophy
s. hyperthecosis
stromatin
stromatolysis
stromic
stromuhr
Ludwig s.
thermo-s.
strong silver protein
Strong vocational interest test

strongyle
Strongylidae
Strongyloidea
Strongyloides
strongyloidiasis
strongyloidosis
strongylosis
Strongylus
S. asini
S. edentatus
S. equinus
S. radiatus
S. ventricosus
S. vulgaris
strontium (Sr)
strontium-85 (^{85}Sr)
strontium-89 (^{89}Sr)
strontium-90 (^{90}Sr)
strontium-87m (^{87m}Sr)
strophanthin
Strophanthus
strophocephaly
strophosomia
structural
s. color
s. formula
s. gene
s. interface
s. isomerism
s. pleiotropy
structuralism
structura oculi accessoriae
structure
accessory s.
accessory visual s.
brush heap s.
chi s.
cointegrate s.
complementary s.
crystal s.
denture-supporting s.
fine s.
gel s.
Holliday s.
primary s.
s. protein
quaternary s.
secondary s.
tertiary s.
tuboreticular s.
structured
s. abstract
s. noise
struma, pl. **strumae**
s. aberrata
s. colloides
Hashimoto s.
ligneous s.
s. lymphomatosa
s. maligna
s. medicamentosa
s. ovarii
Riedel s.
strumiform
strumitis

S

strumous
Strümpell
    S. disease
    S. phenomenon
    S. reflex
Strümpell-Marie disease
struvite
    s. calculus
strychnine
strychninism
Strychnos
Stryker
    S. frame
    S. saw
Stryker-Halbeisen syndrome
STSs
    sequence-tagged site
STS for syphilis (*var. of* standard
  serologic tests for syphilis)
Stuart factor
stuck finger
student
    s. nurse
    S. *t* test
study
    analytic s.
    blind s.
    case control s.
    cohort s.
    cross-over s.
    cross-sectional s.
    diachronic s.
    double blind s.
    ecologic s.
    flow-volume loop s.
    follow-up s.
    Framingham Heart S.
    longitudinal s.
    multivariate s.
    synchronic s.
stump
    s. cancer
    s. hallucination
    s. neuralgia
stun
stunned myocardium
stupe
stupor
    benign s.
    catatonic s.
    depressive s.
    malignant s.
stuporous
    s. catatonia
Sturge-Kalischer-Weber syndrome
Sturge-Weber
    S.-W. disease
    S.-W. syndrome
Sturm
    S. conoid
    S. interval
Sturmdorf operation
stutter
stuttering
    urinary stuttering

stuttering urination
sty, pl. **sties**
    meibomian s.
    zeisian s.
style
stylet, stylette
    endotracheal s.
styliform
styloauricularis
styloauricular muscle
styloglossus muscle
stylohyal
stylohyoid
    s. branch of facial nerve
    s. ligament
    s. muscle
styloid
    s. cornu
    s. process of fibula
    s. process of radius
    s. process of temporal bone
    s. process of third metacarpal bone
    s. process of ulna
    s. prominence
styloiditis
stylolaryngeus
stylomandibular ligament
stylomastoid
    s. artery
    s. foramen
    s. vein
stylomaxillary ligament
stylopharyngeal
    s. branch of glossopharyngeal nerve
    s. muscle
stylopharyngeus muscle
stylopodium
styloradial reflex
stylostaphyline
stylosteophyte
stylus, stilus
    s. tracing
stype
"s"-type cholinesterase
styptic
    s. collodion
    s. colloid
    s. cotton
Stypven time test
styramate
styrax
styrene
styrol
styrone
subabdominal
subabdominoperitoneal
subacetate
subacromial
    s. bursa
    s. bursitis
subacute
    s. bacterial endocarditis (SBE)
    s. combined degeneration of the
      spinal cord
    s. glomerulonephritis

s. granulomatous thyroiditis
s. hepatitis
s. inclusion body encephalitis
s. inflammation
s. lymphocyte thyroiditis
s. migratory panniculitis
s. necrotizing encephalomyelopathy (SNE)
s. necrotizing myelitis
s. nephritis
s. rheumatism
s. sclerosing leukoencephalitis
s. sclerosing panencephalitis (SSPE)
s. spongiform encephalopathy
subadventitial fibrosis
subalimentation
subanal
subanconeus muscle
subaortic
s. lymph node
s. stenosis
subapical segment
subaponeurotic
subarachnoid
s. anesthesia
s. cavity
s. cistern
s. hemorrhage
s. space
subarcuate fossa
subareolar duct papillomatosis
subastragalar amputation
subatomic
subaural
subauricular
subaxial
subaxillary
subbasal
subbrachycephalic
subcaeruleus nucleus
subcalcarine
subcallosal
s. area
s. fasciculus
s. gyrus
subcapital fracture
subcapsular
s. cataract
subcarbonate
subcardinal
subcartilaginous
subcecal fossa
subcellular
subception
subchloride
subchondral
subchorial
s. lake
s. space
subchorionic
subchoroidal
subclass
subclavian
s. artery
s. duct

s. groove
s. loop
s. lymphatic trunk
s. muscle
s. nerve
s. plexus
s. steal
s. steal syndrome
s. sulcus
s. triangle
s. vein
subclavicular
subclavius muscle
subclinical
s. coccidioidomycosis
s. diabetes
s. seizure
subcloning
subcollateral
subcommissural organ
subconjunctival
subconjunctivitis
subconscious
s. memory
s. mind
subconsciousness
subcoracoid bursa
subcoracoid-pectoralis minor tendon syndrome
subcorneal
s. pustular dermatitis
s. pustular dermatosis
subcoronal hypospadias
subcortex
subcortical
s. arteriosclerotic encephalopathy
subcostal
s. angle
s. arch
s. artery
s. groove
s. line
s. muscle
s. nerve
s. plane
subcostalgia
subcostosternal
subcranial
subcrepitant rale
subcrepitation
subcrestal pocket
subcruralis
subcrural muscle
subcrureus
subculture
subcuneiform nucleus
subcurative
subcutaneous (s.c., SQ)
s. acromial bursa
s. bursa of the laryngeal prominence
s. bursa of lateral malleolus
s. bursa of medial malleolus
s. bursa of teres major
s. bursa of tibial tuberosity

S

subcutaneous *(continued)*
s. bursa of tuberosity of tibia
s. calcaneal bursa
s. emphysema
s. fat necrosis of newborn
s. flap
s. implantation
s. infrapatellar bursa
s. mastectomy
s. olecranon bursa
s. operation
s. part of external anal sphincter
s. phycomycosis
s. prepatellar bursa
s. ring
s. tenotomy
s. tissue
s. tissue of penis
s. tissue of perineum
s. transfusion
s. vein of abdomen
s. wound
subcuticular suture
subcutis
subdelirium
subdeltoid
s. bursa
s. bursitis
subdental
subdiaphragmatic
s. abscess
s. pyopneumothorax
subdigastric node
subdorsal
subduce
subdural
s. cavity
s. cleavage
s. cleft
s. hematoma
s. hematorrhachis
s. hemorrhage
s. hygroma
s. space
subendocardial
s. branch of atrioventricular bundle
s. conducting system of heart
s. layer
s. myocardial infarction
subendothelial layer
subendothelium
subendymal
subependymal giant cell astrocytoma
subependymoma
subepidermal, subepidermic
s. abscess
subepithelial
subepithelium
suberic acid
suberosis
subfalcial herniation
subfamily
subfascial prepatellar bursa
subfertility

subfissure
subfolium
subfornical organ (SFO)
subgaleal
s. emphysema
s. hemorrhage
subgallate
subgemmal
subgenus
subgerminal cavity
subgingival
s. calculus
s. curettage
s. space
subglenoid
subglossal
subglottic
subgranular
subgrundation
subhepatic
s. abscess
s. recess
s. space
subhyaloid
subhyoid, subhyoidean
s. bursa
subhypoglossal nucleus
subicteric
subicular
subiculum, pl. **subicula**
s. promontorii
subiliac
subilium
subinfection
subinflammatory
subinguinal
s. fossa
s. triangle
subintimal
subintrant
subinvolution
subiodide
subjacent
subject
subjective
s. assessment data
s. fremitus
s. insomnia
s., objective, assessment, and plan (SOAP)
s. probability
s. psychology
s. sign
s. symptom
s. synonym
s. vertigo
s. vision
subjugal
subkingdom
sublation
sublenticular
s. limb of internal capsule
s. part of internal capsule
sublentiform limb of internal capsule
sublethal

subleukemia
subleukemic leukemia
sublimate
    corrosive s.
sublimation
sublime
sublimed sulfur
subliminal
    s. self
    s. stimulus
    s. thirst
sublimis
sublingual
    s. artery
    s. bursa
    s. caruncula
    s. crescent
    s. cyst
    s. fold
    s. fossa
    s. ganglion
    s. gland
    s. medication
    s. nerve
    s. pit
    s. tablet
    s. vein
sublobular
sublumbar
subluminal
subluxation
    arytenoid s.
sublymphemia
submammary mastitis
submandibular
    s. duct
    s. fossa
    s. ganglion
    s. gland
    s. lymph node
    s. triangle
submarginal
submaxilla
submaxillary
    s. duct
    s. fossa
    s. ganglion
    s. gland
    s. triangle
submedial, submedian
submembranous
submental
    s. artery
    s. lymph node
    s. triangle
    s. vein
    s. vertex projection
    s. vertex radiograph
submentovertex radiograph
submentovertical projection
submerged tonsil
submetacentric chromosome
submicronic
submicroscopic
submitochondrial particle

submorphous
submucosa
submucosal
    s. implant
    s. plexus
submucous laryngeal cleft
subnarcotic
subnasal
    s. point
subnasion
subneural apparatus
subnitrate
subnormal
subnormality
subnotochordal
subnucleus
suboccipital
    s. decompression
    s. muscle
    s. nerve
    s. neuralgia
    s. neuritis
    s. part of vertebral artery
    s. region
    s. triangle
    s. venous plexus
suboccipitobregmatic diameter
suboccluding ligature
subocclusal surface
suboptimal
suborbital
suborder
suboxidation
suboxide
subpapillary
    s. layer
    s. network
subparabrachial nucleus
subparietal sulcus
subpatellar
subpectoral
subpellicular
    s. fibril
    s. microtubule
subpelviperitoneal
subpericardial
subperiodic periodicity
subperiosteal
    s. abscess
    s. amputation
    s. fracture
    s. implant
subperitoneal
    s. appendicitis
    s. fascia
subperitoneoabdominal
subperitoneopelvic
subpetrosal
subpharyngeal
subphrenic
    s. abscess
    s. recess
    s. space
subphylum
subpial

S

subplacental
subplasmalemmal dense zone
subpleural
subplexal
subpopliteal recess
subpreputial
subpubic angle
subpulmonary
subpulmonic effusion
subpyloric
    s. lymph node
    s. node
subpyramidal
subquadricipital muscle
subretinal
subsalt
subsartorial
    s. canal
    s. fascia
subscapular
    s. artery
    s. axillary lymph node
    s. branch of axillary artery
    s. bursa
    s. fossa
    s. muscle
    s. nerve
subscapularis
    s. muscle
subscleral
subsclerotic
subscription
subsegmental atelectasis
subseptate uterus
subserosa
subserous, subserosal
    s. layer
    s. plexus
subsibilant
subsidence
subsidiary atrial pacemaker
subsistence diet
subspinale
subspinous
substage
substance
    s. abuse
    s. abuse disorder
    alpha s.
    anterior perforated s.
    autacoid s.
    bacteriotropic s.
    basophil s.
    basophilic s.
    blood group s.
    blood group-specific s. A and B
    cementing s.
    central gray s.
    central and lateral intermediate s.
    chromidial s.
    chromophil s.
    compact s.
    controlled s.
    cortical s.
    s. dependence

    s. dependence disorder
    exophthalmos-producing s. (EPS)
    filar s.
    gelatinous s.
    glandular s. of prostate
    gray s.
    ground s.
    H s.
    innominate s.
    Kendall s.
    s. of lens of eye
    medullary s.
    müllerian inhibiting s. (MIS)
    muscular s. of prostate
    neurosecretory s.
    Nissl s.
    s. P
    periaqueductal gray s.
    P s. of Lewis
    posterior perforated s.
    pressor s.
    proper s.
    Reichstein s.
    released s.
    reticular s.
    Rolando s.
    Rolando gelatinous s.
    Schwann white s.
    slow-reacting s. (SRS)
    slow-reacting s. of anaphylaxis
     (SRS-A)
    soluble specific s. (SSS)
    specific capsular s.
    spongy s.
    standard s.
    Stilling gelatinous s.
    threshold s.
    tigroid s.
    vasodepressor s.
    white s.
    zymoplastic s.
substance-induced organic mental disorder
substantia, pl. **substantiae**
    s. adamantina
    s. alba
    basal s.
    s. basalis
    s. basophilia
    s. cinerea
    s. compacta
    s. compacta ossium
    s. corticalis
    s. eburnea
    s. ferruginea
    s. fundamentalis
    s. gelatinosa
    s. gelatinosa centralis
    s. glandularis prostatae
    s. grisea
    s. grisea centralis
    s. innominata
    s. intermedia centralis
    s. intermedia lateralis
    s. lentis

s. medullaris
s. muscularis prostatae
s. nigra
s. ossea dentis
s. perforata anterior
s. perforata posterior
s. perforata rostralis
s. propria of cornea
s. propria corneae
s. propria membranae tympani
s. propria of sclera
s. propria sclerae
s. reticularis
s. reticulofilamentosa
s. spongiosa
s. trabecularis
s. vitrea
substernal
s. angle
s. goiter
substernomastoid
substitute
blood s.
plasma s.
volume s.
substituted amide
substitution
generic s.
s. product
stimulus s.
symptom s.
s. therapy
s. transfusion
substitutive therapy
substrate
s. cycle
s. inhibition
insulin receptor s.-1 (IRS-1)
s. specificity
suicide s.
substrate-level phosphorylation
substratum
substructure
implant denture s.
subsulfate
subsuperior segment
subsurface cisterna
subtalar joint
subtarsal
subtemporal decompression
subtendinous
s. bursae of gastrocnemius muscle
s. bursa of iliacus
s. bursa of infraspinatus
s. bursa of latissimus dorsi
s. bursa of sartorius
s. bursa of subscapularis
s. bursa of tibialis anterior
s. bursa of trapezius
s. bursa of triceps brachii
s. iliac bursa
s. prepatellar bursa
subtentorial
subterminal
subtetanic

subthalamic
s. fasciculus
s. nucleus
subthalamus
subthreshold stimulus
subthyroideus
subtilisin
subtilopeptidase
subtotal
s. hysterectomy
s. thyroidectomy
subtraction
energy s.
subtrapezial
subtribe
subtrochanteric
subtrochlear
subtuberal
subtympanic
subumbilical
subungual, subunguial
s. abscess
s. exostosis
s. melanoma
subunit
s. vaccine
suburethral
subvaginal
subvalvar, subvalvular
s. aortic stenosis
subvertebral
subvirile
subvirion
subvitrinal
subvocal speech
subwaking
subzonal
subzygomatic
succagogue
succedaneous
s. dentition
s. tooth
succedaneum
succenturiate placenta
successional lamina
successive contrast
succinate
active s.
s. dehydrogenase
succinate semialdehyde
s. s. dehydrogenase
succinic
s. acid cycle
s. thiokinase
succinimide
succinylacetone
N-**succinyladenylic acid**
succinylcholine
succinyl-CoA
s-CoA ligase
s-CoA synthetase
succinyl-coenzyme A
succinyldicholine
O-**succinylhomoserine (thiol)-lyase**
succinylsulfathiazole

S

succisulfone iminodiethanol
succorrhea
succubus
succuss
succussion
    hippocratic s.
    s. sound
suck
sucking
    s. blister
    s. chest wound
    s. cushion
    s. louse
    s. pad
suckle
suckling reflex
Sucquet
    S. anastomosis
    S. canal
Sucquet-Hoyer
    S.-H. anastomoses
    S.-H. canal
sucralfate
sucrase
sucrate
sucrose
    s. hemolysis test
    s. octaacetate
sucrose α-D-glucohydrolase
sucrosemia
sucrosuria
suction
    s. cup
    s. curettage
    s. drainage
    s. ophthalmodynamometer
    s. plate
    posttussive s.
    Wangensteen s.
suctorial pad
sudamen, pl. sudamina
Sudan
    S. black B
    S. brown
    S. III, IV
    S. red III
    S. virus
    S. yellow
sudanophilia
sudanophilic
sudanophobic
    s. zone
sudation
sudden
    s. deafness
    s. death
    s. infant death syndrome (SIDS)
Sudeck
    S. atrophy
    S. critical point
    S. syndrome
sudomotor
    s. fiber
    s. nerve

sudor
    s. anglicus
sudoresis
sudoriferous
    s. abscess
    s. cyst
    s. duct
    s. gland
sudorific
sudorometer
sudorrhea
suet
    prepared s.
sufentanil citrate
sufficient cause
suffocate
suffocating gas
suffocation
suffocative goiter
suffusion
sugar
    s. acids
    s. alcohol
    s. aldehyde
    amino s.
    beechwood s.
    beet s.
    blood s.
    brain s.
    cane s.
    s. cataract
    corn s.
    deoxy s.
    desoxy s.
    s. ester
    Fischer projection formula of s.
    fruit s.
    gelatin s.
    grape s.
    Haworth conformational formula of cyclic s.
    Haworth perspective formula of cyclic s.
    invert s.
    s. of lead
    malt s.
    manna s.
    maple s.
    milk s.
    nucleoside diphosphate s.
    oil s.
    pectin s.
    reducing s.
    specific soluble s.
    starch s.
    s. tumor
    wood s.
sugar-coated spleen
suggestibility
suggestible
suggestion
    hypnotic s.
    posthypnotic s.

suggestive
>   s. psychotherapy
>   s. therapeutics

suggillation
>   postmortem s.

Sugiura procedure

SUI
>   stress urinary incontinence

suicide
>   s. gesture
>   s. inhibitor
>   physician-assisted s.
>   s. substrate

suicidology

suid herpesvirus

suint

suit
>   anti-G s.

sulbactam

sulbentine

sulcal artery

sulcate

sulci (*pl. of* sulcus)

sulciform

sulcomarginal tract

sulcular
>   s. epithelium
>   s. fluid

sulculus, pl. sulculi

sulcus, pl. sulci
>   alveolobuccal s.
>   alveololabial s.
>   alveololingual s.
>   s. ampullaris
>   ampullary s.
>   s. angularis
>   anterior intermediate s.
>   anterior interventricular s.
>   anterior parolfactory s.
>   anterolateral s.
>   s. anterolateralis
>   s. anthelicis transversus
>   aortic s.
>   s. aorticus
>   s. arteriae occipitalis
>   s. arteriae subclaviae costae primae
>   s. arteriae temporalis mediae
>   s. arteriae vertebralis
>   sulci arteriosi
>   atrioventricular s.
>   s. for auditory tube
>   s. auriculae anterior
>   basilar s.
>   s. basilaris
>   basilar pontine s.
>   s. bicipitalis lateralis
>   s. bicipitalis medialis
>   s. bicipitalis radialis
>   s. bicipitalis ulnaris
>   s. bulbopontis
>   calcaneal s.
>   s. calcanei
>   calcarine s.
>   s. calcarinus
>   callosal s.

callosomarginal s.
s. callosomarginalis
s. caroticus
carotid s.
s. carpi
central s.
central s. of insula
s. centralis
s. centralis insulae
cerebellar sulci
cerebral sulci
sulci cerebri
chiasmatic s.
cingulate s.
s. cinguli
s. of cingulum
circular s. of insula
s. circularis insulae
circular s. of Reil
collateral s.
s. collateralis
s. coronarius
coronary s.
s. corporis callosi
s. of corpus callosum
s. costae
s. costae arteriae subclaviae
costophrenic s.
s. cruris helicis
sulci cutis
dorsal intermediate s.
dorsal median s.
dorsolateral s.
s. ethmoidalis
external spiral s.
fimbriodentate s.
s. fimbriodentatus
s. frontalis inferior
s. frontalis medius
s. frontalis superior
s. frontomarginalis
gingival s.
s. gingivalis
gingivobuccal s.
gingivolabial s.
gingivolingual s.
s. gluteus
s. for greater palatine nerve
habenular s.
s. habenularis
s. hamuli pterygoidei
hippocampal s.
s. hippocampalis
hypothalamic s.
s. hypothalamicus
inferior frontal s.
inferior petrosal s.
inferior temporal s.
s. infraorbitalis
infrapalpebral s.
s. infrapalpebralis
inner spiral s.
s. intermedius anterior
s. intermedius posterior
internal spiral s.

S

sulcus *(continued)*
  interparietal s.
  intertubercular s.
  s. intertubercularis
  s. interventricularis anterior
  s. interventricularis cordis
  s. interventricularis posterior
  intragracile s.
  s. intragracilis
  intraparietal s.
  s. intraparietalis
  intraparietal s. of Turner
  labial s.
  labiodental s.
  s. lacrimalis
  lateral s.
  s. lateralis
  lateral occipital s.
  s. limitans
  s. limitans ventriculi quarti
  limiting s.
  limiting s. of fourth ventricle
  limiting s. of Reil
  lip s.
  longitudinal s. of heart
  lunate s.
  s. lunatus
  malleolar s.
  s. malleolaris
  marginal s.
  s. marginalis
  s. matricis unguis
  medial s. of crus cerebri
  s. medialis cruris cerebri
  median s. of fourth ventricle
  median s. of tongue
  s. medianus linguae
  s. medianus posterior medullae
    oblongatae
  s. medianus posterior medullae
    spinalis
  s. medianus ventriculi quarti
  medullopontine s.
  mentolabial s.
  s. mentolabialis
  middle frontal s.
  middle temporal s.
  s. for middle temporal artery
  Monro s.
  s. musculi subclavii
  s. mylohyoideus
  nasolabial s.
  s. nasolabialis
  s. nervi oculomotorii
  s. nervi petrosi majoris
  s. nervi petrosi minoris
  s. nervi radialis
  s. nervi spinalis
  s. nervi ulnaris
  nymphocaruncular s.
  s. nymphocaruncularis
  nymphohymenal s.
  s. obturatorius
  s. of occipital artery

  s. occipitalis lateralis
  s. occipitalis superior
  s. occipitalis transversus
  occipitotemporal s.
  s. occipitotemporalis
  oculomotor s. of mesencephalon
  s. of the oculomotor nerve
  s. olfactorius
  s. olfactorius cavi nasi
  olfactory s.
  olfactory s. of nasal cavity
  orbital s.
  sulci orbitales
  outer spiral s.
  sulci palatini
  s. palatinus major
  s. palatovaginalis
  paracentral s.
  s. paracentralis
  sulci paracolici
  paraglenoid s.
  s. paraglenoidalis
  sulci paraolfactorii
  parietooccipital s.
  s. parieto-occipitalis
  s. parolfactorius anterior
  s. parolfactorius posterior
  parolfactory sulci
  periconchal s.
  s. for pharyngotympanic tube
  s. popliteus
  postcentral s.
  s. postcentralis
  s. posterior auriculae
  posterior intermediate s.
  posterior interventricular s.
  posterior median s. of medulla
    oblongata
  posterior median s. of spinal cord
  posterior parolfactory s.
  posterolateral s.
  s. posterolateralis
  preauricular s.
  precentral s.
  s. precentralis
  prechiasmatic s.
  s. prechiasmaticus
  s. promontorii cavitatis tympanicae
  s. of promontory of tympanic
    cavity
  s. of pterygoid hamulus
  s. pterygopalatinus
  s. pulmonalis
  pulmonary s.
  rhinal s.
  s. rhinalis
  sagittal s.
  s. of sclera
  s. sclerae
  scleral s.
  sigmoid s.
  s. sinus petrosi inferioris
  s. sinus petrosi superioris
  s. sinus sagittalis superioris
  s. sinus sigmoidei

s. sinus transversi
skin sulci
s. spinosus
s. spiralis externus
s. spiralis internus
subclavian s.
s. subclavianus
s. subclavius
subparietal s.
s. subparietalis
superior frontal s.
superior longitudinal s.
superior occipital s.
superior petrosal s.
superior temporal s.
supra-acetabular s.
s. supraacetabularis
talar s.
s. tali
s. temporalis inferior
s. temporalis medius
s. temporalis superior
s. temporalis transversus
s. tendinis musculi fibularis longi
s. tendinis musculi flexoris hallucis longi
s. tendinis musculi peronei longi
terminal s.
s. terminalis
s. terminalis atrii dextri
s. terminalis cordis
s. terminalis linguae
terminal s. of tongue
s. test
tonsillolingual s.
transverse occipital s.
s. for transverse sinus
transverse temporal s.
s. tubae auditoriae
Turner s.
tympanic s.
s. tympanicus
s. of umbilical vein
s. for vena cava
s. venae cavae
s. venae cavae cranialis
s. venae subclaviae
s. venae umbilicalis
sulci venosi
s. ventralis
ventrolateral s.
s. for vertebral artery
s. verticalis
vomeral s.
s. vomeralis
s. vomeris
s. vomerovaginalis
sulfa
sulfabenzamide
sulfacetamide
sulfacid
sulfacytine
sulfadiazine
sulfadimethoxine
sulfadimidine

sulfadoxine
sulfaethidole
sulfafurazole
sulfaguanidine
sulfaguine
sulfalene
sulfamerazine
sulfameter
sulfamethazine
sulfamethizole
sulfamethoxazole
sulfamethoxydiazine
sulfamethoxypyridazine
sulfamoxole
***p*-sulfamylacetanilide**
sulfanilamide
***N*-sulfanilylacetamide**
***N*-sulfanilylbenzamide**
sulfaphenazole
sulfapyrazine
sulfapyridine
sulfasalazine
sulfatase
multiple s. deficiency
sulfate
acid s.
active s.
s. adenylyltransferase
codeine s.
dermatan s.
iron s.
polysaccharide s. ester
s. respiration
s. salt of dehydroepiandrosterone (DHEAS)
s. water
sulfathiazole
sulfatidate
sulfatide lipidosis
sulfatides
sulfatidosis
sulfation
sulfhemoglobin
sulfhemoglobinemia
sulfhydrate
sulfhydryl reagent
sulfide
sulfikinase
sulfindigotic acid
sulfinpyrazone
β-sulfinylpyruvic acid
sulfisomidine
sulfisoxazole diolamine
sulfite
s. dehydrogenase
s. oxidase
s. reductase
sulfituria
sulfmethemoglobin
sulfoacid
3-sulfoalanine
sulfobromophthalein sodium
sulfocyanate
sulfocyanic acid
***S*-sulfocysteine**

S

3-sulfogalactosylceramide
sulfogel
sulfohydrate
sulfokinase
sulfolysis
sulfomucin
sulfomyxin sodium
sulfonamide
sulfonate
sulfone
sulfonic acid
sulfonium
    s. ion
    s. salt
sulfonylureas
sulfoprotein
6-sulfoquinovosyl diacylglycerol
sulforhodamine B
sulformethoxine
sulfosalicylic acid
sulfosalicylic acid turbidity test
sulfosol
sulfotransferase
sulfoxide
sulfoxone sodium
sulfur
    s. autotrophy
    s. dioxide
    s. group
    s. iodide
    liver of s.
    s. mustard
    precipitated s.
    roll s.
    soft s.
    sublimed s.
    s. trioxide
    vegetable s.
    washed s.
    s. water
    wettable s.
sulfur-35 (^{35}S)
sulfurated
    s. lime
    s. potash
sulfuret
sulfureted hydrogen
sulfuric
    s. acid
    s. ether
    fuming s. acid
    Nordhausen s. acid
    s. oxide
sulfurous
    s. oxide
    sulfurous acid
sulfuryl
sulfydrate
sulindac
sulisobenzone
Sulkowitch reagent
sulpiride
sulthiame

Sulzberger-Garbe
    S.-G. disease
    S.-G. syndrome
summating potential
summation
    s. beat
    s. gallop (S$_7$)
    s. of stimuli
summer
    s. asthma
    s. diarrhea
    s. itch
    s. prurigo
    s. rash
Sumner sign
sump
    s. drain
    s. syndrome
sun
    s. protection factor (SPF)
    s. stroke
sunburn
sundowning
sunflower cataract
sunflower seed oil
sunscreen
sunstroke
superabduction
superacidity
superacromial
superactivity
superacute
superalimentation
superanal
superantigen
superciliary
    s. arch
    s. ridge
supercilium, pl. **supercilia**
supercoiling
superconducting magnet
superdicrotic
superdistention
superduct
superego
supereruption
superexcitation
superextension
superfatted soap
superfetation
superficial
    s. angioma
    s. back muscle
    s. brachial artery
    s. branch
    s. branch of the lateral plantar nerve
    s. branch of medial circumflex femoral artery
    s. branch of the medial plantar artery
    s. branch of the radial nerve
    s. branch of the superior gluteal artery

s. branch of the transverse cervical artery
s. branch of the ulnar nerve
s. burn
s. cardiac plexus
s. cerebral vein
s. cervical artery
s. cervical nerve
s. circumflex iliac artery
s. circumflex iliac vein
s. cleavage
s. dorsal sacrococcygeal ligament
s. dorsal vein of clitoris
s. dorsal vein of penis
s. ectoderm
s. epigastric artery
s. epigastric vein
s. external pudendal artery
s. fascia
s. fascia of penis
s. fascia of perineum
s. fascia of scrotum
s. fibular nerve
s. flexor muscle of finger
s. gray layer of superior colliculus
s. head of flexor pollicis brevis
s. implantation
s. inguinal lymph node
s. inguinal pouch
s. inguinal ring
s. investing fascia of perineum
s. lamina
s. lateral cervical lymph node
s. layer
s. layer of deep cervical fascia
s. layer of the levator palpebrae superioris
s. layer of temporal fascia
s. linear keratitis
s. lingual muscle
s. lymph vessel
s. middle cerebral vein
s. origin
s. palmar arterial arch
s. palmar artery
s. palmar branch of radial artery
s. palmar venous arch
s. parotid lymph node
s. part of anterior compartment of forearm
s. part of external anal sphincter
s. part of masseter muscle
s. part of parotid gland
s. part of posterior compartment of leg
s. perineal pouch
s. perineal space
s. peroneal nerve
s. posterior sacrococcygeal ligament
s. punctate keratitis
s. reflex
s. spreading melanoma
s. temporal artery
s. temporal branch of auriculotemporal nerve

s. temporal plexus
s. temporal vein
s. transverse metacarpal ligament
s. transverse metatarsal ligament
s. transverse muscle of perineum
s. transverse perineal muscle
s. volar artery
superficialis volae
superflexion
superfuse
superfusion
supergenual
superhelicity
superimposed
    s. eclampsia
    s. preeclampsia
superimpregnation
superinduce
superinfection
superinvolution
superior
    s. aberrant ductule
    s. alveolar nerve
    s. anastomotic vein
    s. angle of scapula
    s. articular facet of atlas
    s. articular pit of atlas
    s. articular process
    s. articular process of sacrum
    s. articular surface of atlas
    s. articular surface of tibia
    s. aspect
    s. auricular muscle
    s. azygoesophageal recess
    s. basal vein
    s. belly of omohyoid muscle
    s. border
    s. border of body of pancreas
    s. border of pancreas
    s. border of petrous part of temporal bone
    s. border of scapula
    s. border of spleen
    s. border of suprarenal gland
    s. branch
    s. branch of the oculomotor nerve
    s. branch of the pubic bone
    s. branch of the right and left inferior pulmonary veins
    s. branch of the superior gluteal artery
    s. branch of the transverse cervical nerve
    s. bursa of biceps femoris
    s. carotid triangle
    s. central tegmental nucleus
    s. cerebellar artery
    s. cerebellar artery syndrome
    s. cerebellar peduncle
    s. cerebral vein
    s. cervical cardiac branch of vagus nerve
    s. cervical cardiac nerve
    s. cervical ganglion
    s. choroid vein

S

superior *(continued)*
s. cistern
s. clunial nerve
s. colliculus
s. costal facet
s. costal pit
s. costotransverse ligament
s. dental arch
s. dental branch of superior dental plexus
s. dental nerve
s. dental plexus
s. dental rami
s. duodenal flexure
s. duodenal fold
s. duodenal fossa
s. duodenal recess
s. epigastric artery
s. epigastric vein
s. esophageal sphincter
s. extensor retinaculum
s. extremity
s. extremity of kidney
s. eyelid
s. facet of trochlear of talus
s. fascia of pelvic diaphragm
s. fibular retinaculum
s. fovea
s. frontal convolution
s. frontal gyrus
s. frontal sulcus
s. ganglion of glossopharyngeal nerve
s. ganglion of vagus nerve
s. gastric lymph node
s. gemellus muscle
s. gingival branch of superior dental plexus
s. gluteal artery
s. gluteal nerve
s. gluteal vein
s. hemorrhagic polioencephalitis
s. hemorrhoidal artery
s. hemorrhoidal plexus
s. hemorrhoidal vein
s. horn of falciform margin of saphenous opening
s. horn of thyroid cartilage
s. hypogastric plexus
s. hypophysial artery
s. ileocecal recess
s. intercostal artery
s. intercostal vein
s. internal parietal artery
s. labial artery
s. labial branch of facial artery
s. labial branch of infraorbital nerve
s. labial vein
s. laryngeal artery
s. laryngeal cavity
s. laryngeal nerve
s. laryngeal vein
s. laryngotomy

s. lateral brachial cutaneous nerve
s. lateral genicular artery
s. ligament of epididymis
s. ligament of incus
s. ligament of malleus
s. limb
s. limb of ansa cervicalis
s. limbic keratoconjunctivitis
s. lingular artery
s. lingular branch of lingular branch of superior lobar left pulmonary artery
s. lingular bronchopulmonary segment S IV
s. lobar artery
s. lobe of (right/left) lung
s. longitudinal fasciculus
s. longitudinal muscle of tongue
s. longitudinal sinus
s. longitudinal sulcus
s. macular arteriole
s. macular venule
s. margin of cerebral hemisphere
s. maxillary nerve
s. medial genicular artery
s. mediastinum
s. medullary velum
s. member
s. mesenteric artery
s. mesenteric artery syndrome
s. mesenteric ganglion
s. mesenteric lymph node
s. mesenteric plexus
s. mesenteric vein
s. nasal concha
s. nasal retinal arteriole
s. nasal retinal venule
s. nasal venule of retina
s. nuchal line
s. oblique muscle
s. oblique muscle of head
s. occipital gyrus
s. occipital sulcus
s. occipitofrontal fasciculus
s. olivary complex
s. olivary nucleus
s. olive
s. omental recess
s. ophthalmic vein
s. orbital fissure
s. palpebral arterial arch
s. palpebral vein
s. paraplegia
s. parietal gyrus
s. parietal lobule
s. part of diaphragmatic surface of liver
s. part of duodenum
s. part of lingular vein
s. part of vestibular ganglion
s. part of vestibulocochlear nerve
s. pelvic aperture
s. peroneal retinaculum
s. petrosal sinus
s. petrosal sulcus

s. pharyngeal constrictor muscle
s. phrenic artery
s. phrenic lymph node
s. phrenic vein
s. pole
s. pole of kidney
s. pole of testis
s. polioencephalitis
s. posterior serratus muscle
s. pubic ligament
s. pubic ramus
s. pulmonary sulcus tumor
s. quadrigeminal brachium
s. radioulnar joint
s. recess of lesser peritoneal sac
s. recess of omental bursa
s. recess of tympanic membrane
s. rectal artery
s. rectal lymph node
s. rectal plexus
s. rectal vein
s. rectus muscle
s. renal segment
s. retinaculum of extensor muscle
s. root of ansa cervicalis
s. sagittal sinus
s. salivary nucleus
s. salivatory nucleus
s. segment
s. segmental artery
s. segmental artery of kidney
s. semilunar lobule
s. suprarenal artery
s. surface of cerebellar hemisphere
s. surface of talus
s. tarsal muscle
s. tarsus
s. temporal convolution
s. temporal fissure
s. temporal gyrus
s. temporal line of parietal bone
s. temporal retinal arteriole
s. temporal retinal venule
s. temporal sulcus
s. temporal venule of retina
s. thalamostriate vein
s. thoracic aperture
s. thoracic artery
s. thyroid artery
s. thyroid notch
s. thyroid plexus
s. thyroid tubercle
s. thyroid vein
s. tibial articulation
s. tibiofibular joint
s. tracheobronchial lymph node
s. transverse scapular ligament
s. triangle sign
s. trunk of brachial plexus
s. turbinated bone
s. tympanic artery
s. ulnar collateral artery
s. vein of cerebellar hemisphere
s. vein of vermis
s. vena cava

s. vena cava syndrome
s. vermian branch of superior
 cerebellar artery
s. vesical artery
s. vestibular area
s. vestibular nucleus
s. wall of orbit
superiority complex
superlactation
superligamen
supermedial
supermotility
supernatant fluid
supernormal
s. conduction
s. recovery phase
supernumerary
s. breast
s. kidney
s. mamma
s. organ
s. placenta
supernutrition
superolateral
s. cerebral surface
s. face of cerebral hemisphere
s. surface of cerebrum
superomedial margin
superovulation
superoxide dismutase (SOD)
superparasite
superparasitism
superpetrosal
supersaturate
supersaturated solution
superscription
supersonic
s. ray
s. wave
superstructure
implant denture s.
supertension
supertraction conus
supervoltage
supinate
supination
s. of the foot
s. of the forearm
s. reflex
supinator
s. crest of ulna
s. jerk
s. longus reflex
s. muscle
supine
s. hypotensive syndrome
s. position
suppedania
supplemental
s. air
s. groove
s. lobe
s. ridge
supplementary
s. menstruation

S

supplementary *(continued)*
 s. motor area epilepsy
 s. motor cortex
support
 basic life s.
 s. medium
supporter
supporting
 s. area
 s. cell
 s. reaction
 s. reflex
supportive psychotherapy
suppository
 glycerin s.
suppressed menstruation
suppression
 s. amblyopia
 fixation s.
 immune s.
 intergenic s.
 intragenic s.
suppressor
 amber s.
 s. cell
 s. mutation
 s. tRNA
suppressor-sensitive mutant
suppurant
suppurate
suppuration
suppurative
 s. appendicitis
 s. arthritis
 s. cerebritis
 s. choroiditis
 s. encephalitis
 s. gingivitis
 s. hepatitis
 s. hyalitis
 s. inflammation
 s. mastitis
 s. necrosis
 s. nephritis
 s. periodontitis
 s. pleurisy
 s. pneumonia
 s. pulpitis
 s. synovitis
supra-acetabular
 s. groove
 s. sulcus
supra-acromial
supra-anal
supra-arytenoid cartilage
supra-auricular point
supra-axillary
suprabuccal
suprabulge
supracallosal gyrus
supracardinal
supracerebellar
supracerebral
supracervical hysterectomy

suprachiasmatic
 s. artery
 s. nucleus
suprachoroid
 s. lamina of sclera
 s. layer
suprachoroidea
supraciliary
supraclavicular
 s. lymph node
 s. muscle
 s. part of brachial plexus
 s. triangle
supraclavicularis
supraclinoid aneurysm
supracollicular sphincter
supracondylar
 s. fracture
 s. process of humerus
supracondyloid
supracostal
supracotyloid
supracrestal
 s. line
 s. plane
supracristal
 s. plane
supradiaphragmatic
supraduction
supraduodenal artery
supraepicondylar process
supragingival calculus
supraglenoid
 s. tubercle (of scapula)
supraglottic
 s. laryngectomy
supraglottitis
suprahepatic space
suprahisian block
suprahyoid
 s. branch of lingual artery
 s. gland
 s. muscle
suprainguinal
suprainterparietal bone
supraintestinal
supralemniscal nucleus
supraliminal
supralumbar
supramalleolar
supramammary
supramammillary nucleus
supramandibular
supramarginal
 s. convolution
 s. gyrus
supramastoid
 s. crest
 s. fossa
supramaxilla
supramaxillary
supramaximal stimulus
suprameatal
 s. pit

s. spine
s. triangle
supramental
supramentale
supranasal point
supraneural
supranormal
s. conduction
s. excitability
supranuclear
s. lesion
s. paralysis
supraocclusion
supraoptic
s. artery
s. nucleus
s. nucleus of hypothalamus
s. recess
supraopticohypophysial tract
supraorbital
s. arch
s. artery
s. foramen
s. margin
s. nerve
s. neuralgia
s. notch
s. point
s. reflex
s. ridge
s. vein
supraorbitomeatal plane
suprapatellar
s. bursa
s. reflex
suprapelvic
supraperiosteal implant
supraphysiologic, supraphysiological
suprapineal recess
suprapleural membrane
suprapubic
s. cystotomy
s. lithotomy
suprapyloric
s. lymph node
s. node
suprarenal
s. body
s. capsule
s. cortex
s. gland
s. impression on liver
s. medulla
s. plexus
s. vein
suprascapular
s. artery
s. ligament
s. nerve
s. notch
s. vein
suprascleral
suprasellar cyst
supraspinal
supraspinalis muscle

supraspinatus
s. muscle
s. syndrome
supraspinous
s. fossa
s. ligament
s. muscle
suprastapedial
suprasternal
s. bone
s. notch
s. plane
s. pulsation
s. space
suprastyloid crest of radius
suprasylvian
suprasymphysary
supratemporal
supratentorial
suprathoracic
supratonsillar
s. fossa
s. recess
supratragic tubercle
supratrochlear
s. artery
s. nerve
s. vein
supraturbinal
supratympanic
supraumbilical reflex
supravaginal part of cervix
supravalvar
s. aortic stenosis-infantile
hypercalcemia syndrome
s. aortic stenosis syndrome
s. stenosis
supravalvular stenosis
supraventricular
s. crest
s. extrasystole
s. tachycardia
supraversion
supravesical fossa
supravital stain
supreme
s. concha
s. intercostal artery
s. intercostal vein
s. nasal concha
s. turbinated bone
suprofen
sural
s. artery
s. communicating branch of
common fibular nerve
s. communicating branch of
common peroneal nerve
s. nerve
s. region
suralimentation
suramin sodium
surdocardiac syndrome
surface
acromial articular s. of clavicle

surface *(continued)*
s. anatomy
anterior s.
anterior s. of arm
anterior articular s. of dens
anterior s. of cornea
anterior s. of elbow
anterior s. of eyelid
anterior s. of forearm
anterior s. of iris
anterior s. of kidney
anterior s. of leg
anterior s. of lens
anterior s. of lower limb
anterior s. of maxilla
anterior s. of patella
anterior s. of petrous part of
   temporal bone
anterior s. of prostate
anterior s. of radius
anterior s. of suprarenal gland
anterior talar articular s. of
   calcaneus
anterior s. of thigh
anterior s. of ulna
anterior s. of uterus
anteroinferior s. of pancreas
anterolateral s. of arytenoid cartilage
anterolateral s. of (shaft of)
   humerus
anteromedial s. of shaft of humerus
anterosuperior s. of body of
   pancreas
approximal s. of tooth
articular s.
articular s. of acromion
articular s. of arytenoid cartilage
articular s. of mandibular fossa of
   temporal bone
articular s. on calcaneus for cuboid
   bone
articular s. of patella
arytenoidal articular s. of cricoid
auricular s. of ilium
auricular s. of sacrum
axial s.
balancing occlusal s.
basal s.
buccal s.
calcaneal articular s. of talus
carpal articular s. of radius
s. catalysis
cerebral s.
s. coil
colic s. of spleen
contact s. of tooth
costal s.
costal s. of lung
costal s. of scapula
cuboid articular s. of calcaneus
decayed, missing, and filled s.
   (DMFS, dmfs)
denture basal s.
denture foundation s.

denture impression s.
denture occlusal s.
denture polished s.
diaphragmatic s.
distal s. of tooth
dorsal s.
dorsal s. of digit
dorsal s. of sacrum
dorsal s. of scapula
s. epithelium
external s.
external s. of cochlear duct
external s. of cranial base
external s. of frontal bone
external s. of parietal bone
facial s. of tooth
fibular articular s. of tibia
gastric s. of spleen
glenoid s.
gluteal s. of ilium
grinding s.
incisal s.
inferior articular s. of atlas
inferior articular s. of tibia
inferior s. of cerebellar hemisphere
inferior cerebral s.
inferior s. of petrous part of
   temporal bone
inferior s. of tongue
inferolateral s. of prostate
infratemporal s. of (body of)
   maxilla
infratemporal s. of greater wing of
   sphenoid
interlobar s. of lung
internal s.
internal s. of cranial base
internal s. of frontal bone
internal s. of parietal bone
interproximal s. of tooth
intestinal s. of uterus
lateral s.
lateral s. of arm
lateral s. of fibula
lateral s. of finger
lateral s. of leg
lateral s. of lower limb
lateral malleolar s. of talus
lateral s. of ovary
lateral s. of testis
lateral s. of tibia
lateral s. of toe
lateral s. of zygomatic bone
lingual s. of tooth
lunate s. of acetabulum
malleolar articular s. of fibula
malleolar articular s. of tibia
masticating s.
masticatory s.
maxillary s. of greater wing of
   sphenoid bone
maxillary s. of palatine bone
medial s.
medial s. of arytenoid cartilage
medial cerebral s.

medial s. of cerebral hemisphere
medial s. of fibula
medial s. of lung
medial s. of ovary
medial s. of testis
medial s. of tibia
medial s. of toes
medial s. of ulna
mediastinal s. of lung
mesial s. of tooth
s. microscopy
middle talar articular s. of
  calcaneus
s. mucous cell of stomach
nasal s. of maxilla
nasal s. of palatine bone
navicular articular s. of talus
occlusal s. of tooth
orbital s.
palatine s. of horizontal plate of
  palatine bone
palmar s. of finger
patellar s. of femur
pelvic s. of sacrum
Petzval s.
plantar s. of foot
plantar s. of toe
popliteal s. of femur
posterior s.
posterior s. of arm
posterior articular s. of dens
posterior s. of arytenoid cartilage
posterior s. of cornea
posterior s. of elbow
posterior s. of eyelids
posterior s. of fibula
posterior s. of forearm
posterior s. of iris
posterior s. of kidney
posterior s. of leg
posterior s. of lens
posterior s. of lower limb
posterior s. of pancreas
posterior s. of petrous part of
  temporal bone
posterior s. of prostate
posterior s. of radius
posterior s. of scapula
posterior s. of shaft of humerus
posterior s. of suprarenal gland
posterior talar articular s.
posterior s. of thigh
posterior s. of tibia
posterior s. of ulna
renal s. of spleen
renal s. of suprarenal gland
right and left pulmonary s. of
  heart
sacropelvic s. of ilium
sternal articular s. of clavicle
sternocostal s. of heart
subocclusal s.
superior articular s. of atlas
superior articular s. of tibia
superior s. of cerebellar hemisphere

superior s. of talus
superolateral cerebral s.
superolateral s. of cerebrum
symphysial s. of pubis
talar articular s. of calcaneus
temporal s.
s. tension
s. tension theory of narcosis
tentorial s.
s. thalamic vein
s. thermometer
thyroid articular s. of cricoid
  (cartilage)
tympanic s. of cochlear duct
urethral s. of penis
ventral s. of digit
vesical s. of uterus
vestibular s. of cochlear duct
vestibular s. of tooth
visceral s. of liver
visceral s. of the spleen
working occlusal s.
surface-active
surfactant
nonionic s.
zwitterionic s.
surfactant-specific protein
surgeon
attending s.
dental s.
s. general
S. General's Office (SGO)
genitourinary s.
oral s.
surgeon's knot
surgery
ambulatory s.
aseptic s.
closed s.
cosmetic s.
craniofacial s.
Doctor of S. (ChD)
Doctor of Dental S. (DDS)
endolymphatic sac s.
esthetic s.
functional endoscopic sinus s.
  (FESS)
keratorefractive s.
laparoscopic s.
laparoscopically assisted s.
left ventricular volume reduction s.
lung volume reduction s.
major s.
Master of Dental S. (M.D.S.)
microscopically controlled s.
minimally invasive s.
minor s.
Mohs micrographic s.
open heart s.
oral s.
orthognathic s.
orthopedic s.
plastic s.
reconstructive s.
skull base s.

S

surgery *(continued)*
    stereotactic s.
    thoracoscopic s.
    transsexual s.
    ventricular reduction s.
    video-assisted thoracic s. (VATS)
surgical
    s. abdomen
    s. anatomy
    s. anesthesia
    s. appliance
    s. ciliated cyst
    s. diathermy
    s. emphysema
    s. eruption
    s. erysipelas
    s. ligation
    s. maggot
    s. microscope
    s. neck of humerus
    s. orthodontics
    s. pathology
    s. prosthesis
    s. rod
    s. silk
    s. splint
    s. template
surging faradism
surrenal
surrogate
    mother s.
    s. mother
surround
    acoustic s.
sursumduction
sursumversion
surveillance
    immune s.
    immunological s.
    post-marketing s.
survey
    field s.
    s. line
    skeletal s.
surveying
surveyor
survival
    s. analysis
    s. time
susceptibility
    s. cassette
    s. testing
suspended animation
suspension
    amorphous insulin zinc s.
    chromic phosphate ^{32}P colloidal s.
    Coffey s.
    s. colloid
    crystalline insulin zinc s.
    extended insulin zinc s.
    insulin zinc s.
    s. laryngoscopy
    magnesia and alumina oral s.

    prompt insulin zinc s.
    s. stability
suspensoid
suspensory
    s. bandage
    s. ligament of axilla
    s. ligament of breast
    s. ligament of clitoris
    s. ligament of Cooper
    s. ligament of duodenum
    s. ligament of esophagus
    s. ligament of eyeball
    s. ligament of gonad
    s. ligament of lens
    s. ligament of ovary
    s. ligament of penis
    s. ligament of testis
    s. ligament of thyroid gland
    s. muscle of duodenum
    s. retinaculum of breast
sustained
    s. action tablet
    s. pulse
sustentacular
    s. cell
    s. fiber of retina
sustentaculum, pl. **sustentacula**
    s. lienis
    s. tali
susurrus
    s. aurium
Sutter blood group
Sutton
    S. disease
    S. nevus
    S. ulcer
sutura, pl. **suturae**
    s. coronalis
    suturae cranii
    s. ethmoidolacrimalis
    s. ethmoidomaxillaris
    s. frontalis
    s. frontalis persistens
    s. frontoethmoidalis
    s. frontolacrimalis
    s. frontomaxillaris
    s. frontonasalis
    s. frontozygomatica
    s. incisiva
    s. infraorbitalis
    s. intermaxillaris
    s. internasalis
    s. interparietalis
    s. lacrimoconchalis
    s. lacrimomaxillaris
    s. lambdoidea
    s. metopica
    s. nasofrontalis
    s. nasomaxillaris
    s. notha
    s. occipitomastoidea
    s. palatina mediana
    s. palatina transversa
    s. palatoethmoidalis
    s. palatomaxillaris

s. parietomastoidea
s. plana
s. sagittalis
s. serrata
s. sphenoethmoidalis
s. sphenofrontalis
s. sphenomaxillaris
s. spheno-orbitalis
s. sphenoparietalis
s. sphenosquamosa
s. sphenovomeriana
s. sphenozygomatica
s. squamoparietalis
s. squamosomastoidea
s. temporozygomatica
s. zygomaticofrontalis
s. zygomaticomaxillaris
s. zygomaticotemporalis

sutural

s. bone
s. cataract
s. ligament

suture

s. abscess
absorbable surgical s.
Albert s.
apposition s.
approximation s.
atraumatic s.
blanket s.
bridle s.
Bunnell s.
buried s.
button s.
catgut s.
coaptation s.
cobbler's s.
Connell s.
continuous s.
control release s.
coronal s.
cranial s.
Cushing s.
Czerny s.
Czerny-Lembert s.
delayed s.
dentate s.
doubly armed s.
Dupuytren s.
end-on mattress s.
ethmoidolacrimal s.
ethmoidomaxillary s.
Faden s.
false s.
far-and-near s.
figure-of-8 s.
frontal s.
frontoethmoidal s.
frontolacrimal s.
frontomaxillary s.
frontonasal s.
frontozygomatic s.
Frost s.
Gély s.
glover s.

Gould s.
Gussenbauer s.
Halsted s.
harmonic s.
implanted s.
incisive s.
infraorbital s.
intermaxillary s.
internasal s.
interparietal s.
interrupted s.
Jobert de Lamballe s.
s. joint
lacrimoconchal s.
lacrimomaxillary s.
lambdoid s.
Lembert s.
lens s.
s. ligature
locking s.
mattress s.
median palatine s.
metopic s.
nasomaxillary s.
nerve s.
neurocentral s.
nonabsorbable surgical s.
occipitomastoid s.
palatoethmoidal s.
palatomaxillary s.
Paré s.
parietomastoid s.
Parker-Kerr s.
persistent frontal s.
petrosquamous s.
plane s.
pledgetted s.
premaxillary s.
purse-string s.
quilted s.
relaxation s.
retention s.
sagittal s.
secondary s.
serrate s.
shotted s.
sphenoethmoidal s.
sphenofrontal s.
sphenomaxillary s.
sphenooccipital s.
spheno-orbital s.
sphenoparietal s.
sphenosquamous s.
sphenovomerine s.
sphenozygomatic s.
spiral s.
squamomastoid s.
squamoparietal s.
squamous s.
subcuticular s.
temporozygomatic s.
tendon s.
tension s.
transfixion s.
transverse palatine s.

S

suture *(continued)*
    tympanomastoid s.
    uninterrupted s.
    wedge-and-groove s.
    zygomaticomaxillary s.
    zygomaticotemporal s.
suturectomy
suxamethonium
Suzanne gland
SV
    simian virus
SV40
    simian vacuolating virus No. 40
Sv
    sievert
SV40-adenovirus hybrid
Svedberg
    S. equation
    S. unit
    S. unit of flotation
swab
swage
swallow
    Gastrografin s.
    hypaque s.
    somatic s.
    s. syncope
    visceral s.
swallowing
    s. reflex
    s. threshold
Swan-Ganz catheter
Swann antigen
swan-neck deformity
Sw^a antigen
swarming
sweat
    s. duct
    s. gland
    s. gland carcinoma
    night s.
    s. pore
    red s.
    s. test
sweating test
sweaty feet syndrome
Swedish
    S. gymnastics
    S. movement
sweep
sweet
    s. balm
    s. birch oil
    S. disease
    s. precipitate
swelling
    albuminous s.
    arytenoid s.
    brain s.
    Calabar s.
    cloudy s.
    fugitive s.
    genital s.
    hunger s.

    labial s.
    labioscrotal s.
    lateral lingual s.
    levator s.
    Neufeld capsular s.
    scrotal s.
    Spielmeyer acute s.
swim bladder
swimmer's
    s. ear
    s. itch
swimming
    s. pool conjunctivitis
    s. pool granuloma
swine
    s. encephalitis virus
    s. erysipelas
    s. fever virus
    s. influenza
    s. influenza viruses
    s. vesicular disease
swineherd's disease
swinepox virus
swinging light test
Swiss
    S. cheese endometrium
    S. mouse leukemia virus
    S. type agammaglobulinemia
switch
    class s.
switching
    class s.
    s. site
swollen
    s. belly disease
    s. belly syndrome
Swyer-James-MacLeod syndrome
Swyer-James syndrome
Swyer syndrome
sycosis
Sydenham
    S. chorea
    S. disease
Sydney
    S. crease
    S. crease
    S. line
    S. line
syllabic speech
syllable-stumbling
sylvatic
    s. plague
Sylvest disease
sylvian
    s. angle
    s. aqueduct
    s. cistern
    s. fissure
    s. line
    s. point
    s. valve
    s. ventricle
symballophone
symbion, symbiont

symbiosis
    dyadic s.
    mutualistic s.
    triadic s.
symbiote
symbiotic
    s. fermentation phenomenon
symblepharon
    anterior s.
    posterior s.
symbol
symbolia
symbolism
symbolization
symbrachydactyly
Syme
    S. amputation
    S. operation
Symington anococcygeal body
symmelia
Symmers clay pipestem fibrosis
symmetric
    s. adenolipomatosis
    s. asphyxia
    s. distal neuropathy
    s. disulfide
    s. fetal growth restriction
symmetrical gangrene
symmetry
    inverse s.
sympathectomy
    chemical s.
    periarterial s.
    presacral s.
sympathetectomy
sympathetic
    s. agent
    s. amine
    s. blockade
    s. branch to submandibular ganglion
    s. formative cell
    s. ganglia
    s. heterochromia
    s. hormone
    s. hypertonia
    s. imbalance
    s. iridoplegia
    s. iritis
    s. nerve
    s. nervous system
    s. ophthalmia
    s. part of autonomic division of peripheral nervous system
    s. plexuses
    s. reflex dystrophy
    s. root of ciliary ganglion
    s. root of otic ganglion
    s. root of pterygopalatine ganglion
    s. root of sublingual ganglion
    s. root of submandibular ganglion
    s. saliva
    s. segment
    s. symptom
    s. trunk
    s. uveitis

sympathetoblast
sympathic
sympathicectomy
sympathicoblast
sympathiconeuritis
sympathicopathy
sympathicotonia
sympathicotonic
sympathicotripsy
sympathicotropic cell
sympathin
sympathism
sympathizer
sympathizing eye
sympathoadrenal
sympathoblast
sympathochromaffin cell
sympathogonia
sympatholytic
sympathomimetic amine
sympathy
symperitoneal
symphalangism, symphalangy
symphyseotome (*var. of* symphysiotome)
symphyseotomy (*var. of* symphysiotomy)
symphyses
symphysial, symphyseal
    s. surface of pubis
symphysic
    s. teratosis
symphysion
symphysiotome, symphyseotome
symphysiotomy, symphyseotomy
symphysis
    intervertebral s.
    s. intervertebralis
    s. mandibulae
    mandibular s.
    manubriosternal s.
    s. manubriosternalis
    mental s.
    s. mentalis
    s. menti
    pericardial s.
    pubic s.
    s. pubica
    s. pubis
    s. sacrococcygea
    s. xiphosternalis
symplasmatic
symplast
sympodia
symport
symporter
symptom
    abstinence s.
    accessory s.
    accidental s.
    assident s.
    Baumès s.
    Bolognini s.
    cardinal s.
    s. complex
    concomitant s.
    constitutional s.

S

symptom *(continued)*
deficiency s.
Demarquay s.
Epstein s.
equivocal s.
first rank s. (FRS)
Fischer s.
s. formation
Gordon s.
s. group
incarceration s.
induced s.
local s.
localizing s.
Macewen s.
negative s.
objective s.
pathognomonic s.
positive s.
Pratt s.
presenting s.
rainbow s.
reflex s.
Schneider first rank s.
schneiderian first rank s.
s. score
Sklowsky s.
subjective s.
s. substitution
sympathetic s.
Trendelenburg s.
Uhthoff s.
Wartenberg s.
withdrawal s.
symptomatic
s. epilepsy
s. erythema
s. fever
s. headache
s. myeloid metaplasia
s. nanism
s. neuralgia
s. porphyria
s. pruritus
s. reaction
s. tetany
s. treatment
s. varicocele
symptomatology
symptomatolytic
symptomolytic
symptosis
sympus
s. apus
s. dipus
s. monopus
Syms tractor
synadelphus
synanamorph
synanastomosis
synandrogenic
synanthem, synanthema
synaphoceptors
synapse, pl. **synapses**

axoaxonic s.
axodendritic s.
axosomatic s.
electrotonic s.
pericorpuscular s.
synapsin I
synapsis
synaptic
s. bouton
s. cleft
s. conduction
s. ending
s. phase
s. resistance
s. terminal
s. trough
s. vesicle
synaptinemal complex
synaptology
synaptonemal complex
synaptophysin
synaptosome
synarthrodia
synarthrodial joint
synarthrophysis
synarthrosis, pl. **synarthroses**
syncanthus
syncaryon
syncephalus asymmetros
syncephaly
syncheilia
syncheiria
synchilia
synchiria
synchondrodial joint
synchondroseotomy
synchondrosis, pl. **synchondroses**
anterior intraoccipital s.
s. arycorniculata
arycorniculate s.
cranial synchondroses
synchondroses cranii
s. epiphyseos
synchondroses intersternebrales
s. intraoccipitalis anterior
s. intraoccipitalis posterior
s. manubriosternalis
neurocentral s.
petrooccipital s.
s. petro-occipitalis
posterior intraoccipital s.
sphenoethmoidal s.
s. sphenoethmoidalis
sphenooccipital s.
s. spheno-occipitalis
s. sphenopetrosa
sphenopetrosal s.
sphenopetrous s.
sternal s.
synchondroses sternales
s. xiphosternalis
synchondrotomy
synchorial
synchronia
synchronic study

s. aortitis
s. cirrhosis
s. fever
s. leukoderma
s. meningoencephalitis
s. nephritis
s. osteochondritis
s. roseola
s. tooth
s. ulcer
syphiloderm, syphiloderma
syphiloid
syphilologist
syphilology
syphiloma of Fournier
syr
syrupus
Syriac ulcer
syrigmus
syringadenoma
syringadenosus
syringe
air s.
chip s.
control s.
Davidson s.
dental s.
fountain s.
hypodermic s.
Luer s.
Luer-Lok s.
Neisser s.
probe s.
ring s.
Roughton-Scholander s.
rubber-bulb s.
syringeal
syringectomy
syringes (*pl. of* syrinx)
syringitis
syringoadenoma
syringobulbia
syringocarcinoma
syringocele
syringocystadenoma papilliferum
syringocystoma
syringoencephalomyelia
syringoid
syringoma
chondroid s.
syringomeningocele
syringomyelia
syringomyelic
s. dissociation
s. hemorrhage
syringomyelocele
syringomyelus
syringopontia
syringotome
syringotomy
syrinx, pl. **syringes**
syrosingopine
syrup, sirup
ipecac s.
syrupus (syr)

syrupy
syssarcosic
syssarcosis
syssarcotic
system
absolute s. of unit
absorbent s.
alimentary s.
anterolateral s.
arch-loop-whorl s. (ALW)
association s.
autonomic nervous s.
Bethesda s.
blood group s.
blood-vascular s.
bulbosacral s.
cardiovascular s.
caudal neurosecretory s.
centimeter-gram-second s. (CGS)
central nervous s. (CNS)
cerebrospinal s.
charge transfer s.
chromaffin s.
circulatory s.
closed s.
colloid s.
complement s.
conducting s. of heart
craniosacral nervous s.
cytochrome s.
cytochrome P-450 s.
dermoid s.
digestive s.
ecological s.
electron-transport s.
endocrine s.
endomembrane s.
esthesiodic s.
exterofective s.
extrapyramidal motor s.
feedback s.
foot-pound-second s. (FPS, fps)
gamma motor s.
genital s.
genitourinary s.
geographic information s.
glandular s.
haversian s.
health information s.
hematopoietic s.
hepatic portal s.
heterogeneous s.
hexaxial reference s.
His-Tawara s.
homogeneous s.
hypophyseoportal s.
hypophysial portal s.
hypophysioportal s.
hypothalamohypophysial portal s.
hypoxia warning s.
immune s.
indicator s.
information s.
integumentary s.
intermediary s.

S

system (*continued*)
  International S. of Units (SI)
  interofective s.
  involuntary nervous s.
  kallikrein s.
  kinetic s.
  limbic s.
  linnaean s. of nomenclature
  lymphatic s.
  lymphoid s.
  s. of macrophages
  masticatory s.
  metameric nervous s.
  meter-kilogram-second s.
  metric s.
  mononuclear phagocyte s. (MPS)
  muscular s.
  nervous s.
  neuromuscular s.
  nonspecific s.
  occlusal s.
  oculomotor s.
  open s.
  O-R s.
    oxidation-reduction system
  oxidation-reduction s. (O-R system)
  parasympathetic nervous s.
  patient care information s. (PCIS)
  pedal s.
  periodic s.
  peripheral nervous s.
  picture archive and
    communication s. (PACS)
  Pinel s.
  portal s.
  pressoreceptor s.
  projection s.
  properdin s.
  Purkinje s.
  redox s.
  renal portal s.
  renin-angiotensin s.
  renin-angiotensin-aldosterone s.
  reproductive s.
  respiratory s.
  reticular activating s. (RAS)
  reticuloendothelial s. (RES)
  second signaling s.
  skeletal s.
  somesthetic s.
  static s.
  stomatognathic s.
  subendocardial conducting s. of
    heart
  sympathetic nervous s.
  T s.
  thoracolumbar s.
  thoracolumbar nervous s.
  triaxial reference s.
  urinary s.
  urogenital s.
  uropoietic s.
  vascular s.
  vegetative nervous s.

  vertebral-basilar s.
  vertebral venous s.
  visceral motor s.
  visceral nervous s.
  Zaffaroni s.
systema
  s. alimentarium
  s. cardiovasculare
  s. conducens cordis
  s. digestorium
  s. genitalia
  s. lymphaticum
  s. lymphoideum
  s. nervosum
  s. nervosum autonomicum
  s. nervosum centrale
  s. nervosum periphericum
  s. respiratorium
  s. skeletale
  s. urinarium
  s. urogenitale
systematic
  s. anatomy
  s. bacteriology
  s. desensitization
  s. name
systematization
systematized delusion
Système International d'Unités
systemic
  s. anaphylaxis
  s. anatomy
  s. autoimmune disease
  s. blastomycosis
  s. capillary leak syndrome
  s. chondromalacia
  s. circulation
  s. death
  s. febrile disease
  s. heart
  s. hyalinosis
  s. lupus erythematosus (SLE)
  s. mastocytosis
  s. myelitis
  s. poisoning
  s. scleroderma
  s. sclerosis
  s. vascular resistance
  s. venous hypertension
systemoid
systole
  aborted s.
  atrial s.
  auricular s.
  electrical s.
  electromechanical s.
  extras.
  late s.
  premature s.
  ventricular s.
systolic
  s. bruit
  s. click
  s. gallop
  s. gallop rhythm

s. gradient
s. honk
s. murmur
s. pressure
s. shock
s. thrill
s. time interval
s. whoop

systolic/diastolic ratio
systolometer
systremma
syzygial
syzygiology
syzygium
syzygy

S

τ (*var. of* tau)
θ (*var. of* theta)
T
    tesla
    tocopherol
        T agglutinogen
        T antigen
        T cell
        T cell antigen receptor
        T cytotoxic cell (Tc)
        T enzyme
        T fiber
        T group
        T helper cell (Th)
        T helper subset 1 cell
        T helper subset 2 cell
        T lymphocyte
        T myelotomy
        T system
        T tube
        T tubule
        T wave
2,4,5-T
    2,4,5-trichlorophenoxyacetic acid
T_3
    3,5,3-triiodothyronine
T_4
    thyroxine
T
    absolute temperature
T_m
    temperature midpoint
t
    temperature
        t distribution
        t test
t_m
    temperature midpoint
TA
    terminologia anatomica
Ta
    tantalum
tabanid
Tabanidae
Tabanus
tabardillo
tabatière anatomique
tabby cat striation
tabella, pl. **tabellae**
tabes
    t. infantum
    t. mesenterica
tabescence
tabescent
tabetic
    t. arthropathy
    t. crisis
    t. cuirass
    t. dissociation
    t. neurosyphilis
tabetiform
tabic

tabid
tablature
table
    Aub-DuBois t.
    contingency t.
    examining t.
    external t. of calvaria
    Gaffky t.
    inner t. of skull
    internal t. of calvaria
    life t.
    occlusal t.
    operating t.
    outer t. of skull
    t. salt
    tilt t.
    vitreous t.
tablespoon
tablet
    buccal t.
    compressed t.
    dispensing t.
    enteric coated t.
    hypodermic t.
    prolonged action t.
    sublingual t.
    sustained action t.
    t. triturate
taboo, tabu
tabular
tabule
tabun
T.A.B. vaccine
Tac antigen
Tacaribe
    T. complex of viruses
    T. virus
tache
    t. blanche
    t. laiteuse
tachistoscope
tachogram
tachograph
tachography
tachometer
tachy-
tachyarrhythmia
tachyauxesis
tachybradycardia syndrome
tachycardia
    atrial chaotic t.
    atrioventricular junctional t.
    auricular t.
    AV junctional t.
    bidirectional ventricular t.
    Coumel t.
    double t.
    ectopic t.
    t. en salves
    essential t.
    t. exophthalmica
    fetal t.

T

tachycardia *(continued)*
  junctional t.
  multifocal atrial t. (MAT)
  nodal t.
  orthostatic t.
  paroxysmal t.
  reflex t.
  sinus t.
  supraventricular t.
  ventricular t.
  t. window
tachycardia-bradycardia syndrome
tachycardiac
tachycardic
tachycrotic
tachykinin
tachypacing
tachyphylaxis
tachypnea
  transient t. of the newborn
tachyrhythmia
tachysterol
tachysystole
tachyzoite
tacrine
tactile
  t. agnosia
  t. anesthesia
  t. cell
  t. corpuscle
  t. disk
  t. elevation
  t. fremitus
  t. hallucination
  t. hyperesthesia
  t. image
  t. meniscus
  t. organ
  t. papilla
  t. sense
taction
tactometer
tactor
tactual
  T. Performance Test
TAD
  transient acantholytic dermatosis
tadpole-shaped pupil
Taenia
  T. africana
  T. armata
  T. crassicollis
  T. demerariensis
  T. dentata
  T. equina
  T. hominis
  T. hydatigena
  T. madagascariensis
  T. minima
  T. ovis
  T. philippina
  T. pisiformis
  T. quadrilobata
  T. saginata

  T. solium
  T. taeniaeformis
taenia
Taeniarhynchus
taeniasis
taeniid
Taeniidae
taenioid
Taeniorhynchus
Taenzer stain
TAF
  tumor angiogenic factor
tag
  anal skin t.
  epiploic t.'s
  sentinel t.
  skin t.
tagatose
tagged atom
tagliacotian
Tagliacozzi
Tahyna virus
tail
  t. bone
  t. bud
  t. of caudate nucleus
  t. of dentate gyrus
  t. of epididymis
  t. fold
  t. of helix
  t. of pancreas
  t. sheath
  t. vertebrae
tailgut
tailor's
  t. cramp
  t. muscle
Tait law
Taiwan Dobrava-Belgrade virus
Taka-diastase
Takahara disease
Takayama stain
Takayasu
  T. arteritis
  T. disease
  T. syndrome
talalgia
talar
  t. articular surface of calcaneus
  t. sulcus
talc operation
talcosis
  pulmonary t.
talcum
talion
  t. dread
talipedic
talipes
  t. calcaneovalgus
  t. calcaneovarus
  t. calcaneus
  t. cavus
  t. equinovalgus
  t. equinovarus
  t. equinus

t. plantaris
t. planus
t. transversoplanus
t. valgus
t. varus
Tallerman treatment
tallow
prepared mutton t.
t. soap
talo-
talocalcaneal, talocalcanean
t. interosseous ligament
t. joint
t. ligament
talocalcaneonavicular joint
talocrural
t. articulation
t. joint
talofibular
talonavicular
t. joint
t. ligament
talon cusp
taloscaphoid
talose
talotibial
talus
tamarind
tambour sound
tamed iodine
Tamm-Horsfall
T.-H. mucoprotein
T.-H. protein
tamoxifen citrate
tampon
Corner t.
tamponade, tamponage
cardiac t.
chronic t.
heart t.
tamponing, tamponment
tanacetol, tanacetone
tandem
tangentiality
tangential wound
tangent screen
tangible body macrophage
Tangier disease
tangle
neurofibrillary t.
tank
Hubbard t.
t. respirator
tannase
tannate
tanned red cell
tanner
T. growth chart
T. stage
t. ulcer
tannic acid
tannic acid glycerite
tannin
tannylacetate
tantalum (Ta)

tantalum bronchography
tantrum
tanycyte
tanyphonia
TAP
tap
heel t.
mitral t.
pericardial t.
pleural t.
spinal t.
tape
adhesive t.
tapered bougie
tapeta (*pl. of* tapetum)
tapetochoroidal
tapetoretinal degeneration
tapetoretinopathy
tapetum, pl. **tapeta**
t. alveoli
t. nigrum
t. oculi
tapeworm
taphophilia
taphophobia
Tapia syndrome
tapinocephalic
tapinocephaly
tapioca
tapir mouth
tapotement
tapping
TAPVC
total anomalous pulmonary venous connection
TAPVR
total anomalous pulmonary venous return
Taq polymerase
TAR
thrombocytopenia and absent radius
tar
t. acne
t. camphor
coal t.
t. keratosis
rectified t. oil
tarantism
tarantula
American t.
black t.
European t.
Peruvian t.
taraxacum
Tardieu
T. ecchymosis
T. petechiae
T. spot
tardive
cyanose t.
t. cyanosis
t. dyskinesia
target
t. behavior
t. cell
t. cell anemia

T

target *(continued)*
    t. gland
    t. organ
    t. patient
    t. response
targeting
targretin
Tarin
    T. space
    T. tenia
    T. valve
tariric acid
Tarlov cyst
Tarnier forceps
tarragon oil
tarry cyst
tars- *(var. of* tarso-*)*
tarsal
    t. arch
    t. bone
    t. canal
    t. cartilage
    t. cyst
    t. fold
    t. gland
    t. interosseous ligament
    t. joint
    t. ligament
    t. plate
    t. sinus
    t. tunnel syndrome
tarsale, pl. **tarsalia**
tarsalgia
tarsalis
tarsectomy
tarsectopia, tarsectopy
tarsen
tarsi *(pl. of* tarsus*)*
tarsitis
tarso-, tars-
tarsoclasia, tarsoclasis
tarsoepiphyseal aclasis
tarsomalacia
tarsomegaly
tarsometatarsal
    t. joint
    t. ligament
tarso-orbital
tarsophalangeal reflex
tarsorrhaphy
tarsotarsal
tarsotibial amputation
tarsotomy
tarsus, pl. **tarsi**
    t. inferior
    inferior t.
    t. superior
    superior t.
tartar
    cream of t.
    t. emetic
    soluble t.
tartaric acid
tart cell

tartrate
    acid t.
    normal t.
tartrated antimony
tartrazine
tastant
taste
    after-t.
    t. blindness
    t. bud
    t. bulb
    t. cell
    color t.
    t. corpuscle
    t. deficiency
    franklinic t.
    t. hair
    t. pore
    t. ridge
    voltaic t.
TAT
    thematic apperception test
TATA box
tattoo
    amalgam t.
tau, τ
taurine
taurocholate
taurocholic acid
taurodontism
Taussig-Bing
    T.-B. disease
    T.-B. syndrome
tautomeric
    t. fiber
tautomerism
Tawara node
taxa *(pl. of* taxon*)*
taxanes
taxis
    negative t.
    positive t.
taxon, pl. **taxa**
taxonomic
taxonomy
    chemical t.
    numerical t.
Taxus
Tay cherry-red spot
Taylor
    T. apparatus
    T. back brace
    T. disease
    T. splint
Tay-Sachs disease
TB
    tuberculosis
Tb
    terbium
TBG
    thyroxine-binding globulin
tBoc
    tert-butyloxycarbonyl
TBP
    thyroxine-binding protein

TBPA
> thyroxine-binding prealbumin

TBW
> total body water

Tc
> T cytotoxic cell
> technetium

^{99}Tc
> technetium-99

^{99m}Tc
> technetium-99m
> ^{99m}Tc-dimercaptosuccinic acid
> (DMSA, ^{99m}Tc-DMSA)
> ^{99m}Tc-glucoheptanate

2,3,7,8-TCDD
> 2,3,7,8-tetrachlorodibenzo[b,e][1,4]dioxin

^{99m}Tc-dimercaptosuccinic acid

^{99m}Tc-DMSA
> ^{99m}Tc-dimercaptosuccinic acid

Tγ cell

Tμ cell

T-cell
> T.-c. growth factor
> T.-c. growth factor-1, -2

T-cell–rich, B-cell lymphoma

TCG
> time compensation gain

TCID$_{50}$
> tissue culture infectious dose

^{99m}Tc pyrophosphate

T-dependent antigen

TDF
> testis-determining factor

TDP
> ribothymidine 5′-diphosphate

TdT
> terminal deoxynucleotidyl transferase

TDTH cell

Te
> tellurium

tea
> Hottentot t.
> Jesuit t.
> Mexican t.
> Paraguay t.

teacher's node

teaching hospital

tear
> artificial t.'s
> bucket-handle t.
> crocodile t.'s
> t. film
> t. gas
> Mallory-Weiss t.
> t. sac
> t. stone

tearing

tease

teaspoon

teat

tebutate

technetium (Tc)

technetium-99 (^{99}Tc)

technetium-99m (^{99m}Tc)
> ^{99m}Tc diphosphonate

^{99m}Tc-DTPA
^{99m}Tc sestamibi
^{99m}Tc sulfur colloid

technic

technical error

technician

technique
> airbrasive t.
> air-gap t.
> atrial-well t.
> ballpoint pen t.
> Barcroft-Warburg t.
> Begg light wire differential force t.
> cellulose tape t.
> direct t.
> enzyme-multiplied immunoassay t.
> (EMIT)
> Ficoll-Hypaque t.
> flicker fusion frequency t.
> fluorescent antibody t.
> flush t.
> Hampton t.
> Hartel t.
> high-kV t.
> Ilizarov t.
> immunoperoxidase t.
> indirect t.
> Jerne t.
> Judkins t.
> Knott t.
> long cone t.
> McGoon t.
> Merendino t.
> microetching t.
> Mohs fresh tissue chemosurgery t.
> Ouchterlony t.
> PAP t.
> rebreathing t.
> Rebuck skin window t.
> sealed jar t.
> Seldinger t.
> sterile insect t.
> vacuum pack t.
> washed field t.

technocausis

technologist

technology
> assisted reproductive t.

teclothiazide

tecta (*pl. of* tectum)

tectal
> t. plate
> t. stria

tectiform

Tectiviridae

tectobulbar tract

tectocephalic

tectocephaly

tectology

tectonic keratoplasty

tectoolivary fiber

tectopontine
> t. fiber
> t. tract

tectoreticular fiber

T

tectorial
    t. membrane
tectorium
tectospinal
    t. decussation
    t. tract
tectum, pl. **tecta**
    t. mesencephali
    t. of midbrain
TEDD
    total end-diastolic diameter
teel oil
teeth (*pl. of* tooth)
teething
T-E fistula
teflurane
tegmen, pl. **tegmina**
    t. cruris
    t. mastoideum
    t. tympani
    t. ventriculi quarti
tegmenta (*pl. of* tegmentum)
tegmental
    t. decussation
    t. field of Forel
    t. nucleus
    t. root of tympanic cavity
    t. syndrome
    t. wall of middle ear
    t. wall of tympanic cavity
tegmentotomy
tegmentum, pl. **tegmenta**
    t. mesencephali
    mesencephalic t.
    t. of midbrain
    midbrain t.
    t. of pons
    t. pontis
    t. rhombencephali
    rhombencephalic t.
    t. of rhombencephalon
tegmina (*pl. of* tegmen)
tegument
tegumental, tegumentary
Teichmann crystal
teichoic acids
teichopsia
tel-, tele-, telo-
tela, pl. **telae**
    t. choroidea
    t. choroidea of fourth ventricle
    t. choroidea inferior
    t. choroidea superior
    t. choroidea of third ventricle
    t. choroidea ventriculi quarti
    t. choroidea ventriculi tertii
    t. conjunctiva
    t. elastica
    t. subcutanea
    t. subcutanea penis
    t. subcutanea perinei
    t. submucosa
    t. submucosa pharyngis
    t. subserosa
    t. vasculosa

Teladorsagia davtiani
telalgia
telangiectasia
    calcinosis, Raynaud phenomenon, esophageal motility disorder, sclerodactyly and t. (CREST)
    cephalooculocutaneous t.
    essential t.
    hereditary benign t.
    hereditary hemorrhagic t.
    t. lymphatica
    t. macularis eruptiva perstans
    primary t.
    secondary t.
    spider t.
    t. verrucosa
telangiectasis, pl. **telangiectases**
telangiectatic
    t. angioma
    t. angiomatosis
    t. cancer
    t. fibroma
    t. glioma
    t. lipoma
    t. osteogenic sarcoma
    t. wart
telangioma
telangion
telangiosis
tele- (*var. of* tel-)
telecanthus
telecardiogram
telecardiophone
telecobalt
telediagnosis
telediastolic
telehopsias
telelectrocardiogram
telemeter
telemetry
    cardiac t.
telencephalic
    t. flexure
    t. vesicle
telencephalization
telencephalon
teleology
teleomitosis
teleomorph
teleonomic
teleonomy
teleopsia
teleorganic
telepathine
telepathy
telephone
    t. ear
    t. theory
teleradiography
teleradiology
teleradium
    t. therapy
telereceptor
telergy
teleroentgenography

teleroentgentherapy
telescope
    Hopkins rod-lens t.
telescopic
    t. denture
    t. spectacles
telesis
telesystolic
teletherapy
television microscope
TeLinde operation
telluric
tellurism
tellurium (Te)
telo- (*var. of* tel-)
telocentric chromosome
telodendron
telogen effluvium
teloglia
telognosis
telokinesia
telolecithal
    t. egg
    t. ovum
telomerase
telomere
telomeric R-banding stain
telopeptide
telophase
Telosporea
Telosporidia
telotism
TEM
    triethylenemelamine
temazepam
temper
temperament
temperance
temperate
    t. bacteriophage
    t. virus
temperature (*t*)
    absolute t. (*T*)
    basal body t.
    t. coefficient
    critical t.
    denaturation t. of DNA
    effective t.
    equivalent t.
    eutectic t.
    fusion t. (wire method)
    maximum t.
    mean t.
    melting t.
    melting t. of DNA
    t. midpoint (T_m, t_m)
    minimum t.
    optimum t.
    room t. (RT)
    t. sense
    sensible t.
    t. spot
    standard t.
temperature-compensated vaporizer
temperature-sensitive mutant

template
    t. RNA
    surgical t.
temple
tempolabile
tempora (*pl. of* tempus)
temporal
    t. aponeurosis
    t. apophysis
    t. arteritis
    t. bone
    t. branch of facial nerve
    t. canal
    t. contiguity
    t. cortex
    t. crest of mandible
    t. dispersion
    t. fascia
    t. fossa
    t. horn
    t. line
    t. line of frontal bone
    t. lobe
    t. lobe epilepsy
    t. muscle
    t. plane
    t. pole
    t. pole of cerebrum
    t. process of zygomatic bone
    t. region of head
    t. ridge
    t. squama
    t. surface
    t. vein
    t. venules of retina
temporalis muscle
temporary
    t. base
    t. callus
    t. cartilage
    t. denture
    t. memory
    t. parasite
    t. restoration
    t. stricture
    t. threshold shift
    t. tooth
temporo-
temporoauricular
temporofrontal tract
temporohyoid
temporomalar
temporomandibular
    t. arthrosis
    t. articular disk
    t. articulation
    t. joint
    t. joint dysfunction (TMD, TMJ)
    t. joint pain-dysfunction syndrome
    t. ligament
    t. nerve
temporomaxillary vein
temporo-occipital
temporoparietalis muscle
temporoparietal muscle

T

temporopontine
> t. fiber
> t. tract

temporosphenoid
temporozygomatic suture
tempostabile, tempostable
temps utile
tempus, pl. **tempora**
TEN
> toxic epidermal necrolysis
> t. Horn sign

tenacious
tenacity
> cellular t.

tenaculum, pl. **tenacula**
> t. forceps
> tenacula tendinum

tenalgia crepitans
tenascin
tender
> t. line
> t. point
> t. zones

tenderness
> pencil t.
> rebound t.

tendines (*pl. of* tendo)
tendinitis
tendinoplasty
tendinosuture
tendinous
> t. arch
> t. arch of levator ani muscle
> t. arch of pelvic fascia
> t. arch of soleus muscle
> t. chiasm of the digital tendons
> t. cord
> t. inscription
> t. intersection
> t. intersection of rectus abdominis
> t. opening
> t. sheath of abductor pollicis longus and extensor pollicis brevis muscle
> t. sheath of extensor carpi radialis muscle
> t. sheath of extensor carpi ulnaris muscle
> t. sheath of extensor digiti minimi muscle
> t. sheath of extensor digitorum and extensor indicis muscle
> t. sheath of extensor digitorum longus muscle of foot
> t. sheath of extensor hallucis longus muscle
> t. sheath of extensor pollicis longus muscle
> t. sheath of flexor carpi radialis muscle
> t. sheath of flexor digitorum longus muscle of foot
> t. sheath of flexor hallucis longus muscle
> t. sheath of flexor pollicis longus muscle

> t. sheath of superior oblique muscle
> t. sheath of tibialis anterior muscle
> t. sheath of tibialis posterior muscle
> t. spot
> t. synovitis
> t. xanthoma

tendo, pl. **tendines**
> t. Achillis
> t. Achillis reflex
> t. calcaneus
> t. calcaneus communis
> t. conjunctivus
> t. cricoesophageus
> t. oculi
> t. palpebrarum

tendo-
tendolysis
tendomucin, tendomucoid
tendon
> Achilles t.
> t. advancement
> t. bundle
> calcaneal t.
> t. cell
> central t. of diaphragm
> central t. of perineum
> conjoined t.
> conjoint t.
> coronary t.
> cricoesophageal t.
> Gerlach annular t.
> t. graft
> hamstring t.
> heel t.
> t. recession
> t. reflex
> t. sheath syndrome
> t. suture
> Todaro t.
> t. transplantation
> trefoil t.
> Zinn t.

tendonitis
tendophony
tendosynovitis
tendotomy
tendovaginal
tendovaginitis
> radial styloid t.

tenectomy
tenesmic
tenesmus
ten Horn
tenia, pl. **teniae**
> taeniae acusticae
> t. choroidea
> teniae coli
> colic t.
> t. fimbriae
> t. fornicis
> t. of the fornix
> t. of fourth ventricle
> free t.
> t. hippocampi
> t. libera

medullary teniae
mesocolic t.
t. mesocolica
omental t.
t. omentalis
t. semicircularis
Tarin t.
t. tecta
t. telae
t. terminalis
t. thalami
thalamic t.
teniae of Valsalva
t. ventriculi quarti
t. ventriculi tertii

teniacide
teniafuge
tenial
teniasis
somatic t.

tenicide
teniform
tenifugal
tenifuge
tenioid
teniola
t. corporis callosi

tennis
t. elbow
t. leg
t. thumb

teno-, tenon-, tenont-, tenonto-
tenodesis
tenodynia
tenofibril
tenolysis
tenomyoplasty
tenomyotomy
Tenon
T. capsule
T. space

tenon- (*var. of* teno-)
tenonectomy
tenonitis
tenont- (*var. of* teno-)
tenontitis
tenonto- (*var. of* teno-)
tenontography
tenontology
tenontomyoplasty
tenontomyotomy
tenontoplastic
tenontoplasty
tenophony
tenophyte
tenoplastic
tenoplasty
tenoreceptor
tenorrhaphy
tenostosis
tenosuspension
tenosuture
tenosynovectomy
tenosynovitis
t. crepitans

de Quervain t.
localized nodular t.
pigmented villonodular t.
stenosing t.
villous t.

tenotomy
curb t.
graduated t.
subcutaneous t.

tenovaginitis
tense
t. part of the tympanic membrane
t. pulse

tensile
t. strength
t. stress

tensiometer
tension
arterial t.
t. curve
t. headache
interfacial surface t.
t. line
ocular t. (Tn)
t. pneumopericardium
t. pneumothorax
premenstrual t.
surface t.
t. suture
tissue t.

tension-type headache
tensor, pl. **tensores**
t. fasciae latae muscle
t. muscle of fascia lata
t. muscle of soft palate
t. muscle of tympanic membrane
t. tarsi muscle
t. tympani muscle
t. tympani reflex
t. veli palati muscle

tent
oxygen t.
sponge t.

tentacle
tenth cranial nerve [CN X]
tentorial
t. angle
t. basal branch of internal carotid artery
t. marginal branch of cavernous part of internal carotid artery
t. nerve
t. notch
t. sinus
t. surface

tentorium, pl. **tentoria**
cerebellar t.
t. cerebelli
t. of hypophysis

TEPA
triethylenephosphoramide

tephromalacia
tephrylometer
TEPP
tetraethyl pyrophosphate

T

teprotide
tera-
teras, pl. **terata**
teratic
teratism
terato-
teratoblastoma
teratocarcinoma
teratogen
teratogenesis
teratogenic, teratogenetic
teratogenicity
teratoid tumor
teratologic
teratology
teratoma
    t. orbitae
    sacrococcygeal t.
    triphyllomatous t.
teratomatous cyst
teratophobia
teratosis
    atresic t.
    ceasmic t.
    ectogenic t.
    ectopic t.
    hypergenic t.
    symphysic t.
teratospermia
teratozoospermia
terazosin hydrochloride
terbium (Tb)
terbutaline sulfate
ter in die (t.i.d.)
terebene
terebinthinate
terebinthine
terebinthinism
terebrant, terebrating
terebration
teres, gen. **teretis**, pl. **teretes**
    t. major muscle
    t. minor muscle
terfenadine
tergal
tergum
terminad
terminal
    t. addition enzyme
    amino-t.
    t. artery
    axon t.
    t. bar
    t. bouton
    t. branch of middle cerebral artery
    t. bronchiole
    t. cisternae
    t. crest
    t. deletion
    t. deoxynucleotidyl transferase (TdT)
    t. disinfection
    t. duct carcinoma
    t. endocarditis
    t. filum
    t. ganglion

    t. hair
    t. hematuria
    t. hinge position
    t. ileus
    t. infection
    t. jaw relation record
    t. leukocytosis
    t. line
    t. nerve
    t. nerve corpuscle
    t. notch of auricle
    t. nucleus
    t. oxidase
    t. oxidation
    t. part
    t. plate
    t. pneumonia
    t. redundancy
    t. respiratory unit
    t. sinus
    t. stria
    t. sulcus
    t. sulcus of tongue
    synaptic t.
    t. thread
    t. transferases
    t. vein
    t. ventricle
    t. web
terminatio, pl. **terminationes**
    terminationes nervorum liberae
termination
    t. codon
    t. factor
    selective t.
    t. sequence
    t. signal
term infant
termini (*pl. of* terminus)
Terminologia Anatomica (**TA**)
terminoterminal anastomosis
terminus, pl. **termini**
    C t.
    termini generales
    N t.
termolecular
termone
ternary complex
Ternidens
    t. deminutus
teroxide
terpene
p-terphenyl
terpineol
terpin hydrate
terpinol
terrace
terra japonica
Terrien
    T. marginal degeneration
    T. valve
territoriality
territorial matrix
Terry syndrome

tetraethylmonothionopyrophosphate
tetraethyl poisoning
tetraethyl pyrophosphate (TEPP)
tetraethylthiuram disulfide
tetragastrin
tetraglycine hydroperiodide
tetragon, tetragonum
    t. lumbale
tetragonus
tetrahydric
tetrahydro-
tetrahydrocannabinol (THC)
tetrahydrofolate (THF)
5,6,7,8-tetrahydrofolate dehydrogenase
tetrahydrofolate methyltransferase
tetrahydrofolic acid (FH$_4$)
tetrahydrozoline hydrochloride
Tetrahymena pyriformis
tetraiodophenolphthalein sodium
tetralogy
    Eisenmenger t.
    t. of Fallot
tetramastia
tetramastigote
tetramastous
tetramelus
Tetrameres
tetrameric, tetramerous
tetramethyl acridine
tetramethylammonium iodide
tetramethyldiarsine
tetramethylputrescine
tetranitrol
tetranucleotide
tetraotus
tetraparesis
tetrapeptide
tetraperomelia
tetraphocomelia
tetraplegia
tetraplegic
tetraploid
tetrapus
tetrapyrrole
tetrasaccharide
tetrascelus
tetrasomic
tetraster
tetrastichiasis
tetraterpenes
tetratomic
Tetratrichomonas ovis
tetravalent
tetrazole
tetrazolium
    nitroblue t. (NBT)
tetrazonium salt
tetrodotoxin (TTX)
tetrose
tetrotus
tetroxide
tetter
Teutleben ligament
Texas snakeroot
text blindness

textiform
textural
texture
textus
TGC
    time-varied gain control
TGE virus
TGF
    transforming growth factor
TGFalpha
    transforming growth factor a
TGFbeta
    transforming growth factor b
Th
    T helper cell
Thal
thalam- (*var. of* thalamo-)
thalamectomy
thalamencephalic
thalamencephalon
thalami (*pl. of* thalamus)
thalamic
    t. fasciculus
    t. gustatory nucleus
    t. syndrome
    t. tenia
thalamo-, thalam-
thalamocortical fiber
thalamolenticular
thalamostriate vein
thalamotomy
thalamus, pl. thalami
    dorsal t.
    ventral t.
thalassemia, thalassanemia
    β-δ t.
    α t.
    A$_2$ t.
    beta t.
    F t.
    t. intermedia
    α t. intermedia
    Lepore t.
    t. major
    t. minor
β-δ thalassemia
thalassophobia
thalassoposia
thalassotherapy
thalidomide
thallic
thallium (Tl)
    t.-201 (^{201}Tl)
    t. poisoning
Thallophyta
thallophyte
thallotoxicosis
thallus
Thal procedure
thanato-
thanatobiologic
thanatognomonic
thanatography
thanatoid
thanatology

T

thanatomania
thanatophidia
thanatophobia
thanatophoric dwarfism
thanatos
Thane method
thaumatropy
Thayer-Martin
  T.-M. agar
  T.-M. medium
THC
  tetrahydrocannabinol
Thd
  ribothymidine
thea
theaism
theater
thebaic
thebaine
thebesian
  t. circulation
  t. foramina
  t. valve
  t. vein
theca, pl. **thecae**
  t. cell of stomach
  t. cell tumor
  t. cordis
  t. externa
  t. folliculi
  t. interna
  t. interna cone
  t. lutein cell
  t. tendinis
  t. vertebralis
thecal
  t. whitlow
thecodont
thecoma
thecomatosis
Theden method
Theile
  T. canal
  T. gland
  T. muscle
Theiler
  T. mouse encephalomyelitis virus
  T. original virus
Theileriidae
thein
theinism, theism
thel- (*var. of* thelo-)
thelarche
Thelazia
  t. californiensis
  t. callipaeda
thelaziasis
thele
thelium, pl. **thelia**
thelo-, thel-
thelorrhagia
thematic
  t. apperception test (TAT)
  t. paralogia
  t. paraphasia

thenad
thenal
thenaldine
thenar
  t. eminence
  t. prominence
  t. space
thenen
thenyl
thenyldiamine hydrochloride
Theobald Smith phenomenon
theobroma
  t. oil
theobromine
theomania
theophobia
theophylline
  t. ethylenediamine
  t. sodium glycinate
theorem
  Bayes t.
  Bernoulli t.
  central limit t.
  Gibbs t.
theory
  adsorption t. of narcosis
  aerodynamic t.
  Altmann t.
  Arrhenius-Madsen t.
  atomic t.
  Baeyer t.
  balance t.
  beta-oxidation-condensation t.
  Bohr t.
  Brønsted t.
  Burn and Rand t.
  Cannon t.
  Cannon-Bard t.
  catastrophe t.
  cellular immune t.
  celomic metaplasia t. of
    endometriosis
  chaos t.
  chemiosmotic t.
  cloacal t.
  clonal deletion t.
  clonal selection t.
  cognitive dissonance t.
  colloid t. of narcosis
  darwinian t.
  decay t.
  dipole t.
  duplicity t. of vision
  Ehrlich t.
  t. of electrolytic dissociation
  emergency t.
  enzyme inhibition t. of narcosis
  Flourens t.
  Frerichs t.
  Freud t.
  game t.
  gastrea t.
  gate-control t.
  germ layer t.
  gestalt t.

Haeckel gastrea t.
Helmholtz t. of accommodation
Helmholtz t. of color vision
Helmholtz-Gibbs t.
Helmholtz t. of hearing
Hering t. of color vision
humoral t.
hydrate microcrystal t. of anesthesia
implantation t. of the production of
  endometriosis
incasement t.
information t.
instructive t.
kern-plasma relation t.
Knoop t.
Ladd-Franklin t.
lamarckian t.
learning t.
libido t.
Liebig t.
lipoid t. of narcosis
mass action t.
t. of medicine
membrane expansion t.
Metchnikoff t.
Meyer-Overton t. of narcosis
miasma t.
Miller chemicoparasitic t.
mnemic t.
molecular dissociation t.
monophyletic t.
myoelastic t.
neurochronaxic t.
Ollier t.
omega-oxidation t.
overproduction t.
oxygen deprivation t. of narcosis
Pauling t.
permeability t. of narcosis
phlogiston t.
pithecoid t.
place t.
Planck t.
polyphyletic t.
preformation t.
quantum t.
recapitulation t.
Reed-Frost t. of epidemics
reed instrument t.
reentry t.
resonance t. of hearing
scientific t.
Semon-Hering t.
sensorimotor t.
side-chain t.
somatic mutation t. of cancer
Spitzer t.
stringed instrument t.
surface tension t. of narcosis
telephone t.
thermodynamic t. of narcosis
traveling wave t.
van't Hoff t.
Warburg t.

Wollaston t.
Young-Helmholtz t. of color vision
theotherapy
thèque
therapeusis
therapeutic
  t. abortion
  t. anesthesia
  t. angiography
  t. community
  t. crisis
  t. dose
  t. electrode
  t. fever
  t. group
  t. incompatibility
  t. index
  t. iridectomy
  t. malaria
  t. nihilism
  t. optimism
  t. pessimism
  t. pneumothorax
  t. radiology
  t. range
  t. ratio
therapeutics
  ray t.
  suggestive t.
therapeutist
therapia magna sterilisans
therapist
therapy
  alkali t.
  analytic t.
  anticoagulant t.
  antisense t.
  autoserum t.
  aversion t.
  behavior t.
  client-centered t.
  cognitive t.
  collapse t.
  conditioning t.
  conjoint t.
  convulsive t.
  cytoreductive t.
  depot t.
  diathermic t.
  directly observed t.
  electroconvulsive t. (ECT)
  electroshock t.
  electrotherapeutic sleep t.
  estrogen replacement t.
  extended family t.
  family t.
  fast-neutron radiation t.
  fever t.
  foreign protein t.
  functional orthodontic t.
  gene t.
  geriatric t.
  gestalt t.
  heterovaccine t.
  hormone replacement t. (HRT)

T

therapy *(continued)*
    hyperbaric oxygen t.
    implosive t.
    individual t.
    inhalation t.
    insulin coma t.
    interstitial t.
    intralesional t.
    maintenance drug t.
    marital t.
    marriage t.
    microwave t.
    milieu t.
    myofunctional t.
    nonspecific t.
    occupational t. (OT)
    orthodontic t.
    orthomolecular t.
    oxygen t.
    parenteral t.
    photodynamic t.
    photoradiation t.
    physical t. (PT)
    plasma t.
    play t.
    proliferation t.
    protein shock t.
    psychedelic t.
    psychoanalytic t.
    pulse t.
    quadrangular t.
    radiation t.
    radium beam t.
    rational t.
    reflex t.
    replacement t.
    respiratory t.
    root canal t.
    rotation t.
    salvage t.
    sclerosing t.
    serum t.
    shock t.
    social t.
    social network t.
    solar t.
    specific t.
    substitution t.
    substitutive t.
    teleradium t.
    thrombolytic t.
    thyroid t.
    Time-Line t.
    total push t.
    ultrasonic t.
    viral t.
    x-ray t.
therencephalous
theriaca
therio-
theriomorphism
therm
therm- *(var. of* thermo-)
thermacogenesis

thermal
    t. anesthesia
    t. artifact
    t. burn
    t. capacity
    t. sense
    t. spectrum
thermalgesia
thermalgia
thermanalgesia
thermanesthesia
thermatology
thermelometer
thermesthesia
thermesthesiometer
thermic
    t. sense
    thermic anesthesia
    thermic fever
thermistor
thermo-, therm-
thermoacidophiles
thermoalgesia
thermoanalgesia
thermoanesthesia
thermocauterectomy
thermocautery
thermochemistry
thermochroic
thermochroism
thermochrose
thermochrosis
thermochrosy
thermocoagulation
thermocouple
thermocurrent
thermodiffusion
thermodilution
thermoduric
thermodynamic
    t. potential
    t. theory of narcosis
thermodynamics
thermoelectric
    t. pile
thermoelectricity
thermoesthesia
thermoesthesiometer
thermoexcitory
thermogenesis
    nonshivering t.
    shivering t.
thermogenic, thermogenetic
    t. action
thermogenics
thermogenin
thermogenous
thermogram
thermograph
thermography
    infrared t.
    liquid crystal t.
thermohyperalgesia
thermohyperesthesia
thermohypesthesia

thermohypoesthesia
thermoinhibitory
thermointegrator
thermojunction
thermokeratoplasty
thermolabile opsonin
thermology
thermoluminescence dosimetry
thermolysis
thermolytic
thermomassage
thermometer
    air t.
    axilla t.
    axillary t.
    clinical t.
    differential t.
    gas t.
    resistance t.
    self-registering t.
    spirit t.
    surface t.
    wet and dry bulb t.
thermometric
thermometry
thermoneurosis
thermonuclear
thermopenetration
thermophile, thermophil
thermophilic
thermophobia
thermophore
thermophylic
thermopile
thermoplacentography
thermoplasma, pl. thermoplasmata
Thermoplasma acidophilum
thermoplastic
thermoplegia
thermoprecipitin reaction
thermoreceptor
thermoregulation
thermoregulator
thermoscope
thermoset
thermostable, thermostabile
    t. enzyme
    t. opsonin
    t. opsonin test
thermostat
thermosteresis
thermostromuhr
thermosystaltic
thermosystaltism
thermotactic, thermotaxic
thermotaxis
    negative t.
    positive t.
thermotherapy
thermotic
thermotics
thermotonometer
thermotropism
theroid
therology

thesaurismosis
thesaurismotic
thesaurosis
thesis, pl. theses
theta, θ
    t. antigen
    t. rhythm
    t. wave
thetins
Thezac-Porsmeur method
THF
    tetrahydrofolate
thia-
thiabendazole
thiabutazide
thiacetazone
thialbarbital
thiambutosine
thiamin
    t. chloride unit
    t. hydrochloride
    t. hydrochloride unit
    t. mononitrate
    t. pyridinylase
    t. pyrophosphate (TPP)
thiaminase
    t. I, II
thiamine
thiamphenicol
thiamylal sodium
Thiara
thiazide diabetes
thiazin dye
thiazolidinediones
thiazolsulfone
thick
    t. filament
    t. skin
thickness
    Breslow t.
thiel
Thiemann
    T. disease
    T. syndrome
thiemia
thienamycin
thienyl
thienylalanine
Thiersch
    T. canaliculi
    T. graft
thiethylperazine maleate
thigh
    t. bone
    Heilbronner t.
    t. joint
thigmesthesia
thigmotaxis
thigmotropism
thimerosal
thin
    t. filament
    t. section
    t. skin

T

thinking
    abstract t.
    archaic-paralogical t.
    concrete t.
    creative t.
    magical t.
    prelogical t.
    t. through
thin-layer
    t.-l. chromatography (TLC)
    t.-l. electrophoresis (TLE)
    t.-l. immunoassay
thinning
    shear t.
thio-
thioacid
thioalcohol
thioamide
thioate
thiobarbiturates
thiocarbamide
thiocarlide
thiochrome method
thioclastic cleavage
thioctic acid
thiocyanate
thiocyanic acid
thiocyanogen
    t. number
    t. value
thiodepsipeptide
thiodiphenylamine
thioester
thioesterase
thioesters
thioethanolamine acetyltransferase
thioether
thioflavin
    t. S
    t. T
    t. T stain
thiofuran
thioglucosidase
thioglycerol
thioglycolate, thioglycollate
thioglycolic acid
thioguanine
-thioic acid
thiokinase
thiol
    t. enzyme
    t. ester
thiolase
thiole
thiolesterase
thiolhistidylbetaine
thioltransacetylase A
thiolysis
thiomersal
thiomersalate
thiomethyladenosine
-thione
thionein
thioneine
thionic

thionine
thiono-
thiopanic acid
thiopental sodium
thiophene
thiophenicol
thiopropazate hydrochloride
thioproperazine
thioredoxin reductase
thioridazine hydrochloride
thiosemicarbazide
thiosemicarbazone
thiosulfate
    t. cyanide transsulfurase
    t. sulfurtransferase
    t. thiotransferase
thiosulfuric acid
thiotepa
thiothixene
thiotransacetylase B
2-thiouracil
4-thiouracil
thiourea
thioxanthene
thioxo-
thioxolone
thiphenamil hydrochloride
third
    t. corpuscle
    t. cranial nerve [CN III]
    t. cuneiform bone
    t. disease
    t. eyelid
    t. finger
    t. and fourth pharyngeal pouch
      syndrome
    t. heart sound (S_3)
    t. molar
    t. occipital nerve
    t. ovary
    t. parallel pelvic plane
    t. part of duodenum
    t. peroneal muscle
    t. sound
    t. spacing
    t. temporal convolution
    t. toe [III]
    t. tonsil
    t. trochanter
    t. ventricle
    t. ventriculostomy
third-degree
    t.-d. AV block
    third-degree burn
third-year molar tooth
thirst
    false t.
    t. fever
    insensible t.
    morbid t.
    subliminal t.
    true t.
Thiry fistula
Thiry-Vella fistula
thixolabile

thixotropic fluid
thixotropy
Thogotoviruses
Thoma
    T. ampulla
    T. fixative
    T. law
Thomas splint
Thompson
    T. ligament
    T. test
Thomsen disease
Thomson sign
thonzonium bromide
thonzylamine hydrochloride
thorac- (*var. of* thoraco-)
thoracal
thoracalgia
thoracentesis
thoraces (*pl. of* thorax)
thoracic
    t. aorta
    t. aortic plexus
    t. axis
    t. cage
    t. cardiac branch of thoracic
      ganglia
    t. cardiac branch of vagus nerve
    t. cardiac nerve
    t. cavity
    t. compliance
    t. constriction of esophagus
    t. duct
    t. fistula
    t. ganglia
    t. girdle
    t. gland
    t. goiter
    t. index
    t. inlet
    t. interspinales muscle
    t. interspinal muscle
    t. intertransversarii muscle
    t. intertransverse muscle
    t. kidney
    t. kyphosis
    t. limb
    t. longissimus muscle
    t. lymph node
    t. nerve [T1–T12]
    t. outlet
    t. outlet syndrome (TOS)
    t. part of aorta
    t. part of esophagus
    t. part of iliocostalis lumborum
      muscle
    t. part of peripheral autonomic
      plexuses and ganglia
    t. part of spinal cord
    t. part of thoracic duct
    t. part of trachea
    t. pulmonary branch of thoracic
      ganglia
    t. respiration
    t. rotator muscle

    t. skeleton
    t. spine
    t. splanchnic ganglion
    t. splanchnic nerve
    t. splenosis
    t. stomach
    t. vein
    t. vertebrae [T1–T12]
    t. wall
thoracico- (*var. of* thoraco-)
thoracicoabdominal
thoracicoacromial
thoracicohumeral
thoracic-pelvic-phalangeal dystrophy
thoraco-, thorac-, thoracico-
thoracoabdominal
    t. ectopia cordis
    t. nerve
thoracoacromial
    t. artery
    t. trunk
    t. vein
thoracoappendicular muscle
thoracoceloschisis
thoracocentesis
thoracocyllosis
thoracocyrtosis
thoracodelphus
thoracodorsal
    t. artery
    t. nerve
thoracodynia
thoracoepigastric vein
thoracogastroschisis
thoracolaparotomy
thoracolumbar
    t. aponeurosis
    t. fascia
    t. nervous system
    t. system
thoracolumbosacral orthosis
thoracolysis
thoracomelus
thoracometer
thoracomyodynia
thoracopagus
thoracoparacephalus
thoracopathy
thoracoplasty
    conventional t.
thoracopneumoplasty
thoracoschisis
thoracoscope
thoracoscopic surgery
thoracoscopy
thoracostenosis
thoracosternotomy
    transverse t.
thoracostomy tube
thoracotomy
    anterior t.
    axillary t.
    clamshell t.
    minithoracotomy

T

thoracotomy *(continued)*
    muscle-sparing t.
    posterolateral t.
thoradelphus
thorax, pl. **thoraces**
    barrel-shaped t.
    Peyrot t.
thorium
    t. emanation
Thormählen test
thorn
    t. apple
    t. apple crystal
    dendritic t.
    T. syndrome
    T. test
Thornwaldt
thought
    t. broadcasting
    t. insertion
    t. process disorder
    trend of t.
    t. withdrawal
thread
    terminal t.
threaded implant
threadworm
thready pulse
threatened abortion
three-chambered heart
three-cornered bone
three-day
    t.-d. fever
    t.-d. measles
three-dimensional record
three-glass test
three-headed muscle
three-incision esophagectomy
threonic acid
threonine
    t. deaminase
    t. dehydratase
threose
thresher's lung
threshold
    absolute t.
    achromatic t.
    auditory t.
    t. body
    brightness difference t.
    t. of consciousness
    convulsant t.
    differential t.
    t. differential
    displacement t.
    double-point t.
    erythema t.
    fibrillation t.
    galvanic t.
    t. of island of Reil
    light differential t.
    t. limit value (TLV)
    minimum light t.
    t. of nose

    t. pad
    pain t.
    t. percussion
    phenotypic t.
    relational t.
    renal t.
    t. shift
    speech awareness t.
    speech detection t.
    speech reception t.
    stimulus t.
    t. stimulus
    t. substance
    swallowing t.
    t. trait
    visual t.
    t. of visual sensation
thrill
    diastolic t.
    hydatid t.
    presystolic t.
    systolic t.
thrix
throat
    ears, nose, and t. (ENT)
    eye, ear, nose, and t. (EENT)
    sore t.
throb
thromb- *(var. of* thrombo-)
thrombase
thrombasthenia
    Glanzmann t.
    hereditary hemorrhagic t.
thrombectomy
thrombi *(pl. of* thrombus)
thrombin
    human t.
    t. time
thrombinogen
thrombinogenesis
thrombo-, thromb-
thromboangiitis obliterans
thromboarteritis
thromboasthenia
thromboblast
thromboclastic
thrombocyst, thrombocystis
thrombocytasthenia
thrombocyte
thrombocythemia
thrombocytic series
thrombocytin
thrombocytopathy
thrombocytopenia
    t. and absent radius (TAR)
    autoimmune neonatal t.
    essential t.
    immune t.
    isoimmune neonatal t.
thrombocytopenia-absent radius syndrome
thrombocytopenic purpura
thrombocytopoiesis
thrombocytosis
thromboelastogram
thromboelastograph

thromboembolectomy
thromboembolism
　　pulmonary t. (PTE)
thromboendarterectomy
　　pulmonary t. (PTEA)
thromboendocarditis
thrombogen
thrombogene
thrombogenic
thromboid
thrombokatilysin
thrombokinase
thrombolic
thrombolus
thrombolymphangitis
thrombolysis
　　t. in myocardial infarction (TIMI)
thrombolytic therapy
thrombomodulin
thrombon
thrombonecrosis
thrombopathic syndrome
thrombopathy
　　constitutional t.
thrombopenia
thrombopenic purpura
thrombophilia
thrombophlebitis
　　t. migrans
　　t. saltans
thromboplastid
thromboplastin
thromboplastinogen
thrombopoiesis
thrombopoietin
thrombosed
thrombosin
thrombosis, pl. thromboses
　　atrophic t.
　　cerebral t.
　　compression t.
　　coronary t.
　　creeping t.
　　dilation t.
　　effort-induced t.
　　marantic t.
　　mural t.
　　placental t.
　　plate t.
　　platelet t.
　　posttraumatic arterial t.
　　posttraumatic venous t.
thrombospondin-related adhesive protein
thrombostasis
thrombosthenin
thrombotic
　　t. gangrene
　　t. hydrocephalus
　　t. infarct
　　t. microangiopathy
　　t. thrombocytopenic purpura
　　t. thrombocytopenic purpura and
　　　hemolytic uremic syndrome (TTP-
　　　HUS)

thrombotonin
thromboxane (TX)
　　individual t. (TX)
thrombozyme
thrombus, pl. thrombi
　　agglutinative t.
　　agonal t.
　　antemortem t.
　　ball t.
　　ball-valve t.
　　bile t.
　　currant jelly t.
　　fibrin t.
　　globular t.
　　hyaline t.
　　infective t.
　　laminated t.
　　marantic t., t. thrombus
　　mixed t.
　　mural t.
　　obstructive t.
　　pale t.
　　parietal t.
　　postmortem t.
　　propagated t.
　　red t.
　　secondary t.
　　stratified t.
　　valvular t.
　　white t.
through
　　t. drainage
　　t. transfer imaging
through-and-through
　　t.-a.-t. laceration
　　t.-a.-t. myocardial infarction
throughput
thrush fungus
thuja oil
thujol
thujone
thulium (Tm)
thumb
　　bifid t.
　　t. forceps
　　gamekeeper's t.
　　hitchhiker t.
　　t. lancet
　　t. reflex
　　tennis t.
thumbprinting
thumps
thunderclap headache
thus
thuya
thuyol
Thy
　　thymine
Thygeson disease
thym- (var. of thymo-)
thyme
　　t. camphor
　　t. oil
thymectomy
　　extended t.

T

thymectomy *(continued)*
    maximal t.
    transcervical t.
thymelcosis
thymi *(pl. of* thymus)
thymi- *(var. of* thymo-)
-thymia
thymic
    t. abscess
    t. acid
    t. agenesis
    t. alymphoplasia
    t. branch of internal thoracic artery
    t. corpuscle
    t. hypoplasia
    t. lymphopoietic factor
    t. vein
thymicolymphatic
thymidine (dThd)
    t. 5′-monophosphate
    t. phosphorylase
    thymidine 5′-diphosphate (dTDP)
    t. 5′-triphosphate (dTTP)
    tritiated t.
thymidylate synthase
thymidylic acid
thymin
thymine (Thy)
    t. deoxyribonucleoside
    t. deoxyribonucleotide
    t. dimer
    t. nucleotide
thyminuria
thymitis
thymo-, thym-, thymi-
thymocyte
thymogenic
thymokinetic
thymol
    t. blue
    t. iodide
    t. turbidity test
thymoma
thymonuclease
thymopoietin
thymoprival, thymoprivic, thymoprivous
thymosin
thymoxamine
thymus, pl. **thymi, thymuses**
    t. gland
    t. treatment
thymus-dependent zone
thymus-independent antigen
thyreo-
thyro-, thyr-
thyroacetic acid
thyroadenitis
thyroaplasia
thyroarytenoid muscle
thyrocalcitonin
thyrocardiac disease
thyrocele
thyrocervical trunk
thyrocolloid

thyroepiglottic
    t. ligament
    t. muscle
    t. part of thyroarytenoid muscle
thyrofissure
thyrogenic, thyrogenous
thyroglobulin
thyroglossal
    t. duct
    t. duct cyst
thyroglossal diverticulum *(var. of* thyroid
    diverticulum)
thyrohyal
thyrohyoid
    t. branch of ansa cervicalis
    t. membrane
    t. muscle
thyrohypophysial syndrome
thyroid
    accessory t.
    t. articular surface of cricoid
      cartilage
    t. axis
    t. body
    t. bruit
    t. cartilage
    t. colloid
    t. crisis
    t. diverticulum
    t. eminence
    t. foramen
    t. gland
    t. ima artery
    t. insufficiency
    t. lymph node
    t. storm
    t. suppression test
    t. therapy
    t. toxicosis
    t. vein
thyroidea
    t. accessoria
    t. ima
thyroidectomy
    "chemical" t.
    near-total t.
    subtotal t.
thyroidism
thyroiditis
    autoimmune t.
    chronic atrophic t.
    chronic fibrous t.
    chronic lymphadenoid t.
    chronic lymphocytic t.
    de Quervain t.
    focal lymphocytic t.
    giant cell t.
    giant follicular t.
    Hashimoto t.
    ligneous t.
    lymphocytic t.
    parasitic t.
    Riedel t.
    subacute granulomatous t.
    subacute lymphocyte t.

thyroidology
thyroidotomy
thyroid-stimulating
    t.-s. hormone (TSH)
    t.-s. hormone-releasing factor (TSH-RF)
    t.-s. hormone stimulation test
    t.-s. immunoglobulins (TSI)
thyrointoxication
thyrolaryngeal
thyroliberin
thyrolingual
    t. cyst
    t. duct
thyrolytic
thyromegaly
thyronine
thyropalatine
thyroparathyroidectomy
thyropathy
thyroperoxidase
thyropharyngeal
    t. part of inferior constrictor muscle of pharynx
    t. part of inferior pharyngeal constrictor muscle of pharynx
thyroplasty
thyroprival
thyroprivia
thyroprivic, thyroprivous
thyroprotein
thyroptosis
thyrotomy
thyrotoxic
    t. coma
    t. crisis
    t. encephalopathy
    t. heart disease
    t. myopathy
    t. serum
thyrotoxicosis
    apathetic t.
    t. medicamentosa
thyrotoxin
thyrotroph
thyrotrophic
thyrotrophin
thyrotropic hormone
thyrotropin-producing adenoma
thyrotropin-releasing
    t.-r. factor (TRF)
    t.-r. hormone (TRH)
    t.-r. hormone stimulation test
thyrotropin resistance
thyroxine, thyroxin (T$_4$)
    labeled t.
    radioactive t.
    radiolabeled t.
    t. sodium
thyroxine-binding
    t.-b. globulin (TBG)
    t.-b. prealbumin (TBPA)
    t.-b. protein (TBP)
Thysanosoma actinoides

Ti
    titanium
TIA
    transient ischemic attack
tibia, pl. tibiae
    saber t.
    t. valga
    t. vara
tibiad
tibial
    t. border of foot
    t. collateral ligament
    t. collateral ligament of ankle joint
    t. communicating nerve
    t. crest
    t. intertendinous bursa
    t. nerve
    t. nutrient artery
    t. phenomenon
    t. tarsal tendinous sheath
    t. tuberosity
tibiale posticum
tibialis
    t. anterior muscle
    t. posterior muscle
tibio-
tibiocalcaneal
    t. ligament
    t. part of deltoid ligament
    t. part of medial ligament of ankle joint
tibiocalcanean
tibiofascialis
tibiofemoral index
tibiofibular
    t. articulation
    t. joint
    t. ligament
    t. syndesmosis
tibionavicular
    t. ligament
    t. part of deltoid ligament
    t. part of medial ligament of ankle joint
tibioperoneal
tibioscaphoid
tibiotalar part of medial ligament of ankle joint
tibiotarsal
tic
    convulsive t.
    t. de pensée
    t. douloureux
    facial t.
    glossopharyngeal t.
    habit t.
    local t.
    psychic t.
    rotatory t.
    spasmodic t.
ticarcillin disodium
tick
    t. paralysis
    t. typhus

T

tick-borne
    t.-b. encephalitis (Central European subtype)
    t.-b. encephalitis (Eastern subtype)
    t.-b. encephalitis virus
    t.-b. virus
tickling
ticolubant
tic-tac
    t.-t. rhythm
    t.-t. sound
t.i.d.
    ter in die
tidal
    t. air
    t. drainage
    t. volume (V_T)
    t. wave
tide
    acid t.
    alkaline t.
    fat t.
    red t.
Tiedemann
    T. gland
    T. nerve
tie-over dressing
Tietze syndrome
tiger heart
tight junction
tiglate
tiglian
tiglic acid
tiglyl-CoA
tiglyl-coenzyme A
tigroid
    t. body
    t. fundus
    t. retina
    t. striation
    t. substance
tigrolysis
TIL
    tumor-infiltrating lymphocytes
tilorone
tilt
    pantoscopic t.
    t. table
    t. test
tilting
    t. disk valve
    t. disk valve prosthesis
timbre
time
    activated clotting t. (ACT)
    activated partial thromboplastin t. (aPTT)
    AH conduction t.
    association t.
    biologic t.
    bleeding t.
    circulation t.
    clot retraction t.
    clotting t.
    coagulation t.

    t. compensation gain (TCG)
    concentration × t. (CxT)
    t. constant
    doubling t.
    euglobulin clot lysis t.
    fading t.
    t. of flight
    forced expiratory t. (FET)
    half-t.
    HR conduction t.
    HV conduction t.
    inertia t.
    interatrial conduction t.
    intraatrial conduction t.
    left ventricular ejection t. (LVET)
    t. marker
    PA conduction t.
    partial thromboplastin t. (PTT)
    PH conduction t.
    prothrombin t.
    reaction t.
    recognition t.
    relaxation t.
    repetition t. (TR)
    rise t.
    running t.
    Russell's viper venom clotting t.
    sensation t.
    t. sense
    sinoatrial conduction t. (SACT)
    sinoatrial recovery t. (SART)
    survival t.
    thrombin t.
    tissue thromboplastin inhibition t.
    utilization t.
time-compensated gain
time-gain compensation
time-lapse microscopy
Time-Line therapy
time-varied
    t.-v. gain (TVG)
    t.-v. gain control (TGC)
TIMI
    thrombolysis in myocardial infarction
timnodonic acid
timolol maleate
tin (Sn)
    t. oxide
tin-113 (^{113}Sn)
tinct.
    tinctura
tinctable
tinction
tinctorial
tinctura, pl. **tincturae (tinct., tr.)**
tincture
    alcoholic t.
    ammoniated t.
    belladonna t.
    digitalis t.
    ethereal t.
    glycerinated t.
    green soap t.
    hydroalcoholic t.

tinea
- t. barbae
- t. capitis
- t. circinata
- t. corporis
- t. favosa
- t. glabrosa
- t. imbricata
- t. kerion
- t. manus
- t. nigra
- t. pedis
- t. profunda
- t. sycosis
- t. tonsurans
- t. unguium
- t. versicolor

Tinel sign
tine test
tinfoil
tingibility
tingible
tingle
tingling
- distal t. on percussion

tinidazole
tinnitus
- t. aurium
- t. cerebri
- clicking t.
- Leudet t.

tint
tinted
- t. denture base
- t. vision

tioconazole
tip
- t. of auricle
- t. of ear
- t. of elbow
- t. link
- t. of nose
- t. of posterior horn
- root t.
- t. of tongue
- t. of tooth root
- Woolner t.

tipping
tiprenolol hydrochloride
TIPS
- transjugular intrahepatic portosystemic shunt

Tiselius
- T. apparatus
- T. electrophoresis cell

Tissierella praeacuta
Tissot spirometer
tissue
- adenoid t.
- adipose t.
- areolar t.
- t. basophil
- bone t.
- bronchus-associated lymphoid t. (BALT)
- brown adipose t.
- cancellous t.
- cardiac muscle t.
- cartilaginous t.
- cavernous t.
- chondroid t.
- chromaffin t.
- connective t.
- t. culture
- t. culture infectious dose (TCID$_{50}$)
- dartoic t.
- t. displaceability
- t. displacement
- elastic t.
- epithelial t.
- erectile t.
- fatty t.
- fibrohyaline t.
- fibrous t.
- t. fluid
- Gamgee t.
- gelatinous t.
- gingival t.'s
- granulation t.
- gut-associated lymphoid t. (GALT)
- Haller vascular t.
- hard t.
- hemopoietic t.
- t. hormone
- indifferent t.
- interstitial t.
- investing t.'s
- islet t.
- t. lymph
- lymphatic t., t. tissue
- mesenchymal t.
- mesonephric t.
- metanephrogenic t.
- t. molding
- mucosa-associated lymphoid t. (MALT)
- mucous connective t.
- multilocular adipose t.
- muscular t.
- myeloid t.
- nasion soft t.
- nephrogenic t.
- nervous t.
- nodal t.
- osseous t.
- osteogenic t.
- osteoid t.
- periapical t.
- t. plasminogen activator
- t. registration
- t. respiration
- reticular t.
- retiform t.
- rubber t.
- skeletal muscle t.
- smooth muscle t.
- subcutaneous t.
- subcutaneous t. of penis
- subcutaneous t. of perineum
- t. tension

T

tissue *(continued)*
    t. thromboplastin inhibition time
    trabecular t. of sclera
    t. valve
    t. weighting factor
tissue-bearing area
tissue-specific antigen
tissue-trimming
tissular
titanium (Ti)
    t. dioxide
titer
TITh
    3,5,3-triiodothyronine
titillation
titin
titrant
titratable acidity test
titrate
titration
    colorimetric t.
    formol t.
    potentiometric t.
titubation
Tizzoni stain
Tj antigen
Tl
    thallium
²⁰¹Tl
    thallium-201
TLC
    thin-layer chromatography
TLE
    thin-layer electrophoresis
TLV
    threshold limit value
TM
    transcendental meditation
Tm
    thulium
TMD
    temporomandibular joint dysfunction
TMJ
    temporomandibular joint dysfunction
TMJ syndrome
TM-mode
TMP
    ribothymidylic acid
T-mycoplasma
Tn
    ocular tension
TNF
    tumor necrosis factor
TNM staging
TNP-470
TNT
    trinitrotoluene
toad skin
to-and-fro
    t.-a.-f. anesthesia
    t.-a.-f. murmur
    t.-a.-f. sound
toasted shins

tobacco
    t. heart
    wild t.
tobacco-alcohol amblyopia
Tobia fever
tobramycin
Tobruk splint
tocainide hydrochloride
toco-
tocochromanol-3
tocodynagraph
tocodynamometer
tocograph
tocography
tocol
tocology
tocolytic
tocometer
tocopherol (T)
    mixed t.'s concentrate
tocopherolquinone (TQ)
tocopherylquinone
tocophobia
tocoquinone
tocotrienol
tocotrienolquinone
TOCP
    triorthocresyl phosphate
Todaro tendon
Todd
    T. paralysis
    T. postepileptic paralysis
    T. unit
toddler's
    t. diarrhea
    t. fracture
Tod muscle
toe
    t. clonus
    fourth t. [IV]
    great t. I
    hammer t.
    little t. [V]
    Morton t.
    painful t.
    t. phenomenon
    second t. [II]
    stiff t.
    third t. [III]
    webbed t.'s
toe-drop
toenail
    ingrowing t.
tofenacin hydrochloride
Togaviridae
togavirus
toilet
    pulmonary t.
    t. training
Toison stain
Tokelau ringworm
Toker cell
toko-
tolazamide
tolazoline hydrochloride

tolbutamide test
tolcyclamide
Toldt
    T. fascia
    T. membrane
tolerance
    acoustic t.
    cross t.
    t. dose
    frustration t.
    high dose t.
    immunologic high dose t.
    impaired glucose t.
    individual t.
    t. limit
    nonresponder t.
    pain t.
    species t.
    split t.
    vibration t.
tolerant
tolerize
tolerogen
tolerogenic
tolhexamide
tolmetin
tolnaftate
tolonium chloride
Tolosa-Hunt syndrome
tolpropamine
Tolu balsam
toluene
toluic acid
toluidine
    alkaline t. blue O
    t. blue O
    t. blue stain
toluol
toluoyl
toluylene red
tolyl
Toma sign
-tome
tomentum cerebri
Tomes
    T. fiber
    T. granular layer
    T. process
Tommaselli disease
tomogram
tomograph
tomography
    computed t. (CT)
    computerized axial t. (CAT)
    conventional t.
    dynamic computed t.
    electron beam t. (EBT)
    helical computed t.
    high-resolution computed t. (HRCT)
    hypocycloidal t.
    nuclear magnetic resonance t.
    positron emission t. (PET)
    single photon emission computed t.
     (SPECT)

    spiral computed t.
    trispiral t.
tomolevel
tomomania
-tomy
tonaphasia
tone
    affective t.
    t. color
    t. decay test
    emotional t.
    feeling t.
    fundamental t.
    heart t.'s
    Traube double t.
toner
tongue
    baked t.
    bald t.
    beet-t.
    bifid t.
    black t.
    black hairy t.
    t. bone
    burning t.
    t. of cerebellum
    cleft t.
    coated t.
    t. depressor
    dotted t.
    fissured t.
    furred t.
    geographic t.
    grooved t.
    hairy t.
    hobnail t.
    magenta t.
    mandibular t.
    t. phenomenon
    raspberry t.
    red strawberry t.
    scrotal t.
    smoker's t.
    stippled t.
    strawberry t.
    tongue crib
    tongue-swallowing
    tongue thrust
tongue-tie
tonic
    bitter t.
    t. contraction
    t. control
    t. convulsion
    t. epilepsy
    t. pupil
    t. reflex
    t. seizure
tonic-clonic seizure
tonicity
tonicoclonic
tonin
toning
tonitrophobia
tono-

T

tonoclonic
tonofibril
tonofilament
tonograph
tonography
tonometer
    applanation t.
    Gärtner t.
    Goldmann applanation t.
    Mackay-Marg t.
    Mueller electronic t.
    pneumatic t.
    Schiötz t.
tonometry
tonophant
tonoplast
tonoscillograph
tonotopic
tonotropic
tonsil
    cerebellar t.
    t. of cerebellum
    eustachian t.
    faucial t.
    Gerlach t.
    laryngeal t.'s
    lingual t.
    Luschka t.
    palatine t.
    pharyngeal t.
    submerged t.
    third t.
    tubal t.
tonsilla, pl. **tonsillae**
    t. adenoidea
    t. cerebelli
    t. intestinalis
    t. lingualis
    t. palatina
    t. pharyngealis
    t. tubaria
tonsillar, tonsillary
    t. branch of the facial artery
    t. branch of glossopharyngeal nerve
    t. branch of lesser palatine nerve
    t. calculus
    t. crypt
    t. fossa
    t. fossulae
    t. herniation
    t. ring
tonsillectomy
tonsillitis
    lacunar t.
    Vincent t.
tonsillo-
tonsillolingual sulcus
tonsillolith
tonsillopathy
tonsillotome
tonsillotomy
tonsilolith
tonus
    baseline t.

    myogenic t.
    neurogenic t.
tooth, pl. **teeth**
    t. abrasion
    acoustic teeth
    acrylic resin t.
    anatomic t.
    ankylosed t.
    anterior t.
    t. arrangement
    auditory t.
    t. avulsion
    baby t.
    back t.
    bicuspid t.
    buck t.
    t. bud
    canine t.
    carnassial t.
    t. cement
    cheek t.
    Corti auditory t.
    crossbite t.
    cuspid t.
    cuspless t.
    cutting t.
    dead t.
    decayed, extracted, and filled t.
      (def, DEF)
    decayed, missing, and filled teeth
      (DMF, dmf)
    deciduous t.
    devitalized t.
    extruded t.
    eye t.
    fluoridated t.
    t. form
    fused teeth
    geminated t.
    t. germ
    ghost t.
    green t.
    Horner t.
    Huschke auditory t.
    Hutchinson t.
    impacted t.
    incisor t.
    t. ligation
    metal insert t.
    migrating t.
    milk t.
    molar t.
    mottled t.
    multicuspid t.
    natal t.
    neonatal t.
    nonanatomic t.
    nonvital t.
    normally posed t.
    notched t.
    oral t.
    pegged t.
    permanent t.
    perpetually growing t.
    persistently growing t.

t. plane
plastic t.
t. polyp
posterior t.
premolar t.
primary t.
protruding t.
t. pulp
pulpless t.
t. sac
sclerotic t.
screwdriver t.
second t.
t. socket
spaced t.
stomach t.
succedaneous t.
syphilitic t.
temporary t.
third-year molar t.
t. transplantation
tricuspid t.
tube t.
Turner t.
unerupted t.
vital t.
wisdom t.
zero degree t.
toothache
tooth-and-nail syndrome
tooth-borne base
toothed vertebra
top- (*var. of* topo-)
topagnosis
toper's nose
topesthesia
tophaceous
t. gout
tophus, pl. **tophi**
gouty t.
topica
topical
t. anesthesia
t. anesthetic
Topinard
T. facial angle
T. line
topistic
topo-, top-
topoanesthesia
topognosis, topognosia
topogometer
Topografov virus
topographic anatomy
topography
topoisomerase
Topolanski sign
topology
toponarcosis
toponym
toponymy
topopathogenesis
topophobia
topophylaxis
topotecan

toppling gait
TORCH syndrome
torcular herophili
Torek operation
tori (*pl. of* torus)
toric
t. lens
Torkildsen shunt
tornado epilepsy
Tornwaldt
T. abscess
T. cyst
T. disease
T. syndrome
Toronto formula for pulmonary artery banding
torose, torous
Torovirus
torpent
torpid
torpidity
torpor
torque
torr
torrefaction
torrefy
Torre syndrome
torsade de pointes
torsion
t. of appendage
t. disease of childhood
t. dystonia
extravaginal t.
t. fracture
intravaginal t.
t. neurosis
perinatal t.
t. of testis
t. of a tooth
torsional deformity
torsionometer
torsive occlusion
torsiversion
torso
torsoclusion
Torsten Sjögren syndrome
torticollar
torticollis
benign paroxysmal t. of infancy
congenital t.
dermatogenic t.
dystonic t.
fixed t.
hysterical t.
labyrinthine t.
muscular t.
ocular t.
psychogenic t.
spasmodic t.
tortipelvis
tortuous
Torulopsis
torulus, pl. **toruli**
toruli tactiles
torus, pl. **tori**

T

torus (*continued*)
    t. fracture
    t. frontalis
    t. levatorius
    mandibular t.
    t. mandibularis
    t. manus
    t. occipitalis
    palatine t.
    t. palatinus
    t. tubarius
    t. uretericus
    t. uterinus
TOS
    thoracic outlet syndrome
tosyl
tosylate
total
    t. acidity
    t. anomalous pulmonary venous connection (TAPVC)
    t. anomalous pulmonary venous return (TAPVR)
    t. aphasia
    t. ascertainment
    t. body hypothermia
    t. body water (TBW)
    t. breech extraction
    t. cataract
    t. catecholamine test
    t. cell count
    t. cleavage
    t. communication
    t. cricoid cleft
    t. cystectomy
    t. elasticity of muscle
    t. end-diastolic diameter (TEDD)
    t. end-systolic diameter (TESD)
    t. energy
    t. hematuria
    t. hyperopia (Ht)
    t. joint arthroplasty
    t. keratoplasty
    t. lung capacity
    t. mastectomy
    t. necrosis
    t. parenteral nutrition (TPN)
    t. pelvic exenteration
    t. peripheral resistance (TPR)
    t. placenta previa
    t. push therapy
    t. refractory period
    t. sclerectasia
    t. spinal anesthesia
    t. synechia
    t. transfusion
totem
totemism
totemistic
totipotency, totipotence
totipotent
    t. cell
totipotential protoplasm

touch
    t. cell
    t. corpuscle
    royal t.
toughened silver nitrate
Toupet fundoplication
Tourette
    T. disease
    T. syndrome
Tournay
    T. phenomenon
    T. sign
tourniquet
    Dupuytren t.
    Esmarch t.
    t. poditis
    Rummel t.
    t. test
Tourtual
    T. membrane
    T. sinus
Touton giant cell
Tovell tube
TO virus
Towne
    T. projection
    T. projection radiograph
    T. view
tox- (*var. of* toxico-)
toxalbumins
toxanemia
toxaphene
Toxascaris leonina
toxemia
toxemic
    t. jaundice
    t. retinopathy of pregnancy
toxi- (*var. of* toxico-)
toxic
    t. amaurosis
    t. amblyopia
    t. anemia
    t. cataract
    t. cirrhosis
    t. cyanosis
    t. delirium
    t. dementia
    t. epidermal necrolysis (TEN)
    t. equivalent
    t. goiter
    t. hemoglobinuria
    t. hydrocephalus
    t. megacolon
    t. myocarditis
    t. nephrosis
    t. neuritis
    t. psychosis
    t. retinopathy
    t. shock
    t. shock syndrome (TSS)
    t. tetanus
    t. unit (T.U.)
toxicant
toxicemia

toxicity
    oxygen t.
toxico-, tox-, toxi-, toxo-
Toxicodendron
toxicogenic conjunctivitis
toxicoid
toxicologic
toxicologist
toxicology
toxicopathic
toxicophobia
toxicosis
    endogenic t.
    exogenic t.
    T₃ t.
    thyroid t.
    triiodothyronine t.
toxiferines
toxiferous
toxigenic
toxigenicity
toxilic acid
toxin
    animal t.
    anthrax t.
    Bacillus anthracis t.
    bacterial t.
    bee t.
    botulinus t.
    cholera t.
    Clostridium perfringens alpha t.
    Clostridium perfringens beta t.
    Clostridium perfringens epsilon t.
    Clostridium perfringens iota t.
    cobra t.
    Crotalus t.
    diagnostic diphtheria t.
    Dick test t.
    dinoflagellate t.
    diphtheria t.
    erythrogenic t.
    extracellular t.
    intracellular t.
    limes null dose of diphtheria t. (Lo)
    limes reacting dose of diphtheria t. (Lr)
    normal t.
    plant t.
    scarlet fever erythrogenic t.
    Schick test t.
    Shiga t.
    Shigalike t.
    streptococcus erythrogenic t.
    tetanus t.
    t. unit
toxinic
toxinogenic
toxinogenicity
toxinology
toxinosis
toxiphobia
toxisterol
toxo- (*var. of* toxico-)

Toxocara
    T. canis
    T. mystax
toxocariasis
toxoid
toxon, toxone
toxoneme
toxonosis
toxophil, toxophile
toxophore
toxophorous
Toxoplasma gondii
Toxoplasmatidae
toxoplasmosis
    acquired t.
    congenital t.
toxopyrimidine
Toynbee
    T. corpuscle
    T. muscle
    T. tube
TPA
    12-o-tetradecanoylphorbol 13-acetate
TPHA test
TPH test (*var. of* **Treponema pallidum** immobilization test)
TPI test
TPN
    total parenteral nutrition
TPP
    thiamin pyrophosphate
TPR
    total peripheral resistance
TQ
    tocopherolquinone
TR
    repetition time
tr.
    tinctura
trabecula, pl. trabeculae
    anterior chamber t.
    arachnoid t.
    trabeculae arachnoideae
    trabeculae carneae (of right and left ventricles)
    trabeculae carneae ventriculorum dextri et sinistri
    trabeculae of corpora cavernosa
    trabeculae corporis spongiosi penis
    trabeculae corporum cavernosorum
    trabeculae of corpus spongiosum
    trabeculae cranii
    trabeculae lienis
    trabeculae of lymph node
    trabeculae nodi lymphoidei
    septomarginal t.
    t. septomarginalis
    trabeculae of spleen
    splenic t.
    trabeculae splenicae
    t. testis
trabecular
    t. bone
    t. carcinoma
    t. meshwork

T

trabecular *(continued)*
    t. network
    t. reticulum
    t. tissue of sclera
    t. zone
trabeculate
trabeculated bladder
trabeculation
trabeculectomy
trabeculoplasty
    laser t. (LTP)
trabeculotomy
trace
    t. conditioned reflex
    t. conditioning
    t. element
    t. nutrient
tracer
trache- *(var. of* tracheo-)
trachea, pl. **tracheae**
    saber-sheath t.
    scabbard t.
tracheal
    t. bifurcation
    t. branch
    t. breath sound
    t. carina
    t. cartilage
    t. fenestration
    t. gland
    t. intubation
    t. lymph node
    t. mucosa
    t. ring
    t. triangle
    t. tube
    t. tug
    t. ulceration
    t. vein
    t. wall stripe
trachealgia
trachealis muscle
tracheitis
trachel- *(var. of* trachelo-)
trachelalis
trachelectomy
trachelematoma
trachelian
trachelism, trachelismus
trachelitis
trachelo-, trachel-
trachelobregmatic diameter
trachelocele
tracheloclavicular muscle
trachelomastoid
trachelo-occipitalis
trachelopanus
trachelopexia, trachelopexy
tracheloplasty
trachelorrhaphy
trachelos
tracheloschisis
trachelotomy
tracheo-, trache-

tracheoaerocele
tracheobiliary fistula
tracheobroncheopathia osteoplastica
tracheobronchial
    t. diverticulum
    t. dyskinesia
    t. groove
tracheobronchitis
tracheobronchomegaly
tracheobronchoscopy
tracheocele
tracheoesophageal
    t. fistula
    t. puncture
    t. shunt
    t. speech
tracheolaryngeal
tracheomalacia
tracheomegaly
tracheopathia, tracheopathy
    t. osteoplastica
tracheopharyngeal
tracheophonesis
tracheophony
tracheoplasty
    slide t.
tracheorrhagia
tracheoschisis
tracheoscope
tracheoscopic
tracheoscopy
tracheostenosis
tracheostoma
tracheostomy tube
tracheotome
tracheotomy
    t. hook
    t. tube
Trachipleistophora
trachitis
trachoma
    t. body
    follicular t.
    t. gland
    granular t.
    t. virus
trachomatous
    t. conjunctivitis
    t. keratitis
    t. pannus
trachychromatic
trachyonychia
trachyphonia
tracing
    arrow point t.
    cephalometric t.
    Gothic arch t.
    needle point t.
    stylus t.
tract
    alimentary t.
    anterior corticospinal t.
    anterior pyramidal t.
    anterior raphespinal t.
    anterior spinocerebellar t.

anterior spinothalamic t.
anterior trigeminothalamic t.
anterolateral t.
Arnold t.
association t.
auditory t.
bulboreticulospinal t.
Burdach t.
caerulospinal t.
central tegmental t.
cerebellorubral t.
cerebellothalamic t.
Collier t.
comma t. of Schultze
corticobulbar t.
corticopontine t.
corticospinal t.
crossed pyramidal t.
cuneocerebellar t.
dead t.
deiterospinal t.
dentatothalamic t.
descending t. of trigeminal nerve
digestive t.
direct pyramidal t.
dorsal spinocerebellar t.
dorsal trigeminothalamic t.
dorsolateral t.
fastigiobulbar t.
fastigiospinal t.
Flechsig t.
frontopontine t.
frontotemporal t.
gastrointestinal t.
geniculocalcarine t.
genital t.
t. of Goll
Gowers t.
habenulointerpeduncular t.,
  habenulopeduncular t.
Hoche t.
hypothalamohypophysial t.
iliopubic t.
iliotibial t.
interpositospinal t.
interstitiospinal t.
James t.
lateral corticospinal t.
lateral pyramidal t.
lateral raphespinal t.
lateral reticulospinal t.
lateral spinothalamic t.
lateral vestibulospinal t.
Lissauer t.
Loewenthal t.
mamillothalamic t.
Marchi t.
medial reticulospinal t.
medial vestibulospinal t.
medullary reticulospinal t.
mesencephalic t. of trigeminal nerve
Monakow t.
t. of Münzer and Wiener
nerve t.
occipitocollicular t.

occipitopontine t.
occipitotectal t.
olfactory t.
olivocerebellar t.
olivocochlear t.
olivospinal t.
optic t.
parietopontine t.
pontoreticulospinal t.
posterior spinocerebellar t.
posterior trigeminothalamic t.
posterolateral t.
prepyramidal t.
pyramidal t.
respiratory t.
reticulospinal t.
rubrobulbar t.
rubropontine t.
rubroreticular t.
rubrospinal t.
t. of Schütz
sensory t.
septomarginal t.
solitariospinal t.
solitary t.
sphincteroid t. of ileum
spinal t.
spinal t. of trigeminal nerve
spinocerebellar t.
spinocervical t.
spinocervicothalamic t.
spinoolivary t.
spinoreticular t.
spinotectal t.
spinothalamic t.
spinovestibular t.
spiral foraminous t.
Spitzka marginal t.
sulcomarginal t.
supraopticohypophysial t.
tectobulbar t.
tectopontine t.
tectospinal t.
temporofrontal t.
temporopontine t.
trigeminospinal t.
trigeminothalamic t.
tuberoinfundibular t.
Türck t.
urinary t.
uveal t.
ventral raphespinal t.
ventral spinocerebellar t.
ventral spinothalamic t.
ventral trigeminothalamic t.
vestibulospinal t.
vocal t.
Waldeyer t.

tractellum, pl. **tractella**
traction
t. alopecia
t. atrophy
axis t.
Bryant t.
Buck t.

traction *(continued)*
    t. diverticulum
    t. epiphysis
    external t.
    halo t.
    intermaxillary t.
    internal t.
    isometric t.
    isotonic t.
    maxillomandibular t.
    Russell t.
    skeletal t.
    skin t.
tractor
    Lowsley t.
    Syms t.
    Young prostatic t.
tractotomy
    anterolateral t.
    intramedullary t.
    pyramidal t.
    Schwartz t.
    Sjöqvist t.
    spinal t.
    spinothalamic t.
    trigeminal t.
    Walker t.
tractus
    t. anterolaterales
    t. bulboreticulospinalis
    t. caeruleospinalis
    t. cerebellorubralis
    t. cerebellothalamicus
    t. corticobulbaris
    t. corticopontinus
    t. corticospinalis
    t. corticospinalis anterior
    t. corticospinalis lateralis
    t. descendens nervi trigemini
    t. dorsolateralis
    t. fastigiobulbaris
    t. fastigiospinalis
    t. frontopontinus
    t. habenulointerpeduncularis
    t. iliopubicus
    t. iliotibialis
    t. interpositospinalis
    t. interstitiospinalis
    t. mesencephalicus nervi trigemini
    t. occipitopontinus
    t. olfactorius
    t. olivocerebellaris
    t. olivocochlearis
    t. opticus
    t. parietopontinus
    t. pontoreticulospinalis
    t. posterolateralis
    t. pyramidalis
    t. pyramidalis anterior
    t. pyramidalis lateralis
    t. raphespinalis anterior
    t. raphespinalis lateralis
    t. reticulospinalis
    t. rubrobulbaris

    t. rubropontinus
    t. rubrospinalis
    t. solitariospinalis
    t. solitarius
    t. spinalis nervi trigemini
    t. spinocerebellaris anterior
    t. spinocerebellaris posterior
    t. spinocervicalis
    t. spinoolivaris
    t. spinotectalis
    t. spinothalamicus
    t. spinothalamicus anterior
    t. spinothalamicus lateralis
    t. spinovestibularis
    t. spiralis foraminosus
    t. supraopticohypophysialis
    t. tectobulbaris
    t. tectopontinus
    t. tectospinalis
    t. tegmentalis centralis
    t. temporopontinus
    t. trigeminospinalis
    t. trigeminothalamicus anterior
    t. trigeminothalamicus posterior
    t. tuberoinfundibularis
    t. vestibulospinalis
    t. vestibulospinalis lateralis
    t. vestibulospinalis medialis
trafficking
tragacanth, tragacantha
tragal
    t. lamina
tragi (*pl. of* tragus)
tragicus muscle
tragion
tragomaschalia
tragophonia, tragophony
tragus, pl. **tragi**
    accessory t.
TRAIL.
trained reflex
training
    t. analysis
    assertive t.
    aversive t.
    avoidance t.
    escape t.
    t. group (T group)
    toilet t.
train-of-four stimulus
trainwheel rhythm
trait
    Bombay t.
    categorical t.
    chromosomal t.
    codominant t.
    dominant t.
    dominant lethal t.
    galtonian t.
    intermediate t.
    liminal t.
    marker t.
    mendelian t.
    nonpenetrant t.
    penetrant t.

qualitative t.
recessive t.
sickle cell t.
threshold t.
trajector
tramadol
tramazoline hydrochloride
tram line
trance
t. coma
death t.
induced t.
somnambulistic t.
tranexamic acid
tranquilizer
major t.
minor t.
trans-
transacetylase
transacetylation
transaction
transactional
t. analysis
t. psychotherapy
transacylases
transacylation
transaldolase
transaldolation
transamidation
transamidinases
transamidination
transaminases
transamination
transaudient
transaxial plane
transcalent
transcapsidation
transcapsular gray bridge
transcarbamoylases
transcarbamoylation
transcarboxylases
transcellular
t. fluid
t. transport
t. water
transcendental anatomy
transcendental meditation (TM)
transcervical
t. fracture
t. thymectomy
transcobalamins
transcochlear approach
transcondylar fracture
transcortical
t. aphasia
t. apraxia
transcortin
transcranial radiograph
transcriptase
reverse t.
transcription
reverse t.
transcription-based chain reaction
transcutaneous
transcytosis

transdermic
transduce
transducer
t. cell
piezoelectric t.
ultrasound t.
transducin
transductant
transduction
abortive t.
complete t.
Davis battery model of t.
general t.
high-frequency t.
low-frequency t.
mechanoelectric t.
specialized t.
specific t.
transduodenal sphincterotomy
transection
transesophageal echocardiography
transethmoidal
transfection
transfer
charge t.
t. coping
embryo t.
t. factor
Fourier t.
gamete intrafallopian t. (GIFT)
t. gene
group t.
t. imaging
Jones t.
linear energy t. (LET)
t. RNA
transferase
terminal t.
terminal deoxynucleotidyl t. (TdT)
transferase deficiency galactosemia
transference
counter t.
extrasensory thought t.
t. love
negative t.
t. neurosis
passive t.
positive t.
transferred ophthalmia
transferrin
transferring enzyme
transfix
transfixion suture
transform
Fourier t.
transformant
transformation
cavernous t. of portal vein
cell t.
t. constant
Haldane t.
Lobry de Bruyn-van Ekenstein t.
logit t.
lymphocyte t.

T

transformation (*continued*)
    nodular t. of the liver
    t. zone
transformed lymphocyte
transforming
    t. agent
    t. factor
    t. gene
    t. growth factor (TGF)
    t. growth factor alpha
    t. growth factor beta
transfuse
transfusion
    drip t.
    exchange t.
    exsanguination t.
    fetomaternal t.
    t. hepatitis
    indirect t.
    intramedullary t.
    intrauterine t.
    mediate t.
    t. nephritis
    placental t.
    reciprocal t.
    subcutaneous t.
    substitution t.
    total t.
    twin-twin t.
transgene
transgenesis
transgenic mice
transglottic
transglucosylase
transglutaminase
transglycosidation
transglycosylase
trans-Golgi reticulum
transhiatal esophagectomy
transient
    t. acantholytic dermatosis (TAD)
    t. agammaglobulinemia
    t. albuminuria
    t. equilibrium
    t. erythroblastopenia of childhood
    t. evoked otoacoustic emission
    t. global amnesia
    t. hypogammaglobulinemia of infancy
    t. ischemic attack (TIA)
    t. myopia
    t. retinopathy
    t. tachypnea of the newborn
transiliac
transilient
transillumination
transinsular
transischiac
transisthmian
transition
    cervicothoracic t.
    t. electron
    isomeric t.
    t. mutation

transitional
    t. cell
    t. cell carcinoma
    t. cell papilloma
    t. convolution
    t. denture
    t. epithelium
    t. gyrus
    t. leukocyte
    t. object
    t. zone
    t. zone of lips
transjugular intrahepatic portosystemic shunt (TIPS)
transketolase
transketolation
translabyrinthine approach
translation
    nick t.
translatory movement
translocation
    bacterial t.
    balanced t.
    t. carrier
    t. chromosome
    group t.
    reciprocal t.
    robertsonian t.
    unbalanced t.
translucent
translumbar aortography
transmeatal incision
transmembrane potential
transmethylase
transmethylation factor
transmigration
    direct ovular t.
    external ovular t.
    ovular t.
transmissible
    t. gastroenteritis virus of swine
    t. plasmid
transmission
    duplex t.
    horizontal t.
    iatrogenic t.
    neurohumoral t.
    transovarial t.
    transstadial t.
    vertical t.
transmitted light
transmural
    t. myocardial infarction
    t. pressure
transmutation
transnasal fiberoptic laryngoscopy
transneuronal atrophy
transnexus channel
transocular
transonance
transonic
transorbital
    t. leukotomy
    t. lobotomy
transosseous venography

transovarial transmission
transparent
- t. dentin
- t. septum

transparietal
transpeptidase
transpeptidation
transperitoneal
trans phase
transphosphatases
transphosphorylases
transphosphorylation
transpirable
transpiration
- pulmonary t.

transpire
transplacental
transplant
- Gallie t.
- hair t.
- t. lung syndrome

transplantar
transplantation
- t. antigen
- bone marrow t.
- cardiopulmonary t.
- t. of cornea
- corneal t.
- t. genetics
- heart t.
- heart-lung t.
- pancreaticoduodenal t.
- renal t.
- tendon t.
- tooth t.

transpleural
transporionic axis
transport
- active t.
- t. antibiotic
- axoplasmic t.
- facilitated t.
- t. host
- hydrogen t.
- t. maximum
- t. medium
- t. number
- paracellular t.
- passive t.
- transcellular t.
- vesicular t.

transposable element
transposase
transpose
transposition
- t. of arterial stem
- corrected t. of the great vessels
- t. of the great vessels
- penoscrotal t.

transposon
transpulmonary pressure
transpyloric plane
transsection
transsegmental

transseptal
- t. fiber
- t. orchiopexy

transsexualism
transsexual surgery
transsphenoidal
trans-splicing
transstadial transmission
transsulfurase
transsulfuration
transsynaptic
- t. chromatolysis
- t. degeneration

transtentorial herniation
transthalamic
transthermia
transthoracic
- t. echocardiography
- t. esophagectomy
- t. pacemaker
- t. pressure

transthoracotomy
transthyretin
transudate
transudation
transude
transulfurase
transureteroureteral anastomosis
transureteroureterostomy (TUU)
transurethral
- t. resection
- t. resection syndrome

transvaalin
transvaginal scanning
transvector
transversalis fascia
transversarial part of vertebral artery
transverse
- t. abdominal incision
- t. acetabular ligament
- t. amputation
- t. anthelicine groove
- t. arch of foot
- t. artery of neck
- t. arytenoid muscle
- t. atlantal ligament
- t. auricular muscle
- t. branch of lateral femoral circumflex artery
- t. carpal ligament
- t. cerebral fissure
- t. cervical artery
- t. cervical ligament
- t. cervical nerve
- t. cervical vein
- t. colon
- t. costal facet
- t. crest
- t. crest of internal acoustic meatus
- t. crural ligament
- t. diameter
- t. disk
- t. ductule of epoöphoron
- t. facial artery
- t. facial fracture

transverse *(continued)*
- t. facial vein
- t. fasciculi
- t. fissure of cerebellum
- t. fissure of the right lung
- t. fold of rectum
- t. foramen
- t. fornix
- t. genicular ligament
- t. head
- t. hermaphroditism
- t. horizontal axis
- t. humeral ligament
- t. intermesocolic fossa
- t. lie
- t. ligament of acetabulum
- t. ligament of the atlas
- t. ligament of elbow
- t. ligament of knee
- t. ligament of leg
- t. ligament of pelvis
- t. ligament of perineum
- t. metacarpal ligament
- t. metatarsal ligament
- t. muscle of abdomen
- t. muscle of auricle
- t. muscle of chin
- t. muscle of nape
- t. muscle of thorax
- t. muscle of tongue
- t. myelitis
- t. nasal groove
- t. nerve of neck
- t. occipital sulcus
- t. oval pelvis
- t. palatine fold
- t. palatine ridge
- t. palatine suture
- t. pancreatic artery
- t. part of iliofemoral ligament
- t. part of left branch of portal vein
- t. part of nasalis muscle
- t. part of trapezius muscle
- t. pericardial sinus
- t. perineal ligament
- t. plane
- t. pontine fiber
- t. presentation
- t. process of vertebra
- t. relaxation
- t. rhombencephalic flexure
- t. ridge
- t. ridge of sacrum
- t. scapular artery
- t. section
- t. septum
- t. sinus
- t. sinus of pericardium
- t. tarsal articulation
- t. tarsal joint
- t. temporal convolutions
- t. temporal gyri
- t. temporal sulcus
- t. thoracosternotomy
- t. tibiofibular ligament
- t. vein of face
- t. vein of neck
- t. vein of scapula
- t. velum
- t. vesical fold

transversectomy
transversion mutation
transversocostal
transversospinales muscle
transversospinal muscle
transversourethralis
transversovertical index
transversus
- t. abdominis muscle
- t. menti muscle
- t. nuchae muscle
- t. thoracis muscle

transvestism
transvestite
transvestitism
Trantas dot
Tr^a antigen
tranylcypromine sulfate
TRAP
    twin reversed arterial perfusion sequence
trapezia (*pl. of* trapezium)
trapezial
trapeziform
trapeziometacarpal
trapezium, pl. **trapezia**
- t. bone

trapezius muscle
trapezoid
- t. body
- t. bone
- t. ligament
- t. line
- t. ridge

trapidil
Trapp formula
Trapp-Häser formula
Traube
- T. bruit
- T. corpuscle
- T. double tone
- T. dyspnea
- T. plugs
- T. semilunar space
- T. sign

Traube-Hering
- T.-H. curve
- T.-H. wave

traum- (*var. of* traumato-)
trauma, pl. **traumata**
- birth t.
- t. from occlusion
- occlusal t.
- psychic t.

traumat- (*var. of* traumato-)
traumatic
- t. alopecia
- t. amenorrhea
- t. amnesia

t. amputation
t. anemia
t. anesthesia
t. aneurysm
t. asphyxia
t. bone cyst
t. cataract
t. cervical discopathy
t. dermatitis
t. fever
t. herpes
t. meningocele
t. neurasthenia
t. neuritis
t. neuroma
t. neurosis
t. occlusion
t. orchitis
t. pneumothorax
t. progressive encephalopathy
t. psychosis
t. retinopathy
t. tetanus

traumatism
traumatize
traumato-, traum-, traumat-
traumatogenic occlusion
traumatology
traumatonesis
traumatopathy
traumatopnea
traumatopyra
traumatosepsis
traumatotherapy
Trautmann triangular space
traveler's diarrhea
traveling wave theory
traverse
tray

acrylic resin t.
annealing t.
impression t.

trazodone hydrochloride
Treacher Collins syndrome
treacle
treat
treatment

active t.
Carrel t.
causal t.
conservative t.
Dakin-Carrel t.
t. denture
dietetic t.
empiric t.
endodontic t.
Goeckerman t.
heat t.
insulin coma t.
insulin shock t.
isoserum t.
Kenny t.
light t.
medical t.
Mitchell t.

moral t.
Nauheim t.
palliative t.
preventive t.
prophylactic t.
root canal t.
Schott t.
shock t.
solar t.
symptomatic t.
Tallerman t.
thymus t.
Tweed edgewise t.
Weir Mitchell t.

treble increase at low levels
trefoil

t. polypeptide
t. tendon

trehala
trehalase
trehalose
Treitz

T. arch
T. fascia
T. fossa
T. hernia
T. ligament
T. muscle

Trélat stools
tremacamra
Trematoda
trematode, trematoid
trembles
trembling palsy
tremelloid, tremellose
tremogram
tremograph
tremolabile
tremophobia
tremor

action t.
alcoholic withdrawal t.
alternating t.
alternative t.
benign essential t.
coarse t.
continuous t.
essential t.
familial t.
fine t.
flapping t.
head t.'s
heredofamilial t.
hysterical t.
intention t.
kinetic t.
passive t.
persistent t.
physiologic t.
pill-rolling t.
postural t.
progressive cerebellar t.
psychogenic t.
resting t.
senile t.

T

tremor (continued)
    static t.
    volitional t.
    wing-beating t.
tremorgram
tremorine
tremostable
tremulor
tremulous iris
trench
    t. fever
    t. foot
    t. mouth
Trendelenburg
    T. gait
    T. operation
    T. position
    T. radiograph
    T. sign
    T. symptom
    T. test
trend of thought
trepanation
    t. of cornea
    corneal t.
trephination
trephine biopsy
trephocyte
trepidatio cordis
trepidation
Treponema
    T. carateum
    T. cuniculi
    T. denticola
    T. genitalis
    T. hyodysenteriae
    T. mucosum
    T. pallidum
    T. pallidum hemagglutination test
    T. pallidum immobilization reaction
    T. pallidum immobilization test
    T. pertenue
treponema-immobilizing antibody
treponemal antibody
treponematosis
treponeme
treponemiasis
treponemicidal
treppe
Tresilian sign
tresis
tretinoin
Treves fold
Trevor disease
TRF
    thyrotropin-releasing factor
TRH
    thyrotropin-releasing hormone
TRH-stimulation test (*var. of* thyrotropin-releasing hormone stimulation test)
tri-
triacetic acid
triacetin
triacetylglycerol

triacetyloleandomycin
triacylglycerol lipase
triad
    acute compression t.
    t. asthma
    Beck t.
    Charcot t.
    Fallot t.
    hepatic t.
    Hull t.
    Hutchinson t.
    Kartagener t.
    portal t.
    Saint t.
triadic symbiosis
triage
    economic t.
trial
    t. base
    Bernoulli t.
    t. case
    clinical t.
    t. denture
    t. and error
    t. frame
    t. of labor after cesarean section
    t. lens
    randomized controlled t. (RCT)
triamcinolone
    t. acetonide
    t. diacetate
tri-amelia
triamterene
triangle
    anal t.
    anterior t. of neck
    Assézat t.
    auricular t.
    auscultatory t.
    t. of auscultation
    axillary t.
    Béclard t.
    Bonwill t.
    Burger t.
    Burow t.
    Calot t.
    cardiohepatic t.
    carotid t.
    cephalic t.
    cervical t.
    clavipectoral t.
    Codman t.
    crural t.
    cystohepatic t.
    deltoideopectoral t.
    deltopectoral t.
    digastric t.
    Einthoven t.
    Elaut t.
    t. of elbow
    facial t.
    Farabeuf t.
    femoral t.
    t. of fillet
    frontal t.

Garland t.
Gombault t.
Grocco t.
Grynfeltt t.
Hesselbach t.
inferior carotid t.
inferior lumbar t.
inferior occipital t.
infraclavicular t.
inguinal t.
interscalene t.
Killian t.
Koch t.
Labbé t.
Langenbeck t.
lateral pelvic wall t.
Lesser t.
Lesshaft t.
Lieutaud t.
lumbar t.
lumbocostal t. of diaphragm
lumbocostoabdominal t.
Macewen t.
Malgaigne t.
Marcille t.
muscular t.
occipital t.
omoclavicular t.
omotracheal t.
palatal t.
paravertebral t.
Petit lumbar t.
Philippe t.
Pirogoff t.
posterior t. of neck
pubourethral t.
Reil t.
retromolar t.
sacral t.
t. of safety
Scarpa t.
sternocostal t.
subclavian t.
subinguinal t.
submandibular t.
submaxillary t.
submental t.
suboccipital t.
superior carotid t.
supraclavicular t.
suprameatal t.
tracheal t.
Tweed t.
umbilicomammillary t.
urogenital t.
t. of vertebral artery
vesical t.
Ward t.
Weber t.
Wilde t.
triangular
t. bandage
t. bone
t. cartilage
t. crest

t. disk of wrist
t. fascia
t. fold
t. fossa of auricle
t. fovea of arytenoid cartilage
t. lamella
t. ligament
t. ligament of liver
t. muscle
t. nucleus
t. nucleus of septum
t. part
t. pit of arytenoid cartilage
t. recess
t. ridge
t. uterus
triangularis
triangulum
Triatoma
Triatominae
triaxial reference system
triazolam
triazologuanine
triazolopyridine antidepressant
tribasic
t. calcium phosphate
t. magnesium phosphate
tribasilar synostosis
tribe
tribology
triboluminescence
tribrachia
tribrachius
tribromsalan
tributyrase
tributyrin
tributyrinase
tributyrylglycerol
TRIC agent
tricalcium phosphate
tricarboxylic acid cycle
tricephalus
triceps
t. brachii
t. bursa
t. coxae
t. muscle
t. reflex
t. surae
t. surae reflex
trich- (*var. of* tricho-)
trichalgia
trichangion
trichatrophia
trichauxis
trichi- (*var. of* tricho-)
-trichia
trichiasis
trichilemmal cyst
trichilemmoma
Trichina
trichina, pl. **trichinae**
Trichinella
T. pseudospiralis.
T. spiralis

T

trichinelliasis
Trichinellicae
Trichinelloidea
trichinellosis
trichiniasis
trichiniferous
trichinization
trichinoscope
trichinosis granuloma
trichinous
trichion
trichite
trichloral
trichlorfon
trichloride
trichlormethiazide
trichlormethine
trichloroacetic acid
trichloroethane
trichloroethanol
trichloroethene
trichloroethyl alcohol
trichloroethylene
trichlorofluoromethane
trichloromethane
trichloromonofluoromethane
trichlorophenol
(2,4,5-trichlorophenoxy)acetic acid (2,4,5-T)
tricho-, trich-, trichi-
Trichocephalus
trichochrome
trichocyst
Trichodectes
Trichoderma
trichodiscoma
trichodynia
trichodystrophy
trichoepithelioma
    desmoplastic t.
    hereditary multiple t.
trichoesthesia
trichofolliculoma
trichogen
trichoglossia
trichohyalin
trichoid
tricholemmoma
trichologia
trichology
trichoma
trichomatosis
trichomegaly
trichomonacide
trichomonad
Trichomonadidae
Trichomonas
    T. buccalis
    T. foetus
    T. gallinarum
    T. hominis
    T. ovis
    T. suis
    T. tenax
    T. vaginalis

trichomoniasis vaginitis
trichomycetosis
trichomycosis axillaris
trichonodosis
trichonosis
trichopathic
trichopathophobia
trichopathy
trichophagia
trichophagy
trichophobia
trichophytic
trichophytobezoar
Trichophyton
    T. concentricum
    T. equinum
    T. megninii
    T. mentagrophytes
    T. rubrum
    T. schoenleinii
    T. simii
    T. tonsurans
    T. verrucosum
    T. violaceum
trichophytosis
Trichopleuris
trichopoliodystrophy
trichopoliosis
Trichoptera
trichoptilosis
trichorhinophalangeal syndrome
trichorrhexis
    t. invaginata
    t. nodosa
trichoschisis
trichosis
    t. carunculae
    t. sensitiva
    t. setosa
trichosomatous
Trichosporon
trichosporonosis
trichosporosis
trichostasis spinulosa
trichostrongyle
Trichostrongylidae
trichostrongylosis
Trichostrongylus
    T. axei
    T. capricola
    T. colubriformis
    T. longispicularis
    T. tenuis
    T. vitrinus
Trichothecium
trichothiodystrophy
trichotillomania
trichotomy
trichotoxin
trichotrophy
trichroic
trichroism
trichromat
trichromatic

trichromatism
  anomalous t.
trichromatopsia
trichrome stain
trichromic
trichterbrust
trichuriasis
Trichuris
  T. suis
  T. trichiura
  T. vulpis
tricipital
triclobisonium chloride
triclofenol piperazine
triclofos
tricorn protease
tricornute
tricresol
tricrotic
tricrotism
tricrotous
Tricula
tricuspid, tricuspidal, tricuspidate
  t. area
  t. atresia
  t. incompetence
  t. insufficiency
  t. murmur
  t. orifice
  t. stenosis
  t. tooth
  t. valve
tricyclamol chloride
tricyclic antidepressant
tridactylous
tridentate
trident hand
tridermic
tridermoma
tridigitate
tridihexethyl chloride
tridymite
tridymus
trielcon
trientine hydrochloride
triethanolamine
triethylene glycol
triethylenemelamine (TEM)
triethylenephosphoramide (TEPA)
triethylenetetramine dihydrochloride
triethylenethiophosphoramide
trifacial
  t. nerve
  t. neuralgia
trifid stomach
trifluoperazine hydrochloride
trifluoroacetyl
2,2,2-trifluoroethyl vinyl
5-trifluoromethyldeoxyuridine
trifluperidol hydrochloride
triflupromazine hydrochloride
trifluridine
trifocal lens
trifurcation
trigastric

trigeminal
  t. cave
  t. cavity
  t. crest
  t. decompression
  t. ganglion
  t. impression
  t. lemniscus
  t. nerve [CN V]
  t. neuralgia
  t. pulse
  t. rhizotomy
  t. rhythm
  t. tractotomy
  t. tubercle
trigeminofacial reflex
trigeminospinal tract
trigeminothalamic tract
trigeminus
trigeminy
trigenolline
trigger
  t. area
  ECG t.
  EKG t.
  t. finger
  t. point
  t. zone
triggered activity
triglyceride
trigona (*pl. of* trigonum)
trigonal
trigone
  t. of auditory nerve
  t. of bladder
  cerebral t.
  collateral t.
  deltoideopectoral t.
  fibrous t.
  t. of fillet
  t. of habenula
  habenular t.
  hypoglossal t.
  t. of hypoglossal nerve
  inguinal t.
  t. of lateral lemniscus
  t. of lateral ventricle
  left fibrous t. (of heart)
  lemniscal t.
  Lieutaud t.
  Müller t.
  olfactory t.
  right fibrous t.
  vagal nerve t.
  t. of vagus nerve
  ventricular t.
  vertebrocostal t.
trigonelline
trigonid
trigonitis
trigonocephalic
trigonocephaly
trigonum, pl. **trigona**
  t. auscultationis
  t. caroticum

T

trigonum *(continued)*
    t. cerebrale
    t. cervicale
    t. cervicale anterius
    t. cervicale posterius
    t. clavipectorale
    t. collaterale
    t. colli
    t. colli anterius
    t. colli laterale
    t. cystohepaticum
    t. deltoideopectorale
    t. deltopectorale
    t. femorale
    t. femoris
    trigona fibrosa cordis
    t. fibrosum dextrum
    t. fibrosum sinistrum
    t. habenulae
    t. hypoglossi
    t. inguinale
    t. lemnisci lateralis
    t. lumbale inferius
    t. lumbocostale diaphragmatis
    t. musculare (regionis cervicalis anterioris)
    t. nervi acustici
    t. nervi hypoglossi
    t. nervi vagi
    t. olfactorium
    t. omoclaviculare
    t. omotracheale
    t. palati
    t. parietale laterale pelvis
    t. retromolare
    t. sternocostale
    t. sternocostale diaphragmatis
    t. submandibulare
    t. submentale
    t. vagale
    t. ventriculi
    t. vesicae
trihexosylceramide
trihexyphenidyl hydrochloride
trihybrid
trihydric alcohol
trihydroxyestrin
triiniodymus
triiodide
triiodomethane
triiodothyronine
    t. toxicosis
    t. uptake test
3,5,3′-triiodothyronine (T$_3$, TITh)
triketohydrindene hydrate
triketohydrindene reaction
triketopurine
trilabe
trilaminar blastoderm
trilateral
trilobate, trilobed
trilocular
trilogy
    t. of Fallot

trilostane
trimalleolar fracture
trimastigote
trimeprazine tartrate
trimer
trimester
trimetaphan camsylate
trimetazidine
trimethadione
trimethaphan camsylate
trimethidium methosulfate
trimethobenzamide hydrochloride
trimethoprim
trimethoprim-sulfamethoxazole
trimethylamine
trimethylaminuria
trimethylcarbinol
trimethylene
trimethylethylene
N^ε-trimethyllysine
trimethylomelamine
trimetozine
trimetrexate
trimipramine
trimorphic
trimorphism
trimorphous
trinitrocellulose
trinitroglycerin
trinitrotoluene (TNT)
trinitrotoluol
trinucleotide
triodothyronine
    reverse triodothyronine (RT$_3$)
triokinase
triol
triolein
triophthalmos
triorchism
triorthocresyl phosphate (TOCP)
triose
triosekinase
triosephosphate isomerase
triotus
trioxide
trioxsalen
trioxymethylene
tripalmitin
triparanol
tripelennamine hydrochloride
tripeptidases
tripeptide
triphammer pulse
triphenylmethane dye
triphyllomatous teratoma
Tripier amputation
triplant implant
triple
    t. arthrodesis
    t. A syndrome
    t. bond
    t. helix
    t. phosphate
    t. point
    t. quartan

t. repeat disorder
t. response
t. rhythm
t. screen
t. symptom complex
t. vision
t. X syndrome
triplegia
triplet
nonsense t.
t. oxygen
t. state
triploblastic
triploid
triploidy
triplopia
tripod
t. fracture
Haller t.
vital t.
tripodia
triprolidine hydrochloride
triprosopus
tripsis
triquetrous cartilage
triquetrum
t. bone
triradial, triradiate
triradius
Tris
trishydroxymethylmethylamine
tris-
trisaccharide
tris(hydroxymethyl)aminomethane
tris(hydroxymethyl)methylamine (Tris)
triskaidekaphobia
trismic
trismoid
trismus
t. capistratus
t. nascentium
t. neonatorum
t. sardonicus
trisodium phosphate
trisomic
trisomy
t. C, D syndrome
t. 8, 13, 18, 20, 21 syndrome
trispiral tomography
trisplanchnic
tristearin
trisulcate
tritanomaly
tritanopia
triterpenes
tritiated thymidine
triticeal cartilage
triticeoglossus
triticeous
triticeum
tritium
triton tumor
Tritrichomonas
tritubercular
triturable

triturate
trituration
trityl
trivalence, trivalency
trivalent
trivalve
trivial name
trizonal
tRNA
transfer rna
trocar
Hasson t.
troch
trochiscus
trochanter
greater t.
lesser t.
t. major
t. minor
t. reflex
small t.
t. tertius
third t.
trochanteric, trochanterian
t. bursa
t. bursae of gluteus medius
t. bursae of gluteus minimus
t. crest
t. fossa
t. syndrome
trochanterplasty
trochantin
trochantinian
troche
trochiscus, pl. **trochisci (troch)**
trochlea, pl. **trochleae**
t. femoris
fibular t. of calcaneus
t. fibularis calcanei
t. humeri
t. of humerus
muscular t.
t. muscularis
t. musculi obliqui superioris bulbi
peroneal t. of calcaneus
t. peronealis
trochleae of phalanges of hand and foot
t. phalangis (manus et pedis)
t. of superior oblique (muscle)
t. tali
t. of the talus
trochlear
t. fossa
t. fovea
t. nerve [CN IV]
t. notch
t. nucleus
t. pit
t. process
t. spine
t. synovial bursa
trochleariform
trochlearis
trochleiform

T

trochocardia
trochoid
    t. articulation
    t. joint
trochorizocardia
troglitazone
Troglotrema salmincola
Troisier
    T. ganglion
    T. node
trolamine
Trolard vein
troleandomycin
trolnitrate phosphate
Tröltsch
    T. corpuscle
    T. pockets
    T. recess
Trombicula
    t. akamushi
    t. alfreddugesi
    t. deliensis
trombiculiasis
trombiculid
Trombiculidae
Trombidiidae
tromethamine
Trömner reflex
trona
tropaic acid
tropane
tropate
tropeic acid
tropeine
tropentane
tropeolins
troph- (*var. of* tropho-)
trophectoderm
Tropheryma whippelii
trophic
    t. change
    t. gangrene
    t. hormone
    t. nucleus
    t. syndrome
    t. ulcer
-trophic
trophicity
trophism
tropho-, troph-
trophoblast
    t. interferon
    plasmodial t.
    syncytial t.
trophoblastic
    t. lacuna
    t. operculum
trophoblastin
trophochromatin
trophochromidia
trophocyte
trophoderm
trophodermatoneurosis
trophodynamics
trophoneurosis

trophoneurotic
    t. atrophy
    t. leprosy
trophonucleus
trophoplast
trophospongia
trophotaxis
trophotropic zone of Hess
trophotropism
trophozoite
-trophy
tropia
-tropic
tropic acid
tropical
    t. abscess
    t. acne
    t. anemia
    t. boil
    t. bubo
    t. diarrhea
    t. disease
    t. eczema
    t. eosinophilia
    t. hyphemia
    t. mask
    t. measles
    t. medicine
    t. myositis
    t. pyomyositis
    t. sore
    t. splenomegaly
    t. splenomegaly syndrome
    t. sprue
    t. typhus
    t. ulcer
tropicamide
tropic hormone
tropine
    t. mandelate
    t. tropate
tropism
    negative t.
    positive t.
    viral t.
tropocollagen
tropoelastin
tropometer
tropomyosin
troponin
trough
    gingival t.
    Langmuir t.
    t. sign
    synaptic t.
Trousseau
    T. point
    T. sign
    T. spot
    T. syndrome
Trousseau-Lallemand body
troxerutin
troxidone
true
    t. aneurysm

t. ankylosis
t. cementoma
t. cholinesterase
t. conjugate
t. diverticulum
t. dwarfism
t. glottis
t. hermaphroditism
t. hypertrophy
t. knot
t. lumen
t. muscle of back
t. neurogenic thoracic outlet syndrome
t. pelvis
t. precocious puberty
t. rib [I–VII]
t. thirst
t. vertebra
t. vocal cord

truncal
truncate ascertainment
truncus, pl. **trunci**
t. arteriosus
t. arteriosus communis
t. brachiocephalicus
t. celiacus
t. corporis callosi
t. costocervicalis
t. encephali
t. fascicularis atrioventricularis
t. inferior plexus brachialis
t. linguofacialis
t. lumbosacralis
trunci (lymphatici) intestinales
trunci (lymphatici) lumbales
t. (lymphaticus) bronchiomediastinalis
t. (lymphaticus) jugularis
t. medius plexus brachialis
t. nervi accessorii
persistent t. arteriosus
trunci plexus brachialis
t. pulmonalis
t. subclavius
t. superior plexus brachialis
t. sympathicus
t. thyrocervicalis
t. vagalis

Trunecek sign
trunk
accessory nerve t.
t. of atrioventricular bundle
t.'s of brachial plexus
brachiocephalic (arterial) t.
bronchomediastinal (lymphatic) t.
celiac (arterial) t.
t. of corpus callosum
costocervical (arterial) t.
inferior t. of brachial plexus
intestinal (lymphatic) t.'s
jugular lymphatic t.
linguofacial (arterial) t.
lumbar (lymphatic) t.'s
lumbosacral (nerve) t.
middle t. of brachial plexus

nerve t.
pulmonary t.
subclavian lymphatic t.
superior t. of brachial plexus
sympathetic t.
thoracoacromial t.
thyrocervical t.
vagal nerve t.

trusion
Trusler rule for pulmonary artery banding
truss
truth serum
try-in
trypan blue
trypanicidal
trypanicide
trypanid
trypanocidal
trypanocide
Trypanoplasma
Trypanosoma
    T. avium
    T. brucei
    T. brucei brucei
    T. brucei gambiense
    T. brucei rhodesiense
    T. cruzi
    T. dimorphon
    T. escomelis
    T. gambiense
    T. hominis
    T. ignotum
    T. lewisi
    T. melophagium
    T. rangeli
    T. rhodesiense
    T. theileri
    T. triatomae
    T. ugandense
trypanosomatid
Trypanosomatidae
trypanosome
t. fever
t. stage
trypanosomiasis
acute t.
African t.
American t.
chronic t.
Cruz t.
East African t.
Gambian t.
Rhodesian t.
South American t.
West African t.
trypanosomic
trypanosomicide
trypanosomid
trypanosomosis
trypan red
tryparsamide
trypomastigote
trypsin
crystallized t.

T

trypsin *(continued)*
    t. G-banding stain
    t. inhibitor
α_1-**trypsin inhibitor**
trypsinogen, trypsogen
tryptamine
tryptamine-strophanthidin
tryptic
tryptone
tryptonemia
tryptophan (W)
    t. decarboxylase
    t. desmolase
    t. 2,3-dioxygenase
    t. oxygenase
    t. pyrrolase
    t. synthase
    t. synthetase
tryptophanase
tryptophanuria with dwarfism
tsetse
TSH
    thyroid-stimulating hormone
TSH-RF
    thyroid-stimulating hormone-releasing
    factor
TSH-stimulating test *(var. of* thyroid-
    stimulating hormone stimulation test)
TSI
    thyroid-stimulating immunoglobulins
TSS
    toxic shock syndrome
TSTA
    tumor-specific transplantation antigen
tsutsugamushi
    t. disease
    t. fever
TTP-HUS
    thrombotic thrombocytopenic purpura and
    hemolytic uremic syndrome
TTX
    tetrodotoxin
T.U.
    toxic unit
tuaminoheptane
tuba, pl. **tubae**
    t. acustica
    t. auditiva
    t. auditoria
    t. eustachiana
    t. eustachii
    t. fallopiana
    t. fallopii
    t. uterina
tubage
tubal
    t. abortion
    t. air cell
    t. branch
    t. branch of ovarian artery
    t. branch of the tympanic plexus
    t. branch of the uterine artery
    t. cartilage
    t. colic

    t. dysmenorrhea
    t. extremity of ovary
    t. gland of pharyngotympanic tube
    t. infantilism
    t. ligation
    t. pregnancy
    t. prominence
    t. tonsil
tubatorsion
tube
    Abbott t.
    air t.
    auditory t.
    Babcock t.
    Bouchut t.
    bronchial t.
    Cantor t.
    cardiac t.
    Carlen t.
    t. cast
    cathode ray t. (CRT)
    Celestin t.
    Coolidge t.
    Crookes-Hittorf t.
    t. curare
    digestive t.
    drainage t.
    Durham t.
    empyema t.
    endobronchial t.
    endotracheal t.
    eustachian t.
    fallopian t.
    feeding t.
    Ferrein t.
    field emission t.
    Geiger-Müller t.
    germ t.
    Haldane t.
    intratracheal t.
    Levin t.
    Martin t.
    medullary t.
    Miescher t.'s
    Miller-Abbott t.
    molybdenum target t.
    Moss t.
    nasogastric t.
    nasotracheal t.
    nephrostomy t.
    neural t.
    O'Dwyer t.
    orotracheal t.
    otopharyngeal t.
    pharyngotympanic t.
    photomultiplier t.
    Pitot t.
    pus t.
    rectifier t.
    Rehfuss stomach t.
    Robertshaw t.
    roll t.
    rotating anode t.
    Ruysch t.
    Ryle t.

Sengstaken-Blakemore t.
Southey t.
speaking t.
stomach t.
T t.
test t.
thoracostomy t.
t. tooth
Tovell t.
Toynbee t.
tracheal t.
tracheostomy t.
tracheotomy t.
tympanostomy t.
uterine t.
vacuum t.
Venturi t.
Wangensteen t.
x-ray t.

tubectomy
tubed
t. flap
t. pedicle flap

tuber, pl. **tubera**
t. anterius
ashen t.
calcaneal t.
t. calcanei
t. calcis
t. cinereum
t. cochleae
t. corporis callosi
t. dorsale
eustachian t.
frontal t.
t. frontale
gray t.
t. ischiadicum
t. of ischium
t. maxillae
omental t.
t. omentale hepatis
t. omentale pancreatis
parietal t.
t. parietale
t. radii
t. valvulae
t. vermis
t. of vermis
t. zygomaticum

tuberal nucleus
tubercle
accessory t.
acoustic t.
adductor t. of femur
amygdaloid t.
anatomic t.
anterior t. of atlas
anterior t. of cervical vertebrae
t. of anterior scalene muscle
anterior thalamic t.
anterior t. of thalamus
areolar t.'s
articular t. of temporal bone
ashen t.

auricular t.
t. bacillus
calcaneal t.
Carabelli t.
carotid t.
caseous t.
Chassaignac t.
conoid t.
corniculate t.
crown t.
cuneate t.
cuneiform t.
darwinian t.
deltoid t.
dental t.
dorsal t. of radius
epiglottic t.
fibrous t.
genial t.
genital t.
Gerdy t.
Ghon t.
gracile t.
gray t.
greater t.
hard t.
hyaline t.
iliac t.
t. of iliac crest
inferior thyroid t.
infraglenoid t.
intercolumnar t.
intercondylar t.
intervenous t.
jugular t. of occipital bone
labial t.
lateral t.
lesser t.
Lisfranc t.
Lister t.
Lower t.
mammillary t.
mammillary t. of hypothalamus
marginal t.
medial t.
mental t.
molar t.
Montgomery t.'s
Morgagni t.
Müller t.
nuchal t.
obturator t.
olfactory t.
orbital t.
phallic t.
pharyngeal t.
posterior t.
Princeteau t.
pterygoid t.
pubic t.
t. of rib
Rolando t.
t. of saddle
Santorini t.
scalene t.

T

tubercle *(continued)*
    scalene t. of Lisfranc
    t. of scaphoid
    sinus t.
    soft t.
    superior thyroid t.
    supraglenoid t. (of scapula)
    supratragic t.
    t. of tooth
    t. of trapezium
    trigeminal t.
    t. of upper lip
    wedge-shaped t.
    Whitnall t.
    Wrisberg t.
tubercul- *(var. of* tuberculo-)
tubercula *(pl. of* tuberculum)
tubercular, tuberculated
tuberculation
tuberculid
    nodular t.
    papular t.
    papulonecrotic t.
    rosacea-like t.
tuberculin
    Koch old t.
    purified protein derivative of t.
    (PPD)
    t. test
tuberculin-type hypersensitivity
tuberculitis
tuberculo-, tubercul-
tuberculocele
tuberculochemotherapeutic
tuberculocidal
tuberculoderma
tuberculofibroid
tuberculoid
    t. leprosy
    t. rosacea
tuberculoma
tuberculoopsonic index
tuberculoprotein
tuberculosis (TB)
    adult t.
    aerogenic t.
    anthracotic t.
    arrested t.
    attenuated t.
    basal t.
    cerebral t.
    childhood t.
    childhood type t.
    cutaneous t.
    t. cutis
    t. cutis orificialis
    t. cutis verrucosa
    disseminated t.
    enteric t.
    exudative t.
    generalized t.
    healed t.
    inactive t.
    t. lymphadenitis

    miliary t.
    open t.
    t. papulonecrotica
    postprimary t.
    primary t.
    pulmonary t.
    reactivation t.
    reinfection t.
    secondary t.
    t. vaccine
tuberculostat
tuberculostatic
tuberculous
    t. bronchopneumonia
    t. enteritis
    t. lymphadenitis
    t. meningitis
    t. nephritis
    t. pericarditis
    t. peritonitis
    t. rheumatism
    t. spondylitis
    t. wart
tuberculum, pl. tubercula
    t. adductorium femoris
    t. anterius atlantis
    t. anterius thalami
    t. anterius vertebrarum cervicalium
    tubercula areolae
    t. arthriticum
    t. articulare ossis temporalis
    t. auriculae
    t. calcanei
    t. caroticum
    t. cinereum
    t. conoideum (claviculare)
    t. corniculatum
    t. coronae
    t. costae
    t. cuneatum
    t. cuneiforme
    t. deltoideum
    t. dentis
    t. dorsale radii
    t. epiglotticum
    t. gracile
    t. hypoglossi
    t. iliacum
    t. impar
    t. infraglenoidale (scapulae)
    t. intercondylare (mediale et
    laterale)
    t. intervenosum (atrii dextri)
    t. jugulare ossis occipitalis
    t. labii superioris
    t. laterale (processus posterioris) tali
    t. majus (humeri)
    t. mallei
    t. marginale (ossis zygomatici)
    t. mediale (processus posterioris)
    tali
    t. mentale (mandibulae)
    t. minus (humeri)
    t. molare
    t. musculi scaleni anterioris

t. obturatorium
t. olfactorium
t. orbitale ossis zygomatici
t. ossis scaphoidei
t. ossis trapezii
t. pharyngeum (partis basilaris ossis occipitalis)
t. posterius atlantis
t. posterius vertebrarum cervicalium
t. pubicum
t. sellae
t. septi narium
t. superius
t. supraglenoidale (scapulae)
t. supratragicum
t. thyroideum inferius
t. thyroideum superius
t. of trapezium bone
t. trigeminale
tuberiferous
tuberoinfundibular tract
tuberomammillary nucleus
tuberose
tuberositas
t. coracoidea
t. costalis
t. deltoidea (humeri)
t. glutea
t. iliaca
t. ligamenti coracoclavicularis
t. masseterica
t. musculi serrati anterioris
t. ossis cuboidei
t. ossis metatarsalis primi [I]
t. ossis metatarsalis quinti [V]
t. ossis navicularis
t. phalangis distalis (manus et pedis)
t. pronatoria
t. pterygoidea (mandibulae)
t. radii
t. sacralis
t. tibiae
t. ulnae
t. unguicularis
tuberosity
bicipital t.
calcaneal t.
t. for coracoclavicular ligament
coracoid t.
costal t.
t. of cuboid (bone)
deltoid t.
t. of distal phalanx (of hand and foot)
t. of fifth metatarsal (bone) [V]
t. of first metatarsal (bone) [I]
gluteal t.
greater t. of humerus
iliac t.
infraglenoid t.
ischial t.
lateral femoral t.
lesser t. of humerus
masseteric t.

maxillary t.
medial femoral t.
t. of navicular bone
omental t. of liver
pronator t.
pterygoid t. of mandible
radial t.
t. of radius
t. reduction
sacral t.
scaphoid t.
t. for serratus anterior (muscle)
tibial t.
t. of ulna
ungual t.
tuberous
t. root
t. sclerosis
tubi (*pl. of* tubus)
Tübinger perimeter
tubo-
tuboabdominal pregnancy
tubocurarine chloride
tuboligamentous
tuboovarian
t. abscess
t. pregnancy
tubo-ovarian varicocele
tubo-ovariectomy
tubo-ovaritis
tuboperitoneal
tuboplasty
tuboreticular structure
tubotorsion
tubotympanic, tubotympanal
t. canal
t. recess
tubouterine
t. pregnancy
tubovaginal
tubular
t. adenoma
t. aneurysm
t. carcinoma
t. cyst
t. excretory mass
t. forceps
t. gland
t. maximum
t. respiration
t. vision
tubulature
tubule
Albarran y Dominguez t.
connecting t.
convoluted t. of kidney
convoluted seminiferous t.
dental t.'s
dentinal t.
discharging t.
Henle t.'s
Kobelt t.'s
malpighian t.'s
mesonephric t.
metanephric t.

T

tubule *(continued)*
    paragenital t.
    pronephric t.
    segmental t.
    seminiferous t.
    Skene t.
    spiral t.
    straight seminiferous t.
    straight t. of testis
    T t.
    uriniferous t.
    wolffian t.'s
tubuli *(pl. of* tubulus*)*
tubuliform
tubulin-tyrosine ligase
tubulization
tubuloacinar gland
tubuloalveolar gland
tubulocyst
tubulodermoid
tubuloglomerular feedback
tubulointerstitial nephritis
tubuloneogenesis
tubuloracemose
tubulorrhexis
tubulose, tubulous
tubulus, pl. **tubuli**
    tubuli biliferi
    tubuli contorti
    tubuli dentales
    tubuli epoöphori
    tubuli galactophori
    tubuli lactiferi
    tubuli paroöphori
    t. rectus
    t. renalis contortus
    tubuli seminiferi recti
    tubuli seminiferi recti testi
    t. transversus
tubus, pl. **tubi**
    t. digestorius
    t. medullaris
    t. vertebralis
Tucker-McLean forceps
tuffstone body
tuft
    enamel t.
    malpighian t.
    synovial t.'s
tufted
    t. cell
    t. phalanx
tuftsin
tug, tugging
    tracheal t.
tularemia
    glandular t.
    pulmonary t.
    pulmonic t.
tularemic
    t. chancre
    t. conjunctivitis
    t. pneumonia
tulle gras

Tullio phenomenon
Tulp valve
tumbu dermal myiasis
tumefacient
tumefaction
tumefy
tumentia
tumeric yellow
tumescence
tumescent liposuction
tumid
tumor
    acinar cell t.
    acoustic t.
    acute splenic t.
    adenoid t.
    adenomatoid odontogenic t.
    adipose t.
    ameloblastic adenomatoid t.
    amyloid t.
    t. angiogenic factor (TAF)
    t. antigen
    aortic body t.
    Bednar t.
    benign t.
    blood t.
    t. blush
    borderline ovarian t.
    Brenner t.
    Brooke t.
    brown t.
    t. burden
    calcifying epithelial odontogenic t.
    carcinoid t.
    carotid body t.
    t. cell t.
    cellular t.
    cerebellopontine angle t.
    chromaffin t.
    Codman t.
    collision t.
    connective t.
    dermal duct t.
    dermoid t.
    desmoid t.
    desmoplastic small cell t.
    dysembryoplastic neuroepithelial t.
    eighth nerve t.
    t. embolism
    embryonal t.
    embryonal t. of ciliary body
    embryonic t.
    endocervical sinus t.
    endodermal sinus t.
    endometrioid t.
    Erdheim t.
    Ewing t.
    fecal t.
    fibroid t.
    gastrointestinal autonomic nerve t.
    gastrointestinal stromal t.
    giant cell t. of bone
    giant cell t. of tendon sheath
    glomus jugulare t.
    glomus tympanicum t.

Godwin t.
granular cell t.
granulosa cell t.
Grawitz t.
heterologous t.
hilar cell t. of ovary
histoid t.
homologous t.
innocent t.
interstitial cell t. of testis
islet cell t.
juxtaglomerular cell t.
Klatskin t.
Krukenberg t.
Landschutz t.
Leydig cell t.
Lindau t.
low malignant potential t.
t. lysis syndrome
malignant t.
malignant mixed müllerian t.
  (MMMT)
t. marker
melanotic neuroectodermal t. of
  infancy
Merkel cell t.
mesonephroid t.
mixed mesodermal t.
mixed t. of salivary gland
mixed t. of skin
mucoepidermoid t.
t. necrosis factor (TNF)
t. necrosis factor-alpha
t. necrosis factor-beta
Nelson t.
oil t.
oncocytic hepatocellular t.
organoid t.
Pancoast t.
papillary t.
paraffin t.
phantom t.
phyllodes t.
pilar t. of scalp
Pindborg t.
Pinkus t.
placental site trophoblastic t.
pontine angle t.
potato t. of neck
pregnancy t.
primitive neuroectodermal t.
ranine t.
Rathke pouch t.
retinal anlage t.
Rous t.
sand t.
Sertoli-Leydig cell t.
Sertoli-stromal cell t.
solitary fibrous t.
squamous odontogenic t.
t. stage
steroid cell t.
sugar t.
superior pulmonary sulcus t.
t. suppressor gene

teratoid t.
theca cell t.
triton t.
turban t.
villous t.
t. virus
Warthin t.
Wilms t.
yolk sac t.
Zollinger-Ellison t.
tumoral calcinosis
tumor-associated antigen
tumoricidal
tumorigenesis
  foreign body t.
tumorigenic
tumor-infiltrating lymphocytes (TIL)
tumorlets
tumorous
**tumor-specific transplantation antigen
  (TSTA)**
tumultus cordis
TUNEL
Tunga penetrans
tungiasis
Tungidae
tungstate
  calcium t.
tungsten (W)
  t. arc lamp
  t. carbide
tunic
  Bichat t.
  Brücke t.
  fibrous t. of corpus spongiosum
  fibrous t. of eye
  mucosal t.'s
  mucous t.
  muscular t.'s
  muscular t. of gallbladder
  nervous t. of eyeball
  serous t.
  vascular t. of eye
tunica, pl. **tunicae**
  t. adventitia
  t. albuginea
  t. albuginea of corpora cavernosa
  t. albuginea corporis spongiosi
  t. albuginea corporum cavernosorum
  t. albuginea of corpus spongiosum
  t. albuginea oculi
  t. albuginea ovarii
  t. albuginea of ovary
  t. albuginea of testis
  t. albuginea testis
  t. carnea
  t. conjunctiva
  t. conjunctiva bulbi
  t. conjunctiva palpebrarum
  t. dartos
  t. elastica
  t. externa
  t. externa oculi
  t. externa thecae folliculi
  t. extima

T

tunica (*continued*)
  t. fibromusculocartilaginea bronchi
  t. fibrosa
  t. fibrosa bulbi
  t. fibrosa hepatis
  t. fibrosa lienis
  t. fibrosa renis
  t. fibrosa splenis
  tunicae funiculi spermatici
  Haller t. vasculosa
  t. interna bulbi
  t. interna thecae folliculi
  t. intima
  t. media
  t. mucosa
  t. mucosa bronchi
  t. mucosa cavitatis tympani
  t. mucosa coli
  t. mucosa ductus deferentis
  t. mucosa esophagi
  t. mucosa gastrica
  t. mucosa intestini crassi
  t. mucosa intestini tenuis
  t. mucosa laryngis
  t. mucosa linguae
  t. mucosa nasi
  t. mucosa oris
  t. mucosa pelvis renalis
  t. mucosa pharyngis
  t. mucosa tracheae
  t. mucosa tubae auditivae
  t. mucosa tubae auditoriae
  t. mucosa tubae uterinae
  t. mucosa ureteris
  t. mucosa urethrae femininae
  t. mucosa uteri
  t. mucosa vaginae
  t. mucosa vesicae biliaris
  t. mucosa vesicae felleae
  t. mucosa vesicae urinariae
  t. mucosa vesiculae seminalis
  t. muscularis
  t. muscularis bronchiorum
  t. muscularis coli
  t. muscularis ductus deferentis
  t. muscularis esophagi
  t. muscularis gastrica
  t. muscularis glandulae vesiculosae
  t. muscularis intestini crassi
  t. muscularis intestini tenuis
  t. muscularis partis intermediae
    urethrae masculinae
  t. muscularis partis prostaticae
    urethrae masculinae
  t. muscularis partis spongiosae
    urethrae masculinae
  t. muscularis pelvis renalis
  t. muscularis pharyngis
  t. muscularis recti
  t. muscularis tracheae
  t. muscularis tubae uterinae
  t. muscularis ureteris
  t. muscularis urethrae femininae
  t. muscularis urethrae masculinae
  t. muscularis uteri
  t. muscularis vaginae
  t. muscularis ventriculi
  t. muscularis vesicae biliaris
  t. muscularis vesicae felleae
  t. muscularis vesicae urinariae
  t. nervea
  t. propria
  t. propria corii
  t. propria lienis
  t. reflexa
  t. sclerotica
  t. serosa
  t. serosa coli
  t. serosa esophagi
  t. serosa gastricae
  t. serosa hepatis
  t. serosa intestini crassi
  t. serosa intestini tenuis
  t. serosa pericardii serosi
  t. serosa peritonei
  t. serosa pleurae parietalis
  t. serosa pleurae visceralis
  t. serosa splenis
  t. serosa tubae uterinae
  t. serosa uteri
  t. serosa ventriculi
  t. serosa vesicae biliaris
  t. serosa vesicae felleae
  t. serosa vesicae (urinariae)
  t. spongiosa urethrae femininae
  t. spongiosa vaginae
  t. submucosa
  t. urethrae masculinae
  t. vaginalis communis
  t. vaginalis testis
  t. vasculosa
  t. vasculosa bulbi
  t. vasculosa lentis
  t. vasculosa oculi
  t. vasculosa testis
  t. vitrea

tuning
  t. curve
  t. fork

tunnel
  aortico-left ventricular t.
  carpal t.
  t. cell
  Corti t.
  t. disease
  t. vision

Tuohy needle
T₃ uptake test
turanose
turban tumor
Turbatrix aceti
turbid
turbidimeter
turbidimetric
turbidimetry
turbidity
turbinal
  t. varix
turbinate

turbinated
　　t. body
　　t. bone
　　t. crest
turbinectomy
turbinotome
turbinotomy
turbulence
　　heart rate t.
Türck
　　T. bundle
　　T. column
　　T. degeneration
　　T. tract
Turcot syndrome
turgescence
turgescent
turgid
turgor vitalis
turista
Türk
　　T. cell
　　T. leukocyte
turkey
　　t. gobbler neck
　　t. red
Turkish saddle
Turlock virus
turmeric
turn
Turner
　　T. sulcus
　　T. syndrome
　　T. tooth
turnover
　　t. number
turpentine
　　Canada t.
　　Chian t.
　　t. enema
　　larch t.
　　t. oil
　　t. poisoning
　　rectified t. oil
　　t. spirit
　　Venice t.
　　white t.
turps
turricephaly
TUR syndrome
turunda, pl. **turundae**
tussal
tussicular
tussiculation
tussigenic
tussis
tussive
　　t. fremitus
　　t. syncope
tutamen, pl. **tutamina**
　　tutamina cerebri
　　tutamina oculi
Tuttle proctoscope
TUU
　　transureteroureterostomy

TVG
　　time-varied gain
TWAR
　　Chlamydia pneumoniae
Tweed
　　T. edgewise treatment
　　T. triangle
tweezers
twelfth cranial nerve [CN XII]
twelfth-year molar
twenty-nail dystrophy
twiddler's syndrome
twig
twilight
　　t. state
　　t. vision
twin
　　allantoidoangiopagous t.'s
　　t. cone
　　conjoined asymmetric t.
　　conjoined equal t.
　　conjoined symmetric t.
　　conjoined unequal t.
　　t. crystal
　　dichorial t.'s
　　diovular t.
　　dizygotic t.'s
　　enzygotic t.
　　fraternal t.'s
　　t. helix
　　heterologous t.'s
　　identical t.'s
　　incomplete conjoined t.
　　locked t.'s
　　t. method
　　monoamniotic t.'s
　　monochorial t.'s
　　monovular t.'s
　　monozygotic t.'s
　　parasitic t.
　　t. placenta
　　placental parasitic t.
　　polyzygotic t.
　　t. pregnancy
　　t. reversed arterial perfusion sequence (TRAP)
　　Siamese t.
　　uniovular t.'s
twinge
twinning
twin-twin transfusion
twisted hair
twist form
twitch
two-bellied muscle
two-carbon fragment
two-dimensional
　　t.-d. chromatography
　　t.-d. echocardiography
　　t.-d. immunoelectrophoresis
two-dimension–three-dimension phenomenon
two-glass test
two-headed muscle
Twort-d'Herelle phenomenon

T

Twort phenomenon
two-step exercise test
two-tail test
two-way catheter
TX
　　individual thromboxane
　　thromboxane
TY1-S-33 medium
tybamate
tying forceps
tylectomy
tylion, pl. **tylia**
tyloma
　　tyloma conjunctivae
tylosis, pl. **tyloses**
　　t. ciliaris
　　t. linguae
　　t. palmaris et plantaris
tyloxapol
tymazoline
tympan- (*var. of* tympano-)
tympana (*pl. of* tympanum)
tympanal
tympanectomy
tympani- (*var. of* tympano-)
tympania
tympanic
　　t. air cell
　　t. antrum
　　t. aperture of canaliculus
　　t. attic
　　t. body
　　t. bone
　　t. canal
　　t. canaliculus
　　t. cavity
　　t. enlargement
　　t. ganglion
　　t. gland
　　t. groove
　　t. incisure
　　t. intumescence
　　t. labium of limbus of spiral lamina
　　t. lamella
　　t. lip of limbus of spiral lamina
　　t. lip of spiral limbus
　　t. membrane
　　t. nerve
　　t. notch
　　t. opening of canaliculus for chorda tympani
　　t. opening of eustachian tube
　　t. opening of pharyngotympanic auditory tube
　　t. part of temporal bone
　　t. plate of temporal bone
　　t. plexus
　　t. promontory
　　t. ring
　　t. scute
　　t. sinus
　　t. sulcus
　　t. surface of cochlear duct
　　t. vein
　　t. wall of cochlear duct
tympanichord
tympanichordal
tympanicity
tympanism
tympanites
　　uterine t.
tympanitic resonance
tympanitis
tympano-, tympan-, tympani-
tympanocentesis
tympanoeustachian
tympanogram
tympanohyal bone
tympanomalleal
tympanomandibular
tympanomastoid
　　t. fissure
　　t. suture
tympanomastoidectomy
tympanomastoiditis
tympanometry
tympanophonia, tympanophony
tympanoplasty
tympanosclerosis
tympanosquamosal
tympanosquamous fissure
tympanostapedial
　　t. junction
　　t. syndesmosis
tympanostomy tube
tympanotemporal
tympanotomy
tympanum, pl. **tympana**
tympany
　　Škoda t.
Tyndall
　　T. effect
　　T. phenomenon
tyndallization
type
　　t. A, B behavior
　　t. A, B personality
　　ampullary t. of renal pelvis
　　basic personality t.
　　blood t.
　　branching t. of renal pelvis
　　buffalo t.
　　t. 1, 2 choroidal neovascularization
　　t. culture
　　t. 1, 2, 3, 4 dextrocardia
　　t. 1, 2 diabetes
　　t. 2 diabetes mellitus
　　t. 1 G_{M1} gangliosidosis
　　t. 1, 2, 3, 4, 5, 6, 7 glycogenosis
　　t. IA, IB, II achondrogenesis
　　t. IH mucopolysaccharidosis
　　t. I H/S mucopolysaccharidosis
　　t. I, II cell
　　t. I, II error
　　t. III hypersensitivity reaction
　　t. I, II, III, IV collagen
　　t. I, II, III, IV osteogenesis imperfecta

t. I, II, III, IV, V familial hyperlipoproteinemia
t. I, II, III, V acrocephalosyndactyly
t. II, III, V, VI, VII mucopolysaccharidosis
t. I, II interferon
t. III punctate palmoplantar keratoderma
t. IS mucopolysaccharidosis
t. IVA, B mucopolysaccharidosis
nomenclatural t.
t. species
t. strain
test t.
wild t.

typhinia
typhl- (*var. of* typhlo-)
typhlectasis
typhlectomy
typhlenteritis
typhlitis
typhlo-, typhl-
typhlodicliditis
typhloempyema
typhloenteritis
typhlolithiasis
typhlomegaly
typhlon
typhlopexy, typhlopexia
typhlorrhaphy
typhlosis
typhlostomy
typhlotomy
typho-
typhoid

abdominal t.
ambulatory t.
apyretic t.
t. bacillus
t. bacteriophage
bilious t. of Griesinger
t. cholera
t. fever
fowl t.
latent t.
t. pleurisy
t. pneumonia
provocation t.
t. septicemia
t. vaccine
walking t.

typhoidal
typhoid-paratyphoid A and B vaccine
typholysin
typhomania
typhosepsis
typhous
typhus

Australian tick t.
endemic t.
epidemic t.
European t.
exanthematous t.
flea-borne t.
Indian tick t.

louse-borne t.
Manchurian t.
Mexican t.
mite t.
mite-born t.
t. mitior
murine t.
North Queensland tick t.
prison fever t.
Queensland tick t.
recrudescent t.
Sao Paulo t.
scrub t.
shop t.
Siberian tick t.
tick t.
tropical t.
urban t.
t. vaccine

typical

t. achromatopsia
t. antipsychotic agent
t. drusen
t. pseudocholinesterase

typing

bacteriophage t.
HLA t.

typist's cramp
typus

t. ampullaris pelvis renalis
t. dendriticus pelvis renalis

Tyr
tyraminase
tyramine oxidase
tyrannism
tyremesis
tyrocidin, tyrocidine
Tyrode solution
tyrogenous
Tyroglyphus longior
tyroid
tyroketonuria
tyroma
tyropanoate sodium
Tyrophagus putrescentiae
tyrosinase
tyrosine (Y)

t. aminotransferase
t. iodinase
t. kinase
t. phenol-lyase
t. transaminase

tyrosinemia
tyrosinosis
tyrosinuria
tyrosis
tyrosyluria
tyrothricin
tyrotoxism
Tyrrell fascia
TYSGM-9 medium
Tyson gland
Tyzzeria
Tzanck

T. cell
T. test

T

Tzanck · **Tzanck**

Tzanck
  T. cell

T. test

υ

upsilon

U

unit

U

internal energy

ubihydroquinone
ubiquinol (H$_2$Q, QH$_2$)
ubiquinone
ubiquinone-6 (-Q$_6$)
ubiquinone-10 (-Q$_{10}$)
ubiquitin
ubiquitin-protease pathway
UDP

uridine 5-diphosphate

UDP-*N*-acetylglucosamine:lysosomal enzyme *N*-acetylglucosaminyl-1-phosphotransferase
UDPG

uridine diphosphoglucose

UDPGal

uridine diphosphogalactose

UDPgalactose
UDPgalactose 4-epimerase
UDPGlc

uridine diphosphoglucose

UDP-GlcUA

uridine diphosphoglucuronic acid

UDPglucose
UDPglucose 4-epimerase
UDPglucose-hexose-1-phosphate uridylyltransferase
UDPglucuronate-bilirubinglucuronoside glucuronosyltransferase
UDPglucuronate-bilirubin glucuronosyltransferase
UDPxylose
UFA

unesterified free fatty acid

Uffelmann reagent
UGI

upper gastrointestinal series

Uhl anomaly
Uhthoff

U. sign
U. symptom
U. syndrome

UIP

usual interstitial pneumonia

ukambin
ulcer

acute decubitus u.
anastomotic u.
Buruli u.
chrome u.
chronic u.
Curling u.
decubitus u.
dendritic corneal u.
dental u.
diphtherial u.
distention u.

elusive u.
fascicular u.
Fenwick-Hunner u.
Gaboon u.
gastric u.
gravitational u.
gummatous u.
hard u.
healed u.
herpetic u.
Hunner u.
hypopyon u.
indolent u.
inflamed u.
Mann-Williamson u.
marginal ring u. of cornea
Marjolin u.
Meleney u.
Mooren u.
Oriental u.
penetrating u.
peptic u.
perforated u.
perforating u. of foot
phagedenic u.
phlegmonous u.
pressure u.
recurrent aphthous u.'s
ring u. of cornea
rodent u.
Saemisch u.
serpent u. of cornea
serpiginous u.
serpiginous corneal u.
simple u.
sloughing u.
soft u.
stasis u.
stercoral u.
stomal u.
stress u.
Sutton u.
syphilitic u.
Syriac u.
Syrian u.
tanner's u.
trophic u.
tropical u.
undermining u.
varicose u.
venereal u.
venous u.
Zambesi u.

ulcera (*pl. of* ulcus)
ulcerate
ulcerated
ulceration

tracheal u.

ulcerative

u. colitis
u. pharyngitis
u. stomatitis

U

ulcerogenic
ulceroglandular
ulceromembranous
    u. gingivitis
    u. pharyngitis
ulcus, pl. **ulcera**
ule- (*var. of* ulo-)
ulegyria
ulerythema
    u. ophryogenes
Ulex europaeus
Ullmann
    U. line
    U. syndrome
Ullrich
ulna, pl. **ulnae**
ulnad
ulnar
    u. border of forearm
    u. branch of medial antebrachial
      cutaneous nerve
    u. bursa
    u. clubhand
    u. collateral ligament
    u. collateral ligament of elbow joint
    u. collateral ligament of wrist joint
    u. communicating branch of
      superficial radial nerve
    u. eminence of wrist
    u. extensor muscle of wrist
    u. flexor muscle of wrist
    u. head
    u. margin of forearm
    u. nerve
    u. notch
    u. recurrent artery
    u. reflex
    u. vein
ulnen
ulnocarpal
ulnoradial
ulo-, ule-
uloid
ulotrichous
ultimate
    u. principle
    u. strength
ultimobranchial
    u. body
    u. pouch
ultimum moriens
ultra-
ultrabrachycephalic
ultracentrifugation
ultracentrifuge
ultracytostome
ultradian
    u. rhythm
ultradolichocephalic
ultrafast Pap stain
ultrafilter
ultrafiltration
    u. coefficient
    u. hemodialyzer
ultralente insulin

ultraligation
ultramicroscope
ultramicroscopic
ultramicrotome
ultramicrotomy
ultrashortwave diathermy
ultrasonic
    u. cardiography
    u. cephalometry
    u. cleaning
    u. egg recovery
    u. lithotripsy
    u. microscope
    u. nebulizer
    u. ray
    u. scaler
    u. therapy
    u. waves
ultrasonics
ultrasonogram
ultrasonograph
ultrasonographer
ultrasonography
    Doppler u.
    duplex u.
    endovaginal u.
    gray-scale u.
    real-time u.
ultrasonosurgery
ultrasound
    u. cardiography
    diagnostic u.
    obstetric u.
    u. transducer
ultrastructural anatomy
ultrastructure
ultratherm
ultrathin section
ultraviolet (UV)
    u. A (UVA)
    u. B (UVB)
    u. C (UVC)
    extravital u.
    u. index
    intravital u.
    u. keratoconjunctivitis
    u. lamp
    u. microscope
    u. ray
    u. spectrum
ultromotivity
ultropaque method
ululation
Ulysses syndrome
umber
    u. codon
    u. mutation
umbilical
    u. artery
    u. cord
    u. cyst
    u. duct
    u. fascia
    u. fissure
    u. fistula

u. fossa
u. fungus
u. granuloma
u. hernia
u. notch
u. part of left branch of portal vein
u. prevesical fascia
u. region
u. ring
u. souffle
u. vein
u. vesicle
umbilicate
umbilicated cataract
umbilication
umbilici (*pl. of* umbilicus)
umbilicomammillary triangle
umbilicovesical fascia
umbilicus, pl. **umbilici**
umbo, pl. **umbones**
u. membranae tympani
u. of tympanic membrane
Umbre virus
UMP
uridine 5-monophosphate
u. synthase
un-
unarmed rostellum
unbalanced translocation
uncal
u. artery
u. herniation
unci (*pl. of* uncus)
uncia
unciform
u. bone
u. fasciculus
u. pancreas
unciforme
Uncinaria
uncinariasis
uncinate
u. attack
u. bundle of Russell
u. epilepsy
u. fasciculus of cerebellum
u. fasciculus of Russell
u. fit
u. gyrus
u. pancreas
u. process of cervical vertebra
u. process of ethmoid bone
u. process of first thoracic vertebra
u. process of pancreas
uncinatum
uncipressure
uncombable hair syndrome
uncomfortable level
uncompensated
u. acidosis
u. alkalosis
uncompetitive
u. inhibition
u. inhibitor

uncomplemented
unconditioned
u. reflex
u. response
u. stimulus
unconjugated bilirubin
unconscious
collective u.
u. homosexuality
unconsciousness
unco-ossified
uncouplers
uncoupling factor
uncovertebral joint
uncrossed diplopia
unction
unctuous
uncture
uncus, pl. **unci**
u. band of Giacomini
u. gyri parahippocampalis
undecenoic acid
undecoylium chloride
undecoylium chloride-iodine
undecylenate
undecylenic acid
underachievement
underachiever
underbite
undercut gauge
underdrive pacing
undermining ulcer
undernutrition
undersensing
undershoot
understain
underventilation
underwinding
undescended testis
undetermined nitrogen
undifferentiated
u. cell
u. cell adenoma
u. type fever
undine
undiversion
undoing
undulant fever
undulate
undulating
u. fever
u. membrane
u. pulse
undulipodium, pl. **undulipodia**
unequal
u. cleavage
u. crossing-over
u. pulse
u. retinal image
unerupted tooth
unesterified free fatty acid (FFA, UFA)
uneven crossing-over
unformed visual hallucination
ung

U

ungual
> u. phalanx
> u. tuberosity

unguent

ungues (*pl. of* unguis)

Unguiculata

unguiculate

unguiculus

unguinal

unguis, pl. **ungues**
> u. aduncus
> u. avis
> Haller u.
> u. incarnatus

Ungulata

ungulate

unguligrade

uni-

uniarticular

uniaxial joint

unibasal

Uniblue A

unicameral, unicamerate
> u. bone cyst

unicanalicular sphincter

unicellular
> u. gland
> u. sclerosis

unicentral

unicornous, unicornate, unicornuate

unicorn uterus

unicuspid, unicuspidate

unidentified reading frame (URF)

unidirectional
> u. block
> u. flux
> u. replication

unifamilial

uniflagellate

uniforate

uniform

unigerminal

uniglandular

unilaminar, unilaminate
> u. primary follicle

unilateral
> u. anesthesia
> u. hemianopia
> u. hermaphroditism
> u. hyperlucent lung
> u. lobar emphysema

unilobar

unilocal

unilocular
> u. fat
> u. hemianopia
> u. hydatid cyst
> u. joint

unimolecular reaction

uninducible mutant

uninhibited neurogenic bladder

uninterrupted suture

uninuclear, uninucleate

uniocular

union
> autogenous u.
> faulty u.
> fibrous u.
> primary u.
> secondary u.
> vicious u.

uniovular, unioval
> u. twins

unipennate muscle

unipolar
> u. cell
> u. electrocardiogram
> u. lead
> u. neuron

uniport

uniporter

unipotent

uniseptate

unit (U)
> absolute u.
> alexin u.
> Allen-Doisy u.
> alpha u.'s
> amboceptor u.
> androgen u.
> Ångström u.
> antigen u.
> antitoxin u.
> antivenene u.
> atomic mass u. (amu)
> base u.'s
> bel u.
> Bethesda u.
> biologic standard u.
> bird u.
> Bodansky u.
> British thermal u. (BTU)
> capon u.
> capon-comb u.
> cat u.
> centimeter-gram-second u.
> CGS u.
> u. character
> chlorophyll u.
> chorionic gonadotropin u.
> Clauberg u.
> colony-forming u.
> complement u.
> u. of convergence
> Corner-Allen u.
> coronary care u. (CCU)
> corpus luteum hormone u.
> critical care u.
> CT u.
> Dam u.
> digitalis u.
> diphtheria antitoxin u.
> dog u.
> electromagnetic u. (emu)
> electrostatic u. (esu)
> u. of energy
> epidermal-melanin u.
> equine gonadotropin u.
> estradiol benzoate u.

estrone u.
u. fibril
Fishman-Lerner u.
Florey u.
foot-pound-second u.
u. of force
FPS u.
gravitational u.'s
G u. of streptomycin
u. of heat
hemolysin u., hemolytic u.
heparin u.
Holzknecht u.
Hounsfield u.
Howell u.
insulin u.
intensive care u. (ICU)
u. of intermedin
international u. (IU)
International System of U.'s (SI)
Jenner-Kay u.
Karmen u.
Kienböck u. (X)
King u.
King-Armstrong u.
u. of length
u. of light
L u. of streptomycin
u. of luminous flux
u. of luminous intensity
lung u.
u. of luteinizing activity
u. of magnetic field intensity
u. of magnetic flux intensity
u. of mass
u. membrane
meter-kilogram-second u., MKS u.
Montevideo u.'s
motor u.
mouse u. (m.u.)
u. of ocular convergence
ostiomeatal u.
Oxford u.
u. of oxytocin
u. of penicillin
phosphatase u.
physiologic u.
u. of pitch (mel)
practical u.'s
u. of progestational activity
progesterone u.
prolactin u.
u. of radioactivity
riboflavin u.
roentgen u.
Schwann cell u.
Sherman u.
Sherman-Bourquin u. of vitamin B_2
Sherman-Munsell u.
SI u.'s
Somogyi u.
S u. of streptomycin
Steenbock u.
streptomycin u.'s
Svedberg u.

terminal respiratory u.
tetanus antitoxin u.
thiamin chloride u.
thiamin hydrochloride u.
u. of thyrotrophic activity
Todd u.
toxic u. (T.U.)
toxin u.
USP u.
u. of vasopressin
vitamin A u.
vitamin B_2, B_6 u.
vitamin B_1 hydrochloride u.
vitamin C u.
vitamin D u.
vitamin E u.
vitamin K u.
volume u. (VU)
u. of wavelength
u. of weight
Wood u.'s
u. of work
United States Adopted Names (USAN)
United States Pharmacopeia (USP)
United States Public Health Service (USPHS)
uniting
u. canal
u. cartilage
u. duct
univalence, univalency
univalent antibody
univentricular
u. connection
u. heart
universal
u. antidote
u. appliance
u. donor
u. infantilism
u. solvent
Universal Precautions
unmedullated
unmodified zinc oxide-eugenol cement
unmyelinated
u. fiber
u. nerve
Unna
U. boot
U. disease
U. nevus
U. stain
Unna-Pappenheim stain
Unna-Taenzer stain
Unna-Thost syndrome
unofficial
unpaired
u. allosome
u. chromosome
u. thyroid venous plexus
unphysiologic
unresolved pneumonia
unroofed coronary sinus syndrome
unsanitary

U

unsaturated
- u. alcohol
- u. fat
- u. fatty acid

unsex

unsharp masking

unspecified amino acid (Xaa)

unstable
- u. angina
- u. bladder
- u. colloid
- u. equilibrium
- u. fracture
- u. hemoglobin hemolytic anemia
- u. hemoglobins
- u. lie

unstrained jaw relation

unstriated muscle

unsystematized delusion

unthrifty

ununited fracture

Unverricht disease

unwinding protein

upbeat nystagmus

UPJ
- ureteropelvic junction

upper
- u. abdominal periosteal reflex
- u. airway
- u. dental arcade
- u. esophageal constriction
- u. extremity
- u. extremity of fibula
- u. eyelid
- u. gastrointestinal series (UGI)
- u. GI series
- u. jaw
- u. jaw bone
- u. lateral cutaneous nerve of arm
- u. lid
- u. limb
- u. lip
- u. lobe of lung
- u. motor neuron
- u. motor neuron lesion
- u. pole
- u. pole of testis
- u. subscapular nerve
- u. thoracic splanchnic nerve
- u. uterine segment

up promoter mutation

upregulation

upregulation/downregulation hypothesis

upsiloid

upsilon (υ)

upstream

uptake

Ura
- uracil

urachal
- u. cyst
- u. fistula
- u. fold
- u. ligament

urachus

uracil (Ura)
- u. dehydrogenase
- u. mustard
- u. oxidase
- u. phosphoribosyltransferase

uracil-6-carboxylic acid

Uragoga

uramustine

uranin

uraninite

uranisco- (*var. of* urano-)

uraniscochasm

uranisconitis

uraniscoplasty

uraniscorrhaphy

uraniscus

uranium nephritis

urano-, uranisco-

uranoplasty

uranorrhaphy

uranoschisis

uranostaphyloplasty

uranostaphylorrhaphy

uranostaphyloschisis

uranoveloschisis

uranyl acetate stain

urapidil

uraroma

urarthritis

urate
- u. crystals stain
- u. oxidase

uratemia

urateribonucleotide phosphorylase

uratic

uratolysis

uratolytic

uratoma

uratosis

uraturia

Urbach-Wiethe disease

Urban
- u. cutaneous leishmaniasis
- U. operation
- u. typhus

urceiform

urceolate

Urd
- uridine

ur-defenses

ure-, urea-, ureo-

urea
- u. clearance
- u. clearance test
- u. cycle
- u. frost
- u. nitrogen
- u. peroxide
- u. stibamine

ureagenesis

ureal

Ureaplasma
- *u. urealyticum*

ureapoiesis

urease test
urecholine supersensitivity test
uredema
ureic
ureide
3-ureidohydantoin
3-ureidoisobutyric acid
3-ureidopropionic acid
ureidosuccinic acid
urelcosis
uremia
     hypercalcemic u.
uremic
     u. breath
     u. colitis
     u. coma
     u. lung
     u. pericarditis
     u. pneumonia
     u. pneumonitis
     u. polyneuropathy
uremigenic
ureo- (*var. of* ure-)
ureotele
ureotelia
ureotelic
urerythrin
uresiesthesia
uresis
ureter
     curlicue u.
     ectopic u.
     ileal u.
     postcaval u.
     retrocaval u.
     retroiliac u.
ureteral
     u. branch
     u. colic
     u. ectopia
     u. meatus
     u. opening
     u. reimplantation
ureteralgia
uretercystoscope
ureterectasia
ureterectomy
ureteric
     u. branch
     u. branch of the inferior suprarenal artery
     u. branch of the ovarian artery
     u. branch of the patent part of umbilical artery
     u. branch of the renal artery
     u. branch of the testicular artery
     u. bud
     u. dysmenorrhea
     u. fold
     u. orifice
     u. pelvis
     u. plexus
ureteritis
uretero-
ureterocalicostomy

ureterocele
     ectopic u.
     orthotopic u.
ureterocelorraphy
ureterocolic
ureterocolostomy
ureterocutaneous fistula
ureterocystoplasty
ureterocystoscope
ureterocystostomy
ureteroenteric
ureteroenterostomy
ureterography
ureterohydronephrosis
ureteroileal anastomosis
ureteroileoneocystostomy
ureteroileostomy
ureterolithiasis
ureterolithotomy
ureterolysis
ureteroneocystostomy
ureteronephrectomy
ureteropathy
ureteropelvic
     u. junction (UPJ)
     u. junction obstruction
ureteroplasty
ureteroproctostomy
ureteropyelitis
ureteropyelography
ureteropyeloplasty
ureteropyelostomy
ureteropyosis
ureterorectostomy
ureterorenal reflux
ureterorrhagia
ureterorrhaphy
ureteroscope
ureterosigmoid anastomosis
ureterosigmoidostomy
ureterostenosis
ureterostomy
     cutaneous u.
     cutaneous loop u.
ureterotomy
ureterotrigonoenterostomy
ureteroureteral anastomosis
ureteroureterostomy
ureterovaginal fistula
ureterovesical
     u. junction
     u. obstruction
ureterovesicostomy
urethan, urethane
urethr- (*var. of* urethro-)
urethra
     anterior u.
     female u.
     u. feminina
     male u.
     u. masculina
     membranous u.
     u. muliebris
     penile u.
     posterior u.

U

urethra *(continued)*
    prostatic u.
    spongy u.
    u. virilis
urethral
    u. artery
    u. calculus
    u. carina of vagina
    u. caruncle
    u. crest
    u. crest of female
    u. crest of male
    u. dilation
    u. diverticulum
    u. fever
    u. gland
    u. groove
    u. hematuria
    u. lacuna
    u. opening
    u. papilla
    u. plate
    u. pressure profile
    u. stricture
    u. surface of penis
    u. syndrome
    u. valves
urethralgia
urethrectomy
urethremorrhagia
urethrism, urethrismus
urethritis
    anterior u.
    follicular u.
    gonorrheal u.
    granular u.
    nongonococcal u.
    nonspecific u.
    u. petrificans
    posterior u.
    simple u.
urethro-, urethr-
urethrobulbar
urethrocele
urethrocutaneous fistula
urethrocystometrography
urethrocystometry
urethrocystopexy
urethrodynia
urethrography
urethrometer
urethropenile
urethroperineal
urethroperineoscrotal
urethropexy
urethroplasty
    Cecil u.
urethroprostatic
urethrorectal
urethrorrhagia
urethrorrhaphy
urethrorrhea
urethroscope
urethroscopic

urethroscopy
urethrospasm
urethrostaxis
urethrostenosis
urethrostomy
    perineal u.
urethrotome
urethrotomy
    external u.
    internal u.
    perineal u.
urethrovaginal
    u. fistula
    u. sphincter
urethrovesical angle
urethrovesicopexy
-uretic
URF
    unidentified reading frame
urge incontinence
urgency
    motor u.
    sensory u.
urginea
uri-, uric-, urico-
urian
uric acid
    u. a. oxidase
uric acid infarct
uricase
urico- *(var. of* uri-)
uricolysis
uricolytic index
uricosome
uricosuria
uricosuric
uricotele
uricotelia
uricotelic
uridine (Urd)
    cyclic u. 3′,5′-monophosphate
    (cUMP)
    u. 5′-diphosphate (UDP)
    u. diphosphoxylose
    u. 5′-monophosphate (UMP)
    u. phosphorylase
    u. 5′-triphosphate (UTP)
uridine diphosphogalactose (UDPGal)
    u. d. 4-epimerase
uridine diphosphoglucose (UDPG, UDPGlc)
    u. d. 4-epimerase
uridine diphosphoglucuronic acid (UDP-GlcUA)
uridrosis
    u. crystallina
uridylic acid synthase
uridyltransferase
uriesthesia
urin-, urino-
urinal
urinalysis
urinary
    u. apparatus
    u. bladder

u. calculus
u. cast
u. concentration test
u. cyst
u. exertional incontinence
u. fever
u. fistula
u. nitrogen
u. organ
u. reflex
u. sand
u. schistosomiasis
u. smear
u. stuttering
u. system
u. tract
u. tract infection (UTI)
urinate
urination
stuttering u.
urine
ammoniacal u.
black u.
chylous u.
cloudy u.
crude u.
febrile u.
feverish u.
gouty u.
honey u.
maple syrup u.
milky u.
nebulous u.
residual u.
uriniferous tubule
urinific
uriniparous
urino- (*var. of* urin-)
urinogenital
urinogenous
urinoma
urinometer
urinometry
urinoscopy
urinosexual
urinous
uriposia
uro-
uroammoniac
uroanthelone
urobilin
urobilinemia
urobilin IXα
urobilinogen
urobilinogen IXα
urobilinuria
urocanase
urocanate
u. hydratase
urocanic
urocanic acid
urocanic aciduria
urocanicase
urocele
urocheras

urochesia
urochrome
urochromogen
urocrisia
urocrisis
urocyanin
urocyanogen
urocyanosis
urocyst
urocystic
urocystis
urodynamics
urodynia
uroenterone
uroerythrin
uroflavin
uroflowmeter
urofollitropin
urofuscohematin
urogastrone
urogenital
u. apparatus
u. cleft
u. diaphragm
u. fistula
u. membrane
u. mesentery
u. peritoneum
u. region
u. ridge
u. septum
u. sinus
u. sinus anomaly
u. system
u. triangle
urogenous
uroglaucin
urogonadotropin
urograffin
urogram
intravenous u. (IVU)
urography
antegrade u.
cystoscopic u.
excretory u.
intravenous u.
retrograde u.
urogravimeter
urohematin
urohematoporphyrin
uroheparin
urohypertensin
urokinase
urolagnia
uroleucinic acid, uroleucic acid
urolith
urolithiasis
urolithic
urolithology
urologic, urological
urologist
urology
urolutein
uromelanin
urometer

U

uroncus
uronic acids
uronoscopy
uropathy
    obstructive u.
urophanic
urophein
uropoiesis
uropoietic system
uroporphyrin
    u. I
    u. III
uroporphyrinogen
    u. decarboxylase
    u. III cosynthase
uropsammus
uropterin
uropurpurin
uroradiology
urorectal
    u. fold
    u. membrane
    u. septum
urorosein
urorubin
urorubrohematin
uroschesis
uroscopic
uroscopy
urosemiology
urosepsin
urosepsis
urospectrin
urothelial
    u. carcinoma
    u. papilloma
urothelium
urothion
urothorax
uroxanthin
uroxin
ursodeoxycholic acid
ursodiol
urtica
urticant
urticaria
    acute u.
    u. bullosa
    cholinergic u.
    chronic u.
    u. chronica
    cold u.
    u. endemica
    u. epidemica
    factitious u.
    febrile u.
    giant u.
    heat u.
    u. hemorrhagica
    u. maculosa
    u. medicamentosa
    papular u.
    u. perstans
    u. pigmentosa
    pressure u.

    solar u.
    u. subcutanea
    u. vesiculosa
    vibratory u.
urticarial
    u. fever
    u. vasculitis
urticate
urtication
urushiol oxidase
USAN
    United States Adopted Names
u-score method
Usher syndrome
USP
    United States Pharmacopeia
USPHS
    United States Public Health Service
USP unit
ustilaginism
Ustilago
    U. maydis
    U. zeae
ustulation
usual
    u. interstitial pneumonia (UIP)
    u. interstitial pneumonia of Liebow
usurpation
uta
uter- (*var. of* utero-)
uteri (*pl. of* uterus)
uterine
    u. appendages
    u. artery
    u. atony
    u. calculus
    u. cavity
    u. colic
    u. contraction
    u. dysmenorrhea
    u. extremity of ovary
    u. gland
    u. horn
    u. inertia
    u. insufficiency
    u. opening of uterine tubes
    u. ostium of uterine tubes
    u. part of uterine tube
    u. pregnancy
    u. sinus
    u. sinusoid
    u. souffle
    u. tetanus
    u. tube
    u. tympanites
    u. vein
    u. venous plexus
in utero
utero-, uter-
uteroabdominal pregnancy
uterocervical
uterocystostomy
uteroepichorial membrane
uterofixation
uteroglobin

uteroglobin-adducin
uterolith
uterometer
utero-ovarian varicocele
uteroparietal
uteropelvic
uteroperitoneal fistula
uteropexy
uteroplacental
    u. apoplexy
    u. sinus
uteroplasty
uterosacral
uterosalpingography
uteroscope
uteroscopy
uterotomy
uterotonic
uterotropic
uterotubal
uterotubography
uterovaginal
    u. canal
    u. plexus
uteroventral
uteroverdine
uterovesical
    u. fold
    u. ligament
    u. pouch
uterus, pl. uteri
    u. acollis
    anomalous u.
    arcuate u.
    u. arcuatus
    u. bicornis
    u. bicornis bicollis
    u. bicornis unicollis
    bicornous u.
    bifid u.
    u. bifidus
    biforate u.
    u. biforis
    u. bilocularis
    bipartite u.
    u. bipartitus
    cordiform u.
    u. cordiformis
    Couvelaire u.
    u. didelphys
    double-mouthed u.
    duplex u.
    u. duplex
    gravid u.
    heart-shaped u.
    incudiform u.
    u. incudiformis
    large loop excision of
      transformation zone of the cervix
      of the u. (LLETZ)
    masculine u.
    u. masculinus
    one-horned u.
    u. parvicollis
    septate u.

    u. septus
    subseptate u.
    u. subseptus
    triangular u.
    u. triangularis
    unicorn u.
    u. unicornis
UTI
    urinary tract infection
utility
utilization time
UTP
    uridine 5-triphosphate
utricle
    prostatic u.
    u. of vestibular labyrinth
utricular
    u. cyst
    u. duct
    u. nerve
    u. recess of bony labyrinth
    u. recess of membranous labyrinth
    u. reflex
    u. spot
utriculi (pl. of utriculus)
utriculitis
utriculoampullar nerve
utriculosaccular duct
utriculus, pl. utriculi
    u. prostaticus
utriform
UV
    ultraviolet
UVA
    ultraviolet A
uvaeformis
uva ursi
UVB
    ultraviolet B
UVC
    ultraviolet C
uvea
uveal
    u. part of trabecular reticulum
    u. part of trabecular tissue of
      sclera
    u. staphyloma
    u. tract
uveitic
uveitis, pl. uveitides
    anterior u.
    Förster u.
    Fuchs u.
    heterochromic u.
    intermediate u.
    lens-induced u.
    phacoanaphylactic u.
    phacogenic u.
    posterior u.
    sympathetic u.
uveocutaneous syndrome
uveoencephalitic syndrome
uveoencephalitis
uveomeningitis syndrome
uveoparotid fever

U

uveoscleritis
uviform
uviofast
uviol
uviometer
uvioresistant
uviosensitive
uvitex 2B
uvomorulin
uvul- (*var. of* uvulo-)
uvula, pl. uvuli
    bifid u.
    u. of bladder
    u. cerebelli
    Lieutaud u.
    u. palatina
    palatine u.
    u. of soft palate
    u. [TA] of cerebellum

    uvula [TA] of cerebellum
    u. vermis
    u. vesicae
uvulaptosis
uvularis
uvular muscle
uvulatome
uvulectomy
uvuli (*pl. of* uvula)
uvulitis
uvulo-, uvul-
uvulopalatopharyngoplasty
uvulopalatoplasty
uvuloptosis
uvulotome
uvulotomy
U wave
Uzbekistan hemorrhagic fever

V
gas flow
visual acuity
V antigen
V gene
V lead
V wave

V̇
V_D
physiologic dead space
V_T
tidal volume
V_{O2}
oxygen consumption
V_{CO2}
carbon dioxide elimination
V
volume
V_{max}
maximum velocity
v
velocity
v̄
mixed venous blood

V-2 carcinoma
VA
ventriculoatrial
VA conduction
VA
alveolar ventilation
VAC
ventriculoatrial conduction
vaccenic acid
vaccina
vaccinal
vaccinate
vaccination
vaccinator
vaccine
adjuvant v.
aqueous v.
attenuated v.
autogenous v.
bacillus Calmette-Guérin v.
BCG v.
v. body
Brucella strain 19 v.
Calmette-Guérin v.
cholera v.
crystal violet v.
diphtheria, tetanus, and acellular
pertussis v. (DTaP)
diphtheria toxoid, tetanus toxoid,
and pertussis v. (DPT, DTP)
duck embryo origin v. (DEV)
Flury strain v.
foot-and-mouth disease virus v.'s
Haemophilus influenzae type B v.
Haffkine v.
hepatitis B v.
heterogenous v.
Hib v.

high-egg-passage v., HEP v.
hog cholera v.'s
human diploid cell v. (HDCV)
human diploid cell rabies v.
inactivated poliovirus v. (IPV)
influenza virus v.'s
live v.
live oral poliovirus v.
low-egg-passage v., LEP v.
v. lymph
measles, mumps, and rubella v.
(MMR)
measles virus v.
multivalent v.
mumps virus v.
oil v.
oral poliovirus v. (OPV)
Pasteur v.
pertussis v.
plague v.
pneumococcal v.
poliomyelitis v.'s
poliovirus v.
polysaccharide conjugated v.
polyvalent v.
rabies v.
rabies v., Flury strain egg-passage
rickettsia v., attenuated
Rocky Mountain spotted fever v.
rubella virus v., live
Sabin v.
Salk v.
Semple v.
smallpox v.
split-virus v.
staphylococcus v.
stock v.
subunit v.
T.A.B. v.
tetanus v.
tuberculosis v.
typhoid v.
typhoid-paratyphoid A and B v.
typhus v.
v. virus
whooping-cough v.
yellow fever v.
vaccinia
v. gangrenosa
generalized v.
v. lymph
progressive v.
v. virus
vaccinial
vacciniform
vaccinist
vaccinization
vaccinogen
vaccinogenous
vaccinoid
v. reaction
vaccinostyle

V

vaccinum
VACTERL syndrome
in vacuo
vacuolar
    v. degeneration
    v. nephrosis
vacuolate, vacuolated
vacuolating virus
vacuolation
vacuole
    autophagic v.
    contractile v.
    digestive v.
    parasitophorous v.
vacuolization
vacuome
vacuum
    v. aspirator
    v. casting
    v. desiccator
    v. disk phenomenon
    v. extractor
    v. flask
    v. headache
    v. investing
    v. pack technique
    v. tube
vadum
vagabond's disease
vagal
    v. attack
    v. bradycardia
    v. nerve stimulation
    v. nerve trigone
    v. nerve trunk
    v. part of accessory nerve
vagectomy
vagi (*pl. of* vagus)
vagin- (*var. of* vagino-)
vagina, pl. **vaginae**
    bipartite v.
    v. bulbi
    v. carotica
    v. cellulosa
    v. communis tendinum musculorum fibularium communis
    v. communis tendinum musculorum flexorum (manus)
    v. externa nervi optici
    vaginae fibrosae digitorum manus
    vaginae fibrosae digitorum pedis
    v. fibrosa tendinis
    v. interna nervi optici
    v. masculina
    v. mucosa tendinis
    v. musculi recti abdominis
    vaginae nervi optici
    v. oculi
    v. processus styloidei
    septate v.
    vaginae synoviales digitorum manus
    v. synovialis
    v. synovialis tendinis
    v. synovialis trochleae
    v. tendinis intertubercularis
    v. tendinis musculi extensoris carpi ulnaris
    v. tendinis musculi extensoris digiti minimi
    v. tendinis musculi extensoris hallucis longi
    v. tendinis musculi extensoris pollicis longi
    v. tendinis musculi fibularis longi plantaris
    v. tendinis musculi flexoris carpi radialis
    v. tendinis musculi flexoris hallucis longi
    v. tendinis musculi flexoris pollicis longi
    v. tendinis musculi obliqui superioris
    v. tendinis musculi peronei longi plantaris
    v. tendinis musculi tibialis anterioris
    v. tendinis musculi tibialis posterioris
    vaginae tendinum carpales palmares
    vaginae tendinum carpalium
    vaginae tendinum carpalium dorsalium
    vaginae tendinum digitorum pedis
    v. tendinum musculi extensoris digitorum pedis longi
    v. tendinum musculi flexoris digitorum pedis longi
    v. tendinum musculorum abductoris longi et extensoris brevis pollicis
    v. tendinum musculorum extensoris digitorum et extensoris indicis
    v. tendinum musculorum extensorum carpi radialium
    v. tendinum musculorum fibularium communis
    v. tendinum musculorum peroneorum communis
    vaginae tendinum tarsales anteriores
    vaginae tendinum tarsales fibulares
    vaginae tendinum tarsales tibialis
    vaginae vasorum
vaginal
    v. artery
    v. atresia
    v. celiotomy
    v. column
    v. cornification test
    v. cuff
    v. dysmenorrhea
    v. fornix
    v. gland
    v. hysterectomy
    v. hysterotomy
    v. intraepithelial neoplasia
    v. introitus
    v. laceration
    v. lithotomy
    v. mucification test
    v. mucosa
    v. myomectomy

v. nerve
v. opening
v. orifice
v. part of cervix
v. pool
v. process
v. process of peritoneum
v. process of sphenoid bone
v. process of testis
v. rugae
v. smear
v. synovial membrane
v. venous plexus
vaginapexy
vaginate
vaginectomy
vaginism
vaginismus
posterior v.
vaginitis, pl. **vaginitides**
v. adhesiva
adhesive v.
amebic v.
atrophic v.
v. cystica
desquamative inflammatory v.
v. emphysematosa
Gardnerella v.
nonspecific v.
pinworm v.
senile v.
v. senilis
vagino-, vagin-
vaginoabdominal
vaginocele
vaginodynia
vaginofixation
vaginohysterectomy
vaginolabial
vaginomycosis
vaginopathy
vaginoperineal
vaginoperineoplasty
vaginoperineorrhaphy
vaginoperineotomy
vaginoperitoneal
vaginopexy
vaginoplasty
vaginoscopy
vaginosis
bacterial v.
vaginotomy
vaginovesical
vaginovulvar
Vaginulus plebeius
vagitus uterinus
vago-
vagoaccessorius
vagoglossopharyngeal
vagolysis
vagolytic
vagomimetic
vagotomy
vagotonia
vagotonic

vagotropic
vagovagal
v. reflex
vagrant's disease
vagus, pl. **vagi** (*See also* vagi)
v. area
vagi eminentia
v. nerve [CN X]
v. pulse
valence, valency
v. electron
negative v.
positive v.
valent
Valentin
V. corpuscle
V. ganglion
V. nerve
Valentine
V. position
V. test
valepotriates
valerate
valerian
valerianate
valeric acid
valethamate bromide
valetudinarian
valetudinarianism
valgoid
valgus
valid
validation
consensual v.
validity
concurrent v.
construct v.
content v.
criterion-related v.
face v.
predictive v.
valine
valinomycin
valla (*pl. of* vallum)
vallate
v. papillae
vallecula, pl. **valleculae**
v. cerebelli
v. of cerebellum
epiglottic v.
v. epiglottica
v. sylvii
v. unguis
vallecular dysphagia
Valleix point
valley
v. fever
vallis
vallum, pl. **valla**
v. unguis
valmethamide
valnoctamide
valoid
valproic acid

V

Valsalva
  V. antrum
  V. ligament
  V. maneuver
  V. muscle
  V. sinus
  V. test
value
  acetyl v.
  buffer v.
  buffer v. of the blood
  C v.
  caloric v.
  Hehner v.
  homing v.
  iodine v.
  maturation v.
  normal v.
  pH v.
  phenotypic v.
  predictive v.
  R_f v.
  reference v.
  thiocyanogen v.
  threshold limit v. (TLV)
valva, pl. **valvae**
  v. aortae
  v. atrioventricularis dextra
  v. atrioventricularis sinistra
  v. ileocecalis
  v. mitralis
  v. tricuspidalis
  v. trunci pulmonalis
valval, valvar
valvate
valve
  Amussat v.
  anal v.'s
  anterior urethral v.
  aortic v.
  atrioventricular v.'s
  AV v.'s
  ball v.
  Bauhin v.
  Béraud v.
  bicuspid v.
  bileaflet v.
  biologic v.
  Björk-Shiley v.
  Blom-Singer v.
  Bochdalek v.
  Braune v.
  Carpentier-Edwards v.
  caval v.
  congenital v.
  coronary v.
  v. of coronary sinus
  eustachian v.
  v. of foramen ovale
  Gerlach v.
  Guérin v.
  Heister v.
  Heyer-Pudenz v.
  Hoboken v.'s
  Huschke v.

ileocecal v.
ileocolic v.
v. of inferior vena cava
Kerckring v.'s
Krause v.
left atrioventricular v.
Mercier v.
mitral v.
Morgagni v.'s
nasal v.
v. of navicular fossa
nonrebreathing v.
O'Beirne v.
v. of oval foramen
parachute mitral v.
porcine v.
posterior urethral v.'s
prosthetic v.
pulmonary v.
v. of pulmonary trunk
pulmonic v.
rectal v.
reducing v.
right atrioventricular v.
Rosenmüller v.
semilunar v.
spiral v. of cystic duct
Starr-Edwards v.
sylvian v.
Tarin v.
Terrien v.
thebesian v.
tilting disk v.
tissue v.
tricuspid v.
Tulp v., Tulpius v.
urethral v.'s
v. of Varolius
venous v.
v. of vermiform appendix
vesicoureteral v.
v. of Vieussens
Vieussens v.
valveless
valviform
valvoplasty
valvotomy
  v. knife
  mitral v.
  rectal v.
valvula, pl. **valvulae**
  Amussat v.
  valvulae anales
  v. bicuspidalis
  valvulae conniventes
  v. foraminis ovalis
  v. fossae navicularis
  Gerlach v.
  v. lymphatica
  v. processus vermiformis
  v. semilunaris
  v. semilunaris anterior valvae trunci
    pulmonalis
  v. semilunaris dextra valvae aortae

v. semilunaris dextra valvae trunci pulmonalis
v. semilunaris posterior valvae aortae
v. semilunaris sinistra valvae aortae
v. semilunaris sinistra valvae trunci pulmonalis
v. semilunaris tarini
v. sinus coronarii
v. spiralis
v. tricuspidalis
v. venae cavae inferioris
v. venosa
v. vestibuli
valvular
v. endocarditis
v. incompetence
v. insufficiency
v. prolapse
v. regurgitation
v. sclerosis
v. thrombus
valvule
Foltz v.
lymphatic v.
valvulitis
rheumatic v.
valvuloplasty
valvulotome
valvulotomy
valyl
vampire bat
van
v. Bogaert encephalitis
v. Buchem syndrome
v. Buren disease
v. Buren sound
v. Deen test
v. den Bergh test
v. der Hoeve syndrome
v. der Velden test
v. der Waals forces
v. Ermengen stain
v. Gieson stain
v. Helmont mirror
v. Horne canal
V. Lohuizen syndrome
V. Slyke apparatus
V. Slyke formula
vanadate
vanadic acid
vanadium
v. group
vancomycin
vandal root
vanilla
vanillate
vanillic acid
vanillin
vanillism
vanillylmandelic acid (VMA)
vanillylmandelic acid test
vanished testis syndrome
vanishing
v. cream

v. lung
v. lung syndrome
van't
v. Hoff equation
v. Hoff law
v. Hoff theory
vapor
anesthetic v.
v. density
v. pressure
vaporization
vaporize
vaporizer
flow-over v.
temperature-compensated v.
vaporthorax
vapotherapy
Va/Q
ventilation/perfusion ratio
Vaquez disease
variability
baseline v. of fetal heart rate
beat-to-beat v. of fetal heart rate
variable
continuous random v.
v. coupling
v. deceleration
dependent v.
discrete random v.
independent v.
intermediate v.
intervening v.
mixed discrete-continuous random v.
moderator v.
random v.
v. region
variable-interval reinforcement schedule
variance
ball v.
v. ratio
variant
v. angina pectoris
v. hemoglobin
inherited albumin v.'s
L-phase v.'s
variate
variation
continuous v.
varication
variceal
varicella
v. encephalitis
v. gangrenosa
varicellation
varicella-zoster virus
varicelliform
varicelloid
v. smallpox
Varicellovirus
varices (*pl. of* varix)
variciform
varico-
varicoblepharon
varicocele
ovarian v.

V

varicocele *(continued)*
    symptomatic v.
    tubo-ovarian v.
    utero-ovarian v.
varicocelectomy
varicography
varicoid
varicomphalus
varicophlebitis
varicose
    v. aneurysm
    v. bronchiectasis
    v. eczema
    v. ulcer
    v. vein
varicosis, pl. **varicoses**
varicosity
varicotomy
varicula
varicule
variegate porphyria
variegation
variola
    v. benigna
    v. hemorrhagica
    v. major
    v. maligna
    v. miliaris
    v. minor
    v. pemphigosa
    v. sine eruptione
    v. vaccine, variola v.
    v. vaccinia
    v. vera
    v. verrucosa
    v. virus
variolar
variolate
variolation
variolic
varioliform
variolization
varioloid
variolous
variolovaccine
varix, pl. **varices**
    v. anastomoticus
    aneurysmal v.
    cirsoid v.
    conjunctival v.
    esophageal v.
    gelatinous v.
    lymph v.
    turbinal v.
varnish (dental)
Varolius, Varolio
Varolius sphincter
varus
vas, pl. **vasa**
    v. aberrans hepatis, pl. vasa
      aberrantia hepatis
    v. aberrans of Roth
    vasa aberrantia
    v. afferens, pl. vasa afferentia

    v. anastomoticum
vasa brevia
    v. capillare
vasa chylifera
    v. collaterale
    v. deferens, pl. vasa deferentia
    v. efferens, pl. vasa efferentia
Ferrein vasa aberrantia
Haller v. aberrans
vasa lymphatica
    v. lymphaticum
    v. lymphaticum afferens
    v. lymphaticum efferens
    v. lymphaticum profundum
    v. lymphaticum superficiale
vasa nervorum
vasa previa
    v. prominens ductus cochlearis
vasa recta
vasa recta renis
vasa sanguinea auris internae
vasa sanguinea choroideae
vasa sanguinea intrapulmonalia
vasa sanguinea retinae
    v. sanguineum
    v. spirale
vasa vasorum
vasa vorticosa

vas-
vasa aberrantia hepatis (*pl. of* vas
    aberrans hepatis)
vasa afferentia (*pl. of* vas afferens)
vasa deferentia (*pl. of* vas deferens)
vasa efferentia (*pl. of* vas efferens)
vasal
vascula (*pl. of* vasculum)
vascular
    v. bud
    v. cataract
    v. circle
    v. circle of optic nerve
    v. cones
    v. dementia
    v. dentin
    v. fold of the cecum
    v. gland
    v. headache
    v. keratitis
    v. lacuna
    v. lamina of choroid
    v. layer
    v. layer of choroid coat of eye
    v. layer of eyeball
    v. layer of testis
    v. leiomyoma
    v. meninx
    v. murmur
    v. nerve
    v. organ of lamina terminalis
    v. papillae
    v. pedicle
    v. plexus
    v. polyp
    v. ring
    v. sclerosis

v. cava inferior
v. caval foramen
v. cava superior
venae cavernosae penis
venae centrales hepatis
v. centralis glandulae suprarenalis
v. centralis retinae
v. cephalica
v. cephalica accessoria
v. cephalica antebrachii
venae cerebelli
v. cervicalis profunda
venae choroideae oculi
v. choroidea inferior
v. choroidea superior
venae ciliares anteriores
venae circumflexae femoris laterales
venae circumflexae femoris mediales
v. circumflexa humeri anterior
v. circumflexa humeri posterior
v. circumflexa iliaca profunda
v. circumflexa iliaca superficialis
v. colica dextra
v. colica media
v. colica sinistra
v. colli profunda
venae columnae vertebralis
v. comitans
v. comitans of hypoglossal nerve
v. comitans nervi hypoglossi
venae comitantes
venae conjunctivales
venae cordis
v. cordis magna
v. cordis media
venae cordis minimae
v. cordis parva
v. cornus posterioris
v. coronaria ventriculi
v. cutanea
v. cystica
venae digitales dorsales pedis
venae digitales palmares
venae digitales plantares
v. diploica
venae directae laterales
venae dorsales clitoridis superficiales
venae dorsales linguae
venae dorsales penis superficiales
v. dorsalis clitoridis profunda
v. dorsalis corporis callosi
v. dorsalis penis profunda
venae ductuum semicircularium
v. emissaria, pl. venae emissariae
v. emissaria condylaris
v. emissaria mastoidea
v. emissaria occipitalis
v. emissaria parietalis
venae encephali occipitales
venae epigastricae superiores
v. epigastrica inferior
v. epigastrica superficialis
venae episclerales
v.(e) posterior(es) ventriculi sinistri
venae esophageae

venae ethmoidales
v. facialis
v. facialis anterior
v. facialis communis
v. facialis posterior
v. faciei profunda
v. femoralis
v. fenestrae cochleae
venae fibulares
venae frontales
v. gastrica dextra
venae gastricae breves
v. gastrica sinistra
v. gastro-omentalis dextra
v. gastro-omentalis sinistra
venae geniculares
venae gluteae inferiores
venae gluteae superiores
v. gyri olfactorii
v. hemiazygos
v. hemiazygos accessoria
venae hemispherii cerebelli
superiores
venae hemorrhoidales inferiores
venae hemorrhoidales mediae
v. hemorrhoidalis superior
venae hepaticae
venae hepaticae dextrae
venae hepaticae intermediae
venae hepaticae mediae
venae hepaticae sinistrae
v. hypogastrica
v. ileocolica
v. iliaca communis
v. iliaca externa
v. iliaca interna
v. iliolumbalis
inferior v. cava (IVC)
venae inferiores cerebelli
venae inferiores cerebri
v. inferior vermis
v. innominata
venae insulares
venae intercapitulares
venae intercostales anteriores
venae intercostales posteriores
v. intercostalis superior dextra
v. intercostalis superior sinistra
v. intercostalis suprema
venae interlobares renis
venae interlobulares hepatis
venae interlobulares renis
v. intermedia antebrachii
v. intermedia basilica
v. intermedia cephalica
v. intermedia cubiti
venae internae cerebri
v. intervertebralis
venae jejunales et ilei
v. jugularis anterior
v. jugularis externa
v. jugularis interna
venae labiales anteriores
venae labiales posteriores
v. labialis inferior

V

vena (*continued*)
v. labialis superior
venae labyrinthi
v. lacrimalis
v. laryngea inferior
v. laryngea superior
v. lateralis ventriculi lateralis
v. lienalis
v. lingualis
v. lingularis
v. lobi medii
venae lumbales
v. lumbalis ascendens
v. magna cerebri
v. mammaria interna
v. maxillaris, pl. venae maxillares
v. medialis ventriculi lateralis
v. mediana antebrachii
v. mediana basilica
v. mediana cephalica
v. mediana cubiti
v. media profunda cerebri
venae mediastinales
v. media superficialis cerebri
venae medullae oblongatae
venae medullae spinalis
venae membri inferioris
venae membri superioris
venae meningeae
venae meningeae mediae
venae mesencephalicae
v. mesenterica inferior
v. mesenterica superior
venae metacarpeae dorsales
venae metacarpeae palmares
venae metatarseae dorsales
venae metatarseae plantares
v. modioli communis
venae musculophrenicae
venae nasales externae
v. nasofrontalis
venae nuclei caudati
v. obliqua atrii sinistri
v. obturatoria, pl. venae obturatoriae
v. occipitalis
v. ophthalmica inferior
v. ophthalmica superior
v. ovarica dextra
v. ovarica sinistra
v. palatina externa
venae palpebrales
venae palpebrales inferiores
venae palpebrales superiores
venae pancreaticae
venae pancreaticoduodenales
venae paraumbilicales
venae parietales
venae parotideae
venae pectorales
venae pedunculares
venae perforantes
venae pericardiacae
venae pericardiacophrenicae
venae peroneae

v. petrosa
venae pharyngeae
venae phrenicae superiores
v. phrenica inferior
venae pontis
v. pontomesencephalica
v. pontomesencephalica anterior
v. poplitea
v. portae hepatis
v. portalis
v. posterior corporis callosi
v. posterior septi pellucidi
v. preauricularis
v. precentralis cerebelli
venae prefrontales
v. prepylorica
venae profundae cerebri
venae profundae clitoridis
venae profundae penis
v. profunda femoris
v. profunda linguae
venae pudendae externae
v. pudenda interna
venae pulmonales
v. pulmonalis inferior dextra
v. pulmonalis inferior sinistra
v. pulmonalis superior dextra
v. pulmonalis superior sinistra
venae radiales
v. recessus lateralis ventriculi quarti
venae rectae
venae rectales inferiores
venae rectales mediae
v. rectalis superior
venae renales
v. retromandibularis
venae retroperitoneales
v. revehens, pl. venae revehentes
venae sacrales laterales
v. sacralis mediana
v. saphena accessoria
v. saphena magna
v. saphena parva
v. scalae tympani
v. scalae vestibuli
v. scapularis dorsalis
venae sclerales
venae scrotales anteriores
venae scrotales posteriores
venae sigmoideae
venae spinales
v. spiralis modioli
venae cavernosae of spleen
v. splenica
venae stellatae
v. sternocleidomastoidea
venae striatae
v. stylomastoidea
v. subclavia
venae subcutaneae abdominis
v. sublingualis
v. submentalis
venae superficiales cerebri
v. superficialis
superior v. cava

venae superiores cerebelli
venae superiores cerebri
v. superior vermis
v. supraorbitalis
v. suprarenalis dextra
v. suprarenalis sinistra
v. suprascapularis
venae supratrochleares
venae temporales profundae
venae temporales superficiales
v. temporalis media
v. terminalis
v. testicularis dextra
v. testicularis sinistra
venae thalamostriatae inferiores
v. thalamostriata superior
v. thoracica interna
v. thoracica lateralis
v. thoracoacromialis
v. thoracoepigastrica
venae thymicae
v. thyroidea ima
v. thyroidea inferior
v. thyroidea media
v. thyroidea superior
venae tibiales anteriores
venae tibiales posteriores
venae tracheales
venae transversae cervicis
venae transversae colli
v. transversa faciei
v. transversa scapulae
venae tympanicae
venae ulnares
v. umbilicalis
v. uncalis
venae uterinae
v. ventricularis inferior
v. vertebralis
v. vertebralis accessoria
v. vertebralis anterior
venae vesicales
venae vestibulares (anterius et posterius)
v. vitellina
venae vorticosae
venacavography
venae advehentes (*pl. of* vena advehens)
venae emissariae (*pl. of* vena emissaria)
venae maxillares (*pl. of* vena maxillaris)
venae obturatoriae (*pl. of* vena obturatoria)
venae revehentes (*pl. of* vena revehens)
Ven antigen
venation
vene-
venectasia
venectomy
veneer
venenation
veneniferous
venenosalivary
venenosity
venenous

venereal
v. bubo
v. disease
v. lymphogranuloma
v. sore
v. ulcer
v. wart
venereology
venereophobia
venesection
Venezuelan
V. equine encephalomyelitis
V. equine encephalomyelitis virus
V. hemorrhagic fever
veni- (*var. of* veno-)
Venice turpentine
venin
venipuncture
Venn diagram
veno-, veni-
venocaval filter
venoclysis
venofibrosis
venogram
venography
splenic portal v.
transosseous v.
vertebral v.
venom
v. hemolysis
kokoi v.
Russell's viper v.
venomosalivary
venomotor
venooclusive disease of the liver
venoperitoneostomy
venopressor
venorespiratory reflex
venosclerosis
venose
venosinal
venosity
venostasis
venostat
venostomy
venotomy
venous
v. angioma
v. angle
v. artery
v. blood
v. capillary
v. circle of mammary gland
v. congestion
v. embolism
v. foramen
v. gangrene
v. groove
v. heart
v. hum
v. hyperemia
v. insufficiency
v. lake
v. ligament
v. malformation

V

venous (*continued*)
v. murmur
v. occlusion plethysmography
v. plexus
v. plexus of bladder
v. plexus of canal of hypoglossal nerve
v. plexus of foramen ovale
v. pulse
v. return
v. segment of the kidney
v. sinus
v. sinus of sclera
v. star
v. stasis
v. ulcer
v. valve
venous-stasis retinopathy
venovenostomy
vent
venter
v. anterior musculi digastrici
v. frontalis musculi occipitofrontalis
v. inferior musculi omohyoidei
v. occipitalis musculi occipitofrontalis
v. posterior musculi digastrici
v. superior musculi omohyoidei
ventilate
ventilation
airway pressure release v.
alveolar v. ($\dot{V}$A)
artificial v.
assist-control v.
assisted v.
bag v.
continuous positive pressure v. (CPPV)
controlled v.
controlled mechanical v. (CMV)
high-frequency v.
intermittent mandatory v. (IMV)
intermittent positive pressure v. (IPPV)
inverse-ratio v.
liquid v.
mandatory minute v.
manual v.
maximum voluntary v. (MVV)
mechanical v.
v. meter
negative pressure v.
noninvasive positive pressure v.
permissive hypercapnic v.
pressure-controlled v.
pressure-support v.
proportional assist v.
pulmonary v.
synchronized intermittent mandatory v. (SIMV)
wasted v.
ventilation/perfusion mismatch
ventilation/perfusion ratio ($\dot{V}$a/$\dot{Q}$)
ventilation-perfusion scan

ventilator
cuirass v.
ventilatory compliance
ventplant
ventrad
ventral
v. acoustic stria
v. anterior nucleus of thalamus
v. aortas
v. apron prepuce
v. border
v. branch
v. decubitus
v. funiculus
v. gland
v. hernia
v. horn
v. intermediate nucleus of thalamus
v. lateral geniculate nucleus
v. lateral nucleus of thalamus
v. mesocardium
v. mesogastrium
v. nucleus of thalamus
v. nucleus of trapezoid body
v. pallidum
v. pancreas
v. part of intertransversarii laterales lumborum muscle
v. part of pons
v. plate
v. plate of neural tube
v. posterior intermediate nucleus of thalamus
v. posterior nucleus of thalamus
v. posterolateral nucleus of thalamus
v. posteromedial nucleus of thalamus
v. premammillary nucleus
v. primary rami of cervical spinal nerve
v. primary rami of lumbar spinal nerve
v. primary rami of sacral spinal nerve
v. primary rami of thoracic spinal nerve
v. primary ramus of spinal nerve
v. principal nucleus
v. rami of cervical nerve
v. rami of lumbar nerve
v. rami of sacral nerve
v. rami of thoracic nerve
v. ramus of spinal nerve
v. raphespinal tract
v. root of spinal nerve
v. sacrococcygeal ligament
v. sacrococcygeal muscle
v. sacrococcygeus muscle
v. sacroiliac ligament
v. spinocerebellar tract
v. spinothalamic tract
v. splanchnic artery
v. striatum
v. surface of digit
v. tegmental decussation

v. thalamic peduncle
v. thalamus
v. tier thalamic nucleus
v. trigeminothalamic tract
v. white column
v. white commissure
ventralis
ventral paraflocculus
ventricle
Arantius v.
cerebral v.'s
v. of cerebral hemisphere
v. of diencephalon
double outlet right v.
Duncan v.
fifth v.
fourth v.
laryngeal v.
lateral v.
left v.
Morgagni v.
parchment right v.
v. of rhombencephalon
right v.
right and left v.'s of heart
single v.
sixth v.
sylvian v.
v. of Sylvius
terminal v.
third v.
Verga v.
Vieussens v.
Wenzel v.
ventricose
ventricular
v. aberration
v. afterload
v. aneurysm
v. artery
v. assist device
v. band of larynx
v. bigeminy
v. bradycardia
v. capture
v. complex
v. conduction
v. diastole
v. diverticulum
v. escape
v. extrasystole
v. fibrillation
v. filling pressure
v. fluid
v. flutter
v. fold
v. fusion beat
v. gradient
v. inhibited pulse generator
v. late potential
v. layer
v. ligament
v. loop
v. plateau
v. preexcitation

v. preload
v. reduction surgery
v. rhythm
v. septal defect
v. septum
v. standstill
v. synchronous pulse generator
v. systole
v. tachycardia
v. triggered pulse generator
v. trigone
ventricularis
ventricularization
ventricular ponderance
ventriculectomy
partial left v.
ventriculi (*pl. of* ventriculus)
ventriculitis
ventriculo-
ventriculoatrial (VA)
v. conduction (VAC)
ventriculocisternostomy
ventriculography
radionuclide v.
ventriculomastoidostomy
ventriculonector
ventriculophasic
ventriculoplasty
reduction left v.
ventriculopuncture
ventriculoradial dysplasia
ventriculoscopy
ventriculostomy
third v.
ventriculosubarachnoid
ventriculotomy
ventriculus, pl. ventriculi
v. cordis dexter/sinister
v. dexter
v. laryngis
v. lateralis
v. quartus
v. quintus
v. sinister
v. terminalis
v. tertius
ventriduct
ventriduction
ventro-
ventrobasal
v. complex
v. nuclei
ventrocystorrhaphy
ventrodorsad
ventroinguinal
ventrolateral
v. nucleus
v. sulcus
ventromedial
v. nucleus
v. nucleus of hypothalamus
ventromedian
ventroptosis, ventroptosia
ventroscopy
ventrotomy

V

Venturi
- V. effect
- V. meter
- V. tube

venula, pl. **venulae**
- v. macularis inferior
- v. macularis superior
- v. medialis retinae
- v. nasalis retinae inferior
- v. nasalis retinae superior
- venulae rectae of kidney
- venulae rectae renis
- venulae stellatae
- v. temporalis retinae inferior
- v. temporalis retinae superior

venular

venule
- high endothelial postcapillary v.'s
- inferior macular v.
- inferior nasal v. of retina
- inferior nasal retinal v.
- inferior temporal v. of retina
- inferior temporal retinal v.
- medial v. of retina
- nasal v.'s of retina
- pericytic v.
- postcapillary v.'s
- stellate v.
- straight v.'s of kidney
- superior macular v.
- superior nasal v. of retina
- superior nasal retinal v.
- superior temporal v. of retina
- superior temporal retinal v.
- temporal v.'s of retina

venulous

VER
- visual evoked response

verapamil

veratric acid

veratridine

veratrine

Veratrum
- *v. album*
- *v. viride*

verbal
- v. agraphia
- v. apraxia
- v. autopsy

verbigeration

verbomania

verdigris

verdine

verdoglobin

verdohemochrome

verdohemoglobin

verdoperoxidase

Veress needle

Verga ventricle

verge
- anal v.

vergence
- v. of lens

Verheyen star

Verhoeff elastic tissue stain

vermes (*pl. of* vermis)

vermi-

vermian fossa

vermicidal

vermicide

vermicular
- v. colic
- v. movement
- v. pulse

vermiculation

vermicule

vermiculose, vermiculous

vermiculus

vermiform
- v. appendage
- v. appendix
- v. process

vermifugal

vermifuge

vermilion
- v. border
- v. zone

vermilionectomy

vermin

verminal

vermination

verminous
- v. abscess
- v. appendicitis
- v. ileus

vermis, pl. **vermes**

vermix

vernal
- v. catarrh
- v. conjunctivitis
- v. encephalitis
- v. keratoconjunctivitis

Verner-Morrison syndrome

Vernet syndrome

Vernier acuity

vernix
- v. caseosa

Verocay body

vero cytotoxin

Veronal

verruca, pl. **verrucae**
- v. digitata
- v. filiformis
- v. peruana, v. peruviana
- v. plana
- v. plana juvenilis
- v. plana senilis
- v. plantaris
- seborrheic v.
- v. senilis
- v. simplex
- v. vulgaris

verruca peruviana (*var. of* verruca peruana)

verruciform

verrucose

verrucosis
- lymphostatic v.

verrucous
- v. carcinoma

v. endocarditis
v. hemangioma
v. hyperplasia
v. nevus
v. vegetations
v. xanthoma
verruga
v. peruana
versicolor
version
bimanual v.
bipolar v.
cephalic v.
combined v.
external cephalic v.
internal cephalic v.
internal podalic v.
pelvic v.
podalic v.
postural v.
Potter v.
spontaneous v.
Wright v.
versive seizure
vertebra, pl. **vertebrae**
basilar v.
block vertebrae
butterfly v.
v. C1$_{c2}$
caudal vertebrae
cervical vertebrae [C1–C7]
vertebrae cervicales [C1–C7]
vertebrae coccygeae [Co1–Co4]
coccygeal vertebrae [Co1–Co4]
codfish vertebrae
cranial v.
v. dentata
dorsal vertebrae
false v.
first cervical v.
hourglass vertebrae
H-shape vertebrae
ivory v.
vertebrae lumbales [L1–L5]
lumbar vertebrae [L1–L5]
v. magna
odontoid v.
picture frame v.
v. plana
v. prominens
rugger jersey v.
vertebrae sacrales [S1–S5]
sacral vertebrae [S1–S5]
second cervical v.
vertebrae spuriae
tail vertebrae
vertebrae thoracicae [T1–T12]
thoracic vertebrae [T1–T12]
toothed v.
true v.
v. vera
vertebral
v. arch
v. artery
v. body

v. border of scapula
v. canal
v. column
v. defects, anal atresia, tracheoesophageal fistula with esophageal atresia, and radial and renal anomalies (VATER)
v. epidural space
v. foramen
v. formula
v. fusion
v. ganglion
v. groove
v. line of pleural reflection
v. nerve
v. notch
v. part of the costal surface of the lungs
v. part of diaphragm
v. plexus
v. polyarthritis
v. pulp
v. region
v. rib
v. vein
v. venography
v. venous plexus
v. venous system
vertebral-basilar system
vertebrarium
Vertebrata
vertebrate
v. hormone
vertebrated
v. catheter
v. probe
vertebrectomy
vertebro-
vertebroarterial
v. foramen
vertebrochondral
v. rib
vertebrocostal
v. trigone
vertebrofemoral
vertebroiliac
vertebromediastinal recess
vertebropelvic ligament
vertebrosacral
vertebrosternal
v. rib
vertex, pl. **vertices**
v. cordis
v. of cornea
v. corneae
corneal v.
v. presentation
vertical
v. aspect
v. axis
v. banded gastroplasty
v. crest of internal acoustic meatus
v. dimension
v. elastic
v. growth phase

V

vertical *(continued)*
   v. heart
   v. hymen
   v. illumination
   v. index
   v. muscle of tongue
   v. nystagmus
   v. opening
   v. osteotomy
   v. overlap
   v. parallax
   v. plate
   v. retraction syndrome
   v. strabismus
   v. transmission
   v. vertigo
verticalis
vertices (*pl. of* vertex)
verticil
verticillate
Verticillium
verticomental
verticosubmental view
vertiginous
vertigo, objective vertigo
   aural v.
   benign paroxysmal positional v.
   Charcot v.
   chronic v.
   endemic paralytic v.
   epidemic v.
   height v.
   horizontal v.
   hysterical v.
   laryngeal v.
   lateral v.
   mechanical v.
   nocturnal v.
   ocular v.
   organic v.
   paralyzing v.
   physiologic v.
   positional v.
   positional v. of Bárány
   postural v.
   sham-movement v.
   subjective v.
   vertical v.
   visual v.
vertometer
verumontanum
very low density lipoprotein (VLDL)
vesalianum
Vesalius
   V. bone
   V. foramen
   V. vein
vesic- (*var. of* vesico-)
vesica, pl. **vesicae**
   v. biliaris
   v. fellea
   v. prostatica
   v. urinaria

vesical
   v. calculus
   v. diverticulum
   v. fistula
   v. gland
   v. hematuria
   v. lithotomy
   v. nervous plexus
   v. reflex
   v. surface of uterus
   v. triangle
   v. vein
vesicalis anus
vesicant
vesicate
vesicating gas
vesication
vesicle
   acoustic v.
   acrosomal v.
   air v.
   allantoic v.
   amniocardiac v.
   auditory v.
   blastodermic v.
   cerebral v.
   cervical v.
   coated v.
   encephalic v.
   forebrain v.
   germinal v.
   v. hernia
   hindbrain v.
   lens v.
   lenticular v.
   malpighian v.'s
   matrix v.'s
   midbrain v.
   ocular v.
   ophthalmic v.
   optic v.
   otic v.
   pinocytotic v.
   primary brain v.
   seminal v.
   synaptic v.
   telencephalic v.
   umbilical v.
vesico-, vesic-
vesicoabdominal
vesicobullous
vesicocele
vesicocervical
vesicoclysis
vesicocolic fistula
vesicocutaneous fistula
vesicointestinal
   v. fistula
vesicolithiasis
vesicoprostatic
vesicopubic
vesicopustular
vesicopustule
vesicorectal
vesicorectostomy

vesicosigmoid
vesicosigmoidostomy
vesicospinal
vesicostomy
vesicotomy
vesicoumbilical
    v. ligament
vesicoureteral
    v. reflux
    v. valve
vesicourethral
    v. canal
vesicouterine
    v. fistula
    v. ligament
    v. pouch
vesicouterovaginal
vesicovaginal
    v. fistula
vesicovaginorectal
    v. fistula
vesicovisceral
vesicula, pl. **vesiculae**
    v. fellis
    v. ophthalmica
    v. seminalis
    v. umbilicalis
vesicular
    v. appendages of epoophoron
    v. appendices of uterine tube
    v. breath sound
    v. exanthema of swine virus
    v. follicle
    v. keratitis
    v. keratopathy
    v. murmur
    v. ovarian follicle
    v. rale
    v. resonance
    v. respiration
    v. rickettsiosis
    v. stomatitis
    v. stomatitis virus
    v. transport
    v. venous plexus
vesiculate
vesiculation
vesiculectomy
vesiculitis
vesiculo-
vesiculobronchial
vesiculocavernous
    v. respiration
vesiculography
vesiculopapular
vesiculoprostatitis
vesiculotomy
vesiculotubular
vesiculotympanic
vesiculotympanitic resonance
Vesiculovirus
Vesling line
vesp.
    vesper
vesper (vesp.)

vessel
    absorbent v.
    afferent v.
    anastomosing v.
    anastomotic v.
    blood v.
    capillary v.
    chyle v.
    collateral v.
    corkscrew v.
    deep lymph v.
    efferent v.
    hairpin v.'s
    v.'s of internal ear
    lacteal v.
    lymph v.'s
    lymphatic v.'s
    nutrient v.
    superficial lymph v.
    v.'s of vessels
    vitelline v.'s
vestibula (*pl. of* vestibulum)
vestibular
    v. anus
    v. apparatus
    v. aqueduct
    v. area
    v. blind sac
    v. branch of labyrinthine artery
    v. canal
    v. cecum of the cochlear duct
    v. crest
    v. fissure of cochlea
    v. fold
    v. fossa
    v. ganglion
    v. gland
    v. hair cell
    v. labium of limbus of spiral lamina
    v. labyrinth
    v. lamella (of osseous spiral lamina)
    v. ligament
    v. lip of limbus of spiral lamina
    v. lip of spiral limbus
    v. membrane
    v. nerve
    v. neurectomy
    v. neuronitis
    v. nuclei
    v. nystagmus
    v. organ
    v. part of vestibulocochlear nerve
    v. root
    v. root of vestibulocochlear nerve
    v. schwannoma
    v. screen
    v. surface of cochlear duct
    v. surface of tooth
    v. wall of cochlear duct
    v. window
vestibularis
vestibulate

V

vestibule
>aortic v.
>buccal v.
>esophagogastric v.
>gastroesophageal v.
>labial v.
>v. of larynx
>v. of mouth
>nasal v.
>v. of nose
>v. of omental bursa
>oral v.
>Sibson aortic v.
>v. of vagina

vestibulitis
vestibulo-
vestibulocerebellar ataxia
vestibulocerebellum
vestibulocochlear
>v. artery
>v. nerve [CN VIII]
>v. nucleus
>v. organ

vestibulo-equilibratory control
vestibuloocular reflex
vestibulopathy
>idiopathic bilateral v.
>migraine-related v.

vestibuloplasty
vestibulospinal
>v. reflex
>v. tract

vestibulotomy
vestibulourethral
vestibulum, pl. **vestibula**
>v. aortae
>v. bursae omentalis
>v. laryngis
>v. nasi
>v. oris
>v. pudendi
>v. vaginae

vestige
>v. of ductus deferens
>v. of processus vaginalis
>v. of vaginal process

vestigial
>v. fold
>v. muscle
>v. organ

vestigium, pl. **vestigia**
>v. processus vaginalis

vesuvin
Veterans Administration hospital
veterinarian
veterinary
>v. medicine

Vi
>Vi antibody
>Vi antigen

via, pl. **viae**
viability
viable
>v. cell count

viae (*pl. of* via)

vial
vibesate
vibrating line
vibration
>v. syndrome
>v. tolerance

vibrative
vibrator
vibratory
>v. massage
>v. sensibility
>v. urticaria

Vibrio
>v. *alginolyticus*
>v. *cholerae*
>El Tor v.
>v. *fetus*
>v. *fluvialis*
>v. *furnissii*
>v. *hollisae*
>v. *metschnikovii*
>v. *mimicus*
>Nasik v.
>v. *parahaemolyticus*
>v. *sputorum*
>v. *vulnificus*

vibrio
Vibrion septique
vibriosis, pl. **vibrioses**
vibrissa, pl. **vibrissae**
vibrissal
vibrocardiogram
vibromasseur
vibrotherapeutics
Viburnum prunifolium
vicarious
>v. hypertrophy
>v. menstruation

vicine
vicious
>v. cicatrix
>v. circle
>v. union

Vicq
>V. d'Azyr bundle
>V. d'Azyr centrum semiovale
>V. d'Azyr foramen

Victoria blue
Victoria orange
vidarabine
video-assisted thoracic surgery (VATS)
videoendoscope
videoendoscopy
video fluoroscopy
videokeratoscope
vidian
>v. artery
>v. canal
>v. nerve
>v. vein

Vierra sign
Vieth-Müller circle
Vieussens
>V. ansa
>V. anulus

V. centrum
V. foramina
V. ganglia
V. isthmus
V. limbus
V. loop
V. ring
V. valve
V. vein
V. ventricle

view

axial v.
base v.
v. box
Caldwell v.
half axial v.
Judet v.
long axis v.
Stenvers v.
Towne v.
verticosubmental v.
Waters v.

vigabatrin
vigil

coma v.

vigilambulism
vigilance
villi (*pl. of* villus)
villin
villitis
villose
villositis
villosity
villous

v. adenoma
v. atrophy
v. carcinoma
v. papilloma
v. placenta
v. tenosynovitis
v. tumor

villus, pl. **villi**

anchoring v.
arachnoid villi
chorionic villi
floating v.
free v.
intestinal villi
villi intestinales
villi pericardiaci
pericardial villi
peritoneal villi
villi peritoneales
pleural villi
villi pleurales
primary v.
secondary v.
synovial villi
villi synoviales
tertiary v.

vimentin
vinblastine sulfate
Vinca

V, alkaloid
V, *rosea*

vincaleucoblastine
Vincent

V. angina
V. bacillus
V. disease
V. infection
V. spirillum
V. tonsillitis

vincristine sulfate
vinculin
vinculum, pl. **vincula**

v. breve digitorum manus
v. breve of finger
v. linguae
vincula lingulae cerebelli
long v.
v. longum digitorum manus
v. longum of finger
v. preputii
short v.
vincula tendinea of digits of hand
and foot
vincula tendinum digitorum manus
et pedis
vincula of tendons

vindesine
Vineberg procedure
vinegar

v. eel
mother of v.
pyroligneous v.
wood v.

vinic
vinous

v. liquor

vinyl

v. carbinol
v. chloride

vinylbenzene
vinylene
vinylidene
violaceous
violence

domestic v.

violet

Hoffman v.
visual v.

violinist's cramp
viomycin
viosterol
VIP

vasoactive intestinal polypeptide

viper

Russell's v.

Viperidae
VIPoma
Vipond sign
viprynium embonate
viraginity
viral

v. cystitis
v. dysentery
v. encephalomyelitis
v. envelope
v. gastroenteritis

V

viral *(continued)*
    v. hemagglutination
    v. hemorrhagic fever
    v. hemorrhagic fever virus
    v. hepatitis
    v. hepatitis type A, B, C, D, E
    v. load
    v. neutralization
    v. pericarditis
    v. probe
    v. strand
    v. therapy
    v. tropism
    v. wart
Virchow
    V. angle
    V. cell
    V. corpuscle
    V. crystal
    V. disease
    V. node
    V. psammoma
Virchow-Hassall body
Virchow-Holder angle
Virchow-Robin space
viremia
vires (*pl. of* vis)
virga
virgin
    v. generation
    v. silk
virginal
    v. membrane
Virginia snakeroot
virginity
virgophrenia
viricidal
viricide
-viridae
viridans
    v. hemolysis
    v. streptococci
virile
    v. member
virilescence
virilia
virilism
    adrenal v.
virility
virilization
virilizing
-virinae
virion
viripotent
viroid
virologist
virology
viropexis
virtual
    v. endoscopy
    v. focus
    v. image
virucidal
virucide

virucopria
virulence
virulent
    v. bacteriophage
    v. bubo
    v. phage mutant
viruliferous
viruria
virus, pl. **viruses**
    v. A, B, C hepatitis
    Abelson murine leukemia v.
    adenoassociated v. (AAV)
    adenoidal-pharyngeal-conjunctival v.
    adenosatellite v.
    AIDS-related v. (ARV)
    Akabane v.
    amphotropic v.
    Andes v.
    animal viruses
    A-P-C v.
    Argentine hemorrhagic fever v.
    attenuated v.
    Aujeszky disease v.
    Australian X disease v.
    avian encephalomyelitis v.
    avian influenza v.
    avian lymphomatosis v.
    avian neurolymphomatosis v.
    avian pneumoencephalitis v.
    avian viral arthritis v.
    B v.
    B19 v.
    bacterial v.
    Barmah Forest v.
    Bayou v.
    Bittner v.
    BK v.
    Black Creek Canal v.
    v. blockade
    bluetongue v.
    Bolivian hemorrhagic fever v.
    Borna disease v.
    Bornholm disease v.
    bovine leukemia v. (BLV)
    bovine leukosis v.
    bovine papular stomatitis v.
    bovine virus diarrhea v.
    Bunyamwera v.
    Bwamba v.
    CA v.
    California v.
    canine distemper v.
    Capim v.
    Caraparu v.
    Catu v.
    CELO v.
    Central European tick-borne encephalitis v.
    C group viruses
    Chagres v.
    chicken embryo lethal orphan v.
    chickenpox v.
    chikungunya v.
    Coe v.
    cold v.

Colorado tick fever v.
Columbia S. K. v.
common cold v.
contagious ecthyma (pustular
  dermatitis) v. of sheep
contagious pustular stomatitis v.
Côte-d'Ivoire virus
cowpox v.
Crimean-Congo hemorrhagic fever v.
croup-associated v.
cytopathogenic v.
defective v.
delta v.
dengue v.
distemper v.
DNA v.
dog distemper v.
duck hepatitis v.
duck influenza v.
duck plague v.
Duvenhage v.
eastern equine encephalomyelitis v.
EB v.
Ebola v.
Ebola v. Côte-d'Ivoire
Ebola v. Reston
Ebola v. Sudan
Ebola v. Zaire
ECHO v.
ECMO v.
ecotropic v.
ECSO v.
ectromelia v.
EEE v.
EMC v.
emerging v.
encephalitis v.
v. encephalomyelitis
encephalomyocarditis v.
enteric viruses
enteric cytopathogenic human
  orphan v.
enteric cytopathogenic monkey
  orphan v.
enteric cytopathogenic swine
  orphan v.
enteric orphan viruses
enzootic encephalomyelitis v.
ephemeral fever v.
epidemic gastroenteritis v.
epidemic keratoconjunctivitis v.
epidemic myalgia v.
epidemic parotitis v.
epidemic pleurodynia v.
Epstein-Barr v. (EBV)
FA v.
fibrous bacterial v.
filamentous bacterial v.
filtrable v.
fixed v.
Flury strain rabies v.
FMD v.
foamy v.
foot-and-mouth disease v.
Four Corners v.

Friend v.
Friend leukemia v.
GAL v.
gallus adenolike v.
gastroenteritis v. type A, B
GB v.
German measles v.
Germiston v.
goatpox v.
Graffi v.
green monkey v.
Gross leukemia v.
Guama v.
Guanarito v.
Guaroa v.
HA1, HA2 v.
hand-foot-and-mouth disease v.
Hantaan v.
helper v.
hemadsorption v. type 1, 2
Hendra v.
v. hepatitis
hepatitis A v. (HAV)
hepatitis B v. (HBV)
hepatitis C v. (HCV)
hepatitis D v.
hepatitis delta v. (HDV)
hepatitis E v. (HEV)
hepatitis G v. (HGV)
herpes simplex v. (HSV)
herpes zoster v.
hog cholera v.
horsepox v.
human immunodeficiency v. (HIV)
human immunodeficiency v.-1 (HIV-
  1)
human immunodeficiency v.-2 (HIV-
  2)
human T-cell lymphoma/leukemia v.
human T-cell lymphotropic v.
human T lymphotrophic v.
v. III of rabbits
Ilhéus v.
inclusion conjunctivitis virus-
infantile gastroenteritis v.
infectious ectromelia v.
infectious hepatitis v.
infectious papilloma v.
infectious porcine
  encephalomyelitis v.
influenza virus
insect virus
iridescent v.
Jamestown Canyon v.
Japanese B encephalitis v.
JC v.
Junin v.
K v.
Kasokero v.
Kelev strain rabies v.
v. keratoconjunctivitis
Kilham rat v.
Koongol viruses
Korean hemorrhagic fever v.
Kyasanur Forest disease v.

virus *(continued)*

La Crosse v.
lactate dehydrogenase v.
Lassa v.
latent rat v.
LCM v.
louping-ill v.
Lucké v.
Lunyo v.
lymphadenopathy-associated v.
 (LAV)
lymphocytic choriomeningitis v.
lymphogranuloma venereum v.
Machupo v.
malignant catarrhal fever v.
mammary cancer v. of mice
mammary tumor v. of mice
Marburg v.
Marek disease v.
marmoset v.
masked v.
Mason-Pfizer v.
Mayaro v.
measles v.
Menangle v.
Mengo v.
milker's nodule v.
mink enteritis v.
MM v.
Mokola v.
molluscum contagiosum v.
Moloney v.
monkey B v.
monkeypox v.
mouse encephalomyelitis v.
mouse hepatitis v.
mouse leukemia viruses
mouse mammary tumor v.
mouse parotid tumor v.
mouse poliomyelitis v.
mousepox v.
mouse thymic v.
mucosal disease v.
mumps v.
murine sarcoma v.
Murray Valley encephalitis v.
Murutucu v.
MVE v.
myxomatosis v.
naked v.
ND v.
negative strand v.
Negishi v.
neonatal calf diarrhea v.
neurotropic v.
Newcastle disease v.
New York v.
Nipah v.
non-A, non-B hepatitis v.
nonoccluded v.
Norwalk v.
occluded v.
Omsk hemorrhagic fever v.
oncogenic v.

o'nyong-nyong v.
orf v.
Oriboca v.
ornithosis v.
orphan v.
Pacheco parrot disease v.
pantropic v.
papilloma v.
pappataci fever viruses
parainfluenza viruses
paravaccinia v.
parrot v.
Patois v.
pharyngoconjunctival fever v.
phlebotomus fever viruses
plant viruses
pneumonia v. of mice
poliomyelitis v.
polyoma v.
porcine hemagglutinating
 encephalomyelitis v.
Powassan v.
pseudocowpox v.
pseudolymphocytic
 choriomeningitis v.
pseudorabies v.
psittacosis v.
Puumala v.
PVM v.
quail bronchitis v.
Quaranfil v.
rabbit fibroma v.
rabbit myxoma v.
rabbitpox v.
rabies v.
rabies v., Flury strain
rabies v., Kelev strain
Rauscher leukemia v.
REO v.
respiratory enteric orphan v.
respiratory syncytial v.
Reston v.
Rida v.
Rift Valley fever v.
RNA v.
RNA tumor v.
Ross River v.
Rous-associated v. (RAV)
Rous sarcoma v. (RSV)
Rs v.
Rubarth disease v.
rubella v.
rubeola v.
Russian autumn encephalitis v.
Russian spring-summer
 encephalitis v.
Sabia v.
Salisbury common cold viruses
salivary gland v.
sandfly fever viruses
San Miguel sea lion v.
Semliki Forest v.
Sendai v.
Seoul v.
serum hepatitis v.

sheep-pox v.
shipping fever v.
Shope fibroma v.
Shope papilloma v.
Simbu v.
simian v. (SV)
simian vacuolating v. No. 40
  (SV40)
Sindbis v.
Sin Nombre v.
slow v.
smallpox v.
snowshoe hare v.
soremouth v.
Spondweni v.
St. Louis encephalitis v.
street v.
Sudan v.
swine encephalitis v.
swine fever v.
swine influenza viruses
swinepox v.
Swiss mouse leukemia v.
Tacaribe v.
Tahyna v.
Taiwan Dobrava-Belgrade v.
temperate v.
Teschen disease v.
Tete viruses
TGE v.
Theiler mouse encephalomyelitis v.
Theiler original v.
tick-borne v.
tick-borne encephalitis v.
TO v.
Topografov v.
trachoma v.
transmissible gastroenteritis v. of
  swine
tumor v.
Turlock v.
Umbre v.
vaccine v.
vaccinia v.
vacuolating v.
varicella-zoster v.
variola v.
VEE v.
Venezuelan equine
  encephalomyelitis v.
vesicular exanthema of swine v.
vesicular stomatitis v.
viral hemorrhagic fever v.
visceral disease v.
visna v.
VS v.
WEE v.
Wesselsbron disease v.
western equine encephalomyelitis v.
West Nile encephalitis v.
v. X disease
xenotropic v.
Yaba v.
Yaba monkey v.
yellow fever v.

Zaire v.
Zika v.
-virus
virus-associated hemophagocytic syndrome
viruses (*pl. of* virus)
virusoid
virus shedding
virus-transformed cell
vis, pl. **vires**
  v. conservatrix
  v. a fronte
  v. a tergo
  v. vitae, v. vitalis
viscance
viscera (*pl. of* viscus)
viscerad
visceral
  v. anesthesia
  v. arch
  v. brain
  v. cavity
  v. cleft
  v. crisis
  v. disease virus
  v. disorder
  v. epilepsy
  v. fascia
  v. inversion
  v. larva migrans
  v. layer
  v. layer of serous pericardium
  v. layer of tunica vaginalis of
    testis
  v. leishmaniasis
  v. lymph node
  v. lymph node of abdomen
  v. mesoderm
  v. motor fiber
  v. motor neuron
  v. motor system
  v. muscle
  v. nerve
  v. nervous system
  v. node
  v. nuclei of oculomotor nerve
  v. pelvic fascia
  v. pericardium
  v. peritoneum
  v. plate
  v. pleura
  v. pleurisy
  v. sense
  v. skeleton
  v. surface of liver
  v. surface of the spleen
  v. swallow
  v. traction reflex
visceralgia
viscerimotor
viscero-
viscerocranium
  cartilaginous v.
  membranous v.
viscerogenic
  v. reflex

V

viscerograph
visceroinhibitory
visceromegaly
visceromotor
    v. reflex
visceroparietal
visceroperitoneal
visceropleural
visceroptosis, visceroptosia
viscerosensory
    v. reflex
visceroskeletal
visceroskeleton
viscerosomatic
viscerotome
viscerotomy
viscerotonia
viscerotrophic
    v. reflex
viscerotropic
viscid
viscidity
viscidosis
viscoelasticity
viscoelastic retardation
viscometer
viscosimeter
viscosimetry
viscosity
    absolute v.
    anomalous v.
    apparent v.
    dynamic v.
    kinematic v.
    newtonian v.
    relative v.
viscotoxins
viscous
viscum
viscus, pl. **viscera**
visibility acuity
visible spectrum
vision
    achromatic v.
    binocular v.
    blue v.
    central v.
    chromatic v.
    colored v. (VC)
    cone v.
    direct v.
    double v.
    facial v.
    green v.
    halo v.
    haploscopic v.
    indirect v.
    multiple v.
    night v.
    oscillating v.
    peripheral v.
    photopic v.
    red v.
    rod v.
    scotopic v.

    stereoscopic v.
    subjective v.
    tinted v.
    triple v.
    tubular v.
    tunnel v.
    twilight v.
    yellow v.
visiting nurse
visna virus
visual
    v. acuity (V)
    v. agnosia
    v. alexia
    v. angle
    v. aphasia
    v. area
    v. aura
    v. axis
    v. blackout
    v. cortex
    v. cycle
    v. efficiency
    v. evoked potential
    v. evoked response (VER)
    v. extinction
    v. field
    functional v. loss
    v. image
    v. inattention
    v. inspection with acetic acid
    v. orbicularis reflex
    v. organ
    v. pathway
    v. pigment
    v. projection
    v. purple
    v. receptor cell
    v. threshold
    v. vertigo
    v. violet
    v. yellow
visualize
visual-kinetic dissociation
visual-spatial agnosia
visuoauditory
visuognosis
visuomotor
visuopsychic
visuosensory
visuospatial
visuscope
vita glass
vital
    v. capacity
    v. center
    v. force
    v. index
    v. knot
    v. node
    v. pulp
    v. sign
    v. spirit
    v. stain
    v. statistics

v. tooth
v. tripod
vitalism
vitalistic
vitality
v. test
vitalize
vitalometer
vital red
vitals
vitamer
vitamin
v. A, A_1, A_2
v. A_1 acid
v. A_1 alcohol
v. A aldehyde
v. A_2 aldehyde
antiberiberi v.
antihemorrhagic v.
antineuritic v.
antirachitic v.
antiscorbutic v.
antisterility v.
v. A unit
v. B_T
v. B_x
v. B, B_1, B_2, B_3, B_4, B_5, B_6, B_{12}, B_T, B_X
v. B_2, B_6 unit
v. B complex
v. B_c conjugase
v. B_1 hydrochloride unit
v. B_{12} neuropathy
v. B_{12} with intrinsic factor concentrate
v. C, D, D_2, D_3, E, F, G, H,K, P, PP, U
coagulation v.
v. C test
v. C unit
v. D–binding protein
v. D milk
v. D-resistant rickets
v. D unit
v. E unit
fat-soluble v.
fertility v.
v. K_2, v. $K_2(30)$
v. K_5
v. K_1, v. $K_1(20)$
v. K_3
v. K_4
v. $K_2(35)$
v. K unit
microbial v.
permeability v.
vitamin $K_1(20)$ (*var. of* vitamin K_1)
vitamin $K_2(30)$ (*var. of* vitamin K_2)
vitellarium
vitelliform
v. degeneration
v. retinal dystrophy
vitellin
vitelline
v. artery

v. cord
v. duct
v. fistula
v. membrane
v. pole
v. reservoir
v. sac
v. vein
v. vessels
vitelliruptive degeneration
vitellogenesis
vitellogenin
vitellointestinal
v. cyst
v. duct
vitellolutein
vitellorubin
vitellose
vitellus
v. ovi
vitiated air
vitiation
vitiliginous
v. choroiditis
vitiligo, pl. **vitiligines**
v. iridis
vitrectomy
anterior v.
posterior v.
vitrein
vitreitis
vitreo-
vitreodentin
vitreoretinal
v. choroidopathy syndrome
v. traction syndrome
vitreoretinopathy
exudative v.
vitreotapetoretinal dystrophy
vitreous
v. body
v. camera
v. cell
v. chamber
v. chamber of eye
v. detachment
v. hernia
v. humor
v. lamella
v. membrane
persistent anterior hyperplastic primary v.
persistent posterior hyperplastic primary v.
primary v.
secondary v.
v. table
tertiary v.
vitreum
vitrification
vitriol
in vitro
vitronectin
vitrosin

Vittaforma
vivarium, pl. **vivaria**
vivax
　　v. fever
　　v. malaria
vivi-
vividialysis
vividiffusion
vivification
viviparity
viviparous
viviperception
vivisect
vivisection
vivisectionist, vivisector
in vivo
Vladimiroff-Mikulicz amputation
VLDL
　　very low density lipoprotein
VMA
　　vanillylmandelic acid
VMA test
V-max
VMC
　　void metal composite
V-MI
　　volpe-manhold index
vocal
　　v. amusia
　　v. cord
　　v. cord nodule
　　v. fold
　　v. fremitus
　　v. ligament
　　v. muscle
　　v. process
　　v. process of arytenoid cartilage
　　v. resonance (VR)
　　v. shelf
　　v. spectrum
　　v. tract
vocal fry
vocalis muscle
Vogel law
Voges-Proskauer reaction
Vogt
　　V. angle
　　V. cephalodactyly
　　V. syndrome
Vogt-Koyanagi syndrome
Vogt-Spielmeyer disease
Vohwinkel syndrome
voice
　　amphoric v.
　　bronchial v.
　　cavernous v.
　　epigastric v.
　　eunuchoid v.
　　v. fatigue syndrome
　　myxedema v.
void
　　flow v.
　　signal v.
voiding
　　v. cystogram

　　v. cystourethrogram (VCUG)
　　v. flow rate
　　v. internal urethral orifice
void metal composite (VMC)
vol.
　　volatile
vola
volar
　　v. carpal ligament
　　v. interosseous artery
　　v. interosseous nerve
volaris
volatile (vol.)
　　v. anesthetic
　　v. fatty acid number
　　v. mustard oil
　　v. oil
volatilization
volatilize
Volhard test
volition
volitional
　　v. tremor
Volkmann
　　V. canal
　　V. cheilitis
　　V. contracture
　　V. spoon
volley
Vollmer test
Volpe-Manhold Index (V-MI)
volsella
volt
　　kiloelectron v.'s (keV)
voltage
voltage-gated channel
voltaic
　　v. taste
voltaism
voltameter
voltampere
voltmeter
Voltolini disease
volume (V)
　　atomic v.
　　v. averaging
　　closing v.
　　distribution v.
　　v. element
　　end-diastolic v.
　　end-systolic v.
　　expiratory reserve v. (ERV)
　　extracellular fluid v. (ECFV)
　　forced expiratory v. (FEV)
　　v. index
　　inspiratory reserve v. (IRV)
　　mean corpuscular v. (MCV)
　　minute v.
　　packed cell v.
　　partial v.
　　residual v. (RV)
　　respiratory minute v. (RMV)
　　resting tidal v.
　　standard v.
　　stroke v.

v. substitute
tidal v. (V$_T$)
v. unit (VU)
volume-controlled respirator
volume-displacement plethysmograph
volumenometer
volume-time curve
volumetric
v. analysis
v. flask
v. solution (VS)
volumometer
voluntary
v. dehydration
v. guarding
v. hospital
v. muscle
v. mutism
v. nystagmus
voluptuous
volute
volutin
v. granule
Volvox
volvulosis
volvulus
cecal v.
gastric v.
mesenteroaxial v.
sigmoid v.
vomeral
v. groove
v. sulcus
vomerine
v. canal
v. cartilage
v. crest of choana
v. groove
vomeris
vomerobasilar
v. canal
vomeronasal
v. cartilage
v. organ
vomerorostral canal
vomerovaginal
v. canal
v. groove
vomit
Barcoo v.
bilious v.
black v.
coffee-ground v.
vomiting
cerebral v.
cyclic v.
dry v.
epidemic v.
fecal v.
v. gas
morning v.
pernicious v.
v. of pregnancy
projectile v.
psychogenic v.

v. reflex
retention v.
stercoraceous v.
vomition
vomiturition
vomitus
v. cruentes
v. marinus
v. niger
von
v. Economo disease
v. Gierke disease
v. Graefe sign
v. Hippel disease
v. Hippel-Lindau syndrome
v. Kossa stain
v. Recklinghausen disease
v. Spee curve
v. Willebrand disease
v. Willebrand factor
Voorhoeve disease
vortex, pl. **vortices**
v. coccygeus
v. cordis
v. corneal dystrophy
Fleischer v.
v. of heart
v. lentis
vortices pilorum
v. vein
Vorticella
vorticose
v. vein
Vossius lenticular ring
vox
v. choleraica
voxel
voyeur
voyeurism
VP
vasopressin
V-pattern
V.-p. esotropia
V.-p. exotropia
VR
vocal resonance
VS
volumetric solution
V-shaped area of esophagus
VS virus
VU
volume unit
vulgaris
vulnerable
v. child syndrome
v. period
v. phase
vulnerary
Vulpian atrophy
vulsella, vulsellum
v. forceps
vulva, pl. **vulvae**
vulvar, vulval
v. dystrophy

V

vulvar *(continued)*
    v. intraepithelial neoplasia
    v. slit
vulvectomy
vulvismus
vulvitis
    chronic atrophic v.
    chronic hypertrophic v.
    follicular v.
vulvo-

vulvocrural
vulvodynia
vulvouterine
vulvovaginal
    v. anus
    v. cystectomy
    v. gland
vulvovaginitis
Vw antigen
V-Y flap

W

tryptophan
tungsten
watt
W chromosome
W factor
W ray
Waardenburg syndrome
Wachendorf
Wachendorf membrane
Wachstein-Meissel stain for calcium-magnesium-ATPase
Wada test
wadding
waddingtonian homeostasis
waddle
waddling gait
wafer
Wagner
W. disease
W. syndrome
WAGR syndrome
waist
waist-hip ratio
waiter's cramp
Walcher position
Waldenström
W. macroglobulinemia
W. purpura
W. syndrome
W. test
Waldeyer
W. fossae
W. gland
W. sheath
W. space
W. throat ring
W. tract
W. zonal layer
Waldeyer
walk
Walker
W. chart
W. tractotomy
walking typhoid
walk-through angina
wall
anterior w. of middle ear
anterior w. of stomach
anterior w. of tympanic cavity
anterior w. of vagina
axial w.'s of the pulp chambers
carotid w. of middle ear
carotid w. of tympanic cavity
cavity w.
cell w.
chest w.
enamel w.
external w. of cochlear duct
inferior w. of orbit
inferior w. of tympanic cavity
jugular w. of middle ear

labyrinthine w. of middle ear
labyrinthine w. of tympanic cavity
lateral w. of middle ear
lateral w. of orbit
lateral w. of tympanic cavity
mastoid w. of middle ear
mastoid w. of tympanic cavity
medial w. of middle ear
medial w. of orbit
medial w. of tympanic cavity
membranous w. of middle ear
membranous w. of trachea
membranous w. of tympanic cavity
nail w.
parietal w.
posterior w. of middle ear
posterior w. of stomach
posterior w. of tympanic cavity
posterior w. of vagina
pulpal w.
splanchnic w.
superior w. of orbit
tegmental w. of middle ear
tegmental w. of tympanic cavity
thoracic w.
tympanic w. of cochlear duct
vestibular w. of cochlear duct
Wallenberg syndrome
wallerian
w. degeneration
w. law
wallet stomach
wall-eye
wall-eyed bilateral internuclear ophthalmoplegia (WEBINO)
Walsh procedure
Walthard cell rest
Walther
W. canal
W. dilator
W. duct
W. ganglion
W. plexus
wandering
w. abscess
w. cell
w. erysipelas
w. goiter
w. kidney
w. liver
w. organ
w. pacemaker
w. pneumonia
Wangensteen
W. drainage
W. suction
W. tube
Wangiella
Wang test
warble
w. botfly
w. fly

W

Warburg
- W. apparatus
- W. old yellow enzyme
- W. respiratory enzyme
- W. theory

Warburg-Dickens-Horecker shunt
Warburg-Lipmann-Dickens-Horecker shunt
Ward-Romano syndrome
Wardrop
Wardrop method
Ward triangle
warfarin sodium
warm
- w. agglutinin
- w. autoantibody

warm-blooded
- w.-b. animal

warm-cold hemolysin
warmup phenomenon
Warren shunt
wart
- anatomic w.
- asbestos w.
- common w.
- digitate w.
- filiform w.
- flat w.
- fugitive w.
- genital w.
- Henle w.'s
- infectious w.
- mosaic w.
- Peruvian w.
- pitch w.
- plane w.
- plantar w.
- postmortem w.
- senile w.
- soot w.
- telangiectatic w.
- tuberculous w.
- venereal w.
- viral w.

Wartenberg symptom
Warthin-Finkeldey cell
Warthin-Starry silver stain
Warthin tumor
wartpox
warty
- w. dyskeratoma
- w. horn

wash
washed
- w. field technique
- w. sulfur

washing soda
washout
- w. cannula
- w. test

Wasmann gland
wasserhelle cell
Wassermann
- W. antibody

- W. reaction
- W. test

Wassermann-fast
wasted ventilation
wasting
- w. disease
- salt w.
- w. syndrome

watchmaker's cramp
Water
- bag of w.
- false w.

water
- w. of adhesion
- alkaline w.
- aromatic w.
- w. aspirator
- autoprotolysis constant of w. (K_w)
- baryta w.
- w. bath
- w. bed
- bitter w.
- bound w.
- bromine w.
- calcic w.
- w. canker
- carbonated w.
- carbon dioxide-free w.
- carbonic w.
- chalybeate w.
- chlorine w.
- w. of combustion
- w. of constitution
- w. of crystallization
- deionized w.
- w. depletion
- distilled w.
- w. diuresis
- w. dressing
- earthy w.
- free w.
- w. gas
- gentian aniline w.
- w. glass
- hard w.
- heavy w.
- indifferent w.
- w. for injection
- w. intoxication
- intracellular w.
- w. itch
- lime w.
- w. of metabolism
- mineral w.
- potable w.
- purified w.
- saline w.
- Selters w., Seltzer w.
- soft w.
- sulfate w.
- sulfur w.
- total body w. (TBW)
- transcellular w.
- w. wheel murmur

water-clear cell of parathyroid

water-drinking test
waterfall
water-hammer pulse
Waterhouse-Friderichsen syndrome
watering-can
    w.-c. perineum
    w.-c. scrotum
Waters
    W. operation
    W. projection
    W. view
    W. view radiograph
watershed
    w. infarction
water-soluble chlorophyll derivatives
Waterston
    W. operation
    W. shunt
water-trap stomach
waterwheel sound
water-whistle sound
watery eye
Watson-Crick helix
Watson-Schwartz test
watt (W)
wave
    A w.
    acid w.
    alkaline w.
    alpha w.
    w. analyzer
    arterial w.
    B w.
    beta w.
    brain w.
    C w.
    cannon w.
    D w.
    delta w.
    dicrotic w.
    electrocardiographic w.
    epsilon w.
    excitation w.
    F w.
    f w., ff w.'s
    fibrillary w.
    fibrillatory w.'s
    flat top w.
    fluid w.
    flutter-fibrillation w.
    w. form
    microelectric w.'s
    mucosal w.
    w. number
    overflow w.
    P w.
    percussion w.
    postextrasystolic T w.
    pulse w.
    Q w.
    R w.
    random w.
    recoil w.
    retrograde P w.
    S w.

    sonic w.
    supersonic w.
    T w.
    theta w.
    tidal w.
    Traube-Hering w.
    U w.
    ultrasonic w.'s
    V w.
    x w.
    y w.
waveform
    pressure w.
wavelength
wavenumber
waveshape
wax
    w. acid
    w. alcohol
    animal w.
    baseplate w.
    bleached w.
    bone w.
    boxing w.
    Brazil w.
    carnauba w.
    casting w.
    Chinese w.
    ear w.
    earth w.
    emulsifying w.
    w. expansion
    w. form
    grave w.
    Horsley bone w.
    inlay w.
    Japan w.
    mineral w.
    w. model denture
    montan w.
    palm w.
    paraffin w.
    w. pattern
    vegetable w.
    white w.
    wool w.
    yellow w.
waxing, waxing-up
wax-tipped bougie
waxy
    w. cast
    w. degeneration
    w. finger
    w. kidney
    w. liver
    w. spleen
Wb
    weber
WBC
    white blood cell
WDHA syndrome
weakness
    directional w.
wean
weaning

W

weanling
wear
    occlusal w.
wear-and-tear pigment
weaver's cough
web
    esophageal w.
    w. eye
    w. of fingers/toes
    laryngeal w.
    terminal w.
Webb antigen
webbed
    w. finger
    w. neck
    w. penis
    w. toes
webbing
Weber
    W. gland
    W. law
    W. organ
    W. paradox
    W. point
    W. sign
    W. stain
    W. syndrome
    W. test for hearing
    W. triangle
weber (Wb)
Weber-Christian disease
Weber-Cockayne syndrome
Weber-Fechner law
WEBINO
    wall-eyed bilateral internuclear
        ophthalmoplegia
Webster
Webster test
Wechsler-Bellevue scale
Wechsler intelligence scale
weddellite
    w. calculus
Wedensky
    W. effect
    W. facilitation
    W. inhibition
wedge
    w. biopsy
    w. bone
    dental w.
    w. pressure
    w. resection
    w. spirometer
wedge-and-groove
    w.-a.-g. joint
    w.-a.-g. suture
wedge-shaped
    w.-s. fasciculus
    w.-s. tubercle
WEE
    western equine encephalomyelitis
weekend hospital
Weeks bacillus
Weeksella
    w. zoohelcum

weeping eczema
WEE virus
Wegener granulomatosis
Wegner
    W. disease
    W. line
Wegner
Weibel
Weibel-Palade body
Weichselbaum coccus
Weidel reaction
Weigert
    W. iodine solution
    W. iron hematoxylin stain
    W. law
    W. stain for actinomyces
    W. stain for elastin
    W. stain for fibrin
    W. stain for myelin
    W. stain for neuroglia
Weigert-Gram stain
weight
    apothecaries w.
    atomic w. (at. wt., AW)
    birth w.
    combining w.
    dry w.
    equivalent w.
    gram-atomic w.
    gram-molecular w.
    molecular w. (mol wt, MW)
    w. sense
weightlessness
Weil
    W. basal layer
    W. basal zone
    W. disease
Weil-Felix
    W.-F. reaction
    W.-F. test
Weill
Weill
Weill-Marchesani syndrome
Weinberg
Weinberg reaction
Weingrow reflex
Weir Mitchell
Weir Mitchell treatment
Weisbach
Weisbach angle
Weismann
weismannism
Weiss
Weiss sign
Weitbrecht
    W. cartilage
    W. cord
    W. fiber
    W. foramen
    W. ligament
Welch bacillus
Welcker angle
welder's
    w. conjunctivitis
    w. lung

well counter
well-differentiated lymphocytic lymphoma
wellness
Wells
Wells syndrome
welt
wen
Wenckebach
    W. block
    W. period
    W. phenomenon
Wenzel ventricle
Wepfer gland
Werdnig-Hoffmann
    W.-H. disease
    W.-H. muscular atrophy
Werlhof disease
Wermer syndrome
Wernekinck
    W. commissure
    W. decussation
Wernekinck, Werneking
Werner
    W. syndrome
    W. test
Wernicke
    W. aphasia
    W. area
    W. center
    W. disease
    W. encephalopathy
    W. field
    W. radiation
    W. reaction
    W. region
    W. sign
    W. syndrome
    W. zone
Wernicke-Korsakoff
    W.-K. encephalopathy
    W.-K. syndrome
Wertheim operation
Werther disease
Wesselsbron
    W. disease
    W. disease virus
    W. fever
West
    W. African fever
    W. African sleeping sickness
    W. African trypanosomiasis
    W. Indian smallpox
    W. Nile encephalitis virus
    W. Nile fever
    W. syndrome
Westberg
Westberg space
Westergren method
Westermark sign
western
    W. blot
    W. blot analysis
    W. blotting
    w. equine encephalomyelitis (WEE)
    w. equine encephalomyelitis virus

Westphal
Westphal-Piltz phenomenon
Westphal pupillary reflex
wet
    w. beriberi
    w. compress
    w. cup
    w. cutaneous leishmaniasis
    w. dream
    w. and dry bulb thermometer
    w. gangrene
    w. lung
    w. nurse
    w. pack
    w. pleurisy
    w. shock
wettable sulfur
wet-technique liposuction
wet-to-dry dressing
Wetzel grid
Wever-Bray phenomenon
Weyers-Thier syndrome
WF
    working formulation for clinical usage
whale finger
Wharton
    W. duct
    W. jelly
wheal
wheal-and-erythema reaction
wheal-and-flare reaction
wheat
    w. germ
    w. gum
wheat germ oil
Wheatstone
Wheatstone bridge
wheel
    Burlew w.
Wheeler
Wheeler-Johnson test
Wheeler method
wheeze
    asthmatoid w.
"w" hernia
whetstone crystal
whewellite
    w. calculus
whey
    alum w.
    w. alum
    w. protein
whiff test
whip bougie
whiplash
    w. injury
    w. retinopathy
Whipple
    W. disease
    W. operation
whipworm
whisky, whiskey
whisper

W

whispered
> w. bronchophony
> w. pectoriloquy

whispering pectoriloquy

whistle
> Galton w.

whistle-tip catheter

whistling
> w. deformity
> w. face syndrome
> w. rale

Whitaker test

White
> w. arsenic
> w. beeswax
> w. bile
> w. blood cell (WBC)
> w. blood cell cast
> w. cell cast
> w. commissure
> w. corpuscle
> w. of eye
> w. fat
> w. fiber
> w. finger
> w. forelock
> w. gangrene
> w. infarct
> w. lead
> w. limbal girdle of Vogt
> w. line
> w. line of anal canal
> w. line of Toldt
> w. matter
> w. mercuric precipitate
> w. muscle
> w. mustard
> w. noise
> w. petrolatum
> w. piedra
> w. pine
> w. pitch
> w. pulp
> w. pulp of spleen
> w. pupillary reflex
> w. rami communicantes
> w. reaction
> w. soft paraffin
> w. sponge nevus
> w. spot
> w. spot disease
> w. substance
> w. thrombus
> w. turpentine
> w. wax
> w. yolk

whitegraft reaction

Whitehead
> W. deformity
> W. operation

white-out syndrome

whitepox

whites

whiting

whitlockite

whitlow
> herpetic w.
> thecal w.

Whitman frame

Whitmore
> W. bacillus
> W. disease

Whitnall tubercle

WHO
> World Health Organization

whole blood

whole-body
> w.-b. counter
> w.-b. titration curve

whoop
> systolic w.

whooping cough

whooping-cough vaccine

whorl
> coccygeal w.
> digital w.
> hair w.'s

whorled
> w. enamel

WI-38 cell

Wickham stria

Widal
> W. reaction
> W. syndrome

wide
> w. dynamic range compression
> w. field ocular
> w. plane
> w. spectrum

wideband

wide-latitude film

widow's peak

width
> orbital w.
> window w.

Wigand maneuver

Wilbrand knee

wild
> w. ginger
> w. mandrake
> w. tobacco
> w. type
> w. yeast

Wilde
> W. cord
> W. triangle

Wilder
> W. diet
> W. sign
> W. stain for reticulum

Wildermuth ear

Wildervanck syndrome

wildfire
> w. rash

wild-type strain

Wilhelmy balance

Wilkie disease

Willett

Willett forceps

Williams
    W. factor
    W. stain
    W. syndrome
Williams-Beuren syndrome
Willis
    W. centrum nervosum
    W. cord
    W. pancreas
    W. paracusis
    W. pouch
Willis
Williston law
willow
Wilms tumor
Wilson
    W. disease
    W. method
    W. muscle
Wilson method
Wilson-Mikity syndrome
windage
windburn
Windigo psychosis
window
    aortic w.
    aorticopulmonary w.
    aortic-pulmonic w.
    aortopulmonary w.
    cochlear w.
    w. level
    lung w.
    mediastinal w.
    oval w.
    round w.
    soft tissue w.
    tachycardia w.
    vestibular w.
    w. width
windpipe
wine
    high w.
    low w.
    red w.
    sherry w.
    w. spirit
wing
    angel w.
    ashen w.
    w. cell
    w. of central lobule
    w. of crista galli
    gray w.
    greater w. of sphenoid (bone)
    w. of ilium
    lesser w. of sphenoid (bone)
    w. of nose
    w. plate
    w. of sacrum
    w. of vomer
wing-beating tremor
winged
    w. catheter
    w. scapula
Winiwarter-Buerger disease

wink
    w. reflex
winking spasm
Winslow
    W. ligament
    W. pancreas
    W. star
winter
    w. eczema
    w. itch
    w. sleep
Winterbottom sign
wintergreen oil
Winternitz sound
Wintersteiner
    W. compound F
    W. rosette
wire
    w. arch
    arch w.
    guide w.
    Kirschner w.
    ligature w.
    separating w.
    w. splint
    wrought w.
wire-loop lesion
wiring
    circumferential w.
    circumzygomatic w.
    continuous loop w.
    craniofacial suspension w.
    Gilmer w.
    Ivy loop w.
    perialveolar w.
    pyriform aperture w.
    Stout w.
Wirsung
    W. canal
    W. duct
wiry
    w. pulse
wisdom tooth
Wiskott-Aldrich syndrome
Wissler syndrome
Wistar rat
witch hazel
witch's milk
withdrawal
    w. reflex
    w. symptom
    w. syndrome
without (s̄)
witkop
Wittigo psychosis (*var. of* Windigo psychosis)
witzelsucht
wobble
    w. base
    w. hypothesis
Wohlfahrtia
wohlfahrtiosis
Wohlfart-Kugelberg-Welander disease
Wolfe graft
Wolfe-Krause graft

W

Wolff
Wolff-Chaikoff
    W.-C. block
    W.-C. effect
wolffian
    w. body
    w. cyst
    w. duct
    w. duct carcinoma
    w. rest
    w. ridge
    w. tubules
Wolff-Parkinson-White syndrome
Wölfler gland
Wolf-Orton body
wolfram, wolframium
Wolfram syndrome (DIDMOD)
Wolfring gland
wolfsbane
Wolinella
Wollaston
    W. doublet
    W. theory
Wolman
    W. disease
    W. xanthomatosis
womb
    falling of the w.
Wood
    W. glass
    W. lamp
    W. light
    W. units
Wood
    w. charcoal
    w. naphtha
    w. spirit
    w. sugar
    w. vinegar
Wood
wood alcohol
woodcutter's encephalitis
wooden resonance
wooden-shoe heart
wood wool
wool
    w. alcohols
    w. fat
    hydrous w. fat
    w. wax
Woolf-Lineweaver-Burk plot
woolly
    w. hair
    w. hair nevus
Woolner tip
woolsorter's
    w. disease
    w. pneumonia
word blindness
word deafness
word salad
Woringer-Kolopp disease
work
workaholic

working
    w. bite
    w. contact
    w. occlusal surface
    w. occlusion
    w. side
    w. side condyle
Working Formulation for Clinical Usage (WF)
working out
working through
workstation
World Health Organization (WHO)
Worm
    w. abscess
    caddis w.
    Manson eye w.
    meal w.
worm bark
wormian
    w. bone
Wormley test
wormseed
wormwood
wort
    St. John's w.
Worth amblyoscope
Woulfe bottle
wound
    abraded w.
    avulsed w.
    w. botulism
    w. clip
    crease w.
    w. dehiscence
    w. fever
    glancing w.
    gunshot w.
    gutter w.
    incised w.
    w. myiasis
    nonpenetrating w.
    open w.
    penetrating w.
    perforating w.
    puncture w.
    septic w.
    seton w.
    stab w.
    subcutaneous w.
    sucking chest w.
    tangential w.
woven bone
W-plasty
W.r.
    wassermann reaction
Wrᵃ
    Wright antigen
wrap
    cardiac muscle w.
wreath
    ciliary w.
Wright
    W. antigen (Wrᵃ)
    W. respirometer

W. stain
W. syndrome
W. version
wrightine
wrinkle
wrinkler muscle of eyebrow
Wrisberg
W. cartilage
W. ganglia
W. ligament
W. nerve
W. tubercle
wrist
w. clonus
w. clonus reflex
w.-drop

w. joint
w. sign
wrist-hand orthosis
writer's cramp
writhing number
writing hand
wrought wire
wryneck
Wuchereria
w. bancrofti
w. malayi
wuchereriasis
Wurster
W. reagent
W. test
Wyburn-Mason syndrome

W

X
- halogen atom
- Kienböck unit
- xanthosine
  - X chromosome
  - X disease
  - X inactivation
  - X zone

X
- reactance
  - x wave

Xaa
- unspecified amino acid

Xan
- xanthine

xanth- (*var. of* xantho-)

xanthelasma
- generalized x.
- x. palpebrarum

xanthematin

xanthemia

xanthene
- x. dye

xanthic

xanthidylic acid

xanthine (Xan)
- x. dehydrogenase
- x. nucleotide
- x. oxidase
- x. ribonucleoside

xanthinol niacinate, xanthinol nicotinate

xanthinuria

xanthism

xanthiuria

xantho-, xanth-

xanthoastrocytoma
- pleomorphic x.

xanthochromatic

xanthochromia

xanthochromic

xanthoderma

xanthodont

xanthogranuloma
- juvenile x.
- necrobiotic x.

xanthogranulomatous
- x. cholecystitis
- x. pyelonephritis

xanthoma
- x. diabeticorum
- x. disseminatum
- eruptive x.
- fibrous x.
- x. multiplex
- x. palpebrarum
- x. planum
- tendinous x.
- x. tuberosum
- x. tuberosum simplex
- verrucous x.

xanthomatosis
- biliary x.

- x. bulbi
- cerebrotendinous x.
- chronic idiopathic x.
- familial hypercholesteremic x.
- generalized plane x.
- normal cholesteremic x.
- Wolman x.

Xanthomonas
- *x. maltophilia*

xanthophyll

xanthoproteic

xanthoproteic acid

xanthoprotein
- x. reaction

xanthopsia

xanthopuccine

xanthosine (X, Xao)
- x. 5′-monophosphate (XMP)
- x. 5′-triphosphate (XTP)

xanthosis

xanthous

xanthurenic acid

xanthuria

xanthyl

xanthylic
- x. acid

Xao
- xanthosine

Xe
- xenon

^{133}Xe
- xenon-133

xemilofiban

xenic culture

xeno-

xenobiotic

xenodiagnosis

xenogeneic
- x. graft

xenogenic

xenogenous

xenograft

xenon (Xe)
- x.-133 (^{133}Xe)

xenon-arc photocoagulator

xenoparasite

xenophobia

xenophonia

Xenopsylla

xenotropic virus

xenyl

xeransis

xerantic

xerasia

xero-

xerochilia

xeroderma
- x. pigmentosum

xerogram

xerography

xeroma

xeromammography

X

xeromenia
xeromycteria
xerophagia, xerophagy
xerophthalmia
xerophthalmus
xeroradiograph
xeroradiography
xerosis
    x. parenchymatosus
xerostomia
xerotic
    x. degeneration
    x. keratitis
xerotripsis
Xg
    Xg antigen
    Xg blood group
X-inactivation
xiph- (*var. of* xipho-)
xiphi- (*var. of* xipho-)
xiphisternal
    x. crunching sound
    x. joint
xiphisternum
xipho-, xiph-, xiphi-
xiphocostal
    x. angle
xiphodynia
xiphoid
    x. cartilage
    x. process
xiphoidalgia
xiphoiditis
xiphopagus
X-linked
    X.-l. agammaglobulinemia
    X.-l. gene
    X.-l. hypogammaglobulinemia
    X.-l. hypogammaglobulinemia with growth hormone deficiency
    X.-l. ichthyosis
    X.-l. inheritance
    X.-l. locus
    X.-l. lymphoproliferative disease
    X.-l. lymphoproliferative syndrome
    X.-l. recessive bulbospinal neuronopathy
XMP
    xanthosine 5-monophosphate
XO
    XO female
    XO gonadal dysgenesis
    XO syndrome
x-omat

X-pattern
    X.-p. esotropia
    X.-p. exotropia
x-radiation
x-ray
    x.-r. dosimetry
    x.-r. generator
    x.-r. microscope
    x.-r. therapy
    x.-r. tube
XTP
    xanthosine 5-triphosphate
XX gonadal dysgenesis
XX male
XXX female
XXY
    XXY male
    XXY syndrome
Xy
    xylose
XY gonadal dysgenesis
Xyl
    xylose
xyl-, xylo-
xylazine
xylene
    x. cyanol FF
xylenol
xylidine
xylitol
    x. dehydrogenase
xylo- (*var. of* xyl-)
xylobiose
xyloidin
xyloketose
xylol
xylometazoline hydrochloride
xylonic acid
xylopyranose
xylose (Xy, Xyl)
    x. test
xylostyptic ether
xylulose
    x. 5-phosphate
    x. reductase
L-xylulosuria
xylyl
    x. bromide
xylylene
xysma
XYY
    XYY male
    XYY syndrome

Y

tyrosine
yttrium
    Y body
    Y cartilage
    Y chromosome

y

y wave

Yaba

    Y. monkey virus
    Y. virus

YAC

yeast artificial chromosome

YAG

yttrium-aluminum-garnet

yang

yanggona

Yangtze

    Y. edema
    Y. Valley fever

yaqona

yaw

mother y.

yawn

yawning

yaws

    bosch y.
    bush y.
    foot y.

Yb

ytterbium

year

disability-adjusted life y.'s (DALYs)
y.'s of potential life lost (YPLL)
quality-adjusted life y.'s (QALY)

yeast

y. artificial chromosome (YAC)
brewers' y.
compressed y.
cultivated y.
dried y.
y. extract agar
y. fungus
primary dried y.
y. RNase
wild y.

yellow

y. atrophy of the liver
y. body
y. bone marrow
y. cartilage
y. corallin
corallin y.
y. disease
y. enzyme
y. fever
y. fever vaccine
y. fever virus
y. fiber
y. hepatization
indicator y.
y. ligament

y. mercury iodide
y. nail
y. nail syndrome
y. precipitate
y. root
y. skin
y. soft paraffin
y. spot
tumeric y.
y. vision
visual y.
y. wax
y. yolk

yerba santa

Yersinia

    Y. *enterocolitica*
    Y. *frederiksenii*
    Y. *intermedia*
    Y. *kristensenii*
    Y. *pestis*
    Y. *pseudotuberculosis*

yersiniosis

pseudotubercular y.

yield

quantum y.
y. strength
y. stress

yin-yang

-yl

-ylene

ylides

Y-linkage

Y-linked

    Y.-l. gene
    Y.-l. inheritance
    Y.-l. locus

yogurt, yoghurt

yohimbine

yoke

alveolar y.'s
y. bone
sphenoidal y.

yolk

y. cell
y. cleavage
y. membrane
y. sac
y. sac carcinoma
y. sac tumor
y. stalk
white y.
yellow y.

Yorke autolytic reaction

Young

    Y. modulus
    Y. prostatic tractor
    Y. rule
    Y. syndrome

Young-Helmholtz theory of color vision

YPLL

years of potential life lost

ypsiliform

Y

Y-shaped
    Y-s. cartilage
    Y-s. ligament
Yt^a antigen
ytterbium (Yb)
yttrium (Y)

    y.-90
    y.-aluminum-garnet (YAG)
Yvon test

Z
 benzyloxycarbonyl
  Z band
  Z chromosome
  Z disk
  Z filament
  Z gene
  Z line

Z
 atomic number

z
 zepto-

Zaffaroni system
zafirlukast
Zaglas ligament
Zahn infarct
Zaire virus
Zambesi ulcer
zanamivir
Zappert counting chamber
Zarit burden interview
Zavanelli maneuver
zea
zearalenone
zeatin
zeaxanthin
zeaxanthol
zebra body
Zeeman effect
ZEEP
 zero end-expiratory pressure
zein
Zeis gland
zeisian
  z. sty
Zeitgeist
Zellweger syndrome
zelophobia
zelotypia
Zenker
  Z. degeneration
  Z. diverticulum
  Z. fixative
  Z. paralysis
zeolite
zeoscope
zepto- (z)
zeptometer (zm)
zero
  absolute z.
  z. degree tooth
  z. end-expiratory pressure (ZEEP)
  z. gravity
  z. time-binding DNA
zero-order reaction
zeta
  z. potential
  z. sedimentation ratio (ZSR)
zetacrit
zetaprotein
zeugmatography
zidovudine

Ziehen
Ziehen-Oppenheim disease
Ziehl-Neelsen stain
Ziehl stain
Ziemann
  Z. dot
  Z. stippling
Zieve
Zieve syndrome
Zika
  Z. fever
  Z. virus
Zimmerlin atrophy
Zimmermann
  Z. corpuscle
  Z. elementary particle
  Z. granule
  Z. reaction
  Z. test
zinc (Zn)
  z. acetate
  z. caprylate
  z. chloride
  z. colic
  z. finger
  z. fume fever
  z. gelatin
  z. iodide
  medicinal z. peroxide
  z. oxide
  z. oxide and eugenol
  z. permanganate
  z. peroxide
  z. phenolsulfonate
  z. phosphate cement
  z. phosphide
  z. stearate
  z. sulfate
  z. sulfate flotation centrifugation
   method
  z. sulfate flotation concentration
  z. sulfocarbolate
  z. superoxide
  z. undecylenate, z. undecenoate
  z. white
zinc-65 (^{65}Zn)
zinciferous
zincoid
zinc undecenoate (*var. of* zinc
 undecylenate)
zingiber
Zinn
  Z. artery
  Z. corona
  Z. ligament
  Z. membrane
  Z. ring
  Z. tendon
  Z. vascular circle
  Z. zonule
zirconium (Zr)

Z

zirconium *(continued)*
- z. granuloma
- z. oxide

Zivert syndrome

zm
- zeptometer

Zn
- zinc

⁶⁵Zn
- zinc-65

zo- *(var. of* zoo-*)*

zoanthropic

zoanthropy

zoetic

zoic

zoite

Zollinger-Ellison
- Z.-E. syndrome
- Z.-E. tumor

Zöllner line

zolpidem

zomepirac sodium

zona, pl. **zonae**
- z. arcuata
- z. ciliaris
- z. corona
- z. dermatica
- z. epithelioserosa
- z. externa medullae renalis
- z. fasciculata
- z. glomerulosa
- z. hemorrhoidalis
- zonae hypothalamicae
- z. incerta
- z. interna medullae renalis
- z. lateralis
- z. medialis
- z. medullovasculosa
- z. ophthalmica
- z. orbicularis (articulationis coxae)
- z. pectinata
- z. pellucida
- z. perforata
- z. periventricularis
- z. pupillaris
- z. radiata
- z. reticularis
- z. striata
- z. tecta
- z. transitionalis analis
- z. vasculosa

zonal
- z. necrosis

zonary
- z. placenta

zonate

zone
- abdominal z.
- anal transitional z.
- androgenic z.
- arcuate z.
- Barnes z.
- z. centrifugation
- cervical z.

cervical z. of tooth
ciliary z.
comfort z.
z.'s of discontinuity
dolorogenic z.
entry z.
ependymal z.
epileptogenic z.
equivalence z.
erogenous z.'s, erotogenic z.'s
fetal z.
gingival z.
Golgi z.
grenz z.
Head z.'s
hemorrhoidal z.
z.'s of hypothalamus
inner z. of renal medulla
intermediate z.
intermediate z. of iliac crest
interpalpebral z.
intertubular z.
isoelectric z.
isopycnic z.
language z.
latent z.
lateral z.
Lissauer marginal z.
Looser z.'s
mantle z.
Marchant z.
marginal z.
medial z.
motor z.
neutral z.
nucleolar z.
Obersteiner-Redlich z.
orbicular z. of hip joint
outer z. of renal medulla
pectinate z.
pellucid z.
peritubular z.
periventricular z.
polar z.
protective z.
pupillary z.
reflexogenic z.
secondary X z.
segmental z.
Spitzka marginal z.
subplasmalemmal dense z.
sudanophobic z.
tender z.'s
thymus-dependent z.
trabecular z.
transformation z.
transitional z.
transitional z. of lips
trigger z.
trophotropic z. of Hess
vascular z.
vermilion z., vermilion transitional z.
Weil basal z.
Wernicke z.

z. 1, 2, 3, 4 of West
X z.
zonesthesia
zoning
zonography
zonoskeleton
zonula, pl. **zonulae**
z. adherens
z. ciliaris
z. occludens
zonular
z. band
z. cataract
z. fiber
z. layer
z. scotoma
z. space
zonule
ciliary z.
Zinn z.
zonulitis
zonulolysis, zonulysis
zoo-, zo-
zooanthroponosis
zooblast
zoo blot analysis
zoochrome
zoodermic
zooerastia
zoofulvin
zoogenesis
zoogeography
zooglea
zoogonous
zoogony
zoograft
zoografting
zooid
zoolagnia
zoolite, zoolith
zoologist
zoology
zoom
zoomania
zoomaric acid
Zoomastigina
Zoomastigophorasida
Zoomastigophorea
zoonosis
direct z.
zoonotic
z. cutaneous leishmaniasis
z. infection
z. potential
zooparasite
zoopathology
zoophagous
zoophile
zoophilia
zoophilic
zoophilism
erotic z.
zoophobia
zoophyte
zooplastic graft

zooplasty
zoosadism
zoosmosis
zoospermia
zoosterol
zootechnics
zootic
zootoxin
zootrophic
zorubicin
zoster
z. encephalomyelitis
geniculate z.
z. immune globulin
zosteriform
zosteroid
zoxazolamine
Z-plasty
Zr
zirconium
Zsigmondy test
ZSR
zeta sedimentation ratio
Z-tract injection
Zubrod scale
Zuckerkandl
Z. body
Z. convolution
Z. fascia
zusammen
zwieback
Zwischenferment
zwittergents
zwitter hypothesis
zwitterionic
z. buffer
z. detergent
z. surfactant
zwitterions
zyg- (*var. of* zygo-)
zygal
z. fissure
zygapophysial, zygapophyseal
z. joint
zygapophysis, pl. **zygapophyses**
z. inferior
z. superior
zygion
zygo-, zyg-
zygoma
zygomatic
z. arch
z. bone
z. border of greater wing of
sphenoid bone
z. branch of facial nerve
z. diameter
z. fossa
z. margin of greater wing of
sphenoid bone
z. nerve
z. process of frontal bone
z. process of maxilla
z. process of temporal bone
z. region

Z

zygomatico-
zygomaticoauricular
    z. index
zygomaticoauricularis
zygomaticofacial
    z. branch of zygomatic nerve
    z. foramen
zygomaticofrontal
zygomaticomaxillary
    z. suture
zygomatico-orbital
    z.-o. artery
    z.-o. foramen
zygomaticosphenoid
zygomaticotemporal
    z. branch of zygomatic nerve
    z. foramen
    z. suture
zygomaticus
    z. major muscle
    z. minor muscle
zygomaxillare
zygomaxillary
    z. point
Zygomycetes
zygomycosis
zygon
zygonema

zygopodium
zygosis
zygosity
zygosperm
zygospore
zygosyndactyly
zygote
zygotene
zygotic
zygotoblast
zygotomere
zymase
zymo-, zym-
zymodeme
zymogen
    z. granule
zymogenesis
zymogenic
    z. cell
zymogenous
zymogram
zymoplastic substance
zymosan
zymoscope
zymosterol
zymotic papilloma
zyxin
ZZ genotype

Common Prefixes, Suffixes, and Combining Forms

a-	not, without, less		bleph/blepharo-	eyelid
ab/abs-	away from		brachi/brachio-	arm
-ac	pertaining to		brady-	slow
acous/acouso-	hearing		bronch/bronchi-	bronchus
acr/acro-	extremity, topmost		bucc/bucco-	cheek
-acusis	hearing condition		carcin/carcino-	cancer
-ad	toward, in the direction of		cardi/cardio-	heart, esophageal opening of stomach
ad-	increase, adherence, motion toward, very		cata-	down
			-cele	pouching, hernia
aden/adeno-	gland		-centesis	puncture for aspiration
adip/adipo-	fat		cephal/cephalo-	head
adren/adreno-	gland		chem/chemo-	chemistry, drug
aer/aero-	air, gas		chlor/chloro-	green
-al	pertaining to		chol-	bile
alge/algesi-	pain		chondrio/ chondro-	cartilage, gristle
-algia	pain			
algio/algo-	pain		chrom/chromato-	color
ambi-	around, on all sides, both		-cidal/cide	killing, destroying
an-	not, without		circum-	around
ankyl/ankylo-	crooked, stiff		cis-	on this side
ante-	before		co-	with, together, in association
anti-	against, opposed to		col/colo/colono-	colon
apo-	separated from, derived from		com-	with, together
-ar	pertaining to		cor-	with, together
arteri/arterio-	artery		crani/cranio-	cranium, skull
arthr/arthro-	joint, articulation		cry/cryo-	cold
articul/articulo-	joint		cycl-	circle, cycle
-ary	pertaining to		cyst/cysti/cysto-	bladder or sac
-ase	enzyme		cyt/cyto-	cell
-asthenia	weakness		-cyte	cell
-ation	process		dactyl/dactylo-	digit (finger or toe)
aut/auto-	self, same		de-	away from, cessation
bacteri/bacterio-	bacteria		derm/dermato-	skin
bi-	twice, double		-desis	binding
bio-	life		dextr/dextro-	right, on the right side
blast/blasto-	germ or bud			

di-	separation
dif-	separation
dis-	separation, taking apart
duodeno-	duodenum
dynamo-	force, energy
-dynia	pain
dys-	bad, difficult
-eal	pertaining to
ec-	out, away
ect-	outer, outside
-ectasis	expansion, dilation
ecto-	outer, outside
-ectomy	excision, removal
-emia	blood condition
encephal/ encephalo-	brain
enter/entero-	small intestine
epi-	upon
erythr/erythro-	red
esthesio-	sensation
eu-	good, well
ex-	out of, away from
exo-	exterior, outward
extra-	outside
fibr/fibro-	fiber
-form	in the form or shape of
-galact/galacto-	milk
-gen	origin or production
gloss/glosso-	tongue
glott/glotto-	opening
gluco-	glucose
glyco-	sugar
gnath/gnatho-	jaw
-gram	recording
-graph	recording instrument
-graphy	process of recording
gyn/gyne/ gyneco/gyno-	woman
hem/hema/ hemat/hemato-	blood
hemi-	one-half
hemo-	blood
hepat/hepatico/ hepato-	liver
hidr/hidro-	sweat
hist/histio/histo-	tissue
hydr/hydro-	water
hyper-	above normal, excessive
hypo-	below normal, deficient
hyster/hystero-	uterus
-ia/iasis	condition
-iatrics	treatment
-iatry	treatment
-ic	pertaining to
-icle	small
-ics	organized knowledge, treatment
ileo-	ileum
infra-	below
inter-	between, among
intra-	within
irid/irido-	iris
ischi/ischio-	ischium
-ism	condition, disease
-ismus	spasm, contraction
iso-	equal, like
-ist	one who specializes in
-ite	the nature of, resembling
-itis	inflammation
-ium	structure, tissue
karyo-	nucleus
kerat/kerato-	cornea
kin/kine/kinesi/ kinesio-	movement
kino-	movement
kyph/kypho-	humped
lacrim/lacrimo-	tear
lact/lacti/lacto-	milk
laryng/laryngo-	larynx
latero-	lateral

lei/leio-	smooth
-lepsis/lepsy	seizure
lepto-	light, slender
leuk/leuko-	white
linguo-	tongue
lip/lipo-	fat
lith/litho-	stone, calculus
log-	speech
-logist	one who specializes in study or treatment of
logo-	speech
-logy	study of
lymph/lympho-	lymph
lys-/lyso-	dissolution
macr/macro-	large, long
-malacia	softening
mast/masto-	breast
meg/mega-	large
megal/megalo-	large
-megaly	large
melan/melano-	black
mening/meningo-	meninges
mes/meso-	middle
meta-	after, behind
-meter	instrument for measuring
-metry	process of measuring
micr/micro-	smallness, one-millionth
mon/mono-	single
morph/morpho-	form, shape
muscul/musculo-	muscle
my/myo-	muscle
myc/myco-	fungus
myel/myelo-	bone marrow, spinal cord
myring/myringo-	eardrum
myx/myxo-	mucus
necr/necro-	death
neo-	new
nephr/nephro-	kidney
neur/neuri/neuro-	nerve

oculo-	eye
odont/odonto-	tooth
odyn/odyno-	pain
-oid	resemblance to
olig/oligo-	few, little
-oma	tumor
-omata	plural of -oma
onco-	tumor, bulk, volume
onych/onycho-	fingernail, toenail
oo-	egg, ovary
oophor/oophoro-	ovary
ophthalm/ophthalmo-	eye
orchi/orchido/orchio-	testis
orth/ortho-	straight, normal, correct
-osis	process, condition, state
osseo-	bony
ossi-	bone
ost/oste/osteo-	bone
ot/oto-	ear
-ous	pertaining to
ovari/ovario/ovi/ovo-	ovary
oxo-	addition of oxygen
oxy-	sharp, acid, acute, oxygen
pachy-	thick
pan/pant/panto-	all, entire
para-	alongside of, abnormal
-paresis	slight paralysis
path/patho-	disease
-pathy	disease
pelv/pelvi/pelvo-	hip bone
-penia	deficiency
per-	through
peri-	around, about
-pexy	fixation
phaco-	lens-shaped

-phage/phagia	eating, devouring
phago-	eating, devouring
-phagy	eating, devouring
pharmaco-	drugs, medicine
pharyng/	pharynx
pharyngo-	
-phil/philia	attraction for
phleb/phlebo-	vein
phob/phobo-	exaggerated fear, sensitivity
phon/phono-	sound
phos-	light
phot/photo-	light
phren/phreni-	diaphragm
phrenico/phreno-	diaphragm
-plasia	formation
-plasty	surgical repair, reconstruction
-plegia	paralysis
pleur/pleura/	rib, pleura
pleuro-	
pneum/pneuma-	air, lung
pneumat/	air, lung
pneumato-	
pod/podo-	foot
-poiesis	production
poly-	multiplicity
post-	after, behind, posterior
pre-	anterior, before
presby/presbyo-	old age
pro-	before, forward
proct/procto-	anus, rectum
psych/psyche/	mind
psycho-	
-ptosis	falling, downward placement
pyel/pyelo-	pelvis
pyo-	pus
pyro-	fever
quadr/quadri-	four
rachi/rachio	spine
radio-	radiation, radius

re-	again, backward
rect/recto-	rectum
ren/reno-	kidney
reticul/reticulo-	net
retro-	backward, behind
rhabd/rhabdo-	rod shaped, striated
rhin/rhino-	nose
-rrhage	burst forth
-rrhagia	discharge
-rrhaphy	surgical suturing
-rrhea	flowing
-rrhexis	rupture
salping/salpingo-	tube
sarco-	muscular, fleshlike
schisto-	split, cleft
schiz/schizo-	split, cleft, division
scler/sclero-	hardness
scoli/scolio-	twisted
-scope	instrument for viewing
-scopy	use of instrument for viewing
semi-	one-half, partly
sial/sialo-	saliva, salivary gland
sigmoid/	sigmoid, sigmoid
sigmoido-	colon
sinistr/sinistro-	left, left side
sito-	food, grain
somat/somatico	body, bodily
/somato-	
spasmo-	spasm
sperma/	semen,
spermato/	spermatozoa
spermo-	
splanchn/	viscera
splanchni-/	
splanchno-	
splen/spleno-	spleen
spondyl/	vertebra
spondylo-	
-stasis	stop, stand
steno-	narrowness, constriction

stheno-	strength, force, power	tox/toxi/toxico/ toxo-	toxin, poison
stom/stoma-	mouth	trache/tracheo-	trachea
stomat/stomato-	mouth	trans-	across, through, beyond
-stomy	creation of opening		
sub-	beneath	trich/trichi/ trichia/tricho-	hair, hairlike structure
super-	in excess, above, superior	-tripsy	crushing
		tympan/ tympano-	eardrum
supra-	above, excessive	-ula/ule	small
sy/syl-	together	ultra-	beyond, excessive
sym-	together	uni-	one
syn-	together	uri/uric/urico-	uric acid
sys-	together	ur/uro-	urine
tachy-	fast	varic/varico-	swollen or twisted vein
thel/thelo-	nipples		
therm/thermo-	heat	vas-/vaso-	duct, blood vessel
thorac/thoracico/ thoraco-	chest, thorax	vasculo-	blood vessel
		vesic/vesico-	vesicle
thromb/thrombo-	blood clot	xanth/ xanthomy	yellow, yellowish condition or process of
thyr/thyro-	thyroid gland		
-tic	pertaining to		
toco-	childbirth	zo/zoo-	animal, animal life
-tome	cutting instrument	zym/zymo-	fermentation, enzyme
-tomy	cutting operation		
tono-	tone, tension, pressure		
top/topo-	place, topical		

Ligaments

Shoulder/upper arm
acromioclavicular
collateral ulnar
conoid
coracoacromial
coracoclavicular
coracohumeral
costoclavicular
glenohumeral
inferior transverse
interclavicular
superior transverse
trapezoid

Hand/forearm
annular ligament of radius
collateral ligament of interphalangeal
   articulation
collateral ligament of
   metacarpophalangeal articulation
collateral radial
deep transverse metacarpal
dorsal carpometacarpal
dorsal intercarpal
dorsal metacarpal
dorsal radiocarpal
interosseous intercarpal
interosseous metacarpal
palmar carpometacarpal
palmar intercarpal
palmar ligament of interphalangeal
   articulation
palmar metacarpal
palmar radiocarpal
palmar ulnocarpal
pisohamate
pisometacarpal
quadrate
radial carpal
radiate ligament of wrist

superficial transverse metacarpal
transverse carpal
ulnar carpal

Spine
alar
anterior longitudinal
anterior sacrococcygeal
anterior sacroiliac
apical dental
caudal retinaculum
cruciform ligament of atlas
costotransverse
deep posterior sacrococcygeal
iliofemoral
iliolumbar
interarticular
interspinal
intertransverse
lateral atlantooccipital
lateral sacrococcygeal
lateral costotransverse
lumbocostal
nuchal
posterior longitudinal
sacrospinal
superficial posterior sacrococcygeal
supraspinal
transverse ligament of atlas

Hip/thigh
inguinal
ischiofemoral
ligament of head of femur
round ligament of femur
transverse ligament of acetabulum

Knee/calf
anterior cruciate ligament of knee
anterior ligament of head of fibula
anterior meniscofemoral

Common Professional Titles

BDS	Bachelor of Dental Surgery
BDSc	Bachelor of Dental Science
ChB	Bachelor of Surgery
ChD	Doctor of Surgery
CM	Chirurgiae Magister, Master in Surgery
CMA	Certified Medical Assistant
CMT	Certified Medical Transcriptionist
CNM	Certified Nurse-Midwife
CRNA	Certified Registered Nurse Anesthetist
DC	Doctor of Chiropractic
DDS	Doctor of Dental Surgery
DHy	Doctor of Hygiene
DMD	Doctor of Dental Medicine
DO	Doctor of Osteopathy
DP	Doctor of Podiatry
DPH	Doctor of Public Health
DPM	Doctor of Podiatric Medicine
DrPH	Doctor of Public Health
FAAN	Fellow of the American Academy of Nursing
FACCP	Fellow of the American College of Chest Physicians
FACD	Fellow of the American College of Dentists
FACNM	Fellow of the American College of Nuclear Medicine
FACNP	Fellow of the American College of Nuclear Physicians
FACOG	Fellow of the American College of Obstetricians and Gynecologists
FACP	Fellow of the American College of Physicians
FACR	Fellow of the American College of Radiology
FACSM	Fellow of the American College of Sports Medicine
FCAP	Fellow of the College of American Pathologists
FCCP	Fellow of the College of Chest Physicians
FFR	Fellow of the Faculty of Radiologists (United Kingdom)
FRCP	Fellow of the Royal College of Physicians (England)
FRCP(C)	Fellow of the Royal College of Physicians (Canada)
FRCP(E)	Fellow of the Royal College of Physicians (Edinburgh)
FRCP(Edin)	Fellow of the Royal College of Physicians (Edinburgh)
FRCP(I)	Fellow of the Royal College of Physicians (Ireland)
FRCS	Fellow of the Royal College of Surgeons (England)
FRCS(C)	Fellow of the Royal College of Surgeons (Canada)
FRCS(E)	Fellow of the Royal College of Surgeons (Edinburgh)
FRCS(Edin)	Fellow of the Royal College of Surgeons (Edinburgh)
FRCS(I)	Fellow of the Royal College of Surgeons (Ireland)

Appendix 4

FRS	Fellow of the Royal Society
FRSC	Fellow of the Royal Society (Canada)
LRCP	Licentiate of the Royal College of Physicians (England)
LRCP(E)	Licentiate of the Royal College of Physicians (Edinburgh)
LRCP(I)	Licentiate of the Royal College of Physicians (Ireland)
LRFPS	Licentiate of the Royal Faculty of Physicians and Surgeons
LRSC	Licentiate of the Royal College of Surgeons (England)
LRSC(E)	Licentiate of the Royal College of Surgeons (Edinburgh)
LRSC(I)	Licentiate of the Royal College of Surgeons (Ireland)
MRCP	Member of the Royal College of Physicians (England)
MRCP(E)	Member of the Royal College of Physicians (Edinburgh)
MRCP(I)	Member of the Royal College of Physicians (Ireland)
MRCS	Member of the Royal College of Surgeons (England)
MRCS(E)	Member of the Royal College of Surgeons (Edinburgh)
MRCS(I)	Member of the Royal College of Surgeons (Ireland)
PhD	Doctor of Philosophy
PharmD	Doctor of Pharmacy
RD	Registered Dietician
RDH	Registered Dental Hygienist
RN	Registered Nurse
RPh	Registered Pharmacist